ACSM'S RESOURCE MANUAL

FOR
GUIDELINES FOR EXERCISE TESTING AND PRESCRIPTION

Fourth Edition

SENIOR EDITOR

Jeffrey L. Roitman, EdD, FACSM
Director, Cardiac Rehabilitation
Research Medical Center
Kansas City, Missouri

SECTION EDITORS

Matt Herridge, PhD
Cardiac Rehabilitation Department
Charleston Area Medical Center
Charleston, West Virginia

Moira Kelsey, RN, MS
Clinical Coordinator
Division of Thoracic and Cardiovascular Surgery
Ohio State University Medical Center
Columbus, Ohio

Thomas P. LaFontaine, PhD
Manager
WELLAWARE Disease Prevention and Community
 Wellness Program
Boone Hospital Center
Columbia, Missouri

Lydia Miller, MS, RCEP
Co-Director of Cardiac Rehabilitation
Georgetown Hospital
Georgetown, Texas

Michael Wegner, PhD, FACSM
Medical Liason
KOS Pharmaceutical Inc.
Miami Lakes, Florida

Mark A. Williams, PhD, FACSM
Professor of Medicine
Division of Cardiology
Director, Cardiovascular Disease Prevention and
 Rehabilitation
Cardiac Center of Creighton University
Omaha, Nebraska

Tracy York, MS
Director of Operations
Lake Austin Spa Resort
Austin, Texas

ACSM'S RESOURCE MANUAL

FOR
GUIDELINES FOR EXERCISE TESTING AND PRESCRIPTION

Fourth Edition

AMERICAN COLLEGE OF SPORTS MEDICINE

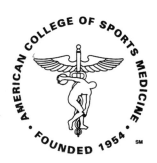

LIPPINCOTT WILLIAMS & WILKINS
A **Wolters Kluwer** Company
Philadelphia • Baltimore • New York • London
Buenos Aires • Hong Kong • Sydney • Tokyo

Editor: Peter Darcy
Managing Editor: Matthew J. Hauber
Marketing Manager: Christen DeMarco
Production Editor: Lisa JC Franko
Compositor: Maryland Composition
Printer: Courier Corporation

Printed in the United States of America
First Edition, 1988
Second Edition, 1993
Third Edition, 1998
Fourth Edition, 2001

Library of Congress Cataloging-in-Publication Data

American College of Sports Medicine.
    ACSM's resource manual for Guidelines for exercise testing and prescription / American College of Sports Medicine.—4th ed. /
senior editor, Jeffrey L. Roitman ; section editors, Matt Herridge
. . . [et al.].
        p. ; cm.
    Includes bibliographical references and index.
    ISBN 0-7817-2525-9
    1. Exercise therapy—Handbooks, manuals, etc.   2. Exercise tests—
Handbooks, manuals, etc. I. Title: Resource manual for Guidelines
for exercise testing and prescription. II. Roitman, Jeffrey L. III.
Herridge, Matt. IV. American College of Sports Medicine. Guidelines
for exercise testing and prescription. V. Title.
    [DNLM: 1. Exercise Test. 2. Exercise—physiology. 3. Exercise Therapy.
4. Exertion.   WE 103 A5125g 1991 Suppl. 2001]
RM725 .R42 2001
615.8'2—dc21   00-053506

The publishers have made every effort to trace the copyright holders for borrowed material. If they have inadvertently overlooked any, they will be pleased to make the necessary arrangements at the first opportunity.

To purchase additional copies of this book, call our customer service department at **(800) 638-3030** or fax orders to **(301) 824-7390**. International customers should call **(301) 714-2324**.

To purchase additional copies of this book or for information concerning American College of Sports Medicine certification and suggested preparatory materials, call **(800) 486-5643**.

01 02 03 04 05
1 2 3 4 5 6 7 8 9 10

FOREWORD

It is an honor and a privilege for me to introduce to you the fourth edition of the *American College of Sports Medicine's Resource Manual for Guidelines for Exercise Testing and Prescription.* This compendium of 80 chapters and accompanying appendices largely represents the fundamental knowledge that must be mastered by candidates applying for ACSM's certifications in preventive and rehabilitative exercise programming. This revision is the product of a prestigious group of scientists, clinicians, and researchers who have painstakingly worked to summarize, in a clear and concise manner, the core material and latest research findings in their respective areas of expertise. Specific sections concerning lifestyle modifications, anatomy and biomechanics, exercise physiology, cardiopulmonary and other chronic diseases, electrocardiography, exercise programming, human development, behavior change, and program implementation have been maintained and improved.

An impressive gain in the management of persons with and without chronic disease has been the establishment of the benefits of regular physical activity and its progressive incorporation into the mainstream of contemporary medical care. Exercise is now accepted as a bona fide preventive and therapeutic measure. However, special deficits or defects resulting from congenital deformities, injury, or disease and the needs and limitations imposed by these conditions must be considered in formulating safe and effective exercise prescription. To this end, we have come to recognize the usefulness of exercise testing in evaluating the cardiorespiratory, hemodynamic, and electrocardiographic responses to physical exertion, both before and after various therapeutic interventions.

In the era of managed, capitated health care, primary care physicians and allied health professionals, such as exercise physiologists, nurses, physical educators, physical therapists, and registered dietitians, will assume an increasingly important role in implementing exercise-based primary and secondary prevention programs. Although hypertension, hyperlipidemia, obesity, and diabetes mellitus may be favorably affected by regular physical activity, optimal health-related outcomes will be achieved only by complementing exercise with education and counseling, medical surveillance and emergency support when appropriate, pharmacotherapy if necessary, and interventions to enhance psychosocial functioning and long-term adherence to lifestyle changes. The latter include assessing the client's readiness for change, providing services that are designed to circumvent or attenuate common barriers to enrollment and adherence (e.g., offering group and home-based programs), keeping goals short-term and attainable, using motivational incentives accruing to periodic exercise testing and risk factor assessment, recruiting spouse and family support of the intervention, and recording goal achievements.

In the new millennium, our changing medical environment will dictate greater individual responsibility to maintain health and prevent disease. This text provides substantial reinforcement for the adoption of exercise as one of the interventions necessary to achieve this objective. Those who master the material in this volume will be especially well prepared to help others help themselves. The challenge is yours!

Barry A. Franklin, PhD, FACSM

PREFACE

The American College of Sports Medicine certification program for exercise professionals began in 1975 with the publication of the first edition of *ACSM's Guidelines for Exercise Testing and Prescription* ("the *Guidelines*") and the subsequent examination of candidates for certification. The first edition of the *Resource Manual for Guidelines for Exercise Testing and Prescription* was published in 1988. The original purpose of this book was to be a companion to the *Guidelines*. This book continues to serve that purpose for fitness professionals who are candidates for certification and for professionals requiring the resources behind the *Guidelines*.

The objectives for certification, the knowledge, skills and abilities, or KSAs, are written to describe a set of minimum competencies that various exercise professionals should possess. They are, therefore, required knowledge, skills, and abilities for successful certification. The KSAs are divided into those associated with the health and fitness track and the clinical track.

The fourth edition of the *Resource Manual* presents background information for the KSAs to assist both professionals in the field and candidates for certification. This edition has been slightly revised from the third edition.

The most significant changes include renumbering of the KSAs consistent with the sixth edition of *ACSM's Guidelines for Exercise Testing and Prescription*, published in 2000. Once again, these have been indexed to chapters at the front of the book. Numbered KSAs, matched by icon to the level of certification, are found at the beginning of each chapter. In this way, the book becomes more user friendly to the professional wishing to find information referring to specific KSAs. This format also enables the reverse indexing of the KSAs; thus, the list in the front contains references to chapters where the KSA may be found.

No single reference can provide all of the answers for professionals or candidates for certification, but the fourth edition of the *Resource Manual* is an authoritative source. The contributors are among the best in their specialty, each a well known researcher or practitioner. The information is current and presents what is known about the topic, we hope in a way that will make it useful to the exercise professional and candidate for certification.

The fourth edition of the *Resource Manual* continues to be a primary reference source for KSAs as well as for information relative to the practice of the fitness professional (both health and fitness and clinical professionals). More broadly, the *Resource Manual* is a reference work for those working in either the clinical or the health and fitness environment for topics relative to exercise physiology, disease management, wellness, prevention of disease, behavioral psychology, program administration, and the wide array of topics that exercise professionals encounter on a daily basis.

ACKNOWLEDGMENTS

The editors thank these individuals who contributed to this book by reviewing manuscripts and providing editorial assistance.

James Allen, MD
Paul A. Becker, MD
Dale R. Bergren, PhD
Jeffrey J. Betts, PhD
Elaine Filusch Betts, PhD, PT
Gordon Blackburn, PhD
Timothy L. Blackburn, MD, FACC
Susan A. Bloomfield, PhD
Michael S. Bolander, PT
Charles J. Brook, MD
William N. Brodine, MD
Ellsworth R. Buskirk, PhD
Brian W. Carlin, MD
Tom Clanton, PhD
Diane Cullen, PhD
Fred Daniels, MS
Bill Day, PhD
Loni Denne, RN, BSN
Robert Doroghazi, MD
Ami M. Drimmer, PhD
Barbara L. Drinkwater, PhD
J. Larry Durstine, PhD
Greg Dwyer, PhD
Joan M. Eckerson, PhD
Daniel E. Hilleman, PharmD
Marigold A. Edwards, PhD
JoAnne M. Eickhoff-Shemek, PhD
Paul S. Fardy, PhD
Rita A. Frickle, MS, RD, LMNT
Andrew W. Gardner, PhD
Richard Gevirtz, PhD
Terry Glenn, PhD, PT
Bill Grantham, MS
Thomas P. Guck, PhD
James Hagberg, PhD
Susan J. Hall, PhD

Larry F. Hamm, PhD
Chad Harris, PhD
Steven H. Herman, PhD
Eric S. Hockstad, MD, FACC
Elizabeth Holford, PhD
Kady Hommel Anderson, MBA
Reed Humphrey, PhD, PT
Dianne R. Jewell, MS, PT
George Kelly, PhD
W. Larry Kenney, PhD
Sean M. Kenniff, MD
Steven J. Keteyian, PhD
Joy A. Kistler, MS
Fred Klinge, MBA
Kenneth L. Knight, PhD
Harold W. Kohl III, PhD
David Lombard, PhD
Ben Londeree, EdD
Terry Marble, PhD, PT
Carol Mayberry, PhD
David A. Mays, PharmD, BCPS
Timothy R. McConnell, PhD
Diane McCullen, PhD
Henry S. Miller, Jr., MD
Geri A. Moore, MA
Byron Nelson, PG
Richard B. Parr, EdD
Robert W. Patton, PhD
Jody Payne, BS
Claire Peel, PhD, PT
Linda S. Pescatello, PhD
Hilary Welch Petrowski
George B. Pierson, MD
Michael Porter, MS
Robin B. Purdie, MS
Janet Walberg Rankin, PhD
Brian Rieger, MS
Scott O. Roberts, PhD
Eric Samaniego, MS
Stuart Sanders, MD

Albert B. Schultz, PhD
Wayne E. Sinning, PhD
Barbara Smith, RN, PhD
L. Kent Smith, MD, MPH
Christine Snow, PhD
Wayne Sotile, PhD
Catherine J. Spangler Perry, RN, MSN
Nick Stergiou, PhD
Kerry Stewart, PhD
Michael H. Stone, PhD
James Stray-Gundersen, MD
Tom R. Thomas, PhD
Janet P. Wallace, PhD
Mary Watson, MS, RD
Michael J. Waxman, MD
Hilary Welch Petrowski, MS
Mary Ellen Wewers, PhD, RN, ANP
Mark A. Williams, PhD
Richard Winett, PhD
Nancy C. Zambraski, MS

Again, I acknowledge the assistance of those who provided support for the time and effort that this book required. The section editors once again have provided the ongoing, day-to-day help with the sections, individual chapters, editing, and contributors that is essential to producing a book such as this. Thanks to D. Mark Robertson, ACSM staff member, for his help with this and many other publications from ACSM. Thanks also to the editors at Lippincott Williams & Wilkins, Pete Darcy, Matt Hauber, Lisa Franko, and Lisa Manhart, who have been patient, supportive, and incredibly helpful to me with their efforts. Mark Williams, PhD, and Hilary Welch Petrowski, MS, both provided invaluable assistance in reading page proofs. I have great appreciation for their role in easing my workload at a critical time. Kay, you are the light of my life. Finally, to all my staff at Research Medical Center, Baptist Medical Center, and Research Belton Hospital, who put up with my complaints and absence, thank you very much.

Contributors

Frank Ancharski, MS
HealthPoint Fitness & Wellness Center
Waltham, Massachusetts

Tony G. Babb, PhD
Institute of Exercise and Environmental Medicine
Presbyterian Hospital of Dallas and UT Southwestern
    Medical Center
Dallas, Texas

Kenneth C. Beck, PhD
Division of Pulmonary and Critical Care Medicine
Mayo Clinic
Rochester, Minnesota

Sue G. Beckham, PhD
Department of Kinesiology
University of Texas at Arlington
Arlington, Texas

Thomas E. Bernard, PhD
College of Public Health
University of South Florida
Tampa, Florida

Valerie Bishop, MS
Cardiac and Pulmonary Rehabilitation
Medical City Dallas
Dallas, Texas

Susan A. Bloomfield, PhD
Department of Health and Kinesiology
Texas A&M University
College Station, Texas

James Blumenthal, PhD
Department of Psychiatry and Behavioral Sciences
Duke University Medical Center
Durham, North Carolina

Sorin Brener, MD
Interventional Cardiology
Cleveland Clinic Foundation
Cleveland, Ohio

Kelly D. Brownell, PhD
Department of Psychology
Yale University
New Haven, Connecticut

Peter H. Brubaker, PhD
Department of Health & Exercise Science
Wake Forest University
Winston-Salem, North Carolina

Cedric X. Bryant, PhD, FACSM
Stairmaster Health & Fitness Institute
Stairmaster Health & Fitness Products
Kirkland, Washington

Jill A. Bush, PhD
Children's Nutritional Research Center
Baylor College of Medicine
Houston, Texas

Graham E. Caldwell, PhD
Exercise Science
University of Massachusetts
Amherst, Massachusetts

Barbara N. Campaigne, PhD
Diabetes Care
Global Scientific Communications
Eli Lilly and Company
Indianapolis, Indiana

Mike Caton, MEd
Millennium Health & Fitness
Colorado Springs, Colorado

Richard Casaburi, PhD, MD
Division of Respiratory and Critical Care Physiology and
    Medicine
Harbor–UCLA Medical Center
Torrance, California

Chris Cole, MD
FitLinx
Stamford, Connecticut

David E. Corbin, PhD, ACSE, FASHA
School of Health, Physical Education, and Recreation
University of Nebraska at Omaha
Omaha, Nebraska

Edward F. Coyle, PhD
Kinesiology and Health Education
The University of Texas at Austin
Austin, Texas

Brent Darden, MS
Winning Habits
Dallas, Texas

J. Mark Davis, PhD
Department of Exercise Science
University of South Carolina
Columbia, South Carolina

Paul G. Davis, PhD
Department of Exercise and Sport Science
University of North Carolina at Greensboro
Greensboro, North Carolina

Rebecca Davis, PhD
University of Maryland
Cooperative Extension
Baltimore, Maryland

Scott R. Demaree, MEd
Human Performance Laboratory
Texas A&M University
College Station, Texas

Gary A. Dudley, PhD
Department of Exercise Science
University of Georgia
Athens, Georgia

J. Larry Durstine, PhD, FACSM, FAACVPR
Department of Exercise Science
University of South Carolina
Columbia, South Carolina

Nestor Fernandez II, MBA
Western Athletic Clubs
University of San Francisco
San Francisco, California

Robert Fitts, PhD
Department of Biology
Marquette University
Milwaukee, Wisconsin

Steven J. Fleck, PhD, FACSM
Department of Sport Science
Colorado College
Colorado Springs, Colorado

Barry A. Franklin, PhD
Beaumont Rehab and Health Center
William Beaumont Hospital
Birmingham, Michigan

Denise M. Fredette, MS, PT
School of Physical Therapy
Texas Women's University
Houston, Texas

Scott Going, PhD
Department of Physiology
The University of Arizona
Tucson, Arizona

Neil F. Gordon, MD, PhD, MPH
Center for Disease Prevention
Savannah, Georgia

Andrew M. Gottlieb, PhD
Cambridge Therapy Center
Palo Alto, California

Mark D. Grabiner, PhD
Department of Biomedical Engineering
Lerner Research Institute
The Cleveland Clinic Foundation
Cleveland, Ohio

James E. Graves, PhD
Department of Exercise Science
Syracuse University
Syracuse, New York

Carlos M. Grilo, PhD
Yale Psychiatric Institute
Yale University School of Medicine
New Haven, Connecticut

Larry R. Gurchiek, DA, ATC
Department of Health and Physical Education
University of South Alabama
Mobile, Alabama

Linda K. Hall, PhD
McConnell Heart Health Center
Columbus, Ohio

Joseph Hamill, PhD
Exercise Science
University of Massachusetts
Amherst, Massachusetts

Julie Hanson-Zuckerman
Institute for Exercise & Environmental Medicine
Presbyterian Hospital of Dallas
Dallas, Texas

Sharon A. Harvey, MA
Cardiac ECG, Stress, and ECG Rehabilitation
The Cleveland Clinic Foundation
Cleveland, Ohio

George Havenith, PhD
Department of Human Sciences
Loughborough University
Loughborough, United Kingdom

Kathryn Hellweg, PhD
Department of Teaching and Learning
Rochester Public Schools
Rochester, Minnesota

David L. Herbert, JD
Herbert & Benson, Attorneys at Law
Canton, Ohio

William G. Herbert, PhD
Human Nutrition, Foods, and Exercise
Virginia Tech
Blacksburg, Virginia

William R. Hiatt, MD
Novartis Professor of Cardiovascular Research
University of Colorado School of Medicine
Denver, Colorado

Michael Holewijn, PhD
Research and Development Department
Netherlands Aeromedical Institute
Soesterberg, The Netherlands

Robert G. Holly, PhD
Department of Exercise Science
University of California
Davis, California

Connie C. W. Hsia, MD
Pulmonary and Critical Care Medicine
University of Texas, Southwestern Medical Center
Dallas, Texas

Reed Humphrey, PhD, PT, FACSM
Physical Therapy, Medical College of Virginia
Virginia Commonwealth University
Richmond, Virginia

Donna Israel, RD, PhD
Fitness Formula Inc.
Richardson, Texas

Bruce D. Johnson, PhD
Division of Pulmonary and Critical Care Medicine
Mayo Clinic and Foundation
Rochester, Minnesota

Leonard A. Kaminsky, PhD, FACSM
School of Physical Education
Ball State University
Muncie, Indiana

Michaela Kiernan, PhD
Department of Medicine
Stanford University School of Medicine
Palo Alto, California

Abby C. King, PhD
Department of Medicine
Stanford University School of Medicine
Palo Alto, California

John E. Kovaleski, PhD, ATC
Department of Health and Physical Education
University of South Alabama
Mobile, Alabama

William J. Kraemer, PhD, FACSM
Human Performance Laboratory
Ball State University
Muncie, Indiana

Thomas P. LaFontaine, PhD, FACSM, FAACVPR
Wellaware
Boone Hospital Center
Columbia, Missouri

John A. Larry, MD

Division of Cardiology
The Ohio State University Medical Center
Columbus, Ohio

Richard W. Latin, PhD

School of Health, Physical Education and Recreation
University of Nebraska at Omaha
Omaha, Nebraska

Michael Lauer, MD

Stress ECG Laboratory
The Cleveland Clinic Foundation
Cleveland, Ohio

John M. Lawler, PhD

Redox Biology Laboratory
Texas A&M University
College Station, Texas

Ben Levine, MD

Institute for Exercise and Environmental Medicine
Presbyterian Hospital of Dallas
Dallas, Texas

Donald A. Mahler, MD

Section of Pulmonary & Critical Care Medicine
Dartmouth Medical School
Lebanon, New Hampshire

Bonita L. Marks, PhD, FACSM

Exercise Science Teaching Laboratory
Department of Exercise and Sport Science
University of North Carolina
Chapel Hill, North Carolina

John E. Martin, PhD

Department of Psychology
San Diego State University
San Diego, California

Philip E. Martin, PhD

Exercise Science and Physical Education
Arizona State University
Tempe, Arizona

Timothy R. McConell, PhD

Cardiac Rehabilitation
Geisinger Health System
Danville, Pennsylvania

Stuart M. McGill, PhD

Department of Kinesiology
Faculty of Applied Health Sciences
University of Waterloo
Waterloo, Ontario, Canada

Victoria McGrath, MS

National Accounts
Netpulse Media Networks
San Francisco, California

Nancy Houston Miller, RN, BS

Stanford Cardiac Rehabilitation Program
Stanford University School of Medicine
Palo Alto, California

Sandra L. Minor, PhD

Public Health
Southern Connecticut State University
New Haven, Connecticut

Aryan Mooss, MD

Division of Cardiology
Creighton University School of Medicine
Omaha, Nebraska

Tinker D. Murray, PhD, FACSM

HPER Department
Southwest Texas State University
San Marcos, Texas

Jonathan Myers, PhD

Cardiovascular Medicine
Stanford University/Palo Alto VAHCS
Palo Alto, California

Frederic J. Pashkow, MD

Heart Institute
The Queen's Medical Center
Honolulu, Hawaii

Albert W. Pearsall IV, MD

Department of Orthopaedics
University of South Alabama Medical Center
Mobile, Alabama

James A. Peterson, PhD

Healthy Learning Videos, Inc.
Monterey, California

Lori L. Ploutz-Snyder, PhD

Exercise Science
Syracuse University
Syracuse, New York

Susan Poindexter, MS, RD, LD

Charleston Area Medical Center
Charleston, West Virginia

Michael L. Pollock, PhD[1]

Center for Exercise Science
University of Florida
Gainesville, Florida
[1]Deceased.

Scott K. Powers, PhD, EdD
Center for Exercise Science
Exercise and Sport Sciences
University of Florida
Gainesville, Florida

Elizabeth J. Protas, PhD, PT
School of Physical Therapy
Texas Woman's University
Houston, Texas

Julie M. Pulcipher, PhD, PT
Department of Rehabilitation Services
Guadalupe Valley Hospital
Seguin, Texas

Judith G. Regensteiner, PhD
University of Colorado School of Medecine
Denver, Colorado

Paul M. Ribisl, PhD
Department of Health and Exercise Science
Wake Forest University
Winston-Salem, North Carolina

Rosemary Riley, PhD, RD
Ross Products Division
Abbott Laboratories
Columbus, Ohio

Jeffrey L. Roitman, EdD, FACSM
Research Medical Center
Baptist Medical Center
Kansas City, Missouri

Robert Scales, PhD
Division of Physical Performance & Development
University of New Mexico
Albuquerque, New Mexico

Stephen F. Schaal, MD
Division of Cardiology
The Ohio State University Medical Center
Columbus, Ohio

James D. Shaffrath, MD
Department of Exercise Science
University of California
Davis, California

Janet M. Shaw, PhD
Department of Exercise and Sport Science
The University of Utah
Salt Lake City, Utah

Sally A. Shumaker, PhD
Bowman Gray School of Medicine
Wake Forest University
Winston-Salem, North Carolina

Wesley E. Sime, PhD, MPH
Health and Human Performance
University of Nebraska-Lincoln
Lincoln, Nebraska

L. Kent Smith, MD, MPH
Arizona Heart Institute
Phoenix, Arizona

Patricia M. Smith, PhD
Department of Health Studies and Gerontology
University of Waterloo
Waterloo, Ontario, Canada

Wayne M. Sotile, PhD
Cardiac Rehabilitation Program
Wake Forest University
Winston-Salem, North Carolina

Barbara H. Southard, MS, RN
Health Management Consultants of Virginia, Inc.
Floyd, Virginia

Douglas R. Southard, PhD, MPH, PAC
Health Management Consultants of Virginia, Inc.
Floyd, Virginia

Ray W. Squires, PhD
Cardiovascular Health Clinic
Division of Cardiovascular Diseases and Internal
    Medicine
Mayo Clinic
Rochester, Minnesota

Linda St. Clair, MS, RD, LD
Highland Hospital Hospital
Charleston, West Virginia

Kerry J. Stewart, EdD
Division of Cardiology
Johns Hopkins University School of Medicine
Baltimore, Maryland

C. Barr Taylor, MD
Department of Psychiatry
Stanford Medical Center
Palo Alto, California

Tom R. Thomas, PhD

Department of Nutritional Sciences
University of Missouri
Columbia, Missouri

Jeff S. Volek, PhD, RD

Exercise and Nutrition Core
The Human Performance Laboratory
Ball State University
Muncie, Indiana

Mitchell H. Whaley, PhD, FACSM

School of Physical Education
Ball State University
Muncie, Indiana

Karen Wheeler, MS, RD, LD

Charleston, West Virginia

Mark A. Williams, PhD

Division of Cardiology
Creighton University School of Medicine
Omaha, Nebraska

Kerri M. Winters, PhD

Department of Health Promotion and Exercise Science
Northern Arizona University
Flagstaff, Arizona

Kara A. Witzke, PhD

Department of Health, Physical Education, and Exercise
   Science
Norfolk State University
Norfolk, Virginia

Linda D. Zwiren, EdD, FACSM

Department of Physical Education, Sport Sciences
Department of Biology
Hofstra University
Hempstead, New York

How to Use This Book

In the section of the front material entitled KSA Listing, the KSAs are printed exactly as they are in *ACSM's Guidelines*. A third column shows the chapter number where material relative to that KSA can be found. In many instances, more than one chapter is listed because information relative to a KSA is found in more than one chapter. Similarly, at the beginning of each chapter there are numbered icons. The icon illustrates the level of certification, and the number can be matched to the individual KSA in the front of the book. This index is not exhaustive in that every single piece of information about a KSA has been indexed. Candidates for certification are encouraged to look through the table of contents and the index seeking additional sources for material that interests them.

This system allows candidates studying for certification to locate information pertinent to a KSA quickly and easily. Individual KSAs can be located by using the table of KSAs at the front and referring to the specific chapter or chapters indexed. Likewise, information concerning the KSAs covered in any chapter can be found at the beginning of the chapter.

ICON KEY

 Group Exercise Leader

 Health Fitness Instructor

 Health Fitness Director

 Exercise Specialist

 Program Director

KSA Listing

Numbering System

The system for numbering KSAs is designed to more specifically denote the *level of certification* (the first number in sequence) and the *content matter* (the second number in the sequence) of the KSA. The system is as follows.

Level of Certification

The first number in the sequence denotes the certification level of the KSA. KSAs numbered 1. are specific to exercise leader; KSAs numbered 2. are specific to health and fitness instructor, and so on. The first numbers denote level of certification as follows:

1. Exercise Leader
2. Health Fitness Instructor
3. Health Fitness Director
4. Exercise Specialist
5. Program Director

Content Matter

The second number in the sequence denotes the content of the KSA. KSAs numbered .1 are related to anatomy and biomechanics; KSAs numbered .2 are related to exercise physiology. The second numbers denote content matter as follows:

.1 Anatomy and biomechanics
.2 Exercise physiology
.3 Human development and aging
.4 Pathophysiology and risk factors
.5 Human behavior and psychology
.6 Health appraisal and fitness testing
.7 Safety and injury prevention
.8 Exercise programming
.9 Nutrition and weight management
.10 Program and administration or management
.11 Electrocardiography

Example

A KSA numbered 1.3. is a KSA for an exercise leader that relates to human development and aging. A KSA numbered 4.4. is for an exercise specialist that relates to pathophysiology and risk factors.

This numbering system allows exact determination of KSAs specific to the level of certification and the content matter.

KSA: Health and Fitness Track

KSA Number	Anatomy and Biomechanics	Chapter
1.1.0	Knowledge of anatomy as it relates to exercise and health.	
1.1.0.1	Knowledge of the basic structures of bone, skeletal muscle, and connective tissues.	9, 34, 44, 54
1.1.0.2	Knowledge of the basic anatomy of the cardiovascular system and respiratory system.	7, 8
1.1.0.3	Ability to identify the major bones and muscles. Major muscles include but are not limited to the trapezius, pectoralis major, latissimus dorsi, biceps, triceps, rectus abdominis, internal and external obliques, erector spinae, gluteus maximus, quadriceps, hamstrings, adductors, abductors, and gastrocnemius.	9
1.1.0.4	Definition of the following terms: supination, pronation, flexion, extension, adduction, abduction, hyperextension, rotation, circumduction, agonist, antagonist, and stabilizer.	44
1.1.0.5	Ability to identify the joints of the body.	11
1.1.1	Knowledge of biomechanical aspects of exercise participation.	44
1.1.1.1	Ability to identify the plane in which each muscle action occurs.	
1.1.1.2	Knowledge of the interrelationships among center of gravity, base of support, balance, stability, and proper spinal alignment.	11, 12

	of expired minute ventilation to oxygen consumption, and ratio of expired minute ventilation to carbon dioxide consumption.	15, 16, 36, 42
5.2.0	Ability to discuss the mechanisms by which functional capacity and cardiovascular, pulmonary, metabolic, endocrine, and neuromuscular adaptations occur in response to exercise testing and training in healthy and various diseased states.	17, 19, 31, 32, 33, 34, 35, 36, 37

KSA NUMBER	HUMAN DEVELOPMENT AND AGING	CHAPTER
1.3.0	Knowledge of the benefits and risks associated with exercise training in prepubescent and postpubescent youth.	58, 60
1.3.1	Knowledge of the benefits and precautions associated with resistance and endurance training in older adults.	53, 59, 61
1.3.2	Ability to describe specific leadership techniques appropriate for working with participants of all ages.	60, 61
2.3.0	Knowledge of the changes that occur during growth and development from childhood to old age.	59, 60, 61
2.3.0.1	Ability to modify cardiovascular and resistance exercises based on age and physical condition.	59, 60, 61
2.3.0.2	Knowledge of and ability to describe the changes that occur in maturation from childhood to adulthood for skeletal muscle, bone structure, reaction time, coordination, heat and cold tolerance, maximal oxygen consumption, strength, flexibility, body composition, resting and maximal heart rate, and resting and maximal blood pressure.	44, 59, 60, 61
2.3.0.3	Knowledge of the effect of the aging process on the musculoskeletal and cardiovascular structure and function at rest, during exercise, and during recovery.	59, 60, 61
2.3.0.4	Ability to characterize the differences in the development of an exercise prescription for children, adolescents, and older participants.	59, 60, 61
2.3.0.5	Knowledge of and ability to describe the unique adaptations to exercise training in children, adolescents, and older participants with regard to strength, functional capacity, and motor skills.	59, 60, 61
2.3.0.6	Knowledge of common orthopaedic and cardiovascular considerations for older participants and the ability to describe modifications in exercise prescription that are indicated.	59, 61
4.3.0	Knowledge of selecting appropriate testing and training modalities according to the age and functional capacity of the individual.	60, 61
4.3.0.1	Ability to select an appropriate test protocol according to the age and functional capacity of the individual.	42, 60, 61
4.3.1	Ability to describe the importance of and appropriate methods for resistance training in older individuals.	53, 61
5.3.0	Ability to explain differences in overall policy and procedures for the inclusion of different age groups in an exercise program.	61
5.3.1	Ability to discuss facility and equipment adaptations necessary for different age groups.	61, 77

KSA NUMBER	PATHOPHYSIOLOGY AND RISK FACTORS	CHAPTER
1.4.0	Knowledge of cardiovascular, respiratory, metabolic, and musculoskeletal risk factors that may require further evaluation by medical or allied health professionals before participation in physical activity.	13, 15, 27, 28, 30, 31, 39
1.4.0.1	Ability to determine risk factors that may be favorably modified by physical activity habits.	26, 29, 30, 32, 35
1.4.0.2	Knowledge to define total cholesterol, high-density lipoprotein (HDL) cholesterol, ratio of total cholesterol to HDL cholesterol, low-density lipoprotein (LDL) cholesterol, triglycerides, hypertension, and atherosclerosis.	2, 26, 27, 30, 32, 35
1.4.0.3	Knowledge of plasma cholesterol levels for adults as recommended by the National Cholesterol Education Program.	1, 30, 35
2.4.0	Knowledge of the pathophysiology of atherosclerosis and how this process is influenced by physical activity.	1, 26, 30
2.4.1	Knowledge of the risk factor concept of coronary artery disease and the influence of heredity and lifestyle on the development of coronary artery disease.	1, 26, 29, 30, 35
2.4.2	Knowledge of the atherosclerotic process, the factors involved in its genesis and progression, and the role of exercise training in treatment.	1, 2, 26, 27, 30, 35
2.4.3	Ability to discuss in detail how lifestyle factors, including nutrition, physical activity, and heredity, influence lipid and lipoprotein profiles.	1, 2, 3, 30, 35
2.4.4	Knowledge of cardiovascular risk factors or conditions that may require consultation with medical personnel before testing or training, including inappropriate changes in resting or exercise heart rate and blood pressure; new onset of discomfort in chest, neck, shoulder, or arm; changes in the pattern of discomfort during rest or exercise; fainting or dizzy spells; and claudication.	16, 29, 32, 33
2.4.5	Knowledge of respiratory risk factors or conditions that may require consultation with medical personnel before testing or training, including asthma, exercise-induced bronchospasm, extreme breathlessness at rest or during exercise, bronchitis, and emphysema.	36, 37, 38, 39
2.4.6	Knowledge of metabolic risk factors or conditions that may require consultation with medical personnel before testing or training, including body weight more than 20% above optimal, body mass index above thyroid disease, diabetes or glucose intolerance, and hypoglycemia.	30, 31
2.4.7	Knowledge of musculoskeletal risk factors or conditions that may require consultation with medical personnel before testing or training, including acute or chronic back pain, osteoarthritis, rheumatoid arthritis, osteoporosis, tendinitis, and low back pain.	13, 34
3.4.0	Ability to define atherosclerosis, the factors causing it, and the interventions that may delay or reverse the atherosclerotic process.	1, 2, 3, 4, 5, 6, 26, 30, 35
3.4.1	Ability to describe the causes of myocardial ischemia and infarction.	27
3.4.2	Ability to describe the pathophysiology of hypertension, obesity, hyperlipidemia, diabetes, chronic obstructive pulmonary diseases, arthritis, osteoporosis, chronic diseases, and immunosuppressive disease.	1, 3, 4, 5, 6, 32, 34, 35, 37

4.5.2	Ability to describe the principles of crisis management and factors influencing coping and learning in illness states.	62, 63, 64
4.5.3	Ability to describe the psychological issues to be confronted by the patient and by family members of patients who have cardiorespiratory disease and/or who have had an acute myocardial infarction or cardiac surgery.	64, 66
4.5.4	Knowledge of the psychological issues associated with an acute cardiac event versus those associated with chronic cardiac conditions.	64
4.5.5	Knowledge of the psychological stages involved with the acceptance of death and dying and ability to recognize when it is necessary for a psychological consultation or referral to a professional resource.	64
5.5.0	Ability to demonstrate an understanding of the need for psychosocial consultation and referral of individuals who exhibit signs of psychological distress.	62, 64
5.5.1	Knowledge of community resources for psychosocial support and behavior modification and outline an example of a referral system.	64, 67
5.5.2	Knowledge of the observable signs and symptoms of anxiety or depressive symptoms secondary to cardiopulmonary disorders.	64

KSA NUMBER	HEALTH APPRAISAL AND FITNESS TESTING	CHAPTER
1.6.1	Knowledge of the importance of a health and medical history.	40, 41
1.6.2	Knowledge of the value of a medical clearance prior to exercise participation.	40, 41
1.6.3	Skill to measure pulse rate accurately both at rest and during exercise.	
2.6.0	Knowledge, skills, and abilities to assess the health status of individuals and the ability to conduct fitness testing.	40, 41
2.6.0.1	Ability to obtain a health history and risk appraisal that includes medical history, family history of cardiac disease, orthopaedic limitations, prescribed medications, activity patterns, nutritional habits, stress and anxiety levels, and smoking and alcohol use.	40, 41, 42, 46
2.6.0.2	Ability to describe the categories of participants who should receive medical clearance prior to administration of an exercise test or participation in an exercise program.	40, 41
2.6.0.3	Ability to identify precautions and contraindications to exercise testing or participation.	40, 42
2.6.0.4	Ability to discuss the limitations of informed consent and medical clearance prior to exercise testing.	40, 42, 75
2.6.0.5	Ability to obtain informed consent.	
2.6.0.6	Ability to explain the purpose and procedures for monitoring clients before, during, and after cardiorespiratory fitness testing.	41, 42
2.6.0.7	Skill in instructing participants in the use of equipment and test procedures.	41, 42
2.6.0.8	Ability to describe the purpose of testing, select an appropriate submaximal or maximal protocol, and conduct an assessment of cardiovascular fitness on the cycle ergometer or the treadmill.	41, 42
2.6.0.9	Skill in accurately measuring heart rate, blood pressure, and obtaining rating of perceived exertion at rest and during exercise according to established guidelines.	
2.6.0.10	Ability to locate and measure skinfold sites, skeletal diameters, and girth measurements used for estimating body composition.	10, 45
2.6.0.11	Ability to describe the purpose of testing, select appropriate protocols, and conduct assessments of muscular strength, muscular endurance, and flexibility.	41, 43, 44, 54
2.6.0.12	Skill in various techniques of assessing body composition.	
2.6.0.13	Knowledge of the advantages, disadvantages, and limitations of the various body composition techniques.	45
2.6.0.14	Ability to interpret information obtained from the cardiorespiratory fitness test and the muscular strength and endurance, flexibility, and body composition assessments for apparently healthy individuals and those with stable disease.	41, 42, 43, 44, 45
2.6.0.15	Ability to identify appropriate criteria for terminating a fitness evaluation and demonstrate proper procedures to be followed after discontinuing such a test.	41
2.6.0.16	Ability to modify protocols and procedures for cardiorespiratory fitness tests in children, adolescents, and older adults.	60, 61
2.6.0.17	Knowledge of common drugs from each of the following classes of medications and ability to describe the principal action and the effects on exercise testing and prescription:	
2.6.0.17.1	Antianginals	
2.6.0.17.2	Antihypertensives	
2.6.0.17.3	Antiarrhythmics	
2.6.0.17.4	Bronchodilators	
2.6.0.17.5	Hypoglycemics	
2.6.0.17.6	Psychotropics	
2.6.0.17.7	Vasodilators	
2.6.0.18	Ability to identify the effects of the following substances on exercise response: antihistamines, tranquilizers, alcohol, diet pills, cold tablets, caffeine, and nicotine.	
2.6.0.19	Skill in techniques for calibration of a cycle ergometer and a motor-driven treadmill.	
3.6.0	Knowledge of the use and value of the results of the fitness evaluation and exercise test for various populations.	41, 42
3.6.1	Ability to design and implement a fitness testing and health appraisal program that includes but is not limited to staffing needs, physician interaction, documentation, equipment, marketing, and program evaluation.	40, 41, 72, 75

2.8.0.9	Ability to explain and implement exercise prescription guidelines for apparently healthy clients, increased-risk clients, and clients with controlled disease.	16, 31, 32, 33, 34, 39, 52, 53
2.8.0.10	Ability to adapt frequency, intensity, duration, mode, progression, level of supervision, and monitoring techniques in exercise programs for patients with controlled chronic disease (heart disease, diabetes mellitus, obesity, hypertension), musculoskeletal problems, pregnancy and/or postpartum period, and exercise-induced asthma.	16, 31, 32, 33, 34, 39
2.8.0.11	Ability to understand the components of an exercise session and the proper sequence (i.e., pre-exercise evaluation, warm-up, aerobic stimulus phase, cool-down, muscular strength and/or endurance, and flexibility).	52
2.8.0.12	Skill in the use of various methods for establishing and monitoring levels of exercise intensity, including heart rate, rate of perceived exertion, and metabolic equivalents.	
2.8.0.13	Knowledge of special precautions and modifications of exercise programming for participation at altitude, various ambient temperatures, humidity, and environmental pollution.	24, 25
2.8.0.14	Ability to design resistive exercise programs to increase or maintain muscular strength and/or endurance.	18, 19, 43, 53
2.8.0.15	Ability to evaluate flexibility and prescribe appropriate flexibility exercises for all major muscle groups.	44, 54
2.8.0.16	Knowledge of the importance of recording exercise sessions and performing periodic evaluations to assess changes in fitness status.	
2.8.0.17	Knowledge of the advantages and disadvantages of implementation of interval, continuous, and circuit training programs.	52, 56
2.8.0.18	Ability to design training programs using interval, continuous, and circuit training programs.	52, 56
2.8.0.19	Ability to discuss the advantages and disadvantages of various commercial exercise equipment in developing cardiorespiratory fitness, muscular strength, and muscular endurance.	53, 77
2.8.0.20	Knowledge of the types of exercise programs available in the community and how these programs are appropriate for various populations.	
4.8.0	Knowledge of the implications (benefits versus risks) of exercise for individuals with coronary artery disease risk factors and for individuals with established stable cardiovascular, pulmonary, metabolic, and/or orthopaedic disorders.	39, 58
4.8.1	Knowledge, skills, and abilities necessary to establish and supervise individualized exercise prescriptions based on medical information and exercise test data, including intensity, duration, frequency, progression, precautions, and type of physical activity for a variety of chronic disease and disability conditions, including, but not limited to the following:	
4.8.1.1	Coronary artery disease, myocardial infarction	16
4.8.1.2	Percutaneous transluminal coronary angiography, stent	
4.8.1.3	Congestive heart failure	
4.8.1.4	Heart transplantation	
4.8.1.5	Chronic obstructive pulmonary disease	39
4.8.1.6	Asthma	39
4.8.1.7	Bronchitis	39
4.8.1.8	Stroke, transient ischemic attack	
4.8.1.9	Diabetes	31
4.8.1.10	Hypertension	32
4.8.1.11	Obesity	55
4.8.1.12	Renal disease, transplantation	
4.8.1.13	Common orthopaedic and neuromuscular conditions	
4.8.2	Ability to modify exercise (type of physical activity, intensity, duration, progression) according to health status.	
4.8.3	Knowledge of basic mechanisms of action of medications that may affect exercise testing and the exercise prescription, including the following:	
4.8.3.1	Beta-adrenergic blockers	
4.8.3.2	Diuretics	
4.8.3.3	Calcium channel blockers	
4.8.3.4	Antihypertensives	
4.8.3.5	Antihistamines	
4.8.3.6	Antihyperglycemics	
4.8.3.7	Psychotropics	
4.8.3.8	Alcohol	
4.8.3.9	Diet pills	
4.8.3.10	Cold tablets	
4.8.3.11	Caffeine	
4.8.3.12	Nicotine	
4.8.4	Ability to discuss warm-up and cool-down phenomena with specific reference to angina and ischemic electrocardiographic changes, arrhythmias, and blood pressure changes and with general reference to cardiovascular, pulmonary, and metabolic diseases.	16, 39
4.8.5	Ability to discuss the appropriate use of static and dynamic exercise for those with cardiovascular, pulmonary, and metabolic disease.	15, 16, 39
4.8.6	Knowledge of the design of a strength and flexibility program for the following individuals or groups:	
4.8.6.1	Cardiovascular disease, pulmonary disease, metabolic disease, musculoskeletal disorders	18, 19, 34, 39
4.8.6.2	Elderly	61

TABLE OF CONTENTS

SECTION ONE

LIFESTYLE AND HEALTH

SECTION EDITOR: Mark A. Williams, PhD, FACSM

1.4.0.3

2.4.0, 2.4.1, 2.4.2, 2.4.3

3.4.0, 3.4.2

5.4.0

CHAPTER **1**

CONCEPTUAL BASIS FOR CORONARY ARTERY DISEASE RISK FACTOR ASSESSMENT IN CLINICAL PRACTICE

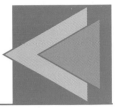

Aryan Mooss and Neil F. Gordon

Cardiovascular disease is the leading cause of death in developed countries and is a major component of the global burden of disease, accounting for 45.6% of deaths (1). In the United States 13.5 million patients have a history of myocardial infarction or angina, and many times that number are at risk for developing coronary heart disease (2). However, the age-adjusted rate of cardiovascular mortality has decreased by 40% in the past 30 years. This decline is attributable to better treatment options and more effective primary and secondary prevention strategies (3).

CORONARY RISK FACTORS

Coronary atherosclerosis is multifactorial in origin. The process begins in childhood and results from an atherogenic milieu, which is the clustering of several genetic, biological, behavioral, and environmental factors collectively known as coronary risk factors. The term *risk factor*, proposed by the Framingham investigators, came with the realization that no known single factor causes coronary atherosclerosis, but a combination of factors can be correlated with the development of coronary heart disease (4). For a risk factor to be clinically useful, it must satisfy the following criteria: strength of association (high odds ratio), consistency (multiple studies confirming the association), temporal relationship (the risk factor must precede the disease over many years), gradient (the greater the level of risk factor, the higher the risk), biological plausibility, and experimental and clinical evidence from human primary and secondary prevention studies (5). From a practical standpoint, modifiability of a risk factor is also a clinically significant attribute.

Two important concepts in risk factor evaluation must be emphasized. First, risk factors, such as elevated cholesterol and hypertension, function in a continuum of increasing risk rather than through all-or-none cutoff values (for example, a cholesterol level of ≥ 200 mg/dL or blood pressure ≥ 140/90). Individuals with cholesterol levels more than 300 mg/dL are at three to five times higher risk

for coronary heart disease than those with cholesterol levels of 200 mg/dL, although only 3–5% of the Framingham population have cholesterol levels of 300 mg/dL or more (6). Similar data for hypertension prove that there is indeed a risk pyramid (7). Those at the top of the pyramid are at the highest risk for disease, but those at the lower levels of the pyramid account for the largest number of cases in the community because they constitute a larger segment of the population. The second important consideration is the multiplicative effect of risk factors; that is, the greater the number of risk factors, the greater the level of risk (Fig. 1.1). For example, a smoker with modest elevation of cholesterol or hypertension is at much higher risk for developing coronary heart disease than a nonsmoker with severe hypertension and high cholesterol. Therefore, a comprehensive risk evaluation of an individual is an essential prerequisite to developing strategies for primary prevention of coronary heart disease.

Risk factors for coronary heart disease are generally classified as shown in Table 1.1. However, a mechanistic classification of risk factors has been proposed for assessment and prevention (Table 1.2) (8). This approach divides coronary risk factors into four categories: (*a*) causal risk factors, (*b*) conditional risk factors, (*c*) predisposing risk factors, and (*d*) plaque burden.

Causal Risk Factors

The major causal risk factors are cigarette smoking, elevated cholesterol (or low levels of low-density lipoprotein [LDL] cholesterol), decreased levels of high-density lipoprotein (HDL), hypertension, and diabetes. The Framingham risk prediction model incorporates these causal risk factors, in addition to age and sex, in assessing the 10-year risk of developing hard end points of coronary heart disease, namely death and myocardial infarction. The exact mechanisms by which these five major causal risk factors initiate atherogenesis are unknown. However, their major role has been established by overwhelming scientific evidence. Moreover, these risk factors

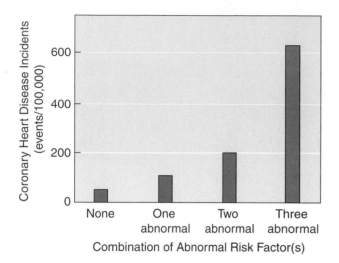

Figure 1.1. Relationship between a combination of abnormal risk factors (cholesterol = 250 mg/dL, systolic blood pressure = 160 mm Hg, smoking = 1 pack of cigarettes/day) and incidence of coronary heart disease. (From Kannel WB, Gordon T. The Framingham Study: an epidemiological investigation of cardiovascular disease. Section 30. Washington, Public Health Service, NIH, DHEW Publication [NIH] 1974;74–599.)

are modifiable by therapeutic modalities. This is in contrast to the conditional and predisposing risk factors, which are controversial for the following reasons: (*a*) Their independent causal role is not firmly established. (*b*) Some of these factors are not modifiable. (*c*) Strong clinical evidence of a beneficial effect from modification of these risk factors is lacking.

Cigarette Smoking

Cigarette smoking is the most preventable cause of death in the United States (9). Autopsy studies have shown that the extent of atherosclerosis is linearly related to the number of cigarettes smoked (Fig. 1.2) (10). The risk also increases in accordance with the number of years of smoking and the depth of inhalation. Nearly 40% of cardiovascular deaths are attributable to cigarette smoking. Smokers have twice the risk of developing coronary heart disease and a twofold to fourfold increased risk of sudden death.

The deleterious effects of smoking are particularly noteworthy in the young. In myocardial infarction survivors under age 40, the most common accompanying risk factor is cigarette smoking. As in men, women who smoke are at increased risk for coronary artery disease (11). Risk doubles in women who smoke as few as one to four cigarettes per day.

Acutely, cigarette smoking accentuates risk by elevating the myocardial oxygen demand (through increases in heart rate and blood pressure), reducing oxygen transport, increasing susceptibility to malignant ventricular arrhythmias, predisposing the coronary artery to spasm, and increasing platelet adhesiveness. Smoking also leads

to endothelial dysfunction (12). In addition, smoking leads to vasoconstriction and loss of endothelial cell integrity, thereby facilitating transport of atherogenic lipoprotein and scavenger cells across the endothelial barrier. Cigarette smokers have increased levels of fibrinogen and reduced fibrinolytic activity (13). Smoking also has a direct effect on serum lipids, decreasing HDL level and increasing LDL and triglyceride levels (14).

Table 1.1. Coronary Artery Disease Risk Factor Thresholds for Use with ACSM Risk Stratification

POSITIVE RISK FACTORS	DEFINING CRITERIA
1. Age	Men ≥ 45 years; women ≥ 55 or premature menopause without estrogen replacement therapy
2. Family history	MI or sudden death before 55 years of age in father or other male first-degree relative before 65 years of age in mother or other female first-degree relative
3. Current cigarette smoking	
4. Hypertension	Blood pressure ≥ 140/90 mm Hg, confirmed by measurements on at least 2 separate occasions, or taking antihypertensive medication
5. Hypercholesterolemia	Total serum cholesterol ≥ 200 mg/dL (5.2 mmol/L) (if lipoprotein profile is unavailable) or HDL < 35 mg/dL (0.9 mmol/L)
6. Diabetes mellitus	Persons with IDDM who are >30 years of age, or have had IDDM for > 15 years, and persons with NIDDM who are >35 years of age should be classified as patients with disease
7. Sedentary lifestyle/ physical inactivity	Persons among the least active 25% of the population, as defined by the combination of sedentary jobs involving sitting for a large part of the day and no regular exercise or active recreational pursuits

NEGATIVE RISK FACTOR	COMMENTS
1. High serum HDL cholesterol	≥ 60 mg/dL (1.6 mmol/L)

It is common to sum risk factors in making clinical judgments. If HDL is high, subtract one risk factor from the sum of positive risk factors, since high HDL decreases risk of coronary artery disease.

Obesity is not listed as an independent positive risk factor because its effects are exerted through other risk factors (e.g., hypertension, hyperlipidemia, diabetes). Obesity should be considered as an independent target for intervention.

IDDM, insulin-dependent diabetes mellitus; NIDDM, non–insulin-dependent diabetes mellitus; HDL, high-density lipoprotein.

Reprinted with permission from ASCM. ASCM's Guidelines for Exercise Testing and Prescription. 6th ed. Philadelphia: Lippincott Williams & Wilkins, 2000.

Table 1.2. Mechanistic Classification of Coronary Risk Factors

1. Causal risk factors
   - Cigarette smoking
   - Elevated levels of cholesterol and low density liprotein
   - Decreased levels of high density lipoprotein
   - Hypertension
   - Diabetes
2. Conditional risk factors
   - Triglycerides
   - Lipoprotein (a)
   - Homocysteine
   - Fibrinogen
   - Tissue plasminogen activator
   - Tissue plasminogen activator inhibitor
   - C-reactive protein
3. Predisposing risk factors
   - Obesity
   - Sedentary lifestyle
   - Behavioral factors
   - Socioeconomic status
   - Ethnicity
   - Male sex
   - Postmenopausal status
   - Family history of premature coronary disease
4. Plaque burden
   - Age
   - Extra coronary vascular disease
   - Coronary calcium score

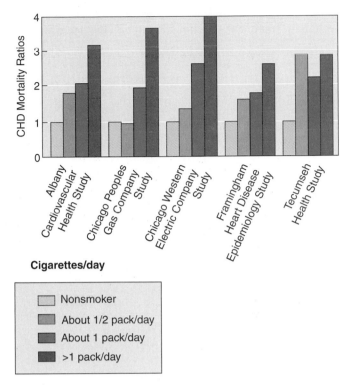

Figure 1.2. Coronary heart disease mortality ratios according to the amount of cigarettes smoked in five populations. (Reprinted with permission from The Pooling project Research Group. Relationship of blood pressure, serum cholesterol, smoking habit, relative weight, and ECG abnormalities to incidence of major coronary events: Final report of the Pooling Project. J Chron Dis 1978;31:202.)

There is overwhelming evidence that stopping smoking reduces the cardiovascular risk substantially, affecting both initial and recurrent coronary heart disease event rates. On an average, the rate can be reduced by 50% within 1 year of cessation of smoking (15). Finally, it has been estimated that approximately 50,000 deaths per year in the United States are caused by passive smoke. Most of these deaths are due to cardiovascular disease (16). A meta-analysis of epidemiological studies related to passive smoking concluded that overall, nonsmokers exposed to environmental smoke had a relative risk of coronary heart disease of 1.25 as compared with that of nonsmokers not exposed to smoke (17).

Cholesterol and Low-Density Lipoproteins

The relationship between cholesterol level and coronary heart disease is continuous and graded (Fig. 1.3) (18). Evidence from animal studies, experimental investigations, epidemiological studies, and clinical trials indicates conclusively that high serum cholesterol is a major cause of coronary heart disease and that lowering cholesterol level reduces the risk (19). About 38 million Americans are estimated to have total cholesterol levels of ≥ 240 mg/dL (2). Cholesterol circulates in the plasma in three sizes of lipoprotein particles, very low density lipoprotein (VLDL) cholesterol, LDL cholesterol, and HDL cholesterol. Total cholesterol is equal to the sum of these three fractions. Coronary heart disease is directly

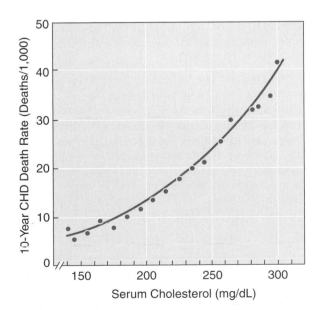

Figure 1.3. Relationship between serum cholesterol level and coronary heart disease death rate. (From Expert Panel on Detection, Evaluation, and Treatment of High Blood Cholesterol in Adults [Adult Treatment Panel II]. Second report of the National Cholesterol Education Program [NCEP] Men Screened for MRFIT Program. NIH Publication No. 93, 1993;361, 662.)

Table 1.3. Treatment Decisions Based on LDL Cholesterol

DIETARY THERAPY		
	INITIATION LEVEL	LDL GOAL
Without CHD and with fewer than 2 risk factors	≥ 160 mg/dL	< 160 mg/dL
Without CHD and with 2 or more risk factors	≥ 130 mg/dL	< 130 mg/dL
With CHD	> 100 mg/dL	≤ 100 mg/dL
DRUG TREATMENT		
	CONSIDERATION LEVEL	LDL GOAL
Without CHD and with fewer than 2 risk factors	≥ 190 mg/dL[a]	< 160 mg/dL
Without CHD and with 2 or more risk factors	≥ 160 mg/dL	< 130 mg/dL
With CHD	≥ 130 mg/dL[b]	≤ 100 mg/dL

[a] In men under 35 years of age and premenopausal women with LDL cholesterol levels 190–219 mg/dL, drug therapy should be delayed except in high-risk patients such as those with diabetes.
[b] In CHD patients with LDL cholesterol levels 100–129 mg/dL, the physician should exercise clinical judgment in deciding whether to initiate drug treatment.
Reprinted from Second Report of the National Expert Panel on Detection, Evaluation, and Treatment of High Blood Cholesterol in Adults (Adult Treatment Panel II). NIH Publication No. 93, 1993.

and linearly related to the levels of total cholesterol and LDL cholesterol and inversely related to the levels of HDL cholesterol. Most of the risk attributed to total cholesterol is explained by the LDL cholesterol concentration (5). Oxidized LDL cholesterol is considered to be a major factor in the pathogenesis of atherosclerosis. The National Cholesterol Education Program Adult Treatment Panel (NCEP-ATP) sets a high priority on LDL cholesterol management (Table 1.3) (20). In the MRFIT Trial, for each 50 mg/dL increase in total cholesterol above 200 mg/dL, coronary heart disease rates doubled (21). Framingham risk prediction model uses total cholesterol (not LDL cholesterol) and HDL cholesterol along with other major risk factors in estimating the risk of coronary events in the asymptomatic individual (22). Several large randomized trials have proved the benefit of cholesterol reduction in primary and secondary prevention trials (23–27).

High-Density-Lipoprotein Cholesterol

A low level of serum HDL cholesterol is an important predictor of coronary heart disease. Several large epidemiological studies suggested that for each 1 mg/dL increase in HDL cholesterol, a 2% decrease in coronary heart disease risk is noted in men and 3% decrease in women (28). The Framingham risk prediction model incorporates HDL cholesterol as a negative risk factor. Furthermore, a low LDL cholesterol level did not eliminate the risk imparted by low HDL cholesterol, while a high HDL cholesterol seemed to offset some of the risk of high LDL cholesterol (Fig. 1.4) (29). HDL cholesterol plays a critical role in reverse cholesterol transport (30). In addition, HDL cholesterol may retard atherogenesis through prevention of LDL cholesterol oxidation and monocyte adhesion to endothelial cells (31). Therapeutic options to increase HDL cholesterol levels include nonpharmacological approaches, such as exercise and moderate alcohol use, and pharmacological agents, including niacin, gemfibrozil, 3-hydroxy-3-methylglutaryl-coenzyme A (HMG-CoA) reductase inhibitors and hormone replacement therapy. The recently published Veterans Affairs High

Figure 1.4. Risk of coronary heart disease risk by high density lipoprotein cholesterol and low density lipoprotein cholesterol levels. (Adapted from Kannel WB, Gordon T. The Framingham Study: an epidemiological investigation of cardiovascular disease. Section 30. Washington, Public Health Service, NIH, DHEW Publication [NIH] 1974;74–599.)

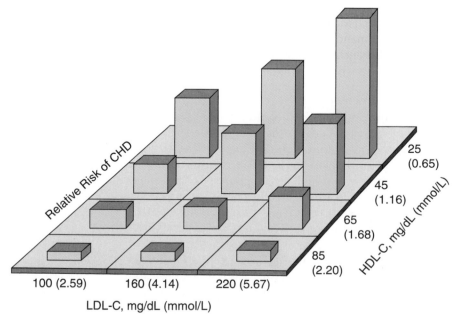

Density Lipoprotein Cholesterol Interventional Trial reported that in men with coronary heart disease and an HDL cholesterol level < 40 mg/dL, gemfibrozil resulted in a significant 24% reduction in death, nonfatal myocardial infarction, and stroke (32).

Hypertension

Nearly 50 million adult Americans have high blood pressure (≥140/90 mm Hg) (33). Data from numerous studies indicate a continuous relationship between blood pressure and cardiovascular risk, with lowest risk for adults with systolic blood pressure below 120 mm Hg and diastolic blood pressure below 80 mm Hg (34). The Framingham risk prediction model incorporates systolic blood pressure as a major risk factor in the occurrence of major coronary events. Elevation of blood pressure causes vascular endothelial dysfunction and injury leading to increased migration of atherogenic elements, including LDL, monocytes, and macrophages. A meta-analysis of the major randomized trials of antihypertensive therapy demonstrated a 42% reduction in the incidence of stroke and 14% reduction in coronary heart disease events (35). Isolated systolic hypertension, defined as systolic blood pressure ≥ 140 mm Hg and diastolic blood pressure <90 mm Hg, is common in men and women over age 65 years and is an independent risk factor for coronary heart disease. A recent meta-analysis suggests that one coronary or cerebral vascular event would be prevented for every 18 patients treated (336). The Joint National Commission–VI (JNC-VI) guidelines recommend a very aggressive approach in the treatment of hypertension, especially in the presence of target organ damage, diabetes, or clinical cardiovascular disease (33).

Blood pressure may be classified as outlined in Table 1.4, and persons with values above normal should be followed up as outlined in Table 1.5. Hypertension is believed to predispose patients to coronary artery disease by both direct vascular injury and adverse effects on the myocardium, which include increased wall stress and myocardial oxygen demand. Although substantial evidence attests to the health benefits of reducing blood pressure, the reduction in coronary artery disease events with antihypertensive therapy has been less than anticipated in most studies. This finding should not detract from the importance of reducing blood pressure but has raised concern about the potentially proatherogenic effects of certain antihypertensive treatments (such as the unfavorable effect of beta-blockers and thiazide diuretics on serum lipids) (37).

Lifestyle modification, including weight reduction, increased physical activity, and moderation of dietary sodium and alcohol intake, are recommended both as definitive and adjunctive therapy for hypertension (33). If blood pressure remains ≥ 140/90 mm Hg despite 3 to 6 months of lifestyle modification, drug therapy should be initiated. This is especially important in individuals with target organ disease and/or other known coronary artery disease risk factors (33). A variety of factors, including

Table 1.4. Classification of Blood Pressure for Adults Age 18 Years and Older[a]

CATEGORY	SYSTOLIC (MM HG)	DIASTOLIC (MM HG)
Normal[b]	< 130	< 85
High normal	130–139	85–89
Hypertension[c]		
STAGE 1 (mild)	140–159	90–99
STAGE 2 (moderate)	160–179	100–109
STAGE 3 (severe)	180–209	110–119
STAGE 4 (very severe)	≥ 210	≥ 120

[a] Not taking antihypertensive drugs and not acutely ill. When systolic and diastolic pressures fall into different categories, the higher category should be selected to classify the individual's blood pressure status. For instance, 160/92 mm Hg should be classified as stage 2, and 180/120 mm Hg should be classified as stage 4. Isolated systolic hypertension (ISH) is defined as SBP ≥ 140 mm Hg and DBP < 90 mm Hg and staged appropriately (e.g., 170/85 mm Hg is defined as stage 2 ISH).
[b] Optimal blood pressure with respect to cardiovascular risk is SBP < 120 mm Hg and DBP < 80 mm Hg. However, unusually low readings should be evaluated for clinical significance.
[c] Based on the average of two or more readings taken at each of two or more visits following an initial screening.
Note: In addition to classifying stages of hypertension based on average blood pressure levels, the clinician should specify presence or absence of target-organ disease and additional risk factors. For example, a patient with diabetes and a blood pressure of 142/94 mm Hg plus left ventricular hypertrophy should be classified as "stage 2 hypertension with target-organ disease (left ventricular hypertrophy) and with another major risk factor (diabetes)." This specificity is important for risk classification and management.

concomitant diseases, demographic characteristics, the use of accompanying drugs that may lead to drug interactions, cost of medication, and metabolic and subjective side effects should be considered in the selection of initial and subsequent antihypertensive drug therapy (33).

Diabetes

Coronary heart disease is also the most common cause of death in patients with type II diabetes, and it contributes significantly to the mortality in type I diabetes. One-fourth of myocardial infarctions occur in patients with diabetes (38). Diabetes is considered a major coronary risk factor, especially in women. Both microvascular and macrovascular disease are strongly associated with diabetes and appear to be major components of the pathogenesis of atherosclerosis in diabetics. The diagnostic criteria for diabetes include a fasting blood sugar level > 126 mg/100 mL and a 2-hour postprandial glucose level > 200 mg/dL (39). Diabetes is associated with a low level of HDL cholesterol and increased levels of VLDL cholesterol and triglycerides. There also appears to be a clustering of other risk factors, including hypertension, obesity, and dyslipidemia, in diabetics. Women with diabetes partially or completely lose their gender-related protection from coronary artery disease (40). The term *syndrome X* is used to describe a cluster of concomitant conditions, namely glucose intolerance, dyslipidemia, hypertension, central

Table 1.5. Recommendations for Follow-up Based on Initial Set of Blood Pressure Measurements for Adults Age 18 and Older

INITIAL SCREENING BLOOD PRESSURE (MM HG)[a]		FOLLOW-UP RECOMMENDED[b]
SYSTOLIC	DIASTOLIC	
< 130	< 85	Recheck in 2 yr
130–139	85–89	Recheck in 1 yr[c]
140–159	90–99	Confirm within 2 mo
160–179	100–109	Evaluate or refer to source of care within 1 mo
180–209	110–119	Evaluate or refer to source of care within 1 wk
≥ 210	≥ 120	Evaluate or refer to source of care immediately

[a] If the systolic and diastolic categories are different, follow recommendation for the shorter time follow-up (e.g., 160/85 mm Hg should be evaluated or referred to source of care within, 1 month).
[b] The scheduling of follow-up should be modified by reliable information about past blood pressure measurements, other cardiovascular risk factors, or target-organ disease
[c] Consider providing advice about lifestyle modifications (see Chapter 3).

obesity, and hyperinsulinemia. The common defect in this risk factor clustering is insulin resistance.

The importance of diabetes as a major coronary risk factor is further recognized by the JNC-VI guideline on the management of hypertension, which considers the presence of diabetes equal to the presence of clinical cardiovascular disease (33). Furthermore, the mortality from coronary heart disease in patients with type II diabetes may be as high as that in nondiabetic individuals with previous myocardial infarction (41). In the Diabetes Control and Complication Trial (DCCT), aggressive management of diabetes with tight glycemic control reduced the rate of microvascular complications in type I diabetes (42). Although DCCT was not primarily an event trial, intensive therapy reduced major cardiovascular events by 41%. The United Kingdom Prospective Diabetes Study (UKPDS) group reported that intensive blood glucose control reduced diabetes-related microvascular disease in type II diabetes, and there was a strong trend in favor of reduced risk of myocardial infarction (43). The UKPDS showed that in obese patients, intensive therapy reduced diabetes-related death, myocardial infarction, and all-cause mortality (44). The UKPDS group and Hypertension Optimal Treatment (HOT) study reported that aggressive control of blood pressure (target blood pressure <150/85 mm Hg in UKPDS and <130/85 mm Hg in HOT) resulted in less morbidity and mortality in type II diabetes (45, 46).

Conditional Risk Factors

Conditional risk factors are those that are associated with an increased risk of coronary heart disease but whose causal link has not been proved with certainty. The possible reasons causal link is uncertain include the following: (a) Compared to the causal risk factors, the atherogenic potential may be weak. (b) The prevalence of these risk factors may not be enough to detect a significant independent effect in epidemiological studies. The conditional risk factors include elevated triglyceride level and a group of novel or emerging risk factors, including lipoprotein-a, homocysteine, coagulation factors, such as fibrogen and plasminogen activator inhibitor-1, and C-reactive protein.

In considering the clinical utility of a new marker for coronary heart disease and risk assessment, three important issues must be considered. First, there must be a reliable assay technique for the marker of interest. Second, there must be consistency in the prospective epidemiological studies, indicating that the novel marker of interest can be detected in the individual before the onset of clinical disease. Third, there must be evidence that assessment of the new risk factor adds to the ability to predict the risk independent of conventional risk factors. Another issue to be considered in the evaluation of novel risk factors is modifiability. To date there is no conclusive evidence that modifying these new risk factors improves outcomes in primary or secondary prevention scenarios.

Triglycerides

The importance of triglycerides as a coronary risk factor remains speculative. The correlation between plasma triglyceride level and coronary heart disease observed in univariate analysis tends to weaken or disappear when adjusted for HDL cholesterol levels. The Prospective Cardiovascular Munster Study and the Lipid Research Clinic follow-up study found positive correlations between high triglyceride level and coronary heart disease, although no independent predictive value for triglycerides was found (47, 48). LDL cholesterol, HDL cholesterol, diabetes, insulin resistance, and obesity confound the association of triglycerides to coronary artery disease. However, very high triglyceride levels caused by genetic defects such as familial lipoprotein lipase deficiency are not associated with atheroma or coronary artery disease. No primary or secondary prevention trials specifically addressing triglyceride reduction and coronary artery disease risk are available. Nevertheless, the National Cholesterol Education Program Adult Treatment Panel classifies triglyceride levels as normal (< 200 mg/dL), borderline high (200–399 mg/dL), high (400–999 mg/dL), and very high (≥1,000 mg/dL) and recommends that patients with triglyceride levels ≥ 200 mg/dL be counseled to reduce body weight, increase exercise, decrease fat intake, quit smoking, and limit alcohol intake (20).

Homocysteine

Homocysteine is an amino acid formed during methionine metabolism. In the normal individual, fasting plasma homocysteine level is 5–15 μmol/L. Homocysteine levels increase with aging; menopause; chronic renal insufficiency; vitamin B_6, B_{12}, and folate deficiency; and cardiac transplantation (49). A meta-analysis of 27 studies indicated that increased homocysteine levels are associated with an increased risk of coronary artery disease, peripheral arterial disease, stroke, and venous thromboembolism (50). Increased homocysteine levels seem to predict mortality in patients with known coronary artery disease (51). High levels of homocysteine are associated with endothelial dysfunction, enhanced platelet aggregation, and vascular smooth muscle proliferation. Folate supplementation may be effective in reducing homocysteine levels. The clinical usefulness of measuring homocysteine levels as part of cardiovascular risk evaluation is uncertain because of nonstandardized assay technique, inconsistent epidemiological studies, and lack of additive value to total and HDL cholesterol. Moreover, prospective randomized studies proving the beneficial effects of increased folic acid intake in the setting of primary or secondary prevention are lacking.

Lipoprotein-a

Data regarding the risk of cardiovascular disease associated with elevated lipoprotein-a (Lp-a) levels conflict. Prospective investigations suggest an important role of Lp-a in major coronary events (52). However, in the Physician Health Study, Lp-a levels failed to predict cardiovascular events (53). Race has also been suggested to affect Lp-a level, which might be expected to affect risk. However, although blacks generally have higher Lp-a concentrations than whites, this does not seem to translate into an increased risk of coronary heart disease (49). Lifestyle interventions do not appear to lower Lp-a levels, and niacin is the only conventional lipid agent known to lower Lp-a. Estrogen replacement may also be beneficial (54, 55).

Fibrinogen

Elevated levels of fibrinogen have been shown to correlate with myocardial infarction and stroke, probably as a result of enhanced blood viscosity and increased thrombogenicity. The prospective epidemiological studies correlating increased fibrinogen level to coronary heart disease are consistent, and they indicate that fibrinogen levels provide an independent risk prediction over and above that provided by HDL cholesterol levels. A meta-analysis of six prospective epidemiological studies confirms the association of increased fibrinogen level with subsequent myocardial infarction or stroke (49). Fibrinogen levels are generally higher in men than women and smokers than nonsmokers (49). Physical inactivity and elevated triglycerides are also associated with increased fibrinogen levels (56). Nonetheless, the assay techniques for fibrinogen levels are not standardized, and the clinical utility of measuring fibrinogen levels as part of risk factor screening is unproved.

Tissue Plasminogen Activator

Increased levels of tissue plasminogen activator (t-PA) and plasminogen activator inhibitor-1 have been associated with enhanced risk of coronary artery disease. Insulin resistance and hypertriglyceridemia are also associated with increased plasminogen activator inhibitor levels. For t-PA and plasminogen activator inhibitor, nonstandardized assay techniques and lack of independent prognostic value beyond total cholesterol and HDL levels limit the clinical utility. Furthermore, angiotensin-converting enzyme inhibitors may enhance plasma fibrinolytic variables (49).

C-Reactive Protein

C-reactive protein is an acute phase reactant and a marker for underlying systemic inflammation. Several studies have established an association between C-reactive protein and various manifestations of atherosclerosis. Of the novel risk factors, C-reactive protein is the only one that has met all three criteria for clinical utility of novel risk factors, namely standardized assay techniques, consistent prospective epidemiological studies correlating the level of C-reactive protein with coronary heart disease risk, and independent predictive value beyond that obtained by other conventional risk factors (Fig. 1.5) (57). However, the pathophysiological role of C-reactive protein in atherosclerosis is unclear. The presence of C-reactive protein immunoreactivity has been demonstrated in the unstable coronary plaque (58). No available therapy specifically reduces high C-reactive protein levels, although it is of interest that baseline concentrations of high C-reactive protein levels seem to modulate the efficacy of aspirin and HMG coenzyme A reductase inhibitors. Data from two double-blind randomized clinical trials suggest that relative efficacy of aspirin and statins may be greater in persons with evidence of underlying inflammation as assessed by levels of C-reactive proteins (59, 60).

Predisposing Risk Factors

Obesity, physical inactivity, various behavioral characteristics, poor socioeconomic status, male gender, family history of premature coronary artery disease, postmenopausal status, and aging are considered predisposing risk factors. This classification is the result of either their effect on causal or conditional risk factors or their as yet unrecognized independent effect on the development of coronary heart disease. Clearly, the presence of some predisposing risk factors intensifies certain causal risk factors; for example, obesity worsens insulin resistance and thereby increases the risk of vascular disease. However, modification of risk factors such as obesity and physical inactivity may reduce the coronary heart disease event rate, although again, it is uncertain whether the beneficial effects are independent of favorable influences on causal or conditional risk factors.

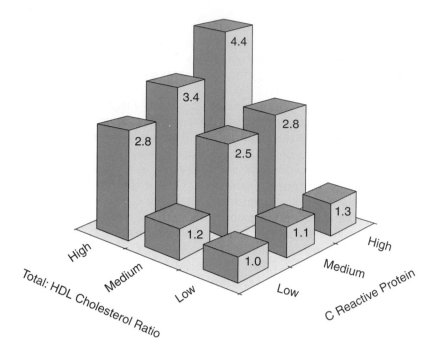

Figure 1.5. Relative risks of first myocardial infarction among apparently healthy men associated with high, middle, and low tertiles of the total cholesterol:high density lipoprotein ratio and high, middle, and low tertiles of C-reactive protein. (Adapted with permission from Circulation 1998;97:2009.)

Obesity

The prevalence of obesity in the U.S. appears to have increased substantially during the past decade, and one in three adults is now considered overweight (61). Obesity contributes to many adverse health outcomes, and obesity-related conditions are estimated to contribute to 300,000 deaths annually in the United States (62). Obesity is associated with an accentuated risk of cardiovascular disease (Fig. 1.6). Analysis of the relationship between obesity and coronary artery disease is difficult because of its association with other risk factors, in particular physical inactivity, hypertension, hyperlipidemia, and diabetes. However, recent reports from the Framingham Heart Study support the independence of obesity as a risk factor for coronary artery disease (63). In syndrome X, visceral or central abdominal obesity, high triglyceride levels, low HDL cholesterol levels, insulin resistance, and hypertension are metabolically linked. This form of obesity is relatively common and is associated with a markedly increased risk of coronary artery disease.

No studies have specifically evaluated the effect of weight loss on coronary artery disease events. Comprehensive programs that incorporate behavioral modalities to increase physical activity and improve diet have been shown to induce weight loss sufficient to produce significant cardiovascular health benefits in many obese individuals. In this respect, even modest weight loss of 5–10% of initial body weight has positive benefits on coronary artery disease risk factors, and weight loss of this magnitude may be realistic for many individuals (64).

Unfortunately, improvements in coronary artery disease risk factors are not maintained if weight is regained, and most of those who lose a significant amount of weight regain the lost weight within a relatively short time. Recognition of the need for long-term and perhaps lifelong treatment has led certain experts to embrace the concept of long-term drug therapy, as is used in other chronic diseases. A national task force on the prevention and treatment of obesity, however, recently concluded that until more long-term data are available, pharmacotherapy cannot be recommended for routine use in obese individuals, although it may be helpful in carefully selected patients (65).

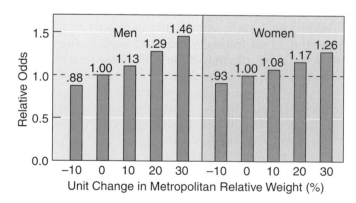

Figure 1.6. The relative odds of developing cardiovascular disease corresponding to degree of change in relative weight between age 25 years and entry into the Framingham Study. The odds ratios reflect adjustments for the effects of relative weight at age 25 years and risk factor levels at exam 1. (With permission from Hubert HB, et al. Obesity as an independent risk factor for cardiovascular disease: a 26-year follow-up of participants in the Framingham Heart Study. Circulation 1983;67:968.)

Physical Inactivity

Epidemiological criteria have been used to establish a relationship between physical activity and coronary artery disease, with the following principles having been met:

1. Consistency. The association has been documented in a variety of settings and populations, with the better-designed studies showing the strongest associations.
2. Strength. The relative risk of coronary artery disease associated with physical inactivity is comparable with that observed for cigarette smoking, hypercholesterolemia, and hypertension.
3. Temporal sequencing. Physical inactivity has been observed to predate the diagnosis of coronary artery disease.
4. Dose response. The risk of coronary artery disease increases as physical activity decreases.
5. Biologic plausibility (66).

However, the precise mechanism by which physical inactivity predisposes persons to coronary artery disease has yet to be fully elucidated. Positive results of activity include the following:

1. Improvement of the balance between myocardial oxygen supply and demand at a given submaximal exercise intensity
2. Decreased platelet aggregation and enhanced fibrinolysis
3. Reduced susceptibility to malignant ventricular arrhythmias
4. Improved endothelial-mediated vasomotor tone
5. Beneficial effect on other coronary artery disease risk factors

Regarding the beneficial effect on other coronary artery disease risk factors, regular physical activity has been shown to lower resting systolic and diastolic blood pressure, reduce serum triglyceride levels, increase serum HDL cholesterol levels, and enhance glucose tolerance and insulin sensitivity (66, 67). However, despite this evidence, millions of U.S. adults remain essentially sedentary. Indeed, the number of individuals who are inactive is substantially greater than the number who smoke cigarettes, have hypercholesterolemia, or have hypertension. Thus, the overall effect of stimulating Americans to lead a more physically active lifestyle could lower coronary artery disease rates more than by reducing any other single risk factor (68).

Behaviorial Characteristics

The psychosocial factors associated with risk of coronary artery disease include the so-called type A personality, hostility, depression, chronic stress produced by situations with high demand and low control, and social

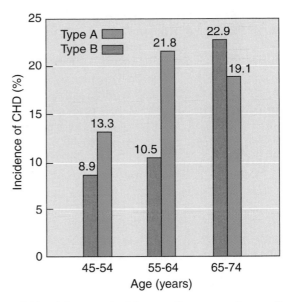

Figure 1.7. Eight-year incidence of coronary heart disease among men by the Framingham Type A and B behavior patterns. (With permission from Haynes SG, Feinleib M, Kannel WB. The relationship of psychosocial factors to coronary heart disease in the Framingham Study. III. Eight-year incidence of coronary heart disease. Am J Epidemiol 1980;111:37.)

isolation (Fig. 1.7) (69). Psychosocial factors are postulated to accentuate the risk via two major mechanisms. First, they may exert a detrimental influence by direct mechanisms that primarily include neuroendocrine effects, such as changes in catecholamine and serotonin levels. Second, they may indirectly accentuate risk by influencing adherence to lifestyle recommendations and compliance with drug therapy. Interventions of potential benefit include behavior modification, biofeedback, meditation, exercise, and when indicated, pharmacotherapy.

Postmenopausal Status

Coronary artery disease manifests itself approximately a decade later in women than in men. Nevertheless, it remains the leading cause of death among women in the United States. The role of hormone replacement therapy in postmenopausal women is uncertain. The postmenopausal estrogen–progesterone intervention trials have established the efficacy of hormone replacement therapy in raising HDL cholesterol levels and decreasing levels of LDL cholesterol, total cholesterol, and fibrinogen (70). Nonetheless, beneficial effects on coronary heart disease end points have not been found (71).

Unmodifiable Risk Factors

Male gender, family history of premature coronary artery disease, low socioeconomic status, and age are risk factors that are not amenable to intervention. Recognition of them is nonetheless important for helping to reduce the risk of future cardiac events and should be considered when attempting to match the level of management with the level of risk (72).

Plaque Burden

The concept of the atherosclerotic plaque itself being a risk factor is new and is based on the observation that once atherosclerotic plaque reaches a certain stage of development, coronary events continue to occur in spite of controlling other conventional risk factors (8). In the conventional sense, plaque burden is not a risk factor for the disease; rather, it is the disease. The extent of coronary atherosclerosis, that is, plaque burden, is a powerful predictor of coronary events (73). Intracoronary ultrasound and coronary angiography (which generally underestimates the extent of disease) can be used to assess the extent of coronary atherosclerosis. In the clinical setting, age, vascular disease in extra coronary vascular beds, and coronary calcium score measured by electron beam computed tomography (EBCT) can be used as surrogate markers of plaque burden. Most coronary risk prediction models, for example the Framingham model, incorporate age as a major risk factor based on the observation that extent of coronary atherosclerosis is greater in the older person than in the younger one. There is a high correlation between severity of atherosclerosis in the coronary and carotid vessels (74). Measurement of the thickness of the carotid intima media by ultrasonography predicts major coronary events independent of other risk factors (75). EBCT can be used to measure the amount of calcium in the coronary atherosclerotic plaque, and the calcium score reflects the extent of disease (76). A recent prospective study suggests that EBCT may be highly effective in predicting cardiovascular events (77). Both carotid ultrasound and EBCT have the potential to replace age in risk prediction models, although more studies are needed.

GLOBAL RISK ASSESSMENT IN THE ASYMPTOMATIC INDIVIDUAL

Patients with known coronary heart disease are at significant risk for future coronary events, and this risk can be reduced by well-accepted secondary prevention strategies (78). However, in the setting of primary prevention, strategies to reduce risk may in some cases be less clear. The controversy regarding primary prevention strategies can be attributed to two observations: (*a*) The absolute cardiovascular risk in asymptomatic individuals with coronary risk factors is generally low, making aggressive prevention strategies generally not cost effective. (*b*) Most coronary events in a community occur in individuals with only mild to moderate elevation of risk factors. The individuals with marked elevation of risk factors, namely cholesterol or blood pressure, constitute only a minority of the total population. Therefore, strategies aimed at identifying high-risk individuals have an effect for the individual but only minimal usefulness in preventing cardiovascular events for the community.

By using the concept of assessment of global risk, the various risk prediction models can provide a quantitative estimate of the risk of coronary events. For example, patients with stable angina have an average risk of nonfatal myocardial infarction or death of approximately 20% over the next 10 years (8). Such individuals, whose event rate is expected to be 20% or greater in 10 years, are considered high risk, and aggressive secondary prevention strategies are appropriate. Thus, in an individual with no known coronary heart disease but in whom the risk prediction model suggests a 10 year event rate of 20% or greater, it is logical to consider the same aggressive strategies in an attempt at primary prevention.

On the contrary, the use of a single risk factor guideline, such as the most recent National Cholesterol Education Program (NCEP) guideline, increases the potential for overestimation or underestimation of individual coronary heart disease risk. For example, a 46-year-old man with a total cholesterol of 260 mg/dL, HDL of 34 mg/dL, and LDL of 160 mg/dL and no other coronary risk factors has a 10-year risk of developing coronary heart disease of approximately 10%. In contrast, a 55-year-old diabetic hypertensive man with a history of smoking and total cholesterol of 191 mg/dL, HDL of 34 mg/dL, and LDL mg/dL of 131 mg/dL has a 10-year coronary heart disease risk of approximately 27%. Using the NCEP guidelines, the first man would qualify for drug treatment of hypercholesterolemia, but the second one would not.

A global risk prediction model takes into account all known major risk factors for coronary heart disease and gives a quantitative estimate of coronary event rate. The most widely used global risk prediction instrument is the Framingham model that incorporates age, sex, systolic blood pressure, diabetes, total cholesterol, HDL, and cigarette smoking (Table 1.6) (22). In the original Framingham Risk Prediction model, left ventricular hypertrophy was also included (79). However, in the more recent Framingham Prediction model, left ventricular hypertrophy was excluded because it was thought that hypertension is a confounding variable for left ventricular hypertrophy and that adding left ventricular hypertrophy and blood pressure might overpredict risk. Although the Framingham model was derived from the white population of Framingham, Massachusetts, its accuracy has been verified in other populations in the United States, including Hispanics, African-Americans, and Hawaiians.

The European Joint Task Force Risk Chart, developed in collaboration with the European Society of Cardiology, European Atherosclerosis Society, European Society of Hypertension, and other agencies, incorporates age, sex, systolic blood pressure, total cholesterol, smoking status, and diabetes in its model while adjusting for family history of premature coronary artery disease, increased triglycerides, and decreased HDL (80). Other risk prediction models are primarily based on the Framingham Risk

Table 1.6. Scoring for Global Risk Assessment (Adjusted Framingham Scoring)

RISK FACTOR	RISK POINTS		ADDING UP THE POINTS		
	MEN	WOMEN			
Age, yr			Age___ Cholesterol___		
<34	−1	−9	Diabetes___ HDL Cholesterol___		
35–39	0	−4	Smoker___ Blood Pressure___		
40–44	1	0			
45–49	2	3	Total___		
50–54	3	6			
55–59	4	7	ABSOLUTE RISK (HARD CHD), %		
60–64	5	8			
65–69	6	9	RISK POINTS	MEN	WOMEN
70–74	7	10			
Total cholesterol, mg/dL			1	2	1
<160	−3	−2	2	3	2
169–199	0	0	3	4	2
200–239	1	1	4	5	2
240–279	2	2	5	6	2
≥280	3	3	6	7	2
HDL cholesterol, mg/dL			7	9	3
<35	2	5	8	13	3
35–44	1	2	9	16	3
45–49	0	1	10	20	4
50–59	−1	0	11	25	7
≥60	−2	−3	12	30	8
Blood pressure, mm Hg			13	35	11
<120	0	−3	14	45	13
120–129	0	0	15		15
130–139	1	1	16		18
140–159	2	2	17		20
>160	3	3			
Plasma glucose, mg/dL					
<110	0	0			
110–126	1	2			
>126	2	4			
Smoker					
No	0	0			
Yes	2	2			

With permission from *Circulation* 1999;100:991.

Function with some modifications. Although the original Sheffield Table used the same variables as the European Joint Task Force, the modified Sheffield and the New Zealand model incorporate the ratio of total cholesterol to HDL rather than total cholesterol alone, improving specificity in identifying high-risk individuals while maintaining high sensitivity (81, 82).

► SUMMARY

Aggressive primary prevention strategies are appropriate for individuals at high risk for coronary heart disease as indicated by (*a*) presence of vascular disease in noncoronary vascular beds, (*b*) asymptomatic coronary atherosclerosis indicated by EBCT, (*c*) patients with type II diabetes, and (*d*) individuals with a 20% risk of having coronary events based on Framingham prediction models. The universal strategy of lifetime primary prevention can be applied at a community level irrespective of the individual coronary risk profile; this strategy includes smoking cessation, a NCEP/American Heart Association Step I diet, weight loss in those who are overweight (ideal body mass index 21–25 kg/m^2) and moderate exercise for 30–60 minutes three to four times weekly. Coronary heart disease has been and continues to be a major public health problem in the United States and other western countries. Even though there are many risk factors for coronary heart disease, the major or causal risk factors continue to be highly prevalent, and aggressive primary strategies aimed at controlling these risk factors are likely to lead to further decreases in the mortality and morbidity from this lethal disease.

References
1. World Health Report 1997. Geneva: World Health Organization, 1997.

2. American Heart Association. Heart and Stroke Facts: 1994 Statistical Supplement. Dallas: American Heart Association, 1994.

3. Miller M, Vogel RA. The practice of coronary artery disease prevention. 1st ed. Baltimore: Williams & Wilkins, 1996:2.

4. Kannel WB, Dawber TR, Kagan A, et al. Factors of risk in the development of coronary heart disease: Six-year follow-up experience. Ann Intern Med 55:33–50, 1961.

5. Pasternak RC: Grundy SM, Levy D, Thompson PD. Spectrum of risk factors for coronary heart disease. J Am Coll Cardiol 27:978–990, 1996.

6. Gastelli WB, Anderson K, Wilson PW, Levy D. Lipids and risk of coronary heart disease: The Framingham Study. Ann Epidemiol 2:23–28, 1992.

7. Stamler J, Stamler R, Neaton JD. Blood pressure systolic and diastolic, and cardiovascular risk: years population data. Arch Intern Med 153:598–615, 1993.

8. Grundy SM. Primary prevention of coronary heart disease. Circulation 100:988–998, 1990.

9. McGinnis JM, Foege WH. Actual causes of death in the United States. JAMA 270:2207–2212, 1993.

10. McGill HC Jr. The cardiovascular pathology of smoking. Am Heart J 115:250–257, 1988.

11. Willett WC, Green A, Stampfe MJ, et al. Relative and absolute excess risk of coronary heart disease among women who smoke cigarettes. N Engl J Med 317:1303–1309, 1987.

12. Reinders JH, Brinkman HA, VanMourik JA, DeGroot PG. Cigarette smoke impairs endothelial cell prostacyclin production. Atherosclerosis 6:15–23, 1986.

13. Allen RA, Klauf TC, Brommer EJ. Effect of chronic smoking on fibrinolysis. Atherosclerosis 5:443–450, 1985.

14. Craig WY, Palomaik GE, Haddow JE. Cigarette smoking and serum lipid and lipoprotein concentrations: An analysis of published data. BMJ 298:784–788, 1989.

15. Daly LE, Mulcahy R, Graham IM, Hickey M. Long term effect on mortality of stopping smoking after unstable angina and myocardial infarction. BMJ 287:324–326, 1983.

16. Glantz SA, Parmley WW. Passive smoking and heart disease: Epidemiology, physiology and biochemistry. Circulation 83:1–12, 1991.

17. He J, Vupputuri S, Allen K, et al. Passive smoking and the risk of coronary heart disease—a meta-analysis of epidemiologic studies. N Engl J Med 340:920–926, 1999.

18. MRFIT Research Group. Multiple risk factor changes and mortality results. JAMA 248:1465–1477, 1982.

19. American Heart Association, National Heart, Lung and Blood Institute. The cholesterol facts: A summary of the evidence relating to dietary fat, serum cholesterol and coronary heart disease. Circulation 81:1721–1733, 1990.

20. Expert Panel on Detection, Evaluation and Treatment of High Blood Cholesterol in Adults. Summary of the Second Report of the National Cholesteral Education Program (NCEP) Expert Panel on Detection, Evaluation, and Treatment of High Blood Cholesterol in Adults (Adult Treatment Panel II). JAMA 269:3015–3023, 1993.

21. Stamler J, Wentworth D, Neaton JD. Is relationship between serum cholesterol and risk of premature death from coronary heart disease continuous and graded? JAMA 256:2823–2828, 1986.

22. Wilson PWF, D'Agostino RB, Levy D, et al. Prediction of coronary heart disease using risk factor categories. Circulation 97:1837–1847, 1998.

23. Sacks F, Pfeffer M, Moye L, et al. Effect of pravastatin on coronary events after myocardial infarction in patients with average cholesterol levels. N Engl J Med 335:1001–1009, 1996.

24. Tonkin AM. Management of the long term intervention with pravastatin in ischemic heart disease study. Am J Cardiol 76:107C–112C, 1995.

25. Scandinavian Simvastatin Survival Study Group. Baseline serum cholesterol and treatment effect in the Scandinavian Simvastatin Survival Study. Lancet 345:1274–1275, 1995.

26. Shepherd J. The Western Scotland Coronary Prevention Study: a trial of cholesterol reduction in Scottish men. Am J Cardiol 76:113C–117C, 1995.

27. Bowns JR, Clearfield M, Weiss S, et al. Primary prevention of acute coronary events with lovastatin in men and women with average cholesterol levels. Results of AFCAPS/TEXCAPS. JAMA 279:1615–1622, 1998.

28. Harper CR, Jacobson TA. New prospective on the management of low levels of high density lipoprotein cholesterol. Arch Intern Med 159:1049–1057, 1999.

29. Gordon T, Castelli WP, Hjortland MC, et al. High density lipoprotein as a protective factor against coronary heart disease. Am J Med 62:707–714, 1997.

30. Tall AR. Plasma high density lipoproteins. J Clin Invest 86:379–384, 1990.

31. Maier JA, Barcengi HL, Pagan IF, et al. The protective role of high density lipoprotein on oxidized low density lipoprotein induced U937/endothelial cell interactions. Eur J Biochem 221:35–41, 1994.

32. Rubins HB, Robins SJ, Collins D, et al. Gemfibrozil for the secondary prevention of coronary heart disease in men with low levels of HDL cholesterol. N Engl J Med 341:410, 1999.

33. The Sixth Report of the Joint National Committee on Prevention, Detection, Evaluation and Treatment of High Blood Pressure. National High Blood Pressure Education Program. National Institutes of Health.

National Heart, Lung, and Blood Institute. NIH Publication 98-4080, 1997.

34. Stamler J, Neaton J, Wentworth D. Blood pressure and risk of fatal coronary heart disease. Hypertension 13:2–12, 1993.

35. Collins R, Petor, MacMahon S, et al. Blood pressure stroke and coronary heart disease. Lancet 335:827–838, 1990.

36. Mulrow CD, Cornell JA, Herrera CR, et al. Hypertension in the elderly: Implications and generalized ability of randomized trials. JAMA 272:1932–1938, 1994.

37. Roberts WC. Blood lipid levels and antihypertensive therapy. Am J Cardiol 60:33E–35E, 1987.

38. Butler WJ, Ostrander LD, Carman WJ, Lamphiear DE. Mortality from coronary heart disease in the Tecumseh Study: Long term effects of diabetes mellitus, glucose intolerance and other risk factors. Am J Epidemiol 1985 121:541–547.

39. Report of the Expert Committee on the Diagnosis and Complications of Diabetes Mellitus. Diabetes Care 20:1183–1197, 1997.

40. Bierman EL. George Lyman Duff Memorial Lecture. Atherogenesis in diabetes. Arterioscler Thromb 12:647–656, 1992.

41. Haffner SM, Lehto S, Ronnemaa T, et al. Mortality from coronary heart disease in subjects with type II diabetes and nondiabetic subjects with and without prior myocardial infarction. N Engl J Med 339:229–234, 1998.

42. DCCT Research Group. The effect of intensive treatment of diabetes on the development and progression of long term complication of insulin dependent diabetes mellitus. N Engl J Med 329:977–986, 1993.

43. UKPDS Group. Intensive blood glucose control with sulfonylureas or insulin compared with conventional treatment and risk of complications in patients with type II diabetes. Lancet 352:837–853, 1998.

44. UKPDS Group. Effect of intensive glucose control with metformin on complications in overweight patients with type II diabetes. Lancet 352:854–865, 1998.

45. UKPDS Group. Tight blood pressure control and risk of macro and microvascular complications in type II diabetes. BMJ 317:703–713, 1998.

46. Hanson I, Jarchett A, Carruths SG, et al. Effects of intensive blood pressure lowering and low dose aspirin in patients with hypertension, the HOT Study Group. Lancet 351:1755–1762, 1998.

47. Assman G, Schulte H. Triglycerides and atherosclerosis: results from the prospective cardiovascular Munster Study. Atheroscler Rev 22:51–57, 1991.

48. Criqui MH, Heis SG, Kohn R, et al. Plasma triglycerides level and mortality from coronary heart disease. N Engl J Med 328:1220–1225, 1993.

49. Kullo IJ, Gau GT, Tajik AJ. Novel risk factors for atherosclerosis. Mayo Clin Proc 75:369–380, 2000.

50. Boushey CJ, Beresford AS, Omenn GS, Motulsky AG. A quantitative assessment of plasma homocysteine as a risk factor for vascular disease. JAMA 274:1049–1057, 1995.

51. Nygar DO, Nordrehaug JE, Refsum H, et al. Plasma homocysteine levels and mortality in patients with coronary artery disease. N Engl J Med 337:230–236, 1997.

52. Cremer P, Nagel D, Labort B, et al. Lipoprotein-a as predictor of myocardial infarction in comparison to fibrinogen LDL cholesterol and other risk factors. Eur J Clin Invest 24:444–445, 1994.

53. Redker PM, Henneken CM, Stampfer MJ. Prospective study of lipoprotein-a and the risk of myocardial infarction. JAMA 270:2195–2199, 1993.

54. Superko HR. Beyond LDL cholesterol reduction. Circulation 94:2351–2354, 1996.

55. Bostom AG, Cuppies LA, Jenner JL, et al. Elevated plasma lipoprotein(a) and coronary heart disease in men aged 55 years and younger: A prospective study. JAMA 276:544–548, 1996.

56. Yang XC, Jing TY, Resnick LM, et al. Relation of hemostatic risk factors to other risk factors for coronary heart disease and to sex hormones in men. Arterioscler Thromb Vasc Biol 13:467–471, 1993.

57. Ridker PM. Evaluating novel cardiovascular risk factors. Ann Intern Med 130:1933–1937, 1999.

58. Burke AP, Farb A, Mannan P, et al. C-reactive protein is expressed in unstable macrophage rich atherosclerotic plaque. Circulation 96(Suppl 1-I):I–492, 1997.

59. Ridker PM, Cushman M, Stampfer M, et al. Inflammation, aspirin and the risk of cardiovascular disease in apparently healthy men. N Engl J Med 336:973–979, 1997.

60. Ridker PM, Rifai N, Pfeffer MA, et al. Inflammation, pravastatin and the risk of coronary events after myocardial infarction in patients with average cholesterol levels. Circulation 98:838–944, 1998.

61. Kuezmarski RJ, Flegal KM, Campbell SM, et al. Increasing prevalence of overweight among US adults. JAMA 272:205–211, 1994.

62. Pi-Sunyer FX. Medical hazards of obesity. Ann Intern Med 110:655–660, 1993.

63. Hubert HB, Feineib M, McNamara PM, et al. Obesity as an independent risk factor for cardiovascular disease: A 26-year follow-up of participants in the Framingham Heart Study. Circulation 67:968–977, 1983.

64. Blackburn GL, Rosofsky W. Making the connection between weight loss, dieting, and health: The 10% solution. Weight Control Dig 2:121–127, 1992.

65. National Task Force on the Prevention and Treatment of Obesity. Long-term pharmacotherapy in the management of obesity. JAMA 276:1907–1915, 1996.

66. Fletcher GF, Balady G, Blair SN, et al. Statement on Exercise: Benefits and recommendations for physical activity programs for all Americans: A statement for health professionals by the Committee on Exercise

and Cardiac Rehabilitation of the Council on Clinical Cardiology, American Heart Association. Circulation 94:857–862, 1996.

67. Pate RR, Pratt M, Blair SN, et al. Physical activity and public health: A recommendation from the Centers for Disease Control and Prevention and the American College of Sports Medicine. JAMA 273:402–407, 1995.

68. Caspersen CJ, Heath GW. The risk factor concept of coronary heart disease. In: ACSM's Resource Manual for Guidelines for Exercise Testing and Prescription. 2nd ed. Philadelphia: Lea & Febiger, 1993:151–167.

69. Pasternak RC, Grundy SM, Levy D, et al. Task Force 3. Spectrum of risk factors for coronary heart disease. J Am Coll Cardiol 27:978–990, 1996.

70. Writing Group for the PEPI Trial. Effects of estrogen and estrogen-progesterone regimen on heart disease risk factors in postmenopausal women. JAMA 273:199–208, 1995.

71. Hulley S, Grady D, Bush T, et al. Randomized trial of estrogen plus progestin for secondary prevention of coronary heart disease in postmenopausal women. JAMA 280:605–613, 1998.

72. Fuster V, Pearson TA. 27th Bethesda Conference. Matching the intensity of risk factor management with the hazard for coronary disease events. J Am Coll Cardiol 27:957–1047, 1996.

73. Ringquist I, Fisher LD, Mock M, et al. Prognostic valve of angiographic indices of coronary artery disease from the coronary artery surgery study. J Clin Invest 71:1854–1866, 1998.

74. Crouse JR. Carotid and coronary atherosclerosis: What are the connections? Postgrad Med 90: 175–179, 1991.

75. Hodis HN, Mack WJ, LaBree I, et al. The role of carotid arterial intima-media thickness in predicting clinical coronary events. Ann Intern Med 128: 262–269, 1998.

76. Rumberger JA, Schwartz RS, Simons DB. Relation of coronary calcium determined by EBCT and lumina narrowing determined by autopsy. Am J Cardiol 74: 1169–1173, 1994.

77. Arad Y, Spadaro LA, Goodman K, et al. Predictive value of EBCT of the coronary arteries. Circulation 93:1951–1953, 1996.

78. Smith SC Jr, Blair SN, Criqui MH, et al. Preventing heart attack and death in patients with coronary artery disease. Circulation 92:1–4, 1995.

79. Wilson PW. Established risk factors in coronary artery disease, the Framingham Study. Am J Hypertension 7:7S–12S, 1994.

80. Wood D, DeBacker G, Furgoman O, et al. Prevention of coronary heart disease in clinical practice. Eur Heart J 19:1434–1503, 1998.

81. Ramsay LE, Haqiu, Jackson PR, et al. Targeting lipid lowering drug therapy for primary prevention of coronary artery disease: an updated Sheffield table. Lancet 348:387–388, 1996.

82. Dyslipidemia Advisory Group on Behalf of the Scientific Committee of the National Heart Foundation of New Zealand. N Z Med J 109:224–232, 1996.

1.4.0.2

2.4.2, 2.4.3

3.4.0, 3.4.0

4.4.17

5.4.2

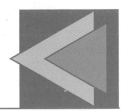

CHAPTER **2**

EPIDEMIOLOGY OF PHYSICAL ACTIVITY, PHYSICAL FITNESS, AND SELECTED CHRONIC DISEASES

Mitchell H. Whaley and Leonard A. Kaminsky

Based on the observed health-related benefits associated with increased physical activity, several health organizations have published position papers calling for efforts to increase public awareness and to establish recommendations for the appropriate quantity and quality of physical activity for adults (1–3). These position statements were based on the continually increasing volume of scientific literature that demonstrates the inverse association between sedentary lifestyle and morbidity or mortality from a number of chronic diseases. The purpose of this chapter is to review the association between sedentary habits and the risk of chronic disease and to review the most recent physical activity recommendations in light of this evidence.

PHYSICAL ACTIVITY VERSUS CARDIORESPIRATORY FITNESS

Prior to reviewing the relationships between levels of physical activity and/or cardiorespiratory fitness resulting from exercise, and chronic illnesses, it is important to review the operational definitions of these two terms (3a). First, the term *physical activity* refers to "any bodily movement produced by skeletal muscles that results in energy expenditure" and therefore may include both occupational and leisure physical activity. In contrast, exercise, considered a subclass of physical activity, is defined as "planned, structured, and repetitive bodily movement done to improve or maintain one or more components of physical fitness." Too often the terms physical activity and exercise are used interchangeably, when indeed both the characteristics of the action taken and the benefits that result may be different. It is particularly important for health care professionals to use these terms correctly to avoid confusion when reviewing the scientific basis and recommendations for increasing physical activity and exercise levels.

MEASUREMENT OF LEISURE TIME PHYSICAL ACTIVITY AND CARDIORESPIRATORY FITNESS

Most studies that assess the association between physical activity habits or fitness levels and the risk of disease include a measure of leisure time physical activity (LTPA) and/or cardiorespiratory fitness (CRF). Studies that assess LTPA have commonly used a single self-reported measure of LTPA at baseline, although some recent studies have included measures of LTPA at both baseline and during the follow-up period (4–10). This latter study design allows for the opportunity to assess the impact of changes in physical activity habits across time on disease and mortality risk. Unfortunately, the considerable variability among assessment instruments used to quantify LTPA must be considered when comparing results between the studies (11–13). Physical activity habits are usually converted to either an estimate of total energy expenditure (e.g., kilocalories per day or week) or a physical activity index for which individuals are assigned to LTPA categories based on a combination of type, amount, and intensity of self-reported physical activity.

However, a number of other studies have used a measure of CRF as a basis for analysis. Because of the difficulties associated with imprecise measures of CRF, only studies that included maximal exercise testing will be presented in this review (12, 14–21); the exception is a recent report of the assessment of change in CRF during the follow-up period using submaximal leg cycle exercise testing (22). However, one limitation of such testing is the impact of a genetic component associated with CRF that probably accounts for 10–50% of fitness level (23). Consequently, CRF should appropriately be viewed as a result of both hereditary factors and habitual physical activity patterns.

Finally, although LTPA and CRF are of particular interest, it is well established that risk of chronic diseases is multifactorial. Thus, numerous factors besides LTPA or CRF contribute to the risk of developing a chronic disease.

Where possible these other factors (confounders) should be controlled for within the analysis despite the argument that various risk factors (e.g., hypercholesterolemia, hypertension, obesity) are actually intermediates between a sedentary lifestyle and the development of some chronic diseases and as such should not be adjusted for when assessing the association between inactivity and development of disease (8). The reader of this text is encouraged to consider the specific measure of LTPA or CRF employed within each study and to adjust for confounders when comparing risk estimates among the available studies.

LTPA/CRF AND CARDIOVASCULAR DISEASE/CORONARY HEART DISEASE

A number of population-based observational studies have linked a sedentary lifestyle or low fitness to greater risk of morbidity and mortality from cardiovascular disease (CVD) or more specifically coronary heart disease (CHD). Reviews of early research concluded that CHD risk for sedentary individuals was approximately double that of more physically active individuals and discovered strong inverse relationships between physical activity or fitness and CHD (24, 25). More recent reviews have called for further delineation of the physical activity dose-response relationship to morbidity and mortality from CHD, more research that includes women, and investigation of whether adoption of a more active lifestyle or improvements in CRF confer protection from CHD inferred by earlier studies (26–29). Recent studies provide new insight regarding these topics, and a summary of the study designs and important findings from these papers are presented in Table 2.1. Several of these recent papers are follow-up reports to earlier analyses within the same cohort (6, 7, 9, 13, 22, 30–38).

With few exceptions, the results described in Table 2.1 are consistent with the finding of a twofold greater risk for CHD among the most inactive as compared to more active men and women (25, 32, 34). Furthermore, a number of studies comparing all-cause mortality (largely influenced by CVD death) or CVD/CHD morbidity and mortality rates among multiple ordinal categories of LTPA reported some form of inverse dose-response association to quantity (total energy expended) and/or quality (intensity) of LTPA (8, 10, 15, 30, 31, 39–42). While the issue of dose response is supported in most studies, several studies summarized in Table 2.1 reported that more vigorous physical activity was necessary to reduce risk of CHD or all-cause death (12, 30, 31, 43).

Until recently, few studies assessed the association between physical activity and all-cause or CVD death in women, and the available data did not clearly support a protective effect of an active lifestyle (14, 25, 34, 37). However, several recent studies that assessed physical activity habits in large cohorts of women support the basis

for a protective effect of increasing amounts of LTPA (8, 10, 40–42). Most of these studies reported an inverse graded association similar to that observed in studies on men.

Several recent studies of physical fitness and CHD are also summarized in Table 2.1. Each of the studies reported an independent inverse relationship between fitness and CHD/CVD (12, 18, 21). These results, derived from studies that included objective measures of CRF, strengthen the findings from earlier studies of men and extend the findings to women (16,18, 44). Comparisons among multiple ordinal fitness categories have also been made to evaluate the question of the optimal level of CRF for protection from CHD. Based on the available studies of fitness and CHD/CVD, it appears that a fitness level below 8 or 9 metabolic equivalents (METs) represents a threshold for middle-aged men that is associated with significantly greater risk. Because only one study provided fitness data for women, the thresholds presented in Table 2.2 are reasonable until more data on women become available.

Change in Physical Activity or Fitness

Results from recent reports that used measures of LTPA or CRF during a follow-up period to assess change in physical activity habits or fitness level provide further support for the positive role of exercise in reducing risk of chronic illnesses. Two reports from the Harvard Alumni Study indicate similar associations between change in physical activity habits and mortality risk; a 41% lower risk of CHD mortality during the follow-up period was seen in subjects who took up moderately vigorous physical activity (> 4.5 METs intensity) compared to those who never engaged in such activity. In addition, these studies indicated a 28% decrease in all-cause mortality risk in men who increased their total energy expenditure during leisure time to more than 1500 kcal/week (6, 7). Also, men who became less active during the follow-up period had a small but statistically greater mortality risk (13%) than those who were inactive at both assessments (7). These results have been supported in more recent studies on men and women (8–10). In addition, data from the Aerobics Center Longitudinal Study demonstrated that men considered physically fit at two examinations had a 67% and 78% lower risk of all-cause and CVD mortality, respectively, than those who were unfit at both examinations (17). An additional study of Norwegian men confirms the protective effect for an increase in fitness level (22).

LTPA/CRF AND CANCER

Cancer is the second leading cause of death for adult men and women in the United States. Several recent review papers have discussed the available epidemiological studies related to physical activity and/or fitness and risk

Table 2.1. Recent Prospective Studies of LTPA/CRF and All-Cause, CVD, and CHD Mortality

REFERENCE	DESIGN	COHORT	CHD END POINT	MAJOR FINDINGS
Blair et al., 1989 (18)	Mean 8-yr follow-up CRF, maximal treadmill time CRF quintiles	ACLS Men (10,224) Women (3,120)	Fatal CVD n = 66 men, 7 women	RR = 7.9^a (−8.8, −3.3)^b for men. RR = 9.3^b (−5.1, 0.5)^b for women for low vs two highest quintiles of fitness.
Morris et al., 1990 (43)	9-yr follow-up Wk recall of LTPA VAE frequency	British civil servants cohort 9,376 men	Fatal & Nonfatal CHD n = 287 fatal	Aged 45–54 yr: RR^c fatal = 0.25 (0.07, 0.93); nonfatal = 0.37 (0.15, 0.77) for frequent VAE vs no VAE.
	VAE > 7.5 kcal/min; > 6 METs; >65% VO$_{2max}$	Aged 45–64 yr at baseline Reported frequent VAE	n = 459 nonfatal	Aged 55–64 yr: RR^c fatal = 0.53 (0.21, 1.32) & nonfatal = 0.43 (0.19, 1.01) for frequent VAE vs no VAE.
	PA categories			Data taken from Table 7.
Leon and Connett, 1991 (13)	10.5-yr follow-up Minnesota LTPA Q PA Tertiles (T1–T3)	MRFIT cohort 12,138 men Aged > 35–57 yr at baseline	Fatal CHD n = 518	RR^d fatal CHD = 0.75 (0.59, 0.96) for middle group vs least active; 0.82 (0.65, 1.03) for most active vs least active. No dose-response for quantity of LTPA for fatal CHD.
Lindsted et al., 1991 (11)	26-yr follow-up Single PA question 2 PA categories	Seventh Day Adventist cohort 9,484 men Aged > 30 yr at baseline Mixture of health status	Fatal CHD n = 1351	RR^e = 0.55 (0.38, 0.78) for moderately active men compared to less active at age 50; remained significant up to age 70 years. Association was not statistically significant for higher levels of activity.
Arraiz et al., 1992 (14)	7-yr follow-up LTPA CHS-PAI PA categories	Canadian Men & women combined Aged 30–64 yr at baseline	Fatal CVD n = 256	RR^f = 0.8 (0.4, 1.4), 0.3 (0.1, 0.9), 0.8 (0.4, 1.4) for inactive, moderate, active groups compared to very active group. Data from Table 4.
Hein et al., 1992 (15)	17-yr follow-up Single PA question PA categories	4,999 men Aged 40–59 yr at baseline engaged in "conditioning" activities	Fatal CHD n = 266 (171 Mls)	RR^g = 1.6 (1.14, 2.21) low vs high groups. No difference in CHD among upper 3 or 4 PA groups.
Sandvik et al., 1993 (21)	Mean 15.9-yr follow-up CRF, maximal leg cycle test CRF, difference in PWC^h	Norwegian 1,960 men Aged 40–59 yr at baseline	Fatal CVD n = 143 (127 Mls or SD)	RR^a = 0.41 (0.20, 0.84) for high vs low quartile. Dose-response (Q2–3 vs Q4) was clearest after the first 7 yr of follow-up. PA was not independently related to CVD.
Paffenbarger et al., 1993, 1994 (6, 7)	9-yr follow-up from 2nd assessment Harvard PAI Change in moderately vigorous LTPA Change in total PAI	Harvard alumni 10,269 healthy men (1993 paper); 14,786 healthy men (1994 paper) Aged 45–84	130 fatal CHD 2,343 deaths through 1988	RR of CHD^i = 0.77 (0.58, 0.96) and 0.71 (0.55, 0.96) for those who maintained or took up moderately vigorous sports (≥4.5 METs). RR of death^i = 0.72 (0.64, 0.82) and 0.77 (0.69, 0.85) for men who increased to or maintained ≥ 1500 kcal/wk of LTPA across assessments.
Lakka et al., 1994 (12)	4.9-yr follow-up Modified Minnesota LTPA Q PA Tertiles CRF, maximal leg cycle test CRF, VO$_{2max}$	Eastern Finnish 1,453 men Aged 42–60 yr at baseline Mixture of health status	Fatal & nonfatal Mls n = 41	LTPA: RR^d = 0.34 (0.12, 0.94) for those with > 2.2 hr/wk of "conditioning" activities vs those with lesser amounts. LTPA: nonconditioning activities were not protective. CRF: RR^d = 0.35 (0.13, 0.92) high vs low fit third; > 2.7 (1 min^{-1}).

Table 2.1. *(Continued)*

REFERENCE	DESIGN	COHORT	CHD END POINT	MAJOR FINDINGS
Rodriquez et al., 1994 (32)	23-yr follow-up Framingham PAI PA tertiles	Honolulu Heart Program 7,074 men Aged 45–68 yr at baseline Free of CHD	Fatal & nonfatal CHD n = 340 (fatal) n = 789 (combined)	RR fatal^d = 0.85 (0.65, 1.13) for high vs low PA tertile. RR Combined fatal & nonfatal^d = 0.95 (0.80, 1.14) for high vs low active tertile. No protective effect for middle tertile for either end point.
Sherman et al., 1994 (34)	16-yr follow-up Framingham PAI PA quartiles	Framingham 1,404 women Aged 50–74 yr at baseline Free of CVD	Fatal CVD n = 106	No relationship between PA and CVD morbidity/mortality.
Shaper et al., 1994 (33)	9-yr follow-up Unique PAI 6 PA categories	British Regional Heart Study 5,695 men Aged 40–59 yr at baseline Mixture of health status Normotensive/1806 hypertensive	Fatal & nonfatal CHD n = 125 (fatal) n = 186 (nonfatal)	Normotensive men RR^d = 0.5 (0.2, 0.9) for moderate/moderately vigorous vs inactive; RR = 0.5 (0.2, 1.1) for vigorous vs inactive. Hypertensive men RR^d = 0.5 (0.2, 0.9) for moderate/moderately vigorous vs inactive; RR = 1.2 (0.5, 2.7) for vigorous vs inactive. Data are from Table 3.
Lee et al., 1995 (30)	24-yr follow-up Harvard PAI PA Quintiles Vigorous vs nonvigorous PA	Harvard alumni 17,321 men Free of CVD, cancer and COPD Mean age 46 yr at baseline	3728 all-cause deaths	Graded inverse relation between total PA and mortality. RR^i for quintiles of increasing PA were 1.00, 0.94, 0.95, 0.91 and 0.91 (P [trend] < .05). RR^i for quintiles of increasing VIG PA were 1.00, 0.88, 0.92, 0.87 and 0.87 (P [trend] = .007). Vigorous PA but not nonvigorous PA associated with longevity.
Blair et al., 1995 (17)	Mean 4.9-yr follow-up CRF, maximal treadmill test Change in CRF	ACLS 9,777 men Aged 20–82 at baseline Healthy & unhealthy	Fatal CVD n = 87	RR^a = 0.48 (0.31, 0.74) for unfit-fit; 0.22 (0.12, 0.39) for fit-fit compared to unfit-unfit.
Haappanen et al., 1996 (39)	10-yr follow-up Unique PA instrument converted to (kcal/wk) 4 PA ordinal categories	1,072 Finnish men Aged 35–63 at baseline Mixture of health status	168 all-cause deaths 93 fatal CVD	Dose response across 4 categories with most active (> 2,100 kcal/wk) as referent group: RR for fatal CVD^j for 1500–2,100 kcal/wk = 1.59 (0.56, 4.49); RR for 800–1,500 kcal/wk = 0.99 (0.34, 2.87); RR for least active (< 800 kcal/wk) = 3.58 (1.45, 8.85). P [trend] < .001.
Lissner et al., 1996 (8)	20-yr follow-up Unique PA index with 3 ordinal categories for baseline PA data Baseline and 6-yr change in PAI	Gothenburg Prospective Study of Women 1,267 healthy women	147 all-cause deaths for baseline PA analysis 105 all-cause deaths for 6-yr change in PA analysis	Age-adjusted RR for all-cause death with least active as the referent group were 0.56 (0.39–0.82) for the middle and 0.45 (0.24, 0.86) for most active. RR^k for change in PAI of 1 unit = 0.67 (0.49, 0.92) reflecting an inverse, graded association between decrease in PA and death.

of cancer and concluded that there was significant evidence to support an inverse association between physical activity and colon cancer. However, no consistent relationships were demonstrated between physical activity and cancers of the rectum, lung, breast, pancreas, or other sites (45–47). Three other studies also reported inconsistent results in describing associations between mortality from combined-sites cancer and either physical activity or

Table 2.1. *(Continued)*

REFERENCE	DESIGN	COHORT	CHD END POINT	MAJOR FINDINGS
Kushi et al., 1997 (40)	7-yr follow-up Single PA question & unique PA instrument yielding 3 ordinal PA categories	Iowa Women's Health Study 32,763 healthy postmenopausal women Aged 55–69 yr	674 CVD deaths	RR for CVD death[l] with least active as the referent group were 0.86 (0.63–1.17) for middle group and 0.55 (0.38, 0.81) for most active (P [trend] = .002). Inverse, graded associations for all cause and CVD deaths were also observed within frequency of moderate PA (< 6 METs) or vigorous (≥ 6 METs).
Fried et al., 1998 (42)	5-yr follow-up Unique PA instrument of energy expended per wk in moderate or vigorous exercise 5 ordinal PA categories	Cardiovascular Health Study 5201 older men and women > 65 yr of age; mean age 73 yr 57% of cohort were women	646 all cause deaths	RR for all cause death[d] with least active as referent group were 0.78 (0.60, 1.00) for 68–473 kcal/wk; 0.81 (0.63, 1.05) for 473–980; 0.72 (0.55, 0.93) for 981–1890; and 0.56 (0.43, 0.74) for > 1890 kcal/wk (P [trend] < .005). Inverse association between physical activity and all-cause death independent of gender.
Hakim et al., 1998 (38)	12-yr follow-up Walking distance per day 4 walking categories: lower < 1 mi/day; middle 1–2 mi/day; high > 2 mi/day	Honolulu Heart Program 707 nonsmoking men Aged 61–81 at baseline	208 all cause deaths 54 CVD deaths (combined CHD & stroke)	RR for all cause death[m] for lower vs higher = 1.8 (1.2, 2.7); RR for lower vs moderate distance = 1.5 (1.1, 2.1); RR for moderate vs higher distance = 1.1 (0.8, 1.7) with P [trend] = 0.01. RR for CVD death[n] for lower vs higher = 2.6 (0.7, 10.3); RR for lower vs moderate distance = 1.1 (0.4, 2.5); RR for moderate vs higher distance = 2.5 (0.7, 8.6) with P [trend] = 0.32.
Kujala et al., 1998 (41)	16-yr follow-up Unique PA instrument 3 PA categories	Finnish Twin Cohort 7925 men; 7977 women Aged 25–64 at baseline Healthy at baseline	1253 all cause deaths n = 319 CHD deaths (237 men; 82 women)	RR for all-cause death[n] with least active as referent group were 0.80 (0.69, 0.91) for occasional exercisers and 0.76 (0.59, 0.98) for conditioning exercisers (> 6 sessions per month of vigorous exercise). P [trend] = .002
Wannamethee et al., 1998 (9)	3-yr follow-up from 2nd assessment Unique PAI Change in PA patterns	British Regional Heart Study 4,311 men Aged 40–59 yr at baseline Mixture of health status	Fatal CVD n = 93	Least active at each assessment as referent group: Most active at each assessment had RR[o] = 0.37 (0.21, 0.63); those who decreased PA during FU had RR 5 0.98 (0.55, 1.74); those who increased PA during FU had RR 0.53 (0.28, 0.98).
Erikssen et al., 1998 (22)	7-yr follow-up from 2nd assessment CRF, submax bike test Change in PWC	1428 Norwegian men Aged 40–60 yr Free of CVD	n = 120 fatal CVD	RR of CVD[d] = 0.47 (0.26, 086) for those who increased CRF vs those who had greatest decline in CRF during follow-up.

fitness (11, 18, 48). However, the most recent and largest of these studies using combined-sites cancer as the end point reported a significant inverse trend across fitness categories for men, with the least fit men more than twice as likely to die of any cancer as the most fit men (48). Unfortunately, the relationship was less clear in women.

A number of more prospective studies have further addressed the association between LPTA or fitness and cancers from specific sites; they are summarized in Table 2.3. Results of five of six studies support the inverse association between LPTA and colon cancer risk found in earlier reports (4, 45–47, 49–52). Despite the dissimilar physical

Table 2.1. *(Continued)*

REFERENCE	DESIGN	COHORT	CHD END POINT	MAJOR FINDINGS
Manson et al., 1999 (10)	8-yr follow-up Unique PA instrument converted to five ordinal wkly MET-hr groups Quntiles of walking distance Change in total PA	Nurses Health Study 72,488 healthy women Aged 40–65 at baseline	Fatal & nonfatal CHD 645 cases (475 nonfatal Mls; 170 deaths from CHD)	RR for fatal/nonfatal CHD[p] for quintiles of increasing MET-hr per wk were 1.00, 0.88, 0.81, 0.74 and 0.66 (P [trend] = 0.002). For women not reporting vigorous exercise, RR[cp] of CHD for quintiles of increasing walking distance were 1.00, 0.78, 0.88, 0.70 and 0.65 (P [trend] = .02). Faster walking pace associated with lower risk For initially sedentary women, the RR[p] of CHD for quintiles of increased PA during follow up were 1.00, 0.85, 0.79, 0.67 and 0.71 (P [trend] = .03).
Lee and Paffenbarger, 2000 (31)	15-yr follow-up Harvard PAI PA Quintiles Light (< 4 METs), moderate (4-<6 METs) vs vigorous (≥ 6 METs) PA	Harvard alumni 13,485 men Free of CVD, cancer, COPD Mean age 57.5 yr at baseline in 1977	2,539 all-cause deaths	RR[q] for quintiles of increasing total PA were 1.00, 0.80, 0.74, 0.80 and 0.73 (P [trend] < .001). No reduction in risk for quintiles of light PA RR[q] for quintiles of increasing moderate PA: 1.00, 1.05, 0.89, 0.82 and 0.97 (P [trend] = .07). RR[q] for quintiles of increasing vigorous PA: 1.00, 0.89, 0.82, 0.82 and 0.77 (P [trend] < .001).

VAE, vigorous aerobic exercise; RR, relative risk; LTPA, leisure time physical activity; PA, physical activity; PAI, Physical Activity Index; GXT, graded exercise test; PWC, physical work capacity; CHS, Canadian Health Survey; HTN, hypertension; MI, myocardial infarction; SD, sudden death. (Values in parentheses indicate the 95% confidence intervals for the risk ratio.)

[a] R adjusted for age only, although additional adjustments for other factors had little effect.

[b] 95% confidence intervals for linear trend slope.

[c] RR adjusted for age, family history of CVD, height, BMI, smoking, hypertension, diabetes, and angina.

[d] RR adjusted for age and other major CHD risk factors.

[e] RR adjusted for age, sex, BMI and smoking.

[f] RR adjusted for race, smoking, education, medical illness, BMI, marital status, and dietary pattern.

[g] RR adjusted for age, social class, and smoking.

[h] Difference in PWC: PWC calculated as the sum of all workloads completed, and the difference between the observe and expected PWC was used as the measure of fitness.

[i] RR adjusted for age, cigarette smoking, hypertension, and BMI.

[j] RR adjusted for age, initial health status, marital status, employment status, and smoking.

[k] RR adjusted for adulthood activity index, initial age, and baseline and 6-yr changes in smoking. TGs, BMI, weight-to-height ratio, DBP.

[l] RR adjusted for age, age at menarche, age at menopause, age at first live birth, alcohol intake, total energy intake, smoking status ERT, BMI, BMI at age 18, weight-to-height ratio, first degree female relative with cancer, HTN, diabetes, education level, and marital status.

[m] RR adjusted for age, TC, HDL, HTN, diabetes, alcohol use, overall PA index, and preference for a Japanese diet.

[n] RR adjusted for age, sex, smoking, occupational group, and use of alcohol.

[o] RR adjusted for age, smoking status, social class, BMI, and self-perception of health.

[p] RR adjusted for age, smoking, BMI, menopausal status, ERT, family history of MI before age 60, multivitamin supplement use, alcohol intake, history of hypertension, history of hypercholesterolemia, and aspirin use.

[q] Adjusted for age, BMI, cigarette smoking, alcohol consumption, and family history of early death.

activity assessment instruments among these recent studies, the average relative risk of colon cancer among the most sedentary men was approximately double that of the most active men. While one study reported a similar reduction in colon cancer risk in women, two other studies failed to show an association between physical activity and colon cancer in this group (51–53).

The results of prospective studies assessing the association between other site-specific cancers and LTPA or fitness have been mixed. Five of eight studies in Table 2.3

Table 2.2. MET Values[a] for Low and High Cardiorespiratory Fitness (CRF) for Adult Men and Women

AGE CATEGORY	MEN (LOW-HIGH FITNESS)	WOMEN (LOW-HIGH FITNESS)
20–39 years	10.1–13.4	7.1–11.1
40–49 years	9.1–12.5	6.6–9.7
50–59 years	8.4–11.7	6.0–8.9
60+ years	7.0–10.5	5.4–8.0

[a] Based on fitness categories as described by Blair SN, Kohl HW, Paffenbarger RS, et al. Physical fitness and all-cause mortality: prospective study of healthy men and women. *JAMA* 262:2395–2402, 1989. Reprinted with permission from Whaley MH, Blair SN. Epidemiology of physical activity, physical fitness and coronary heart disease. *J Cardiovasc Risk* 2:289–295, 1995.

reported a reduction in risk of prostatic cancer in men with increasing physical activity, but these results generally applied to only the most active or fit men or to specific stages of prostate cancer (5, 20, 53, 54). Three studies reported no significant differences related to physical activity, while one reported an increased risk for active men (49, 55–57). Three studies listed in Table 2.3 found no association between LTPA and rectal cancer (4, 49, 53). Three of six studies found an inverse association between LTPA and cancer of the breast, with the protective effect most likely to be in postmenopausal women (53, 58–62). Three of four studies assessing the association between physical activity and incident lung cancer reported an inverse relationship for men, but results were less clear in women (49, 53, 63, 64). In addition, no association was observed between LPTA and cancers of the cervix, stomach, and urinary bladder (49, 53).

In conclusion, the results from the most recent studies of LTPA/CRF and cancer provide support for an inverse association for risk of cancers of the colon in men but not women. When combined with results of studies reviewed previously, the evidence also confirms absence of any association between LTPA and rectal cancer (46). At present, the relationships between LTPA/CRF and other site-specific cancers remain unclear and should continue to be a focus of future prospective studies, particularly in women.

LTPA/CRF AND NON–INSULIN-DEPENDENT DIABETES MELLITUS

Non–insulin-dependent diabetes mellitus (NIDDM) affects some 12 million people in the United States and is a major risk factor for CVD morbidity and mortality. Several recent prospective epidemiological studies have assessed the association between physical activity or fitness and risk of developing NIDDM. A brief summary of each study is presented in Table 2.4. Each of these studies included results from multivariate analyses in which other variables that might confound the relationship between

activity or fitness and NIDDM (e.g., body mass index, traditional CHD risk factors, alcohol consumption) were taken into consideration. Seven of the available studies included male cohorts, and three included women (19, 65–72). In addition, eight of the studies used self-reported physical activity habits as the variable, while two assessed the risk of NIDDM as a function of physical fitness (19, 65–72).

Although the available studies differed significantly in the method of quantifying LTPA or physical fitness, collectively the reports support the finding of an inverse relationship between LTPA and risk of development of NIDDM for both men and women. In addition, the studies that included more elaborate measures of LTPA or a measure of physical fitness also reported stronger associations between inactivity or low fitness and the risk of NIDDM (19, 65, 67, 69). Two studies assessed change in physical activity habits during the follow-up period, and both reported a decreased risk of NIDDM in inactive individuals who adopted a more active lifestyle (70, 72). As is the case with several other chronic diseases, future studies should focus on further defining the relationship between the quantity and quality of physical activity and risk of NIDDM.

LTPA/CRF AND STROKE

Stroke is the third leading cause of death in the United States. Unfortunately, a recent review of physical activity and stroke found that the available data were "equivocal concerning the role that physical activity and physical fitness may play in the risk of stroke" (73). Nine recent prospective epidemiological studies assessed the association between self-reported LPTA and risk of stroke. A brief summary of each study is presented in Table 2.5 (11, 74–81). Of the nine studies reviewed here, all included a cohort of men, while three also included a cohort of women (76, 78, 81).

In summary, the majority of the studies have not supported a dose-response association between LTPA and stroke in men or women. Three of the four studies that reported some amount of protection reported a U-shaped curve across LTPA categories, suggesting that moderate amounts of activity were associated with a reduction in stroke risk (11, 76, 79). Studies that assessed subtype of stroke within their cohort (i.e., hemorrhagic versus thromboembolic) suggested more of a protective effect from hemorrhagic stroke. Of the three studies that assessed stroke risk in women, none reported a protective effect (76, 78, 81). Therefore, consistent with the findings from the Surgeon General's report, "the existing data do not unequivocally support an association between physical activity and risk of stroke" (3). Future studies focusing more attention on stroke subtypes and different populations, particularly women and African-Americans, may provide more insight into the role activity may play in risk of stroke.

Table 2.3. Recent Prospective Studies of LTPA/Physical Fitness and Cancer

REFERENCE	DESIGN	COHORT	CANCER END POINT	MAJOR FINDINGS
Albanes et al., 1989 (53)	10-yr follow-up 2 questions PA recall (recreational & nonrecreational PA) 3 PA categories	NHANES I 5,138 men; 7,407 women Aged 25–74 yr at baseline	Colorectum, lung, prostate, breast, cervix n = 460 combined male cases 399 combined female cases	Nonrecreational activity: RR 1.8[a] (1.4, 2.4) for least active vs most active men for combined sites; strongest relationship seen for lung cancer with RR 2.0 (1.2, 3.5) for least active vs most active men. Recreational activity: RR 1.8 (1.0, 3.3) for prostate for most active vs least active men. No significant associations for women.
Severson et al., 1989 (49)	11-yr follow-up Framingham PAI PA tertiles	7,858 Japanese men in Hawaii Aged 46–68 yr at baseline	Colon, rectum, stomach, lung, prostate, urinary bladder n = 929 combined cases	RR[b] = 0.56 (0.39, 0.80) and 0.71 (0.51, 0.99) for the middle and most active tertiles compared to the lowest active for colon cancer. Incidence of cancer at other sites was not associated with PAI.
Ballard-Barbash et al., 1990 (51)	Up to 28-yr follow-up Framingham PAI PA tertiles	Framingham 1,906 men; 2,308 women Mean age 50 ± 9 yr at baseline	Large-bowel cancer n = 152 cases	RR[c] = 1.4 (0.8–2.6) and 1.8 (1.0–3.2) for men in the middle and lowest PAI tertiles (compared to the most active tertile), respectively. No significant associations for women.
Lee et al., 1991 (4)	23-yr follow-up Change in Harvard PAI 3 PAI categories (< 1000, 1000–2500, > 2500 kcal/wk of LTPA)	Harvard alumni 17,719 men Aged 30–79 yr at baseline	Colon, rectal n = 225 cases n = 44 cases	Increased activity taken at either assessment alone was not related to incidence of cancer. RR[d] for colon cancer = 0.50 (0.27, 0.93) and 0.52 (0.28, 0.94) for men in highest and middle PAI categories at both assessments compared to least active men. No association between PAI and rectal cancer.
Lee et al., 1992 (5)	23-yr follow-up Harvard PAI (analysis 2) Change in PAI (analysis 1) 3 or 4 PAI categories	Harvard alumni 17,719 men Aged 30–79 yr at baseline	Prostate n = 419 cases (analysis 2) n = 221 cases (analysis 1)	RR[e] = 0.12 (0.02, 0.89) for those expending > 4000 kcal/wk vs < 1000 kcal/wk at both assessment points (1962–66 & 1977). RR[e] = 0.53 (0.29, 0.95) for men aged > 70 yr expending > 4000 kcal/wk at either assessment (1962–66 or 1977). No evidence of dose–response relationship.
Dorgan et al., 1994 (58)	Up to 27-yr follow-up Framingham PAI PA quartiles	Framingham 2,307 women	Breast n = 117 cases	No association found between PA and breast cancer.
Giovannucci et al., 1995 (50)	About 5-yr follow-up Unique PA index (MET hr/wk) PA quintiles	Health Professionals Study 47,723 men Aged 40–75 yr at baseline	Colon cancer, adenomas n = 203 colon cancer cases n = 586 adenoma cases	RR[f] = 0.53 (0.32, 0.88) for the most active quintile vs least active quintile. P [weight-to-height trend across quintiles] = .03.
Oliveria et al., 1996 (20)	Follow-up to 1990 questionnaire CRF quartiles PA quartiles (<1000 with 1000 kcal/wk increases	ACLS 12,975 men Aged 20–80 yr at baseline	Prostate n = 94 cases	RR[g] = 0.26 (0.10, 0.63) for most fit quintile vs least fit quintile. P [trend across CRF quartiles] = .004 P [trend across LTPA quartiles] = .826

CURRENT PHYSICAL ACTIVITY RECOMMENDATIONS

The American College of Sports Medicine (ACSM) and a number of other organizations have established recommendations for exercise programs that are useful for both the prevention and rehabilitation of chronic diseases. ACSM's *Guidelines for Exercise Testing and Prescription*, first published in 1975 and now in its sixth edition, and the ACSM position stand on the quality and quantity of exer-

Table 2.3. *(Continued)*

REFERENCE	DESIGN	COHORT	CANCER END POINT	MAJOR FINDINGS
Kampert et al., 1996 (48)	8-yr follow-up CRF quintiles	ACLS 25,341 men; 7,080 women Aged 20–88 yr at baseline	All-sites cancer n = 179 men; 44 women	RR[h] for quintiles of increasing CRF in men: 1.00, 0.54 (0.35, 0.84, 0.56 (0.36, 0.87), 0.59 (0.38, 0.90) and 0.36 (0.21, 0.61). P [trend] < .001. RR for quintiles of increasing CRF in women: 1.00, 0.63 (0.26, 1.54, 0.76 (0.32, 1.80), 0.38 (0.14, 1.03) and 0.47 (0.18, 1.22). P [trend] = .07.
Thune et al., 1997 (59)	Median 13.7-yr follow-up Unique PA instrument with 3 ordinal categories for leisure activity Change in LTPA	25,624 women Aged 20–54 at baseline	Breast n = 351 cases	RR[i] with all women for categories of increasing activity: 1.00; 0.93 (0.71, 1.22) for moderate activity and 0.63 (0.42, 0.95) for regular exercise. P [trend] = .04. RR lowest for consistently active but lean (BMI < 22.8) women (RR = 0.23; CI = 0.09, 0.60).
Martinez et al., 1997 (52)	Range 6–12-yr follow-up Unique PA instrument converted to wkly MET-hr quintiles PA quintiles	Nurses Health Study 89, 448 women 30–55 yr at baseline	Colon n = 47 cases	RR[j] for quintiles of increasing activity: 1.00, 0.71 (0.44, 1.15, 0.78 (0.50, 1.20), 0.67 (0.42, 1.07) and 0.54 (0.33, 0.90). P [trend] = .03. Inverse association mostly related to cancer of the distal colon.
Thune and Lund, 1997 (63)	Range 13–19-yr follow-up Unique PA instrument with 3 ordinal categories for leisure activity	53,242 men; 25,274 women Aged 20–49 yr at baseline	Lung n = 402 men; 41 women	RR[k] with men for categories of increasing activity: 1.00; 0.75 (0.60, 0.94) and 0.71 (0.52, 0.97). P [trend] = .01. RR with women for categories of increasing activity: 1.00; 0.91 (0.48, 1.71) and 0.99 (0.35, 2.78). P [trend] = .88.
Cerhan et al., 1997 (57)	9-yr follow-up Unique PA instrument 3 ordinal categories	Iowa Rural Health Study 1,155 elderly men Mean age 73.5 yr at baseline	Prostate n = 69 cases	RR[l] with least active as referent were 1.5 (0.8, 2.8) and 1.9 (1.0, 3.5) for moderate and high PA, respectively (P = .05).
Rockhill et al., 1998 (61)	6-yr follow-up Unique PA instrument converted to wkly MET-hr 5 ordinal categories	Nurses Health Study II 104,468 women Aged 25–42 yr at baseline	Breast n = 372 cases	RR[m] for increasing PA groups 1.0; 1.1 (0.8, 1.4), 1.1 (0.8, 1.4), 1.0 (0.8, 1.4) and 1.1 (0.8, 1.5).
Sesso et al., 1998 (60)	29 years follow-up Harvard PA Index PA tertiles (< 500, 500–999 and ≥ 1000 kcal/wk	Univ. Penn Health Study 1,566 women Mean age 45.5 at baseline	Breast n = 109 cases	RR[n] for increasing PA within entire cohort with < 500 as referent group were 0.92 (0.58, 1.45) and 0.73 (0.46, 1.14); P [trend] = 0.17. RR for increasing PA for postmenopausal women 0.95 (0.58, 1.57) and 0.49 (0.28, 0.86); P [trend] = .02.
Hartman et al., 1998 (55)	9-yr follow-up Single question for leisure-time PA 3 ordinal categories	ATBC Cancer Study 29,133 Finnish male smokers Aged 50–69 yr at baseline	Prostate n = 317 cases	RR[o] for combined middle & high activity categories vs least active group was 0.9 (0.73, 1.14). Within employed men: RR for combined middle & high activity categories vs least active group was 0.7 (0.46, 0.94).
Giovannucci et al., 1998 (54)	8-yr follow-up Unique PA index (MET-hr/wk) PA quintiles	Health Professionals Study 47,542 men Aged 40–75 yr	Prostate n = 1362 cases	No relationship observed between quintiles of total PA or vigorous PA and total prostate cancer (P = .88 and .59, respectively). RR[p] > 3 hr/wk vigorous activity reduced risk of metastatic prostate cancer = 0.46 (0.24, 0.89).

Table 2.3. *(Continued)*

REFERENCE	DESIGN	COHORT	CANCER END POINT	MAJOR FINDINGS
Rockhill et al., 1999 (62)	16-yr follow-up Unique PA instrument converted to wkly MET-hr at baselines and averaged across 10 years 5 ordinal categories	Nurses Health Study 85,364 women Aged 30–55 yr at baseline	Breast n = 3137 cases	For baseline PA: RR[q] for increasing PA groups were 1.0; 1.03 (0.90, 1.17), 0.97 (0.88, 1.07), 0.90 (0.80, 1.01) and 0.89 (0.80, 0.98). P [trend] = .004. For 10 yr averaged PA: RR for increasing PA groups were 1.0; 0.88 (0.79, 0.98), 0.89 (0.81, 0.99), 0.85 (0.77, 0.94) and 0.82 (0.70, 0.97). P [trend] = .004.
Lee et al., 1999 (64)	16-yr follow-up Harvard PA Index 4 ordinal PA categories	Harvard alumni 13,905 men Mean age 58.3 yr	Lung n = 245	RR[r] for categories of increasing kcal/wk with least active as the referent: 0.87 (0.64–1.18), 0.76 (0.52, 1.11) and 0.61 (0.41, 0.89); P [trend] = .008. Inverse trends also reported for distance walked (P [trend] = .01) and energy expended in activities ≥4.5 METs (P [trend] = .046).
Liu et al., 2000 (56)	11 years follow-up 2 PA questions; Frequency of vig ex 4 PA categories: < 1/wk, 1x/wk, 2–4x/wk, and 5x/wk	Physicians Health Study 22,071 men Aged 40–84 at baseline	Prostate n = 982 cases	No relationship observed for frequency of vigorous PA and prostate cancer (P = .28). RR[s] for increasing frequency of vigorous activity with < 1/wk as referent: 1.02 (0.82, 1.26), 1.07 (0.90, 1.27) and 1.11 (0.90, 1.36).

CRF, cardiorespiratory fitness; LTPA, leisure time physical activity; PA, physical activity; PAI, physical activity index; RR, relative risk; SD, sudden death.

[a] RR adjusted for age, but additional adjustment for confounders did not alter the findings.

[b] RR adjusted for age and BMI.

[c] Results were unchanged after adjustment for BMI, serum TC, alcohol, and other potentially confounding variables.

[d] RR adjusted for age.

[e] RR adjusted for age; based on only 1 case in alumni who were highly active (> 4000 kcal/wk) at both assessments.

[f] RR adjusted for age, BMI, history of polyp diagnosis, parental history of colorectal cancer, pack-yr smoking, aspirin use, intake of folate, methone, alcohol, dietary fiber, red meat, and total energy.

[g] RR adjusted for age, BMI, and smoking status.

[h] Adjusted for age, examination year, cigarette smoking, chronic illnesses, and electrocardiographic abnormalities.

[i] Adjusted for age, BMI, height, parity, and county of residence.

[j] Adjusted for age, cigarette smoking, family history of colorectal cancer, BMI, postmenopausal hormone use, aspirin use, intake of red meat, and alcohol consumption.

[k] Adjusted for age, geographic region, smoking habits (i.e., type and number of cigarettes smoked, years smoked), and BMI.

[l] Adjusted for age, BMI, number of cigarettes.

[m] Adjusted for age at baseline, age at menarche, history of benign breast disease, family history of breast cancer, recent alcohol consumption, height, oral contraception use, and parity and age at first birth.

[n] Adjusted for age and BMI.

[o] Adjusted for intervention groups, age, smoking, prior history of benign prostate enlargement, and urban residence.

[p] Adjusted for age, history of vasectomy, history of diabetes, smoking, height, dietary fat, calcium, monosaccharide fructose, lycopene, and non-vigorous activity.

[q] Adjusted for age at baseline, age at menarche, history of benign breast disease, family history of breast cancer, recent alcohol consumption, height, oral contraception use, parity and age at first birth, BMI at age 18, menopausal status, and postmenopausal hormone use.

[r] Adjusted for age, BMI, and smoking.

[s] Adjusted for age, treatment group, cigarette smoking, alcohol intake, height, history of diabetes mellitus, history of elevated cholesterol, history of HTN, and multivitamin use.

cise, first published in 1978 and now in its third revision, are well accepted as primary resources for exercise programs (82, 83). The remainder of this chapter is devoted to the various organizational recommendations pertaining to physical activity.

Evidence for the relationship between physical activity and chronic disease has been steadily mounting for the past 30 years. Over this period, appreciation for the benefits of various forms of physical activity has increased. However, clear and concise recommendations for physi-

Table 2.4. Recent Prospective Studies of LTPA and Non–Insulin-Dependent Diabetes Mellitus

Reference	Design	Cohort	NIDDM End Point	Major Findings
Manson et al., 1991 (71)	8-yr follow-up 2 PA questions; Frequency of vig ex 2 PA categories	Nurses Health Study 87,253 women Aged 34–59 yr at baseline	Survey; physician diagnosed n = 1,303 cases	RR^a = 0.83 (0.74, 0.93) for women who reported vig ex at least 1× wk vs those who reported no vig ex. 56% reported no vig ex.
Helmrich et al., 1991 (65)	14-yr follow-up Harvard PAI Kcal/wk deciles	Univ. Penn Health Study 5,990 men Aged 39–68 yr at baseline	Survey n = 202 cases	Inverse gradient across PA deciles with approx. 50% drop in risk comparing the low (< 500) to high (> 3500 kcal/wk) decile. RR^b = 0.94 (0.90, 0.98) for each increase in 500 kcal/wk in PAI.
Manson et al., 1992 (66)	5-yr follow-up 2 PA questions Frequency of vig ex 2 PA categories	Physicians Health Study 21,271 men Aged 40–84 yr at baseline	Survey of physicians n = 285 cases	RR^c = 0.71 (0.54, 0.94) for men who reported vig ex at least 1× wk vs those who reported no vig ex. 27% reported no vig ex.
Jackson et al., 1992 (19)	Ave 4.5-yr follow-up Max TM time (CRF) 3 PF categories	ACLS 13,636 men; 4,828 women	Survey; physician diagnosed n = 67 male cases n = 22 female cases	RR = 4.0 (1.53, 10.4) for low vs high fit men. RR = 1.4 (0.51, 3.71) for low vs high fit women.
Burchfiel et al., 1995 (67)	6-yr incidence rate Framingham PAI PA quintiles a combination of quality and quantity of PA	Honolulu Heart Program 6,815 men Aged 45–80 yr at baseline	Diabetic medication use during follow-up exam n = 391	Inverse gradient across quintiles (P < .001). RR^d = 0.49 (0.34, 0.72) for high vs low quintile of PA.
Perry et al., 1995 (68)	12.8-yr follow-up Unique PA index 6 ordinal categories	British Regional Heart Study 7,097 healthy men Aged 40–59 yr at baseline	Physician diagnosed n = 178 cases	RR^e for NIDDM = 0.4 (0.2, .08) for those reporting moderate amounts of PA compared to inactive men.
Lynch et al., 1996 (69)	4-yr follow-up Minnesota LTPA Q: MET and duration thresholds Max bike test (CRF); CRF quartiles	Kuopio Heart Disease Study 897 men (751 with CRF data) Aged 40–65 yr at baseline	Elevated FBG or OGTT or diabetic medication use n = 46 cases	RR^f for NIDDM for < vs ≥ 5.5 METs with at least 40 min/wk was 0.44 (0.22, 0.88). No protective effect for lesser intensity or duration. RR for NIDDM across CRF quartiles with least fit as referent group: 0.77 (0.32, 1.85); 0.26 (0.08, 0.82) and 0.15 (0.03, 0.79).
Hu et al., 1999 (72)	8-yr follow-up Unique PA instrument converted to five ordinal wkly MET-hr groups Quintiles of walking distance Change in total PA	Nurses Health Study 70,102 women Aged 40–65 yr at baseline	Survey incorporating diagnostic information on symptoms & FPG measures or diabetic medication use n = 1419 cases	Baseline PA quintiles with least active as referent group: RR^g for 0.84 (0.72, 0.97), 0.87 (0.75, 1.02), 0.77 (0.65, 0.91), 0.74 (0.62, 0.89) with P [trend] = .002. When no vigorous PA, P [inverse trend across quintiles of walking] = .01. RR for those who increased PA during follow-up = 0.71 (0.55, 0.93).
Okada et al., 2000 (70)	16-yr follow-up 2 PA categories based on frequency of regular exercise (< 1× wk vs ≥ 1× wk) Change in PA habits	Osaka Health Survey 6,013 Japanese men Aged 35–60 yr at baseline	Physical Examination n = 444 cases	RR^h of NIDDM = 0.75 (0.61, 0.93) for those reporting regular exercise ≥1× wk compared with less active men. Compared to < 1× wk, RR of NIDDM = 0.80 (0.64, 0.99) for 1–2×, and 0.55 (0.34, 0.87) for 3–4× wkly exercise. RR of NIDDM for regular activity at both assessments compared to least active at both was 0.63 (0.47, 0.86).

CRF, cardiorespiratory fitness; LTPA, leisure time physical activity; PA, physical activity; PAI, physical activity index; RR, relative risk; vig ex, vigorous exercise; BMI, body mass index; NIDDM, non–insulin-dependent diabetes; CHD, coronary heart disease; HTN, hypertension; BP, blood pressure.
[a] Adjusted for age, BMI, family history of NIDDM, and follow up interval.
[b] Adjusted for age, BMI, history of HTN, and parental history of NIDDM.
[c] Adjusted for age, BMI, total cholesterol, smoking, BP, history of hypertension, alcohol consumption, aspirin, and beta-carotene assignment.
[d] Adjusted for age, BMI, and other CHD risk factors.
[e] Adjusted for age, BMI, CHD status, alcohol intake, smoking, systolic blood pressure, HDL, heart rate, and uric acid.
[f] Adjusted for age, BMI, BP, lipids, parental history of NIDDM, and alcohol consumption.
[g] Adjusted for age, BMI, smoking, menopausal status, parental history of NIDDM, and alcohol consumption.
[h] Adjusted for age, BMI, alcohol consumption, smoking, BP, and parental history of NIDDM.

Table 2.5. Recent Prospective Studies of LTPA and Stroke

REFERENCE	DESIGN	COHORT	STROKE END POINT	MAJOR FINDINGS
Harmsen et al., 1990 (74)	Mean 11.8-yr follow-up Occupational & LTPA 4-point scale reduced to 2 groups for analysis	Swedish 9,998 men Aged 47–55 yr at baseline	Fatal & nonfatal stroke n = 230 cases	No association for combined and type-specific stroke.
Lindsted et al., 1991 (11)	26-yr follow-up Single multiple choice question (4 possible responses) 3 PA categories	Seventh Day Adventist 9,484 men Aged > 30 yr at baseline	Fatal cerebrovascular diseases n = 410 cases	RR^a = 0.78 (0.61, 1.00) and 0.94 (0.65, 1.36) for moderate and high activity groups compared to low active group.
Wannamethee et al., 1992 (75)	9.5-yr follow-up Unique PAI 6 PA categories	British Regional Heart Study 7,735 men Aged 40–59 yr at baseline	Fatal & nonfatal stroke n = 128 cases	RR^b = 0.50 and 0.20 for moderately and vigorously active compared to inactive men (P trend = .008). Association remained after excluding men reporting regular vigorous sporting activity.
Abbott et al., 1994 (77)	22-yr follow-up Framingham PAI 3 PA categories Age-stratified analysis	Honolulu Heart Program 7,530 men Aged 45–68 yr at baseline Analyses at left exluding men with HTN, diabetes, LVH	Hem. TE Annual exam. hospital records, death cert. n = 537 cases (373 TE; 129 Hem; 35 unknown)	Age-adjusted association between PA & Hem stroke for older men (32.1, 37.6 & 10.1 incidence rates × 1000) (P [trend] = .001). In nonsmokers: RR = 2.8^c (1.2, 6.7) Least vs most; RR = 2.4 (1.0, 5.7) Middle vs most for TE stroke. RR = 3.7^c (1.3, 10.4) Least vs most; RR = 2.2 (0.8, 6.4) Middle vs most for Hem stroke. No significant trends for younger men or those who smoked.
Kiely et al., 1994 (76)	18-yr follow-up Framingham PAI PA tertiles from exam 11–12	Framingham 1,228 men; 1,676 women in 2nd analysis (mean age, 63 yr)	Biennial exam diagnoses n = 107 male cases; n = 127 female cases	RR = 0.41^d (0.24, 0.69) and 0.53^d (0.34, 0.84) for middle and high PA tertiles relative to the low PA tertile for men. No significant associations in women in multivariate model.
Gillum et al., 1996 (78)	Mean 11.6-yr follow-up Unique PA Index 3 ordinal categories	NHANES I 5852 men and women Aged 45–74 at baseline	Fatal and nonfatal stroke confirmed by death certificate n = 623 cases	No association between stroke and recreational activity after adjustment for potential confounders.
Lee and Paffenbarger, 1998 (79)	11–13-yr follow-up Harvard PAI 5 energy expenditure groups	Harvard alumni 11,130 men Aged 43–88 at baseline	Fatal and nonfatal stroke Self-reported n = 378 cases	RR^e for increasing categories of PA were 1.0, 0.76 (0.59, 0.98), 0.54 (0.38, 0.76), 0.78 (0.53, 1.15) and 0.82 (0.58, 1.14); P [trend] = .05. RR for walking > 20 km/wk = 0.71 (0.52, 0.96).
Lee et al., 1999 (80)	11.1-yr follow-up Frequency of vigorous exercise 4 ordinal categories	Physician's Health Study 21,823 men Aged 40–84 at baseline	Fatal and nonfatal stroke confirmed by medical records n = 533 cases	RR^f for total stroke for increasing frequency of vigorous PA: 1.0; 0.81 (0.61, 1.07), 0.88 (0.70, 1.10) and 0.86 (0.65, 1.13) with P [trend] = .25. Null results across PA frequency groups for either ischemic (P [trend] = .81) or hemorrhagic stroke (P [trend] = .10).
Evenson et al., 1999 (81)	7.2-yr follow-up Baecke Questionnaire PA quartiles in sport, leisure, work	ARICS 6,219 men; 8,296 women Aged 45–64 yr at baseline	Ischemic stroke confirmed by medical records n = 189 cases	No significant association between leisure time PA and ischemic stroke.

HTN, hypertension; LTPA, leisure time physical activity; LVH, left ventricular hypertrophy; PA, physical activity; PAI, physical activity index; RR, relative risk; Hem, hemorrhagic; TE, thromboembolic; BMI, body mass index; CHD, coronary heart disease; MI, myocardial infarction.

[a] Adjusted for age, smoking, education, medical illnes, BMI, marital status, and dietary patterns.

[b] Adjusted for age, CHD risk factors, heavy drinking, and preexisting ischemic heart disease or stroke.

[c] Adjusted for age, systolic blood pressure, total cholesterol, alcohol intake, serum glucose, serum uric acid, and hematocrit.

[d] Adjusted for age, BMI, other CHD risk factors.

[e] Adjusted for age, smoking, alcohol intake, early parental death.

[f] Adjusted for age, cigarette smoking, alcohol intake, history of angina, hypertension, hypercholesterolemia, diabetes, BMI, parental history of MI (< 60 yr).

cal activity were not available until recently. In the 1990s, four significant pronouncements concerning physical activity and health were made. The first was the announcement in 1992 by the American Heart Association that physical inactivity was considered a major risk factor for heart disease (1). Although this report substantiated the importance of physical activity, it did not provide specific recommendations for activity programs. The first such report to provide specific recommendations was the 1995 public health statement issued by the Centers for Disease Control and Prevention (CDC) and the ACSM. The essence of the new recommendations is captured in the following excerpt from the report:

> *Every US adult should accumulate 30 minutes or more of moderate-intensity physical activity on most, preferably all, days of the week. This recommendation emphasized the benefits of moderate-intensity physical activity and of physical activity that can be accumulated in relatively short bouts. Adults who engage in moderate-intensity—i.e., enough to expend approximately 200 calories per day—can expect many of the health benefits, described herein (2).*

Although the authors of this report clearly stated that their intention was for these recommendations to complement the exercise prescription guidelines from the ACSM, their message was misconstrued by many. Unfortunately, a message that the majority of health benefit could be derived from moderate-intensity physical activity, with little or no additional benefits from exercise involvement, was promoted. Later that year, the National Institutes of Health convened a consensus development conference on physical activity and health (84). The statement published from this conference addressed the issue of the benefits of higher intensity activity. Some of the conclusions from this conference were as follows:

> *Children and adults alike should set a goal of accumulating at least 30 minutes of moderate-intensity physical activity on most, and preferably all, days of the week . . . . Even those who currently meet these daily standards may derive additional health and fitness benefits by becoming more physically active or including more vigorous activity.*

The United States Surgeon General issued the fourth significant report, *Physical Activity and Health*, in 1996 (3). This report was thorough in its review of the scientific evidence related to physical activity and health. The major recommendations issued were as follows:

> *Significant health benefits can be obtained by including a moderate amount of physical activity on most, if not all days of the week . . . . Additional health benefits can be gained through greater amounts of physical activity. People who can maintain a regular regimen of activity that is of longer duration or of more vigorous intensity are likely to derive greater benefit.*

These recent reports allow health care professionals to present a more complete menu of physical activity choices to clients and patients. Often the traditional exercise prescription recommendations were viewed as an all-or-none type of program (i.e., the only option). Now it is clear that health benefits, albeit not necessarily physical fitness benefits, may be obtained by involvement in a wider array of general physical activity patterns. These new recommendations have several unique aspects related to an emphasis on moderate intensity, moderate amounts, and accumulated bouts of physical activity. An overview of these unique aspects are explored in the following section.

Characteristics of Physical Activity

One of the major features of these recent physical activity recommendations is that health benefits can be obtained with efforts of only moderate intensity. This level of intensity was observed to be the threshold in many epidemiological studies like those reviewed earlier in the chapter. However, in these studies, as indicated in Table 2.6, the use of moderate intensity has been assigned to a wide range of intensities. Some studies used the term *moderate physical activity* when referring to the middle of a distribution of quantity of activity (i.e., kcal/week); others used the term *moderate* in the context of intensity (e.g., light, moderate, or vigorous intensity). Based on the measure of LTPA used within a study, it was often difficult to

Table 2.6. Comparison of Physical Activity Intensify Classification Schemes

REFERENCE	CLASSIFICATION	INTENSITY	
Durnin and Passmore (84a)	Moderate	Men	$\sim$ 4.0–5.9 METs
		Women	$\sim$ 2.8–4.3 METs
Bouchard et al. (84b)	Moderate	Young	< 9.0 METs
		Middle-aged	< 7.0 METs
		Old	< 5.0 METs
		Very old	< 2.8 METs
Taylor et al. (84c)	Heavy	> 50% $\dot{V}O_{2max}$	
Paffenbarger et al. (85)	Light	5 kcal/min	
	Mixed	7.5 kcal/min	
	Vigorous	10 kcal/min	
Leon et al. (84d)	Moderate	4.5–5.5 kcal/min	
Paffenbarger et al. (6) and Helmrich et al. (65)	Moderately vigorous	$\geq$ 4.5 METs	
Kohl et al. (84e)	Moderate	4 METs	
Morris et al. (43)	Vigorous	> 7.5 kcal/min or > 65% $\dot{V}O_{2max}$	
Lee et al. (30)	Nonvigorous (light to moderate)	< 6 METs	
	Vigorous	$\geq$ 6 METs	

METs, metabolic equivalents.

distinguish between moderate intensity and moderate amounts of LTPA. Many of the studies that focused more on moderate amounts (a middle group within the analysis) showed a lower risk (for the study end point) in the intermediate group. However, in studies that provided a clear analysis of the intensity question, a number have reported that vigorous LTPA was more protective against the chronic disease end point or was associated with lower mortality risk (30, 31, 85).

The CDC/ACSM physical activity recommendation defined moderate intensity as 3 to 6 METs. The recommendations equate the 3- to 6-MET intensity range with common activities such as brisk walking (3 to 4 mph), cycling for pleasure or transportation (< 10 mph), swimming (moderate effort), conditioning exercises (general calisthenics), racket sports, table tennis, golf (pulling cart or carrying clubs), fishing (standing, casting), canoeing leisurely (2 to 3.9 mph), mowing lawn (power mower), and home repair (painting). One concern with this definition is that the MET range provided represents an absolute intensity level. A "moderate" range can be quite broad in terms of relative intensity (i.e. percent $\dot{V}O_{2max}$ of percent heart rate range) given the large range of functional capacity across genders and age groups. For example, using the values for the lowest quintile of physical fitness for men and women aged 20 to more than 60 years (Institute for Aerobic Research), a 3-MET activity spans a relative intensity range of 29–50%, and a 6-MET activity spans 57–102% of $\dot{V}O_{2max}$ (82). The Surgeon General's report recognized this concern and recommended a classification scheme for physical activity based on relative intensity as shown in Table 2.7. This table also provides corresponding absolute intensity values based on an average functional capacity value for men for each of four age groups. Estimates for absolute intensities for women are obtained by subtracting 1–2 METs from the men's values.

Another major feature of the physical activity recommendations is the importance of the total quantity of activity. The Surgeon General's report concluded that "activity leading to an increase in daily expenditure of approximately 150 kilocalories/day (equivalent to about 1000 kilocalories/week) is associated with substantial health benefits." The CDC/ACSM statement recommended a daily expenditure of approximately 200 kilocalories/day. The support for these caloric expenditure goals is derived from a number of the epidemiological studies that suggest 1500 kcal/week as the threshold level for benefit. A question worthy of consideration is how many minutes of this level of activity would be required to achieve the 150–200 kcal/day goal. The CDC/ACSM statement provides a conversion factor estimate of 4 to 7 kcal/min for the 3- to 6-MET intensity range, which can be used to estimate the time required. The Surgeon General's report provides the following formula relative to the 150-kcal recommendation:

$$\text{Minutes} = \frac{150 \text{ kcal} \times 60 \text{ min/hr}}{\text{METs (kcal/kg/hr)} \times \text{kg}}$$

A number of factors influence the actual rate of energy expenditure and thus the time it requires to meet the 150–200 kcal/day goal. However, it is clear that the least fit individuals involved in activities at the lower end of the moderate intensity range require more than 30 minutes per day to achieve the goal.

The other major feature of all three of the recent physical activity recommendations is the recognition that intermittent physical activity (as short as 10 minutes per bout) is an appropriate means to attain the recommended quantity of daily activity. Support for the beneficial effects of intermittent physical activity comes from the body of studies reviewed earlier in the chapter. It is likely that many of the studies summarized in Tables 2.1 and 2.3–2.5 used physical activity assessment instruments that probably captured a considerable amount of

Table 2.7. Classification of Physical Activity Intensity Based on Endurance-Type Physical Activity Lasting Up to 60 Minutes

	RELATIVE INTENSITY (%)		ABSOLUTE INTENSITY (METs)			
	$\dot{V}O_{2max}$ OR HEART RATE RESERVE	MAXIMAL HEART RATE	AGE (YR)			
INTENSITY			YOUNG (20–39)	MIDDLE-AGED (40–64)	OLD (65–79)	VERY OLD (80+)
Very light	< 25	< 30	< 3.0	< 2.5	< 2.0	≤ 1.25
Light	25–44	30–49	3.0–4.7	2.5–4.4	2.0–3.5	1.26–2.2
Moderate	45–59	50–69	4.8–7.1	4.5–5.9	3.6–4.7	2.3–2.95
Hard	60–84	70–89	7.2–10.1	6.0–8.4	4.8–6.7	3.0–4.25
Very hard	≥ 85	≥ 90	≥ 10.2	≥ 8.5	≥ 6.8	≥ 4.25
Maximal*	100	100	12.0	10.0	8.0	6.0

METs, metabolic equivalents; *Maximal values are mean values achieved during maximal exercise in healthy adults.
Modified from U.S. Department of Health and Human Services. Physical Activity and Health: A Report of the Surgeon General. Atlanta: Centers for Disease Control and Prevention, National Center for Chronic Disease Prevention and Health Promotion, 1996.
Absolute intensity values are based on mean values for men of that age group as represented by the maximal value. It is recommended that corresponding absolute intensity values for women be derived by subtracting 1–2 METs from the values for men.

intermittent physical activity for the study participants. However, most of the studies analyzed a given amount of total physical activity (kcal/week), and thus could not directly contrast the health benefits of intermittent versus continuous physical activity. The CDC/ACSM statement also cited two experimental studies that support the benefit of intermittent exercise (86, 87). However, whether the results from these studies that employed intermittent vigorous exercise bouts (e.g., running) support the notion of health benefits associated with accumulated bouts of moderate-intensity physical activity is debatable. Two more recent studies assessed benefits of accumulated moderate-intensity physical activity (i.e., brisk walking), and while the results suggested similar improvements in fitness for intermittent versus continuous physical activity, the fitness improvement subsequent to the training programs was small (about 5–10% increase in $\dot{V}O_{2max}$) (88, 89). Certainly more research is required on this topic.

In summary, it is now recognized that the intensity threshold for health benefits is lower (moderate intensity) than that required for fitness benefits. Additionally, it is clear that the relationship between the dose (activity amount) and the response (health benefit) is generally linear, suggesting that those who participate in activities with more vigorous intensities or accumulate greater quantities of physical activity will obtain more health benefit.

► SUMMARY

It is well established that sedentary lifestyle or low cardiorespiratory fitness independently increases morbidity and mortality from several of the most prevalent chronic diseases. Based on the available evidence, it may also be concluded that there is an inverse dose-response gradient of risk across categories of either LTPA or CRF. The physical activity gradient, and perhaps the CRF gradient, in most of the studies is the result of a combination of varying levels of both quality and quantity of habitual physical activity. Thus, it is not possible at present to definitively describe the dose-response association of intensity of physical activity to disease risk, and it may well be that no single optimal dose of physical activity yields protection from each of the chronic diseases reviewed within the chapter.

References

1. American Heart Association. Statement on Exercise. Benefits and recommendations for physical activity programs for all Americans. Circulation 86:340–344, 1992.
2. Pate RR., Pratt M, Blair SN, et al. Physical activity and public health: A recommendation from the Centers for Disease Control and Prevention and the American College of Sports Medicine. JAMA 273:402–407,1995.
3. U.S. Department of Health and Human Services. Physical Activity and Health: A Report of the Surgeon General. Atlanta: Centers for Disease Control and Prevention, National Center for Chronic Disease Prevention and Health Promotion, 1996.
3a. Caspersen CJ, Powell KE, Christenson GM. Physical activity, exercise, and physical fitness. Public Health Reports 100:125–131,1985.
4. Lee IM, Paffenbarger RS, Hsieh CC. Physical activity and risk of developing colorectal cancer among college alumni. J Natl Cancer Inst 83:1324–1329,1991.
5. Lee IM, Paffenbarger RS, Hsieh CC. Physical activity and risk of prostatic cancer among college alumni. Am J Epidemiol 135:169–179, 1992.
6. Paffenbarger RS, Hyde RT, Wing AL, et al. The association of changes in physical-activity level and other lifestyle characteristics with mortality among men. N Engl J Med 328:538–545, 1993.
7. Paffenbarger RS, Kampert JB, Lee IM, et al. Changes in physical activity and other lifeway patterns influencing longevity. Med Sci Sports Exerc 26:857–865, 1994.
8. Lissner L, Bengtsson C, Bjorkelund C, Wedel H. Physical activity levels and changes in relation to longevity: A prospective study of Swedish women. Am J Epidemiol 143:54–62, 1996.
9. Wannamethee SG, Shaper AG, Walker M. Changes in physical activity, mortality, and incidence of coronary heart disease in older men. Lancet 351:1603–1608, 1998.
10. Manson JE, Hu FB, Rich-Edwards JW, et al. A prospective study of walking as compared with vigorous exercise in the prevention of coronary heart disease in women. N Engl J Med 341:650–658, 1999.
11. Lindsted KD, Tonstad S, Kuzma JW. Self-report of physical activity and patterns of mortality in Seventh-Day Adventist men. J Clin Epidemiol 44:355–364,1991.
12. Lakka TA, Venalainen JM, Rauramaa R, et al. Relation of leisure-time physical activity and cardiorespiratory fitness to the risk of acute myocardial infarction. N Engl J Med 330:1549–1554, 1994.
13. Leon AS, Connett J. Physical activity and 10.5 year mortality in the Multiple Risk Factor Intervention Trial (MRFIT). Int J Epidemiol 20:690–697, 1991.
14. Arraiz GA, Wigle DT, Mao Y. Risk assessment of physical activity and physical fitness in the Canadian Health Survey Mortality Follow-up Study. J Clin Epidemiol 45:419–428, 1992.
15. Hein HO, Suadicani P, Gyntelberg F. Physical fitness or physical activity as a predictor of ischaemic heart disease? A 17-year follow-up in the Copenhagen Male Study. J Intern Med 232:471–479, 1992.
16. Slattery ML, Jacobs DR. Physical fitness and cardiovascular disease mortality: The US Railroad Study. Am J Epidemiol 127:571–580, 1988.
17. Blair SN, Kohl HW, Barlow CE, et al. Changes in physical fitness and all-cause mortality: a prospective study of healthy and unhealthy men. JAMA 273:1093–1098, 1995.
18. Blair SN, Kohl HW, Paffenbarger RS, et al. Physical fitness and all-cause mortality: A prospective study of healthy men and women. JAMA 262:2395–2401, 1989.
19. Jackson S, Barlow C, Brill P, Blair S. The association between physical fitness and non-insulin dependent diabetes in men and women. Med Sci Sports Exerc 24:S61, 1992.
20. Oliveria SA, Kohl HW, Trichopoulos D, Blair SN. The asso-

ciation between cardiorespiratory fitness and prostate cancer. Med Sci Sports Exerc 28:97–104, 1996.

21. Sandvik L, Erikssen J, Thaulow E, et al. Physical fitness as a predictor of mortality among healthy, middle-aged Norwegian men. N Engl J Med 328:533–537, 1993.

22. Erikssen G, Liestol K, Bjornholt J, et al. Changes in physical fitness and changes in mortality. Lancet 352:759–762, 1998.

23. Bouchard C, Dionne FT, Simoneau J, Boulay MR. Genetics of aerobic and anaerobic performances. In: Holloszy JO, ed. Exercise and Sports Science Reviews. Baltimore: Williams & Wilkins, 1992:27–58.

24. Berlin JA, Colditz A. A meta-analysis of physical activity in the prevention of coronary heart disease. Am J Epidemiol 132:612–627, 1990.

25. Powell KE, Thompson PD, Caspersen CJ, Kendrick JS. Physical activity and the incidence of coronary heart disease. Annu Rev Public Health 8:253–287, 1987.

26. Blair SN. Physical activity, fitness, and coronary heart disease. In: Bouchard C, Shepard RJ, Stephens T, eds. Physical Activity, Fitness, and Health. Champaign, IL: Human Kinetics 1994:579–590.

27. Haskell WL. Health consequences of physical activity: Understanding and challenges regarding dose-response. Med Sci Sports Exerc 26:649–660, 1994.

28. Morris JN. Exercise in the prevention of coronary heart disease: Today's best buy in public health. Med Sci Sports Exerc 26:807–814, 1994.

29. Whaley MH, Blair SN. Physical activity, physical fitness and coronary heart disease. J Cardiovasc Risk 2:289–295, 1995.

30. Lee IM, Hsieh CC, Paffenbarger RS. Exercise intensity and longevity in men: The Harvard Alumni Health Study. JAMA 273:1179–1184, 1995.

31. Lee IM, Paffenbarger RS. Associations of light, moderate and vigorous intensity physical activity with longevity: The Harvard Alumni Health Study. Am J Epidemiol 151:293–299, 2000.

32. Rodriguez BL, Curb JD, Burchfiel CM, et al. Physical activity and 23-year incidence of coronary heart disease morbidity and mortality among middle-aged men. Circulation 89:2540–2544, 1994.

33. Shaper AG., Wannamethee G, Walker M. Physical activity, hypertension and risk of heart attack in men without evidence of ischaemic heart disease. J Hum Hypertens 8:3–10, 1994.

34. Sherman SE., D'Agostino RB, Cobb JL, Kannel WB. Physical activity and mortality in women in the Framingham Heart Study. Am Heart J 128:879–884, 1994.

35. Donahue RP, Abbott RD, Reed DM, Yano K. Physical activity and coronary heart disease in middle-aged and elderly men: The Honolulu Heart Program. Am J Public Health 78:683–885, 1988.

36. Kannel WB, Sorlie P. Some health benefits of physical activity: The Framingham Study. Arch Intern Med 139:857–861, 1979.

37. Blair SN, Kohl HW, Barlow CE. Physical activity, physical fitness, and mortality in women: Do women need to be active? J Am Coll Nutr 12:368–371, 1993.

38. Hakim AA, Petrovitch H, Burchfiel CM, et al. Effects of walking on mortality among nonsmoking retired men. N Engl J Med 338:94–99, 1998.

39. Haapanen N, Miilunpalo S, Vuori I, et al. Characteristics of leisure time physical activity associated with decreased risk of premature all-cause and cardiovascular disease mortality in middle-aged men. Am J Epidemiol 143:870–880, 1996.

40. Kushi LH, Fee RM, Folsom AR, et al. Physical activity and mortality in postmenopausal women. JAMA 277:1287–1292, 1997.

41. Kujala UM, Kaprio J, Sarna S, Koskenvou M. Relationship of leisure-time physical activity and mortality: The Finnish Twin Cohort. JAMA 279:440–444, 1998.

42. Fried LP, Kronmal RA, Newman AB, et al. Risk factors for 5-year mortality in older adults: The Cardiovascular Health Study. JAMA 279:585–592, 1998.

43. Morris JN, Clayton DG, Everitt MG, et al. Exercise in leisure time: Coronary attack and death rates. Br Heart J 63:325–334, 1990.

44. Ekelund LG., Haskell WL, Johnson JL, et al. Physical fitness as a predictor of cardiovascular mortality in asymptomatic North American men: The Lipid Research Clinics Mortality Follow-up Study. N Engl J Med 319:1379–1384, 1988.

45. Kohl HW, LaPorte RE, Blair SN. Physical activity and cancer: An epidemiological perspective. Sports Med 6:222–237, 1988.

46. Lee IM. Physical activity, Fitness and Cancer. In: Bouchard C, Shepard RJ, Stephens T, eds. Physical Activity, Fitness, and Health. Champaign, IL: Human Kinetics, 1994:814–831.

47. Shephard RJ. Exercise in the prevention and treatment of cancer: An update. Sports Med 15:258–280, 1993.

48. Kampert J, Blair S, Barlow C, Kohl H. Physical activity, physical fitness, and all-cause and cancer mortality: A prospective study of men and women. Ann Epidemiol 6:452–457, 1996.

49. Severson RK, Nomura AMY, Grove JS, Stemmermann GN. A prospective analysis of physical activity and cancer. Am J Epidemiol 130:522–529, 1989.

50. Giovannucci E, Ascherio A, Rimm EB, et al. Physical activity, obesity, and risk for colon cancer and adenoma in men. Ann Intern Med 122:327–334, 1995.

51. Ballard-Barbash B, Schatzkin A, Albanes D, et al. Physical activity and risk of large bowel cancer in the Framingham Study. Cancer Res 50:3610–3613, 1990.

52. Martinez M, Giovannucci E, Spiegelman D, et al. Leisure-time physical activity, body size, and colon cancer in women. J Natl Cancer Inst 89:948–955, 1997.

53. Albanes D, Blair A, Taylor PR. Physical activity and risk of cancer in the NHANES I population. Am J Public Health 79:744–750, 1989.

54. Giovannucci E, Leitzmann M, Spiegelman D, et al. A prospective study of physical activity and prostate cancer in male health professionals. Cancer Res 58:5117–5122, 1998.

55. Hartman TJ, Albanes D, Rautalahti M, et al. Physical activity and prostate cancer in the alpha-tocopherol-beta-carotene (ATBC) cancer prevention study (Finland). Cancer Causes Control 9:11–18, 1998.

56. Lui S, Lee IM, Linson P, et al. A prospective study of physical activity and risk of prostate cancer in US physicians. Int J Epidemiol 29:29–35, 2000.

57. Cerhan JR, Torner JC, Lynch CF, et al. Association of smoking, body mass, and physical activity with risk of prostate

cancer in the Iowa 65+ Rural Health Study. Cancer Causes Control 8:229–238, 1997.

58. Dorgan JF, Brown C, Barrett M, et al. Physical activity and risk of breast cancer in the Framingham Heart Study. Am J Epidemiol 139:662–669, 1994.

59. Thune I, Brenn T, Lund E, Gaard M. Physical activity and the risk of breast cancer. N Engl J Med 336:1269–1275, 1997.

60. Sesso HD, Paffenbarger RS, Lee IM. Physical activity and breast cancer risk in the College Alumni Health Study (United States). Cancer Causes Control 9:433–439, 1998.

61. Rockhill B, Willett WC, Hunter DJ, et al. Physical activity and breast cancer risk in a cohort of young women. J Natl Cancer Inst 90:1155–1160, 1998.

62. Rockhill B, Willett WC, Hunter DJ, et al. A prospective study of recreational physical activity and breast cancer risk. Arch Intern Med 159:2290–2296, 1999.

63. Thune I, Lund E. The influence of physical activity on lung-cancer risk: A prospective study of 81,516 men and women. Int J Cancer 70:57–62, 1997.

64. Lee IM, Sesso HD, Paffenbarger RS. Physical activity and risk of lung cancer. Int J Epidemiol 28:620–625, 1999.

65. Helmrich SP, Ragland DR, Leung RW, Paffenbarger RS. Physical activity and reduced occurrence of non-insulin-dependent diabetes mellitus. N Engl J Med 325:147–152, 1991.

66. Manson JE, Nathan DM, Krolewski AS, et al. A prospective study of exercise and incidence of diabetes among US male physicians. JAMA 268:63–67, 1992.

67. Burchfiel CM, Sharp DS, Curb JD, et al. Physical activity and incidence of diabetes: The Honolulu Heart Program. Am J Epidemiol 141:360–368, 1995.

68. Perry IJ, Wannamethee SG, Walker MK, et al. Prospective study of risk factors for development of non-insulin dependent diabetes in middle-aged men. BMJ 310:560–564, 1995.

69. Lynch J, Helmrich SP, Lakka TA, et al. Moderately intense physical activities and high levels of cardiorespiratory fitness reduce the risk of non-insulin-dependent diabetes mellitus in middle-aged men. Arch Intern Med 156:1307–1314, 1996.

70. Okada K, Hayashi T, Tsumura K, et al. Leisure-time physical activity at weekends and the risk of Type 2 diabetes mellitus in Japanese men: The Osaka Health Survey. Diabetes Med 17:53–58, 2000.

71. Manson JE, Rimm EB, Stampfer MJ, et al. Physical activity and incidence of non-insulin-dependent diabetes mellitus in women. Lancet 338:774–778, 1991.

72. Hu FB, Sigal RJ, Rich-Edwards JW, et al. Walking compared with vigorous physical activity and risk of type 2 diabetes in women: a prospective study. JAMA 282:1433–1439, 1999.

73. Kohl HW, McKenzie JD. Physical activity, fitness and stroke. In: Bouchard C, Shepard RJ, Stephens T, eds. Physical Activity, Fitness, and Health. Champaign, IL: Human Kinetics, 1994:609–621.

74. Harmsen P, Rosengren A, Tsipogianni A, Wilhelmsen L. Risk factors and stroke in middle-aged men in Goteborg, Sweden. Stroke 21:223–229, 1990.

75. Wannamethee SG, Shaper AG. Physical activity and stroke in British middle-aged men. BMJ 304:597–601, 1992.

76. Kiely DK, Wolf PA, Cupples LA, et al. Physical activity and stroke risk: The Framingham Study. Am J Epidemiol 140:608–620, 1994.

77. Abbott RD, Rodriquez BL, Burchfiel CM, Curb JD. Physical activity in older middle-aged men and reduced risk of stroke: The Honolulu Heart Program. Am J Epidemiol 139:881–893, 1994.

78. Gillum RF, Mussolino ME, Ingram DD. Physical activity and stroke incidence in women and men: The NHANES I Epidemiologic Follow-up Study. Am J Epidemiol 143:860–869, 1996.

79. Lee IM, Paffenbarger RS. Physical activity and stroke incidence: The Harvard Alumni Health Study. Stroke 29:2049–2054, 1998.

80. Lee IM, Hennekens CH, Berger K, et al. Exercise and risk of stroke in male physicians. Stroke 30:1–6, 1999.

81. Evenson KR, Rosamond WD, Cai J, et al. Physical activity and ischemic stroke risk: The Atherosclerosis Risk in Communities Study. Stroke 30:1333–1339, 1999.

82. American College of Sports Medicine. ACSM's Guidelines For Exercise Testing and Prescription. 6th ed. Baltimore: Lippincott Williams & Wilkins, 2000.

83. American College of Sports Medicine. The recommended quantity and quality of exercise for developing and maintaining cardiorespiratory and muscular fitness, and flexibility in healthy adults. Med Sci Sports Exerc 30:975–991, 1998.

84. National Institutes of Health. NIH Consensus Statement: Physical Activity and Cardiovascular Health. 13(3):1–33, 1995.

84a. Durnin JVGA, Passmore R. Energy, Work and Leisure. London: Heinmann, 1967.

84b. Bouchard C, Shepard RJ. Physical activity and health: The model and key concepts. In: Bouchard C, Shepard RJ, Stephens T, eds. Physical Activity, Fitness, and Health. Champaign, IL: Human Kinetics, 1994:77–88.

84c. Taylor HL, Jacobs DR, Shucker B, et al. A questionnaire for the assessment of leisure time physical activities. J Chron Dis 31:741–755, 1978.

84d. Leon AS, Connett J, Jacobs OR, Rauramaa R. Leisure-time physical activity levels and risk of coronary heart disease and death. JAMA 258:2388–2395, 1987.

84e. Kohl HW, Blair SN, Paffenbarger RS, et al. A mail survey of physical activity habits as related to measured physical fitness. Am J Epidemiol 127:1228–1238, 1988.

85. Paffenbarger RS, Hyde RT, Wing AL, Hsieh CC. Physical activity, all-cause mortality, and longevity of college alumni. N Engl J Med 314:605–613, 1986.

86. Debusk RF, Stenestrand U, Sheehan M, Haskell WL. Training effects of long versus short bouts of exercise in healthy subjects. Am J Cardiol 65:1010–1013, 1990.

87. Ebisu T. Splitting the distance of endurance running: On cardiovascular endurance and blood lipids. Jpn J Phys Educ 30:37–43, 1985.

88. Jakicic JM, Wing RR, Butler BA, Robertson RJ. Prescribing exercise in multiple short bouts versus one continuous bout: Effects on adherence, cardiorespiratory fitness, and weight loss in overweight women. Int J Obes 19:893–901, 1995.

89. Murphy MH, Hardman AE. Training effects of short and long bouts of brisk walking in sedentary women. Med Sci Sports Exerc 30:152–157, 1998.

2.4.3   3.4.0, 3.4.2   5.4.1

CHAPTER **3**

DIET AND CHRONIC DISEASE

Susan Poindexter, Linda St. Clair, and Karen Wheeler

The foods we eat affect our health throughout our life. In addition to providing essential nutrients for growth and development, foods can supply substances that either contribute to or protect against chronic disease. Such diseases as cancer, osteoporosis, diabetes, hypertension, heart disease, and obesity can be profoundly affected by diet. The purpose of this chapter is to examine the relationship of diet to the development of chronic disease.

CANCER

A large body of evidence supports the theory that foods and nutrients can either increase or decrease risk of cancer. Between 30% and 40% of all cases of cancer are preventable with appropriate diet, physical activity, and maintenance of appropriate body weight (1). The introduction of carcinogens into the body through food seems to have less of an impact on cancer risk than the protective effect imparted by numerous protective chemicals in foods, which can inhibit the cancer process. People consume foods and drinks rather than isolated chemicals from foods. Hence, overall dietary patterns, rather than specific isolated chemicals in foods, are best considered when discussing associations between nutrition and cancer.

Energy Balance

Humans derive energy (calories) from food and use this energy in various human metabolic processes both at rest and during physical activity. Consuming excess calories in relation to level of metabolic activity results in an accumulation of excess body fat and commonly an increase in body weight, body mass index, and mass (1). Cancers of the breast, endometrium, and kidney are associated with high body mass. Maintaining energy balance at a healthy weight is associated with reduced cancer risk. High levels of physical activity reduce the risk of colon cancer (1).

Vegetables and Fruits

There is a strong and consistent pattern showing that diets high in fruit and vegetable (especially vegetable) content decrease the risk of development of many cancers (1). Diets high in dark green, leafy vegetables protect against lung, stomach, mouth, and pharyngeal cancers. Diets high in cruciferous vegetables (broccoli, Brussels sprouts, cauliflower, cabbage) protect against colorectal and thyroid cancers. Diets high in allium vegetables (onion, garlic, leeks, and chives), tomatoes, and citrus protect against stomach cancer. Diets high in carrots protect against lung, stomach, and bladder cancer (1). In addition, various compounds in vegetables and fruits may serve as anticarcinogens that slow the rate of tumor growth or spread (Tables 3.1 and 3.2).

Antioxidants

Antioxidants are dietary components that can protect DNA and cell membranes against oxidative damage from carcinogens. Carotenoids, especially beta-carotene, vitamin C, vitamin E, and selenium, have potent antioxidant abilities. Intakes of carotenoids and vitamin C are highly correlated with vegetable and fruit intake. These nutrients may serve as markers for the overall anticarcinogenic potential of foods and drinks. There is no evidence of harm from high amounts of diet-derived antioxidants. On the other hand, increased risk of lung cancer has been noted in smokers taking beta-carotene supplements (2).

Red Meat

Red meat (beef, pork, and lamb) has been positively associated with increased risk of colorectal cancer. In particular, red meats from domesticated rather than wild animals appear culpable, possibly because of their fatty acid content. Other contributing factors may include protein, iron, or N-nitrosamine compounds produced from meat in the large bowel of humans (1).

Non–meat eaters have decreased incidence of cancer in general (2). This effect may result from inclusion of a large amount and wide array of plants, as well as the ex-

Table 3.1. Phytochemical-Rich Foods

Phytochemical	Where Found
Beta-carotene	Carrots, sweet potatoes, pumpkin, winter squash, cantaloupe, mango, papaya
Lutein	Green vegetables
Lycopene	Tomatoes
Vitamin C	Citrus, leafy green vegetables, broccoli, tomato, strawberries, melon
Vitamin E	Vegetable oils, whole grains
Selenium	Plant foods from high-selenium soil
Isothiocyanates, indole-3-carbinol	Cruciferous vegetables
Allium compounds	Onion, garlic, leeks, chives
Coumarin	Citrus
d-Limonene	Oil from peel of citrus fruit
Quercetin	Red wine, tea

clusion of meat, though others have reported no protective effect from total vegetarianism (3). Therefore, a plant-based diet that includes small amounts of animal product may offer anticancer protection without the need for total vegetarianism.

Alcohol

Alcohol is an addictive drug rather than a food, but is consumed regularly as part of many diets. Worldwide consumption varies from 0–25% of calorie intake. Exam-

Table 3.2. Dietary Recommendations for Cancer Prevention (1)

1. Body mass index should be maintained between 18.5 and 25. Weight gain during adulthood should remain less than 11 pounds.
2. Consume year-round a variety of vegetables and fruits, other than roots, tubers, legumes, and grains (see next item), providing 7% or more of calories or totaling 15–30 oz, or five portions, per day.
3. Consume 20–30 oz, or seven servings per day, of other plant foods, minimally processed (including roots, tubers, legumes, and grains), providing 45–60% of total calories. Refined sugars should be limited to less than 10% of total calories.
4. Alcohol consumption is not recommended. If consumed, alcohol should be limited to 1 serving for women and 2 servings for men. A serving is 3 oz wine, 1 oz distilled spirits, or 8 oz beer.
5. Limit red meat to less than 3 oz/day. Fish, poultry, and nondomesticated meats are preferable.
6. Limit total fat to 15–30% of calories.
7. Limit intake of fatty foods.
8. Salt from all sources should amount to less than 6 g/day.
9. Perishable foods should be safely stored or refrigerated to minimize fungal contaminants and mycotoxins.
10. When levels of food additives, contaminants, or other residues are properly regulated in food and drinks, their presence is not known to be harmful. In economically developing countries, where there may be insufficient regulation, these may be a health hazard.
11. Cook meat and fish at low temperatures. Do not eat charred food or burned meat juices. Consume only occasionally meat or fish that has been grilled over direct flame.

ples of 25% of calorie intake are a bottle of wine, 2 liters of beer, or 200 ml of spirits in a 2000-calorie/day diet. This level of heavy drinking increases risk of cancer of the mouth, pharynx, larynx, esophagus, liver, colon, rectum, and breast (1).

Microbial Contaminants

Aflatoxins are a type of mycotoxin, which is a metabolite of molds. They are most problematic in hot, damp climates with poor storage facilities, where food, especially grains, are stored for long periods. Aflatoxins increase the risk of primary liver cancer (1).

Salt and Refrigeration

Refrigeration has reduced the need for salt as a preservative. The daily human requirement for sodium has been estimated to be 115–500 mg/day, with estimates of average intake at 5–20 times that amount. Excessive salt intake has been associated with stomach cancer (1).

Other Dietary Factors

There is insufficient evidence to show convincing or a probable association between the macronutrients protein, fat, or carbohydrate and increased or decreased risk of cancer. Neither has evidence strongly linked milk, other dairy products, poultry, fish, or eggs to cancer risk. However, some studies have suggested increased risk from saturated fat, very hot drinks, and grilling or barbecuing of meats (1).

Beneficial associations have been reported between reduced risk of cancers and green tea, blueberries, red grape juice, folate, and calcium, low-fat and high-fiber diets, and soy phytoestrogens (4–6). More research is needed to substantiate these associations before public health recommendations can be made about these foods and cancer risk.

Recommendations with regard to cancer prevention and nutritional supplements should be made with extreme caution. Results from the Alpha-Tocopherol, Beta-Carotene Cancer Prevention Trial suggested that beta-carotene supplementation in male smokers is associated with significantly increased risk of lung cancer (2).

OSTEOPOROSIS

Osteoporosis is characterized by low bone mass, structural deterioration, and increased fragility of bone tissue. Those who have not developed peak bone density in early life are at particular risk for developing osteoporosis late in life. Half of the bone mass is developed during the teen years (7). Nutritional factors have a significant influence on the cause of osteoporosis. Consuming adequate amounts of calcium and vitamin D during adolescence and early adulthood is essential to reach peak bone mass (8).

Calcium

Insufficient calcium in the diet over a lifetime can contribute significantly to the development of osteoporosis. Many people do not consume even half the amount of calcium needed to maintain healthy bones. During adolescence, teen years, and early adulthood, the recommended amount of calcium intake is 1200–1500 mg/day.

Dairy products are the most calcium-dense food in the U.S. diet. Drinking three 8-oz glasses of skim milk each day can easily supply almost all of the daily requirement of calcium for most age groups, including the elderly (9). Calcium supplementation in the form of pills or fortified foods (soy products, juices, cereals, and breads) can supply calcium to those intolerant of dairy products. However, calcium intake recommendations do vary throughout the life cycle (Table 3.3).

Calcium supplementation may be particularly effective in populations with a low calcium intake. Supplementation of 500 mg/day to adolescents may produce about 4% gain in skeletal calcium. Supplementation of 800 mg/day may prevent bone loss in postmenopausal women and hip and vertebral fractures in the elderly (11).

Vitamin D

Adequate vitamin D is necessary for absorption of calcium. With daily exposure to the sun, most people can synthesize enough vitamin D on the skin. Vitamin D production may not be adequate in the elderly, in those who are housebound, and during the winter, when there is relatively little exposure to the sun. Vitamin D supplementation in the elderly may prevent hip fractures (11).

Other Nutritional Factors Affecting Bone Health

Observational epidemiological studies suggest that a high protein intake is associated with bone density loss (11). High intakes of sodium and alcohol may also contribute to bone density loss (12, 13). Dietary phytate, oxalate, and caffeine intake may have a small negative effect on calcium absorption and retention (11).

DIABETES

Diabetes is a major cause of mortality and morbidity, yet the management of diabetes and the prevention of complications have been difficult to achieve in the diabetic population. Type I diabetes is an autoimmune disease in which the pancreatic beta-cells are destroyed. Medical nutrition therapy is an essential component of successful management of type I diabetes, but dietary habits are not associated with the development of type I diabetes.

Type II diabetes affects approximately 200 million people worldwide. More than 90% of diabetics have type II diabetes. It progresses through the stages of onset of insulin resistance, impaired glucose tolerance, hyperglycemia, and finally, the clinical diagnosis of diabetes. Dietary habits, specifically excessive calorie intake, are closely associated with the development of type II diabetes (14).

While type II diabetes has a strong familial tendency, the search for a genetic basis for insulin resistance is still under way (14). Since type II diabetes usually has a long prediabetic phase, the early institution of treatment during this period of insulin resistance and impaired glucose tolerance may delay or prevent progression toward disease. Lifestyle modification and pharmacological intervention can contribute to the management of insulin resistance and the prevention of type II diabetes (14).

Lifestyle Modification

Obesity, particularly that associated with an elevated waist-to-hip ratio, is an independent risk factor for the development of insulin resistance and type II diabetes. Acute reduction of calorie intake, irrespective of weight loss, has been shown to improve insulin sensitivity (14, 15). Severely obese human subjects with impaired glucose tolerance can be prevented from developing diabetes with significant weight loss (16). Weight loss is critical and leads to improvement in glucose tolerance, insulin sensitivity, and reduction in lipid levels (14). In the hypertensive diabetic patient, weight loss also promotes decreased blood pressure (14).

Dietary excesses of glucose and fat can cause insulin resistance in muscle and fat tissue (17). High fat consumption, especially high saturated fat, significantly predicts conversion of insulin resistance to type II diabetes, even after controlling for obesity (18). Several studies have demonstrated that combining a low-fat, low-calorie diet with increased physical activity reduces the rate of conversion of impaired glucose tolerance to diabetes (14). Factors that may protect against the development of type

Table 3.3. Calcium Intake Recommendations

NATIONAL ACADEMY OF SCIENCES, 1997 (9)		NATIONAL INSTITUTES OF HEALTH, 1994 (10)	
LIFE STAGE	CALCIUM, MG/DAY	LIFE STAGE	CALCIUM, MG/DAY
1–3	500	1–10	800–1200
4–8	800		
9–13	1300		
14–18	1300	11–24	1200–1500
19–30	1000		
31–50	1000	25–50	1000
51–70	1200	51+ women not on ERT	1500
70+	1200	65+	1500
Pregnant or lactating	1000	Pregnant or lactating	1200–1500
14–18	1300		
19–50	1000		

ERT, estrogen replacement therapy.

II diabetes include increased consumption of vitamin C, fruits, vegetables, potatoes, legumes, and fish (18,19).

HYPERTENSION

Dietary factors that may negatively or positively influence hypertension include sodium intake, alcohol consumption, and intake of fruits, vegetables, and low-fat dairy products. Obesity is also a major risk factor for hypertension that will be addressed later in this chapter.

Sodium Intake

The American Heart Association recommends a sodium intake of not more than 2400 mg/day for all individuals (20). Significantly reducing or eliminating processed foods can most readily accomplish this. In addition, research has suggested that sensitivity to sodium is increased in individuals who are obese; thus, limiting sodium intake is particularly important in this group, particularly among adolescents (21). Obesity activates the sympathetic nervous and renin–angiotensin systems, leading to insulin resistance and hyperinsulinemia. These changes have been related to sodium retention. Conversely, sodium sensitivity appears to be decreased after weight loss (22). Consequently, a diet and exercise program that produces weight loss and reduces sodium intake is recommended for control of high blood pressure.

Alcohol Consumption

Numerous investigators have explored the relationship between alcohol consumption and high blood pressure. Potential mechanisms for the relationship include a direct pressor effect of alcohol on the vessel wall, sensitization of resistance vessels to pressor substances, stimulation of the sympathetic nervous system, and increased production of adrenocorticoid hormones. The evidence from observational and experimental studies suggests that a reduction in alcohol intake is effective in lowering blood pressure in individuals with hypertension as well as individuals with normal blood pressure levels. It is appropriate to include a reduced intake of alcohol as a component in an overall strategy to prevent hypertension. Habitual alcohol intake should not exceed two drinks per day (23).

Intake of Fruits, Vegetables, and Low-Fat Dairy Products

Evidence suggests that individuals who consume diets rich in fruits and vegetables (8 to 10 servings), low-fat dairy products (approximately 3 servings from the dairy group), and reduced saturated and total fat content substantially lowered their blood pressure (24). Furthermore, blood pressure may be reduced even in individuals without hypertension, suggesting that such a diet may be effective preventing hypertension (23). In individuals with hypertension, the reduction in blood pressure of

such a dietary intervention has demonstrated effectiveness similar to that observed in trials of drug monotherapy for mild hypertension (23). However, this dietary approach should complement rather than replace previously discussed dietary recommendations.

CORONARY HEART DISEASE AND ABNORMAL LIPIDS

Dietary factors that may positively or negatively influence the development of coronary heart disease (CHD) or various lipid levels include dietary saturated fat and cholesterol, monounsaturated fats, polyunsaturated fats, trans-fatty acids, omega-3 fatty acids, fiber, alcohol, and soy protein. Obesity, which is also a risk factor for CHD and which can be affected by diet, is discussed later in this chapter.

Fats and Cholesterol

Fats are grouped into three broad categories: saturated, monounsaturated, and polyunsaturated. These designations refer to the types of bonds that hold the carbon atom chains together (25). In the case of saturated fats, single bonds are present between all the carbon atoms. Saturated fats are most abundant in animal products but can be found in fairly large amounts in certain plant oils, such as palm and coconut oils. Most are solid or semisolid at room temperature except for the tropical oils, such as palm oil, palm kernel oil, and coconut oil (25). Saturated fats raise the level of low-density lipoprotein (LDL) cholesterol in the blood. Cholesterol, however, is found exclusively in animal products. Diet intervention trials have linked increased saturated fat intake with increased serum cholesterol levels (26). The American Heart Association recommendations for daily dietary fat and cholesterol intakes are listed in Table 3.4 (22). The Step I guidelines were developed for the U.S. population. Persons with a history of CHD or high cholesterol should reduce saturated fat intake to 7% or less of total calories

Table 3.4. Recommended Intake as Percent of Total Calories

NUTRIENT	STEP I DIET	STEP II DIET
Total fat	30% or less	30% or less
Saturated fatty acids	8–10%	7% or less
Polyunsaturated fatty acids	Up to 10%	Up to 10%
Monounsaturated fatty acids	Up to 15%	Up to 15%
Carbohydrate	55% or more	55% or more
Protein	Approximately 15%	Approximately 15%
Cholesterol	Less than 300 mg per day	Less than 200 mg per day
Total Calories	To achieve and maintain desired weight	

and cholesterol intake to less than 200 mg per day, as directed by Step II guidelines (22).

Monounsaturated fatty acids have one double bond in the fatty acid chain. Olive oil and canola oil contain high amounts of monounsaturated fat. Two oils that have become more recently available to the public, high-oleic safflower oil and high-oleic sunflower oil, also belong in this category (25). Monounsaturated fats have been demonstrated to lower LDL cholesterol levels while maintaining or even raising high-density lipoprotein (HDL) levels.

Polyunsaturated fats have two or more double bonds. Oils that contain a high percentage of polyunsaturated fats include corn, safflower, peanut, cottonseed, soybean, fish, walnut, and flaxseed oil. All polyunsaturated oils are liquid at room temperature (25). Research indicates that the various polyunsaturated oils can have dramatically different effects on health depending on the ratio of omega-3 to omega-6 fatty acids (25). Omega-3 refers to the fatty acid that has its first double bond between the third and fourth carbon atom, while the omega-6 fatty acid has its first double bond between the sixth and seventh carbon atom. Omega-3 fatty acids (including fish, flaxseed, canola, walnut, and soybean oils) and omega-6 fatty acids (including corn, safflower, sunflower, cottonseed, soybean, peanut, sesame, rapeseed, borage, and primrose oils) are converted to hormonelike substances called eicosanoids (25,27). Many chronic diseases are characterized by an excess of eicosanoids resulting from the conversion of omega-6 fatty acids (25). The Lyon Heart Study demonstrated that decreasing the ratio of omega-6 to omega-3 fatty acids to 4 to 1 resulted in a 76% lower risk of death from cardiovascular disease and reduced the incidence of heart failure, heart attack, and stroke (25). The typical western diet contains approximately 14 to 20 times as much omega-6 fatty acids as omega-3 fatty acids (25).

Trans-Fatty Acids

Fatty acids are the building blocks of oils and other fats. Hydrogenation rearranges the molecular bonds on fatty acids, transforming them into look-alike molecules called trans-fatty acids (25). Trans-fatty acids behave in many ways like saturated fat, including raising LDL cholesterol. But they are even more destructive than saturated fat, because they also lower the HDL cholesterol (25). Avoiding or limiting use of margarine, processed foods, and commercially baked or fried foods containing hydrogenated oils decreases trans-fatty acid intake.

Fiber

Soluble fiber increases the excretion of cholesterol in the bile (28). To increase intake of soluble fiber, include or increase servings of fruits (especially those with high pectin content, such as apples, strawberries, and citrus), vegetables, oats, oat bran, and beans. Insoluble fiber passes quickly through the body, adding bulk to the stool and preventing constipation. Wheat bran is a good source of insoluble fiber (29).

Alcohol

Several consensus groups have concluded that moderate alcohol consumption (1 to 2 drinks per day) reduces the overall risk of cardiovascular disease, but the basis for the protective effect of alcohol remains unclear. Data also suggest that a moderate intake of wine may protect against CHD (25, 30). Alcohol consumption beginning in middle age (ages 35 to 69) might suffice, while averting much of the risk of accidents and cancer associated with drinking (31). Additional recommendations for alcohol consumption:

- Don't start consuming alcohol if you don't already.
- If you do consume alcohol, do so in moderation.
- If you have any health problems or are taking any prescription medications, talk with your doctor about whether drinking is safe for you (32).

Soy Protein

The U.S. Food and Drug Administration (FDA) has approved the health claim for soy protein, noting that when included in a low-fat and low-cholesterol diet, soy protein can lower total blood cholesterol and LDL cholesterol levels without adversely affecting HDL cholesterol levels (33, 34). The FDA stated, "in order to claim the healthy effects of soy, a product must contain 6.25 g of soy protein or more, be low-fat (less than 3 g), be low in saturated fat (less than 1 g) and low in cholesterol (less than 20 mg)" (33). The FDA concluded, "The effect of soy on blood lipids is due to the protein component per se and not any one particular physiologically active component, including isoflavones" (33, 35). Soybeans, soy nuts, textured soy protein, soy milk, tofu, and tempeh are examples of soy protein foods. Soy sauce and soy oil do not qualify for the protective claim.

OBESITY

The steady increase in the number of Americans who are obese is a major public health concern, since obesity is associated with several chronic diseases (36, 37). The prevalence of obesity among adults 20 years of age or older is estimated to be 54.9% overall (59.4% for men and 50.7% for women). This represents a 25% increase in the prevalence of obesity over the past 3 decades (36). Excessive body fat substantially increases the risk of morbidity from hypertension, type II diabetes, gallbladder disease, osteoarthritis, dyslipidemia, coronary artery disease, sleep apnea, other respiratory problems, and some forms of cancer (38–40). The mean estimate for deaths attributable to obesity in the United States is 324,940 per year (41).

Accumulation of excess body fat is a complex condition that can be attributed to several factors, including genetic, biochemical, psychological, physiological conditions and physical inactivity. The increased prevalence of obesity in the United States reflects a change in lifestyle patterns influenced by an overabundance of food choices, decreased opportunities and motivation for physical activity, and a decline in cigarette smoking (42). Approximately 24% of American adults are completely sedentary and 54% spend inadequate time in physical activity (43).

Treatment of obesity is generally recommended to reduce health risks. Small reductions in body weight (as little as 10–15%) have been associated with significant improvements in hyperglycemia, insulin resistance, sleep apnea, osteoarthritis, hyperlipidemia, and hypertension (44, 45). However, weight loss is often short term, and regaining weight is a significant problem for most who lose weight initially (46). Finally, not all weight loss is associated with reduced incidence of mortality. In fact, there is evidence to suggest that the highest mortality rates occur in adults who have either lost excessive weight or gained excessive weight (47).

Many types of weight loss and weight management programs are available, including very low calorie diets, gastric bypass surgery, and pharmacotherapy (48). These types of programs are commonly expensive, and results have not been impressive (46, 49). It has been estimated that $30 billion to $50 billion dollars are spent annually on weight loss gimmicks and remedies (50). A more conservative means for achieving healthy body weight recommended by the American Dietetic Association Guidelines includes adoption of a healthful eating style with an energy intake that does not exceed expenditure (51). At least 30 minutes of moderate physical activity, as noted in the Dietary Guidelines for Americans, is recommended (52, 53). Weight management interventions should include cognitive-behavioral methods that may include counseling about self-esteem and body image and how to cope with societal pressure to reduce to an unrealistic weight (50).

► SUMMARY

Research associating eating style with chronic disease is abundant. While a cause-and-effect relation is difficult to prove, this chapter provides valuable guidelines regarding day-to-day food choices that can affect health outcome. Dietary intake plays a major role in the ability to fight against chronic diseases, such as cancer, osteoporosis, diabetes, hypertension, heart disease, and obesity.

References
1. World Cancer Research Fund, American Institute for Cancer Research. Food, Nutrition, and the Prevention of Cancer: a Global Perspective. American Institute for Cancer Research, Washington, DC, 1997.
2. The Alpha Tocopherol, B Carotene Cancer Prevention Study Group. The effect of vitamin E and B carotene on the incidence of lung cancer and other cancers in male smokers. N Engl J Med 330:1029–1035, 1994.
3. Fraser GE. Associations between diet and cancer, ischemic heart disease, and all-cause mortality in non-Hispanic white California Seventh-Day Adventists. Am J Clin Nutr 70(3S):532S–538S, 1999.
4. Key TJ, Fraser GE, Thorogood M, et al. Mortality in vegetarians and non-vegetarians: A collaborative analysis of 8300 deaths among 76,000 men and women in five prospective studies. Publ Health Nutr 1:33–41, 1998.
5. Garay CA, Engstrom PF. Chemoprevention of colorectal cancer: Dietary and pharmacological approaches. Oncology 13:89–97, 1999.
6. Strauss L, Santti R, Saarinen N, et al. Dietary phytoestrogens and their role in hormonally dependent disease. Toxicol Lett 102–103:349–354, 1998.
7. Power ML, Heaney RP, Kalkwarf HJ, et al. The role of calcium in health and disease. Am J Obstet Gynecol 181:1560–1569, 1999.
8. Standing Committee on the Scientific Evaluation of Dietary Reference Intakes, Food and Nutrition Board, Institute of Medicine. Dietary Reference Intakes for Calcium, Phosphorus, Magnesium, Vitamin D, and Fluoride. Washington, DC: National Academy Press, 1997.
9. Heaney RP, McCarron DA, Dawson-Hughes B, et al. Dietary changes favorably affecting bone remodeling in older adults. J Am Dietetic Assoc 99:1228–1233, 1999.
10. National Institutes of Health. Optimal Calcium Intake. NIH Consensus Statement. Bethesda, MD: National Institutes of Health, 12:4, 1994.
11. Lau EM. Nutrition and osteoporosis. Curr Opin Rheumatol 10:368–372, 1998.
12. Packard PT, Heaney RP. Medical nutrition therapy for patients with osteoporosis. J Am Dietetic Assoc 97:414–417, 1997.
13. Deal CL. Osteoporosis: Prevention, diagnosis, and management. Am J Med 102:35S–39S, 1997.
14. Goldberg RB. Prevention of type II diabetes. Med Clin North Am 82:805–821, 1998.
15. Cheah JS. Management of obesity in NIDDM (non-insulin-dependent diabetes mellitus). Singapore Med J 39:380–384, 1998.
16. Long SD, O'Brien K, MacDonald KG Jr, et al. Weight loss in severely obese subjects prevents the progression of impaired glucose tolerance to Type II diabetes mellitus. Diabetes Care 17:372–375, 1994.
17. Proietto J, Filippis A, Nakhla C, Clark S. Nutrient-induced insulin resistance. Mol Cell Endocrinol 151:143–149, 1999.
18. Feskens EJM, Stengard J, Virtanen SM, et al. Dietary factors determining diabetes and impaired glucose tolerance: A 20-year follow-up of the Finnish and Dutch cohorts of the Seven Countries Study. Diabetes Care 18:1104–1111, 1995.
19. Diabetes Prevention Research Group. The Diabetes Prevention Program: Design and methods for a clinical trial in the prevention of type II diabetes. Diabetes Care 22: 623–634, 1999.
20. www.americanheart.org.

21. Rocchini AP, Key J, Bondie D, et al. The effects of weight loss on the sensitivity of blood pressure to sodium in obese adolescents. New Engl J Med 321:580–585, 1989.

22. He J, Ogden L, Vupputuri S, et al. Dietary sodium intake and subsequent risk of cardiovascular disease in overweight adults. JAMA 282:2027–2033, 1999.

23. National High Blood Pressure Education Program, National Institutes of Health. Working Group Report on Primary Prevention of Hypertension. NIH Pub 93–2669, 1993.

24. Appel L, Moore T, Obarzanek E, et al. A clinical trial of the effects of dietary patterns on blood pressure. N Engl J Med 336:1117–1122, 1997.

25. Simopoulos A, Robinson J. The Omega Diet. Harper-Collins, 1999:9–45.

26. Renaud S, Paul T. Cretan Mediterranean diet for prevention of coronary heart disease. Am J Clin Nutr 61(Suppl):1360S–1367S, 1995.

27. Schaefer E, Lichtenstein A, Lamon-Fava S, et. al. Body weight and LDL cholesterol changes after consumption of a low fat ad libitum diet. JAMA 274:1450–1455, 1995.

28. Ornish D. Dr. Dean Ornish's Program of Reversing Heart Disease. New York: Ivy, 1996:273.

29. Ornish D. Everyday Cooking with Dr. Dean Ornish. New York: HarperCollins, 1997:70.

30. Klatsky A, Armstrong M, Friedman G. Red wine, white wine, liquor, and beer and the risk of coronary hospitalizations. J Am Coll Cardiol 29(Suppl 76A), 1997.

31. Thun MJ, Peto R, Lopez AD, et al. Alcohol consumption and mortality among middle-aged and elderly US adults. N Engl J Med 337:1705–1713, 1997.

32. Alcohol and Heart Disease. Heart Watch. N Engl J Med 2000; 7/6/00

33. Hasler C. Public Health Implications of the Soy Protein Health Claim. Soy Connection Winter:1, 1999–2000.

34. American Heart Association. 1999 Heart Facts. Dallas: AHA, 1999.

35. Balmir F, Staack R, Jeffery E, et al. An extract of soy flour influences serum cholesterol and thyroid hormones in rats and hamsters. J Nutr 126:3046–3053, 1996.

36. Flegal KM, Carroll MD, Kuczmarski RJ, Johnson CL. Overweight and obesity in the United States: prevalence and trends, 1960–1994. Int J Obes Relat Metab Disord 22:39–47, 1998.

37. Mokdad AH, Serdula MK, Dietz WH, et al. The spread of the obesity epidemic in the United States, 1991–1998. JAMA 282:1519–1522, 1999.

38. Pi-Sunyer FX. Medical hazards of obesity. Ann Intern Med;119(7, Part 2):655–660, 1993.

39. Must A, Spadano J, Coakley EH, et al. The disease burden associated with overweight and obesity. JAMA 282:1523–1529, 1999.

40. Ernst ND, Obarzanek E, Clark MB, et al. Cardiovascular health risks related to overweight. J Am Dietet Assoc 97(Suppl 7):S47–51, 1997.

41. Allison DB, Fontaine KR, Manson JE, et al. Annual deaths attributable to obesity in the United States. JAMA 282:1530–1538, 1999.

42. Pi-Sunyer FX. The fattening of America. JAMA 272:238–239, 1994.

43. Pate RR, Pratt M, Blair SN, et al. Physical activity and public health: A recommendation from the Centers for Disease Control and Prevention and the American College of Sports Medicine. JAMA 273:402–407, 1995.

44. Pi-Sunyer FX. Short-term medical benefits and adverse effects of weight loss. Ann Intern Med 119(7, Part 2):722–726, 1993.

45. Higgins M, D'Agostino R, Kannel W, Cobb J. Benefits and adverse effects of weight loss: Observations from the Framingham Study. Ann Intern Med 19(7,Part 2):758–763, 1993.

46. National Institutes of Health Technology Assessment Conference Panel. Methods for voluntary weight loss and control. Ann Intern Med 119(7, Part 2):764–770, 1993.

47. Andres R, Muller DC, Sorkin JD. Long-term effects of change in body weight on all-cause mortality: A review. Ann Intern Med 119(7, Part 2):737–743, 1993.

48. National Heart, Lung and Blood Institute Expert Panel on the Identification, Evaluation, and Treatment of Overweight and Obesity in Adults. Executive summary of the clinical guidelines on the identification, evaluation, and treatment of overweight and obesity in adults. J Am Dietet Assoc 98:1178–1191, 1998.

49. Levy AS, Heaton AW. Weight control practices of U.S. adults trying to lose weight. Ann Intern Med 119(7, Part 2):661–666, 1993.

50. The painful business of losing weight. Economist Aug 30, 1997:45.

51. American Dietetics Association. Weight management: Position of the American Dietetic Association, J Am Diet Assoc 97:71–74, 1997.

52. Van Horn L, Donato K, Kumanyika S, et al. The dietitian's role in developing and implementing the first federal obesity guidelines. J Am Dietet Assoc 98:1115–1117, 1998.

53. US Department of Agriculture, US Department of Health and Human Services. Dietary Guidelines for Americans. 4th ed. Home and Garden Bulletin 232. Washington, DC: USDA, 1995.

Suggested Reading

Glade MJ. Food, nutrition, and the prevention of cancer: A global approach. Nutrition 15:523–526, 1999.

National Institutes of Health, Osteoporosis and Related Bone Diseases, National Resource Center. Osteoporosis overview. *www.osteo.org/osteo.html* 1–9, 1999.

American Diabetes Association. Nutrition recommendations and principles for people with diabetes mellitus. Diabetes Care 23(S1):543–546, 2000.

CHAPTER **4**

TOBACCO EXPOSURE AND CHRONIC ILLNESS

Bonita L. Marks

The use of tobacco products is one of the most detrimental modifiable risk factors. Elimination of tobacco use can significantly reduce the risk of a variety of chronic illnesses. Exposure to environmental tobacco smoke has been proven to be deleterious to health and to cause chronic disease. The purposes of this chapter are (*a*) to review the epidemiology of tobacco use, (*b*) to present the potential pathological mechanisms leading to various health conditions, and (*c*) to provide suggestions for the reduction of chronic illnesses related to tobacco consumption.

PREVALENCE OF TOBACCO USE AND ITS HEALTH IMPACT

Cigarette smoking contributes to more than 400,000 preventable premature deaths annually from cardiopulmonary diseases, suggesting that smoking is responsible for one of five deaths annually in the United States (1). Approximately 90% of lung cancers, 80% of emphysema, 75% of bronchitis, and 30% of coronary heart disease (CHD) is attributable to smoking. Though relative risk of smoking for lung cancer is higher, the absolute risk is greatest for CHD (2). Furthermore, several meta-analyses have reported that nonsmokers exposed to environmental tobacco smoke (ETS) have a 1.2–1.3 relative risk (see Morbidity and Mortality section later in this chapter for explanation of relative risk) of developing CHD. Both active smoking and passive exposure to ETS demonstrate similar dose-response relationships for increased risk (3, 4). A variety of chronic illnesses known to be caused or exacerbated by tobacco use and ETS exposure are listed in Table 4.1.

Since the 1960s great progress has been made in reducing cigarette smoking in the United States. Smoking prevalence dropped from 42.4% in 1965 to 24.7% in 1997. The decline has coincided with the 1964 Surgeon General's report linking lung cancer to smoking, with increases in tobacco taxation and cost of tobacco products, and with a general movement toward the adoption of

Table 4.1. Chronic Illnesses Caused or Exacerbated by Active Tobacco Use or Passive Smoking

Immune system	Cancers: lung, esophagus, larynx, breast, oral and nasal cavities, pancreas, bladder; rheumatoid arthritis; hepatitis B interaction
Cardiovascular system	Heart disease, hypertension, stroke, peripheral vascular disease
Metabolic system	Diabetes, chronic liver disease
Pulmonary system	Emphysema, chronic bronchitis, asthma, sinusitis
Reproductive system	Infertility, ectopic pregnancy, spontaneous abortion, low birth weight, placenta previa, abruptio placentae, infant mortality
Other conditions	Peptic ulcer, periodontal disease

healthier lifestyles. However, the general decline in the prevalence of cigarette smoking has been accompanied by a 68% increase in cigar smoking since 1993. Additionally, smokeless tobacco use has remained constant at 5.5% prevalence among men and 1.5% prevalence among women, with use highest in high school–aged white boys. Despite the decrease in overall smoking prevalence, 48 million Americans remain active cigarette smokers, at an estimated health care cost in excess of $50 billion dollars (1).

In contrast to the decline in cigarette smoking for the general population, cigarette smoking among high school students has been on the rise. During the 1970s and 1980s the average prevalence was approximately 30%, and smoking actually decreased in high school seniors. Smoking prevalence increased by 6.5% from 1991 to 1997; the increase was particularly high among whites (1). Data indicate that in 1997 smoking prevalence in adult men and women was similar, with 24.7 million men and 22.3 million women claiming to be smokers. Smoking was greatest in the 18–24-year-old age cohort (28.7%) and lowest in the cohort of those over 65 years old (12%). Smoking prevalence among minorities was

41

highest among American Indians and Alaska Natives (34.1%) and lowest among Asians and Pacific Islanders (16.9%). Smoking prevalence among African-Americans and Hispanics was approximately 25% and 20% respectively. For all ethnic groups, those in the lowest socioeconomic groups demonstrated the highest smoking prevalence rate, approximately 34% (5).

Smoking-related health problems in Eastern Europe and Asia indicate a disproportionate number of deaths from cardiovascular diseases since the early 1990s. In Russia, almost two-thirds of men smoke, more than 50% of both men and women have elevated blood pressure, and one-third exhibit elevated cholesterol levels (6). It is estimated that two-thirds of Chinese men are smokers and that in China tobacco use causes more than 2 million deaths each year (7).

MORBIDITY AND MORTALITY

Smokers have more chronic diseases, such as peptic ulcer disease, sinusitis, chronic bronchitis, and chronic emphysema, than those who have never smoked (8). Furthermore, smokers exhibit greater frequency of small-airway obstructions and associated symptoms than nonsmokers, with decreased lung capacity and other respiratory problems seen even in teenagers who smoke (9). It has also been suggested that the negative health effects due to cigarette smoking are most pronounced in those who have concomitant health problems or other cardiovascular risk factors (10).

A method commonly used for determining the risks associated with smoking is *relative risk ratio*, that is, the ratio of the occurrence rate of events (morbidity or mortality) of smokers compared with the same rates in nonsmokers. A ratio greater than 1 indicates increased risk; 1, the same risk; and less than 1, less risk than nonsmokers. Data indicate that the age at which one starts to smoke, along with the frequency of smoking, strongly increases the mortality ratio of smokers (8). Smoking is associated with a 2.1–2.6 relative risk ratio for all causes of death and a 3.6–4.7 relative risk of death from CHD (10, 11). Additionally, a strong association between cigarette smoking and death from cancer, chronic bronchitis, and tuberculosis has been demonstrated (12). Males who smoked approximately 35 cigarettes per day demonstrated a death rate from cancer of 315/100,000, whereas the cancer-related mortality for nonsmokers was 7/100,000. The leading causes of death in cigarette smokers are CHD, lung cancer, chronic obstructive pulmonary disease, and cancer of the larynx (13). As with morbidity data, ex-smokers have lower overall mortality directly related to the number of years of abstention. After 15 years of total cessation from smoking, the mortality ratio between ex-smokers and nonsmokers is similar (8).

COMPONENTS OF TOBACCO SMOKE

Tobacco smoke contains more than 4000 chemicals, 60 of which have been identified as carcinogenic. The most hazardous components identified in the smoke include hydrogen cyanide, nicotine, and carbon monoxide (14). Hydrogen cyanide causes lung damage by injuring the cilia, which act as a filter for the lungs, thereby impairing resistance to infection (13). It also diminishes oxidative metabolism by impairing aerobic enzymatic pathways.

Nicotine is the addictive component in tobacco. It has paradoxical effects and influences the sympathetic and parasympathetic nervous systems and the central nervous system. Nicotine is quickly absorbed from the respiratory tract, buccal mucous membranes, and skin. Its influence causes the release of catecholamines, resulting in increased heart rate and blood pressure, constriction of the systemic blood vessels, decreased peristalsis and tone in the gastrointestinal tract, release of glucose by the liver, constricted bronchi, stomach secretions, and an increase in resting and activity metabolism (15, 16). Increased heart rate coupled with vasoconstriction increases the risk of myocardial ischemia, angina, and ventricular arrhythmias in patients with CHD (17).

Carbon monoxide also has a significant impact. Because hemoglobin has an affinity for both oxygen and an even greater affinity for carbon monoxide, there is a tendency for carbon monoxide to combine with hemoglobin to form carboxyhemoglobin (COHb). COHb competes with oxygen for binding sites on hemoglobin, which limits the oxygen-carrying capacity of hemoglobin, hence availability of oxygen to the tissues, particularly the myocardium (17). Normal blood COHb levels for nonsmokers range from 0.5–2%, whereas the COHb blood levels in smokers commonly exceed 2% and can reach 15% or higher (14). It is possible that the resulting ischemia and the increase in carbon monoxide level in the blood provide the basis for ventricular irritability and reduce the threshold for ventricular arrhythmias, including ventricular tachycardia and ventricular fibrillation (13). Prolonged exposure to carbon monoxide also increases erythropoiesis, thereby increasing blood viscosity and risk of clotting (18). The combination of nicotine and increased carbon monoxide reduces plasma high-density lipoproteins (HDLs), increases platelet adhesion, and increases fibrinogen and homocysteine levels—all of which increase the risk of thrombotic events and stroke (19, 20).

Nicotine and carbon monoxide are also present in ETS, which is a combination of mainstream smoke (MSS) exhaled during active smoking and sidestream smoke (SSS), which is delivered from the burning end of the cigarette into the environment. Because cigarettes burn at higher temperatures during inhalation, combustion is more complete, and as a result, some of the toxic components of the smoke are eliminated. Conversely, the SSS that passive smokers inhale contains higher concentrations of these toxic components (3). For instance, the carbon monoxide content of SSS is 2.5 times greater than in MSS and similarly, the nicotine content is 1.3 to 2.6 times greater in SSS (14). However, SSS contains less hydrogen cyanide than does MSS. Nonetheless, ETS contains many of the same properties (some to a greater degree) as smoke inhaled directly by active smokers. Thus, similar physiological effects and negative health consequences should be expected from passive smoking (21, 22).

ATHEROSCLEROSIS: HEART DISEASE AND STROKE

Atherosclerosis is accumulation of plaque in the arterial wall. Progression of the disease eventually leads to a decrease in the vessel lumen size, and ultimately blood flow is obstructed. This disease is the leading cause of death in the United States and other "western culture" nations (19). About 30% of CHD-related deaths in the United States are attributed to smoking, and level of risk is dose related. Smoking doubles the risk of stroke and increases risk of peripheral vascular disease (23–25). This risk appears to be a function of the number of packs of cigarettes per day times the number of years of smoking (pack-year history) (24, 25). It has also been suggested that passive smoking increases risk of stroke (22, 24–26).

Homocysteine, a natural amino acid, is believed to activate the coagulation system and may adversely affect the arterial endothelium (27). Hence, elevated homocysteine (>12 μmol/L) appears to increase risk of heart disease and stroke (19). Though elevated homocysteine levels may be due to dietary deficiencies, specifically in folate, B_6 and B_{12}, smokers also have increased levels of homocysteine (28–30).

Fibrinogen is a precursor in the coagulation process (15). Elevated fibrinogen, seen in active smokers, is a risk factor for heart disease and stroke (21). Normal fibrinogen levels are approximately 2.7 g/L (31), while smokers commonly have fibrinogen levels ranging between 3 and 4.3 g/L (32–34). Second-hand smoke causes increased fibrinogen levels (> 3 g/L) (33). An increase in fibrinogen level of as little as 0.15 g/L has been shown to increase CHD risk by 20%. Fibrinogen levels to return to "normal" after 5 years of cessation from smoking (34).

Evidence suggests that some factors associated with increased risk of disease may be reversed upon quitting smoking and that quitting for 2 years results in a nearly 50% reduction of risk of many chronic diseases. After 5 years of smoking cessation, patients in both the Framingham Heart Study (35) and the Nurses Health Study (36) demonstrated a normalized risk ratio for stroke. However, Tell et al. (37) reported that stroke risk reduction was also dose dependent, in that former light smokers (less than a pack a day) had the normal stroke risk, whereas former heavy smokers remained at greater risk for stroke than nonsmokers (37). Pipe and cigar smokers

had the same risk ratios as light cigarette smokers (38).

HYPERTENSION

Hypertension (HTN) is defined as arterial pressure at rest greater than or equal to 140 mm Hg systolic and/or 90 mm Hg diastolic. It is known that smoking causes an acute as well as a chronic increase in blood pressure, predisposing the smoker to hypertension and end organ damage (39, 40). The basis for the interaction of smoking and HTN is unclear; however, possible mechanisms include nicotine-induced nervous system stimulation, chemoreceptor stimulation, and vasopressin release (41). The Atherosclerosis Risk in Communities (ARIC) study, a 3-year population-based project consisting of 16,000 people 45–64 years of age, reported that atherosclerosis progressed 1.6 times as fast in smokers with HTN as in smokers without HTN or ex-smokers (39). Consequently, heart disease is the most common cause of death in smokers with HTN, increasing risk twofold to threefold (42).

CHRONIC OBSTRUCTIVE PULMONARY DISEASE

Tobacco exposure and nicotine exposure have been shown to be associated with the development of bronchitis, emphysema, and asthma. Although the shortness of breath common to smokers is probably due in part to lack of regular physical activity, tobacco smoke and nicotine exposure cause decreased functioning of the cilia on the respiratory epithelial cells, resulting in accumulation of debris in the respiratory passageways. Smoke irritation causes increased fluid secretions into the bronchioles and swelling of the epithelial lining, both of which further compromise lung function and result in bronchitis (15).

Most chronic smokers exhibit some degree of emphysema, which results in loss of compliance and elasticity of the lungs. Emphysema progresses to obstruction of the terminal bronchi and finally destruction of the alveolar walls (15). Recent research suggests that the inflammatory process responsible for causing chronic bronchitis in smokers may have a different pathogenesis from the traditional bronchitis episode. When compared to patients with chronic bronchitis who did not smoke, smokers with chronic bronchitis had a significantly higher infiltration rate of macrophages, neutrophils, eosinophils, mast cells, and T lymphocytes in the bronchi, indicating an immune system that may be more susceptible to respiratory disorders (43).

The prevalence of asthma is also significantly increased in smokers, with acute attacks triggered by both active smoking and environmental tobacco smoke. Furthermore, the Third National Health and Nutrition Examination Survey (1988–1994) determined that ETS significantly increased the incidence of asthma, chronic bronchitis, and wheezing episodes in very young children. In addition, maternal prenatal smoking resulted in adjusted odds ratios of 1.8 and 2.2 for asthma and chronic bronchitis, respectively (44).

CANCER

Cigarette smoking causes 1 in 5 deaths from cancer, and the risk of developing lung cancer is 10 times greater for smokers than nonsmokers. Smoking has also been linked to cancer of the larynx, pharynx, oral cavity, esophagus, pancreas, and bladder (3). The combination of smoking and alcohol use or smoking and coffee or tea use has been shown to increase risk of pancreatic cancer (45, 46). Pipe smoking is specifically associated with lip cancer, although the risk of lung cancer is lower, since pipe smokers tend to not inhale as deeply as cigarette smokers (3).

Use of smokeless tobacco is neither benign nor a safe alternative to smoking. The nicotine exposure from a single chew is equivalent to smoking one cigarette (47). Furthermore, smokeless tobacco users have four times the risk for oral and pharyngeal cancers as nonusers (48). Three-quarters of more than 30,000 new cases of oral and pharyngeal cancers that develop annually in the U.S. have been directly attributed to tobacco use. The mean survival rate for this type of cancer is 50% after 5 years (49). There is strong evidence that exposure to ETS also causes lung cancer. It has been reported that nonsmokers living with a smoker have a 24–26% excess risk of developing lung cancer. The relative risk is not significantly different between genders, and the risk increases by 23% for every 10 cigarettes smoked per day (50).

Although the data are less definitive, relative risk of breast cancer appears to be greater for women who have smoked (51, 52). Furthermore, breast cancer seems to develop at an earlier age for smokers than in nonsmokers. even when adjustments for age, family history of breast cancer, and breast-feeding are made.

OBESITY

It is well documented that smokers are less active, eat less nutritiously, and usually weigh less than nonsmokers (29, 53). Also, there is a general perception in the public sector, particularly among smokers, that upon quitting smoking, people gain weight. However, when controlled for confounding variables, data do not support a relationship between smoking and/or smoking cessation and measures of obesity, including body mass index (BMI) and mortality (54, 55). Similarly, parallel increases in mean BMI over 10 years for smokers, ex-smokers, and nonsmokers have been reported, further suggesting that weight gain pattern is independent of smoking status (56, 57).

Obesity combined with smoking, however, has been shown to be an independent risk factor for thromboem-

bolic events. Men have a relative risk of 3.9 for a thromboembolic event if waist circumference exceeds 100 cm and an additional 2.8 relative risk if they smoke at least 15 cigarettes a day (58). Women who smoke have more upper body fat, thus increased cardiovascular risk. Furthermore, this regional body fat decreases when these women quit smoking, even though they had an overall weight gain (59). Additional research indicates that cigarette smoking combined with obesity increases stroke rate by 72% (60). Finally, data suggest that in women with cancer, obesity may accelerate cancer growth (61, 62).

DIABETES

Diabetes is the seventh leading cause of death due to medical complications and associated heart disease, stroke, hypertension, and end-stage renal disease. Furthermore, non–insulin-dependent diabetes (NIDDM) is also influenced by lifestyle risk factors, such as physical inactivity and obesity (63). The association of smoking and upper body fat deposition is a marker for insulin resistance, elevated plasma glucose concentrations, and diabetes (64). Furthermore, the Nurses Health Study demonstrates a positive association between smoking and NIDDM. Women who are heavy smokers have a relative risk of 1.42 for NIDDM compared with nonsmokers (65). Smoking can and does exacerbate medical problems associated with diabetes.

▶ **SUMMARY: FUTURE DIRECTIONS**

Despite efforts to educate tobacco users about the associated health risks, surveys indicate that most smokers do not think they are at increased risk for heart disease or cancer. Even among smokers who reported having hypertension, angina, or a family history of myocardial infarctions, fewer than half perceive their risk of myocardial infarction as greater than average (66). While smoking cessation should certainly be the ultimate goal, mortality and disease risk can be lowered when smokers change to filtered cigarettes and tar yields lower than 15 mg/cigarette or decrease tobacco consumption (67). In conclusion, smokers and smokeless tobacco users continue to require education regarding the harmful effects of tobacco use and must be encouraged to modify smoking behavior with the ultimate intent of permanently ceasing the use of tobacco products.

References
1. Centers for Disease Control and Prevention. Tobacco use—United States, 1900–1999. JAMA 292:2202–2204, 1999.
2. U.S. Department of Health, Education, and Welfare. The Smoking Digest: Progress Report on a Nation Kicking the Habit. Bethesda, MD: National Cancer Institute,1977:5–34.
3. Law MR, Morris JK, Wald NJ. Environmental tobacco smoke

exposure and ischaemic heart disease: an evaluation of the evidence. BMJ 315:973–980, 1997.

4. He J, Vupputuri S, Allen K, et al. Passive smoking and the risk of coronary heart disease: A meta-analysis of epidemiologic studies. N Engl J Med 340:920–926, 1999.

5. Centers for Disease Control and Prevention. Cigarette smoking among adults—United States, 1997. JAMA 282:2115–2116, 1999.

6. Grim CE, Grim CM, Petersen JR, Li J, et al. Prevalence of cardiovascular risk factors in the Republic of Georgia. J Hum Hyperten 13:243–247, 1999.

7. Chen Z, Xu Z, Collins R, et al. Early health effects of the emerging tobacco epidemic in China: A 16-year prospective study. JAMA 278:1500–1504, 1997.

8. Mangan G, Golding J. Psychopharmacology of Smoking. London: Cambridge University, 1984.

9. Niewohner D, Kleinerman J, Rice D. Pathologic changes in the peripheral airways of young cigarette smokers. N Engl J Med, 291:755–758, 1974.

10. Kannel WB. Update on the role of cigarette smoking in coronary artery disease. Am Heart J 101:319–328, 1981.

11. Friedman G, Dales L, Ury, H. Mortality in middle-aged smokers and nonsmokers. N Engl J Med 300:213–217, 1979.

12. Doll R, Hill AB. Mortality of British doctors in relation to smoking: Observations on coronary thrombosis. Natl Cancer Inst Monogr 19:205–268, 1966.

13. US Department of Health, Education, and Welfare. Smoking and Health: A Report of the US Surgeon General. Rockville, MD: HEW, Public Health Service, Office of the Assistant Secretary for Health, Office on Smoking and Health, 1979.

14. National Cancer Institute. Cancer Facts: Environmental Tobacco Smoke. Bethesda, MD: NCI, 1995:171–199.

15. Guyton AC, Hall JE. Textbook of Medical Physiology. 9th ed. Philadelphia: WB Saunders, 1996:225, 463–469, 773, 780, 873, 1066.

16. Marks BL, Perkins KA. The effects of nicotine on metabolic rate. Sports Med 10:277–285, 1990.

17. Leon AS. Scientific rationale for preventive practice in atherosclerotic and hypertensive cardiovascular disease. In: Pollock ML, Schmidt DH, eds. Heart Disease and Rehabilitation. Champaign, IL: Human Kinetics, 1995:141–151.

18. Lowe GDO, Drummond MM, Forbes CD, Barbenel JC. The effects of age and cigarette-smoking on blood plasma viscosity in men. Scott Med J 25:13–17, 1980.

19. Harpel PC. Homocysteine, atherogenesis, and thrombosis. Fibrinolysis Proteolysis 11(Suppl 1):77–80, 1997.

20. Krobot K, Hense HW, Cremer P, et al. Determinants of plasma fibrinogen: Relation to body weight, waist-to-hip ratio, smoking, alcohol, age, and sex. Arterioscler Thromb 12:780–788, 1992.

21. Taylor AE, Johnson DC, Kazemi H. Environmental tobacco smoke and cardiovascular disease: A position paper from the Council on Cardiopulmonary and Critical Care. American Heart Association. Circulation 86:699–702, 1992.

22. Glantz SA, Parmley WW. Passive smoking and heart disease: Mechanisms and risk. JAMA 273:1047–1053, 1995.

23. Ockene IS, Miller NH. Cigarette smoking, cardiovascular disease, and stroke: A statement of healthcare professionals from the American Heart Association. Circulation 96:3243–3247, 1997.

24. Aldoori MI, Rahman SH. Smoking and stroke: A causative role: Heavy smokers with hypertension benefit most from stopping. BMJ 317:962–963, 1998.

25. Gorelick PB, Sacco RL, Smith DB, et. al. Prevention of a first stroke: A review of guidelines and a multidisciplinary consensus statement from the National Stroke Association. JAMA 281:1112–1120, 1999.

26. Valkonen M, Kuusi T. Passive smoking induces atherogenic changes in low-density lipoproteins. Circulation 29:2012–2016, 1998.

27. Lipton SA, Kim WK, Choi YB, et al. Neurotoxicity associated with dual actions of homocysteine at the N-methyl-dopaspartate receptor. Proc Natl Acad Sci U S A 94:5923–5928, 1997.

28. Godin CS, Crooks PA. In vivo depletion of S-adenosyl-L-homocysteine and S-adenosyl-L-methionine in guinea pig lung after chronic S-(-)-nicotine administration. Toxicol Lett 31(1):23–29, 1986.

29. Johnson RK, Wang MQ, Smith MJ, Connolly G. The association between parental smoking and the diet quality of low-income children. Pediatrics 97:312–317, 1996.

30. Dalery K, Lussier-Cacan S, Selhub J, et al. Homocysteine and coronary artery disease in French Canadian subjects: relation with vitamins B_{12}, B_6, pyridoxal phosphate, and folate. Am J Cardiol 75:1107–1111, 1995.

31. Hathaway WE, Goodnight SH. Disorders of Hemostasis and Thrombosis: A Clinical Guide. New York: McGraw-Hill, 1993:30–37.

32. Kannel WB. Influence of fibrinogen on cardiovascular disease. Drugs 54(Suppl 3):32–40, 1997.

33. Dobson AJ, Alexander HM, Heller RF, Lloyd DM. Passive smoking and the risk of heart attack or coronary death. Med J Aust 154:793–797, 1991.

34. Meade TW, Imeson J, Stirling Y. Effects of changes in smoking and other characteristics on clotting factors and the risk of ischaemic heart disease. Lancet 2:986–988, 1987.

35. Wolf PA, D'Agostina RB, Kannel WB, et al. Cigarette smoking as a risk factor for stroke: The Framingham study. JAMA 259:1026–1029, 1988.

36. Colditz GA, Bunita R, Stampfer JM, et al. Cigarette smoking and risk of stroke in middle-aged women. N Engl J Med 18:937–941, 1988.

37. Tell GS, Polak JF, Ward BJ, et al. Relation of smoking with carotid artery wall thickness and stenosis in older adults: The cardiovascular health study. Circulation 90:2905–2909, 1994.

38. Wannamathee SG, Shaper AG, Wincup PH, Walker M. Smoking cessation and the risk of stroke in middle aged men. JAMA 274:155–160, 1995.

39. Howard G, Wagenknecht LE, Burke GL, et al. Cigarette smoking and progression of atherosclerosis: The Atherosclerosis Risk in Communities (ARIC) study. JAMA 279:119–124, 1998.

40. Verdecchia P, Schillaci G, Borgioni C, et al. Cigarette smoking, ambulatory blood pressure and cardiac hypertrophy in essential hypertension. J Hypertens 13:1209–1215, 1995.

41. Kochar MS, Bindra RS. The additive effects of smoking and hypertension. Postgrad Med 100:147–148, 151–154, 159–160, 1996.

42. Sleight P. Smoking and hypertension. Clin Exper Hypertens 15:1181–1192, 1993.

43. Saetta M, Turato G, Facchini FM, et al. Inflammatory cells in the bronchial glands of smokers with chronic bronchitis. Am J Respir Crit Care Med 156:1633–1639, 1997.

44. Gergen PJ, Fowler JA, Maurer KR, et al. The burden of environmental tobacco smoke exposure on the respiratory health of children 2 months through 5 years of age in the United States: Third national health and nutrition examination survey, 1988–1994. Pediatrics 101(2):E8, 1998.

45. Talamini G, Bassi C, Falconi M, et al. Alcohol and smoking as risk factors in chronic pancreatitis and pancreatic cancer. Digest Dis Sci 44:1303–1311, 1999.

46. Mori M, Hariharan M, Anandakumar M, et al. A case-control study on risk factors for pancreatic disease in Kerala, India. Hepatogastroenterology 46:(25):25–30, 1999.

47. Schroeder KL, Soller HA, Chen MS, et al. Screening for smokeless tobacco-associated lesions: Recommendations for dental practitioners. J Am Dent Assoc 116:388, 1988.

48. Winn DM, Blot WJ, Shy CM, et al. Snuff dipping and oral cancer among women in the southern United States. N Engl J Med 304:745–759, 1981.

49. Marwick C. Increasing use of chewing tobacco, especially among younger persons, alarms Surgeon General. JAMA 269:195, 1993.

50. Hackshaw AK, Law MR, Wald NJ. The accumulated evidence on lung cancer and environmental tobacco smoke. BMJ 315:9980–9988, 1997.

51. Palmer JR, Rosenberg L. Cigarette smoking and the risk of breast cancer. Epidemiol Rev 5:145–156, 1993.

52. Bennicke K, Conrad C, Sabroe S, Sorensen HT. Cigarette smoking and breast cancer. BMJ 310:1431–1433, 1995.

53. Rodin J, Wack J. The relationship between cigarette smoking and body weight: A health promotion dilemma. In: Matarazzo J, ed. Behavioral Health. New York: Wiley, 1984:671–690.

54. Sempos CT, Durazo-Arvizu R, McGee DL, et al. The influence of cigarette smoking on the association between body weight and mortality: The Framingham Heart Study revisited. Ann Epidemiol 8:289–300, 1998.

55. Chyou PH, Burchfiel CM, Yano K, et al. Obesity, alcohol consumption, smoking and mortality. Ann Epidemiol 7:311–317, 1997.

56. Simmons, G, Jackson R, Swinburn B, Yee RL. The increasing prevalence of obesity in New Zealand: Is it related to recent trends in smoking and physical activity? N Z Med J 109(1018):90–92, 1996.

57. Boyle CA, Dobson AJ, Egger G, Magnus P. Can the increasing weight of Australians be explained by the decreasing prevalence of cigarette smoking? Int J Obes Rel Metab Dis 18(1):55–60, 1994.

58. Hansson PO, Eriksson H, Welin L, et al. Smoking and abdominal obesity: Risk factors for venous thromboembolism among middle-aged men: "The study of men born in 1913." Arch Intern Med 159:1886–1890, 1999.

59. Lissner L, Bengtsson C, Lapidus L, Bjorkelund C. Smoking initiation and cessation in relation to body fat distribution based on data from a study of Swedish women. Am J Publ Health 82:273–275, 1992.

60. Shinton R. Lifelong exposures and the potential for stroke prevention: The contribution of cigarette smoking, exercise, and body fat. J Epidemiol Community Health 51:138–143, 1997.

61. Daniell HW, Tam E, Filice A. Larger axillary metastases in obese women and smokers with breast cancer: An influence by host factors on early tumor behavior. Breast Cancer Res Treat 25:192–201, 1993.

62. Kirschner CV, Yordan EL, DeGeest K, Wilbanks GD. Smoking, obesity, and survival in squamous cell carcinoma of the vulva. Gynecol Oncol 56(1):79–94, 1995.

63. Leon AS. Diabetes. In: Skinner JS, ed. Exercise Testing and Exercise Prescription for Special Cases. 2nd ed. Philadelphia: Lea & Febiger, 1993:153–183.

64. Rimm EB, Chan J, Stampfer MJ, et al. Prospective study of cigarette smoking, alcohol use, and the risk of diabetes in men. BMJ 310:555–559, 1995.

65. Rimm EB, Manson JE, Stampfer MJ, et. al. Cigarette smoking and the risk of diabetes in women. Am J Public Health 83:211–214, 1993.

66. Ayanian JZ, Cleary PD. Perceived risks of heart disease and cancer among cigarette smokers. JAMA 281:1019–1021, 1999.

67. Tang JL, Morris JK, Wald NJ, et. al. Mortality in relation to tar yield of cigarettes: A prospective study of four cohorts. BMJ 311:1530–1533, 1995.

CHAPTER **5**

INFLUENCE OF EMOTIONAL DISTRESS ON CHRONIC ILLNESS

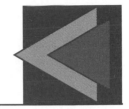

Robert Scales and James Blumenthal

Chronic illnesses such as cardiovascular disease (CVD), cancer, chronic obstructive pulmonary disease (COPD), and diabetes account for more than 70% of deaths in the United States (1). Consequently, the alleviation of chronic illness is a priority of the Year 2010 Health Objectives for the nation (2). Chronic illnesses typically progress through a series of stages of increasing morbidity. The physical limitations and emotional issues surrounding the illness can devastate the quality of life. The causes of many chronic illnesses remain obscure, and a complete cure is seldom achieved. The influence of emotional distress on chronic illness is underrecognized compared to other risk factors, despite a rapidly growing body of evidence showing an underlying relationship between psychosocial factors and chronic disease progression (3).

This chapter reviews epidemiological and clinical research investigating the relationship between emotional distress and chronic illness. The chapter addresses the following questions: Do psychosocial factors cause chronic illness in those who are free from disease? Will psychosocial factors exacerbate the illness in someone already diagnosed with disease? Is it the illness that causes the psychosocial disorder? Does chronic illness progress because of other risk factors that have been negatively influenced by psychosocial factors? Clearly, a great deal more investigation in this area is needed. However, as this review shows, there are enough convincing data to herald the message to heath care providers that more serious attention should be given to the evaluation and care associated with the emotional aspects of health.

This chapter is directed to the exercise professional who may have a limited background in psychology and the mental health aspects of disease prevention. It is intended to serve as a quick reference guide for those who need relevant information for professional and public education. The chapter does not provide a comprehensive review of the psychosocial literature associated with chronic illness. Instead, it focuses on the major chronic illnesses that account for most of the morbidity and mortality in an adult population. This includes CVD, cancer,

COPD, asthma, diabetes, chronic pain, and rheumatoid arthritis. Emphasis is given to three psychosocial domains recently identified in the Surgeon General's Report on Mental Health: (*a*) life stress, (*b*) depression, and (*c*) anxiety (4). Other psychosocial factors worthy of review but beyond the scope of this chapter include personality traits and social isolation. These factors have been reviewed elsewhere (4–7).

LIFE STRESS

Stressful life events in adulthood include the breakup of intimate personal relationships, death of a family member or friend, economic hardship, role conflict, work overload, racism and discrimination, poor physical health, accidental injuries, and intentional assaults of physical safety (8–10). Stressful life events in adulthood may also reflect the past. Severe trauma in childhood, including sexual and physical abuse, may persist as a stressor into adulthood or may make the individual particularly vulnerable to ongoing stress (11). Every individual exhibits a unique response to stressful life events that includes some combination of physiological, cognitive, emotional, and behavioral characteristics (12).

DEPRESSION

Depression takes a monumental toll through human suffering, lost productivity, and suicide. Moreover, when unrecognized, it can result in unnecessary health care use. Depression ranks among the top 10 causes of disability worldwide (13). Major depression is the best-known mood disorder, but there are others, including bipolar disorder (one or more episodes of mania) and dysthymia (a chronic but milder form of major depression) (4). Episodes of major depression are characterized by depressed mood and a markedly decreased interest in all activities, persisting for at least 2 weeks and accompanied by at least four of the following additional symptoms: changes in appetite, sleep disturbance, fatigue, psychomotor retardation or agitation, feelings of guilt or worthlessness, difficulty concentrating, and suicidal thoughts. It is estimated that depression will rank as the second major cause of disability worldwide in the year 2020 (14).

The causes of depression are not fully known. It may be triggered by stressful life events, stressful social conditions (e.g., poverty and discrimination), neurochemical imbalances, and maladaptive cognitions. Depression is twice as common in women as men. A host of pharmacological and psychosocial interventions can effectively reduce depression (4).

ANXIETY

Anxiety disorders are the most prevalent mental disorders in adults (15). The anxiety disorders also affect twice as many women as men. This includes panic disorder, phobias, obsessive-compulsive disorder, posttraumatic stress disorder, and generalized anxiety disorder. Underlying this heterogeneous group of disorders is a state of heightened arousal or fear in relation to stressful events or feelings. The biological manifestations of anxiety, which are grounded in the fight-or-flight response, are unmistakable: they include surge in heart rate, sweating, and tensing of muscles. But this is certainly not the whole picture. Although the full array of biological causes and correlates of anxiety are not yet in our grasp, numerous effective treatments for anxiety disorders now exist. Treatment draws on an assortment of behavioral psychotherapies and pharmacological approaches, administered alone or in combination (4).

CHRONIC ILLNESS

The relationship between these specific aspects of mental health and chronic illness is discussed in this section.

Cardiovascular Disease

Approximately 14 million Americans have coronary artery disease (CAD); 4 million have cerebrovascular disease, and 2 million have peripheral vascular disease (16). Consequently, cardiovascular disease is the most prevalent chronic illness in the United States (2). In reviewing the literature, it is clear that there is more research investigating the relationship between psychosocial factors and CVD than any other chronic illness. Therefore, a large portion of this chapter focuses on the CVD literature.

Evidence indicates a relationship between chronic life stress at work and the development of CVD. In a meta-analysis of five populations numbering more than 12,000 individuals and covering an 18- to 30-year period, work stress was associated with high levels of cholesterol, systolic blood pressure, and smoking behavior (17). Monotonous work, high-paced work, and job burnout have been correlated with an increased incidence of CAD

(18). High-demand jobs with low decision latitude have been associated with a fourfold increased risk of cardiovascular-related death (19). Work stress resulting from high demand and low reward is also reported to be associated with an increase in cardiac events and the progression of carotid atherosclerosis (20–22). Researchers have discovered that in a working population, compared to a nonworking population, there is a 33% increase in relative risk of disease events on Mondays (23). In a more recent study involving a sample of 170,000 men and women, death from CAD was 20% above the daily average on Mondays for those under 50 (24). In the 20-year follow-up of the Framingham Study, the incidence of angina was two times greater among those who exhibited higher levels of worry, dissatisfaction with work, feeling undue time pressure, and competitive drive (25). Together, these studies indicate a strong correlation between this form of chronic stress and the development of CVD, as well as CVD morbidity and mortality.

Some 30 years ago, Holmes and Rahe (8) developed the Recent Life Change Questionnaire to assess the severity of typical stressful life events. The death of a spouse, divorce, and loss of a job were considered high stress, whereas vacations and holidays were given a lower weighting. Elevations in scores on the survey have been found to be associated with myocardial infarction (MI) or sudden cardiac death during a 6-month period preceding these events (26).

In two large studies involving CAD patients, those at higher risk had significantly more socioeconomic difficulties, also lacking social support or social connections to deal with stress (27, 28). The Harvard Mastery of Stress Study, one of the longest prospective studies ever conducted in this field, revealed that severe anxiety and conflict with hostility were accurate predictors of CAD and risk of overall future illness (29).

Studies on animals and humans have determined that psychological stress has an adverse effect on the cardiovascular system (30–36). The mechanism by which stress may influence atherogenesis involves a complex interaction of sympathetic arousal, hypothalamic stimulation, and adrenergic and neurohormonal responses that lead to increased blood pressure, increased circulating catecholamine levels, and increased platelet activity (37–39). The resulting increased shearing forces of blood on the arterial wall lead to endothelial injury and arterial wall damage. Thus, chronic exposure to psychological stress promotes the development of atherosclerosis, which may result in vasospasm, myocardial ischemia, coronary artery occlusion, myocardial infarction, and increased incidence of ventricular arrhythmia, a known risk factor for sudden cardiac death (40–42). Rozanski et al. (7) show these pathophysiological mechanisms in a schematic diagram (Fig. 5.1).

The 1-month community-based prevalence of major depression episodes is approximately 5% (43). However,

PHYSIOLOGIC
EFFECTS

CLINICAL
CONSEQUENCES

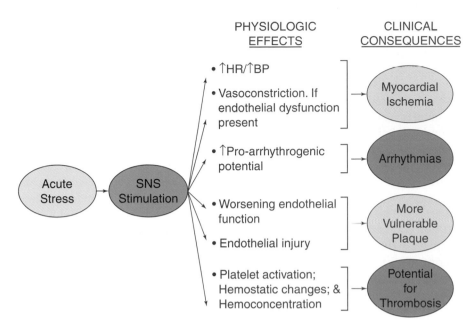

Figure 5.1. Pathophysiological effects of acute psychosocial stress. Sympathetic nervous system (SNS) stimulation emanating from acute stress leads to a variety of effects, ranging from heart rate and blood pressure stimulation to direct effects on coronary vascular endothelium. Clinical consequences of these effects include myocardial ischemia, cardiac arrhythmias, and fostering of more vulnerable coronary plaques and hemostatic changes. These changes form a substrate for development of acute myocardial infarction and sudden cardiac death (with permission from Rozanski A, Blumenthal JA, Kaplan J. Impact of psychological factors on the pathogenesis of cardiovascular disease and implications for therapy. Circulation 99:2192–2217, 1999)

among CAD patients, the prevalence is three times higher. In addition, lower levels of depressive symptoms occur at least as commonly in this patient population (44). Recent epidemiological studies among healthy and CAD populations consistently demonstrate a significant prospective relationship between major depression episodes and the incidence of future cardiac events (45–49). Furthermore, there is evidence supporting the existence of a gradient between the magnitude of depression and future cardiac events (45). Hopelessness, which is a component of depression, has shown a particularly strong link with sudden death and the development of CAD and carotid atherosclerosis (45, 50).

Although conclusions regarding the mechanisms by which psychosocial factors contribute to cardiac events are not definitive, considerable evidence points to several mechanisms likely to be involved in the effect of depression on the prognosis of patients with established CVD. For example, it has been shown that depressed patients exhibit increased sympathetic nervous system outflow and decreased parasympathetic function (51). This can lead to ventricular arrhythmias, platelet activation or aggregation, and increased myocardial oxygen consumption. It is plausible that these kinds of reactions contribute to the pathophysiological processes involved in the development of both CAD and MI. Increased activation of the pituitary adrenal axis in depressed patients has also been shown to produce high levels of cortisol, which can potentiate and prolong the effects of catecholamines (7, 52).

Depression is a predictor of poor adherence to a wide variety of medical treatments (53). An electronic medication monitoring device has demonstrated that elderly patients with major depression are less adherent to taking

medications than nondepressed patients (54). There is evidence that in patients recovering from MI, depression is associated with poor adherence to cardiac rehabilitation and risk factor modification (55). Consequently, depression may indirectly promote the progression of chronic illness by preventing adherence to other treatment regimens, such as healthy eating, physical activity and exercise, taking medications appropriately, abstaining from smoking, stress management, and moderating alcohol consumption.

Depression tends to be underdiagnosed and undertreated in cardiac patients. Fewer than 25% of patients with major depression are recognized as being depressed by their cardiologist or internist, and only about half of patients diagnosed as depressed receive treatment (56). The reasons for this are not clear. It has been suggested that physicians may have difficulty differentiating between the symptoms of depression and those related to the disease (57). Physicians must also weigh the risks of antidepressant medications against their expected benefits (58).

Diabetes

Diabetes is a chronic disease of insulin deficiency and/or resistance to insulin action. In the United States approximately 800,000 people are newly diagnosed each year (59). Diabetes is the leading cause of nontraumatic amputations (about 157,000/year), blindness among working-age adults (about 20,000/year), and end-stage kidney disease (about 30,000/year) (60). Stress, depression, and anxiety are significantly more prevalent among diabetics than the general population (61, 62).

Evidence suggests that stress may precipitate the onset of diabetes or compromise glucose control once the disease is established (63). Glucose toxicity that results from chronic, intermittent stress-induced elevations in blood glucose further compromise pancreatic secretory ability, leading to the progression of the disease (64). However, evidence characterizing the effects of stress in type I diabetes is contradictory. Human studies have shown that stress can stimulate hyperglycemia, hypoglycemia, or have no effect at all on glycemic status in established diabetes. More consistent evidence supports the role of stress in type II diabetes. Evidence from both animal and human studies suggest that individuals with type II diabetes have altered adrenergic sensitivity in the pancreas, which may make them particularly sensitive to stressful life events. Although data for type II diabetes are substantial, no direct evidence demonstrates that stress plays a clinically significant role in the expression or control of the human disease. Few studies have followed patients long enough to allow for making generalizations on clinical outcome. Consequently, more clinical research is needed to determine the degree to which stress affects the onset and course of the disease.

Chronic Obstructive Pulmonary Disease and Asthma

COPD is characterized by airflow obstruction due to chronic bronchitis and emphysema, two diseases that often coexist (2). COPD is the fourth leading cause of death in the United States. Asthma is a lung disease with recurrent exacerbations of airflow constriction, mucus secretion, and chronic inflammation of the airways, resulting in reduced airflow that causes wheezing, coughing, chest tightness, and difficulty breathing. An estimated 15 million Americans have asthma, with an 82% increase in the rate over the past 15 years. Over 50,000 hospitalizations, 5,000 deaths, and more than 133 million days of restricted activity are due to asthma each year (2).

Common psychological reactions among patients with pulmonary disease include anger, frustration, guilt, dependency, and embarrassment (65, 66). However, the most frequently observed psychological symptoms among patients with COPD are depression and anxiety. Studies have reported the prevalence of depression to be anywhere from 26–74% (66–68). Anxiety is another common psychological consequence of COPD. Up to 37% of COPD patients may have one or more panic attacks, as defined by bouts of intense anxiety, physiological arousal, temporary cognitive impairment, and a desire to flee the situation (69). Dyspnea in conjunction with fear of suffocation and death is a source of significant anxiety in this population (66). The emotional arousal of anxiety then increases ventilatory demands on the body, which may lead to hypoxia or hypercapnia. Increased physiological arousal in turn exacerbates anxiety symptoms, which produce greater insufficiency, resulting in a circular pattern that is difficult to break (4). The medical regimen of COPD patients tends to be complex, with an average of six medications per patient (70). Conse-

quently, noncompliance is high, with about half of patients either overusing or underusing their medications (70, 71). Stress reduction strategies, which include relaxation therapy and biofeedback, have demonstrated improvements in the self-management of asthma (72).

Cancer

Cancer is the second leading cause of death in the United States. Approximately 1.25 million Americans are newly diagnosed each year. The four major cancer sites, lung, female breast, prostate, and colon, account for about 54% of these new diagnoses (73). Some researchers believe that stressful life events and chronic depression are associated with the onset of cancer (74–77).

There is ample evidence from human and animal studies demonstrating the downward modulation of immune function concomitant with a variety of stressors (78). Depression has also been demonstrated to cause immune suppression by increasing the synthesis and release of adrenal corticosteroids and by decreasing lymphocyte proliferation and natural killer cell activity (79–81). It is estimated that 20–25% of cancer patients have long-term depression that is commonly unrecognized and untreated (82). However, the evidence of an association between depression and cancer from prospective cohort studies is inconclusive, with findings of both a lack of association and a weak positive relationship (83–88). Therefore, better systematically designed research is needed to elucidate the influence of psychological factors on cancer.

Chronic Pain

Chronic pain is a demoralizing condition that confronts the individual sufferer not only with stress created by pain but with many other continuing stressors that compromise all aspects of the patient's life. Living with chronic pain requires considerable emotional resilience and tends to deplete the individual's emotional reserve (89). Gatchel (90) describes chronic pain as a complex psychophysiological behavior pattern that cannot be broken down into distinct psychosocial and physical components. Instead, pain includes elements of both components. Furthermore, as pain becomes more chronic, the psychosocial factors play an increasingly dominant role in the maintenance of pain behavior and suffering.

Although a relationship is usually found between pain and certain psychological problems, such as depression, the nature of the relationship between the two variables remains inconclusive (91). Some but not all patients develop depression secondary to chronic pain. Others show depression as the primary syndrome, of which pain is a symptom. Moreover, factors that mediate the relationship between depression and pain remain largely unknown (92).

In a study initially evaluating one aspect of this chicken-or-egg question, Polatino et al. (93) assessed 200 patients with chronic low back pain (pain disability present for an average of well over 1 year) for concurrent life-time psychiatric syndromes. They found that 77% of patients met lifetime diagnostic criteria and 59% demonstrated current symptoms for at least one psychiatric diagnosis. The most common of these were major depressive disorder, anxiety disorders, and substance abuse. All of these prevalence rates were significantly higher than in the general population. In patients with a lifetime history of psychiatric syndromes, 54% of those with depression, 95% of those with anxiety disorders, and 94% of those with a substance abuse had these syndromes before the onset of their back pain. These are the first results to suggest that certain psychiatric syndromes may precede chronic low back pain. It appears that a prospective study is needed to substantiate these retrospective-recall results more clearly, since the findings cannot definitively show whether psychopathological disorders in chronic pain patients are consequences of the chronic pain or whether preexisting disorders act as predispositions for pain to become chronic.

Rheumatoid Arthritis

Rheumatoid arthritis (RA) is a chronic systemic autoimmune disorder with no known cause. It is characterized by painful swelling and stiffness of joints. The overall prevalence of RA is approximately 1% in the population. Prevalence increases with age, and in those over 65 years, it may be as high as 5–7%. The severity of joint problems tends to fluctuate over time, with periods of mild activity punctuated by more intense flare-ups. For two-thirds of affected patients, the overall course of the disease is one of progressive deformity and destruction of joints, accompanied by increasing disability (94). RA is more common in women than in men, with a ratio of about 2.5 to 1 (95). The debilitating nature of this disorder, with its associated pain, can interfere with living in a number of ways. As RA progresses, patients may no longer be able to participate in recreational activities and may find their social life curtailed. Not surprisingly, it has been found that RA has a negative influence on quality of life and satisfaction with life (96).

Studies to date have shown that RA can impair mental health (97, 98). Frank et al. (99) estimated that the prevalence of major depression and dysthymia in RA patients was about 18% and 41% respectively, which is higher than in a general population. Reviews of the literature indicate that methodological flaws in the research have weakened any evidence linking various psychological factors with the causes of the disease (97, 100, 101). However, in one study, which attempted to clarify the pathogenic mechanisms associated with the disease, Hendrie et al. (102) investigated the relationships among psychological stress, depressed immune system activity, and the initial manifestation of arthritic symptoms. These investigators compared immunoglobulin levels and life change scores in polyarthritis patients with a history of

joint disease with a duration of less than 6 months. Polyarthritis patients whose immunoglobulin levels were elevated produced a mean life change score for the year preceding initial symptom manifestation that was almost three times that of their counterparts without elevated immunoglobulin levels.

Other researchers have suggested that psychosocial factors may interfere with compliance with the treatment of RA and consequently have an indirect link with the progression of the disease. Estimates of noncompliance with medication in RA patients have ranged from 22–67% (103, 104). Patients with more severe arthritic disease or longer duration of illness may be more likely to be noncompliant than those with relatively mild or recent disease (105).

► SUMMARY

Psychological stress, depression, and anxiety are common among patients living with chronic illness. Skeptics can no longer ignore an abundant amount of evidence strongly linking these factors with the pathogenesis of cardiovascular disease. However, the role of psychosocial factors in the development of other chronic illnesses remains controversial. Future investigations must involve prospective studies that use valid methods to assess the various psychosocial factors and outcomes associated with chronic illness. On the other hand, there is good evidence to indicate that psychosocial factors can have an adverse affect on behavior as regards better-recognized risk factors associated with chronic illness.

Most people with psychosocial issues do not present themselves to mental health services for treatment. Therefore, systems to help non–mental health specialists recognize possible symptoms of emotional distress are needed. Consideration should be given to developing improved liaison relationships with psychological or behavioral specialists to facilitate more specialized interventions when appropriate. In addition, non–mental health specialists should be encouraged to develop skills that will improve their ability to promote healthier behaviors and emotional functioning in the overall treatment of chronic illness.

ACKNOWLEDGMENT

We thank Kelly Conforti, PhD, for her review of the original manuscript.

References
1. National Center for Health Statistics. Births and Deaths. United States, 1995. Monthly Vital Statistics Report, 45 (3) Supp 2. DHHS 96–1120, 1996.
2. US. Department of Health and Human Services, Office of Public Health and Science. Healthy People 2010 Objectives: Draft for public comment. Washington: HHS, Office of Public Health and Science, 1998.

3. McKenna MT, Taylor WR, Marks JS, Koplan JP. Current issues and challenges in chronic disease control. In: Brownson RC, Remington PL, Davis JR, eds. Chronic Disease Epidemiology and Control. Washington: American Public Health Association, 1998:1–26.
4. US Department of Health and Human Services Mental Health: A Report of the Surgeon General. Rockville, MD: HHS, Substance Abuse and Mental Health Services Administration, Center for Mental Health Services, National Institute for Mental Health, National Institute of Mental Health, 1999.
5. Emery CF, Lebowitz KR. Behavioral medicine in pulmonary rehabilitation: Psychological, cognitive, and social factors. In: Hodgkin J, Celli B, Connors G, eds. Pulmonary Rehabilitation. 4th ed. Philadelphia: Lippincott Williams & Wilkins 2000:303–316.
6. Miller TQ, Smith TW, Turner CW, et al. A meta-analytic review of research on hostility and physical health. Psychological Bulletin, 119: 322–348, 1996.
7. Rozanski P, Blumenthal JA, Kaplan J. Impact of psychological factors on the pathogenesis of cardiovascular disease and implications for therapy. Circulation 99:2197–2217, 1999.
8. Holmes T, Rahe R. The social readjustment rating scale. J Psychosom Res 11:213–218, 1967.
9. Krieger N, Rowley DL, Herman AA, et al. Racism, sexism, and social class: Implications for studies of health, disease, and well-being. Am J Prevent Med 9(Suppl):82–122, 1993.
10. Lazarus RS, Folkman S. Stress, appraisal and coping. New York: Springer, 1984.
11. Browne A, Finkelhor D. Impact of child sexual abuse: A review of the research. Psychol Bull 99:66–77, 1986.
12. Sime WE, Eliot RS, Solberg EE. Stress and heart disease. In: Blair S, Painter P, Pate RR, et al., eds. Resource manual for guidelines for exercise testing and prescription. American College of Sports Medicine. 3rd ed. Philadelphia: Lea & Febiger, 1998:43–49.
13. Murray CJL, Lopez AD. Evidence-based health policy: Lessons from the Global Burden of Disease Study. Science 274:740–743, 1996.
14. Murray CJL, Lopez AD. Alternative projections of mortality and disability by cause 1990–2020: Global Burden of Disease Study. Lancet 349:1498–1504, 1997.
15. Regier DA, Farmer ME, Rae DS, et al. Comorbidity of mental disorders with alcohol and other drug abuse: Results from the Epidemiologic Catchment Area (ECA) Study. JAMA 264:2511–2518, 1990.
16. Adams PF, Marano MA. Current estimates from the National Health Interview Survey, 1994. National Center for Health Statistics. Vital Health Stat 10:193, 1995.
17. Pieper C, LaCroix A, Karasek R. The relationship of psychosocial dimensions on work with coronary heart disease. Am J Epidemiol 129: 483–494, 1989.
18. Appels A, Schouten E. Burnout as a risk factor for coronary heart disease. Behav Med 17:53–59, 1991.
19. Karasek RA, Baker D, Marxer F, et al. Job decision latitude, job demands, and cardiovascular disease: A prospective study of Swedish men. Am J Public Health 71:694–705, 1981.
20. Bosma H, Peter R, Siegrist J, Marmot M. Two alternative job stress models and the risk of coronary heart disease. Am J Public Health 88:68–74, 1998.
21. Siegrist J, Peter R, Junge A, et al. Low status control, high effort at work and ischemic heart disease: Prospective evidence from blue-collar men. Soc Sci Med 331:1127–1134, 1990.
22. Lynch JJ, Krause N, Kaplan GA, et al. Work place demands, economic reward, and progression of carotid atherosclerosis. Circulation 96:302–307, 1997.
23. Willich S, Hannelore L, Lewis M, et al. Weekly variation of acute myocardial infarction. Circulation 90:87–93, 1994.
24. Evans C, Chalmers J, Capewell S, et al. "I don't like Mondays": day of the week of coronary heart disease death in Scotland: Study of routine collected data. BMJ 320:218–219, 2000.
25. Eaker ED, Abbott RD, de Knell WB. Frequency of uncomplicated angina pectoris in Type A compared with Type B persons (the Framingham Study). Am J Cardiol 63:1042–1045, 1989.
26. Rahe RH, Romo M, Bennett L, Siltanen P. Recent life changes, myocardial infarction, and abrupt coronary death. Arch Intern Med 133:221–228, 1974.
27. Kaplan GA, Salonsen JT, Cohen RD, et al. Social connections and mortality from all causes and from cardiovascular disease: Prospective evidence from eastern Finland. Am J Epidemiol 128:370–380, 1988.
28. Williams RB, Barefoot JC, Califf RM, et al. Prognostic importance of social and economic resources among medically treated patients with angiographically documented coronary artery disease. JAMA 267:520–524, 1992.
29. Russek LG, King SH, Russek SJ, Russek HI. The Harvard Mastery of Stress Study—35 year follow-up: Prognostic significance of patterns of psychophysiological arousal and adaptation. Psychiatr Med 52:271–285, 1990.
30. Kaplan JR, Manuck SB, Clarkson TB, et al. Social status, environment and atherosclerosis in cynomolgus monkeys. Arteriosclerosis 2, 4:359–368, 1982.
31. Blazer DG. Social support and mortality in an elderly community program. Am J Epidemiol 115, 5:684–694, 1984.
32. Deanfield JE, Shea M, Kensett M, et al. Silent myocardial ischemia due to mental stress. Lancet 2:1001–1005, 1984.
33. Jiang W, Babyak M, Krantz DS, et al. Mental stress-induced myocardial ischemia and cardiac events. JAMA 25:1651–1656, 1996.
34. Krantz DS, Helmers KF, Noel Bairey NC, et al. Cardiovascular reactivity and mental stress-induced myocardial ischemia in patients with coronary artery disease. Psychosom Med 53:1–12, 1991.
35. Orth-Gomer K, Johnson JV. Social isolation and mortality: A six-year follow-up study of a random sample of the Swedish population. J Chronic Dis 40:10:949–957, 1987.
36. Rozanski A, Bairey N, Krantz DS, et al. Mental stress and the induction of silent myocardial ischemia in patients with coronary artery disease. N Engl J Med 318:1005–1012, 1988.
37. Coumel P, Leenhardt A. Mental activity, adrenergic modulation, and cardiac arrhythmias in patients with heart disease. Circulation 83 (Suppl 2): 56–57, 1991.
38. Naesh O, Haedersdal C, Hindberg I, Trap-Jensen J. Platelet activation in mental stress. Clin Physiol 13:299–307, 1993.
39. Verrier RL, Dickerson LW. Autonomic nervous system and

coronary blood flow changes related to emotional activation and sleep. Circulation 83 (Suppl 2):81–89, 1991.

40. Yeung AC, Vekshtein VI, Krantz DS, et al. The effect of atherosclerosis on the vasomotor response of the coronary arteries to mental stress. N Engl J Med 325:1551–1556, 1991.

41. Blumenthal JA, Jiang, W, Waugh RA, et al. Mental stress-induced ischemia in the laboratory and ambulatory ischemia during daily life: Association and hemodynamic features. Circulation 92, 8:2102–2108, 1995.

42. Davis A, Natelson B. Brain-heart interactions: Neurocardiology of arrhythmia and sudden death. Tex Heart Inst J 20:158–169, 1993.

43. Blazer DG, Kessler RC, McGonagle KA, Swartz MS. The prevalence and distribution of major depression in a national community sample: The national co-morbidity survey. Am J Psychiatry 151:979–986, 1994.

44. Hans M, Carney RM, Feedland KE, Skala J. Depression in patients with coronary heart disease: A 12-month follow-up. Gen Hosp Psychiatry 18:61–65, 1994.

45. Anda R, Williamson D, Jones D, et al. Depressed affect, hopelessness, and risk of ischemic heart disease in a cohort of U.S. adults. Epidemiology 4:285–294, 1993.

46. Barefoot JC, Schroll M. Symptoms of depression, acute myocardial infarction, and total mortality in a community sample. Circulation 93:1976–1980, 1996.

47. Barefoot JC, Helms MJ, Mark DB. Depression and long-term mortality risk in patients with coronary artery disease. Am J Cardiol 78:613–717, 1996.

48. Frasure-Smith N, Lesperance F, Talajic M. Depression and 18-month prognosis after myocardial infarction. Circulation 91:999–1005, 1995.

49. Frasure-Smith N, Lesperance F, Junea M, et al. Gender, depression, and one-year prognosis after myocardial infarction. Psychosom Med 61:26–37, 1999.

50. Everson SA, Kaplan GA, Goldberg DE. Hopelessness and 4-year progression of carotid atherosclerosis: The Kuopio ischemic heart disease risk factor study. Arterioscler Thromb Vascul Biol 17:1490–1495, 1997.

51. Vieth RC, Lewis N, Linares OA, et al. Sympathetic nervous system activity in major depression: Basal and desipramine-induced alterations in plasma norepinephrine kinetics. Arch Gen Psychiatry 51, 5:411–422, 1994.

52. Koetnansky R. Catecholamines-corticosteroid interactions. In: Usdin E, Koetnansky R, Kopin IJ, eds. Catecholamines and Stress. Amsterdam: Elsevier/North Holland, 1980:7.

53. Dunbar J. Predictors of patient adherence: Patient characteristics. In: Shumaker SA, Schron EB, Ockene JK, eds. The Handbook of Health Behavior Change. New York: Springer, 1990:348–360.

54. Carney RM, Freedland KE, Eisen SE, et al. Depression is associated with poor adherence to medical treatment regimen in elderly cardiac patients. Health Psychol 14:88–90, 1995.

55. Guiry E, Conroy RM, Hickey N, Mulcahy R. Psychological response to an acute coronary event and its effect on subsequent rehabilitation and lifestyle change. Clin Cardiol 10:256–260, 1987.

56. Mayou R, Foster A, Williamson B. Medical care after myocardial infarction. J Psychosom Res 23:23–26, 1979.

57. Clarke DM. Psychological factors in illness and recovery. N Z Med J 111:410–412, 1998.

58. Carney RM, Freedland KE, Rich MW, Jaffe AS. Depression as a risk factor for cardiac events in established coronary heart disease: A review of possible mechanisms. Ann Behav Med 17, 2:142–149, 1995.

59. Centers for Disease Control and Prevention. National diabetes fact sheet: National estimates and general information on diabetes in the United States. Atlanta: CDC, 1997.

60. Centers for Disease Control and Prevention. Diabetes Surveillance. Atlanta: CDC, 1997.

61. Robinson N, Fuller JH. Role of life events and difficulties in the onset of diabetes mellitus. J Psychosom Res 29:583–591, 1985.

62. Peyrot M, Rubin RR. Levels and risks of depression and anxiety symptomatology among diabetic adults. Diabetes Care 20:585–590, 1997.

63. Surwit RS, Schneider MS, Feinglos MN. Stress and diabetes mellitus. Diabetes Care 15, 10:1413–1422, 1992.

64. Leahy JL. Natural history of beta-cell dysfunction in NIDDM. Diabetes Care, 13: 992–1010, 1990.

65. Guyatt GH, Townsend M, Berman LB, Pugsley SO. Quality of life in patients with chronic airflow limitation. Br J Dis Chest 81:45, 1987.

66. Sandhu HS. Psychosocial issues in chronic obstructive pulmonary disease. Clin Chest Med 7: 629, 1986.

67. Agle DP, Baum GL. Psychological aspects of chronic obstructive pulmonary disease. Med Clin North Am 61: 749, 1977.

68. Isoaho R, Puolijoki H, Huhti E, et al. Chronic obstructive pulmonary disease and cognitive impairment in the elderly. Int Psychogeriatr 8:113, 1996.

69. Porzelius J, Vest M, Nochomovitz M. Respiratory function, cognitions, and panic in chronic obstructive pulmonary patients. Behav Res Ther 30:75, 1992.

70. Dolce JJ, Crisp C, Manzella B, et al. Medication adherence patterns in chronic obstructive pulmonary disease. Chest 99:837, 1991.

71. James PNE, Anderson JB, Prior JG, et al. Patterns of drug taking in patients with chronic airflow obstruction. Postgrad Med J 61:7–10, 1985.

72. Lehrer PM, Sargunaraj D, Hochron S. Psychological approaches to the treatment of asthma. J Consult Clin Psychol 60, 4:639–643, 1992.

73. Landis S, Murray T, Bolden S, Eingo PA. Cancer statistics. Cancer J Clin 48:6–29, 1998.

74. Fras I, Litin EM, Pearson JS. Comparison of psychiatric symptoms in carcinoma of the pancreas with those in some other intra-abdominal neoplasms. Am J Psychiatry 123:1553–1556, 1967.

75. Horne RL, Picard RS. Psychosocial risk factors for lung cancer. Psychosom Med 43:431–438, 1979.

76. Lehrer S. Life change and gastric cancer. Psychosom Med 42:499–502, 1980.

77. Penninx BWJH, Guralnik JM, Pahor M, et al. Chronically depressed mood and cancer risk in older persons. J Natl Cancer Inst 90:1888–1893, 1998.

78. Kiecolt-Glaser JK, Glaser R. Psychoneuroimmunology: Can psychological interventions modulate immunity? J Consult Clin Psychol 60, 4:569–575, 1992.

79. Caroll B, Curtis G, Mendels J. Cerebrospinal fluid and

plasma free cortisol concentrations in depression. Psychosom Med 6:235–244, 1976.

80. Petitto JM, Folds JD, Ozer H, et al. Abnormal diurnal variation in circulating natural killer cell phenotypes and cytotoxic activity in major depression. Am J Psychiatry 149:694–696, 1992.

81. Stein M, Miller AH, Trestman RL. Depression, the immune system, and health and illness: Findings in search of meaning. Arch Gen Psychiatry 48:171–177, 1991.

82. Bottomley A. Depression in cancer patients: A literature review. Eur J Cancer Care 7:181–191, 1998.

83. Levenson JL, Bemis C. The role of psychological factors in cancer onset and progression. Psychosomatics 32, 2:124–134, 1990.

84. Kaplan GA, Reynolds P. Depression and cancer mortality and morbidity: Prospective evidence from the Alameda County Study. J Behav Med 11:1–13, 1988.

85. Zonderman AB, Costa PT Jr, McCrae RR. Depression as a risk for cancer morbidity and mortality in a nationally representative sample. JAMA 262:1191–1195, 1989.

86. Bleiker MA, van der Ploeg HM. Psychosocial factors in the etiology of breast cancer: Review of a popular link. Patient Educ 37:201–224, 1999.

87. Knekt P, Raitasalo R, Heliovaara M, et al. Elevated lung cancer risk among persons with depressed mood. Am J Epidemiol 144:1096–2103, 1996.

88. Linkins RW, Comstock GW. Depressed mood and development of cancer. Am J Epidemiol 132:962–972, 1990.

89. Turk DC. Biopsychosocial perspective on chronic pain. In: Gatchel RJ, Turk DC, eds. Psychological approaches to pain management: A practitioner's handbook. New York: Guilford, 1996:3–32.

90. Gatchel R. Psychological disorders and chronic pain: Cause-effect relationships. In: Gatchel RJ, Turk DC, eds. Psychological Approaches to Pain Management: A Practitioner's Handbook. New York: Guilford, 1996:33–52.

91. Romano JM, Turner JA. Chronic pain and depression: Does the evidence support a relationship? Psychol Bull 97:18–34, 1985.

92. Turk DC, Rudy TE. Toward an empirically derived taxonomy of chronic pain patients: Integration of psychological assessment data. J Consult Clin Psychol 56:233–238, 1988.

93. Polatino PB, Kinney RK, Gatchel RJ, et al. Psychiatric illness and chronic low back pain. Spine 18:66–71, 1993.

94. Walsh JD, Blanchard EB, Kremer JM, Blanchard CG. The psychosocial effects of rheumatoid arthritis on the patient and well partner. Behav Res Ther 37:259–271, 1999.

95. Schumacher HR. Primer on the Rheumatic Diseases. 8th ed. Atlanta: Arthritis Foundation, 1988.

96. Bendtsen P, Hornquist JO. Change and status in quality of life in patients with rheumatoid arthritis. Qual Life Res 1:296–305, 1992.

97. Anderson KO, Bradley LA, Young LD, et al. Rheumatoid arthritis: Review of psychological factors related to etiology, effects and treatment. Psychol Bull 98, 2:358–387, 1985.

98. Young LD. Psychological factors in rheumatoid arthritis. J Consult Clin Psychol 60,4:619–627, 1992.

99. Frank RG, Beck NC, Parker JC, et al. Depression in rheumatoid arthritis. J Rheumatol 15:920–925, 1988.

100. Baum J. A review of psychological aspects of rheumatic diseases. Seminars in Arthritis and Rheumatism, 11:353–361, 1982.

101. Persson LO, Berglund K, Sahlberg D. Psychological factors in chronic rheumatic diseases: A review. Scand J Rheumatol 28:137–144, 1999.

102. Hendrie HC, Paraskevas F, Baragar FD, Adamson JD. Stress, immunoglobulin levels and early polyarthritis. J Psychosom Res 15:337–343, 1971.

103. Ferguson K, Bole GG. Family support, health beliefs, and therapeutic compliance in patients with rheumatoid arthritis. Patient Counsell Health Educ 1:101–105, 1979.

104. Geersten HR, Gray RM, Ward JR. Patient non-compliance within the context of seeking medical care for arthritis. J Chronic Dis 26: 689–698, 1973.

105. Lee P, Tan LJ. Current trends in the treatment of rheumatoid arthritis in general practice. N Z Med J 89:165–167, 1979.

3.4.0, 3.4.2   4.4.3,

CHAPTER **6**

INTEGRATION OF LIFESTYLE BEHAVIORS

Patricia M. Smith and C. Barr Taylor

This chapter describes the integration of lifestyle behavior interventions used in large multifactorial risk reduction trials. Multiple risk factor reduction—that is, simultaneous reduction of factors such as sedentary lifestyle, smoking, hypertension, hyperlipidemia, and obesity—is important because many of the risk factors are interrelated and work synergistically in the development and exacerbation of cardiovascular disease (CVD), and their adverse effects are cumulative.

MULTIFACTORIAL RISK REDUCTION: PRIMARY PREVENTION

Multifactorial risk factor reduction for the primary prevention of CVD originated in the 1970s with the Multiple Risk Factor Intervention Trial (MRFIT). MRFIT, a multisite study involving 22 clinical centers across the United States, focused on the simultaneous reduction of smoking, blood pressure, and blood cholesterol levels (1). Until MRFIT, interventions designed to improve risk factors tended to focus on a single risk factor (i.e., smoking cessation or hypertension or lowering blood cholesterol). The premise behind MRFIT was that simultaneous reduction of several risk factors would result in maximum risk factor change and significant reduction in CVD mortality, nonfatal myocardial infarction (MI), coronary heart disease (CHD) mortality, and all-cause mortality over a 6-year period (1).

MRFIT included more than 12,000 men aged 35–57 who were identified as at high risk for CHD. The men were randomized either to special intervention or to usual sources of health care. The behavioral interventions used in MRFIT (smoking cessation, diet, and compliance with hypertension medication) were designed with close adherence to the principles of behavior change as specified by social learning theory, and they remain among the most comprehensively described interventions in the published scientific literature (2). The interventions, which were multicomponent in design, included group sessions, individual counseling, social support, take-home materials, and highly effective behavioral modifi-

cation techniques (e.g., self-monitoring, goal setting, stimulus control of the environment, systematic desensitization and relaxation, support systems, and feedback). The intervention components were interactive; they included role playing, group discussions, food preparation demonstrations, and potluck dinners. Delivery of the intervention was enhanced by generous use of media materials such as films, cassettes, advertising displays, shopping guides, pamphlets, and cookbooks. Family participation was encouraged. Antihypertensive medications were prescribed as required. The interventions featured multiple follow-up contacts and were delivered by a multidisciplinary team that included nutritionists, psychologists, psychiatrists, physicians, smoking cessation specialists, and health counselors.

The historical perspectives, development of the intervention model and protocol, and a summary of the 4-year results of MRFIT have been presented (3). After 4 years, MRFIT evidenced significant changes in the three risk factors, although the changes fell substantially short of the goals (3). MRFIT also demonstrated that multifactorial risk reduction could reduce CHD mortality in patients free of CHD at baseline. By the 10.5-year follow-up, mortality rates were 10.6% lower for the intervention group than with usual care, and after 16 years, CHD mortality was reduced by 11.4% (4, 5).

Since MRFIT was completed, a number of other primary prevention trials, some occurring in work sites, others at the community level, have focused on primary prevention of CVD. However, few describe their behavioral interventions in sufficient detail to allow replication. Miettinen and Strandberg (6) have reviewed the implications of some of the better-known trials. These authors remain optimistic about the usefulness of multiple risk factor reduction for CVD prevention, although the results of primary prevention trials have been inconsistent. Most notably, prevention has not been consistently obtained even when risk factors have been significantly improved, and differences in risk factor levels between intervention and control groups are often diminished after varying periods of follow-up.

MULTIFACTORIAL RISK REDUCTION: SECONDARY PREVENTION

The remainder of this chapter focuses on the design and delivery of behavioral interventions used in more recent multifactorial risk reduction trials for secondary prevention (i.e., among patients with established CVD). Details of the design and delivery of behavioral interventions used in multifactorial trials are often not presented in a consistent format across published studies. Therefore, it can be difficult to ascertain the components and procedures of the interventions in a way that allows for critical examination and replication of methods and to determine what knowledge, skills, and abilities are required to carry them out. We have therefore developed a series of tables to summarize the information. Five randomized controlled trials that targeted at least two risk factors with behavioral interventions were selected for discussion (7–11).

Investigational Design

The studies included for discussion in this chapter are randomized, controlled secondary prevention trials that monitored risk factor status for at least 1 year after entry into the program. The populations studied ranged in sample size from 48 to 585 (7–11). Participants were predominantly male (76–100%), had an average age of 56

years, and had documented MI (7, 11), atherosclerosis (9, 10), or stable angina pectoris (8). All trials included behavioral interventions to reduce the rate of progression of coronary atherosclerosis (8–10) or prevention of a recurrent MI (7, 11), and half of the trials offered antihypertensive and/or lipid-lowering drug therapy as one of the main components (7, 10, 11). With one exception, the trials were clinic based. The one program that was not clinic based involved a 1-week residential retreat followed by a home-based program (9). The general designs are presented in Table 6.1.

Behavioral interventions for diet and exercise were offered in all studies, and smoking cessation, stress management, and psychosocial interventions such as group support were offered in some but not all of the trials (7–11). Multidisciplinary teams, generally led by physicians, since the study subjects required medical care for cardiovascular disease, delivered the behavioral interventions. Usual-care patients in all of the trials received medical care under the direction of their primary-care physician. Therefore, depending on the usual practice of the physician, many usual-care patients received medication for hypertension and hyperlipidemia, lifestyle risk factor modification advice, and psychosocial intervention for conditions such as depression. Usual-care patients in all studies were also offered annual medical examinations, at

Table 6.1. General Design of Multifactorial Risk Reduction Trials

TRIAL	POPULATION	SELECTION CRITERIA AND PRIMARY TARGET	INTERVENTION LENGTH AND FOLLOW-UP	PROVIDER	THEORETICAL MODEL
WHO 10-year Follow-up, Hämäläinen et al., 1989 (7) Finland	*n* = 375 (IS = 188; UC = 187) *Males:* 80% *Average age:* 54 yr.	*Criterion:* Consecutive nonselected patients treated in hospital for acute MI *Target:* Secondary prevention post MI	*Length:* Intensive contact for 3 mo, close contact for 3 yr *Follow-up:* 1, 2, 3, 6, 10 yr	Multidisciplinary: internist, social worker, psychologist, dietitian, physiotherapist	None specified
Schuler et al., 1992 (8) Germany	*n* = 113 (IS = 56; UC = 57) *Males:* 100% *Average age:* 54 yr	*Criterion:* Stable angina pectoris *Target:* Stop progression of CAD	*Length:* 3 wk on a hospital metabolic ward, 1 yr home based *Follow-up:* 1 yr	Multidisciplinary (not specified)	None specified
Lifestyle Heart Trial, Ornish et al., 1990 (9) United States	*n* = 48 (IS = 28; UC = 20) *Males:* 88% *Average age:* 58 yr	*Criterion:* Angiographically documented CAD *Target:* Stop progression, reverse CAD	*Length:* 1 wk residential retreat, 1 yr home-based program *Follow-up:* 1 yr	Multidisciplinary: stress management–exercise instructor, counselors, nurses, angiographers, chefs, physicians	None specified
SCRIP, Haskell et al., 1994 (10) United States	*n* = 300 (IS = 145; UC = 155) *Males:* 86% *Average age:* 56 yr	*Criterion:* Angiographically defined coronary atherosclerosis *Target:* Reduce rate of progression of coronary atherosclerosis	*Length:* 4 yr *Follow-up:* 4 yr	Multidisciplinary: nurse, dietitian, psychologist, physician. Managed by SCRIP staff in cooperation with private physician	Social learning theory
MULTIFIT DeBusk et al., 1994 (10) United States	*n* = 585 (IS = 293; UC = 292) *Males:* 79% *Average age:* 57 yr	*Criterion:* Hospitalized for MI *Target:* Secondary prevention and disease management	*Length:* 1 yr *Follow-up:* 1 yr	Multidisciplinary: nurse, psychiatrist, cardiologist, lipid specialist, nutritionist	Social learning theory

CAD, coronary artery disease; MI, myocardial infarction: IS, special intervention; SCRIP, Stanford Coronary Risk Intervention Project; UC, usual care.

which time various tests and evaluations regarding risk factor reduction were administered and feedback of results were provided to patients and physicians. Because of the amount of intervention usual-care patients receive in secondary prevention trials, the outcomes of these trials present a very conservative estimate of the effect of behavioral interventions on risk factor reduction.

The primary outcomes varied across the multifactorial trials. They included self-reported adherence to the behavioral regimens, changes in depression or psychosocial functioning, physiological changes including functional capacity, biochemically confirmed smoking status, serum lipid levels, blood pressure, angiograms to determine regression and progression of atherosclerosis, and morbidity and mortality. Across studies, intervention patients had significantly greater changes in most risk factors than did usual-care patients, which provides support for the efficacy of the various interventions. The information provided in the tables summarizes the assessment of the behavioral components of the trials. The original articles provide information on other primary outcomes.

Study Length and Follow-up

The length of time over which an intervention is administered and the frequency and timing of follow-up are important because measurable changes in risk factors take time. Although behavioral interventions often last for a year, the trend is to front-load the intervention for the first few months after recruitment, often with multiple follow-up and clinic visits. The patient is then expected to continue the behavioral regimens at home with less supervision during the remainder of the study.

The WHO trial offered the most extended program: the intervention itself lasted for 3 years (7, 13). All of the trials had a minimum of a 1-year follow-up to the intervention. One of the studies included 4 years of annual follow-ups and another followed participants annually for 10 years (7, 10). Although time is necessary to demonstrate change in risk factors, the rate of risk factor change seems to slow with time, and many of the early differences between the intervention and usual-care groups are attenuated. Although this slowing of risk factor change may be due to regression to the mean, it is more likely due to lack of continued adherence to the behavioral regimens, which may in turn be related to the withdrawal of personal attention and coaching provided by health care specialists during the intervention phase of the trial. Moreover, the pattern of behavior change is believed to cycle and result in relapse many times before a new behavior habit is successfully integrated, and therefore it may take time for risk factor reduction to stabilize.

The success of any program depends on long-term adherence, and efforts to build adherence interventions into the programs are necessary (14). The lesson to be gained from these studies is that although the length of intervention was probably determined more from clinical experi-

ence and other goals unique to the project (e.g., funding), intensive multifactorial risk reduction cannot be achieved without frequent visits spread over at least a year.

Provider

All studies included a multidisciplinary team, which might include a nutritionist–dietitian for the diet component, a clinical psychologist or nurse for the stress reduction and smoking cessation components, and a physician for medications and treadmill testing. Physical therapists and exercise physiologists were used for exercise testing, prescription, and supervision. Nurses or unspecified staff members of the research team who worked in cooperation with the primary-care physician were employed to monitor or manage patients, track medication requirements and symptoms, and refer patients to other medical personnel as necessary (10, 11). The use of multiple health care providers with a broad base of skills and knowledge is critical for success. A multidisciplinary, multicomponent program also requires a fine-tuned system or infrastructure to ensure that patients are moved smoothly through the various components of the program, that they are not lost to follow-up, that necessary liaisons among the various providers are established and maintained, and that patients' needs are met in a timely fashion.

Theory

Only two studies have clearly stated that they followed a theoretical framework in the design of the interventions (10, 11). Both of these studies used Bandura's social learning theory (2). Interventions based on social learning theory focus on helping participants build self-efficacy to change behavior. However, many of the studies incorporated well-known behavior modification techniques in the interventions (e.g., contracts, goal setting, self-monitoring, feedback) that do have antecedents in operant and classical learning theories, although the connection to theory was not specified.

The medical model, involving optimal medical care, physician activation, and medication, dominated in most studies, which put responsibility for change more in the hands of the experts than the patients. Health education appeared to be an unspecified underlying approach to a number of interventions. Although health education is important to decrease knowledge deficits, research to substantiate the relationship between health knowledge and health behavior change and maintenance is lacking.

Multifactorial risk reduction programs should follow a theoretical model in the design of behavioral interventions. The importance of theory lies in its ability to elucidate the underlying biopsychosocial mechanisms involved in change, to clarify what psychosocial variables to use and how to measure them to allow comparison across studies, and to determine systematically what components of an intervention are most effective in bringing about change (15). A good review of theories and intervention approaches to health behavior change has recently been published (16).

Setting

A number of settings were used in these trials (outpatient clinics, home, hospital metabolic wards, and a residential retreat at a hotel), but all had some clinic involvement (7–11). Most settings for the interventions encompassed a combination of clinic and home-based programs. Treadmill testing and educational, nutritional, psychosocial, and smoking cessation counseling at a clinic were common, with patients carrying out the exercise and diet regimens at home.

The relative benefits of the relatively intensive residential program used in two studies remain unclear (8, 9). One advantage of a residential program is control over diet and exercise without noncompliance with prescribed regimens. From a scientific perspective, such information may help elucidate more precisely the effect of lifestyle modification on risk factor profile. However, from an applied perspective, providing meals to patients in residential programs is not equivalent to prescribing diets to individuals who must do their own food shopping and preparation, so the benefit of short-stay residential programs may lie in helping people adapt to a new way of eating. Adherence to behavior change after the initial residential component remains a problem, as it does in all other approaches. Residential programs are possibly more costly and perhaps not as feasible as outpatient programs in terms of dissemination, although that has yet to be determined. It is clear that multifactorial risk reduction can be done in a variety of settings. However, no studies have compared one setting to another relative to efficacy, dissemination, and cost-effectiveness.

BEHAVIORAL INTERVENTIONS

Unfortunately, none of the studies provide sufficient information about the best sequence of intervention or combinations of behaviors to be altered. A variety of sequencing strategies appear to be effective. Behavioral interventions for diet and exercise were offered in all studies, and smoking cessation, stress management, and psychosocial interventions such as group support were offered in some but not all of the trials. The most stringent behavioral intervention featured a rigorous program of lifestyle change involving a low-fat vegetarian diet, light exercise, stress management (daily stretching, breathing exercises, and meditation or prayer, with many of the techniques derived from yoga), smoking cessation, and weekly group support to enhance nurturing relationships (9). Because all studies included diet and exercise interventions, the design of interventions for diet and exercise are studied more closely in the following section, and an overview of these interventions for each study is found in Tables 6.2 and 6.3.

Components of the Behavioral Interventions

All of the studies offered multiple-component programs and frequent contact with several health care providers. The major components included various forms of regular evaluation and assessment, health education, prescribed behavioral goals and regimens, individual or group counseling, behavior change strategies (e.g., relapse prevention training, behavioral modification techniques, exercise logs), medical care, medication (antihypertensive, antiarrhythmic, and lipid lowering), medical examinations, and multimedia delivery of interventions and follow-up. Unfortunately, the type and extent of intervention delivery were not well specified in most studies. Multimedia approaches (e.g., pamphlets, workbooks, videos, audiotapes, telephone follow-up, and personalized, computer-generated guidelines and feedback) are effective if used in a proactive, interactive fashion (17). Many well-designed multimedia materials are readily available from agencies such as the National Cancer Institute; National Heart, Lung, and Blood Institute; and the American Heart Association. Telephone follow-up contact, which is effective, cost-effective, and convenient for patients because they do not have to make so many clinic visits, was underused in most studies. It is important to consider carefully how media can be used most effectively in an interactive, ongoing fashion rather than in a one-time, noninteractive manner.

Multiple-component interventions featuring multiple follow-up contacts by a team of health care providers have been found to be the most effective in changing health behaviors such as smoking (18). Because different people change in different ways, the provision of various opportunities and techniques for change should be considered for programs. However, because different people respond differently to the components, it is difficult to determine the most effective components of any intervention.

Behavioral Prescriptions

The prescriptions for diet, exercise, and psychosocial interventions varied across the studies. In all trials exercise prescription was based on the results of a treadmill test. The range of intensity prescribed was 50–85% of age-adjusted maximum heart rate, duration was 30 to 60 minutes/session for a total of 2 to 3 hours/week, and frequency was 2 to 5 days/week.

The range of prescriptions for the dietary component included low fat (<20% calories/day), low cholesterol (<5–200 mg/day), and high complex carbohydrates (65–75%). Protein intake, when specified, was 15–20% of calories/day. Alcohol and caffeine restrictions and dietary supplements were the exception rather than the rule (7, 9). Some studies specified the use of diet plans such as the one in the National Cholesterol Education Program (NCEP) or the American Heart Association (AHA) Phase 3 (8, 11) which was helpful for understanding the ratio-

Table 6.2. Exercise

TRIAL	COMPONENTS	SETTING	PRESCRIPTION	EVALUATION
WHO 10-year Follow-up, Hämäläinen et al., 1989 (7)	Individually tailored light exercise; exercise supervised in Turku, advised only in Helsinki	Clinic & at home	Intensity determined by cycle ergometer test Details not specified	Adherence, physical working capacity measured at 1, 2, 3, 6, 10 yr post MI
Schuler et al., 1992 (8)	Intensive group training and information in hospital, daily home exercise on cycle ergometer, group information sessions 5×/yr for patients and spouses, exercise log book	Initial 3 wk in hospital metabolic ward Clinic for group exercise Home based for daily exercise	60 min. 2×/wk (group) plus 30 min./day (individual) at 75% MHR	Exercise testing at baseline, 1 yr; attendance at group, daily adherence (log book) at baseline, 3 wk, 3, 6, 12 mo
Lifestyle Heart Trial, Ornish et al., 1990 (9)	Treadmill testing, moderate aerobic exercise, choice of exercise	Initial 1 wk residential retreat, then home based	50–80% HR, minimum 30 min./session, total 3 hr/wk for 1 yr	Questionnaire on type, frequency, duration at baseline, 1 yr
SCRIP, Haskell et al., 1994 (10)	Verbal, written goals; instructions to increase daily activity, exercise endurance; progress tracked by mail, phone	Clinic based Home based		7-day physical activity recall; progress tracked by phone, mail; progress reports by mail; clinic visits 2–3 mo
MULTIFIT, DeBusk et al., 1994 (11)	Treadmill testing, choice of aerobic exercise, portable HR monitor to regulate training intensity during first 8 wk, phone follow-up	Clinic for treadmill Home based exercise	60–85% PHR 30 min/day, 5 days/wk; after 4 wk, 100% PHR or 85% age-predicted MHR	Treadmill in hospital; 3–6 wk post MI; phone follow-up 2 wk, monthly; functional capacity at 6 mo

HR, heart rate; MHR, maximum heart rate; PHR, peak heart rate during treadmill; MI, myocardial infarction; SCRIP, Stanford Coronary Risk Intervention Project.
Some studies differentiate prescription by patient's heart condition (see references).

nale behind the intervention. The most stringent study prescribed a low-fat (<10% calories/day) vegetarian diet (no animal products except egg white and 1 cup per day of nonfat milk or yogurt) (9).

Complete abstinence was the prescription for the smoking interventions. Counseling ranged from educational information only to individualized stop-smoking and relapse prevention programs provided by psychologists and specially trained nurses. Interventions were clearly specified for only two studies (7, 11). The most detailed program described offered in-hospital bedside counseling for post-MI patients, multiple postdischarge telephone follow-up calls to augment the counseling session, take-home materials (videotape, workbook, audiotape), and suggested nicotine replacement therapy for severely addicted patients (11).

Psychosocial interventions involved either group or individual counseling and focused on adaptation to life after a cardiac event and on enhancing interpersonal relationships (8, 9, 11). Topics discussed in counseling included return to work, perceptions of physical ability, anxiety and depression, communication skills, home and work relationships, and strategies for maintaining adherence to risk factor changes. Only two studies specified the psychosocial prescription. In one of these studies, five

group therapy sessions were offered over the 1-year study (8). In the other study, patients attended group sessions for social support with a clinical psychologist twice a week (total of 4 hours/week) for a year (9). Stress management was treated as a separate entity in this study. The prescription involved an additional hour per day of stretching exercises, breathing techniques, meditation or prayer, progressive relaxation, and imagery (9). Many factors, such as motivation and comfort level regarding group therapy, must be considered when incorporating psychosocial interventions into a multifactorial risk reduction program because participants are not specifically seeking psychosocial interventions for their physical conditions. Dropout from psychotherapy may be a problem, especially if frequent attendance is required, and ways to enhance compliance should be considered when developing a psychosocial intervention (12).

Evaluation

Evaluation in this context refers to the behavioral components of the interventions only and does not apply to other end points, such as change in lipid profiles. The method of evaluation, primarily self-report for all behavioral interventions, included exercise logs, smoking status

Table 6.3. Diet

TRIAL	COMPONENTS	SETTING	PRESCRIPTION	EVALUATION
WHO 10-year Follow-up, Hämäläinen et al., 1989 (7)	Health education, nutrition classes, individual counseling	Clinic	Reduce total fat, saturated fat, salt, coffee, energy level if needed. Avoid dietary cholesterol, sugar, big meals, alcohol. Increase polyunsaturated fat, fiber, vitamins, minerals	Not specified
Schuler et al., 1992 (8)	In-hospital teaching, group information sessions 5×/yr for patients, spouses	Initial 3 wk on metabolic ward, then home based	AHA diet Phase 3, <20% fat, <200 mg cholesterol, 15% protein, 65% carbohydrates; polyunsaturated ratio to saturated fat <1	24-hr dietary protocol at baseline, 3 wk, 3, 6, 9, 12 mo
Lifestyle Heart Trial, Ornish et al., 1990 (9)	Low-fat vegetarian diet, cooking classes and meal preparation during retreat, prepared take-out meals available post retreat, weekly support sessions	Initial 1-wk residential retreat, then home based	10% fat, 15–20% protein, 70–75% complex carbohydrates, alcohol limited to 2 units/day, no caffeine; B_{12} supplement	3-day diet diary at baseline, 1 yr
SCRIP, Haskell et al., 1994 (10)	Individualized low-fat, low cholesterol diet; instruction, record review at clinic; verbal, written goals; progress tracked by mail, phone	Clinic and home based	<20% fat, <6% saturated fats, <75 mg cholesterol/day	4-day food records, progress tracked by phone, mail; progress reports by mail; clinic visits every 2–3 mo
MULTIFIT, DeBusk et al., 1994 (10)	Nutritional counseling, nutrition workbook, computer-generated progress reports based on FFQ, prioritized dietary goals, relapse prevention, strategies for dietary maintenance, progress tracked by phone, mail	Home based	NCEP Step 2 diet: low cholesterol, saturated fat	FFQ in hospital, 6, 11, 26 wk after admission; reports mailed to patient within 48–72 hr after FFQ received; questionnaire at 6, 12 mo

AHA, American Heart Association; NCEP, National Cholesterol Education Program; FFQ, food frequency questionnaire; SCRIP, Stanford Coronary Risk Intervention Project.

reports, food frequency questionnaires, and psychosocial questionnaires. The most inconsistent type of assessments was dietary questionnaires ranging from 24-hour recall to 6-month recall. Psychosocial evaluation was not common, and follow-up measurement was specified in only one study (8). The evaluation of compliance remains an important issue in health behavior change. Standardized measurement should be carefully considered not only for internal validity but also to permit comparisons of results across studies.

LIMITATIONS AND FUTURE DIRECTIONS OF MULTIFACTORIAL RISK REDUCTION

The last section of this chapter discusses the future of multifactorial risk reduction interventions in light of cost-effectiveness, generalizability, acceptance, compliance and maintenance, and dissemination.

Cost-Effectiveness

With the advent of managed care, the cost-effectiveness of multifactorial risk reduction has become an important consideration. However, none of these studies provide that data. The cost-effectiveness of individual risk factor reduction (e.g., smoking cessation) has been established and is especially impressive when compared to more invasive and costly medical procedures (19). Using a health care provider, such as a nurse, for managing patients can be a cost-effective method for preventing dropout and enhancing adherence (11, 14). Cost-effectiveness and resource allocation have become important concerns today at work sites and in health care systems and will gain increasing attention in the future (20).

Generalizability

Other questions remain regarding multifactorial risk reduction programs. For example, to whom do they apply? Most trials have focused on white middle-class men, and little is known about the efficacy of such trials with women and nonwhite ethnic groups.

Acceptance

The acceptance of multifactorial risk reduction programs in terms of both the program components and the convenience of participation in an intensive program is another issue. For example, one study prescribed a strict vegetarian diet, and another required multiple clinic visits and blood draws. What is the feasibility of residential programs, which take people away from family, friends, and work? Other questions relate to the use of group versus individual intervention. The group approach may be too general and time consuming and not specific enough to meet the needs of the individual. Certainly individual intervention tailoring was a strength of the Stanford Coronary Risk Intervention Project and MULTIFIT trials, yet the Lifestyle Heart Trial, which achieved equally favorable results, used a group format for the initial residential component of the program (9–11).

Compliance and Maintenance

Compliance and long-term adherence to program components are major concerns in multifactorial risk reduction programs. A major consideration of multifactorial programs is not simply that the participants adopt the desired behaviors but that they maintain them over time. It is therefore imperative that continued attention be focused on enhancing patients' compliance with multiple risk factor reduction.

Dissemination

The feasibility and practicality of multifactorial risk reduction for the general population is not yet determined. How transferable to the community multifactorial risk reduction programs are and whether comprehensive lifestyle changes can be sustained in the general population of people with and without CAD remain unknown. Although there has been great progress in understanding multifactorial risk reduction for CAD and the implementation of behavioral interventions required for preventing or reversing it, many questions regarding dissemination still remain.

▶ SUMMARY

Many lessons have been learned since the inception of multifactorial risk reduction in the 1970s, and researchers continue to refine their methods and interventions. The trials reviewed in this chapter provide some insight to the complexity of the behavioral components of multifactorial risk reduction. Even though the mechanisms are unknown, studies have demonstrated that comprehensive risk factor intervention can lead to significant reduction in risk factor profiles, can reverse coronary atherosclerosis, and may affect long-term, all-cause morbidity and mortality along with coronary morbidity and mortality. Researchers should continue to improve upon design, methods, and implementation and to expand dissemination from the research model to clinical practice and community settings. At the same time, practitioners have adequate models to integrate multifactorial lifestyle programs with existing exercise programs.

References

1. Zukel WJ, Paul O, Schnaper HW. The multiple risk factor intervention trial (MRFIT): I. Historical perspectives. Prev Med 10:387–401, 1981.
2. Bandura A. Social Foundations of Thought and Action: A Social Cognitive Theory. Englewood Cliffs, NJ: Prentice-Hall, 1986.
3. Benfari RC, Sherwin R. Forum: The multiple risk factor intervention trial (MRFIT): The methods and impact of intervention over four years. Prev Med 10:387–553, 1981.
4. Multiple Risk Factor Intervention Trial Research Group. Mortality rates after 10.5 years for participants in the Multiple Risk Factor Intervention Trial. JAMA 263:1795–1801, 1990.
5. Gotto AM. The Multiple Risk Factor Intervention Trial (MRFIT): A return to a landmark trial. JAMA 277:595–597, 1997.
6. Miettinen TA, Strandberg TE. Implications of recent results of long-term multifactorial primary prevention of cardiovascular diseases. Ann Intern Med 24:85–89, 1992.
7. Hämäläinen H, Luurila OJ, Kallio V, et al. Long-term reduction in sudden deaths after a multifactorial intervention programme in patients with myocardial infarction: 10-year results of a controlled investigation. Eur Heart J 10:55–62, 1989.
8. Schuler G, Hambrecht R, Schlierf G, et al. Regular physical exercise and low-fat diet: Effects on progression of coronary artery disease. Circulation 86:1–11, 1992.
9. Ornish D, Brown SE, Scherwitz LW, et al. Can lifestyle changes reverse coronary heart disease? Lancet 336:129–133, 1990.
10. Haskell WL, Alderman EL, Fair JM, et al. Effects of intensive multiple risk factor reduction on coronary atherosclerosis and clinical cardiac events in men and women with coronary artery disease. Circulation 89:975–990, 1994.
11. DeBusk RF, Houston-Miller N, Superko HR, et al. A case-management system for coronary risk factor modification after acute myocardial infarction. Ann Intern Med 120:721–729, 1994.
12. Meichenbaum D, Turk DC. Facilitating Treatment Adherence: A Practitioner's Guidebook. New York: Plenum, 1987.
13. Kallio V, Hämäläinen H, Hakkila J, Luurila OJ. Reduction in sudden deaths by a multifactorial intervention programme after acute myocardial infarction. Lancet 2:1091–1094, 1979.
14. Hill MN, Houston Miller N. Compliance enhancement: A call for multidisciplinary team approaches. Circulation 93:4–6, 1996.
15. Brawley LR. The practicality of using social psychological theories for exercise and health research and intervention. J Appl Sport Psychol 5:99–115, 1993.

16. Elder JP, Ayala GX, Harris S. Theories and intervention approaches to health-behavior change in primary care. Am J Prev Med 17:275–284, 1999.

17. Adler EW. Print That Works: The First Step-by-Step Guide That Integrates Writing, Design, and Marketing. Palo Alto, CA: Bull, 1991.

18. Kottke TE, Battista RN, DeFriese GH, Brekke ML. Attributes of successful smoking cessation interventions in medical practice: A meta-analysis of 39 controlled trials. JAMA 259:2882–2889, 1988.

19. Goldman L, Garber AM, Grover SA, Hlatky MA. Task force 6. Cost-effectiveness of assessment and management of risk factors. J Am Coll Cardiol 27:1020–1030, 1996.

20. Jönsson B. Cost-effectiveness: A new criterion for selecting therapy. J Intern Med 237:1–3, 1995.

Suggested Reading

Miller NH, Taylor CB. Lifestyle Management in Patients with Coronary Heart Disease. Champaign, IL: Human Kinetics Publishers, 1995.

Ornish D. Dr. Dean Ornish's Program for Reversing Heart Disease. New York: Ballantine Books, 1990.

Cardiovascular Disease. (No authors listed.) In Health Behavior Change in Managed Care. Center for Advancement of Health, Washington, DC, 2000. (can be obtained through www.cfah.org.)

SECTION TWO
ANATOMY

SECTION EDITOR: Mark A. Williams, PhD, FACSM

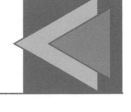

CHAPTER **7**

CARDIOVASCULAR ANATOMY

Tinker D. Murray and Julie M. Pulcipher

The cardiovascular system is a continuous closed arrangement including a pump (the heart) and more than 60,000 miles of conduits (blood vessels) (1). The primary function of the cardiovascular system is to provide an environment for the transport of nutrients and removal of waste products. The cardiovascular system assists with maintenance of homeostasis at rest and during exercise.

The cardiovascular system performs the following specific functions (2–4):

1. Transports oxygenated blood from the lungs to tissues and deoxygenated blood from the tissues to the lungs
2. Distributes nutrients (e.g., glucose, free fatty acids, amino acids) to cells
3. Removes metabolic wastes (e.g., carbon dioxide, urea, lactate) from the periphery for elimination or reuse
4. Regulates pH to control acidosis and alkalosis
5. Transports hormones and enzymes to regulate physiological function
6. Maintains fluid volume to prevent dehydration
7. Maintains body temperature by absorbing and redistributing heat

The following sections provide an overview of the basic structures and functions of the heart and blood vessels.

THE HEART

The adult heart is approximately the size of a fist and weighs between 250 and 350 g (5). The heart is positioned obliquely within the thoracic cavity in a space known as the mediastinum (Fig. 7.1). It is anterior to the vertebral column and posterior to the sternum. The lungs flank the heart bilaterally and slightly overlap it.

The heart has four chambers. The two superior chambers are the atria and the two inferior chambers are the ventricles. The external deep grooves of the heart (called sulci) define the boundaries of the four chambers of the heart (4, 6). The coronary sulcus separates the atria from the ventricles; the interventricular sulcus separates the left and right ventricles (LV, RV). The sulci also contain the major arteries and veins that provide circulation to the heart.

The heart has a base and an apex. The base consists mainly of the left atrium (LA), part of the right atrium (RA), and parts of the proximal portion of the large veins that enter the heart posteriorly. It is located superiorly and near the right sternal border at the level of second and third ribs. The apex of the heart is located inferiorly and to the left of the base at the level of the fifth intercostal space. Approximately two-thirds of the mass of the heart is to the left of the midsternal border. As the heart is palpated at the apex (between the fifth and sixth ribs), the contraction can be easily felt. This is referred to as the point of maximal intensity (PMI) (3).

The heart also has borders. The superior border consists of both atria and the bases of the pulmonary trunk and the aorta. The right border is formed by the RA. The left border consists of the LV and a small part of the LA. The inferior border is formed primarily by the RV and a portion of the LV at the apex.

The heart is rotated to the left in the chest so that the anterior portion of the heart forms the sternocostal surface, which consists mainly of the RA and RV. The diaphragmatic surface consists mainly of the LV where it slopes and rests on the diaphragm.

Tissue Coverings and Layers of the Heart

The heart is covered by a double-walled, loose-fitting membranous sac called the pericardium (Fig. 7.2). The outer wall of the pericardium, the parietal pericardium, has both a fibrous (tough) layer and a serous (smooth) layer. The interior wall is the visceral pericardium, or epicardium. Between the parietal and visceral layers is the pericardial cavity. The pericardial cavity contains pericardial fluid, which acts as a lubricant, reducing friction between the membranes during contractions. If the pericardium becomes inflamed, pericarditis, a condition characterized by painful adhesions, can result.

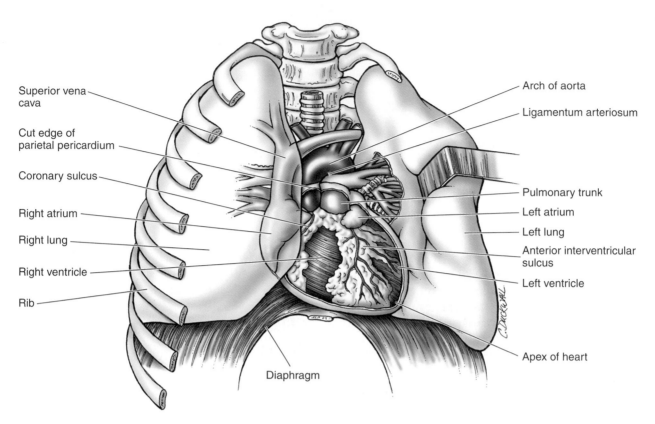

Figure 7.1. Anterior view of the thorax showing the position of the heart in the mediastinum. (Reprinted with permission from Spence AP, Mason EB, eds. Human Anatomy and Physiology. 4th ed. St Paul, MN: West, 1992;595.)

The thickest layer of tissue in the heart is the myocardium. The myocardium is cardiac muscle. Within the myocardium is a network of crisscrossing connective tissue fibers called the fibrous skeleton. This skeleton provides support for the myocardium and the valves of the heart and provides some separation between the atria and the ventricles.

The inner layer of the myocardium is lined with a thin layer of endothelium called the endocardium. The endocardium forms the innermost lining of the walls of the various heart chambers as well as the heart valves. The endocardium joins with the endothelial linings of the blood vessels as they leave and enter the heart (7).

Chambers, Valves, and Blood Flow of the Heart

The heart is two pumps in a single unit with four chambers, or cavities (Fig. 7.3). The right heart (RA and RV) and the left heart (LA and LV) make up the two pumps. The right side of the heart collects blood from the periphery and pumps it through the lungs (pulmonary circuit). The left side of the heart collects blood from the lungs and pumps it throughout the body (systemic circuit) (8–12).

The atria of the heart are separated by the interatrial septum and the ventricles, by the interventricular septum. The LV walls and interventricular septum are two to three times thicker than the RV walls. The atria are smaller and have thinner walls than the ventricles. The thicker myocardium of the ventricles allows the ventricles to pump blood against greater resistance to meet the demand of pumping blood through the systemic circuit. Conversely, the RV has only to pump blood a relatively short distance through the pulmonary circuit.

The heart has four valves whose function is to maintain unidirectional blood flow. The atrioventricular (AV) valves separate the atria from the ventricles. The semilunar valves separate the ventricles from the aorta and pulmonary artery trunk. The AV valves are named for the number of leaflets, or cusps, formed by the endocardium (Fig. 7.4). The right AV valve has three cusps and is called the tricuspid valve, while the left AV valve has only two cusps and is called the bicuspid (or mitral) valve. The tricuspid valve controls the flow of blood from the RA to the RV, while the mitral valve controls blood between the LA and LV. The AV valves are attached to chordae tendineae (strong fibrous bands) and papillary muscles, which arise from folds and ridges of the myocardium within the ventricles. The chordae tendineae and papillary muscles help open the AV valves and prevent them from swinging back into the atria, which would result in retrograde blood flow (13).

7. The LV free wall contracts, the mitral valve closes, and blood flows through the aortic valve into the aorta and its branches, where it is distributed to the coronary circulation and the systemic circulation (13–16).

The Myocardial Blood Supply

Although the interiors of the heart chambers are continuously bathed with blood, only the endocardium is nourished directly, because the myocardium is too thick to permit diffusion to the epicardium. The heart provides the functional supply of blood for the heart via the left and right coronary arteries (LCA, RCA) (Figs. 7.5 and 7.6). The coronary arteries arise from the sinus of Valsalva, at the base of the aorta just above the semilunar valve cusps of the aortic valve (Fig. 7.7).

The LCA angles towards the left side of the heart for about 1 to 2 cm before branching into the left anterior descending (LAD) coronary artery and the circumflex artery (CxA) (17). The LAD artery supplies blood to the interventricular septum and anterior walls of both ventricles. The CxA branches toward the left margin of the heart in the coronary sulcus and supplies blood to the laterodorsal walls of the LA and LV. Both the LAD artery and CxA curve around the left ventricular wall and supply small branches that interconnect (anastomose) with the RCA.

The RCA supplies blood to the right side of the heart as it follows the atrioventricular groove before curving to the back of the heart giving off a posterior interventricular artery (posterior descending artery, or PDA). The RCA and PDA have numerous branches that supply blood to the anterior, posterior, and lateral surfaces of the RV and to the RA.

After blood circuits the coronary artery system, which ends with myocardial capillaries, it is collected by the cardiac veins and travels a path similar to that of the coronary arteries but in the opposite direction. On the posterior aspect of the heart the cardiac veins form an enlarged vessel, the coronary sinus, which empties the blood into the RA. Some smaller anterior cardiac veins also empty directly into the RA.

Cardiac muscle has intrinsic properties that allow it to depolarize and contract without neural stimulation. Cardiac cells interconnect end to end and form intercalated discs (2). These intercalated discs allow electrical impulses to spread from cell to cell and cause the myocardium to act as a single unit or functional syncytium. The components of the heart's conduction system include the sinoatrial (SA) node, the AV node, AV bundle (bundle of His), right and left bundle branches, and the Purkinje fibers (Fig. 7.8).

The electrical impulse, which initiates cardiac contraction, begins at the SA node, or intrinsic pacemaker, of the heart. The cells of the SA node, which lie in the posterior wall of the RA, depolarize spontaneously about 60 to 80

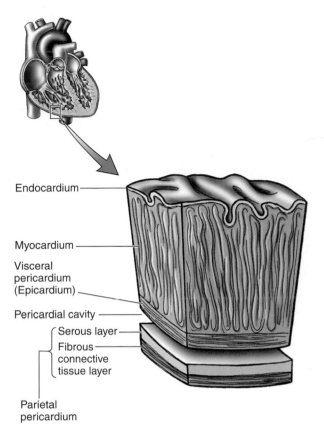

Figure 7.2. The endocardium, myocardium, and pericardium. (Reprinted with permission from Spence AP, Mason EB, eds. Human Anatomy and Physiology. 4th ed. St Paul, MN: West, 1992;596.)

There are two semilunar valves in the heart, each with three cusps. The pulmonic valve lies between the RV and the pulmonary artery. The aortic valve is between the LV and the aorta. The cusps of the semilunar valves prevent the backflow of blood from the arteries to the ventricles.

Blood flow through the heart is accomplished by the following sequence of events, beginning with the return of systemic blood to the RA:

1. Deoxygenated blood flows into the RA via the superior and inferior vena cava, the coronary sinus, and anterior cardiac veins.
2. The RA free wall contracts and blood moves through the tricuspid valve into the RV.
3. The RV free wall contracts, the tricuspid valve closes, and blood flows through the pulmonic valve into the pulmonary arteries and the branches of that system.
4. Blood enters the alveolar capillaries from the pulmonary arteries, where gas exchange occurs.
5. Blood flows back to the LA via the pulmonary veins.
6. The LA free wall contracts and blood flows through the mitral valve and into the LV.

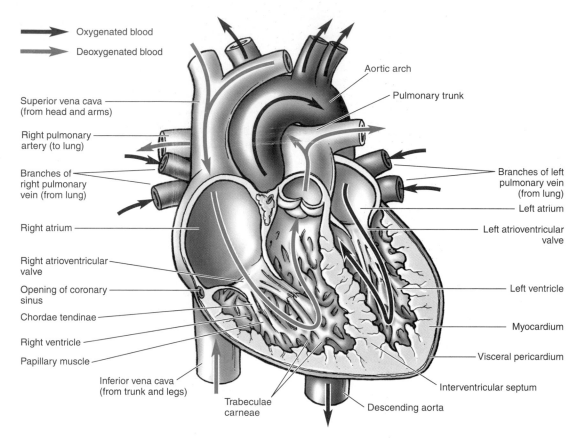

Figure 7.3. Frontal section of the heart. The arrows indicate the path of blood flow through the heart. (Reprinted with permission from Spence AP, Mason EB, eds. Human Anatomy and Physiology. 4th ed. St Paul, MN: West, 1992;600.)

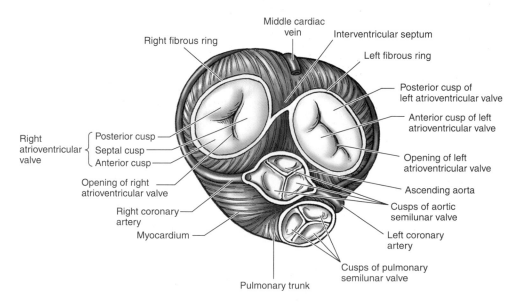

Figure 7.4. Superior view of the heart showing valve openings. (Reprinted with permission from Spence AP, Mason EB, eds. Human Anatomy and Physiology. 4th ed. St Paul, MN: West, 1992;601.)

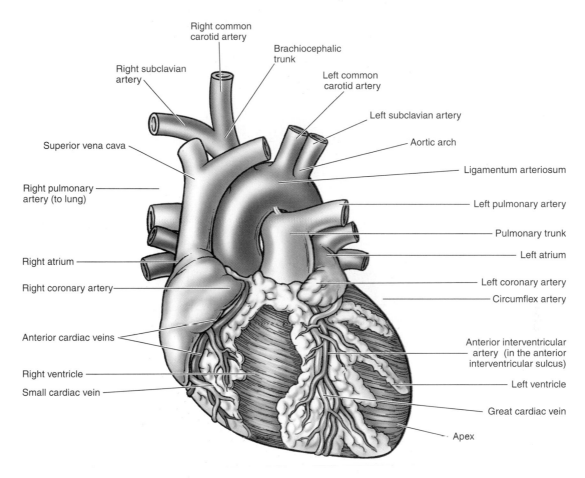

Figure 7.5. Anterior view of the heart. (Reprinted with permission from Spence AP, Mason EB, eds. Human Anatomy and Physiology. 4th ed. St Paul, MN: West, 1992;598.)

times per minute (18). From the SA node, the electrical impulse spreads via internodal gaps through both atria until it reaches the AV node, in the inferior part of the interatrial septum. The electrical impulse is delayed at the AV node for approximately 0.13 seconds to allow the atria to contract and fill the ventricles (18). The impulse then moves rapidly through the bundle of His, through the right and left bundle branches, and through the network of Purkinje fibers in the myocardium of both ventricles. This rapid conduction allows the two ventricles to contract at approximately the same time.

The rate and forcefulness of heart contraction do not depend on intrinsic nerve stimulation but rather are influenced by extrinsic factors, such as autonomic nerve control and hormone activity. Sympathetic nerves stimulate the atria and ventricles of the heart to beat faster (chronotropic effect) and more forcefully (inotropic effect). Parasympathetic nerves (vagi) control the atria and slow the heart rate. Hormones such as norepinephrine and epinephrine stimulate increases in heart rate and force of contraction.

THE BLOOD VESSELS

After blood flows from the heart, it enters the vascular system, which is composed of numerous blood vessels. The blood vessels form a closed system to deliver blood to the tissues; help promote the exchange of nutrients, metabolic wastes, hormones, and other substances with cells; and return blood to the heart.

Arteries carry blood away from the heart (Fig. 7.9). Large arteries branch into smaller arteries and eventually to smaller arterioles. Arterioles branch into capillaries, which allow the exchange of blood with various tissues (e.g., digestive system, liver, kidneys). On the venous side of the circulation, capillaries converge into small venules, which converge to form larger vessels called veins. The largest veins return blood to the heart.

The walls of blood vessel vary in thickness and size because of the presence or absence of one or more layers of tissues (Fig. 7.10). The tunica intima consists of the endothelium and a thin connective-tissue basement membrane. The tunica intima is the only layer common to all of the blood vessels. The internal elastic lamina separates

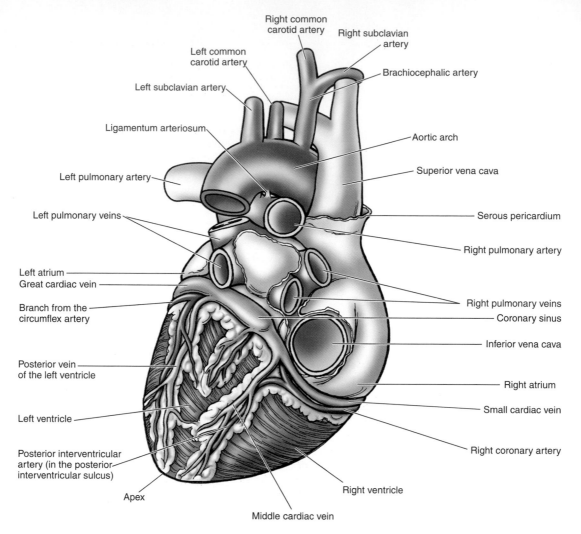

Figure 7.6. Posterior view of the heart. (Reprinted with permission from Spence AP, Mason EB, eds. Human Anatomy and Physiology. 4th ed. St Paul, MN: West, 1992;599.)

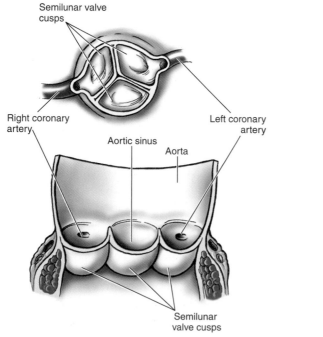

Figure 7.7. The origin of the coronary arteries. (Reprinted with permission from Spence AP, Mason EB, eds. Human Anatomy and Physiology. 4th ed. St Paul, MN: West, 1992;601.)

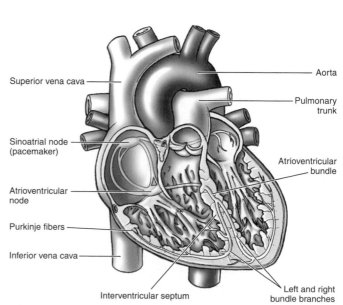

Figure 7.8. The electrical conduction system of the heart. (Reprinted with permission from Spence AP, Mason EB, eds. Human Anatomy and Physiology. 4th ed. St Paul, MN: West, 1992;608.)

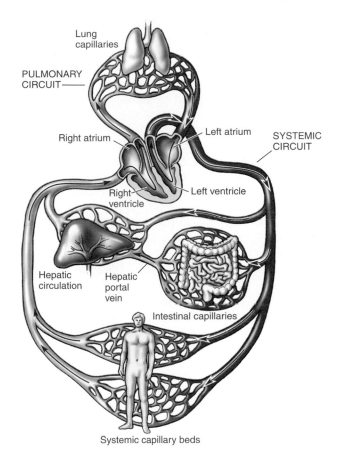

Figure 7.9. Schematic diagram of blood circulation. (Reprinted with permission from Spence AP, Mason EB, eds. Human Anatomy and Physiology. 4th ed. St Paul, MN: West, 1992;604.)

the tunica intima from the middle layer of smooth muscle fibers and elastic fibers, the tunica media. The smooth muscle fibers of the tunica media can be influenced by neural control (parasympathetic and sympathetic nerves), hormones (e.g., acetylcholine, norepinephrine, epinephrine), or local factors (e.g., pH, oxygen levels, carbon dioxide levels), which can cause them to vasoconstrict or vasodilate. The external elastic lamina separates the tunica media from the outermost layer of connective tissue, the tunica adventitia. The adventitia helps attach vessels to surrounding tissues (4).

Arteries can be classified as elastic or muscular or as arterioles according to their size and function. Large arteries like the aorta and those of the pulmonary trunk are called elastic arteries. The tunica media of these vessels is thick and contains many elastic fibers. The elastic nature of these arteries helps maintain pressure within the vessels. Other smaller arteries distribute blood throughout the body. These arteries are called muscular arteries, and their tunica media contains primarily smooth muscle fibers. Muscular arteries are less distensible than elastic arteries. Arterioles have lumens smaller than 0.5 mm, and their tunica media is largely composed of smooth muscle with scattered elastic fibers (4). Arterioles play a major role in regulating blood flow to the capillaries because of their ability to vasoconstrict or vasodilate.

Capillaries form dense networks that branch throughout all tissues. The average capillary is 1 mm in length and 0.01 mm in diameter. This is just large enough for a single red blood cell to pass through (3). Capillaries have extremely thin walls and are the site where the exchange of materials between blood and the interstitial fluid takes place.

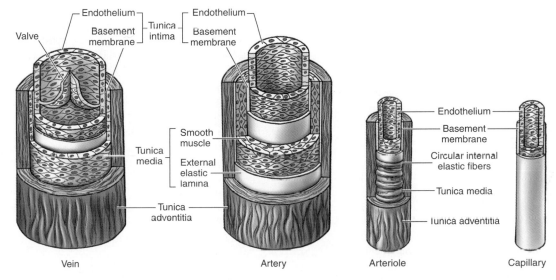

Figure 7.10. Comparison of the structure of blood vessels. (Reprinted with permission from Spence AP, Mason EB, eds. Human Anatomy and Physiology. 4th ed. St Paul, MN: West, 1992;629.)

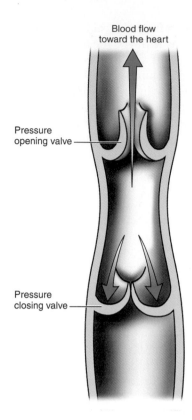

Blood flow
toward the heart

Pressure
opening valve

Pressure
closing valve

Figure 7.11. Valves of a vein. (Reprinted with permission from Spence AP, Mason EB, eds. Human Anatomy and Physiology. 4th ed. St Paul, MN: West, 1992;632.)

Venules, which form from capillaries, consist mainly of tunica intima and tunica adventitia. Veins receive blood from the venules and have the same three tissue layers as arteries. However, the tunica media of the veins is thinner than that found in the arteries. In general, the veins are thinner and more compliant than arteries and act as blood reservoirs. The walls of some veins, such as those in the legs, contain one-way valves that help maintain venous return to the heart by preventing retrograde blood flow even under relatively low pressures (Fig. 7.11). The valves in the veins are made up of folds of tunica intima (endothelium) and are similar in nature to the semilunar valves of the heart.

► SUMMARY

In summary, the cardiovascular system is a closed system of pumps, valves, and conduits that is coordinated to function both anatomically and physiologically to maintain homeostasis. In times of increased cardiovascular work, the system functions in an even more sophisticated manner to meet those demands while it continues to attempt to maintain a homeostatic environment.

References

1. McArdle WD, Katch FI, Katch VL. Essentials of Exercise Physiology. 2nd ed. Baltimore: Lippincott Williams & Wilkins, 1999.
2. Martini F. Fundamentals of Anatomy and Physiology. 3rd ed. Englewood Cliffs, NJ: Prentice-Hall, 1995.
3. Marieb EN. Human Anatomy and Physiology. 3rd ed. Redwood City, CA: Benjamin/Cummings, 1998.
4. Spence AP, Mason EB. Human Anatomy and Physiology. 4th ed. St Paul, MN: West, 1992.
5. Anthony CP, Thibodeau GA. Textbook of Anatomy and Physiology. 11th ed. St Louis: Mosby, 1983.
6. Williams PL, Warwick R, Dyson M, Bannister LH, eds. Gray's Anatomy. 38th ed. London: Churchill Livingstone, 1995.
7. Hole JW. Essentials of Human Anatomy and Physiology. 2nd ed. Dubuque, IA: WC Brown, 1986.
8. Brooks GA, Fahey TD, White TP, Baldwin K. Human Bioenergetics and Its Applications. 3rd ed. Mountain View, CA: Mayfield, 1999.
9. deVries HA, Housh T. Physiology of Exercise for Physical Education, Athletics, and Exercise Science. 5th ed. Madison, WI: WCB Brown and Benchmark, 1994.
10. Fox EL, Bowers RW, Foss ML. The Physiological Basis of Physical Education and Athletics. 5th ed. Madison, WI: WCB Brown and Benchmark, 1993.
11. McArdle WD, Katch FI, Katch VL. Exercise Physiology, Energy, Nutrition, and Human Performance. 4th ed. Baltimore: Williams & Wilkins, 1996.
12. Powers SK, Howley ET. Exercise Physiology: Theory and Application to Fitness and Performance. 3rd ed. Madison, WI: Brown & Benchmark, 1997.
13. Hall-Craggs ECB. Anatomy as a Basis for Clinical Medicine. Baltimore: Williams & Wilkins, 1995.
14. Williams MA. Cardiovascular and respiratory anatomy and physiology: Responses to exercise. In: Baechle TR, ed. Essentials of Strength Training and Conditioning, 2nd ed. Champaign, IL: Human Kinetics, 2000.
15. Montgomery RL. Basic Anatomy for the Health Professions. Baltimore: Urban & Schwarzenberg, 1980.
16. Thibodeau GA, Patton KT, Anthony. CP Anatomy and Physiology. 4th ed. St. Louis: Mosby, 2000.
17. Sokolow M, McIlroy MB. Clinical Cardiology. 2nd ed. Los Altos, CA: Lange Medical, 1979.
18. Wilmore JH, Costill DL. Physiology of Sport and Exercise. 2nd ed. Champaign, IL: Human Kinetics, 1999.

Suggested Reading

Kapit W, Elson LM. The Anatomy Coloring Book. 2nd ed. New York: Pearson Education, 1997.
Moore KL, Agur, AM, Agur, A. Essential Clinical Anatomy. Baltimore: Williams & Wilkins, 1995.
Snell RS. Clinical Anatomy for Medical Students. 5th ed. Baltimore: Lippincott Williams & Wilkins, 1995.

Suggested Web Sites
American College of Cardiology: www.acc.org
American College of Sports Medicine: www.acsm.org
American Heart Association: www.ahmrt.org
Lippincott Williams & Wilkins: www.lww.com

Suggested Key Words for Search Engine Searches
Anatomy and physiology
Cardiovascular anatomy
Coronary anatomy
Human anatomy and physiology

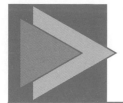

CHAPTER **8**

RESPIRATORY ANATOMY

Donald A. Mahler

This chapter describes the basic anatomy of the respiratory system as it relates to function. Clearly, the anatomy of the respiratory system supports the basic function of exchanging carbon dioxide (CO_2), a byproduct of cellular metabolism, and oxygen (O_2), which is necessary for cellular activity (1). Other important functions include production and metabolism of vasoactive substances and filtering systemic venous blood prior to entry into the left ventricle. The structural components of the respiratory system (Fig. 8.1) are the framework for the corresponding functions of the system (Table 8.1) (2, 3).

CONTROL OF BREATHING

Because respiratory muscles have no intrinsic automaticity, the control of breathing in an awake person results from the interplay of brainstem and cortical respiratory pathways (4). Automatic control structures are located in the brainstem, and voluntary control structures are located in the cerebral cortex.

Automatic Control

The major regions of automatic control are the medullary center and groups of rostral pontine respiratory nuclei. The respiratory neurons in the medulla aggregate into the dorsal respiratory groups (DRG) and ventral respiratory groups (VRG). The DRG contains various types of neurons that initiate inspiration, and the phrenic nerve, which innervates the diaphragm, originates from the DRG. The VRG has various functions, including forced expiration. The pontine respiratory nuclei fine-tune breathing.

Cortical Modulation

Voluntary pathways in the cerebral cortex originate in cortical neurons with efferent projections via spinal pathways to respiratory muscles. Voluntary respiratory activities, such as breath holding, hyperventilation, coughing, singing, and speaking, can override the automatic brainstem respiratory centers. Integration between voluntary (cortical) and automatic (brainstem) respiration occurs by interconnections in the spinal cord (spinal pathways). During sleep and loss of consciousness, automatic control and feedback become dominant for respiration.

Chemoreceptors

The central chemoreceptors in the medulla are activated by changes in arterial CO_2 tension ($PaCO_2$) and pH. These receptors are normally responsible for most of the input to the DRG. At low to moderate altitude, CO_2 is the major stimulus that determines ventilation in healthy individuals. The peripheral chemoreceptors, located at the bifurcation of the carotid arteries, are activated by low arterial oxygen tension (PaO_2) and by increased $PaCO_2$. The peripheral chemoreceptors are important in increasing ventilation when PaO_2 decreases (i.e., at high altitudes).

Mechanoreceptors

Various sensory receptors in the tracheobronchial tree transmit information via the vagal nerve to the DRG and higher respiratory centers. Pulmonary stretch receptors that are slow to adapt are located among smooth muscle cells in both intrathoracic and extrathoracic airways. Their predominant stimulus is lung inflation. Rapidly adapting pulmonary stretch receptors lie among airway epithelial cells, primarily near the region of the carina and in the large bronchi. The major stimuli for rapidly adapting receptors are the rate of lung inflation and various types of endogenous and exogenous agents, including cigarette smoke, relatively benign chemicals, and noxious chemicals. Accordingly, these receptors are also known as irritant receptors. C-fiber endings in the pulmonary interstitial space respond to large hyperinflation and various endogenous agents that may be produced with pulmonary congestion or inflammation. In addition, the chest wall (including diaphragm, intercostal muscles, and ribs) contains muscle spindle receptors that detect muscle stretch and Golgi tendon organs that respond to muscle tension.

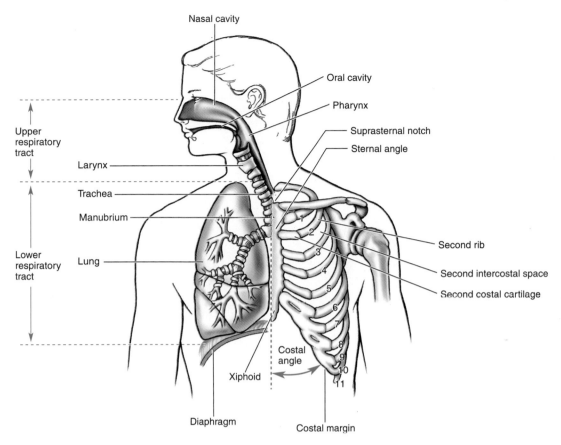

Figure 8.1. The respiratory system consists of an upper respiratory tract (nose, pharynx, and larynx) and a lower respiratory tract (tracheobronchial tree and lungs).

Table 8.1. Structural Components of the Respiratory Tract and Their Corresponding Function

STRUCTURAL COMPONENTS	FUNCTION
Respiratory center	
Peripheral chemoreceptors	Control of breathing
Afferent and efferent nerves	
Upper respiratory tract	
Conducting airways	Distribution of ventilation
Respiratory bronchioles	
Chest wall, respiratory muscles, and pleura	Ventilatory pump
Pulmonary arteries, capillaries, and veins	Distribution of blood flow
Functional respiratory unit	Gas exchange
Mucociliary escalator	Bronchial clearance
Alveolar macrophages	
Lymphatic drainage	Lung clearance and defense

DISTRIBUTION OF VENTILATION

Ventilation of the pulmonary system is accomplished in two major divisions, the upper and lower respiratory tracts.

Upper Respiratory Tract

The upper respiratory tract, which includes the nose, paranasal sinuses, pharynx, and larynx (Fig. 8.2), acts as a conduction pathway for the movement of air into the lower respiratory tract. The function of these structures is to purify, warm, and humidify ambient air before it reaches the gas exchange units. During normal quiet breathing, inspired air is heated to body temperature and the relative humidity is increased to more than 90% during passage through the nose. The pharynx is divided by the soft palate into the nasopharynx and the oropharynx. The epiglottis, located at the base of the tongue, protects the laryngeal opening during swallowing. The larynx contains the vocal cords, which contribute to speech and participate in coughing.

Receptors throughout the upper respiratory tract may initiate a cough response. Coughing is produced by closure of the vocal cords along with contraction of the expiratory muscles to create increased intrathoracic pressures. With sudden opening of the vocal cords, the positive airway pressure forces into the atmosphere air carrying any mucus or particles from the tracheobronchial tree. A cough can move gas from the lung at 10 L/second during the expulsion phase.

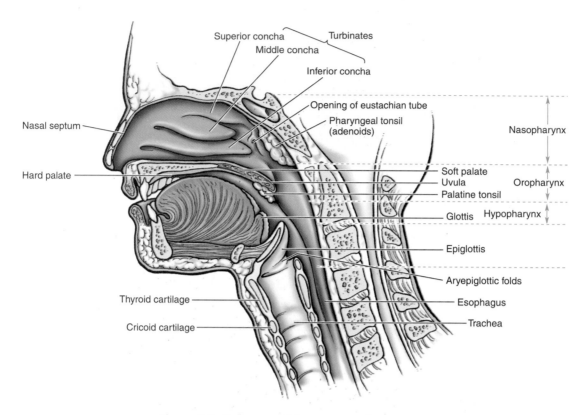

Figure 8.2. Structures of the upper respiratory tract.

Lower Respiratory Tract

The lower respiratory tract begins in the trachea just below the larynx and includes the bronchi, bronchioles, and alveoli (Fig. 8.3). There are approximately 23 generations of airways; the first 16 are conducting airways and the last 7 are respiratory airways ending blindly in approximately 300 million alveoli, which form the gas exchange surface. The structural components of the airways coincide with their functional properties. For example, the volume of the conducting zone is approximately 1 mL of air per pound of body weight and does not contribute to gas exchange, whereas the areas where gas exchange occurs occupy a proportionately greater volume in the lungs.

The trachea begins at the base of the neck and extends approximately 10 to 12 cm to the main carina, where it divides into the right and left main bronchi. It is anterior to the esophagus. The trachea consists of a series of anterior horseshoe-shaped cartilaginous rings and a posterior longitudinal muscle bundle.

The major bronchi contain cartilage that maintains airway patency as well as large numbers of mucus glands that produce secretions in response to irritation, infection, and/or inflammation. In the large airway, irritant receptors, which probably have C-fiber endings, initiate the cough reflex. The right main bronchus divides into three lobar bronchi, upper, middle, and lower. The left main bronchus divides into two lobar bronchi, upper and lower (Fig. 8.4). Fissures separate the two lobes with two

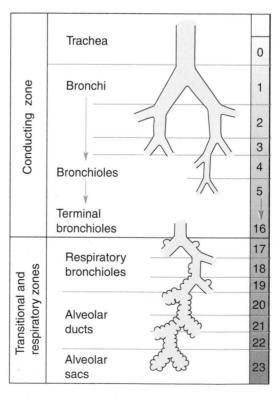

Figure 8.3. Branching of the airways starting from the trachea to the alveolar sacs. There are approximately 23 generations of branching in the tracheobronchial tree.

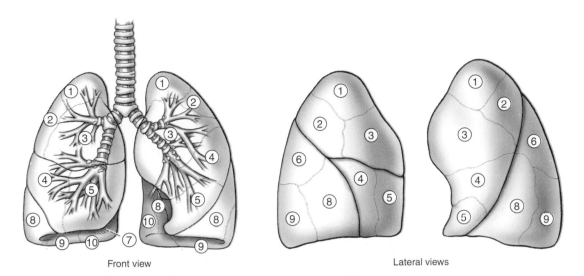

Figure 8.4. Structure of the tracheobronchial tree with corresponding lung segments, which originate from segmental bronchi. The right upper lobe contains segments 1–3, the right middle lobe contains segments 4 and 5, and the right lower lobe contains segments 6–10. The left upper lobe contains segments 1–5, and the left lower lobe contains segments 6–10.

layers of visceral pleura. The lobar bronchi divide into segmental bronchi and segments, 10 on the right and 10 on the left. Columnar cells lining the epithelium (inner lining) of the bronchi consist predominantly of ciliated cells that contain motile cilia, which move or beat in a coordinated manner to move the mucus layer toward the mouth ("mucociliary escalator") (Fig. 8.5). The columnar epithelium is an important barrier for lung defense. Goblet cells interspersed among the ciliated cells secrete mucus.

Segmental bronchi bifurcate further into the terminal bronchioles, which have a diameter of about 1 mm. Beyond the terminal bronchioles are respiratory bronchioles, alveolar ducts, and the alveoli (Fig. 8.3). Air flows through the conducting airways, and at the level of the alveolar ducts and alveoli, movement of air or gas is by diffusion. Transition of the epithelium to squamous cells in alveoli is important to facilitate gas exchange.

VENTILATORY PUMP

The ventilatory pump consists of the chest wall, the respiratory muscles, and the pleural space (Figs. 8.6 and 8.7).

Chest Wall

The chest wall includes muscles of respiration (primarily intercostal muscles) and bones (the spine, ribs, and sternum). The ribs are hinged on the spine by ligaments and cartilage so that the ribs move upward and outward during inspiration and downward and inward during expiration. The hinging movement results in a change in thoracic volume. At rest and at the end of a normal expi-

ration the elastic properties of the chest wall exert an outward (expansion) force, whereas the elastic properties of the lung parenchyma exert an inward (recoil) force. Inspiration (air flow into the lungs) occurs by activation of

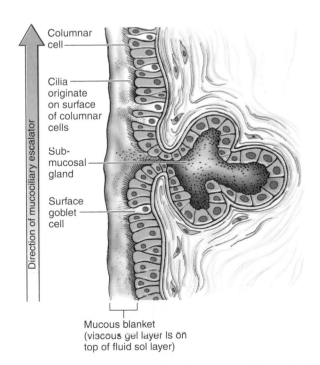

Figure 8.5. Epithelial surface of the bronchial wall contain cilia (fine hair structures that beat in a coordinated manner), columnar cells, goblet cells (which secrete mucus), and mucus (which consists of a viscous gel layer and a fluid sol layer).

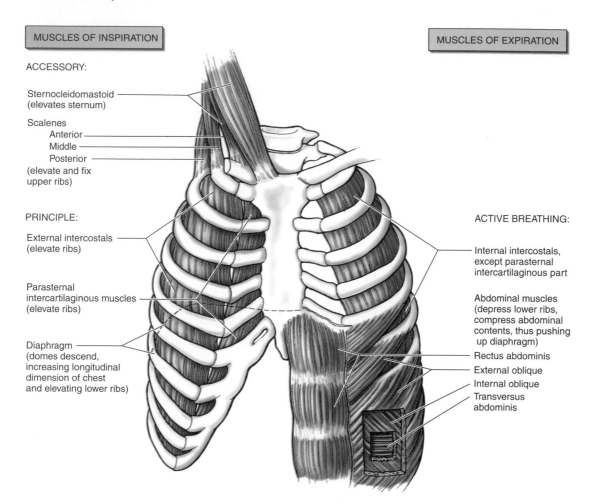

Figure 8.6. The major muscles of respiration. The principal inspiratory muscles, shown on the left, include the diaphragm, external intercostals, and parasternal muscles. The principal expiratory muscles, shown on the right, include the internal intercostals and the abdominal muscles (rectus, transversus, and internal and external obliques).

the respiratory muscles, particularly the diaphragm, which creates a more negative pressure in the pleural space and the lungs. Air enters the lung until the intrapulmonary gas pressure equals atmospheric pressure. During expiration, when the respiratory muscles relax, air flows from the lung into the atmosphere because of the positive pressure generated by the elastic recoil of the lungs.

Respiratory Muscles

The muscles of respiration are the only skeletal muscles essential to life. The muscles of inspiration and expiration are illustrated in Figure 8.6. The diaphragm, the major muscle of inspiration, is innervated by the phrenic nerve, which originates from the third to fifth cervical spinal segments. Spinal cord transection due to injury at or above this level compromises respiratory muscle function and consequently ventilation.

The diaphragm consists of a flat crural portion and vertical muscles called the costal portion. The diaphragm

functions as a piston, with contraction and relaxation of the vertical muscle fibers. With contraction, the crural portion, or dome, moves downward and displaces the abdominal contents so that the abdomen moves outward, as does the chest wall. Expiration is normally passive under quiet breathing because of elastic recoil of the lung; it requires no work. However, during active breathing, when ventilatory requirements are increased (e.g., during exercise) the muscles of expiration are recruited. The major muscles of expiration are the internal intercostals and the abdominal muscles (rectus abdominis, external and internal oblique, and transverse abdominis).

In patients with airflow obstruction (e.g., acute bronchoconstriction in asthma or emphysema), hyperinflation of the lungs stretches the lung tissue and leads to additional elastic recoil, forcing the crural portion of the diaphragm downward and shortening the vertical muscle fibers. This places the diaphragm at a mechanical disadvantage because of the altered length–tension relationship.

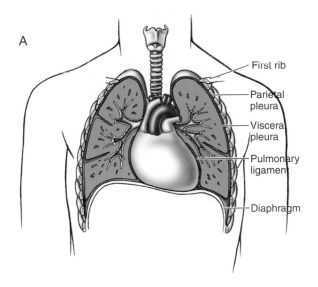

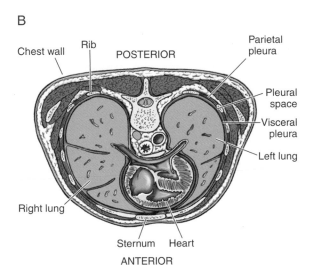

Figure 8.7. Frontal and cross-section views of the chest and lungs shows the pleural layers (visceral and parietal) and the pleural space. With inspiration, negative pressure develops in the pleural space. This allows air to move from the atmosphere into the tracheobronchial tree for gas exchange. The negative intrathoracic pressure also facilitates return of venous blood into the right atrium.

Pleura

The visceral (inner layer) and parietal (outer layer) pleura are thin membranes between the lung and the chest wall; they converge at the lung hila (Fig. 8.7) (5). The pleural space, which lies between the visceral and parietal pleura, contains a small amount of fluid. Because the pleural space is airtight and the chest wall and lung tissue pull against each other across the pleural space, negative pressure is produced at rest. During inspiration both the visceral and parietal pleura expand outward and more negative pressure develops in the pleural space.

Air can enter the pleural space (i.e., pneumothorax) by spontaneous rupture of a subpleural bleb or by trauma to the chest wall (e.g., a fractured rib with penetration of the parietal pleura). With a pneumothorax, the lungs collapse while the chest wall expands because of its intrinsic elastic properties. The parietal pleura contains abundant pain fibers, and irritation of this membrane by a pneumothorax or inflammation produces local chest pain exacerbated by motion of the pleura (e.g., deep inspiration).

DISTRIBUTION OF BLOOD FLOW

The lungs receive blood from the pulmonary arteries, which contain systemic venous blood from the right ventricle, and bronchial arteries, which contain oxygenated blood from the left ventricle. The pulmonary artery trunk emerges from the right ventricle and divides into right and left main pulmonary arteries anterior to the carina of the trachea (Fig. 8.8). The pulmonary arteries divide into branches corresponding to the divisions of the bronchial tree and supply the pulmonary arterioles. The pulmonary circulation is a low-pressure system with a normal mean pressure of approximately 15 mm Hg at rest. The majority of blood flow to the alveoli is derived from the pulmonary circulation, whereas the bronchial arteries supply the walls of the bronchi and bronchioles to the level of the alveoli. Pulmonary arterioles divide into pulmonary

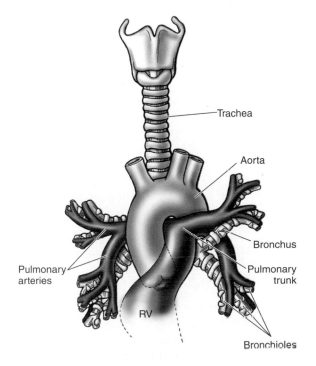

Figure 8.8. The major pulmonary arteries, which originate from the right ventricle (RV). Branches of the pulmonary artery are adjacent to bronchi and bronchioles.

capillaries that form networks in the walls of the alveoli, where gas exchange occurs.

The pulmonary veins carry oxygenated blood from the pulmonary capillaries. These veins converge to form the main pulmonary veins, which empty into to the left atrium. The pulmonary veins also receive blood from the bronchial circulation, which accounts for a right-to-left shunt that normally occurs in the lungs and includes up to 5% of cardiac output.

GAS EXCHANGE

Gas exchange occurs by way of two anatomical structures, the functional respiratory unit and the alveolus. These are described here.

Functional Respiratory Unit

Gas exchange in the lungs occurs at the alveolar–capillary membrane within the anatomical area called the functional respiratory unit (Fig. 8.9). As illustrated in Figure 8.9, a terminal bronchiole enters the center of the functional respiratory unit accompanied by a pulmonary arteriole carrying deoxygenated blood from the body tissues and muscles. The arteriole divides into a rich network of pulmonary capillaries that enter the alveolar walls and drain into pulmonary veins and venules.

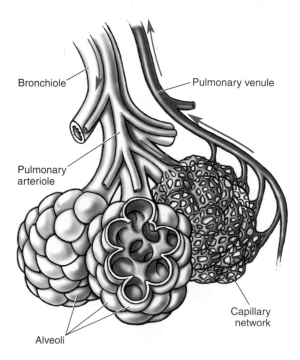

Figure 8.9. The functional respiratory unit. It consists of a bronchiole and corresponding blood supply; pulmonary arteriole carries deoxygenated blood, while pulmonary venule carries oxygenated blood. The rich capillary network supplies the alveoli for the purpose of gas exchange.

Table 8.2. Major Cells of the Alveolus

Alveolar epithelial cells.
Type I covers most of the alveolar surface.
Type II produces surfactant.
Interstitial cells.
Endothelial cells line the pulmonary capillary.
Alveolar macrophages reside within the alveolus, can phagocytose bacteria and particulates.

Alveolus

The alveolus consists of five major cells (Table 8.2). Most of the alveolar surface is covered by a thin layer of type I epithelial cells. The alveolar capillary membrane consists of the alveolar epithelium; the interstitium, containing the basement membrane; and the pulmonary capillary endothelial cells (Fig. 8.10). Type II epithelial cells, found primarily at the junctions of alveolar walls, produce surfactant that consists of a mixture of phospholipids and lipid-binding apoproteins. A thin layer of surfactant lines the alveolus and functions to lower the surface tension in the alveolus. This helps to keep the alveolus open and to prevent collapse.

LUNG CLEARANCE AND DEFENSES

Because the respiratory tract is in direct contact with ambient air and the atmosphere, the lung is at risk for injury from inhalation of particles, gases, and fumes.

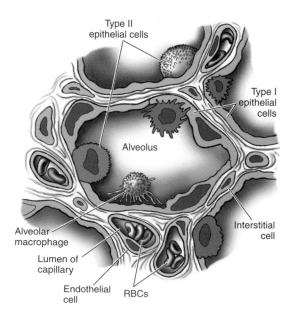

Figure 8.10. The major cells of the alveolus include epithelial cells (types I and II), endothelial cells of the pulmonary capillary, and alveolar macrophages. Also shown are lumen of capillary with red blood cells (RBCs)

Particle Deposition

The deposition of airborne particles into the lungs depends on size, density, travel distance, relative humidity, and breathing pattern. In general, particles greater than 10 μm in diameter settle in the upper respiratory tract. Particles between 2 and 10 μm in diameter are carried in the airstream into the lower respiratory tract, where they settle in the bronchial tree. Particles between 0.5 and 3 μm are deposited in the gas exchange areas (functional respiratory unit).

Mucociliary Escalator

In the main bronchi, ciliated epithelial cells, mucus-producing goblet cells, and mucus glands form the mucociliary apparatus. Inhaled particles may settle on the mucus layer, which is the transport medium for the rhythmic movement of the cilia to move the mucus up the bronchial tree toward the larynx (Fig. 8.5). Material may then be coughed up or swallowed. The transport rate of the mucociliary escalator is about 3 mm/minute, so that approximately 90% of particles directly deposited on the mucus layer are cleared within 2 hours. The velocity of transport of the mucociliary escalator increases from the peripheral to the central airways. Inhalation of toxic fumes, severe air pollution, and exposure to cigarette smoke may disrupt the normal wave patterns or may cause cilia to stop beating (impaired transport).

Alveolar Macrophages

The mucociliary escalator does not extend into the alveolus. Therefore, the principal alveolar defense is the alveolar macrophage. This resident cell can phagocytose (ingest) bacteria and nonliving particulates. Following phagocytosis, bacteria may be killed and enzymes within the cellular lysosomes may digest particles. Alveolar macrophages can also release mediators (cytokines) that recruit and activate other inflammatory cells.

Lymphatic Drainage

A third method of clearance and defense is the lymphatic transport system. Lymphatic vessels in the functional respiratory unit converge in the interlobular septa. Lymphatics also line pulmonary arteries and veins as well as bronchi and converge at the pulmonary hila, where hila lymph nodes are located. Lymphatic fluid from the left and right lungs drains into the thoracic duct and the right lymphatic duct, respectively. These lymphatic vessels enter the systemic venous circulation at the junction of the subclavian and internal jugular veins.

▶ SUMMARY

The respiratory system provides for the exchange of oxygen and carbon dioxide, which is necessary for metabolism. The respiratory anatomy provides the structure for these and other important functions at rest and with physical activity.

References
1. Nilsestuen J. Pulmonary physiology. In: Berghuis P, Cohen N, Decker M, et al., eds. Respiration. Redmond, WA: SpaceLabs, 1992:1–11.
2. Carrin B. Development and structure of the normal human lung. In: Turner-Warwick M, Hodson ME, Corrinm B, Kerr IH, eds. Clinical Atlas: Respiratory Diseases. Philadelphia: Lippincott, 1989:1–14.
3. Staub NC, Albertine KH. Anatomy of the lungs. In: Murray JF, Nadel JA, eds. Textbook of Respiratory Medicine, vol 1. 2nd ed. Philadelphia: Saunders, 1994:3–25.
4. Berger AJ. Control of breathing. In: Murray JF, Nadel JA, eds. Textbook of Respiratory Medicine, vol 1. 2nd ed. Philadelphia: Saunders, 1994:199–218.
5. Light RW. Pleural Diseases. 2nd ed. Philadelphia: Lea & Febiger, 1990:1–7.

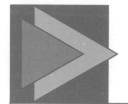

CHAPTER **9**

MUSCULOSKELETAL ANATOMY

Reed Humphrey

A major objective of exercise training is improvement in musculoskeletal fitness. The physiological adaptation of muscle to exercise training may be manifested through improvements in muscle force production, cardiovascular endurance, and resistance to injury. Inherent in designing effective training programs is a thorough understanding of muscle structure and function. This chapter provides a brief overview of the fundamentals of musculoskeletal anatomy. For in-depth study, the reader is referred to a variety of excellent sources (1–5).

BASIC STRUCTURE OF BONE, SKELETAL MUSCLE, AND CONNECTIVE TISSUE

Beyond supporting soft tissue, protecting internal organs, and acting as an important source of nutrients and blood constituents, the bones are the rigid levers for locomotion. The skull, vertebral column, sternum, and ribs are considered the **axial skeleton**; the remaining bones, particularly those of the upper and lower limbs, are considered the **appendicular skeleton**. The major bones of the body are illustrated in Figure 9.1. An outer fibrous layer of connective tissue attaches the bone to muscles, deep fascia, and joint capsules. Just beneath the outer layer is a highly vascular inner layer that contains cells for the creation of new bone. The outer and inner layers that cover the bones constitute the **periosteum**.

The periosteum, continuous with tendons and adjacent articulated structures, anchors muscle to bone. Tendons are likewise continuous with the **epimysium**, the outer layer of connective tissue covering muscle. The macroscopic anatomy of muscle is illustrated in Figure 9.2. Individual skeletal muscles are composed of a varying number of muscle bundles referred to as fasciculi (an individual bundle is a fasciculus). Fasciculi are likewise covered and thus separated by **perimysium**. Individual muscle fibers are enveloped by the **endomysium**. Immediately beneath the endomysium is the thin, membranous **sarcolemma**, the cell membrane that encloses the cellular contents of the muscle fiber, nuclei, local stores of

fat, and glucose (in the form of glycogen), enzymes, contractile proteins, and other specialized structures such as the mitochondria. The major muscles of the body are illustrated in Figures 9.3 and 9.4.

Approximately 5% of skeletal muscle is constituted of the high-energy phosphates, key minerals and energy sources needed for force production; another 20% of muscle composition is protein, principally the contractile elements **myosin**, **actin**, and **tropomyosin**. Water constitutes 75% of muscle composition (6). Physical training results in a significant alteration of these constituents, depending on the specific training stimulus.

Given the wide shift in blood supply shunted to active skeletal muscle during vigorous exercise, a highly competent vascular bed must exist throughout. Likewise, the body has the ability to enhance blood supply through formation of new capillary networks stimulated by physical training that involves endurance or aerobic training.

STRUCTURE AND FUNCTION OF JOINTS IN MOVEMENT

Table 9.1 summarizes commonly used terms of motion, and Figure 9.5 illustrates major movements. Consistent use of these terms is essential to avoid confusion. The effective interaction of bone and muscle to produce movement somewhat depends on joint function. Joints are the articulations between bones, and along with bones and ligaments, they constitute the articular system. **Ligaments** are tough, fibrous connective tissues anchoring bone to bone. Joints are typically classified as **fibrous**, wherein bones are united by fibrous tissue, **cartilaginous** (cartilage or a fibrocartilaginous anchor), or **synovial**, in which a fibrous articular capsule and an inner synovial membrane lining enclose the joint cavity. The cavity is filled with synovial fluid, which provides constant lubrication during human movement to minimize the wearing effects of friction on the cartilaginous covering of the articulating bones. Figure 9.6 illustrates this unique capsular arrangement, which is a critical concern to the exercise specialist. Table 9.2 summarizes the joint classifications and examples in the human body.

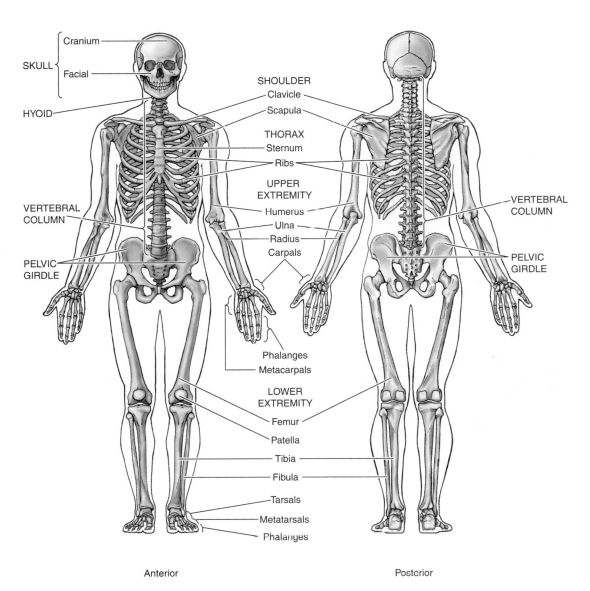

Figure 9.1. Divisions of the skeletal system. (Courtesy of Tortora G, Anagnostakos N. Principles of Anatomy and Physiology. 6th ed. New York: Harper & Row, 1992;163.)

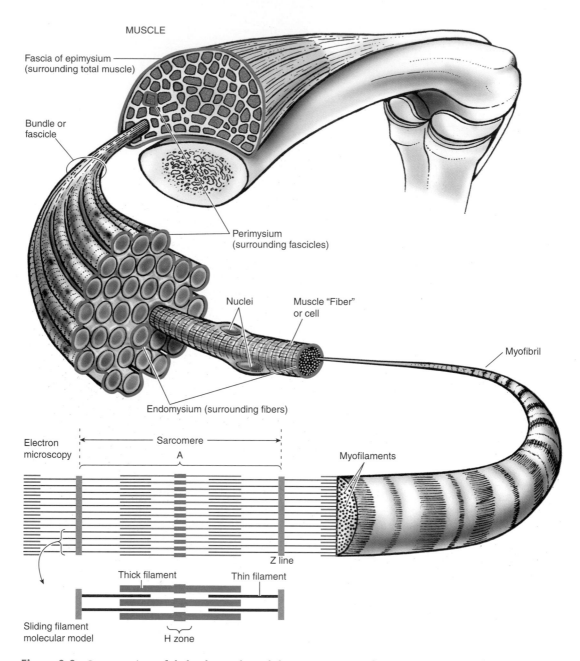

MUSCLE

Fascia of epimysium
(surrounding total muscle)

Bundle or
fascicle

Perimysium
(surrounding fascicles)

Nuclei

Muscle "Fiber"
or cell

Myofibril

Endomysium (surrounding fibers)

Electron
microscopy

Sarcomere

A

Myofilaments

Z line

Thick filament

Thin filament

Sliding filament
molecular model

H zone

Figure 9.2. Cross section of skeletal muscle and the arrangement of its connective tissue wrappings.

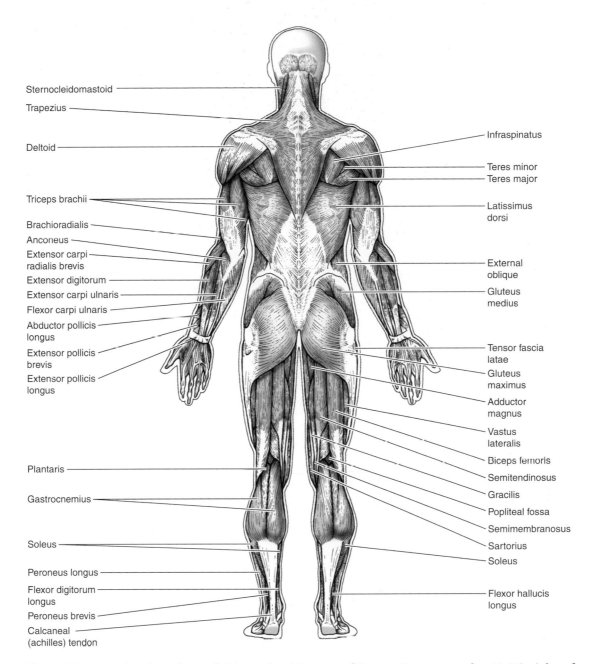

Figure 9.3. Posterior view of superficial muscles. (Courtesy of Tortora G, Anagnostakos N. Principles of Anatomy and Physiology. 6th ed. New York: Harper & Row, 1992;265.)

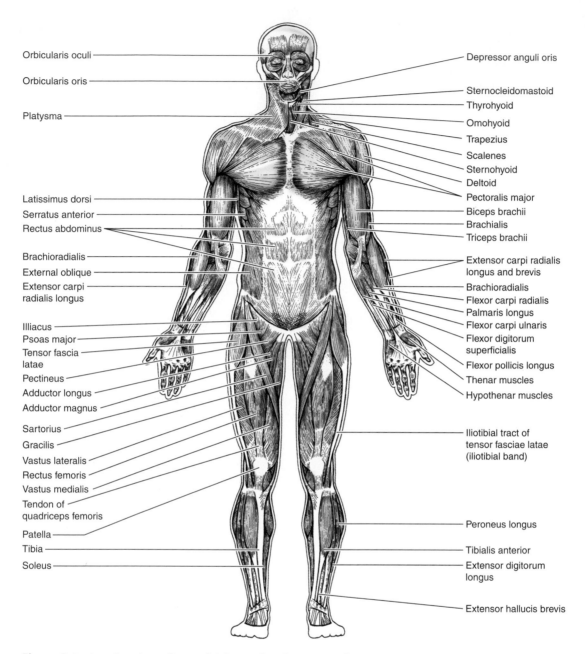

Orbicularis oculi

Orbicularis oris

Platysma

Latissimus dorsi

Serratus anterior

Rectus abdominus

Brachioradialis

External oblique

Extensor carpi
radialis longus

Illiacus

Psoas major

Tensor fascia
latae

Pectineus

Adductor longus

Adductor magnus

Sartorius

Gracilis

Vastus lateralis

Rectus femoris

Vastus medialis

Tendon of
quadriceps femoris

Patella

Tibia

Soleus

Depressor anguli oris

Sternocleidomastoid

Thyrohyoid

Omohyoid

Trapezius

Scalenes

Sternohyoid

Deltoid

Pectoralis major

Biceps brachii

Brachialis

Triceps brachii

Extensor carpi radialis
longus and brevis

Brachioradialis

Flexor carpi radialis

Palmaris longus

Flexor carpi ulnaris

Flexor digitorum
superficialis

Flexor pollicis longus

Thenar muscles

Hypothenar muscles

Iliotibial tract of
tensor fasciae latae
(iliotibial band)

Peroneus longus

Tibialis anterior

Extensor digitorum
longus

Extensor hallucis brevis

Figure 9.4. Anterior view of superficial muscles. (Courtesy of Tortora G, Anagnostakos N. Principles of Anatomy and Physiology. 6th ed. New York: Harper & Row, 1992;266.)

Table 9.1. Commonly Used Terms of Movement

TERM	EXPLANATION OF TERM AND EXAMPLE OF ITS USE
Flexion	*Bending* or decreasing the angle between body parts (e.g., flexing the elbow joint)
Extension	*Straightening* or increasing the angle between body parts (e.g., extending the knee joint).
Abduction	*Moving away from the median plane* (e.g., abducting the upper limb)
Adduction	*Moving toward the median plane* (e.g., adducting the lower limb)
Rotation	*Moving around the long axis* (e.g., medial and lateral rotation of the lower limb)
Circumduction	*Circular movement* combining flexion, extension, abduction, and adduction (e.g., circumducting the upper limb)
Eversion	*Moving the sole of the foot away from the median plane* (e.g., when the lateral surface of the foot is raised)
Inversion	*Moving the sole of the foot toward the median plane* (e.g., when you examine the sole of your foot to remove a splinter
Supination	*Rotating the forearm and hand laterally* so that the palm faces anteriorly (e.g., when a person extends a hand to beg)
Pronation	*Rotating the forearm and hand medially* so that the palm faces posteriorly (e.g., when a person pats a child on the head)
Protrusion	*Moving anteriorly* (e.g., sticking the chin out)
Retrusion	*Moving posteriorly* (e.g., tucking the chin in)

Reprinted with permission from Moore KL. Clinical Oriented Anatomy. 3rd ed., Baltimore: Williams & Wilkins, 1992.

Joints are typically well perfused by numerous arterial branches and are innervated by branches of the nerves supplying the adjacent muscle and overlying skin. Proprioceptive feedback is an important joint sensation, as is pain, owing to the high density of sensory fibers in the joint capsule. This feedback has obvious importance in regulating human movement and in preventing injury.

The degree of movement within a joint is typically called the range of motion (ROM). ROM can be active (AROM), the range that can be reached by voluntary movement, or passive (PROM), the range that can be achieved by external means (e.g., an examiner or device). Joints are typically limited in range by the articulations of bones (as in the limitation of elbow extension by the olecranon process of the ulna), ligamentous arrangement, and soft tissue limitations, as occurs in elbow or knee flexion.

Movement at one joint may influence the extent of movement at adjacent joints, as a number of muscles and other soft tissue structures cross multiple joints. For example, finger flexion decreases in the presence of wrist flexion because muscles that flex both the wrist and fingers cross multiple joints. Tables 9.3 and 9.4 summarize major joint movements and the muscles producing those movements.

MUSCLE FIBER CONTRACTION AND FIBER TYPES

Skeletal muscles are controlled by the central nervous system (CNS) both at higher centers and in individual spinal segments, and by proprioceptive structures (e.g., muscle spindles, Golgi tendon organs) inherent to the muscle and tendon complex. The integration is complex yet remarkably efficient. While it has never been conclusively proved, the preponderance of scientific evidence indicates that when stimulated to contract, muscle tissue shortens or lengthens because the myosin and actin myofilaments slide past each other up to the point of minimum contact without changing individual length. The contact between filaments is known as cross-bridging, and it controls shortening or lengthening of muscles during contractile movements. Table 9.5 summarizes the sliding-filament theory (7). This continual process of forwarding and releasing cross-bridges permits the generation of tension, resulting in concentric (shortening), eccentric (lengthening), or isometric (static) force development. Force production continues as long as the muscle is stimulated, but the ability of the muscle to perform may be limited by intrinsic factors: diminished production of adenosine triphosphate (ATP), decreased pH, and accumulation of metabolic byproducts.

Three common terms describing muscle contraction are **twitch**, **summation**, and **tetanus**. **Twitch** refers to a single brief muscle contraction caused by a single stimulus. **Summation** refers to successive stimuli arriving at a presynaptic terminal at a rate high enough that when summed, they are sufficient to result in muscle contraction. This is known as **temporal summation**. **Spatial summation** occurs when different presynaptic terminals on the same nerve are stimulated at the same time, resulting in contraction. **Tetanus** may be defined as muscle fiber stimulation of such high frequency that it is not able to return to its resting length between contractions (6).

The human body has the ability to perform a wide range of physical tasks combining varying composites of speed, power, and endurance. No single type of muscle fiber possesses the characteristics that would allow optimal performance across this continuum of physical challenges. Rather, muscle fibers possess certain characteristics that result in relative specialization. For example, muscle fasciculi of a specific fiber type are selectively recruited by the body for speed and power tasks of short duration, while others are recruited for endurance tasks of long duration and relatively low intensity. When the challenge requires elements of speed or power but also has an endurance component, yet another type of muscle fiber is recruited.

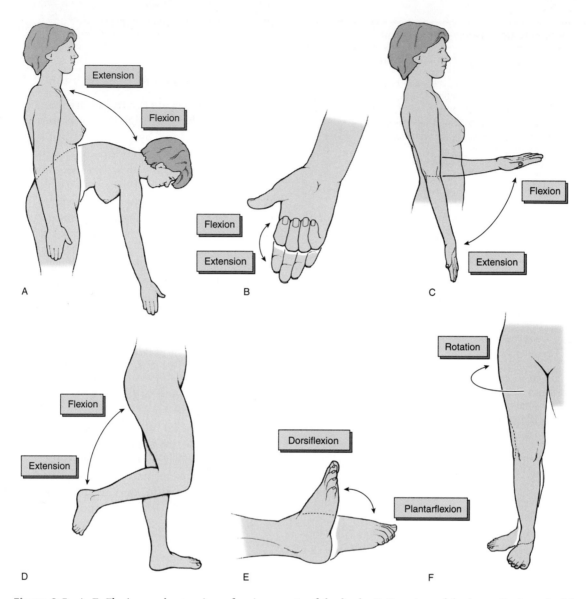

Figure 9.5. **A–E.** Flexion and extension of various parts of the body. **F.** Rotation of the lower limb at the hip joint. (Reprinted with permission from Moore KL. Clinically Oriented Anatomy. 3rd ed. Baltimore: Williams & Wilkins, 1992.)

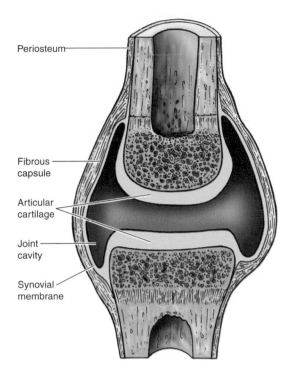

Figure 9.6. A synovial joint. (Reprinted with permission from Moore KL. Clinically Oriented Anatomy. 3rd ed. Baltimore: Williams & Wilkins, 1992.)

Table 9.2. Classification of Joints in the Human Body

JOINT CLASSIFICATION	FEATURES, EXAMPLES
FIBROUS	
Suture	Tight union unique to the skull
Syndesmosis	Interosseous membrane between bones (e.g., the union along the shafts of the radius and ulna, tibia and fibula)
Gomphosis	Unique joint at the tooth socket
CARTILAGINOUS	
Primary (synchondroses; hyaline cartilaginous)	Usually temporary to permit bone growth and typically fuse; some do not (e.g., at the sternum and rib [costal cartilage])
Secondary (symphyses; fibrocartiliaginous	Strong, slightly movable joints (e.g., intervertebral discs, pubic symphysis)
SYNOVIAL	
Plane	Gliding and sliding movements (e.g., acromioclavicular joint)
Hinge (ginglymus)	Uniaxial movements (e.g., elbow, knee extension and flexion)
Ellipsoidal (condyloid)	Biaxial joint (e.g., radiocarpal extension, flexion at the wrist)
Saddle	Unique joint that permits movements in all planes, including opposition (e.g., the carpometacarpal joint of the thumb)
Ball and socket	Multiaxial joints that permit movements in all directions (e.g., hip and shoulder joints)
Pivot	Uniaxial joints that permit rotation (e.g., humeroradial joint)

These different fiber types, to be described more specifically later, should not be thought of as mutually exclusive. In fact, intricate recruitment and switching occurs in muscle over the performance of many tasks, and fibers designed to be optimal for one type of task can contribute to the performance of another. The net result is a functioning muscle that can respond to a wide variety of tasks, and while the composition of the muscle may lend itself to performing best in endurance activities, it still can accomplish speed and power tasks to a lesser degree.

Fortunately, the human body can respond adequately to most physical tasks encountered in everyday living. In the presence of muscle impairment, specific training regimens may restore performance to normal function. Likewise, normal function can be enhanced through exercise training to accomplish physical tasks that are in excess of the demands of daily living, such as athletics (8, 9).

Over the years there has been a fair amount of controversy about the classification of muscle fiber types (10). In addition, there are questions about whether these types can change in response to an intervention such as endurance training (11–14). In either case, there is general agreement that relative to exercise performance, two distinct fiber types—type I (slow twitch) and type II (fast twitch, with their proposed subdivisions)—have been identified and classified by contractile and metabolic characteristics (15, 16). To illustrate the variation in fiber types within the population, Table 9.6 lists fiber type dis-

tribution in elite athletes relative to the normal population.

Type I Muscle Fibers

The characteristics of type I muscle fibers, listed in Table 9.7, are consistent with muscle fibers that resist fatigue. Thus, type I fibers are selected for activities of low intensity and long duration. Within whole muscle, type I motor units asynchronously contract; that is, in addition to their inherent fatigue resistance, endurance is prolonged by the constant switching that occurs to ensure freshly charged muscle as the exercise stimulus continues. Sedentary persons have approximately 50% type I fibers, and this distribution is generally equal throughout the major muscle groups of the body (17). In endurance athletes, the percentage of type I fibers is greater, but this is thought to be largely a genetic predisposition, despite some evidence suggesting that prolonged exercise training can alter fiber type (18, 19).

Table 9.3. Major Movement of the Upper Extremity

REGION	ACTION(S)	PRINCIPAL MUSCLE(S)
Scapula	Fixation	Serratus anterior, pectoralis minor, trapezius, levator scapulae, rhomboids
Upper arm	Flexion	Anterior deltoid, pectoralis major (clavicular head)
	Extension	Latissimus dorsi, pectoralis major (sternocostal head)
	Abduction	Middle deltoid, supraspinatus
	Adduction	Latissimus dorsi, teres major, pectoralis major
	Medial (internal) rotation	Latissimus dorsi, teres major, subscapularis
	Lateral (external) rotation	Infraspinatus, teres minor
Lower arm	Flexion	Biceps brachii, brachialis, brachioradialis
	Extension	Triceps brachii, anconeus
	Supination	Supinator, biceps brachii
	Pronation	Pronator teres, pronator quadratus
Wrist	Flexion	Flexor carpi radialis, palmaris longus, flexor carpi ulnaris, flexor digitorum superficialis
	Extension	Extensor carpi radialis longus and brevis, extensor digitorum, extensor carpi ulnaris
	Adduction	Flexor and extensor carpi ulnaris
	Abduction	Extensor carpi radialis longus and brevis, flexor carpi radialis

Adapted with permission from Moore K, Agur A. Essential Clinical Anatomy. Baltimore: Williams & Wilkins, 1996.

Table 9.4. Major Movement of the Lower Extremity

REGION	ACTION(S)	PRINCIPAL MUSCLE(S)
Abdomen	Flexion and rotation of trunk	External and internal oblique
	Flexion	Rectus abdominis
Back	Laterally bend and rotate head	Splenius (capitus and cervicis), acting unilaterally
	Extension of head and neck	Splenius, acting bilaterally
	Extension of vertebral column	Erector spinae, acting bilaterally (flexion when contracting eccentrically)
	Lateral bending of vertebral column	Erector spinae, acting unilaterally
Thigh	Flexion at hip joint	Iliopsoas
	Extension	Gluteus maximus, hamstrings (semitendinosus, semimembranosus, long head of biceps femoris)
	Abduction and flexion	Tensor fasciae latae, sartorius
	Adduction and medial rotation	Gluteus medius and minimus
	Adduction	Adductor longus, brevis, magnus; gracilis
	Lateral rotation	Piriformis, obturator internis
Lower Leg	Flexion	Hamstrings
	Extension	Quadriceps femoris (rectus femoris; vastus lateralis, medialis, and intermedius)
Foot	Dorsiflexion	Tibialis anterior, extensor digitorum longus; extensor hallucis longus, peroneus tertius
	Plantarflexion	Gastrocnemius, soleus, tibialis posterior, flexor digitorum longus, flexor hallucis longus
	Eversion	Peroneus longus and brevis
	Inversion	Tibialis anterior and posterior

Adapted with permission from Moore K, Agur A. Essential Clinical Anatomy. Baltimore: Williams & Wilkins, 1996.

Essentially, those most successful at endurance activities generally have a high proportion of type I fibers, and this is most likely due to genetic factors supplemented through appropriate exercise training. From a metabolic perspective, type I fibers are those frequently called aerobic, since the generation of energy for continued muscle contraction is met through the ongoing oxidation of available foodstuffs. Thus, with minimal accumulation of anaerobically produced metabolites, continued muscle contraction is favored in type I fibers.

Type II Muscle Fibers

At the opposite end of the continuum, those who achieve the greatest success in power and high-intensity speed tasks usually have a greater proportion of type II muscle fibers distributed through the major muscle groups. Since force generation is so important, type II fibers shorten and develop tension considerably faster than type I fibers (20). These fibers are typically thought of as type IIB fibers, the "classic" fast-twitch fiber.

Metabolically, these fibers are the classic anaerobic fibers, because they rely on energy sources intrinsic to the muscle, not the fuels used by type I fibers. When an endurance component is introduced, such as in events lasting upward of several minutes (800–1500 meter races, for example), a second type of fast-twitch fiber, type IIA, is recruited. As noted in Table 9.7, the type IIA fibers represent a transition of sorts between the needs met by the type I and type IIB fibers. Metabolically, while type IIA fibers have the ability to generate a moderately large amount of force, they also have some aerobic capacity, although not

Table 9.5. Sliding Filament Summary of Muscle Contraction and Relaxation

RESTING MUSCLE

Calcium ions are bound to the SR
Tropomyosin–troponin complex blocks attachment sites for myosin
ATP is bound to myosin heads

MUSCLE CONTRACTION

Nerve impulse exceeding resting potential spreads across sarcolemma and down transverse tubules, causing release of calcium from the SR
Calcium binds with troponin, which permits actin and myosin to form cross bridges
Myosin ATPase is activated, splitting ATP; this transfer of energy causes movement of the myosin cross bridges, generating tension
Cross bridges uncouple when ATP binds to the myosin bridge

RELAXATION

Coupling and uncoupling continue until calcium concentration becomes insufficient
When the nerve impulse ceases, calcium is taken up by the SR: actin and myosin return to a resting state

SR, sarcoplasmic reticulum.

Table 9.6. Muscle Fiber Composition in Selected Populations

SPORT	% TYPE I (SLOW TWITCH)	%TYPE II (FAST TWITCH)
Distance runners	60–90	10–40
Track sprinters	25–45	55–75
Weight lifters	45–55	45–55
Shot putters	25–40	60–75
Nonathletes	47–53	47–53

Reprinted with permission from Powers SK, Howley ET. Exercise Physiology. Dubuque: WC Brown, 1990:160.

Table 9.7. Structural and Functional Characteristics of Slow Twitch (ST) and Fast Twitch (FT$_A$ and FT$_B$) Muscle Fibers

CHARACTERISTICS	ST	FT$_A$	FT$_B$
Neural aspects			
Motor neuron size	Small	Large	Large
Motor neuron recruitment threshold	Low	High	High
Motor nerve conduction velocity	Slow	Fast	Fast
Structural aspects			
Muscle fiber diameter	Small	Large	Large
Sarcoplasmic reticulum development	Less	More	More
Mitochondrial density	High	High	Low
Capillary density	High	Medium	Low
Myoglobin content	High	Medium	Low
Energy substrates			
Phosphocreatine stores	Low	High	High
Glycogen stores	Low	High	High
Triglyceride stores	High	Medium	Low
Enzymatic aspects			
Myosin-ATPase activity	Low	High	High
Glycolytic enzyme activity	Low	High	High
Oxidative enzyme activity	High	High	Low
Functional aspects			
Twitch (contraction) time	Slow	Fast	Fast
Relaxation time	Slow	Fast	Fast
Force production	Low	High	High
Energy efficiency, "economy"	High	Low	Low
Fatigue resistance	High	Low	Low
Elasticity	Low	High	High

Courtesy of Fox EL, Bowers RW, Foss ML. The Physiological Basis of Physical Education and Athletics. 4th ed. Dubuque: WC Brown, 1989:110.

as much as type I fibers. This is a logical and necessary bridge between the types of muscle fibers and the ability to meet the variety of physical tasks imposed. Reference to the existence of the type IIC fiber is necessary in a complete description of human muscle fiber types. The IIC fiber has been described as a rare and undifferentiated muscle fiber type that is probably involved in reinnervation of impaired skeletal muscle (21).

The rapid expansion of information technology has yielded a variety of Internet sites that provide a range of resources for anatomy and radiological correlation. Table 9.8 lists popular sites that were on line at the time of printing. It is by no means exclusive, and the reader is encouraged to search for similar sites.

► SUMMARY

In summary, skeletal muscle profile is composed of varying amounts of type I, IIA, and IIB muscle fibers whose quantity and distribution are largely genetic. While

Table 9.8. Frequently Used Internet Sites for Anatomy

http://www.innerbody.com/htm/body.html—Informative Graphics Corporation
http://www.rad.washington.edu/anatomy/index.html—University of Washington Department of Radiology Exhibits
http://www.imc.gsm.com/—Integrated Medical Curriculum
http://sig.biostr.washington.edu/projects/da/—University of Washington Digital Anatomist Project
http://www.nlm.nih.gov/research/visible/visible human.html—National Institutes of Health Visible Human Project
http://www.radiology.co.uk/xrayfile/xray/index.htm—Scottish Radiological Society
http://www.meddean.luc.edu/lumen/MedEd/GrossAnatomy/anatomy.htm—Loyola University Medical Education Network
http://www.vh.org/Providers/Textbooks/AnatomicVariants/AnatomyHP.html—University of Iowa Virtual Hospital
http://www.vesalius.com/—Versalius Resource for Surgical Education
http://www.anatomy.org/anatomy/index.html—American Association of Anatomists

Table 9.9. Adaptation in Skeletal Muscle Relative to Specific Training Regimens

MUSCLE FIBER TYPE	TYPE I (SLOW TWITCH)		TYPE II (FAST TWITCH)	
VARIABLES	RESISTANCE	ENDURANCE	RESISTANCE	ENDURANCE
% Composition	nc or ?	nc or ?	nc or ?	nc or ?
Fiber size	+	nc or +	++	nc
Contractile property	nc	nc	nc	nc
Oxidative capacity	nc	++	nc	+
Anaerobic capacity	? or +	nc	? or +	nc
Glycogen content	nc	++	nc	++
Capillary density	?	+	?	? or +
Blood flow during work	?	? or +	?	?
Fat oxidation	nc	++	nc	+

nc, no change; ?, unknown; +, moderate increase; ++, large increase. Adapted with permission from Gollnick PD, Sembrowich WI. Adaptations in human skeletal muscle as a result of training. In: Amsterdam E, ed. Exercise and Cardiovascular Health and Disease. New York: Yorke Medical Books, 1977:90; and from McArdle W, Katch F, Katch V. Exercise Physiology. 4th ed. Baltimore: Williams & Wilkins, 1996:334.

the conversion of fiber types through disuse or training and the splitting and/or generation of muscle fibers are somewhat controversial, what is certain about exercise training and fiber type is that metabolic adaptations are significantly enhanced by specific training. These, along with secondary adaptations, are described in Table 9.9.

References

1. Moore KL. Clinically Oriented Anatomy. 3rd Ed. Baltimore: Williams & Wilkins, 1992.
2. Olson TR. A.D.A.M. Student Atlas of Anatomy. Baltimore: Williams & Wilkins, 1996.
3. Agur AMR. Grant's Atlas of Anatomy. 9th ed. Baltimore: Williams & Wilkins, 1991.
4. Moore KL, Agur MR. Essentials of Clinical Anatomy. Baltimore: Williams & Wilkins, 1996.
5. Hall-Craggs ELB. Anatomy as a Basis for Clinical Medicine. 3rd ed. London: Williams & Wilkins, 1995.
6. McArdle WD, Katch F, Katch V. Exercise Physiology: Energy, Nutrition and Human Performance. 4th ed. Baltimore: Williams & Wilkins, 1996.
7. Huxley HE. The structural basis of muscular contraction. Proc R Soc Med 178:131–149, 1971.
8. Coggan AR, Spina RJ, King DS, et al. Skeletal muscle adaptations to endurance training in 60- to 70-yr-old men and women. J Appl Physiol 72:1780–1786, 1992.
9. Jansson E, Kaijser L. Muscle adaptation to extreme endurance training in man. Acta Physiol Scand 100:315, 1977.
10. Armstrong RB. Muscle fiber recruitment patterns and their metabolic correlates. In: Horton ES, Terjunk RL, eds. Exercise, Nutrition and Energy Metabolism. New York: Macmillan, 1988.
11. Gollnick P, Armstrong R, Sembrowich W, et al. Glycogen depletion pattern in human skeletal muscle fiber after heavy exercise. J Appl Physiol 34:615–618, 1973.
12. Chi MMY, Hintz CS, Coyle EF, et al. Effects of detraining on enzymes of energy metabolism in individual human muscle fibers. Am J Physiol 244 (Cell Physiology 13):C276–C287, 1983.
13. Jacobs I, Esbjornsson M, Slyvan C, et al. Sprint training effects on muscle myoglobin, enzymes, fiber types, and blood lactate. Med Sci Sports Exerc 19:368–374, 1987.
14. Jansson E, Sjodin B, Tesch P. Changes in muscle fiber type distribution in man after physical training. Acta Physiol Scand 104:235–237, 1978.
15. Brooke MH, Kaiser KK. Muscle fiber types: How many and what kind? Arch Neurol 23:369–379, 1970.
16. Edstrom L, Nystrom B. Histochemical types and sizes of fibers of normal human muscles. Acta Neurol Scand 45:269–279, 1969.
17. Fox EL, Bowers RW, Foss ML. The Physiological Basis of Physical Education and Athletics. 4th ed. Dubuque: WC Brown, 1989:106–107.
18. Burke F, Cerny F, Costill D, Fink W. Characteristics of skeletal muscle in competitive cyclists. Med Sci Sports Exerc 9:109–112, 1977.
19. Costill D, Daniels J, Evans W, et al. Skeletal muscle enzymes and fiber composition in male and female track athletes. J Appl Physiol 40:149–154, 1976.
20. Vrbova G. Influence of activity on some characteristic properties of slow and fast mammalian muscles. Exerc Sport Sci Rev 7:181–213, 1979.
21. Komi PV, Karlsson J. Skeletal muscle fiber types, enzyme activities and physical performance in young males and females. Acta Physiol Scand 103:210, 1978.

2.1.0.2

2.1.0.3, 2.1.0.4,
4.1.0.1, 4.1.0.2

5.1.1

CHAPTER **10**

SURFACE ANATOMY

Richard W. Latin

Exercise professionals are routinely required to make measurements and assessments based on external body locations or dimensions. Knowledge of basic surface anatomy is essential for determining pulse, electrocardiogram (ECG) lead placements, blood pressure, anthropometric dimensions and for performing cardiopulmonary resuscitation and emergency defibrillations. This chapter presents surface anatomy as it applies to these procedures.

DEFINITIONS OF ANATOMICAL LOCATIONS

The following are terms and their definitions related to anatomical location (1):

1. Anterior (ventral): refers to the front of the body (Fig. 10.1).
2. Anatomical position: the body is erect with feet together and the upper limbs hanging at the sides, palms of the hands facing forward, thumbs facing away from the body, and fingers extended. Typically, all anatomical references are made to the body in this position (Fig. 10.2).
3. Distal: farther away from any reference point (Fig. 10.1).
4. Inferior: away from the head (Fig. 10.2).
5. Lateral: away from the midline of the body (Fig. 10.2).
6. Medial: toward the midline of the body (Fig. 10.2).
7. Posterior (dorsal): refers to the back of the body (Fig. 10.1).
8. Proximal: closer to any point of reference (Fig. 10.1).
9. Superior: toward the head (Fig. 10.2).

DEFINITIONS OF COMMON MOVEMENT TERMS

The following are terms and their definitions related to human movement (2):

1. Abduction: a movement away from the axis or midline of the body when in the anatomical position (Fig. 10.3A, hip abduction).
2. Adduction: a movement toward the axis or midline of the body when in the anatomical position (Fig. 10.3B, hip adduction).
3. Circumduction: a movement in which the distal end of a bone inscribes a circle without the shaft rotating (Fig. 10.4, shoulder circumduction).
4. Extension: a movement that increases the joint angle between two articulating bones (Fig. 10.5, elbow extension).
5. Flexion: a movement that decreases the joint angle between two articulating bones (Fig. 10.5, elbow flexion).
6. Hyperextension: a movement in the direction of extension that positions a joint angle beyond a normal degree of extension (Fig. 10.6, shoulder hyperextension).
7. Pronation: a movement that produces rotation on the axis of a bone. When applied specifically to the forearm, the palm of the hand faces down because the radius rotates on the ulna (Fig 7A, forearm pronation).
8. Rotation: a movement of a segment that produces rotatory action around its own long axis (Fig. 10.8, neck rotation).
9. Supination: a movement that produces rotation on the axis of a bone. When applied specifically to the forearm, the palm of the hand faces up because the radius rotates on the ulna (Fig. 10.7B, forearm supination).

ANATOMICAL SITES FOR ECG LEAD PLACEMENTS

It is important to standardize the method of electrode placement and to select a lead system that provides appropriate ECG monitoring. The Mason-Likar 12-lead ECG system and bipolar lead systems are discussed here.

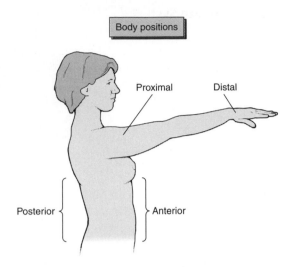

Figure 10.1. Anterior (ventral): the front of the body.

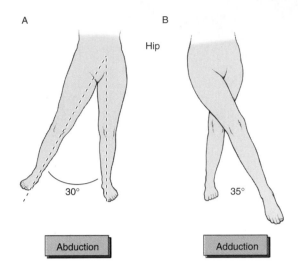

Figure 10.3. A. Abduction: movement away from the superior-inferior axis or mainline of the body when in the anatomical position (hip abduction). **B.** Adduction: movement toward the superior-inferior axis or mainline of the body when in the anatomical position (hip adduction).

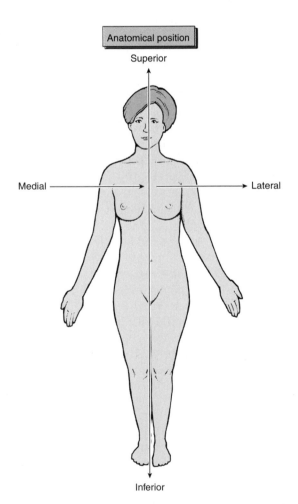

Figure 10.2. Anatomical position: the body is erect with feet together, with the upper limbs hanging at the side, palms or the hands facing forward, thumbs facing away from the body, and fingers extended. Typically all anatomical references to the body relate to this position.

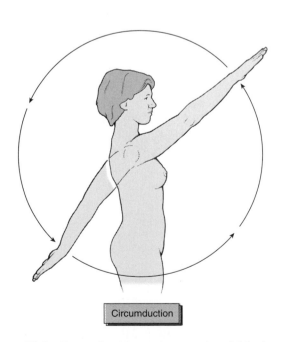

Figure 10.4. Circumduction: movement in which the distal end of a bone inscribes a circle with no shaft rotation (shoulder circumduction).

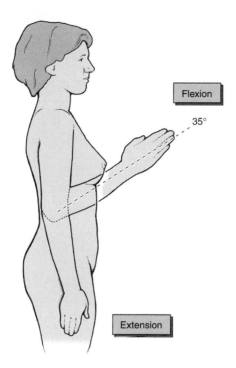

Figure 10.5. Extension: movement that increases the joint angle between two articulating bones (elbow extension).

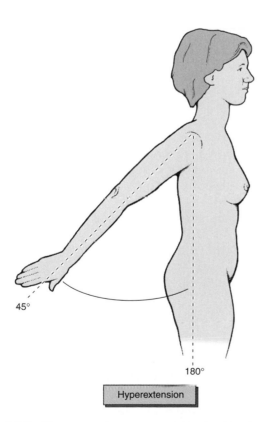

Figure 10.6. Hyperextension: movement in the direction of extension that positions a joint angle beyond normal extension (shoulder hyperextension).

Mason-Likar 12-Lead System

The Mason-Likar 10 electrode placement allows for conventional 12-lead exercise ECG tracings. Electrodes on the torso replace the standard limb electrodes inside the ankles and wrists. The location of these electrodes can be seen in Figure 10.9 and are described next (3, 4):

1. Right arm: upper right arm–chest region immediately below the distal end of the clavicle.
2. Left arm: upper left arm–chest region immediately below the distal end of the clavicle.
3. Right leg: lower right abdominal region immediately above the iliac crest, midclavicular line, at the level of the navel.
4. Left leg: lower left abdominal region immediately above the iliac crest, midclavicular line, at the level of the navel.

If leg electrodes must be moved because of excessive subcutaneous fat or electrical interference from electrode belt box friction, avoid placing them on the rib cage or regions of less body fat on the torso. Any alteration in recommended positions should be noted.

The location of the precordial (V) electrodes, also shown in Figure 10.9, are described next (5):

1. V_1: on the right sternal border in the fourth intercostal space. The fourth intercostal space can be found by locating the right sternoclavicular joint and placing the index finger in the space immediately below the first rib. This is the first intercostal space. Proceed down the sternum until the fourth space is found.
2. V_2: on the left sternal border in the fourth intercostal space.
3. V_3: at the midpoint on a straight line between V_2 and V_4.
4. V_4: on the fifth intercostal space, midclavicular line.
5. V_5: on the anterior axillary line, immediately horizontal to V_4.
6. V_6: on the midaxillary line, immediately horizontal to V_4 and V_5.

Bipolar Lead Systems

Bipolar lead systems are commonly used for exercise tests when extensive ECG data are not required, such as with physical fitness exercise testing or determination of exercise heart rate. There are numerous bipolar lead configurations. One conventional electrode placement is CM-5, in which the negative electrode is placed at the manubrium and the positive electrode at precordial lead V_5. The manubrium lies at the proximal articulations of the clavicles with the sternum. The locations of these and other bipolar leads may be seen in Figure 10.9.

A

B

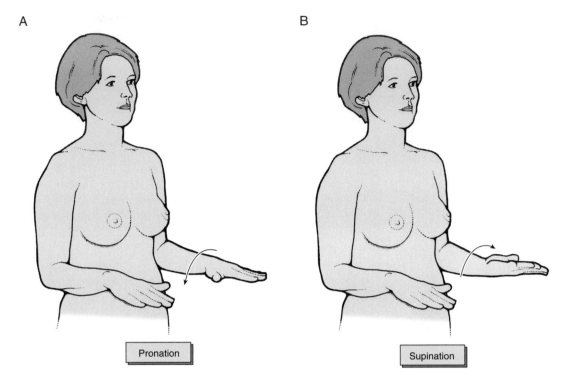

Pronation

Supination

Figure 10.7. A. Pronation: movement that produces rotation on the axis of a bone. When applied specifically to the forearm, the palm of the hand faces down (forearm pronation). **B.** Supination: movement that produces rotation on the axis of a bone. When applied specifically to the forearm, the palm of the hand faces up (forearm supination).

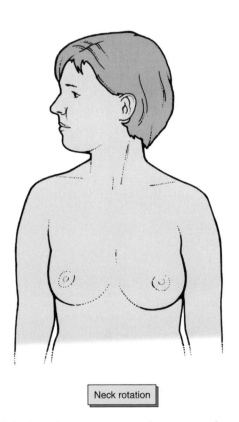

Neck rotation

Figure 10.8. Rotation: movement of a segment that produces rotatory action around its own long axis (neck rotation).

ANATOMICAL SITES FOR BLOOD PRESSURE DETERMINATION

Measurement of arterial blood pressure before, during, and after an exercise test is routine. The most common method used is brachial artery auscultation. This technique requires the use of a stethoscope; a manometer, which may be either aneroid or mercury; and an inflatable cuff of the appropriate width and length. Recommended cuff and bladder dimensions are the following (6):

1. Child (arm girth 13–20 cm): 8 cm wide × 27.5 cm long
2. Adult (arm girth 24–32 cm): 14 cm wide × 54 cm long
3. Large adult: (arm girth 32–42 cm): 17 cm wide × 63 cm long

Most cuffs have an arterial reference indicator near the center of the cuff, which is placed securely over the brachial artery. The lower edge of the cuff should be approximately 1 inch above the antecubital space on the frontal aspect of the elbow. The brachial artery courses through a groove formed by the bifurcation of the triceps and biceps brachii muscles on the medial aspect (inside) of the arm. It should be palpated with the first two fingers at the medial antecubital space, as this is the location for

A

B

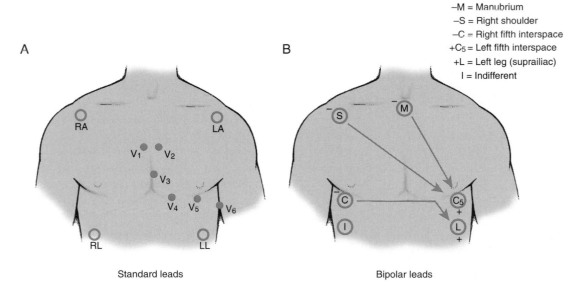

−M = Manubrium
−S = Right shoulder
−C = Right fifth interspace
+C₅ = Left fifth interspace
+L = Left leg (suprailiac)
I = Indifferent

Standard leads

Bipolar leads

Figure 10.9. Lead Placement. **A.** Standard placement. **B.** Bipolar placement.

the diaphragm of the head of the stethoscope. The stethoscope head should be held firmly in this position with moderate pressure. Generally there are nominal differences in blood pressures taken on right or left arms. In addition, novices find it helpful in taking blood pressures during exercise tests to mark the location of the stethoscope head for quick repositioning. The positions of the stethoscope head and pressure cuff are shown in Figure 10.10.

ANATOMICAL SITES FOR PERIPHERAL PULSES

Exercise professionals may measure peripheral pulses to obtain an index of resting heart rate, training bradycardia, or aerobic exercise intensity. Large, superficial arteries are preferred for pulse determination, since they are easily palpable. Two conventional palpation sites are the common carotid and radial arteries.

Carotid Pulse

The right and left common carotid arteries are located on the anterior portion of the neck in the groove formed by the larynx (Adam's apple) and the sternocleidomastoid muscles (large muscles on the lateral sides of the neck) just below the mandible (lower jaw) (1). The carotid pulse is taken by placing the first two fingers in the groove and pressing gently inward. An illustration of this site and technique may be seen in Figure 10.11. Take care when using this site, since baroreceptors in the carotid sinus may be sensitive to pressure and result in a reduction in heart rate in some individuals (7, 8). In extreme cases blood flow may be occluded to the point that light-headedness or fainting occurs. This is probably a concern

mainly when taking the pulse immediately after exercise, less so at rest or during activity (9).

Radial Pulse

The radial artery courses deep on the lateral (thumb side) aspect of the forearm and becomes superficial near the distal head of the radius (1). Gently pressing the first two fingers over this distal region palpates the radial

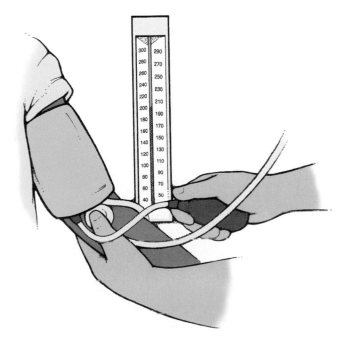

Figure 10.10. Positions of the stethoscope head and pressure cuff.

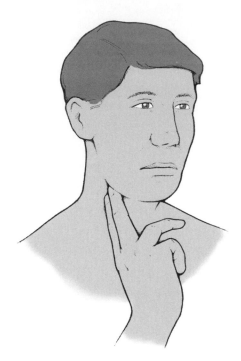

Figure 10.11. The carotid pulse, taken by placing the first two fingers in the groove and pressing gently inward.

pulse. Figure 10.12 illustrates this location. Radial pulses may be difficult to obtain in individuals with large amounts of subcutaneous fat over the palpation site.

Other Pulse Sites

Pulses may be taken at any arterial site. The location and palpation of the brachial artery was presented in the section on blood pressure. Other arterial palpation sites

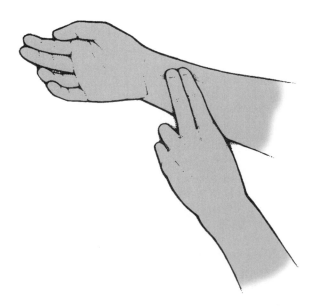

Figure 10.12. Palpation of the radial pulse. Place the first two fingers over this region and gently press.

include temporal (temple region of skull), popliteal (behind the knee), femoral (inguinal fold of groin), and dorsal pedis (top of foot). Lower extremity pulses may provide information regarding the adequacy of peripheral blood flow.

Taking Pulses

The number of seconds a pulse is counted depends on the purpose of the pulse count and the degree of accuracy needed. For instance, during a 6-second pulse count, an error of 1 beat translates to an error of 10 beats per minute (bpm); during a 10-second count, a one-beat error equals a 6-bpm error; and during a 15-second count, a one-beat error means a four-bpm error. At rest and during exercise, 15-second pulse counts are advisable, although it is difficult to obtain a pulse count during many forms of exercise. Therefore, the exerciser may have to stop and take a pulse immediately post exercise. Because heart rates decrease quickly after exercise, a 6-second or 10-second pulse count is suggested.

ANATOMICAL SITES FOR ANTHROPOMETRIC MEASUREMENTS

Anthropometry is the science of measuring the human body using external body dimensions. These measures include weight, height, skinfold thickness, and body diameters, lengths, and girths. In the case of body composition (the distribution of fat and fat-free tissue), what may be measured externally is related to the distribution of fat to fat-free tissue. Therefore, estimations of body composition can be obtained using two or three simple measurements. Equations predicting body composition based on anthropometric measurements are only estimates of values that would be attained with a laboratory technique (10). Selected locations for these assessments are presented here.

Skinfold Thickness

Approximately 50% of body fat is subcutaneous. Therefore, differences in skinfold thickness may be used to estimate the total amount of body fat. All skinfolds should be taken on the right side. Two to three measurements should be obtained at each site, averaging those that are within 1 mm of one another. The following are anatomical locations for selected skinfold sites (5):

1. Abdominal: vertical fold 2 cm to the right of the umbilicus (Fig. 10.13).
2. Biceps: vertical fold on the anterior aspect of the arm over the belly of the biceps muscle 1 cm above the level used to mark the triceps site (Fig. 10.14).
3. Chest–pectoral: diagonal fold half the distance between the anterior axillary line and the nipple (men) or one-third of the distance between the anterior axillary line and the nipple (women) (Fig. 10.15).

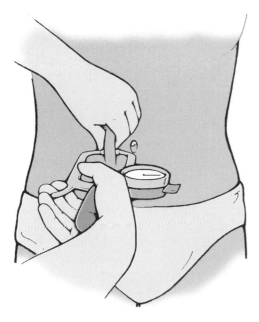

Figure 10.13. Abdominal: vertical fold 2 cm to the right of the umbilicus.

4. Medial calf: vertical fold at the maximum girth of the calf on the midline of the medial border (Fig. 10.16).
5. Midaxillary: vertical fold on the midaxillary line at the level of the xiphoid process of the sternum (Fig. 10.17).
6. Subscapular: diagonal fold (45° angle) 1 to 2 cm below the inferior angle of the scapula (Fig. 10.18).
7. Suprailiac: diagonal fold in line with the natural an-

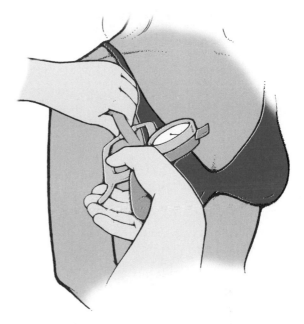

Figure 10.15. Chest–pectoral: diagonal fold half the distance between the anterior axillary line and the nipple (men) or one-third of the distance between the anterior axillary line and the nipple (women).

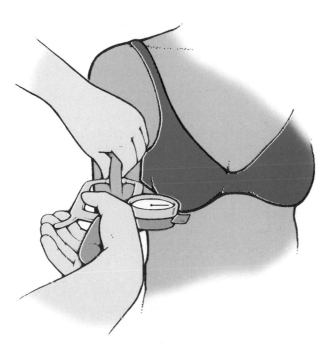

Figure 10.14. Biceps: vertical fold on the anterior aspect of the arm over the belly of the biceps muscle; 1 cm above the level used to mark the triceps site.

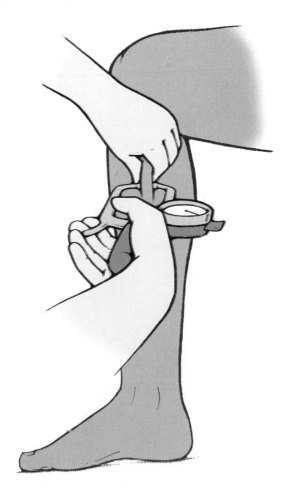

Figure 10.16. Medial calf: vertical fold at the maximum girth of the calf on the midline of the medial border.

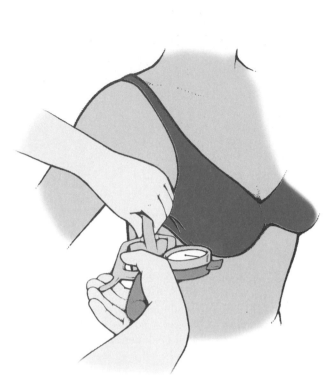

Figure 10.17. Midaxillary: vertical fold on the midaxillary line at the level of the xiphoid process of the sternum.

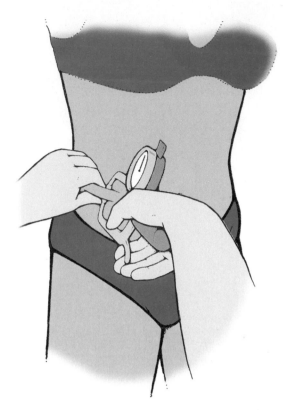

Figure 10.19. Suprailiac: diagonal fold in line with the natural angle of the iliac crest taken in the anterior axillary line immediately superior to the iliac crest.

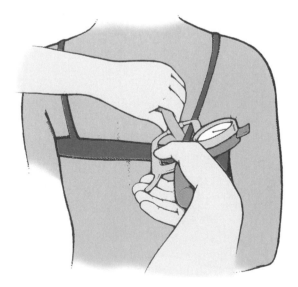

Figure 10.18. Subscapular: diagonal fold (45°) 1 to 2 cm below the inferior angle of the scapula.

gle of the iliac crest taken in the anterior axillary line immediately superior to the iliac crest (Fig. 10.19).

8. Thigh: vertical fold on the anterior midline of the thigh midway between the proximal border of the patella and the inguinal fold (Fig. 10.20).

Triceps: vertical fold on the posterior midline of the upper arm halfway between the acromion and olecranon processes, with the arm held freely to the side (Fig. 10.21).

Body Circumferences

All girths should be taken on the right side of the body with a tension-regulated fiberglass or metal tape. Two to three measurements should be obtained at each site, averaging those that are within 1 cm of one another. The following are anatomical locations for selected girth sites (5):

1. Abdomen: at the level of the umbilicus (Fig. 10.22).
2. Arm: with the subject's arm to the side of the body, midway between the acromion and olecranon processes (Fig. 10.23).
3. Calf: at the maximum girth between the knee and ankle joint (Fig. 10.24).

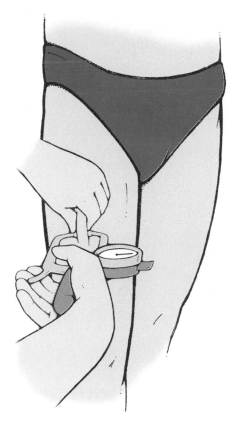

Figure 10.20. Thigh: vertical fold on the anterior midline of the thigh, midway between the proximal border of the patella and the inguinal fold.

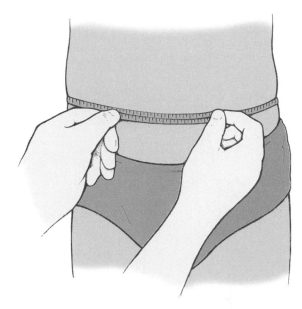

Figure 10.22. Abdomen: at the level of the umbilicus.

4. Forearm: with the arms hanging down but slightly away from the trunk and palms facing forward at the maximum forearm girth (Fig. 10.25).
5. Hips: at the maximal girth of the hips or buttocks region, whichever is larger (above the gluteal fold) (Fig. 10.26).
6. Thigh: with the subject's legs slightly apart, at the maximal girth of the thigh (below the gluteal fold) (Fig. 10.27).
7. Waist: at the narrowest part of the torso (above the umbilicus and below the xiphoid process (Fig. 10.28).

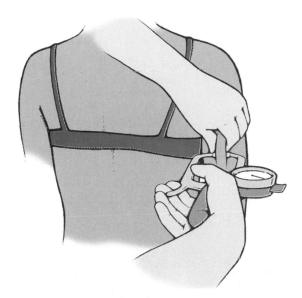

Figure 10.21. Triceps: vertical fold on the posterior midline of the upper arm halfway between the acromion and the olecranon processes, with the arm held freely at the side.

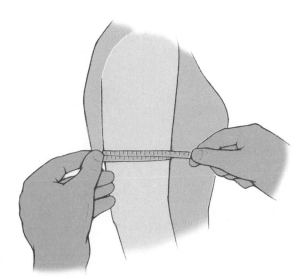

Figure 10.23. Arm: midway between the acromion and olecranon processes with the arm in anatomical position.

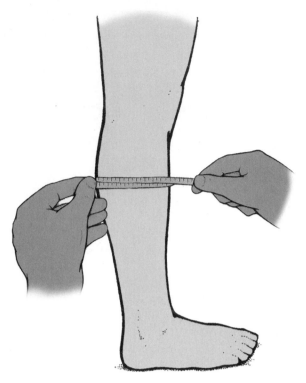

Figure 10.24. Calf: at the maximum girth between the knee and ankle joint.

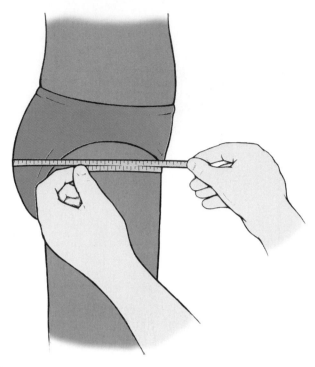

Figure 10.26. Hips: at the maximal girth of the hips or buttocks region above the gluteal fold.

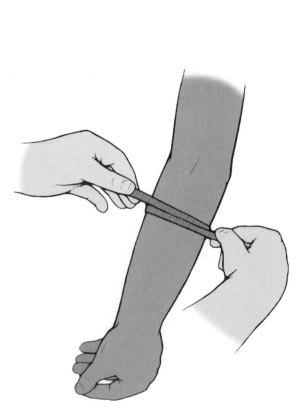

Figure 10.25. Forearm: at maximum forearm girth with the arms hanging down and slightly away from the trunk, palms facing forward.

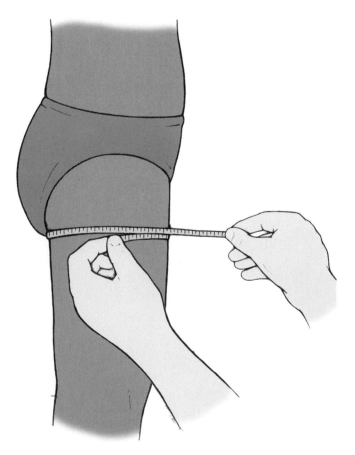

Figure 10.27. Thigh: at the maximal girth of the thigh below the gluteal fold with the legs slightly apart.

ANATOMICAL LANDMARKS FOR CARDIOPULMONARY RESUSCITATION AND ELECTRICAL DEFIBRILLATION

In rare instances exercise professionals have to manage a cardiac emergency. All such personnel should be trained in cardiopulmonary resuscitation (CPR) and institutional procedures for handling emergencies. These skills should be routinely practiced. The following are descriptions of landmarks used for CPR and electrical defibrillation.

CPR

The American Heart Association (11) recommends the following procedures to determine the correct hand position for cardiac compressions. Trace along the lower border of the rib cage with the middle and index fingers up to the xiphoid notch. The middle finger should be placed in the notch and the index finger next to it to avoid placing any direct compressive force on the xiphoid process. The heel of the opposite hand should be positioned next to the index finger on the body of the sternum. Once the hand is positioned, the heel of the other hand is placed on top of it. The rescuer should compress the chest vertically with the fingers interlaced. The correct hand position is shown in Figure 10.29.

Electrical Defibrillation

The standard placement for defibrillation electrodes is one immediately to the right of the upper part of the sternum below the clavicle and the other to the left and 1–2 inches below the left nipple with the electrode center in the midaxillary line. These sites may be seen in Figure

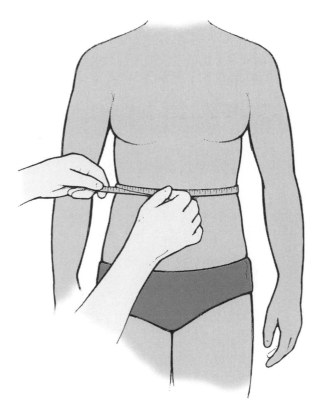

Figure 10.28. Waist: at the narrowest part of the torso (above the umbilicus and below the xiphoid process).

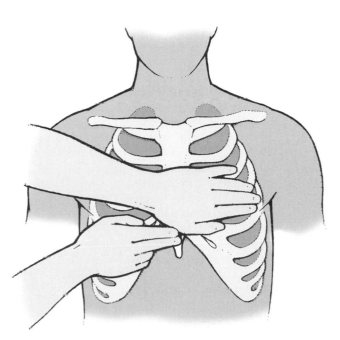

Figure 10.29. The correct hand position for cardiac compressions.

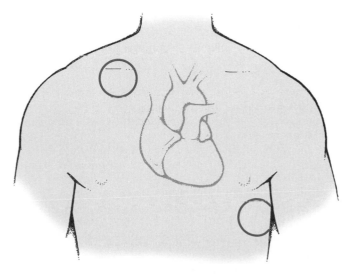

Figure 10.30. The standard placement for defibrillation electrodes. One is applied immediately to the right of the upper part of the sternum below the clavicle and the other to the left of the nipple with the electrode center in the midaxillary line.

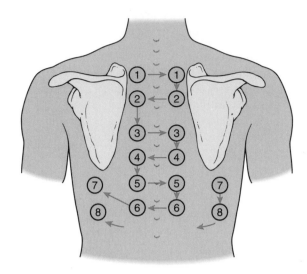

Figure 10.31. Standard regions for auscultation for lung sounds.

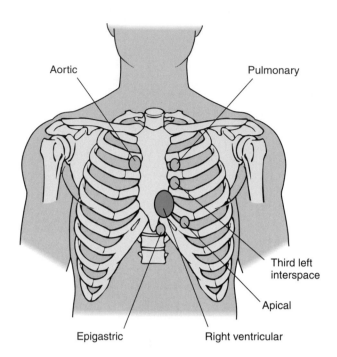

Figure 10.32. Standard regions for auscultation for heart sounds.

10.30. Another acceptable configuration is the anterior electrode over the left apex of the heart and the posterior one in the right infrascapular region. When performing defibrillation on individuals with permanent pacemakers, avoid placing electrodes near the pacemaker generator to circumvent damage or malfunction (11).

Auscultation Regions of the Chest

Exercise professionals may be required to perform auscultation of the chest to listen to heart and lung sounds and murmurs. Standard regions for auscultating the chest for lung sounds can be seen in Figure 10.31, and regions for the heart can be seen in Figure 10.32 (12).

References
1. Spence AP, Reading MA: Basic Human Anatomy. 3rd ed. Redwood, CA: Benjamin/Cummings, 1991.
2. Cooper JM, Adrian M, Glassow RB. Kinesiology. St. Louis: Mosby, 1982.
3. Hanson P. Clinical exercise testing. In: Strauss RH, ed. Sports Medicine. Philadelphia: Saunders, 1984.
4. Froelicher VF, Myers J. Exercise and the Heart. Philadelphia: Saunders, 2000.
5. American College of Sports Medicine. Guidelines for Exercise Testing and Prescription. 6th ed. Baltimore: Williams & Wilkins, 2000.
6. Prisant LM, Alpert BS, Robbins CB, et al. American National Standard for nonautomated sphygmomanometry. Am J Hypertension 8:210–213, 1995.
7. White JR. EKG changes using carotid artery for heart rate monitoring. Med Sci Sports 9:88, 1977.
8. Boone T, Frentz KL, Boyd NR. Carotid palpation at two exercise intensities. Med Sci Sports Exerc 17:705, 1985.
9. Gardner GW, Danks DI, Scharfsienin L. Use of carotid pulse for heart rate monitoring. Med Sci Sports 11:111, 1979.
10. Lohman TG, Roche AF, Martorell R, eds. Anthropometric Standardization Reference Manual. Champaign, IL: Human Kinetics, 1991.
11. Handley AJ, Becker LB, Allen M, et al. Single-rescuer adult basic life support. Circulation 95:2174–2179, 1997.
12. Schull, P, ed. Assessment Made Incredibly Easy. Springhouse, PA: Springhouse, 1997.

Suggested Reading
Ellestad MH. Stress Testing: Principles and Practice. 4th ed. Philadelphia: Davis, 1995.

Golding LA, Meyers CR, Sinning WE, eds. Y's Way to Physical Fitness. Champaign, IL: Human Kinetics, 1989.

Marieb EN. Human Anatomy and Physiology, 4th ed. Redwood, CA: Benjamin/Cummings, 1992.

Maud PJ, Foster C, eds. Physiological Assessment of Human Fitness. Champaign, IL: Human Kinetics, 1995.

Nieman DC. Exercise Testing and Prescription. 4th ed. Mountain View, CA: Mayfield, 1998.

Reid JG, Thomson JM. Exercise Prescription for Fitness. Englewood Cliffs, NJ: Prentice-Hall, 1985.

Wilmore J, Costill D. Physiology of Sport and Exercise. 2nd ed. Champaign, IL: Human Kinetics, 1999.

SECTION THREE
BIOMECHANICS

SECTION EDITOR: Mark A. Williams, PhD, FACSM

CHAPTER **11**

MECHANICAL LOAD ON THE BODY

Joseph Hamill and Graham E. Caldwell

Biomechanics is the application of the principles of physics to the study of biological systems. A common focus of the discipline is the application of mechanics to human movement. While the human body is composed of a number of types of tissue, each one of these tissues is subjected to forces during motion. The forces to which these tissues are exposed are generally called loading, a collective term describing all external forces acting on the system.

BIOMECHANICAL PRINCIPLES

Forces and Torques

For movement of a segment of the body to occur, a force must be applied. A **force** is an interaction of two objects that produces a change in the state of motion of an object. A force may cause an object to move, to accelerate or decelerate, to change direction of movement, or to stop. A force has four characteristics, two of which are its vector quantities of magnitude and direction. The remaining two characteristics are the line of action and the point of application of the force. The point of application of a force is the location at which the force acts on the body. The line of action is the line passing through the point of application in the direction of the action. The unit of force is the newton. In most situations, multiple forces act concurrently on either a segment or the total body. In these cases, vector addition can be used to determine the magnitude and direction of a net force that is the sum of all concurrent forces. If an object is not moving but is static, the sum of the concurrent forces is equal to zero.

Depending upon how forces are applied, they may cause specific types of motion called (*a*) pure translation, or straight line motion; (*b*) pure rotation, or angular motion; or (*c*) general motion, which is a combination of translation and rotation. When a force is applied so that its line of action is directly through the center of mass of an object, the resulting motion is pure translation. When

pure translation occurs, all points of the mass move through the same distance in the same interval.

For pure rotation to take place, two equal and opposite forces must act at a distance from an axis of rotation and not through the center of mass of the body. The product of a force and the perpendicular distance from the line of action of the force to the axis of rotation (the **moment arm**) is called a **moment of force**, or **torque**. The most common unit of torque is the newton-meter (n·m). Each of the two forces results in a torque about the same axis of rotation, with each causing translation and rotation. Since the forces act in opposite directions, the translation from each force cancels the other. Pure rotation, however, results because each torque produces a rotation in the same direction. The pairs of forces arranged to produce pure rotation are a **force couple**.

In causing both translation and rotation, a force must be applied such that the line of action passes through any point other than the center of mass of a free body. Such a force, an eccentric force, results in a torque. A single force causing a torque results in both rotation and translation in the direction of the force application or general motion of the body. In most instances, the forces that act on the human body and result in movement are of this type. If the body is not free, rotation takes place when a force line of action does not pass through the axis of rotation at which the body is constrained. For example, muscles crossing a joint produce forces that cause segments to rotate about the joint.

Newton's Laws of Motion

The three laws of motion promulgated by Sir Isaac Newton (1642–1727) describe the interaction of forces on a body that result in movement. The first law is the **law of inertia**, which states, "a body continues in its state of rest, or of uniform motion in a straight line, unless a force acts upon it." Mathematically, this law can be expressed as follows: If $\Sigma F = 0$, then mv = constant; that is, if the sum of the forces acting on a body is zero, the product of mass

107

and velocity, known as linear momentum, does not change. For human motion the mass (m) is a constant, which means that the velocity (v) does not change. To produce motion of an object that is at rest, a force must be applied. Likewise, to stop or alter a motion, a force must be applied to the object. The inertia of an object describes the resistance to motion and is directly related to the amount of matter (mass) of the object.

The second law, the **law of acceleration**, states, "a body acted on by an external force moves such that the force is equal to the time rate of change of linear momentum." This gives us the expression $F = \Delta(mv) \div \Delta t$, where F is the net force, $\Delta(mv)$ is the change in linear momentum, and Δt is the change in time. However, mass is usually a constant, and the net force results in a change in velocity ($m\Delta v$). Therefore, this law is probably more commonly expressed as "a force applied to an object causes an acceleration ($\Delta v \div \Delta t$) of the object that is proportional to the force and inversely proportional to the mass of the object." This statement results in the well-known expression $F = ma$, where F is the net force acting on the object, m is the mass of the object, and a is the resulting acceleration of the object. This statement provides a cause-and-effect relationship. The force, F, can be thought of as the cause and the result can be thought of as the acceleration of the mass the force acts upon, ma.

Newton's third law, the **law of action–reaction**, states, "for every action there is an equal and opposite reaction." This law can be expressed mathematically as: $F_{AB} = -F_{BA}$. When objects A and B interact, object A produces an effect on B. In turn, the second object, B, produces an equal and opposite effect on A. This law illustrates that forces never act in isolation but always in pairs. For example, during locomotion, the foot exerts a force each time it contacts the ground. The ground, however, exerts an equal and opposite force on the foot. The force that the ground exerts on the individual is referred to as the **ground reaction force**.

FORCES ACTING DURING HUMAN MOVEMENT

Forces result from the interaction of biological systems and their environment. These forces have many classifications; those that are most often considered in the analysis of human movement are described next.

Body Weight

Gravity is the attractive force of the earth on an object, and the magnitude of this attraction is the **body weight** of the object. Since body weight is a force, it is measured in newtons. Body weight is proportional to mass because it is the product of the mass of the object and the acceleration due to gravity (9.81 m/s^2).

Ground Reaction Force

Contact between the human body and another object (e.g., catching a ball, carrying a suitcase, wearing ankle weights) results in the application of an **external force** on the human body, an example of Newton's law of action and reaction. A common external force is the **ground reaction force**, which is provided by the surface upon which the human moves. The ground reaction force changes in magnitude, direction, and point of application during the contact period with the surface and can be measured with a force platform. The ground reaction force can be resolved into orthogonal components, the vertical, anteroposterior, and mediolateral components. These components have a greater magnitude during running than during walking; the magnitude is also affected by the running speed (1). The ground reaction force is the net force acting at the center of an individual's mass; it reflects the force necessary to accelerate the total body center of mass.

Joint Reaction Force

In biomechanical analyses, a single segment is often examined isolated from other segments. In this case, the **joint reaction force** acting across a joint must be considered. According to Newton's third law, equal and opposite forces must act on each of the segments that constitute the joint. In most situations the magnitude of the joint reaction force is unknown but can be calculated given the appropriate kinematic, kinetic, and anthropometric data (2). The joint reaction force does not, however, reflect the actual force between the articular surfaces of the joint. This force, known as the **bone-on-bone force**, is the sum of the joint reaction force and the muscle, tendon, and ligament forces pulling the joint together. The bone-on-bone force is difficult to calculate because the joint reaction force must be combined with individual muscle and ligamentous forces that can only be estimated with computer models (3, 4).

Friction

Friction is a force acting parallel to two surfaces in contact; it acts in the opposite direction of the motion or impending motion (Fig. 11.1). **Translational friction** determines how much horizontal force is required to cause one surface to slide over the other surface. The friction force (F_f), which is proportional to the normal force between the surfaces, is expressed as $F_f = \mu N$, where μ is the **coefficient of friction** and N is the **normal force** (force perpendicular to the surface). The coefficient of friction is a dimensionless number, with larger numbers indicating a greater interaction between the surfaces. The maximum coefficient of friction of the impending motion is the static coefficient of friction; it is greater than the dynamic coefficient of friction measured when movement actually occurs. **Rotational friction** determines how much force

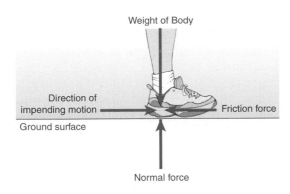

Figure 11.1. Translational friction force during foot contact of a running stride.

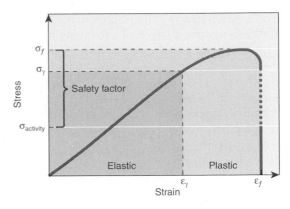

Figure 11.2. An idealized stress-strain curve. The elastic region is bounded by the yield point (designated by ϵ_y, σ_y). The plastic region is bounded by the yield point and the failure point (designated by ϵ_f, σ_f). The stress of normal activity is much less than either the yield or failure point. The difference between the yield and failure points is the safety factor. (Reprinted with permission from Biewener AA, ed. Biomechanics: Structures and Systems. Oxford, UK: Oxford University Press, 1992.)

must be applied as a torque to cause one surface to pivot on another. Rotational friction does not have a coefficient of friction but relies on the relative value of the **free moment of rotation** between the two surfaces. The free moment is generally calculated from force platform parameters and is defined as the moment about the vertical axis positioned at the center of pressure. The translational and rotational components of friction are not independent parameters.

Elastic Force

Elastic forces are generated by the tendency of a deformed material to return to its original state. The amount that a material can be stretched depends on the nature of the material and the magnitude of the force that stretches it. This relationship is described in the following equation: $\mathbf{F} = \mathbf{kx}$, where $\mathbf{F}$ is the force that stretches the material, $\mathbf{k}$ is the stiffness of the material, and $\mathbf{x}$ is the amount that the material was stretched. The stiffness of the material, ($\mathbf{k}$), ranges from very stiff (hard to deform) to very compliant (easy to deform).

The elasticity of biomaterials such as muscle, tendon, and ligament can be tested and the results plotted on a **stress–strain curve**. Stress (σ) is defined as the force per unit area, or the load; it is expressed in newtons/cm^2. Strain (ϵ) is defined as the change in length divided by the initial length and is expressed as a percent. Figure 11.2 illustrates an idealized stress–strain curve. When a biomaterial is stressed and remains below its yield point, that is, within its **elastic region**, it undergoes no permanent change. However, stressing the material so much that it is stretched into its **plastic region** makes permanent changes to the structure of the material. If the deformation continues, the material ultimately fails. The stress point in normal activity is generally much less than the yield point, and thus the difference between the stress point of normal activity and the failure point is regarded as the safety factor (5). Biomaterials that can be stretched are like a spring and can impart a force while they are deformed from their original length. This force, which is due to the potential energy stored in the spring, is referred to as an elastic force (6, 7).

Muscle Force

The role of muscles in the human body is to exert forces on the skeleton that result in a desired segmental posture or motion. A muscle is attached to the skeleton at its origin and insertion so that it spans one or more joints. A muscle can generate only a pulling or tensile force, but it pulls on both segments to which it is attached. When a muscle produces force, it also produces torque, because its line of action forms a moment arm with the joint axis of rotation. The moment arm depends on the joint geometry and in general changes as a function of the joint angle. The muscle torque tends to cause both segments to rotate around the joint crossed by the muscle.

The amount of force that a muscle can exert depends on the excitation it receives from the neural system and on mechanical factors related to length and velocity. The **force–velocity** relationship dictates that the magnitude of force depends on the rate of length change or velocity (8). When a muscle shortens (concentric contraction), the force generated is less than that of an isometric contraction (no change in length; velocity = 0) for the same level of muscle excitation. As the velocity of shortening increases, the amount of force that can be generated decreases. During eccentric (muscle lengthening) contractions, the generated force is greater than that of an isometric contraction. The **force–length** relationship indicates the isometric force that a muscle can exert at different muscle lengths for the same level of excitation (9). At an intermediate optimal length the muscle can produce its greatest force, with reductions in force capability as the muscle attains shorter or longer lengths.

Muscles rarely work in isolation because there are multiple muscles crossing most joints. In many biomechanical analyses, it is assumed that the muscle torque acting across a joint is the net torque of all individual muscles crossing the joint. For example, if the total summed torque from all flexor muscles is greater than the total torque from all extensor muscles, the net torque is flexor. The **net muscle torque** can be calculated using an inverse dynamics approach (10). Researchers and clinicians often assess joint function by determining the net torque that can be generated at each joint angle during an isometric contraction. These **torque–angle** curves illustrate that the torque varies as a function of joint angle (11, 12). The optimal joint angle, at which the net torque is the greatest, is a function of the muscle force–length relations and the moment arm–joint angle relations. The net joint torque can also be assessed as a function of joint angular velocity (13). The **torque–angular velocity** function is dictated by the muscle force–velocity and moment arm–joint angle relations. Instantaneous net muscle torque can also be calculated throughout the time course of dynamic human movements.

To compute the force in individual muscles requires a detailed musculoskeletal model in which the muscles, joints, skeleton, and nervous system are explicitly represented (4, 14). Muscles are often represented by Hill-type muscle models that combine an active contractile component (CC) with a passive series elastic component (SEC). (8) The CC responds to signals from the nervous system by producing force according to the force–velocity and force–length relations. This force is expressed across the SEC, which responds by extending according to its stress–strain curve. An optimization criterion or neural control model dictates the excitation signal each muscle receives, and the Hill models predict the force level of each individual muscle. Some researchers have placed force transducers directly on the tendon to measure muscle forces directly, but this technique is limited because of its invasive nature (15).

APPLICATIONS TO HUMAN MOVEMENT

It has been suggested that there is an optimal window of loading that healthy individuals should maintain and that loading above this window presents the risk of injury (16). However, this window has not been defined, and it is difficult to estimate the load on the body for various activities (17). Nevertheless, the result of the loading on the body depends on three factors: the magnitude of the force, the rate at which the force is applied, and the repetition of load application. During normal activity, the **magnitude of the force** on tissue is within a range that will not cause tissue (e.g., bone) to fail, as in trauma, and in fact, this magnitude of force can be associated with positive effects, particularly when **rate at which the force is applied** is also considered (18). The greater the rate of

loading, the more load can be withstood before failure. Loading rate is clinically relevant because it determines both the fracture pattern and the surrounding soft tissue damage at fracture.

The third factor is **load repetition**. Again, load repetition generally does not result in injury during normal activity, although it has been suggested that repeated impacts such as the collision of the foot with the ground during locomotion can result in microtrauma. To this point it has been reported that repeated impacts can cause trabecular microfractures and cartilage and knee joint degeneration that is consistent with osteoarthritis (19–21).

The human body has a number of mechanisms by which load is attenuated. These include structures such as the fat pads on the plantar surface of the foot, articular cartilage in the joints and bone, and soft tissue surrounding the bone. There are also particular motions of the segments that attenuate shock. In the lower extremity, these include knee flexion, subtalar pronation, and ankle dorsiflexion. Under normal conditions these motions are effective. However, it has been suggested that structural abnormalities in conjunction with repeated activity patterns result in injury. A person with a structural abnormality such as a forefoot varus, for example, has a greater likelihood of excessive motion at the subtalar joint (22). Excessive motion of the subtalar joint has been linked to soft tissue injuries of the knee (23). This research suggests that structural abnormalities cause a mistiming of the lower extremity joint actions, resulting in soft tissue injury. These injuries are not specifically related to the load imposed but are in response to the load imposed on misaligned structures.

One particular source of loading on the body is the ground reaction force. Figure 11.3 illustrates the vertical ground reaction force component during heel–toe running. The first peak on this curve, occurring within 50 ms of contact, is a high-frequency peak (>5 Hz), the **passive peak** or the **impact peak** (24). It is relatively high in magnitude; the loading rate is also very high. The second is a low-frequency peak (<5 Hz), the **active peak.** The active peak is a high-magnitude peak but with a relatively low loading rate. The impact peak has been related to both lower extremity injuries and further orthopaedic problems.

The vertical ground reaction force component has been reconstructed from positional data to gain a better understanding of the impact peak (25). Using this method, researchers partitioned the vertical ground reaction force component and related the contributions of various body segments to the total force. It was illustrated that the passive peak of the vertical component was mainly borne by the lower extremity of the support leg. Therefore, the lower extremity of the support leg was the major shock-bearing and shock-absorbing structure during running.

The impact force resulting from the collision of the foot and the ground produces acceleration in the body

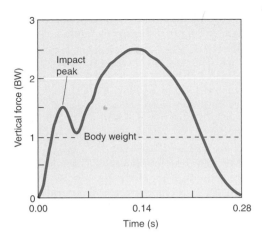

Figure 11.3. Vertical ground reaction force component during heel–toe running.

that is transmitted throughout the skeletal system in the form of a **shock wave**. This shock wave travels through the skeletal system much as a sound wave travels through a solid object, taking about 10 ms to reach the head. As the wave travels through the body, it is attenuated by the body structures and by the kinematics of the body. Figure 11.4 illustrates profiles of the impact shock on the distal medial tibia and the head during the support phase of a running stride. In these profiles, the input shock, measured in gravities (where $1\ G - 9.81\ m/s^2$), has a peak of 4 G, while the peak shock at the head is approximately 1 G.

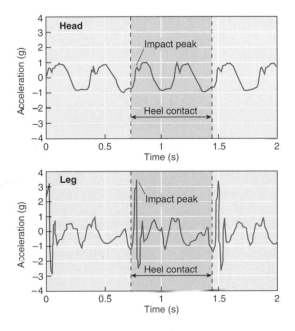

Figure 11.4. Impact shock on the leg and the corresponding shock on the head during heel–toe running.

The importance of attenuating the shock wave before it reaches the head may also have implications for the motor control of gait. If the level of the shock wave is not adequately attenuated, the shock wave may affect motion of the head. The head houses both the visual and the vestibular systems, which contribute environmental information that is essential for the organization of efficient gait. It has been postulated that an unattenuated shock wave would disrupt these systems and possibly impair the control of the locomotor pattern (26).

A number of factors influence the load on the body during locomotion. Increases in load can be seen in increased locomotor speed, in increased stride length at a constant speed, and in activities that produce high peak impact forces, such as running downhill. In downhill running, the center of mass of the runner falls a greater distance, resulting in a harder impact, and the lower extremity must absorb this added shock. The primary mechanism for attenuating this added impact is increased flexion of the knee during the initial portion of the support phase (27). Controlling this increased flexion are the quadriceps muscles of the anterior thigh. Although the quadriceps are knee extensors, they act eccentrically during this portion of support. Repeated eccentric activity over a prolonged period, such as with downhill running, has been related to myofibril and connective tissue damage. This damage has been linked to delayed-onset muscle soreness (28).

It would appear that altering kinematics may reduce the impact force to the system. As was suggested previously, increasing the degree of knee flexion is one possibility. However, there are trade-offs to this strategy. As an example, increasing the knee flexion angle at midstance (so-called Groucho running) indeed reduces the impact shock on the body; the shock transmission from the ankle to the head is decreased to less than 20% of its original value (29). However, the cost of such a strategy is an increased rate of energy use to the point that this style of running is responsible for a 50% increase in steady-state oxygen consumption.

The load on the human body may appear to be deleterious to the various tissues, but loading can also be beneficial. Bone has the ability to alter its size, shape, and structure to meet the demands of loads. Thus, bone can gain or lose cancellous and cortical tissue in response to the level of the stress placed on it. For example, body weight and bone mass are positively correlated (30). Increasing body weight increases bone mass because the added weight constitutes an added mechanical stress on the bone. On the other hand, prolonged weightlessness, such as that of space travel, has been found to decrease bone mass (31). Similarly, when there is a partial or total immobilization of the lower extremity, the limb is not subjected to the normal mechanical stresses, and bone is absorbed.

▶ **SUMMARY**

Force is the interaction of an object with its surroundings. Newton's three laws of motion form the basis for classical mechanics and explain the interactions between objects. The mechanical load on the human system is defined as the sum of the external forces on the system. The forces that constitute the load on the system depend on how the system is defined. For the most part, these are (*a*) body weight, (*b*) ground reaction force, (*c*) joint reaction force, (*d*) elastic force, and (*e*) muscle force.

External forces applied to the body (loading) depend on three factors: the magnitude of the force, the rate at which the force is applied, and the repetition of load application. The load on the system can have both a deleterious effect, causing injury or degeneration of the musculoskeletal system, and a beneficial effect, such as in the remodeling of bone. Fortunately, in the case of the former, the human body has a number of mechanisms by which load can be attenuated.

References

1. Munro CF, Miller DI, Fuglevand AJ. Ground reaction forces in running: A reexamination. J Biomech 20:147–155, 1987.
2. Winter DA. Moments of force and mechanical power in jogging. J Biomech 16:91–97, 1983.
3. An KN, Kwak BM, Chao EY, Morrey BF. Determination of muscle and joint forces: A new technique to solve the indeterminate problem. J Biomech Eng 106:364–367, 1984.
4. Caldwell GE, Chapman AE. The general distribution problem: A physiological solution which includes antagonism. Hum Move Sci 10:355–392.
5. Biewener AA, ed. Biomechanics: Structures and Systems. Oxford, UK: Oxford University Press, 1992.
6. Asmussen E, Bonde-Peterson F. Apparent efficiency and storage of elastic energy in human muscles during exercise. Acta Physiol Scand 92:537–545, 1974.
7. Komi PV, Bosco C. Utilization of stored elastic energy in leg extensor muscles by men and women. Med Sci Sports Exerc 10:261–265, 1978.
8. Hill AV. The heat of shortening and the dynamic constants of muscle. Proc R Soc 126:136–195, 1938.
9. Gordon AM, Huxley AF, Julian JF. The variation in isometric tension with sarcomere length in vertebrate muscle fibres. J Physiol 184:170–192, 1966.
10. Paul JP. Bioengineering studies of the forces transmitted by joints, 2. In: Kenedi RM, ed. Biomechanics and Related Bioengineering Topics. Oxford, UK: Pergamon Press, 1965.
11. Marsh E, Sale DG, McComas AJ, Quinlan J. The influence of joint position on ankle dorsiflexion in humans. J Appl Physiol 51:160–167, 1981.
12. Sale DG, Quinlan J, Marsh E, et al. Influence of joint position on ankle plantar flexion in humans. J Appl Physiol 52:1636–1642, 1982.
13. Wilkie DR. The relation between force and velocity in human muscle. J Physiol 110:249–280, 1950.
14. Crowninshield RD, Brand RA. A physiologically based criterion of muscle force prediction in locomotion. J Biomech 14:793–801, 1981.
15. Gregor RJ, Komi PV, Jarvinen M. Achilles tendon forces during cycling. Int J Sport Med 8:9–14, 1987.
16. Nigg BM, Cole GK, Bruggeman GP. Impact forces during heel–toe running. J Appl Biomech 11:407–432, 1995.
17. Forwood MR, Burr DB. Physical activity and bone mass: Exercise in futility? Bone Min 21:89–112, 1993.
18. Nordin M, Frankel VH. Basic Biomechanics of the Musculoskeletal System. 2nd ed. Philadelphia: Lea & Febiger, 1989.
19. Simon SR, Radin EL, Paul IL, Rose RM. The response of joints to impact loading: 2. In vivo behavior of subchondral bone. J Biomech 5:267–272, 1972.
20. Radin E L, Parker HG, Pugh JW, et al. Response of joints to impact loading: 3. J Biomech 6:51–57, 1973.
21. Voloshin A, Wosk J. An in vivo study of low back pain and shock absorption in the human locomotor system. J Biomech 15:21–27, 1982.
22. Holt KG, Hamill J. Running injuries and treatment: A dynamic approach. In: Sammarco GJ, ed. Rehabilitation of the Foot and Ankle. St. Louis: Mosby, 1995:241–258.
23. Hamill J, Bates BT, Holt KG. Timing of lower extremity joint actions during treadmill running. Med Sci Sports Exerc 24:807–813, 1992.
24. Nigg BM. Biomechanical aspects of running. In: Nigg BM, ed. Biomechanics of Running Shoes. Champaign, IL: Human Kinetics, 1986:1–25.
25. Bobbert MF, Yeadon MR, Nigg BM. Calculation of vertical ground reaction force estimates during running from positional data. J Biomech 24:1095–1105, 1991.
26. Hamill J, Derrick TR, Holt KG. Shock attenuation and stride frequency during running. Hum Move Sci 14:45–60, 1995.
27. Buczek FL, Cavanagh PR. Stance phase knee and ankle kinematics and kinetics during level and downhill running. Med Sci Sports Exerc 22:669–677, 1990.
28. Schwane JA, Johnson SR, Vandenakker CB, Armstrong RB. Delayed-onset muscular soreness and plasma CPK and LDH activities after downhill running. Med Sci Sports Exerc 15:51–56, 1983.
29. McMahon TA, Valiant G, Frederick EC. Groucho running. J Appl Physiol 62:2326–2337, 1987.
30. Exner GU, Prader A, Elasser U, et al. Bone densitometry using computed tomography: 1. Selected determination of trabecular bone density and other bone mineral parameters. Normal values in children and adults. Br J Radiol 52:14–23, 1979.
31. Rambaut PC, Johnston RS. Prolonged weightlessness and calcium loss in man. Acta Astronautica 6:1113–1122, 1979.

CHAPTER **12**

BIOMECHANICS AND PHYSIOLOGY OF POSTURE AND GAIT

Mark D. Grabiner and Philip E. Martin

Maintenance of posture and locomotion are, to varying degrees, critical components of all land-based exercise and athletic activities. The biomechanics and physiology of posture and locomotion have been among the most extensively studied of human activities. This chapter (*a*) introduces the exercise professional to biomechanical and physiological issues associated with postural control and gait and (*b*) provides a basis for understanding the experimental methods used to make quantitative biomechanical and physiological measurements associated with postural control and gait, the outcome variables, the interpretation of the variables, and the limitations of the interpretations. The reference list provides sources through which detailed treatment of many of the concepts may be explored. The first part of this chapter presents a framework of biomechanical fundamentals as they relate to the biomechanics of postural control and postural stability. The second part of this chapter presents some of the basic relationships between the biomechanics and physiology of gait, specifically as they relate to the topic of economy.

POSTURAL CONTROL AND STABILITY

The human tasks that include standing, walking, and running share many common neuromuscular and biomechanical mechanisms to which other motor tasks are subservient. Two of these mechanisms are postural control and stability.

Postural Control

Postural control is the ability to predict, detect, and encode changes in posture; select and adapt a response; and execute the response within the biomechanical constraints of the body and the physical constraints of the environment (1). The extent to which these processes are effective manifests as postural stability. Three common conditions during which the postural control system must function include maintaining postural stability against the force of gravity; maintaining postural stability

in the presence of self-initiated motions, such as lifting a weight; and maintaining postural stability in response to externally applied loads or forces, such as walking into a fixed object.

Postural control depends on the vestibular, visual, and somatosensory systems, which provide feedback to the central nervous system (CNS). This feedback, processed by the CNS, is used to generate muscle activation signals necessary for postural corrections. The vestibular (and otolith) system feedback, housed in the inner ear, provides information related to head position and motion with respect to gravity. The visual system provides information related to head position and motion relative to an external coordinate system. The somatosensory system provides information related to the position and motion of joints. Mechanoreceptors in the skin, for example those in the plantar surface of the foot, provide information regarding pressure that is used to accommodate postural sway that occurs while standing.

The systems that provide postural feedback are redundant. The CNS must decode the incoming signals to determine the status of the system. For example, for a person in a car, the movement of another vehicle detected with peripheral vision indicates only general motion. Often one cannot immediately determine whether the perceived motion is that of the vehicle in which one is seated or that of the second vehicle. However, without shifting the gaze, the person can use feedback from the vestibular and sensorimotor systems to determine whether the perceived motion can be attributed to motion of the vehicle in which the person is riding.

Postural Stability

The term stability broadly refers to whether a system (body) returns to its original stable position or motion or another stable position or motion after it is subjected to a perturbation (disturbance). In humans, the term postural stability generally refers to standing upright. It has traditionally been characterized as a relationship between the center of gravity or center of pressure (measured, for example, with a force plate) and the base of support. The base of support is defined by the size and shape of the contact area defined by the body segments that are in contact with the supporting surface. If the horizontal center of gravity or center of pressure is within the boundaries of the base of support, the basic requirement for static postural stability is satisfied.

The location of the center of gravity is a function of the mass of the body and the manner in which the mass is distributed or oriented. For example, the center of gravity shifts anteriorly and superiorly when the shoulder joint flexes 90°. From a practical standpoint, estimation of the location of the center of gravity can be time consuming and associated with error. Fortunately, the use of force plates makes the quantification of static postural stability fairly straightforward. Quantifying postural stability using force plate data relies to a great extent on determining the center of pressure rather than the center of gravity. The center of pressure is the location on the surface of a force plate through which the resultant force acts. Motion of the center of pressure reflects but does not mirror motion of the center of gravity. However, when the center of pressure lies within the boundaries of the base of support, the basic requirements for static postural stability are satisfied.

Numerous laboratory and clinical tests are available for measuring postural control and postural stability, although there are numerous challenges (2). Laboratory tests have been criticized as having little clinical application and in some cases little biomechanical application. On the other hand, clinical tests have been criticized as having less than satisfactory sensitivity. An example of such difficulties is the general acceptance that physiological changes associated with normal aging result in an increase in the amplitude of static postural sway and that increased postural sway is associated with the increased incidence of falling in older adults. Recent scientific investigation does not necessarily support these contentions. Postural sway and measures of static and dynamic measures of postural control were found to be weakly correlated to the ability of healthy older men and women to recover their balance when subjected to large postural perturbations that required stepping responses (3). These findings demonstrate that the association between increased age-related postural sway and the increased incidence of falling in older adults is not entirely causal. In particular, the data generally suggest that the extent to which the subject becomes posturally unstable as a result of a postural insult is independent of whether the stepping response, if required, will be successful.

Dynamic Posturography

Clinically, it is important to assess the status of the vestibular, visual, and somatosensory components of the postural control system, individually and as an integrated whole. A measurement standard for this purpose is called dynamic posturography (4). Dynamic posturography uses a computer-controlled platform on which the subject stands. A visual surround that provides a consistent visual stimulus to the subject and at the same time visually isolates the subject from the environment encloses the platform. Both the platform on which the subject stands and the visual surround may be moved, under control of the computer. Motion of the platform and the visual surround alters the fidelity of the sensory feedback and thus influences postural stability. Systematic manipulation of the feedback allows derivation of the relative contribution of each feedback system to postural stability.

The sensory organization test (SOT) assesses the three sensory systems that contribute to postural control by manipulating the visual and support surface conditions. There are six conditions in the SOT:

- Eyes open, fixed support surface. During this test, all sensory systems contribute to postural control.
- Eyes closed, fixed support system. During this test the contribution of the visual system to postural control is eliminated.
- Sway-referenced vision, fixed support surface. During this test the contribution of the visual system to postural control is inaccurate.
- Sway-referenced support surface, normal vision. During this test the contribution of the somatosensory system to postural control is inaccurate.
- Eyes closed, sway-referenced support surface. During this test the contribution of the visual and somatosensory systems to postural control are eliminated and inaccurate, respectively.
- Sway-referenced vision and support surface: During this test the contribution of the visual and somatosensory systems to postural control are inaccurate.

An equilibrium quotient (EQ) for each system manipulation is computed and used as an index of postural stability. Systematic reduction of sensory feedback has a substantial effect on the EQ, and age amplifies the effects of the SOT conditions. Diminishing somatosensory feedback (sway referencing) results in a larger reduction of the EQ than does eliminating visual feedback. The largest EQ reduction appears to be elicited when the vestibular system is taxed to the greatest extent.

The balance strategy score (BSS) is also computed for the SOT conditions. The BSS relates to the motor pattern used by a subject to maintain postural stability after a postural perturbation. There are three basic motor strategies for correction of anteroposterior postural perturbations: the ankle strategy, the hip strategy, and the stepping strategy. The specific strategy selected by normal adults depends on the surface upon which the subject is standing and the magnitude of the perturbation. The ankle strategy, which is the most commonly implemented, controls body sway by generating moments about the ankle joint.

The ankle strategy is effective when the support surface is large and firm enough to resist the ankle's movements. Normally the ankle strategy is used to counteract perturbations that are applied slowly and that have low magnitude. An ankle strategy is most useful when the amplitude of body sway does not approach the limit of stability, the point at which a loss of balance is likely. A hip strategy is used in response to larger, more rapidly applied perturbations occurring when the support surface is compliant or smaller than the surfaces of the feet. A hip strategy is employed quite often when a loss of balance is imminent. When neither ankle nor hip strategy can restore postural stability, a stepping response is executed. If executed correctly, the stepping response establishes a new base of support and restores posture stability.

Lastly, dynamic posturography includes a motor coordination test (MCT). During the MCT, large anterior and posterior translations and toes-up and toes-down rotations are applied to the subject. This is achieved by causing the platform on which the subject stands to translate and rotate, respectively. The purpose of the MCT is to assess the activation of the lower extremity and trunk muscles that are stretched by the platform motion and to assess which muscles contribute to the restoration of postural stability. For example, an ankle strategy in response to a perturbation that rotates the subject forward (a backward surface translation) is associated with a distal-to-proximal activation pattern of the posterior ankle, thigh, and trunk muscles. However, a hip strategy associated with a perturbation in the same direction elicits activation of anterior trunk and thigh muscles. Both normal aging and neuromuscular disorders can substantially affect the sequence of muscle activation in response to specific perturbations and the activation latencies (from perturbation to onset of muscle activation).

While dynamic posturography measures postural stability during static upright posture and is considered a gold standard, true measurement of dynamic postural stability is elusive. This is because the easily quantified criterion for static stability (center of pressure within the boundaries of the base of support) is not easily applied to dynamic conditions. For example, during walking, specifically during the swing phase of gait, the center of pressure falls outside of the boundaries of the support foot for up to 80% of the time. A body is considered dynamically stable if active and passive disturbances can be predicted and detected, if responses to the disturbances can be selected, and if the selected responses can be executed. However, unlike static postural stability, dynamic stability has not been defined mathematically. Given that most falls and injuries occur during gait, ascending or descending stairs, or rising from chairs, it seems reasonable, if not expedient, to include dynamic motor tasks in the description of postural stability (1).

The numerous measurement techniques, instruments, and variables confront the exercise practitioner with a problem: the availability of many expedient measurement methods and the inability to generalize from constrained testing conditions to conditions of daily living. Guidelines that are useful in decision making have been developed. The guidelines govern the selection of the task or tasks, perturbation or perturbations, and outcome variables (5). The tasks should represent the normal spectrum of movement and in particular should challenge the postural control system. Similarly, the selection of the perturbation should be based upon the extent to which the system is challenged and to which type of feedback is provided regarding the performance of the postural control system. Outcome variables should be selected according to the ability to identify performance deficits and provide diagnostic information. However, these recommendations represent the ideal and serve as a goal for research. For the exercise professional, they serve as a reminder that effective measurement, interpretation, and application of postural control data are difficult.

RELATIONSHIPS BETWEEN ECONOMY AND LOCOMOTION BIOMECHANICS

Three major considerations influence the relationship between economy and locomotion biomechanics. These include interindividual variation in movement economy, speed of movement, and stride length and rate. Each of these will be discussed in this section.

Interindividual Variation in Movement Economy

Economy is measured by the steady-state oxygen consumption for a given submaximal task. This measure of the aerobic demand is typically normalized to the body mass of the individual, particularly for tasks in which upright posture must be maintained and body weight supported by the musculature. This measure is expressed as milliliters of oxygen consumed per unit of body mass (usually in kilograms) per minute of exercise. Occasionally economy is expressed per unit of distance traveled (e.g., milliliters per kilometer per kilogram) when comparing the economy for different speeds of movement, such as different walking or running speeds. Numerous research reports have demonstrated that the economy of motion for a given task tends to vary widely among individuals. It should be stressed that this between-individual variation in economy is independent of neurological and musculoskeletal deficiencies and diseases that may have large deleterious effects on movement economy.

In describing normal variation in economy among a group of young, healthy adults by correlating the aerobic demands observed for one task against those for another task, Daniels et al. noted that individuals clearly were neither economical nor uneconomical for all types of physical activity (6). Economy tends to be task specific and thus may be governed in part by biomechanical factors that define the movement technique used by an individual to perform a certain task.

Despite the commonly held belief that biomechanical factors help to explain economy differences between individuals, the extent to which these differences can be attributed to biomechanics is not well defined. Assuming that selected biomechanical factors are related to movement economy, the subsequent question is whether lasting changes in movement patterns can be produced so that movement economy is improved. The following sections highlight the observed relationships between movement economy and a few selected kinematic, kinetic, and structural factors and the practical implications of these relationships for measuring economy and prescribing exercise. The reader is referred to published reviews for further information on the topic (7–9).

Speed of Movement

The speed at which an individual moves is one of the simplest and most fundamental biomechanical descriptors of movement. As an example, preferred walking speed is a good indicator of the debilitating effects caused by knee injury and of the general decline in physical performance capabilities of elderly adults (10, 11). Thus, preferred walking speed should not be overlooked as one simple marker that offers insight into the movement capabilities of individuals, especially those whose exercise capacity has been limited by disease, injury, and/or normal aging. The average preferred walking speed of healthy young adults is approximately 1.45 m/second, while that for healthy elderly adults (approximately 70 years of age) is about 1.3 m/second. The preferred walking speed of young and old adults has also been shown to be subtly associated with physical activity status. Individuals pursuing a physically active lifestyle tend to walk slightly faster (approximately 0.1 to 0.2 m/second faster) than sedentary individuals (12).

It is obvious that increasing the speed of movement results in increased rates of oxygen consumption for both walking and running. Altering the speed of walking or running is one of the most common ways of modifying the intensity of the task in exercise evaluations. Many economy comparisons between individuals or groups presented in the research literature have been made at fixed speeds of walking or running, with aerobic demand expressed in milliliters per minute per kilogram. Any confounding effect of speed on economy comparisons is eliminated through use of a common test speed. On the other hand, having subjects walk or run at a preferred speed during an economy or biomechanical evaluation of gait has the appeal of assessing them under exercise conditions that are typical for them and that are within their exercise capabilities.

One problem of using preferred speeds of locomotion during gait evaluations is that there is a speed-related confounder that cannot be ignored. From an economy perspective, a U-shaped speed–economy relationship (Fig. 12.1) for walking exists when aerobic demands for a wide range of walking speeds are expressed relative to distance traveled (milliliters of oxygen per kilogram per kilometer). In other words, there is a speed of walking (approximately 1.25 to 1.35 m/second) for adults that minimizes the aerobic demand required to walk a given distance (12, 13). At walking speeds both higher and lower than this intermediate speed, the cost to traverse a given distance is increased. This effect of speed is most apparent at particularly low and high speeds of walking. For example, Ralston (13) observed that energy expenditure (calories per kilogram per meter) was minimized at approximately 1.25 m/second but that the speed–energy expenditure curve was nearly flat at approximately 1.1 to 1.4 m/second.

Figure 12.1. The aerobic demand to walk a given distance (milliliters per kilogram per kilometer) is affected substantially by walking speed. The most economical walking speed is approximately 1.25 to 1.35 m/second. In contrast, the aerobic demand to run a given distance is affected minimally by speed.

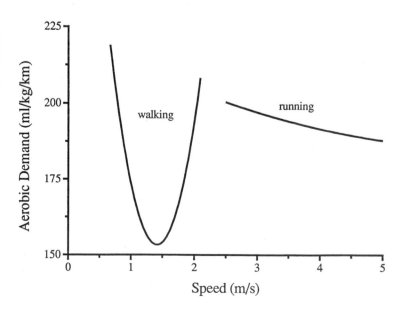

In contrast to walking, the energy cost to run a given distance is reasonably similar for a given individual across a range of running speeds. While Figure 12.1 suggests that there is a subtle decline in the aerobic demand per kilometer traveled as running speed increases, the slope of the speed–economy curve for running can vary somewhat from slightly negative, as shown, to slightly positive, depending on the individual subject, specific subject group, and range of speeds examined. The important point is that the speed confounder is far less of a concern when assessing running economy if the energy demand is met aerobically.

From a biomechanics perspective, comparing gait patterns becomes particularly challenging when comparisons are not being made at a common walking or running speed. The reason for this is that nearly all kinematic and kinetic descriptors of gait are speed dependent. For example, it is well established that as walking speed increases, factors such as stride length, joint angular velocities, peak values for ground reaction forces and net moments about joints of the lower extremity, and activation levels of numerous leg muscles all tend to increase, while other factors, such as stride time and related temporal descriptors of the gait pattern, tend to decrease. Thus, while existing technology and methods offer the potential to describe a wide range of biomechanical characteristics of walking or running patterns, assessing specific deficiencies in gait is compromised or at least substantially complicated by the absence of speed control.

Stride Length and Rate

Stride length is defined as the distance traveled by the body during one full cycle of motion (e.g., from the instant of left foot contact until the subsequent left foot contact). Stride rate or cadence, which is the reciprocal of stride time, indicates the number of strides completed per unit of time. The average speed or velocity of walking or running is simply the product of stride length and stride rate.

The effect that stride length and rate have on gait economy during steady-state, submaximal exercise lends itself to simple experimental assessment because of this relationship and the ability to control velocity by using a treadmill. The protocol used most frequently entails determining first the preferred stride length and rate for a particular velocity, then the steady-state aerobic demand assessments at a series of stride length and rate combinations that deviate from the preferred condition. This is accomplished by having an individual match the stepping rate to an audible signal so that desired stride rate and stride length are produced. This experimental manipulation produces a curvilinear stride length/rate–economy curve (Fig. 12.2). The aerobic demand of walking or running at a controlled speed tends to increase nonlinearly as optimal (preferred) stride length or rate either increases or decreases (14).

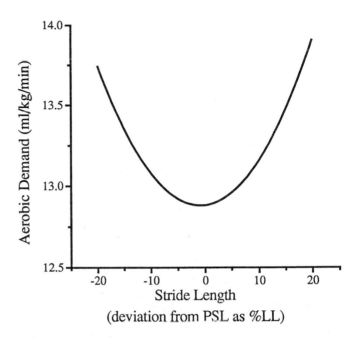

Figure 12.2. Stride length and rate strongly affect the aerobic demand for walking (shown here). For most individuals, as stride length either increases or decreases (hence stride rate decreases or increases, respectively) from the preferred stride length (PSL), expressed as a percentage of leg length (%LL), aerobic demand increases.

The preferred and most economical stride length–rate combinations are usually in close agreement with one another, suggesting that most individuals naturally achieve their optimal stride length and rate through some unknown mechanism. One practical implication of this outcome is that a coach is generally ill-advised to manipulate stride length and rate for the purpose of improving economy and running performance unless aerobic demand data specifically confirm an uneconomical running pattern (14, 15). In addition, research suggests that there is no significant relationship between the most economical stride length and leg length, indicating that it is not possible to predict the most economical stride length from physical dimensions.

The reason for the U-shaped stride length/rate–economy response is probably associated with fundamental muscle force- and power-generating capabilities. Fundamental mechanical properties of muscle indicate that the force-generating capacity of muscle falls nonlinearly as the velocity of shortening increases (16). When plotting power (the product of muscle force and the velocity of shortening) as a function of the velocity of shortening, the capacity of muscle to generate power is greatest when muscle fiber velocity is approximately one-third of maximum shortening velocity. Changes in stride length and rate require concomitant changes in the rates of muscle lengthening and shortening, the rate of force development, and the demand for muscular power output, all of which should affect aerobic demand.

MOVEMENT KINETICS: GROUND REACTION FORCES AND MECHANICAL POWER

Movement kinetics are affected by two major factors. These are ground reaction forces and mechanical power, which are discussed in this section.

Ground Reaction Forces

Gait specialists have extensively studied the ground reaction force, which reflects the net effect of muscular action and segment accelerations while the body is in contact with the ground. There is surprisingly little research, however, that provides insight into the relationships between gait economy and ground reaction force features. Existing research suggests only moderate to weak relationships between economy and characteristics of ground reaction force (17). Economical runners exhibit significantly lower first peaks in the vertical component of the ground reaction force and tend to have small anteroposterior and vertical peak forces and a heel-striking pattern. It is speculated that the need to provide cushioning during early contact may have an important effect on the demands placed on the muscles, which in turn may affect economy. When landing on the forefoot, a person may need to rely more heavily on musculature to cushion the impact. In contrast, the footwear and skeletal structures of a heel striker may play greater roles in cushioning and supporting the body during early contact.

Mechanical Power

Aerobic demand represents a global measure of the physiological demand of walking or running. One example of a global estimate of muscular effort from a biomechanics perspective is mechanical power output. Assuming that a substantial portion of the aerobic demand of gait is associated with muscles performing mechanical work (i.e., actively shortening or lengthening), mechanical power should be an effective predictor of gait economy. This is certainly true when the aerobic demand and mechanical power are studied for a wide range of walking or running speeds. As walking or running speed increases, both aerobic demand (milliliters per minute per kilogram) and mechanical power increase in direct proportion to speed. This is not surprising, since both aerobic demand and power output are viewed as markers of exercise intensity. Research has shown, however, that measures of mechanical power explain only a small amount of the interindividual variation in gait economy when examining a single speed of walking or running (18). This may be because a multitude of factors, biomechanical and otherwise, affect gait economy and the relative importance of these factors is likely to vary from individual to individual. In addition, methods of estimating mechanical power output of the body have their own limitations that limit their accuracy as an estimate of muscular effort.

FLEXIBILITY AND GAIT ECONOMY

One fundamental component of physical fitness is musculoskeletal flexibility. Intuitively, one would speculate that good flexibility, particularly within the trunk and lower extremities, would improve gait economy. This notion is consistent with a widely held view that increasing flexibility is desirable for optimal running performance and may also contribute to reduced incidence of certain types of musculoskeletal injury. Conversely, reduced flexibility may result in a modified gait pattern (e.g., short stride length and high stride rate) that is not economical or in increased muscular effort to produce the same gait pattern because of increased resistance to motion near the extremes of the range of motion (19). This interpretation is compatible with the observations that (*a*) gait economy is known to be adversely affected by advancing age in adults and by lower-extremity orthopaedic pathologies and (*b*) musculoskeletal flexibility tends to decline with old age and joint pathologies.

Interestingly, however, Gleim et al. (20) found that high "non-pathologic musculoskeletal tightness" was modestly related to lower aerobic demands (i.e., better economy) during walking and jogging. The average aerobic demand for the third of the study sample that was determined to be the most flexible was approximately 10% higher than that for the least flexible third of the sample. It was speculated that less flexible individuals may benefit economically from greater elastic energy contributions and a reduced need to use active musculature to neutralize unproductive or undesired movements (19, 20). These rather limited and counterintuitive observations suggest a need for additional research on the specific effects of musculoskeletal flexibility on gait economy in various subject populations.

MODIFICATION OF ECONOMY THROUGH TRAINING AND MOVEMENT EDUCATION

The preceding discussions should leave the reader with the impression that the association between gait kinematics and kinetics and economy is complex and far less definitive than intuition or common beliefs may suggest. Nevertheless, it is possible through careful testing to identify individuals who display uneconomical gait patterns, such as runners who overstride excessively. From an economy perspective, such individuals may clearly benefit from changes in their pattern of motion. However, there are conflicting findings from studies attempting to describe the effect of training and education on movement economy (15, 21–22). From these limited analyses, it is apparent that the question regarding the ability to make significant improvements in economy through biomechanical training remains unanswered.

► SUMMARY

For the exercise professional, biomechanics and physiology are two of the bricks in the foundation of the science of exercise. These two disciplines have considerable overlap relative to postural control and gait. This chapter briefly presents this overlap by first linking the physiology of the postural control system to the mechanics of static and dynamic postural stability and then linking gait economy to the biomechanics of walking and running. Some of the uncertainties associated with each area that affect the utility of the measures for the exercise professional are identified. These uncertainties are related to the technology and models used to collect and analyze research data, the complexity and disparity of human motor performance, and the trade-off between cost and accessibility for various methods of assessment. These uncertainties provide an impetus for continued research and development that ultimately will yield practical applications.

References

1. Horak FB, Shupert CL, Mirka A. Components of postural dyscontrol in the elderly: A review. Neurobiol Aging 10:727–738, 1989.
2. Berg K. Balance and its measure in the elderly: A review. Physiother Can 41:240–246, 1989.
3. Owings TM, Pavol MJ, Foley KT, Grabiner MD. Measures of postural stability are not predictors of recovery from large postural disturbances in healthy older adults. J Am Geriatr Soc 48:42–50, 2000.
4. Wolfson L, Whipple R, Derby CA, et al. A dynamic posturography study of balance in healthy elderly. Neurology 42:2069–2075, 1992.
5. Patla AE, Frank JS, Winter DA. Balance control in the elderly: Implications for clinical assessment and rehabilitation. Can J Public Health 83:S29–S33, 1992.
6. Daniels JT, Scardina NJ, Foley P. VO2 submax during five modes of exercise. In: Bachl N, Prokop L, Sucket R, eds. Proceedings of the World Congress on Sports Medicine. Vienna: Urban & Schwartzenberg, 1984:604–615.
7. Cavanagh PR, Kram R. Mechanical and muscular factors affecting the efficiency of human movement. Med Sci Sports Exerc 17:326–331, 1985.
8. Martin PE, Morgan DW. Biomechanical considerations for economical walking and running. Med Sci Sports Exerc 24:467–474, 1992.
9. Anderson T. Biomechanics and running economy. Sport Med 22:76–89, 1996.
10. Andriacchi TP, Ogle JA, Galante JO. Walking as a basis for normal and abnormal gait measurements. J Biomech 10:261–268, 1977.
11. Himann JE, Cunningham DA, Rechnitzer PA, Patterson DH. Age-related changes in speed of walking. Med Sci Sports Exerc 20:161–166, 1988.
12. Martin PE, Rothstein DE, Larish DD. Effects of age and physical activity status on the speed-aerobic demand relationship of walking. J Appl Physiol 73:200–206, 1992.
13. Ralston HJ. Energy-speed relation and optimal speed during level walking. Arbeitsphysiologica 17:277–283, 1958.
14. Cavanagh PR, Williams KR. The effect of stride length variation on oxygen uptake during distance running. Med Sci Sport Exerc 14:30–35, 1982.
15. Morgan DW, Martin PE, Craig M, et al. Effect of stride length optimization on the aerobic demand of running. J Appl Physiol 77:245–251, 1994.
16. Hill AV. The maximum work and mechanical efficiency of human muscles, and their most economical speed. J Physiol 56:19–41, 1922.
17. Williams KR, Cavanagh PR. Relationship between distance running mechanics, running economy, and performance. J Appl Physiol 63:1236–1245, 1987.
18. Martin PE, Heise GD, Morgan DW. Interrelationships between mechanical power, energy transfers, and walking and running economy. Med Sci Sports Exerc 25:508–515, 1993.
19. Craib MW, Mitchell VA, Fields KB, et al. The association between flexibility and running economy in sub-elite male distance runners. Med Sci Sports Exerc 28:737–743, 1996.
20. Gleim GW, Stachenfeld NS, Nicholas JA. The influence of flexibility on the economy of walking and jogging. J Orthop Res 8:814–823, 1990.
21. Lake MJ, Cavanagh PR. Six weeks of training does not change running mechanics or improve running economy. Med Sci Sports Exerc 28:860–869, 1996.
22. Messier SP, Cirillo KJ. Effects of a verbal and visual feedback system on running technique, perceived exertion and running economy in female novice runners. J Sport Sci 7:113–126, 1989.

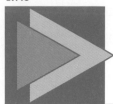

CHAPTER **13**

LOW BACK EXERCISES: PRESCRIPTION FOR THE HEALTHY BACK AND RECOVERY FROM INJURY

Stuart M. McGill

Low back and abdominal exercises are prescribed for a variety of reasons, but primarily for rehabilitation of the injured low back, prevention of injury, and/or as a component of fitness training programs. The objective of exercise prescription is to stress both damaged tissue and other healthy supporting tissues to promote tissue repair while avoiding further excessive loading that can exacerbate existing structural weakness. While knowledge of tissue forces during exercise is important to avoid further injury, choosing the optimal load requires a blend of art and science. In general, the most effective exercise programs are designed to train the motor control system to activate the spine stabilizers, then progress to endurance training, and finally to initiate enhancement of strength and flexibility. The professional challenge is to make wise decisions from the balance of laboratory and clinical experience. This chapter describes the causes of low back injuries and the scientific support for certain types of exercises to train the low back, the specific exercises documented to challenge muscle, enhance performance, and minimize spine loading. It also discusses several caveats for exercise prescription to enhance the chance of positive outcome.

EXERCISE AND LOW BACK PAIN

The reported effectiveness of various training and rehabilitation programs for the low back is quite variable, with some claiming great success and others reporting no success or even negative results (1, 2). In fact, some training programs appear to harm the lower back of some individuals. This tissue damage has been attributed to excessive torso flexion, disadvantageous muscle lengths in some postures, inappropriate orientation of internal structures of the torso with respect to the legs, and other factors (3–7). The discrepancy regarding the effectiveness and safety of exercise programs in various reports may be due to the prescription of inappropriate exercises caused by a lack of understanding of the tissue loading that results during various tasks (8). Exercise professionals sometimes unknowingly formulate programs that create excessive loads and exacerbate the damage. While specific exercises have been recommended in the past for their capacity to maximize muscle activity, virtually none have been examined for safety by quantifying individual spine tissue forces (9, 10). The exercises reviewed in this chapter have been evaluated on a tissue-loading injury criterion.

Many studies report loss of strength, flexibility, and endurance associated with low back injury. However, whether these deficits are the cause or the result of low back injury is not distinguishable from these data, which makes findings open to misinterpretation. Very few longitudinal studies are available, although one such study clearly demonstrated that "more fit" firefighters had fewer injuries than "less fit" peers (11).

Several hypotheses can be considered to explain the general role of exercise on maintaining low back tissue health and optimizing the repair process. Powerful evidence demonstrates that exercise does the following:

- Stimulates tissue hypertrophy
- Slows (possibly reverses) several degenerative conditions
- Enhances the nutritional benefit to the disc
- Is efficacious in treating the injured back compared to surgical intervention, bed rest, or simple flexibility programs (12–15)

In addition, the success of a carefully formulated exercise program that includes progressive stabilization exercise routines, emphasizing muscle cocontraction with the spine in a neutral posture, has been documented (16). While hip flexibility has been shown to be important, spine flexibility has never been shown to enhance the outcome of low back exercise programs for those with low back injury or to reduce the risk of future injury in healthy populations.

ANATOMY

The lumbar spine is composed of five vertebrae, each separated by intervertebral discs and two facet joints posteriorly. While the vertebrae are often considered rigid and most of the motion takes place in the discs, both the discs and vertebrae act as shock absorbers (Fig. 13.1) (17). The ligaments (not shown in Figure 13.1) connect adjacent vertebrae and become strained at the end range of spine motion. Some specific functional aspects of the anatomy are discussed later.

With standing, there is a natural curve in the low back called the lordotic curve. It is a common misconception that hyperlordosis (an extended lumbar spine) is linked to low back pain. Rather, standing hypolordosis and hyperlordosis are indications of biological variability and are problematic only in the most extreme cases. Nonetheless, certain individuals may develop inappropriate muscle balance and flexibility about the hips, low back, and knees that can result in increased loading of these areas during the performance of both athletic and daily activi-

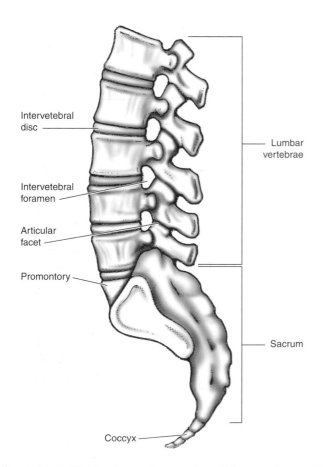

Intervetebral disc

Intervetebral foramen

Articular facet

Promontory

Lumbar vertebrae

Sacrum

Coccyx

Figure 13.1. The lumbar spine consists of five vertebrae with intervening discs. It has a normal lordotic curve, which is a position of elastic equilibrium and lowest stress. (Adapted with permission from White AM, Anderson R, eds. Conservative Care of Low Back Pain. Baltimore: Williams & Wilkins, 1991.)

ties if the level of lordosis is not controlled. Avoiding the end range of motion in the spine during activity can reduce the risk of several types of injury.

HOW SPECIFIC INJURIES OCCUR

Understanding the cause of injury is important for appropriate prescription of exercise and the development of injury avoidance strategies. There is a tendency among those reporting or describing the back injury to identify a single specific event as the cause of the damage, such as lifting and twisting with a box. This description of low back injury is common, particularly among the occupational and medical community, who are often required to identify a single event when filling out injury report forms. However, relatively few low back injuries occur from a single event; rather, the culminating injury event was preceded by a history of excessive loading that gradually reduced the level of tolerance to tissue failure (18). Thus other scenarios in which subfailure loads can result in injury are probably more important but not reported. For example, the ultimate failure of a tissue (i.e., injury) can result from accumulated trauma produced by either repeated application of load (and failure from fatigue) or a sustained load that is applied for long duration or repetitively applied (and failure from deformation and strain). Thus, the injury process may not always be associated with loads of high magnitude. Injury to specific low back structures is described next.

Vertebrae

A number of studies over the years demonstrate that a neutral spine under compressive load results in bony failure, specifically end-plate fracture occurring together with damage to underlying trabeculae (Fig 13.2) (19, 20). Furthermore, repeated loading reduces the ultimate strength so that bony failure occurs at lower levels (21). Disc herniation is an extremely rare occurrence when the spine motion unit is compressed in a neutral posture (i.e., neutral lordotic curve, not flexed, laterally bent, or twisted). High-velocity compression often results in catastrophic vertebral burst fractures, although this is not associated with nonimpact exercise (22).

Disc Herniation

Disc herniation from a one-time application of load is extremely difficult to produce in the laboratory, although it has been described with the application of compression to a spine deviated into hyperflexion and lateral bending (23). Herniation is more consistently produced during many cycles of combined compression, flexion, and torsional loading, and it tends to occur in younger specimens with no visible gross signs of degeneration (24–26). Epidemiological data also link herniation with sedentary occupations and sitting (27). Older discs appear not to have enough fluid to flow, leading to herniation, and

Figure 13.2. End plate fracture **(A)** and intrusion of nuclear material (shown at the tip of the scalpel) into the vertebral body **(B)** from compressive loading of a spine in a neutral posture. These are porcine specimens from the University of Waterloo laboratory.

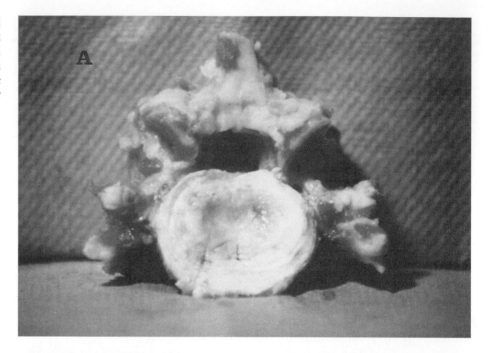

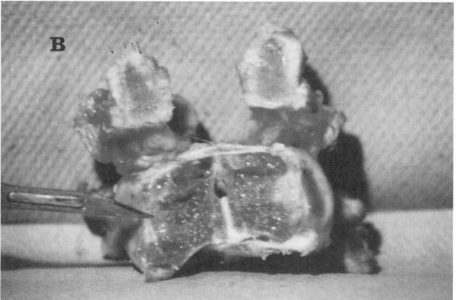

older spines appear not to exhibit classic extrusion of nuclear material, but rather are characterized by delamination of the anulus layers and radial cracks, which appear to progress with repeated loading (28, 29). In summary, it appears that disc herniation is the result of cyclic loading, or prolonged and sustained loading, in deviated spine postures. The notion that disc herniation in an occupational or athletic setting is the result of a single event appears unlikely to be accurate.

Ligaments

A similar story unfolds with bony failure and ligamentous injury. It has been noted that soft tissue injuries are

most common during high-energy traumatic events, such as automobile collisions (30). Other research in both human and animal specimens loaded at slow load rates in bending and shear suggest that most frequently excessive tension in the longitudinal ligaments results in avulsion (tearing away) or bony failure as the ligament pulls some bone away near its attachment (31, 32). Slow strain rates produce mainly ligament avulsion injuries and faster strain rates result in mainly ligamentous failure to the fiber bundles in the middle region of the ligament.

Another clinical report found that approximately 20% of cadaveric spines possessed visibly ruptured interspinous ligaments (in their middle, not at their bony attachment) and that dorsal and ventral positions, together with supraspinous, remained intact (33). Given the oblique fiber direction of the interspinous complex (Fig. 13.3), a very likely scenario to damage this ligament would be slipping, falling, and landing on the buttocks (causing a high ligament loading rate), driving the pelvis forward on impact, and creating a posterior shearing of the lumbar joints when the spine is fully flexed. The interspinous ligament is a major load-bearing tissue in this example of high-energy loading, in which anterior shear displacement is combined with full flexion (34).

Given the available data, it would appear that torn ligaments of the spine during lifting or other nonimpact activities, particularly to the interspinous complex, is more uncommon than common. It appears much more likely that ligament damage occurs during a more traumatic event, such as a fall with direct impact on the spine, which leads to joint laxity and acceleration of subsequent arthritic changes. The possibility of crushing the inter-

spinous ligament complex in forced hyperextension (hyperlordosis) has also been noted (22).

Facets and Neural Arch

The facets and neural arch appear to withstand moderate shearing load and fail under shear loading and torsional loading and hyperextension (35, 36). Failure of the neural arch and pars interarticularis is common among athletes who rapidly cycle between flexion and extension (such as gymnasts and cricket bowlers), suggesting that strain reversal of the flexible arch promotes fatigue and eventually failure (37, 38).

LUMBAR POSTURE AND INJURY AVOIDANCE

Many injuries are associated with the end of range of motion of the spine. Thus, it appears that a neutral spine curvature may reduce the risk of many injuries. Shifts in tissue loading, as predicted from a modeling approach,

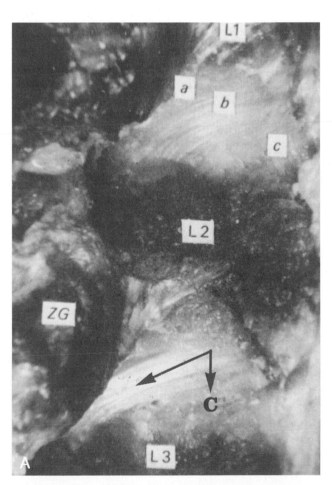
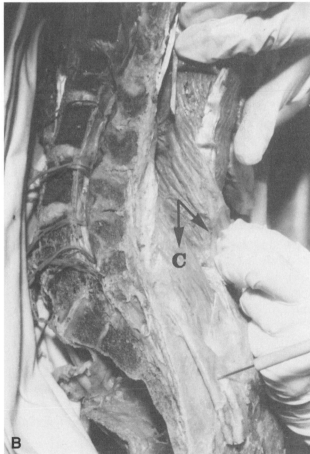

Figure 13.3. A. The interspinous ligament (*C, arrows*) imposes an anterior shear when strained in flexion. **B.** Pars lumborum fibres of iliocostalis lumborum and longissimus thoracis create a posterior shear force on the superior vertebrae. The oblique line of action of the muscle and ligament is shown compared to the compressive axis (C). (A reprinted with permission from Heylings DJ. Supraspinous and interspinous ligaments of the human lumbar spine. J Anat 123:127–131, 1978.)

have dramatic effects on shear loading of the intervertebral column and injury risk. First, the dominant direction of some of the small muscles acting on the spine can produce a posterior shear force on the superior vertebra. In contrast, the interspinous ligament complex generates forces in the opposite direction that impose an anterior shear force on the superior vertebra. During this type of activity, spine posture determines the interplay between passive tissues (ligaments) and muscles, which ultimately modulates the risk of several types of injury. For example, if a load is held in the hands with the spine fully flexed (thus achieving little activity, and tension, in the extensors) and with all spinal joints motionless so that the low back moment remains the same, the ligaments seem to add to the anterior shear, which is of concern relative to risk of injury. However, if a more neutral lumbar curve posture is adopted and the extensor musculature is activated at the same time, there is support for the anterior shearing action of gravity on the upper body and hand-held load, which reduces shear load. In this example, the spine is at much greater risk for shear injury than compressive injury, simply because the spine is fully flexed, or at the end range of motion. Finally, it appears that a fully flexed spine fails at about 20–40% lower compressive load than when not fully flexed.

In summary, evidence from tissue-specific injury generally supports the notion of a neutral lumbar curve when performing loading tasks to minimize the risk of low back injury. There is no evidence to support conscious effort to perform pelvic tilts (i.e., hyperlordosis or lumbar flexion) to prevent injury during lifting or exertion.

METHODS TO EVALUATE SPECIFIC EXERCISES

It is important to understand the applications, and conversely the limitations, of scientific laboratory approaches for investigating tissue loading in vivo that are used to quantify better exercises. Basically, two types of methods are used: (*a*) obtaining individual tissue forces and (*b*) specific data collection procedures with human subjects. Because the low back system is an extremely complex mechanical structure and direct measurement of tissue forces in vivo is not feasible, the only tenable option for tissue load prediction is to use sophisticated modeling approaches. However, several issues must be addressed, including the amount of anatomical detail, reconciliation of the inherent variability of the many unknown forces among the significant load-bearing structures, and prediction of loads in deep and inaccessible muscles and supporting ligaments (39–41).

SCIENCE AND LOW BACK EXERCISE

The following example illustrates the need for quantitative analysis in evaluating the safety of certain exercises (41–43). There has been considerable emphasis on the need to perform sit-ups and other flexion exercises with the knees flexed. Several hypotheses have suggested that this disables the psoas and/or changes the line of action of psoas. Recent magnetic resonance imaging (MRI) data demonstrate that psoas line of action does not change due to lumbar or hip posture except at the lumbosacral joint, as the psoas laminae attach to each vertebrae and follow the changing orientation of spine (44). There is no doubt that psoas shortens with the flexed hip, modulating force production.

But the question remains, is there a reduction in spine load with the legs bent? Recent data suggested no major difference in lumbar load as the result of bending the knees (45). However, excessive compressive loads during any type of sit-up certainly raise a question of safety. This type of quantitative analysis is necessary to demonstrate that the issue of performing sit-ups using bent knees or straight legs is probably not as important as whether to prescribe sit-ups at all.

EXERCISE RECOMMENDATIONS

The following exercises have been formally evaluated and selected according to tissue loading evidence and knowledge of how injury occurs to specific tissues. It is not possible to recommend universally only those low back exercises with the highest muscle challenge and the lowest compressive cost indices. Several exercises are required to train all of the muscles of the lumbar torso, and the exercises that best suit the individual depend on a number of variables, such as fitness level, training goals, any history of spinal injury, and other factors specific to the individual. However, depending on the purpose of the exercise program, several principles apply. For example, an individual beginning a postinjury program is better advised to avoid loading the spine throughout the range of motion, while a trained athlete may indeed achieve higher performance levels by doing so.

Selection of the following exercises is guided by safety, that is, minimizing spine loading during muscle challenge. Therefore, a neutral spine curve (neither hyperlordotic nor hypolordotic) while the spine is under load is emphasized. A general rule is to preserve the normal low back curve (similar to that of upright standing). A caveat for this generalization is that the curve may be modified by patients to enter or maintain a pain-free zone while performing these exercises. Performing a pelvic tilt during some of these exercises has been recommended, but as stated previously, it is not justified, since pelvic tilt increases spine tissue loading and takes the spine out of static–elastic equilibrium. Therefore, it is unwise to recommend the pelvic tilt during challenges to the spine. Exercises in the following sections have been evaluated and chosen according to tissue loading evidence and the knowledge of how injury occurs to specific tissues.

Aerobic Exercise

The mounting evidence supporting the role of aerobic exercise both in reducing the incidence of low back injury and in the treatment of low back patients is quite convincing (11, 41). Recent investigation into loads sustained by the low back tissues during walking confirm very low levels of supporting tissue load coupled with mild but prolonged activation of the supporting musculature (46). Epidemiological evidence also clarifies the effects of aerobic exercise. A large study examined age-related changes to the lumbar spine of elderly people as a function of life-long activity level (12). Those who were runners had no differences in spine changes measured from MRI images, while weight lifters and soccer players were characterized with more disc degeneration and bulges.

Flexibility Exercise

Emphasis on spine flexibility depends on the injury history and exercise or fitness goals. Generally, for the injured back, spine flexibility should not be emphasized until the spine has stabilized and has undergone strength and endurance conditioning. Despite the notion held by some, few quantitative data support a major emphasis on trunk flexibility to improve back health and lessen the risk of injury. In fact, some exercise programs that included loading of the torso throughout the range of motion (in flexion–extension, lateral bend, or axial twist) had negative results, and greater spine mobility has, in some cases, been associated with low back problems (8, 47–50). Furthermore, spine flexibility has been shown to have little predictive value for future low back problems (49, 51). The most successful programs emphasize trunk stabilization throughout exercise with a neutral spine and mobility at the hips and knees (16, 52, 53).

For these reasons, specific torso flexibility exercises should be limited to unloaded flexion extension (the cat stretch) for those concerned with safety or for nonathletes (spine flexibility may be more desirable in athletes who have never had a back injury). The spine may be cycled through full flexion and extension in a slow, smooth motion (Fig. 13.4). Emphasizing a neutral spine throughout, hip and knee flexibility may be achieved with the following maneuvers: hip mobility, standing hip extension, standing hip flexion, and slow lunges (Figs. 13.5 and 13.6).

Strength and Endurance Exercise

While it is well documented that those who have had back injuries have lower muscle strength and endurance performance, very few studies have linked reduced strength and endurance with the risk of a subsequent first-time low back injury. The few results available suggest that endurance has a much greater prophylactic value

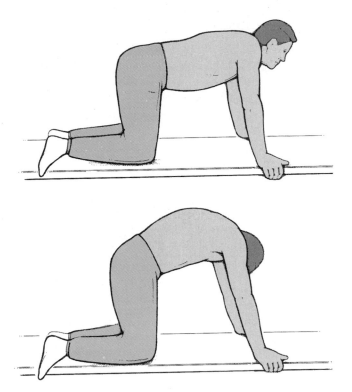

Figure 13.4. The cat stretch is performed by slowly cycling from full spine flexion to full extension. Spine mobility is emphasized rather than pressing at the end range of motion. This exercise provides motion for the spine with very low loading of the intervertebral joints.

than strength (54). Furthermore, emphasis on endurance should precede specific strengthening exercise in a gradual progressive exercise program (i.e., longer-duration, lower-intensity exercises).

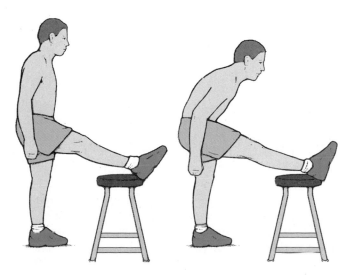

Figure 13.5. Hip mobility is enhanced with standing flexion and extension. *Left,* the correct neutral spine. *Right,* an **incorrect flexed spine.**

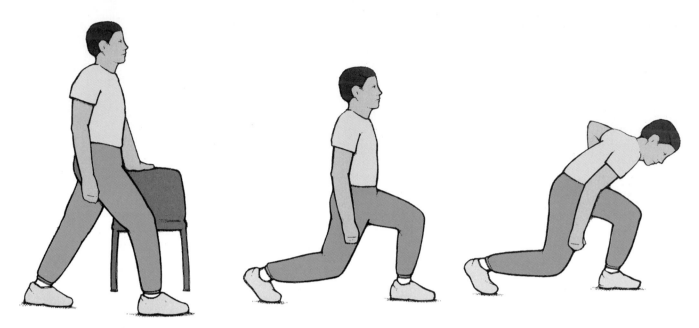

Figure 13.6. Hip mobility, strength, and endurance are challenged with slow lunges. The torso remains upright throughout the lunge effort, while emphasis is placed on a neutral spine curve during hip exercises to focus the stretch over the hip and knee joints (*center*). *Right*, The **incorrect flexed spine.**

Abdominal Exercise: Anterior and Lateral

No single abdominal exercise challenges all of the abdominal musculature; more than one exercise is required. Calibrated intramuscular and surface electromyogram evidence suggests that the various types of curl-ups challenge mainly rectus abdominis, while psoas and obliques (internal and external oblique, transverse abdominis) activity is low (41, 45). Sit-ups, both straight leg and bent knee, are characterized by higher psoas activation and higher low back compression, while leg raises cause even higher activation and spine compression (Table 13.1).

The challenge to the psoas is lowest during curl-ups, followed by higher levels during the horizontal isometric side support. While bent-knee sit-ups were characterized by larger psoas activation than straight-leg sit-ups, the highest psoas activity is observed during leg raises and hand-on-knee flexor isometric exertions. It is interesting to note that the press-heels sit-up, which has been hypothesized to activate hamstrings and neurally inhibit psoas, actually increased psoas activation (55). Active hamstrings create a hip extensor moment requiring more hip flexor activity from the psoas, resulting in a higher compressive penalty on the spine.

An exercise that is not often performed but that has merit is the horizontal side bridge, which challenges the lateral obliques without high lumbar compressive loading. In addition, this exercise produces high activation levels in the quadratus lumborum which is a significant stabilizer of the spine (56). Graded activity in the rectus abdominis and in each of the components of the abdominal wall changes with each of these exercises, demon-

Table 13.1. Low Back Moment, Muscle Activity, and Lumbar Compressive Load During Several Types of Abdominal Exercises

	MUSCLE ACTIVATION		
MOMENT (NM)	RECTUS ABDOMINIS (% MVC)	EXTERNAL OBLIQUE	COMPRESSION (N)
Straight-leg sit-up	148	121	~70	3506
Bent-leg sit-up	154	103	70	3350
Curl-up, feet anchored	92	87	45	2009
Curl-up, feet free	81	67	38	1991
Quarter sit-up	114	78	42	2392
Straight-leg raise	102	57	35	2525
Bent-leg raise	82	35	24	1767
Cross-knee curl-up	112	89	67	2964
Hanging straight leg	107	112	90	2805
Hanging bent leg	84	78	64	3313
Isometric side bridge	72	48	50	2585

MVC contractions were isometric. Activation values higher than 100% are often seen during dynamic exercise.

strating that there is no single best task for the abdominals. Several other clinically relevant findings are as follows:

1. Psoas activation is dominated by hip flexion demands, and psoas activity is not consistent with either lumbar sagittal moment (flexor–extensor torque) or spine compression demands, although there is some question regarding the often-cited idea that the psoas is a lumbar spine stabilizer.
2. Quadratus lumborum activity is consistent with lumbar sagittal moment and compression demands, suggesting a larger role in stabilization.
3. Psoas activation is relatively high (greater than 25% maximal voluntary contraction) during push-ups, suggesting cautious concern for the low back injured.

A good choice for abdominal exercises in the early stages of training or rehabilitation consists of several variations of curl-ups for rectus abdominis and isometric horizontal side bridge (with the body supported by the knees and upper body supported by one elbow on the floor) to challenge the abdominal wall in a way that imposes minimal compressive penalty to the spine. Supporting the body with the feet rather than the knees can increase the level of challenge with the isometric horizontal side support.

Specific recommended low back exercises (Figs. 13.7 and 13.8) include the curl-up with the hands under the low back, which stabilizes the pelvis and assists in preserving a neutral lumbar curvature, and the horizontal isometric side bridge (again with the spine in a neutral curve), using either the knees or feet for support.

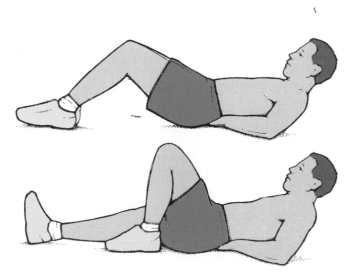

Figure 13.7. The curl-up, in which the head and shoulders are raised off the ground with the hands under the lumbar region to help stabilize the pelvis and support the neutral spine curve (*top*). A variation is to bend only one leg while the other straight leg assists in pelvic stabilization and preservation of a neutral lumbar curve (*bottom*).

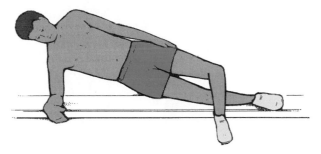

Figure 13.8. The horizontal isometric side bridge. Supporting the lower body with the knees on the floor reduces the demand further for those who are more concerned with safety. Supporting the body with the feet increases the muscle challenge and spine load.

Back Extensors Exercise

Most traditional extensor exercises are characterized by high spine loads, which result from externally applied compressive and shear forces from either free weights or resistance machines. The single-leg extension hold on the hands and knees minimizes external loads on the spine but produces spine extensor moment (and small isometric twisting moments) that activates the extensors (Fig. 13.9). Activation is sufficiently high on one side of the extensors to facilitate training, but the total spine load is reduced, since the contralateral extensors are producing lower forces. Switching legs trains both sides of the extensors. Leg extension with simultaneous contralateral arm raise increases the unilateral extensor muscle challenge but also significantly increases lumbar compression.

The common exercise of lying prone on the floor and raising the upper body and legs off the floor is contraindicated for anyone at risk for low back injury or reinjury. In this task the lumbar region pays a high compression penalty to a hyperextended spine, which transfers load to the facets and crushes the interspinous ligament (noted earlier as an injury mechanism). This type of data illustrates that exercise professionals must design programs with a wide range of objectives and with detailed attention to the effects of such exercises on back health.

The Use of Abdominal Belts

A review of the effects of wearing an abdominal belt is summarized in the following:

1. Those who have never had a back injury appear to have no additional protective benefit from wearing a belt.
2. It appears that those who have had an injury while wearing a belt are at risk for a more severe injury.
3. Belts give people the perception that they can lift more and may in fact enable them to lift more.
4. Belts appear to increase intra-abdominal pressure and blood pressure.
5. Belts appear to change the lifting styles of some people, either increasing or decreasing the load on the spine (57).

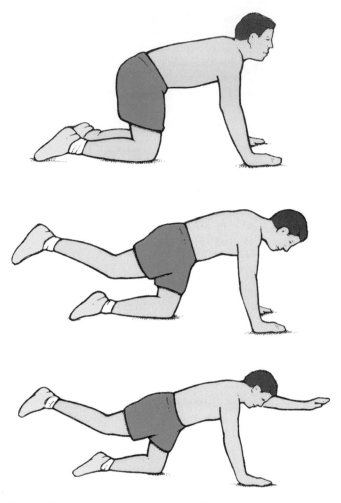

Figure 13.9. Single-leg extension holds, done on the hands and knees, produce mild extensor activity and lower spine compression (<2500N). Raising the contralateral arm increases extensor muscle activity, but also spine compression to levels over 3000N.

In summary, given the assets and liabilities to belt wearing, they are not recommended for routine exercise.

EXERCISE PRESCRIPTION GUIDELINES FOR THE LOW BACK

The following is a list of general caveats for prescribing low back exercises:

1. While there is a common belief that exercise sessions should be performed at least three times per week, it appears that low back exercises have the most beneficial effect when performed daily (58).
2. The axiom no pain, no gain does not apply when exercising the low back, particularly when applied to weight training.
3. While specific low back exercises are described in this chapter, general exercise programs that also combine cardiovascular components, such as walking, have been shown to be more effective in both rehabilitation and injury prevention (46).
4. Diurnal variation in the fluid level of the intervertebral discs changes the stresses on the disc throughout the day: discs are more hydrated early in the morning after rising from bed. It would be very unwise to perform full-range spine motion while under load shortly after rising from bed (22).
5. Low back exercises performed for maintenance of health need not emphasize strength, employing high-load, low-repetition tasks. Rather, more repetitions of less demanding exercises assist in the enhancement of endurance and strength. There is no doubt that back injury can occur during seemingly low-level demands, such as picking up a pencil, and that the risk of injury from motor control error can occur. While the chance of motor control errors resulting in inappropriate muscle forces can increase with fatigue, there is also evidence documenting the changes in passive tissue loading with fatiguing lifting (59). Given that endurance has more protective value than strength, strength gains should not be overemphasized at the expense of endurance (54).
6. There is no such thing as an ideal set of exercises for everyone. Training objectives, including reducing the risk of injury, optimizing general health and fitness, or maximizing athletic performance must be identified. While science cannot evaluate the optimal exercises for each situation, the combination of science and clinical experiential wisdom must be used to enhance low back health and/or specific performance.
7. Patience and compliance are important aspects of all low back exercise programs. Increased function and reducing pain may not occur for up to 3 months (60).

ACKNOWLEDGMENT

I wish to acknowledge the help of several colleagues who have contributed to the collection of works reported here: Daniel Juker, MD; Craig Axler, MSc; Jacek Cholewicki, PhD; Michael Sharratt, PhD; John Seguin, MD; Vaughan Kippers, PhD; Jack Callaghan, PhD; and Robert Norman, PhD. Also, the continual financial support from the Natural Science and Engineering Research Council, Canada, has made this series of work possible.

References

1. Koes BW, Bouter LM, Beckerman H, et al. Physiotherapy exercises and back pain: A blinded review. BMJ 302:1572–1576, 1991.
2. Faas A. Exercises: Which ones are worth trying, for which patients, and when? Spine 12:2874–2879, 1996.
3. Nachemson A, Morris JM. Invivo measurements of intradiscal pressure. J Bone Joint Surg 46A:1077–1080, 1964.
4. Nachemson A. The load on lumbar disks in different positions of the body. Clin Orthop 45:107–112, 1966.

5. Halpern AA, Bleck EE. Sit-up exercises: An electromygraphic study. Clin Orthop 145:172–178, 1979.

6. Vincent WJ, Britten SD. Evaluation of the curl-up: A substitute for the bent knee sit-up. J Phys Ed Rec Feb:74–75, 1980.

7. Jette M, Sidney K, Cicutti N. A critical analysis of sit-ups: A case for the partial curl-up as a test of abdominal muscular endurance. Can J Phys Ed Rec Sept-Oct:4–9, 1984.

8. Malmivaara A, Hakkinen U, Aro T, et al. The treatment of acute low back pain: Bed rest, exercises, or ordinary activity? N Engl J Med 332:351–355, 1995.

9. Walters CE, Partridge MJ. Electromyographic study of the differential action of the abdominal muscles during exercise. Am J Phys Med 36:259–268, 1957.

10. Flint MM. Abdominal muscle involvement during performance of various forms of sit-up exercises: Electromyographic study. Am J Phys Med 44:224–234, 1965.

11. Cady LD, Bischoff DP, O'Connell ER, et al. Strength and fitness and subsequent back injuries in firefighters. J Occup Med 21:269–272, 1979.

12. Videman T, Sarna S, Crites-Battie M, et al. The long term effects of physical loading and exercise lifestyles on back-related symptoms, disability, and spinal pathology among men. Spine 20(b):669–709, 1995.

13. Videman T. Experimental models of osteoarthritis: The role of immobilization. Clin Biomech 2:223–229, 1987.

14. Holm S, Nachemson A. Variations in the nutrition of the canine intervertebral disc induced by motion. Spine 8:866–874, 1983.

15. Richardson C, Jull G, Hodges P, Hides J. Therapeutic Exercise for Spinal Segmental Stabilization in Low Back Pain. Edinburgh: Churchill Livingstone, 1999.

16. Saal JA, Saal JS. Nonoperative treatment of herniated lumbar intervertebral disc with radiculopathy: An outcome study. Spine 14:431–437, 1989.

17. Roaf R. A study of the mechanics of spinal injuries. J Bone Joint Surg 42B:810, 1960.

18. McGill SM. ISB Keynote Lecture. The biomechanics of low back injury: Implications on current practice in industry and the clinic. J Biomech 30:465–475, 1997.

19. Brinkmann P, Biggemann M, Hilweg D. Prediction of the compressive strength of human lumbar vertebrae. Clin Biomech 4(Suppl 2), 1989.

20. Fyhrie DP, Schaffler MB. Failure mechanisms in human vertebral cancellous bone. Bone 15:105–109, 1994.

21. Hansson TH, Keller T, Spengler D. Mechanical behaviour of the human lumbar spine. 2: Fatigue strength during dynamic compressive loading. J Orthop Res 5:479–487, 1987.

22. Adams MA, Dolan P. Recent advances in lumbar spine mechanics and their clinical significance. Clin Biomech 10:3–19, 1995.

23. Adams MA, Hutton WC. Prolapsed Intervertebral disc: A hyperflexion injury. Spine 7:184–191, 1982.

24. Gordon SJ, Yang KH, Mayer PJ, et al. Mechanism of disc rupture: A preliminary report. Spine 16:450–456, 1991.

25. Yang KH, Byrd AJ, Kish VL, et al. Annulus fibrosus tears: An experimental model. Orthop Trans 12:86–87, 1988.

26. Adams MA, Hutton WC. Gradual disc prolapse. Spine 10:524–531, 1985.

27. Videman T, Nurminen M, Troup JD. Lumbar spinal pathology in cadaveric material in relation to history of back pain: Occupation and physical loading. Spine 15:728–740, 1990.

28. Wilder DG, Pope MH, Frymoyer JW. The biomechanics of lumbar disc herniation and the effect of overload and instability. J Spine Dis 1:16–32, 1988.

29. Goel VK, Monroe BT, Gilbertson LG, et al. Interlaminar shear stresses and laminae-separation in a disc: Finite element analysis of the L3-L4 motion segment subjected to axial compressive loads. Spine 20:689–698, 1995.

30. King AI. Injury to the thoraco-lumbar spine and pelvis. In: Nahum AM, Melvin JW, eds. Accidental Injury, Biomechanics and Presentation. New York: Springer-Verlag, 1993.

31. Noyes FR, De Lucas JL, Torvik PJ. Biomechanics of ligament failure: An analysis of strain-rate sensitivity and mechanisms of failure in primates. J Bone Joint Surg 56A:236–253, 1974.

32. Yoganandan H, Pintar R, Butler J, et al. Dynamic response of human cervical spine ligaments. Spine 14:1002–1110, 1989.

33. Rissanen PM. The surgical anatomy and pathology of the supraspinous and interspinous ligaments of the lumbar spine with special reference to ligament ruptures. Acta Orthop Scand (46 Suppl), 1960.

34. Heylings DJ. Supraspinous and interspinous ligaments of the human lumbar spine. J Anat 123:127–131, 1978.

35. Cripton P, Berlemen U, Visarino H, et al. Response of the lumbar spine due to shear loading. In: Injury Prevention Through Biomechanics. Symposium proceedings, May 4–5, Wayne State University, 1985.

36. Adams MA, Hutton WC. The relevance of torsion to the mechanical derangement of the lumbar spine. Spine 6:241–248, 1981.

37. Wiltse LL, Widell EM, Jackson DW. Fatigue fracture: The basic lesion in isthmic spondylolisthesis. J Bone Joint Surg 57A:17–22, 1975.

38. Hardcastle P, Annear P, Foster D. Spinal abnormalities in young fast bowlers. J Bone Joint Surg 74B:421–425, 1992.

39. McGill SM. A myoelectrically based dynamic three-dimensional model to predict loads on lumbar spine tissues during lateral bending. J Biomech 25:395–414, 1992.

40. Cholewicki J, McGill SM. Mechanical stability of the in vivo lumbar spine: Implications for injury and chronic low back pain. Clin Biomech 11:1–15, 1996.

41. Juker D, McGill SM, Kropf P, et al. Quantitative intramuscular myoelectric activity of lumbar portions of psoas and the abdominal wall during a wide variety of tasks. Med Sci Sports Exerc 30(2):301–310, 1998.

42. Callaghan J, Gunning J, McGill SM. Relationship between lumbar spine load and muscle activity during extensor exercises. Phys Ther 78(1):8–18, 1998.

43. Axler CT, McGill SM. Choosing the best abdominal exercises based on knowledge of tissue loads. Med Sci Sports Exerc 29:804–811, 1997.

44. Santaguida L, McGill SM. The psoas major muscle: A three dimensional mechanical modelling study with respect to the spine based on MRI measurement. J Biomech 28(3):339–345, 1995.

45. McGill SM. The mechanics of torso flexion: Sit ups and standing dynamic flexion manoeuvres. Clin Biomech 10:184–192, 1995.

46. Nutter P. Aerobic exercise in the treatment and prevention of low back pain. Occup Med 3:137–145, 1988.

47. Callaghan JP, Patla A, McGill SM. 3D analysis of spine loading during gait. Proceedings of American Society for Biomechanics meeting, Atlanta, GA. Oct. 17–19, 1996.

48. Nachemson A. Newest knowledge of low back pain: A critical look. Clin Orthop 279:8–20, 1992.

49. Biering-Sorensen F. Physical measurements as risk indicators for low back trouble over a one year period. Spine 9:106–109, 1984.

50. Burton AK, Tillotson KM, Troup JD. Variation in lumbar sagittal mobility with low back trouble. Spine 14:584–590, 1989.

51. Battie MC, Bigos SJ, Fischer LD, et al. The role of spinal flexibility in back pain complaints within industry: A prospective study. Spine 15:768–773, 1990.

52. Bridger RS, Orkin D, Henneberg M. A quantitative investigation of lumbar and pelvic postures in standing and sitting: Interrelationships with body position and hip muscle length. Int J Ind Ergonom 9:235–244, 1992.

53. McGill SM, Norman RW. Low back biomechanics in industry: The prevention of injury. In: Grabiner MD, ed. Current Issues of Biomechanics. Champaign, IL: Human Kinetics, 1992.

54. Luoto S, Heliovaara M, Hurri H, et al. Static back endurance and the risk of low back pain. Clin Biomech 10:323–324, 1995.

55. Spring H. Kraft: Theorie und Praxis. New York: Thieme Stuttgardt, 1990.

56. McGill SM, Juker D, Kropf P. Quantitative intramuscular myoelectric activity of quadratus lumborum during a wide variety of tasks. Clin Biomech 11:170–172, 1996.

57. McGill SM. Abdominal belts in industry: A position paper on their assets, liabilities and use. Am Ind Hyg Assoc J 54:752–754, 1993.

58. Mayer TG, Gatchel RJ, Kishino N, et al. Objective assessment of spine function following industrial injury: A prospective study with comparison group and one-year follow up. Spine 10:482–493, 1985.

59. Potvin JR, Norman RW. Can fatigue compromise lifting safety: Proc. NACOB II. The Second North American Congress on Biomechanics, August 24–28, 1992:513–514.

60. Manniche C, Hesselsoe G, Bentzen L, et al. Clinical trial of intensive muscle training for chronic low back pain. Lancet 24:1473–1476, 1988.

SECTION FOUR

EXERCISE PHYSIOLOGY

SECTION EDITORS: *Thomas P. LaFontaine, PhD, FACSM, and*
Michael Wegner, PhD

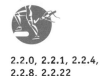

1.2.1, 1.2, 1.2.4   2.2.0, 2.2.1, 2.2.4,   4.2.1.1
                         2.2.8, 2.2.22

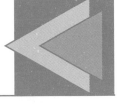

CHAPTER **14**

FUNDAMENTALS OF EXERCISE METABOLISM

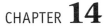

Scott R. Demaree, Scott K. Powers, and John M. Lawler

At rest, a 70-kg human has an energy expenditure of about 1.2 kcal/minute; less than 20% of resting energy expenditure is attributed to skeletal muscle. However, almost all changes occurring in the body during exercise are related to the increase in energy metabolism largely within the contracting skeletal muscle. For example, cardiac output and heart rate increase as a direct linear function of whole-body metabolism. To meet the demands on the heart there is a fourfold increase in myocardial blood flow and oxygen consumption.

During intense exercise, total energy expenditure may increase 15–25 times above resting values, resulting in a caloric expenditure of approximately 18–30 kcal/minute. Most of this increase is used to provide energy for exercising muscles, which may increase energy requirement by a factor of 200 (1). Therefore, daily caloric expenditure can be changed dramatically by simply altering the amount of physical activity performed during a day. The focus of this chapter is on muscle bioenergetics and exercise metabolism. A detailed review of bioenergetics and exercise metabolism is provided in the suggested reading section of this chapter.

ENERGY FOR MUSCULAR CONTRACTION

Adenosine Triphosphate

The energy released through hydrolysis of the high-energy compound adenosine triphosphate (ATP) to form adenosine diphosphate (ADP) and inorganic phosphate (Pi) powers skeletal muscle contractions. This reaction is catalyzed by the enzyme myosin ATPase:

$$ATP \xrightarrow{\text{(myosin ATPase)}} ADP + Pi + energy$$

The amount of ATP directly available in muscle at any time is small, so it must be resynthesized continuously if exercise lasts for more than a few seconds. Muscle fibers contain the metabolic machinery to produce ATP by three pathways: creatine phosphate (CP), rapid glycolysis, and aerobic oxidation of nutrients to carbon dioxide and water.

Creatine Phosphate

The CP system transfers high-energy phosphate from CP to rephosphorylate ATP from ADP as follows:

$$ADP + CP \xrightarrow{\text{(creatine kinase)}} ATP + C$$

This system is rapid because it involves only one enzymatic step (i.e., one chemical reaction); however, CP exists in finite quantities in cells, so the total amount of ATP that can be produced is limited. Oxygen is not involved in the rephosphorylation of ADP to ATP in this reaction, so the CP system is considered anaerobic (without oxygen).

Rapid Glycolysis

When glycolysis is rapid, it is capable of producing ATP without involvement of oxygen. Glycolysis, the degradation of carbohydrate (glycogen or glucose) to pyruvate or lactate, involves a series of enzymatically catalyzed steps (Fig. 14.1). The net energy yield of glycolysis, without further oxidation through aerobic metabolism, is two or three ATPs through substrate level phosphorylation. The net production is two ATPs when glucose is the substrate and three ATPs when glycogen is the substrate. Although glycolysis does not use oxygen and is considered anaerobic, pyruvate can readily participate in aerobic production of ATP when oxygen is available in the cell. Therefore, in addition to being an anaerobic pathway capable of producing ATP without oxygen, glycolysis can also be considered the first step in the aerobic degradation of carbohydrate.

Lactic Acid

Historically, rising blood lactate levels during exercise have been considered an indication of increased anaerobic metabolism within the contracting muscle because of a lack of oxygen. If oxygen is not available in the mitochondria to accept hydrogen released during glycolysis, pyruvate must accept hydrogen to form lactate as an end product so that glycolysis can proceed. However, the hypoxia theory is controversial. Whether the end product of glycolysis is pyruvate or lactate also depends on other fac-

133

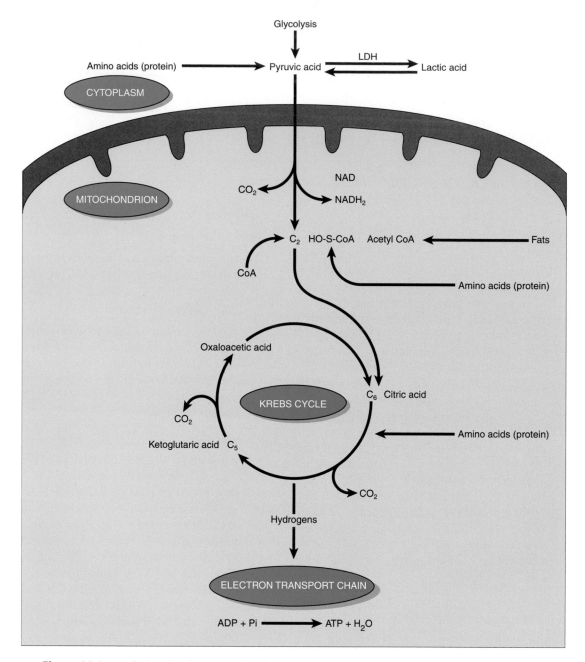

Figure 14.1.   Relationship between glycolysis, the Krebs cycle, and the electron transport chain.

tors, including muscle fiber type and how fast glycolysis is proceeding. If glycolytic flux is extremely rapid, hydrogen production may exceed the transport capability of the shuttle mechanisms that move hydrogen from the cytoplasm (called sarcoplasm in muscle) into the mitochondria, where oxidative phosphorylation occurs without true hypoxia. When glycolytic hydrogen production exceeds the mitochondrial transport capability, pyruvate must again accept the hydrogens to form lactate so glycolysis can continue. During exercise, epinephrine (adrenaline) levels in the blood are elevated, which stim-

ulates muscle glycogenolysis (breakdown of glycogen for fuel), increasing the rate of glycolysis. At rest and during low exercise intensities (<40% of maximal aerobic capacity), slow-twitch muscle fibers are recruited predominantly. As the exercise intensity increases, more fast-twitch fibers are recruited. This recruitment pattern has an important influence on lactic acid production. Conversion of pyruvate to lactate and vice versa is catalyzed by the enzyme lactate dehydrogenase (LDH), which exists in several forms (isozymes). Fast-twitch muscle fibers contain an LDH isozyme that favors the formation of lactate, whereas slow-twitch fibers contain an LDH form that promotes less conversion of pyruvate to lactate or even conversion of lactate to pyruvate. Therefore, more lactate formation occurs in fast-twitch fibers during exercise simply because of the type of LDH isozyme present, independent of oxygen availability in the muscle. Finally, fast-twitch fibers have higher activities of glycolytic enzymes than do slow-twitch fibers, indicating a greater potential of substrate flux through glycolysis.

In summary, debate over the mechanism or mechanisms responsible for muscle lactate production during exercise continues. It seems possible that any one or a combination of these possibilities (or lack of oxygen) may provide an explanation for muscle lactate production during exercise. The most important consequence of elevated lactic acid levels is the contribution to muscle fatigue. However, blood lactate can also be used as a fuel by muscles and other tissues during and following exercise. Lactate concentrations can rise in the blood only when the rate of lactate production begins to exceed its removal. A detailed discussion of this topic is available from other sources (2–5).

Aerobic Oxidation

The final metabolic pathway for ATP production combines two complex metabolic processes, the Krebs cycle and electron transport chain; it resides inside the mitochondria. Oxidative phosphorylation uses oxygen as the final hydrogen acceptor to form water and ATP. Unlike glycolysis, aerobic metabolism can use fat, protein, and carbohydrate as substrates to produce ATP. The interaction of these nutrients is illustrated in Figure 14.1.

Conceptually, the Krebs cycle can be considered a primer for oxidative phosphorylation. Entry into the Krebs cycle begins with the combination of acetyl-coenzyme A (CoA) and oxaloacetic acid to form citric acid. The primary function of the Krebs cycle is to remove hydrogens from four of the reactants involved in the cycle. The electrons from these hydrogens follow a chain of cytochromes (electron transport chain) in the mitochondria, and the energy released from this process is used to rephosphorylate ADP to form ATP. Oxygen is the final acceptor of hydrogen to form water, and this reaction is catalyzed by cytochrome oxidase (Fig. 14.1). Oxidation of carbohydrates via the Krebs cycle and the electron transport chain results in a total of 36 ATPs per unit of glucose substrate or 38 ATPs per unit of glycogen substrate. A more detailed review of oxidative phosphorylation can be found in other sources (6).

Fat Metabolism

Oxidation of fat, which provides acetyl-CoA as substrate for the Krebs cycle, is possible through aerobic metabolism. Glycolysis can also interact with the Krebs cycle in the presence of oxygen by the conversion of pyru-vate to form acetyl-CoA. Fat or triglycerides are lipids broken down to fatty acids and glycerol by hormone-sensitive lipase, which is inhibited by insulin and activated by catecholamines (epinephrine and norepinephrine) and growth hormone. Glycerol can be metabolized through glycolysis or used to make glucose. Free fatty acids enter the blood to be used as fuel in a process known as beta-oxidation, or they may be used as a precursor in the production of many substances, such as cholesterol. Fat metabolism and transport in the blood have important influences on many health-related problems, such as obesity and heart disease. Fatty acids must be activated using ATP and CoA and transported via the carnitine shuttle system to enter the mitochondria for oxidation. In the mitochondrial matrix, beta-oxidation proceeds sequentially by cleaving off two carbon atoms at a time, forming acetyl-CoA, the substrate for the Krebs cycle. A 16-carbon fatty acid such as palmitate yields 129 ATPs.

REGULATION OF BIOENERGETIC PATHWAYS

The bioenergetic pathways that result in production of cellular ATP are under precise control. This control is achieved by regulation of one or more regulatory (allosteric) enzymes, which catalyze one-way reactions. Rate-limiting enzymes in each of the aforementioned bioenergetic pathways can be up-regulated or down-regulated, depending on demand for ATP. In other words, cellular modulators regulate the catalytic activity of allosteric enzymes. Two of the most important modulators of bioenergetic regulatory enzymes are cellular concentrations of ATP and ADP. For example, CP breakdown is regulated by creatine kinase activity. Creatine kinase activity is elevated when cytoplasmic concentrations of ADP increase and ATP levels decrease. Conversely, high cellular ATP levels inhibit creatine kinase activity. This type of negative feedback control is common among bioenergetic pathways in the muscle fiber.

The rate-limiting enzyme in glycolysis is phosphofructokinase (PFK). PFK falls early in the glycolytic pathway, and similar to the regulation of creatine kinase, PFK activity is increased by a rise in cellular ADP concentration and a decrease in ATP levels. PFK activity is inhibited by a variety of factors, including high cellular concentrations of hydrogen ions, citrate, and ATP.

Although oxidative phosphorylation is under complex control, it is clear that cellular levels of ATP, ADP, and Ca^{2+} regulate key enzymes in the Krebs cycle (i.e., isocitrate dehydrogenase) and electron transport chain (i.e., cytochrome oxidase). An increase in cellular levels of ADP promotes oxidative phosphorylation and high concentrations of ATP inhibit this process, which is similar to the control schemes presented for the CP system and glycolysis. A more detailed discussion of oxidative phosphorylation is available (6).

METABOLIC RESPONSES TO EXERCISE

The importance of the interaction of the aforementioned metabolic pathways in the production of ATP during exercise should be emphasized. In reality the energy to perform most types of exercise does not come from a single source but from a combination of anaerobic and aerobic sources (Fig. 14.2). The contribution of anaerobic sources (CP system and glycolysis) to exercise energy metabolism is inversely related to the duration and intensity of the activity. The shorter and more intense the activity, the greater the contribution of anaerobic energy production, whereas the longer the activity and the lower the intensity, the greater the contribution of aerobic energy production. Although proteins can be used as a fuel for aerobic exercise, carbohydrates and fats are the primary energy substrates during exercise in a healthy, well-fed individual. In general, carbohydrates are used as the primary fuel at the onset of exercise and during high-intensity work (7–9). However, during prolonged exercise of low to moderate intensity (longer than 30 minutes), a gradual shift from carbohydrate toward an increasing reliance on fat as a substrate occurs (Fig. 14.3) (9, 10). The greatest amount of fat use occurs at about 60% of maximal aerobic capacity (VO$_{2max}$). A detailed discussion outlining the interplay of substrates during exercise is available from several sources (7–14). A brief discussion of the metabolic response to various types of exercise follows.

Short-Term, High-Intensity Exercise

The energy to perform short-term, high-intensity exercise (5 to 60 seconds' duration), such as weight lifting or sprinting 400 meters, comes primarily from anaerobic pathways. Whether the ATP–CP system or glycolysis dominates the ATP production depends on the duration of the muscular effort. In general, energy for all activities lasting less than 5 seconds comes from the ATP–CP system. In contrast, energy to perform a 20-meter sprint (30 seconds) would come from a combination of the ATP–CP system and anaerobic glycolysis, with glycolysis predominating. The transition from the CP system to glycolysis is not abrupt but rather a gradual shift from one pathway to another as the duration of the exercise increases.

As illustrated in Figure 14.2, exercise bouts lasting longer than 45 seconds use a combination of the CP system, glycolysis, and oxidative phosphorylation. For example, the energy required to sprint 400 meters (60 seconds) comes primarily (about 70%) from anaerobic pathways, while the remaining ATP production is provided by aerobic metabolism. The principal fuel used during this type of exercise is carbohydrate (glycogen) stored in muscle (15).

Transition from Rest to Light Exercise

In the transition from rest to light exercise, oxygen uptake kinetics follow a monoexponential pattern, reaching

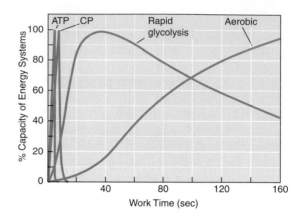

Figure 14.2.   Interaction between anaerobic and aerobic energy sources during exercise including ATP, creatine phosphate, rapid glycolysis, and aerobic (oxidative phosphorylation). Note that energy to perform short-term high intensity exercise comes primarily from anaerobic sources whereas energy for muscular contraction during prolonged exercise comes from aerobic metabolism.

a steady state generally within 1–4 minutes (Fig. 14.4) (16). The time required to reach a steady state increases at higher work rates and is longer in untrained individuals than in aerobically trained individuals. Because oxygen uptake does not increase instantaneously to steady state at the onset of exercise, it is implied that anaerobic energy sources contribute to the required VO$_2$ at the beginning of exercise. Indeed, evidence suggests that both the CP system and glycolysis contribute to the overall production of ATP at the onset of muscular work (17). Once a steady state is obtained, however, the ATP requirements are met by aerobic metabolism. The term oxygen deficit has been used to describe inadequate oxygen consumption at the

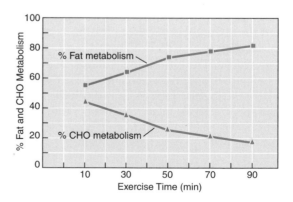

Figure 14.3.   Alterations in substrate utilization during prolonged submaximal (<60% V̇O$_2$max) exercise. CHO = carbohydrate. (With permission from Powers S, Byrd R, Tulley R, et al. Effects of caffeine ingestion on metabolism and performance during graded exercise. *Eur J Appl Physiol* 50:301, 1983.)

onset of exercise (Fig. 14.4). Similar to short-term heavy exercise, the principal fuel used during the transition from rest to light exercise is muscle glycogen (13).

Prolonged Submaximal Exercise

Steady-state VO_2 can usually be maintained during 10 to 60 minutes of submaximal continuous exercise. This rule has two exceptions. First, prolonged exercise in a hot and humid environment results in a steady drift upward of VO_2 during the course of exercise (18). Second, continuous exercise at a high relative work load results in a slow rise in VO_2 across time similar to that observed during exercise in a hot environment. In both cases, this drift probably occurs because of a variety of factors, such as rising body temperature and increasing blood catecholamines (19, 20).

As depicted in Figure 14.3, both carbohydrate and fat are used as substrates during prolonged exercise. During prolonged low- and moderate-intensity exercise, there is a gradual shift from carbohydrate metabolism to the use of fat as a substrate. Explanations for this metabolic shift include the following: fatty acids inhibit the Krebs cycle, leading to accumulation of citrate, which lowers PFK activity. This causes reduced uptake and oxidation of glucose. Carbohydrate metabolism regulates fat metabolism during exercise (21). The onset of exercise of low to moderate intensity produces a high glycolytic flux that slowly diminishes. The resulting glycolytic intermediates inhibit the carnitine transport system, thus preventing long-chain fatty acids from entering mitochondria for oxidation. Other factors that can affect the relative contribution of fat versus carbohydrate as energy substrate during prolonged exercise are nutritional status of the individual and the state of training.

Progressive Incremental Exercise

Figure 14.5 illustrates the oxygen uptake during a progressive incremental exercise test. Note that oxygen up-

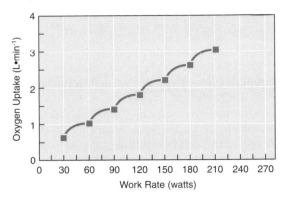

Figure 14.5. Changes in oxygen uptake as a function of work rate during incremental exercise.

take increases linearly with work rate until VO_{2max} is reached. After reaching a steady state, ATP used for muscular contraction during the early stages of an incremental exercise test comes primarily from aerobic metabolism. However, as the exercise intensity increases, blood levels of lactate rise (Fig. 14.6). Although much controversy surrounds this issue, many investigators believe that this lactate inflection point is a point of increasing reliance upon anaerobic metabolism brought about by the increased recruitment of nonoxidative fast-twitch muscle fibers.

Although the precise terminology is controversial, this sudden increase in blood lactate levels—termed the anaerobic threshold or lactate threshold—has important implications for the prediction of performance and perhaps exercise prescription. For example, it has been shown that the anaerobic threshold, used in combination with other physiological variables (i.e., VO_{2max}), is a useful predictor of success in distance running (22, 23). The lactate threshold may also prove to be a marker of the transition from moderate to heavy exercise for subjects and thus useful in exercise prescriptions.

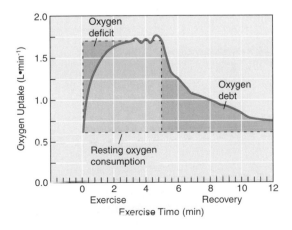

Figure 14.4. Oxygen uptake dynamics at onset and offset of exercise. See text for details.

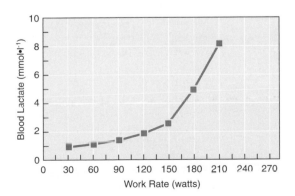

Figure 14.6. Changes in blood lactate concentrations as a function of work rate during incremental exercise.

Recovery From Exercise

Oxygen uptake remains elevated above resting levels for several minutes during recovery from exercise (Fig. 14.4). This elevated postexercise oxygen consumption has traditionally been termed the oxygen debt, but more recently the term elevated postexercise oxygen consumption (EPOC) has been applied (19). In general, postexercise metabolism is higher following high-intensity exercise than after light or moderate work. Furthermore, postexercise VO$_2$ remains elevated longer after prolonged exercise than after shorter-term exertion. The mechanisms to explain these observations are probably linked to the fact that both high-intensity and prolonged exercise result in higher body temperatures, greater ionic disturbance, and higher plasma catecholamines than in light or moderate short-term exercise (19).

MEASUREMENT OF METABOLISM AND OXYGEN CONSUMPTION

Traditionally, whole-body metabolism is measured using one of two strategies: direct or indirect calorimetry (24). The principles behind these two strategies can be explained by the following relationship:

$$Foodstuffs + O_2 \rightarrow Heat + CO_2 + H_2O$$
(Indirect calorimetry)   *(Direct calorimetry)*

Heat is liberated as a consequence of cellular respiration and cell (e.g., muscular) work. Thus, heat production by the body allows a direct assessment of metabolism. Direct calorimetry requires that a subject be placed in an airtight chamber. As heat is released, the temperature inside the chamber rises. Typically, a circulating jacket of water used to transfer heat to the environment allows a means of determining the metabolic rate in joules or kilocalories.

Although direct calorimetry is a precise technique, construction of large chambers for measurement of metabolic rate in humans is prohibitively expensive. Also, heat produced by exercise equipment can complicate measurements using direct calorimetry. The principle of indirect calorimetry uses the measurement of oxygen consumption (VO$_2$) to determine metabolic rate. Using this method, metabolic rate in kilocalories can be estimated using the following formula:

metabolic rate (kcal/minute) =
$$VO_2 \ (L/minute) \times [4.0 + RQ]$$

The most common method of measuring oxygen consumption uses open-circuit spirometry (Fig. 14.7). Volume of inspired oxygen is measured using a dry gas me-

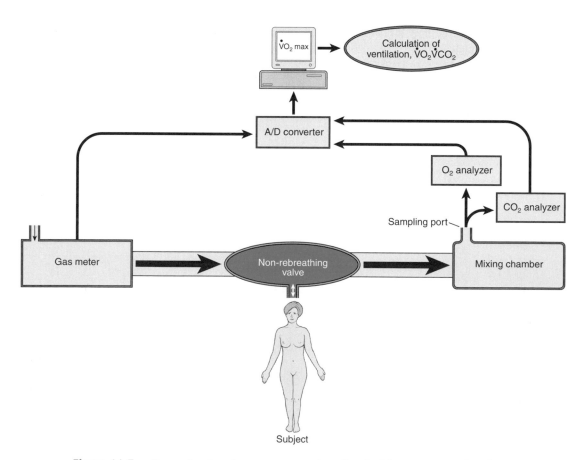

Figure 14.7. Open-circuit spirometry system interfaced with computer technology.

ter, turbine, or pneumatic. A one-way valve directs air through the mouth. Gas fractions are sampled and measured by oxygen and carbon dioxide analyzers on the expired side. Typically, analog voltages from the gas meter and analyzers are converted to digital information and fed into a microcomputer with VO_2 calculated using the Haldane transformation of the Fick equation:

$$VO_2 = V_I \times F_IO_2 \, V_I \times ([1 - F_EO_2 - F_ECO_2] / [1 - F_IO_2 - F_ICO_2]) \times F_EO_2$$

where V_I = inspired ventilation
$\quad F_IO_2$ = inspired oxygen fraction = 0.2093
$\quad F_ICO_2$ = inspired carbon dioxide fraction = 0.0003
$\quad F_EO_2$ = expired oxygen fraction
$\quad F_ECO_2$ = expired carbon dioxide fraction

ENERGY COST OF ACTIVITIES

The energy cost of many types of physical activity has been established. Appendix A lists some physical activities and their associated energy expenditures expressed in kilocalories per minute. Activities that are vigorous and involve large muscle groups usually result in more energy expended than those activities that use small muscle mass or require limited exertion. The estimates of energy expenditure listed in Appendix A were obtained by measuring oxygen cost of these activities in an adult population.

Clinicians often use the term metabolic equivalent (MET) to describe exercise intensity. A single MET is equivalent to the amount of energy expended during 1 minute of rest. Therefore, exercise at a metabolic rate that is five times the resting VO_2 rate is equivalent to 5 METs. In a strict sense, the absolute energy expenditure during exercise at a 5-MET intensity depends on the body size of the individual (i.e., a large person is likely to have a larger resting VO_2 than a small person). For simplicity, individual differences in resting energy expenditures are often overlooked, and 1 MET is considered equivalent to a VO_2 of 3.5 mL/kg/minute; hence, 1 MET represents an energy expenditure of approximately 1.2 kcal/minute for a 70-kg person.

▶ **SUMMARY**

Exercise metabolism is a reflection of each metabolic pathway as it contributes to the increased energy demands of activity and work. Substrates for energy production include carbohydrate, fat, and protein. The mix of these substrates during exercise metabolism depends on the intensity and duration of exercise and the conditioning of the individual.

References

1. Armstrong R. Biochemistry: Energy liberation and use. In: Strauss RS, ed. Sports Medicine and Physiology. Philadelphia: Saunders, 1979.
2. Graham T. Mechanisms of blood lactate increase during exercise. Physiologist 27:299, 1984.
3. Katz A, Sahlin K. Oxygen in regulation of glycolysis and lactate production in human skeletal muscle. Exerc Sport Sci Rev 18:1, 1990.
4. Richardsen RS, Noyszewsky EA, Leogh JS, Wagner PD. Lactate efflux from exercising human skeletal muscle: Role of intracellular P_{O_2}. J Appl Physiol 85:627, 1998.
5. Stainsby W, Brooks C. Control of lactic acid metabolism in contracting skeletal muscles during exercise. Exerc Sport Sci Rev 18:29, 1990.
6. Senior A. ATP synthesis by oxidative phosphorylation. Physiol Rev 68:177, 1988.
7. Gollnick P, Riedy M, Quintinskie J, Bertocci L. Differences in metabolic potential of skeletal muscle fibres and their significance for metabolic control. J Exp Biol 115:191, 1985.
8. Gollnick P. Metabolism of substrates: Energy substrate metabolism during exercise and as modified by training. Fed Proc 44:353, 1985.
9. Newsholme E. The control of fuel utilization by muscle during exercise and starvation. Diabetes 28(Suppl 1):1, 1979.
10. Powers S, Riley W, Howley E. Comparison of fat metabolism between trained men and women during prolonged aerobic work. Res Q Exerc Sport 51:427, 1980.
11. Holloszy J, Coyle E. Adaptations of skeletal muscle to endurance exercise and their metabolic consequences. J Appl Physiol 56:831, 1984.
12. Holloszy J. Utilization of fatty acids during exercise. In: Taylor AW, Gollnick PD, Green HJ, et al., eds. Biochemistry of Exercise VII. Champaign, IL: Human Kinetics, 1990.
13. Stanley W, Connett R. Regulation of muscle carbohydrate metabolism during exercise. FASEB J 5:2155, 1991.
14. Bonen A, McDermott J, Tan M. Glucose transport in muscle. In: Taylor AW, Gollnick PD, Green HJ, et al., eds. Biochemistry of Exercise VII. Champaign, IL: Human Kinetics, 1990.
15. Powers S, Byrd R, Tulley R, et al. Effects of caffeine ingestion on metabolism and performance during graded exercise. Eur J Appl Physiol 50:301, 1983.
16. Powers S, Dodd S, Beadle R. Oxygen uptake kinetics in trained athletes differing in VO_{2max}. Eur J Appl Physiol 54:306, 1985.
17. diPrampero P. Boutellier U, Pietsch P. Oxygen deficit and stores at onset of muscular exercise in humans. J Appl Physiol 55:146, 1983.
18. Powers S, Howley E, Cox R. Ventilatory and metabolic reactions to heat stress during prolonged exercise. J Sports Med 22:32, 1982.
19. Gaesser G, Brooks C. Metabolic bases of excess post-exercise oxygen consumption: A review. Med Sci Sports Exerc 16:29, 1984.
20. Powers S, Howley E, Cox R. A differential catecholamine response during prolonged exercise and passive heating. Med Sci Sports Exerc 14:435, 1982.
21. Coyle EF, Jeukendrup AE, Wagonmakers AJM, Saris WHM. Fatty acid oxidation is directly regulated by carbohydrate metabolism during exercise. Am J Physiol 273:E268, 1997.
22. Farrell PA, Wilmore JH, Coyle EF, et al. Plasma lactate accumulation and distance running performance. Med Sci Sports Exerc 11:338, 1979.
23. Powers S, Dodd S, Deason R, et al. Ventilatory threshold, running economy and distance running performance of trained athletes. Res Q Exerc Sport 51:179, 1983.

24. Powers SK, Howley ET. Exercise Physiology. Madison, WI: Brown & Benchmark, 1994.

Suggested Reading

Brooks G, Fahey T, White T, Baldwin K. Exercise Physiology: Human Bioenergetics and its Applications. Mountain View, CA: Mayfield, 2000.

Holloszy J. Muscle metabolism during exercise. Arch Phys Med Rehab 63:231, 1982.

Mathews C, van Holde K. Biochemistry. Redwood City, CA: Benjamin Cummings, 1990.

McArdle W, Katch F, Katch V. Exercise Physiology. Philadelphia: Lea & Febiger, 1991.

Powers S, Howley E. Exercise Physiology: Theory and Application to Fitness and Performance. Dubuque: William C. Brown, 1996.

1.2.1, 1.2.6   2.2.1, 2.2.2, 2.2.12,   4.2.0.2, 4.2.0.3, 4.2.0.6,
                  2.2.14, 2.2.15, 2.6.0.14   4.2.1.1, 4.2.2.1, 4.2.2.2,
                                     4.2.3, 4.2.3.2, 4.2.3.3

CHAPTER **15**

NORMAL CARDIORESPIRATORY RESPONSES TO ACUTE AEROBIC EXERCISE

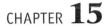

Barry A. Franklin

The energy requirements of exercising human muscle may increase substantially in the transition from rest to maximal physical exertion. Because the available stores of adenosine triphosphate (ATP) are limited and capable of providing energy to maintain vigorous activity for only several seconds, ATP must be constantly resynthesized to provide continuous energy production (Fig. 15.1). Therefore, exercising muscle must possess a large capacity for increasing metabolic rate to produce sufficient ATP so that increased activity can continue. Energy production relies heavily on the respiratory and cardiovascular systems for the delivery of oxygen and nutrients and for the removal of waste products to maintain the internal equilibrium of cells.

The purpose of this chapter is to review the normal cardiorespiratory responses to acute aerobic exercise with specific reference to energy systems, hemodynamics, posture, maximal oxygen consumption ($\dot{V}O_{2max}$), the anaerobic threshold, dynamic versus isometric exertion, arm versus leg exercise, myocardial oxygen consumption, and the effects of physical conditioning. This information is vital to the understanding of the role of exercise physiology in the interpretation of diagnostic and functional exercise testing and the prescription of exercise in health and disease.

ENERGY SYSTEMS FOR EXERCISE

Adenosine triphosphate (ATP) is broken down enzymatically inside cells into adenosine diphosphate (ADP) and phosphate (P) to provide energy for muscle contraction and the generation of force, as summarized by the reaction:

$$ATP + H_2O \rightarrow ADP + P + energy$$

Although not all ATP is formed aerobically, the amount of ATP yielded by anaerobic glycolysis is extremely small (Table 15.1) (1). Nevertheless, anaerobic mechanisms provide a rapid source of ATP, which is particularly important at the beginning of any exercise bout and during

high-intensity activity that can only be sustained for a brief period. As duration of exercise increases, the relative contribution of anaerobic energy sources decreases (Fig. 15.2) (2).

The aerobic system requires adequate delivery and use of oxygen and uses glycogen, fats, and proteins as energy substrates. It can sustain high rates of ATP production for muscular energy. The relative contribution of anaerobic and aerobic metabolism depends on oxygen consumption (respiration), delivery (cardiovascular), and use (muscular extraction) at rates commensurate with the energy demands of activity.

ACUTE CARDIORESPIRATORY RESPONSES TO EXERCISE

Many cardiorespiratory and hemodynamic mechanisms function collectively to support increased aerobic requirements of physical activity. The overall effect of changes in heart rate (HR), stroke volume, cardiac output, blood flow, blood pressure, arteriovenous oxygen difference, and pulmonary ventilation is to oxygenate blood that is delivered to the active tissues.

Heart Rate

Heart rate increases in a linear fashion with the work rate and oxygen uptake during dynamic exercise. The increase in HR during exercise occurs primarily at the expense of diastole (filling time), rather than systole (Fig. 15.3) (3). Thus, at high exercise intensities, diastolic time may be so short as to preclude adequate ventricular filling. The magnitude of the HR response is related to age, body position, fitness, type of activity, the presence of heart disease, medications, blood volume, and environmental factors such as temperature and humidity. In contrast to systolic blood pressure, which usually increases with age, maximum attainable HR decreases with age. The equation, 220 − age, provides an approximation of the maximum HR in healthy men and women, but the variance for any fixed age is considerable (standard deviation about ± 10 beats/minute).

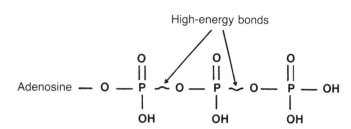

Triphosphate

High-energy bonds

Figure 15.1. Simplified structure of an ATP molecule. The symbol represents the high-energy bonds.

Stroke Volume

The stroke volume (SV) (volume of blood ejected per heart beat) is equal to the difference between end diastolic volume (EDV) and end systolic volume (ESV). The former is determined by HR, filling pressure, and ventricular compliance, whereas the latter depends on two variables: contractility and afterload. Thus, a greater diastolic filling (preload) will increase SV. In contrast, factors that resist ventricular outflow (afterload) will result in a reduced SV.

Stroke volume at rest in the upright position generally varies between 60 and 100 mL/beat among healthy adults, while maximum SV approximates 100 to 120 mL/beat. During exercise, SV increases curvilinearly with the work rate until it reaches near maximum at a level equivalent to approximately 50% of aerobic capacity, increasing only slightly thereafter (4). Within physiological limits, enhanced venous return increases EDV, stretching cardiac muscle fibers and increasing force of contraction (Frank-Starling mechanism); thus ejection fraction may increase. Ejection fraction is defined by the following:

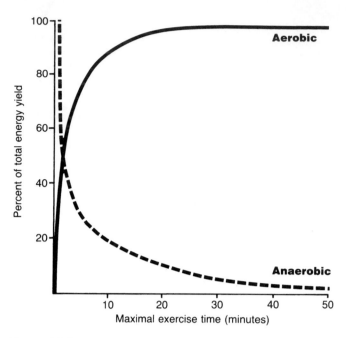

Figure 15.2. Relative contribution of aerobic and anaerobic metabolism during physical activity of increasing duration. In intense activities lasting 1.5 to 2 minutes, the ATP-CP and lactic acid energy systems generate approximately 50% of the energy, while aerobic metabolism supplies the remainder. A distance runner, on the other hand, derives essentially 98% of his energy from aerobic metabolism during a 50-minute training run.

Table 15.1. Characteristics of the Two Mechanisms by Which ATP is Formed

Mechanism	Food or Chemical Fuel	Oxygen Required?	Relative ATP Yield
Anaerobic			
Phosphocreatine	Phosphocreatine	No	Extremely limited
Glycolysis	Glycogen (glucose)	No	Extremely limited
Aerobic			
Krebs cycle and electron transport system	Glycogen, fats, proteins	Yes	Large

Adapted with permission from Mathews DK, Fox EL. The Physiological Basis of Physical Education and Athletics, 3rd ed. Philadelphia: Saunders, 1981.

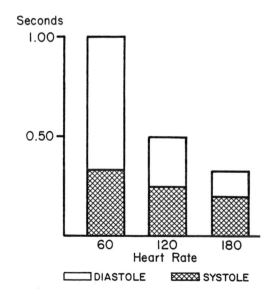

Figure 15.3. Relationship of systolic and diastolic time to HR. Since coronary blood flow predominates during diastole, with increased HR, as during exercise, diastolic (perfusion) time is disproportionately shortened. (Adapted with permission from Dehn MM, Mullins CB. Physiologic effects and importance of exercise in patients with coronary artery disease. J Cardiovasc Med 2:365–387, 1977.)

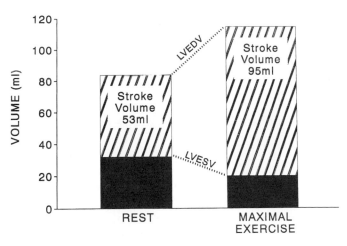

Figure 15.4. Changes in stroke volume from rest to maximal upright exercise is shown in young, healthy men. LVEDV, left ventricular end-diastolic volume; LVESV, left ventricular end-systolic volume. (Adapted with permission from Poliner LR, Dehmer GJ, Lewis SE, et al. Left ventricular performance in normal subjects: A comparison of the responses to exercise in the upright and supine position. Circulation 62:528–534, 1980.)

$$ejection\ fraction = [SV/EDV] \times 100$$

Ejection fraction is normally 65% ± 8%, resulting from both the Frank-Starling mechanism and decreased ESV (Fig. 15.4) (5). The latter is due to increased ventricular contractility, secondary to catecholamine mediated sympathetic stimulation. The magnitude of these changes depends on several variables, including ventricular function, body position, and the intensity of exercise. Moreover, at a higher HR, stroke volume may actually decrease because of the disproportionate shortening in diastolic filling time (Fig. 15.3) (3, 6).

Cardiac Output

The product of SV and HR determines cardiac output. Cardiac output in healthy adults increases linearly with increased work rate, from a resting value of approximately 5 L/minute to a maximum of about 20 L/minute during upright exercise. However, maximum values of cardiac output depend on many factors, including age, posture, body size, presence of cardiovascular disease, and the level of physical conditioning. At exercise intensities up to 50% VO_{2max}, the increase in cardiac output is facilitated by increases in HR and SV (4). Thereafter, the increase results almost solely from the continued rise in HR.

Arteriovenous Oxygen Difference

Oxygen extraction by tissues reflects the difference between oxygen content of arterial blood (about 20 mL O_2/100 mL/dL at rest) and the oxygen content of venous blood (about 15 mL O_2/dL), yielding a typical arteriovenous oxygen difference (CaO$_2$ − CvO$_2$) at rest of 5 mL O_2/dL. This approximates a use coefficient of 25%. During exercise to exhaustion, the mixed venous oxygen content typically decreases to 5 mL/dL blood or lower, thus widening the arteriovenous oxygen difference from 5 to 15 mL/dL blood, corresponding to a use coefficient of 75% (4).

Blood Flow

At rest, 15–20% of the cardiac output is distributed to the skeletal muscles; the remainder goes to visceral organs, the heart, and the brain (7). However, during exercise as much as 85–90% of the cardiac output is selectively delivered to working muscle and shunted away from the skin and the splanchnic, hepatic, and renal vascular beds. Myocardial blood flow may increase four to five times with exercise, whereas blood supply to the brain is maintained at resting levels (8).

Blood Pressure

There is a linear increase in systolic blood pressure (SBP) with increasing levels of exercise, approximating 8 to 12 mm Hg per metabolic equivalent (MET), where 1 MET = 3.5 mL O_2/kg/minute. Maximal values typically reach 190 to 220 mm Hg (9). Nevertheless, maximal SBP should not be greater than 260 mm Hg (10). Diastolic blood pressure (DBP) may decrease slightly or remain unchanged; thus, pulse pressure (SBP minus DBP) generally increases in direct proportion to the intensity of exercise.

Because blood pressure is directly related to cardiac output and peripheral vascular resistance, it provides a noninvasive way to monitor the inotropic performance, or pumping capacity, of the heart. Until automated devices are adequately validated, the blood pressure response to exercise should be taken manually with a cuff and a stethoscope (10). A SBP that fails to rise or falls with increasing work loads may signal a plateau or decrease in cardiac output, respectively (11). Exercise testing should be terminated in persons demonstrating exertional hypotension (SBP toward the end of a test decreasing below baseline standing level and/or SBP decreasing 20 mm Hg or more during exercise after an initial rise). This response has been shown to correlate with myocardial ischemia, left ventricular dysfunction, and an increased risk of cardiac events during follow-up (12). In one study, men with a maximal SBP below 140 mm Hg had a 15-fold increase in the annual rate of sudden death compared with those whose pressures exceeded 200 mm Hg (13).

Pulmonary Ventilation

Pulmonary ventilation ($\dot{V}_E$), the volume of air exchanged per minute, generally approximates 6 L/minute at rest in the average sedentary adult male. At maximal exercise, however, V_E often increases 15- to 25-fold over resting values. During mild to moderate exercise intensities, $\dot{V}_E$ is increased primarily by increasing tidal volume, whereas increases in the respiratory rate are more important to augment $\dot{V}_E$ during vigorous exercise. For the most part, the increase in pulmonary ventilation is directly proportional to the increase in somatic oxygen consumed ($\dot{V}O_2$) and carbon dioxide produced ($\dot{V}CO_2$). However, at a critical exercise intensity (usually 47% to 64% of the $\dot{V}O_{2max}$ in healthy untrained individuals and 70–90% of the $\dot{V}O_{2max}$ in highly trained subjects), $\dot{V}_E$ increases disproportionately relative to $\dot{V}O_2$, paralleling the abrupt nonlinear increases in serum lactate and $\dot{V}CO_2$ (14, 15). This suggests that pulmonary ventilation is perhaps regulated more by the requirement for carbon dioxide removal than by oxygen consumption and that ventilation is not normally a limiting factor to aerobic capacity.

POSTURAL CONSIDERATIONS

Posture has an effect on venous return and preload, particularly during brief bouts of physical exertion. At rest, EDV is highest when the body is recumbent. It decreases progressively as one shifts into sitting and standing postures, respectively. During exercise in the supine position, EDV remains largely unchanged. Thus, alterations in preload have little influence in increasing SV in this type of exercise. During exercise in the upright posture, EDV increases at intensities less than 50% $\dot{V}O_{2max}$. However, at higher exercise intensities, end-diastolic and SVs may decrease in some subjects (16, 17).

Prolonged upright exercise at a constant work rate places an increasing load on the heart (cardiovascular drift). Although the aerobic requirement of the exercise does not change, there is a progressive decrease in venous return, leading to a reduction in SV and a progressive rise in HR. The resulting tachycardia may be attributed, at least in part, to alterations in sympathetic blood flow control mechanisms, increased shunting of blood to the periphery (skin) for cooling, and decreased central blood volume (particularly in warm environments).

MAXIMAL OXYGEN CONSUMPTION

The most widely recognized measure of cardiopulmonary fitness is the aerobic capacity, or $\dot{V}O_{2max}$. This variable is defined physiologically as the highest rate of oxygen transport and use that can be achieved at maximal physical exertion. Somatic oxygen consumption ($\dot{V}O_2$) may be expressed mathematically by a rearrangement of the Fick equation:

$$\dot{V}O_2 = HR \times SV \times (a - vDO_2)$$

where: $\dot{V}O_2$ = oxygen consumption (mL/kg/min)
Heart rate = heart rate (bpm)
Stroke volume = stroke volume (mL/beat)
$(a - vDO_2)$ = arteriovenous oxygen difference

Thus, it is apparent that both central (i.e., cardiac output) and peripheral (i.e., arteriovenous oxygen difference) regulatory mechanisms affect the magnitude of body oxygen consumption.

Typical circulatory data at rest and during maximal exercise in a healthy, sedentary 30-year-old man and a similarly aged world-class endurance athlete are shown in Table 15.2. The absolute resting oxygen consumption (250 mL/minute) divided by body weight (70 kg) gives the resting energy requirement, 1 MET (about 3.5 mL/kg/minute). This expression of resting $\dot{V}O_2$, believed to originate from the work of Balke (18), is extremely important in exercise physiology, being independent of body weight and aerobic fitness. Furthermore, multiples of this value are often used to quantify respective levels of energy expenditure. For example, running at a 6-mph pace requires 10 times the resting energy expenditure; thus the aerobic cost is 10 METs, or 35 mL/kg/minute.

The 10-fold increase in oxygen transport and use in the sedentary individual is contrasted by a 23-fold increase in the endurance athlete, corresponding to a $\dot{V}O_{2max}$ of 35 mL/kg/minute and 80 mL/kg/minute, respectively. Increased aerobic capacity in trained athletes appears primarily as the result of increased maximal cardiac output, because of a greater increment in HR and SV rather than

Table 15.2. Hypothetical Circulatory Data at Rest and During Maximal Exercise for a Sedentary Man and a World-Class Endurance Athlete: 30-Year-Old Subjects

Condition	Oxygen Consumption (L/min)	(mL/kg/min)	Cardiac Output (L/min)	Heart Rate (beats/min)	Stroke Volume (mL/beat)	Arteriovenous Oxygen Difference (mL/dL blood)
Sedentary man (70 kg)						
Rest	0.25	3.5	6.1	70	87	4.0
Maximal exercise	2.50	35.0	17.7	190	93	14.0
World-class endurance athlete (70 kg)						
Rest	0.25	3.5	6.1	45	136	4.0
Maximal exercise	5.60	80.0	35.0	190	184	16.0

an increased peripheral extraction of oxygen. Because there is little variation in maximal HR and maximal systemic arteriovenous oxygen difference with training, $\dot{V}O_{2max}$ virtually defines the pumping capacity of the heart. Therefore, it is of major importance in the cardiovascular evaluation of the individual.

$\dot{V}O_{2max}$ may be expressed on an absolute or relative basis, that is, in liters per minute, reflecting total body energy output and caloric expenditure (i.e., 1 L ~ 5 kcal), or by dividing this value by body weight in kilograms. Because large persons usually have a large absolute oxygen consumption by virtue of larger muscle mass, the latter allows a more equitable comparison between individuals of different body mass. This variable, when expressed as milliliters of oxygen per kilogram of body weight per minute or as METs, is widely considered the single best index of physical work capacity or cardiorespiratory fitness (19).

Determination of the $\dot{V}O_{2max}$

Maximal oxygen consumption is usually determined by measuring the volume and oxygen content of expired air, corrected to standard temperature and pressure dry (STPD), using the following equation:

$$\dot{V}O_2 = \dot{V}_E \, (F_IO_2 - F_EO_2)$$

where: $\dot{V}_E$ = expired air (L/minute)

F_EO_2 = directly measured fraction oxygen in expired air

F_IO_2 = directly measured fraction oxygen in inspired air (normally 0.2093)

Traditionally, $\dot{V}O_2$ has been measured using an open circuit or Douglas bag technique. However, several auto-mated systems are available to measure $\dot{V}O_2$ and related respiratory variables during exercise testing.

Because it is often inconvenient to measure the $\dot{V}O_{2max}$ directly, physiologists have sought to estimate aerobic capacity from the peak treadmill speed and grade, or cycle ergometer work rate, expressed as kilogram meters per minute. The conventional Bruce test is perhaps the most familiar and widely employed treadmill protocol with normative data on oxygen consumption so that aerobic capacity may be estimated from the workload attained (Fig. 15.5) (20). However, when a multistage protocol, like Bruce, is used to predict the $\dot{V}O_{2max}$, aerobic capacity may be markedly overestimated (21). One recent advance in test methodology that can overcome many of the limitations of incremental exercise is ramping (22, 23). Ramp protocols involve a nearly continuous and uniform increase in aerobic requirements that replaces the staging used in conventional exercise tests. With ramping, the gradual increase in demand allows a steady rise in cardiopulmonary responses.

ANAEROBIC (VENTILATORY) THRESHOLD

The onset of metabolic acidosis during exercise, traditionally determined by serial measurements of blood lactate, can be noninvasively determined by assessment of expired gases during exercise testing, specifically pulmonary ventilation ($\dot{V}_E$) and carbon dioxide production ($\dot{V}CO_2$) (24). Theoretically, gas exchange anaerobic threshold (AT) signifies the peak work rate or oxygen consumption at which the energy demands exceed circulatory ability to sustain aerobic metabolism. The physiology underlying the AT may be attributed, at least in part, to buffering of lactic acid by sodium bicarbonate in the

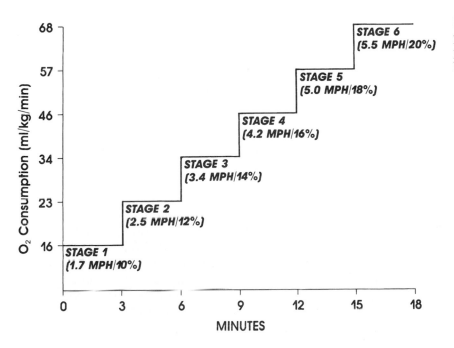

Figure 15.5. The standard Bruce treadmill protocol showing progressive stages (speed, percentage grade) and the corresponding aerobic requirement, expressed as mL/kg/minute.

blood, so that carbon dioxide is released in excess of that produced by muscle metabolism, providing an additional stimulus for ventilation. These biochemical alterations are summarized by the following reaction:

$$HLa \quad + \quad Na \, HCO_3 \quad \rightarrow \quad Na \, La$$
$$\text{(Lactic acid)} \quad \text{(sodium bicarbonate)} \quad \text{(sodium lactate)}$$
$$+ \, H_2 \, CO_3 \, + \, H_2O \, + \, CO_2$$
$$\text{(carbonic acid)}$$

Accordingly, values for $\dot{V}_E$ and carbon dioxide production increase out of proportion to the intensity of exercise performed (Fig. 15.6), suggesting an abrupt increase in serum lactate (14). This method correlates well with the lactate method and obviates measurement of lactate in repeated blood samples. An increase in the ventilatory equivalent for oxygen ($\dot{V}_E/\dot{V}O_2$) during exercise without a

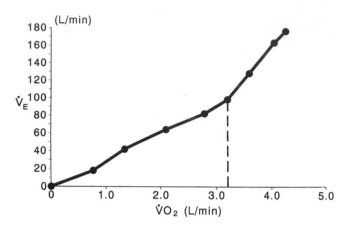

Figure 15.7. Relationship between intensity of exercise ($\dot{V}O_2$) and simultaneous, abrupt nonlinear increase in minute ventilation, signifying the anaerobic threshold. In this subject, the break point occurred at 3.20 L/minute, corresponding to 75% of measured $\dot{V}O_{2max}$ (4.25 L/minute).

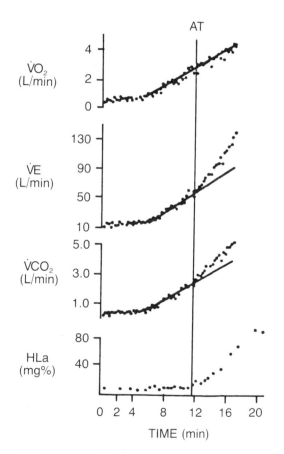

Figure 15.6. Relationship between intensity of exercise (oxygen consumption, $\dot{V}O_2$) and simultaneous, abrupt nonlinear increases in serum lactate (HLa), carbon dioxide production ($\dot{V}CO_2$), and pulmonary ventilation ($\dot{V}_E$) occurring at the anaerobic threshold (AT). Exercise was initiated at minute 4. (Adapted with permission from Davis JA, Vodak P, Wilmore JH, et al. Anaerobic threshold and maximal aerobic power for three modes of exercise. J Appl Physiol 41:544–550, 1976.)

corresponding change in the ventilatory equivalent for carbon dioxide ($\dot{V}_E/\dot{V}CO_2$) has also been reported to be sensitive and reliable for determining the AT (25). There is, however, controversy surrounding the mechanisms responsible for the AT (26). Increased lactate production may result from mechanisms not related to inadequate oxygen delivery. Another theory is that inflections in $\dot{V}_E$ and $\dot{V}CO_2$ are due to inadequate buffering at a fixed metabolic intensity, even when lactate production and oxygen uptake continue to rise linearly.

The AT from respiratory gas measurements is often expressed as a percentage of the $\dot{V}O_{2max}$. For example, a highly trained athlete with a $\dot{V}O_{2max}$ of 4.25 L/minute whose break point in $\dot{V}_E$ occurs at 3.20 L/minute has an AT corresponding to 75% of aerobic capacity (Fig. 15.7). This athlete should be able to maintain exercise intensities below 75% of $\dot{V}O_{2max}$ using a predominance of aerobic processes. Moreover, such exertion should be accomplished without inducing a significant increase in blood lactic acid and muscle fatigue. Although the AT typically corresponds to 55% ± 8% of the $\dot{V}O_{2max}$ in healthy untrained individuals, it normally occurs at a higher percentage of the $\dot{V}O_{2max}$ (i.e., 70–90%) in physically trained subjects (14, 15).

The $\dot{V}O_{2max}$ is recognized as an important predictor of performance in endurance events. However, several studies now suggest that the highest percentage of the $\dot{V}O_{2max}$ that can be used over an extended duration without incurring significant increase in arterial lactate may be an even more important determinant of cardiorespiratory performance (15, 27). This suggests that the AT may be critical in determining optimal pace during endurance events.

DYNAMIC (ISOTONIC) VERSUS ISOMETRIC (STATIC) EXERTION

Dynamic, or isotonic, activity (physical exertion characterized by rhythmic, repetitive movements of large muscle groups) results in increased oxygen consumption and HR that parallels the intensity of activity, as well as an increase in SV. There is a concomitant progressive increase in SBP with maintenance of or a slight decrease in DBP, thus an increasing pulse pressure.

Blood is shunted from the viscera to working skeletal muscle, where increased oxygen extraction increases systemic a-vDO$_2$. Thus, dynamic exercise imposes a volume load on the myocardium, which is the basis for a cardiac training effect. In contrast, isometric exertion involves sustained muscle contraction against a fixed load or resistance with no change in length of the involved muscle group or joint motion.

The cardiovascular response to isometric exertion is apparently mediated by a neurogenic mechanism (28). Activities involving less than 20% of the maximum voluntary contraction (MVC) of the involved muscle group evoke a modest increase in SBP, DBP, and HR. During contractions greater than 20% of the MVC, HR increases in relation to the tension exerted and there is an abrupt and precipitous increase in SBP. The SV remains essentially unchanged except at high levels of tension (>50% MVC), where it may decrease. The result is a moderate increase in cardiac output, which is nevertheless high for the accompanying magnitude of increased metabolism. Despite the increased cardiac output, blood flow to the non-contracting muscle does not significantly increase, probably because of reflex vasoconstriction. The combination of vasoconstriction and increased cardiac output causes a disproportionate rise in systolic, diastolic, and mean blood pressure. Thus, a significant pressure load is imposed on the heart, presumably to increase perfusion to the active (contracting) skeletal muscle. A comparison of the relative hemodynamic responses to dynamic and isometric exercise is shown in Table 15.3.

The magnitude of the pressor response to isometric exertion depends on tension exerted relative to the greatest possible tension in the muscle group (% MVC), as well as muscle mass involved (29, 30). Thus, a relatively mild isometric contraction by weakened upper extremities may evoke an excessive pressor response. The increased myocardial demands are camouflaged by the relatively low aerobic requirements, so the usual warning signs of overexertion (tachycardia, sweating, dyspnea) may be absent. In persons who have an ischemic left ventricle, a marked pressure increase may lead to threatening ventricular arrhythmias, significant ST-segment depression, angina pectoris, ventricular decompensation, and in rare instances, sudden cardiac death (31).

ARM VERSUS LEG EXERCISE

At a fixed power output (kg/minute or watts [W]), HR, SBP, and DBP, the product of the HR times SBP (rate times pressure), V$_E$, $\dot{V}O_2$, respiratory exchange ratio, and blood lactate concentration are higher, while SV and AT (the latter expressed as a percentage of aerobic capacity) are lower during arm exercise than leg exercise (32). Since cardiac output is nearly the same in arm and leg exercise at a fixed oxygen uptake, elevated blood pressure during arm exercise is believed to reflect increased peripheral vascular resistance. During maximal effort, physiological responses are usually greater during leg exercise than arm exercise, except when subjects are limited in ability to perform leg work by neurological, vascular, or orthopaedic impairment of the lower extremities (33).

The disparity in cardiorespiratory and hemodynamic response to arm exercise versus leg exercise at identical work rates appears to be due to several factors. Mechanical efficiency (i.e., the ratio between the output of external work and caloric expenditure, or $\dot{V}O_2$) is lower during arm exercise than leg exercise (33). This may reflect the involvement of smaller muscle groups and the static effort required with arm work, which increases $\dot{V}O_2$ but does not affect the external work output. The higher rate–pressure product and estimated myocardial oxygen consumption at a fixed external work rate for arm work compared with leg work (Fig. 15.8) is believed to reflect increased sympathetic tone during arm exercise, perhaps mediated by reduced SV with compensatory tachycardia, concomitant isometric contraction, vasoconstriction in the nonexercising leg muscles, or all of these factors (34).

$\dot{V}O_{2max}$ during arm exercise in men and women generally varies between 64% and 80% of leg $\dot{V}O_{2max}$ (32). Similarly, maximal cardiac output is lower during arm exercise than leg exercise, whereas the maximal HR, SBP, and rate–pressure product are comparable or slightly lower during arm exercise. The latter, however, has relevance to arm exercise training recommendations, particularly training intensity. Accordingly, an arm exercise prescription that assumes a maximal heart rate equivalent to

Table 15.3. Comparison of the Relative Hemodynamic Responses to Dynamic and Static Exertion

	DYNAMIC (ISOTONIC)	STATIC (ISOMETRIC)
Cardiac output	++++	+
Heart rate	++	+
Stroke volume	++	0
Peripheral resistance	−	+++
Systolic blood pressure	+++	++++
Diastolic blood pressure	0 −	++++
Mean arterial pressure	0 +	++++
Left ventricular work	Volume Load	Pressure Load

+, increase; − decrease; 0, unchanged.

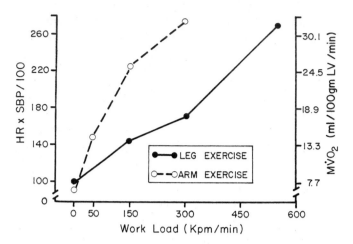

Figure 15.8. Mean rate–pressure product and estimated myocardial oxygen consumption (MV̇O₂) during arm (*broken line*) and leg (*solid line*) exercise. MV̇O₂ is estimated from its hemodynamic correlates, heart rate (HR) multiplied by systolic blood pressure (SBP). (Adapted with permission from Schwade J, Blomqvist CG, Shapiro W. A comparison of the response to arm and leg work in patients with ischemic heart disease. Am Heart J 94:203–208, 1977.)

leg exercise testing may result in an overestimation of the training HR. As a general guideline, the prescribed HR for leg training should be reduced by approximately 10 bpm for arm training (35).

MYOCARDIAL OXYGEN CONSUMPTION

Determinants of myocardial oxygen consumption (MV̇O₂) include HR, myocardial contractility, and the tension or stress developed in the ventricular wall. Wall tension reflects a combination of SBP and ventricular volume and is inversely related to myocardial wall thickness (Fig. 15.9). During exercise, increased HR is the major contributor to increased myocardial oxygen demand. In contrast, oxygen supply is primarily facilitated by increased coronary blood flow, enabled by decreased coronary vascular resistance with only a modest increase in an already substantial myocardial oxygen difference.

Several investigators have reported excellent correlations between measured MV̇O₂, (expressed as milliliters of oxygen per 100 g of left ventricle per minute), HR and rate–pressure product; where $MV̇O_2 = 0.28\,HR - 14$ (r = 0.88) or $MV̇O_2 = ([0.14 \times HR \times SBP]/100) - 6.3)$ (r = 0.92) (36, 37). HR alone is limited in ability to assess MV̇O₂, especially when SBP is markedly elevated; this may occur during upper extremity work involving isometric or isodynamic efforts.

Exercise-induced angina and significant ST-segment depression (≥1 mm) usually occur at the same rate–pressure product in an individual with ischemic heart disease. This suggests the existence of an ischemic threshold at which myocardial oxygen demand exceeds myocardial oxygen supply. The rate–pressure product also provides an estimate of maximal workload that the left ventricle can perform. It has been suggested that an adequate

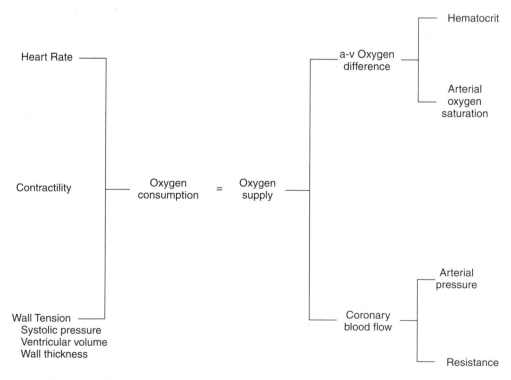

Figure 15.9. Determinants of myocardial oxygen demand and supply.

rate–pressure product during maximal exercise is greater than 25,000; however, this may be influenced by age, clinical status, and medications, especially beta-blockers (10).

References

1. Mathews DK, Fox EL. The Physiological Basis of Physical Education and Athletics, 3rd ed. Philadelphia: Saunders, 1981.
2. Astrand PO, Rodahi K. Textbook of Work Physiology. New York: McGraw-Hill, 1970:304.
3. Dehn MM, Mullins CB. Physiologic effects and importance of exercise in patients with coronary artery disease. J Cardiovasc Med 2:365–387, 1977.
4. Mitchell JH, Blomqvist G. Maximal oxygen uptake. N Engl J Med 284:1018–1022, 1971.
5. Poliner LR, Dehmer CJ, Lewis SE, et al. Left ventricular performance in normal subjects: A comparison of the responses to exercise in the upright and supine position. Circulation 62:528–534, 1980.
6. Ferguson RJ, Faulkner JA, Julius S, et al. Comparison of cardiac output determined by CO_2 rebreathing and dye-dilution methods. J Appl Physiol 25:450–454, 1968.
7. Rowell I.B. Circulation. Med Sci Sports 1:15–22, 1969.
8. Zobi EG, Talmers FN, Christensen RC, et al. Effect of exercise on the cerebral circulation and metabolism. J Appl Physiol 20:1289–1293, 1965.
9. Naughton J, Haider R. Methods of exercise testing. In: Naughton JP, Hellerstein HK, Mohler IC, eds. Exercise Testing and Exercise Training in Coronary Heart Disease. New York: Academic, 1973:79.
10. ACSM. Guidelines for Exercise Testing and Prescription. 5th ed. Baltimore: Williams & Wilkins, 1995:97.
11. Comess KA. Fenster PE. Clinical implications of the blood pressure response to exercise. Cardiology 68:233–244, 1981.
12. Franklin BA. Diagnostic and functional exercise testing: Test selection and interpretation. J Cardiovasc Nurs 10:8–29, 1995.
13. Irving JB, Bruce RA, DeRouen TA. Variations in and significance of systolic pressure during maximal exercise (treadmill) testing: Relation to severity of coronary artery disease and cardiac mortality. Am J Cardiol 39:841–848, 1977.
14. Davis JA, Vodak P, Wilmore JH, et al. Anaerobic threshold and maximal aerobic power for three modes of exercise. J Appl Physiol 41:544–550, 1976.
15. Costill DL. Physiology of marathon running. JAMA 221:1024–1029, 1972.
16. Ginzton LE, Conant R, Brizendine M, et al. Effect of long-term high intensity aerobic training on left ventricular volume during maximal upright exercise. J Am Coll Cardiol 14:364–371, 1989.
17. Concu A, Marcello C. Stroke volume response to progressive exercise in athletes engaged in different types of training. Eur J Appl Physiol 66:11–17, 1993.
18. Balke B. Experimental studies on the functional capacities of middle-aged and aging persons. J Okla Med Assoc 54:120–123, 1961.
19. Buskirk E, Taylor HL. Maximal oxygen intake and its relation to body composition, with special reference to chronic physical activity and obesity. J Appl Physiol 2:72–78, 1957.
20. Bruce RA, Kusumi F, Hosmer D. Maximal oxygen intake and nomographic assessment of functional aerobic impairment in cardiovascular disease. Am Heart J 85:546–562, 1973.
21. Franklin BA. Pitfalls in estimating aerobic capacity from exercise time or workload. Appl Cardiol 14:25–26, 1986.
22. Myers J, Buchanan N, Walsh D, et al. Comparison of the ramp versus standard exercise protocols. J Am Coll Cardiol 17:1334–1342, 1991.
23. Myers J, Buchanan N, Smith D, et al. Individual ramp treadmill: Observations on a new protocol. Chest 101:236S–241S, 1992.
24. Wasserman K, Whipp BJ, Koyal SN, et al. Anaerobic threshold and respiratory gas exchange during exercise. J Appl Physiol 35:236–243, 1973.
25. Davis JA, Frank MH, Whipp BJ, et al. Anaerobic threshold alterations caused by endurance training in middle-aged men. J Appl Physiol 46:1039–1046, 1979.
26. Brooks CA. Anaerobic threshold: Review of the concept and directions for future research. Med Sci Sports Exerc 17:22–31, 1985.
27. Costill DL, Thomason H, Roberts E. Fractional utilization of the aerobic capacity during distance running. Med Sci Sports Exerc 5:248–252, 1973.
28. Lind AR, Taylor SH, Humphreys PW, et al. The circulatory effects of sustained voluntary muscle contraction. Clin Sci 27:229–244, 1964.
29. Lind AR, McNichol GW. Muscular factors which determine the cardiovascular responses to sustained and rhythmic exercise. Can Med Assoc J 96:706–715, 1967.
30. Mitchell JH, Payne FC, Saltin B, et al. The role of muscle mass in the cardiovascular response to static contractions. J Physiol 309:45–54, 1980.
31. Atkins JM, Matthews OA, Blomqvist CG, et al. Incidence of arrhythmias induced by isometric and dynamic exercise. Br Heart J 38:465–471, 1976.
32. Franklin BA. Exercise testing, training and arm ergometry. Sports Med 2:100–119, 1985.
33. Fardy PS, Webb D, Hellerstein HK. Benefits of arm exercise in cardiac rehabilitation. Phys Sportmed 5:30–41, 1977.
34. Schwade J, Blomqvist CG, Shapiro W. A comparison of the response to arm and leg work in patients with ischemic heart disease. Am Heart J 94:203–208, 1977.
35. Franklin BA, Vander L, Wrisley D, et al. Aerobic requirements of arm ergometry: Implications for exercise testing and training. Phys Sportsmed 11:81–90, 1983.
36. Kitamura K, Jorgenson CR, Gobel FL, et al. Hemodynamic correlates of myocardial oxygen consumption during upright exercise. J Appl Physiol 32:516–522, 1972.
37. Nelson RR, Gobel FL, Jorgensen CR, et al. Hemodynamic predictors of myocardial oxygen consumption during static and dynamic exercise. Circulation 50:1179–1189, 1974.

1.2.2, 1.2.3, 1.2.6

2.2.1, 2.2.2, 2.2.12, 2.2.14,
2.2.15, 2.2.17, 2.6.0.14

4.2.0.2, 4.2.0.3, 4.2.0.6,
4.2.1.1, 4.2.2.1, 4.2.2.2,
4.2.3, 4.2.3.2, 4.2.3.3

CHAPTER **16**

ABNORMAL CARDIORESPIRATORY RESPONSES
TO ACUTE AEROBIC EXERCISE

Barry A. Franklin

Three types of exercise can be used to stress the circulatory and ventilatory systems: dynamic, isometric, and a combination of the two (isodynamic). Dynamic exercise is associated with a volume load on the heart and appropriate increases in cardiac output and oxygen uptake. Isometric exercise, on the other hand, imposes a disproportionate pressure load on the left ventricle relative to the somatic aerobic requirements. Surprisingly, superimposing static on dynamic effort appears to attenuate the cardiovascular stress, because the relationship between myocardial oxygen supply and demand is favorably altered.

The acute cardiorespiratory responses to these forms of exercise have both immediate value for evaluating the suitability of physical activity, and prognostic implications in regard to morbidity and mortality. These data extend the clinical information obtained from other sources (history and physical examination, resting electrocardiogram [ECG], blood chemistry profile). They can be used to identify the primary mechanism underlying exercise intolerance, and to assess a change in clinical status or the effectiveness of various interventions (1). The latter may include exercise training, pharmacotherapy, or revascularization procedures such as angioplasty or coronary artery bypass surgery. In this chapter, normal and abnormal cardiorespiratory responses to acute aerobic exercise will be reviewed, with specific reference to clinical exercise testing, the value of gas exchange data, associated ECG and hemodynamic responses, symptoms, isometric and isodynamic exertion, and patients with chronic disease.

CLINICAL EXERCISE TESTING

Dynamic exercise testing is one of the most common evaluations performed in the assessment of persons with known or suspected coronary artery disease (CAD). The test is based primarily on the ECG response to exercise. One millimeter or more of ST segment depression at 80 ms beyond the J point is considered an indicator of myocardial ischemia (2). However, other variables, including angina pectoris, threatening ventricular arrhythmias,

exertional hypotension, and aerobic fitness, expressed as exercise duration, metabolic equivalents (METs), or peak power output (kilogram meters per minute) are also related to subsequent cardiovascular morbidity and mortality. In addition, recent studies suggest that blood lactate concentration at peak exercise appears to be a strong independent predictor of CAD in men (3, 4).

Unfortunately, the conventional exercise ECG has significant limitations in the diagnosis of occult CAD (5), with an approximate sensitivity and specificity of 75% and 85%, respectively. In some persons, exercise-induced ST segment depression suggests myocardial ischemia and underlying heart disease when in fact no disease is present. This scenario, termed a false-positive response, occurs predominantly in populations with a low pretest likelihood of CAD (e.g., young adults, asymptomatic women). Conversely, when a patient is found to have significant CAD and fails to demonstrate exercise-induced ST segment depression, the test is classified as a false-negative test.

Pretest and Posttest Probability of Coronary Disease

Probability tables based on age, gender, the presence of major coronary risk factors (cigarette smoking, hypertension, abnormal lipid/lipoprotein profile, sedentary lifestyle) and related clinical information (ECG, family history) can be used to estimate likelihood ("Bayesian" analysis) of having significant CAD even before an exercise test (6). However, the most meaningful and profound alterations in pretest probability of CAD are caused by symptoms. Atypical angina pectoris raises the pretest probability of significant angiographic coronary disease to 50% in a middle-aged man or postmenopausal woman, whereas typical angina raises it to 90% (7).

These estimates are helpful in deciding whether a diagnostic exercise test is clinically warranted and in clarifying the posttest likelihood of CAD. When the pretest risk of CAD is high, as is the case with a history of typical angina, or very low, as in asymptomatic patients or those with nonanginal pain, a normal or abnormal exercise ECG response has little influence on the posttest likelihood of disease. Accordingly, exercise testing has the greatest impact in persons with an intermediate likelihood of CAD, that is, in those with atypical angina. For example, probability tables suggest that a 55-year-old man with exertional jaw and back pain (atypical angina) has a 59% likelihood of significant CAD before exercise testing. After an exercise ECG, posttest likelihood of CAD is either 90% or 30%, according to the presence or absence, respectively, of significant ST segment depression (8). Thus, applying Bayesian analyses allows the need for additional diagnostic studies (e.g., exercise testing with myocardial perfusion imaging, exercise echocardiography) to be defined more intelligently.

Value of Gas Exchange Data: Differential Diagnosis

The value of clinical exercise testing is not limited to assessing potential indices of myocardial ischemia, suggesting significant CAD. By permitting simultaneous assessment of respiratory gas exchange data, which has been simplified by the availability of computerized systems, cardiopulmonary exercise testing can be especially helpful in the differential diagnosis of exertional dyspnea and fatigue (1). Moreover, in patients with coexistent cardiovascular and pulmonary disease, it can be used to identify the dominant factor limiting exercise tolerance. Differences in body size, muscle mass, age, gender, habitual level of activity, and physical conditioning account for much of the physiological variation in maximal oxygen consumption ($\dot{V}O_{2max}$). It is adversely affected by disease and disuse (10). Decreases in aerobic capacity are often subtle; thus, it is possible for a large percentage of the $\dot{V}O_{2max}$ to be lost before the ability to perform daily activities becomes noticeably compromised (Fig. 16.1) (11).

With cardiopulmonary exercise testing, it is now possible to evaluate and classify chronic heart failure objectively on the basis of oxygen consumption at the anaerobic (ventilatory) threshold (AT) and at maximal exercise ($\dot{V}O_{2max}$). Weber and Janicki (12) demonstrated that treadmill $\dot{V}O_{2max}$ correlates with cardiac reserve, expressed as the maximum cardiac index (Table 16.1). Others, however, suggest that the accuracy and generalizability of this classification scheme is limited, because it is necessary to relate aerobic performance to expected values for matched healthy individuals. Bruce et al. (13) developed the concept of functional aerobic impairment (FAI) for this purpose. The FAI is the percentage difference between observed $\dot{V}O_{2max}$ (measured directly or estimated), and the $\dot{V}O_{2max}$ predicted for a healthy person of the same age, gender, and habitual activity status. Average predicted values of $\dot{V}O_{2max}$ according to age for active and sedentary men and women are shown in Table 16.2.

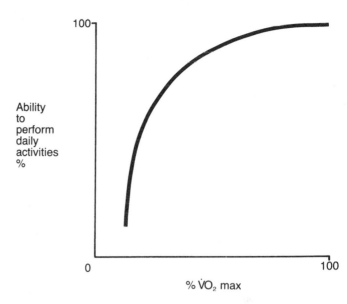

Figure 16.1. The reserve physiological capacity of the oxygen transport system is such that it is possible for much of the aerobic capacity ($\dot{V}O_{2max}$) to be lost before the demands of daily living become compromised. This appears to be true particularly among sedentary individuals. (Adapted with permission from Jones NL, Campbell EJM. Clinical Exercise Testing. Philadelphia: Saunders, 1981:2.)

FAI can be calculated from the following formula:

$$\%FAI = \frac{Predicted\ \dot{V}O_{2max} - Observed\ \dot{V}O_{2max}}{Predicted\ \dot{V}O_{2max}} \times 100$$

The normal value for the FAI is 0%; this indicates that the $\dot{V}O_{2max}$ is 100% of the age- and gender-predicted value and that there is no functional impairment. Negative values for FAI signify above-average fitness. The degree of FAI can be categorized as mild (27%–40%), moderate (41%–54%), marked (55%–68%), and extreme (>68%). The concept of FAI is particularly useful in making serial evaluations of individuals as well as comparisons with peers.

Table 16.1. Weber's Classification of Functional Impairment in Aerobic Capacity and Anaerobic Threshold

Class	Severity	$\dot{V}O_{2MAX}$ (ML/KG/MIN)	AT ($\dot{V}O_{2MAX}$, ML/KG/MIN)
A	mild to none	>20	>14
B	mild to moderate	16–20	11–14
C	moderate to severe	10–16	8–11
D	severe	6–10	5–8
E	very severe	<6	<4

Adapted from Weber KT, Janicki JS. Cardiopulmonary exercise testing for evaluation of chronic cardiac failure. Am J Cardiol 55(Suppl A): 22A–31A, 1985.

Table 16.2. Average $\dot{V}O_{2max}$ Values for Healthy Active and Sedentary Men and Women According to Age

AGE (YEARS)	MEN		WOMEN	
	ACTIVE 69.7 − (0.612 × YEARS)	SEDENTARY[a] 57.8 − (0.445 × YEARS)	ACTIVE 42.9 − (0.312 × YEARS)	SEDENTARY[a] 42.3 − (0.356 × YEARS)
20	57.5	48.9	36.7	35.2
22	56.2	48.0	36.0	34.5
24	55.0	47.1	35.4	33.8
26	53.8	46.2	34.8	33.0
28	52.6	45.3	34.2	32.3
30	51.3	44.5	33.5	31.6
32	50.1	43.6	32.9	30.9
34	48.9	42.7	32.3	30.2
36	47.7	41.8	31.7	29.5
38	46.4	40.9	31.0	28.8
40	45.2	40.0	30.4	28.1
42	44.0	39.1	29.8	27.3
44	42.8	38.2	29.2	26.6
46	41.5	37.3	28.5	25.9
48	40.3	36.4	27.9	25.2
50	39.1	35.6	27.3	24.5
52	37.9	34.7	26.7	23.8
54	36.7	33.8	26.1	23.1
56	35.4	32.9	25.4	22.4
58	34.2	32.0	24.8	21.7
60	33.0	31.1	24.2	20.9
62	31.8	30.2	23.6	20.2
64	30.5	29.3	22.9	19.5
66	29.3	28.4	22.3	18.8
68	28.1	27.5	21.7	18.1
70	26.9	26.7	21.1	17.4

$\dot{V}O_{2max}$ for any age can be predicted using these regression equations from reference #13.
[a] Defined as subjects who do not exert themselves sufficiently to develop sweating at least once a week.

Several approaches have been suggested for the differential diagnosis of exercise intolerance (exertional dyspnea), using gas exchange data to identify the predominant circulatory or ventilatory limitation (1). One widely recognized method examines $\dot{V}O_{2peak}$ and AT as a function of the predicted $\dot{V}O_{2max}$ and considers these variables in sequential fashion, as shown in Fig. 16.2 (14, 15). If $\dot{V}O_{2peak}$ is $\geq$ 85% of the predicted value, exertional symptoms are likely to be attributed to anxiety, obesity, mild cardiopulmonary disease, or combinations thereof. If $\dot{V}O_{2peak}$ is low and AT and "breathing reserve" are normal, exertional intolerance is likely to be due to poor effort, deconditioning, or coronary disease. In contrast, this scenario coupled with a low breathing reserve suggests a ventilatory limitation. As expected, low $\dot{V}O_{2peak}$ and low AT are attributed to circulatory impairment or mixed lesions, depending on the normality of the breathing reserve. This algorithm is attractive in scope, but clearly depends on the validity of the formulas used to classify these variables.

ECG RESPONSES TO EXERCISE TESTING

ECG responses to graded exercise tests should be interpreted according to the magnitude and configuration of ST segment displacement and the presence of supraventricular and ventricular dysrhythmias. Such information is useful in evaluating clinical status as well as the efficacy of selected interventions, including coronary revascularization and medications.

ST Segment Depression

Traditionally, exercise-induced ST segment depression (especially > 1 mm horizontal or downsloping) has been considered diagnostic of myocardial ischemia and suggestive of CAD. McHenry et al. found the ST segment index, that is, the algebraic sum of the ST J segment depression in millimeters and the ST slope in millivolts per second, to be a valid and reliable method to assess exercise-induced myocardial ischemia, as confirmed by angiographically-documented CAD (16). A negative index (i.e., < 0) is considered abnormal, provided that the magnitude of ST segment depression (from the baseline to the J point) is at least 1.0 mm (Fig. 16.3). Recently, exercise-induced QRS prolongation has also been shown to be a marker of myocardial ischemia in patients with CAD (17).

ST Segment Elevation

Although ST segment elevation is an infrequent (0.1% prevalence) and often disregarded ECG response, it is widely regarded as an ominous finding, especially in the absence of a previous Q wave infarction. The finding usually reflects wall motion abnormalities and associated left ventricular dysfunction in patients with a history of myocardial infarction and/or Q waves in the lead corresponding to the ST segment elevation (18, 19). However, exercise-induced ST segment elevation in the absence of a previous myocardial infarction (not over diagnostic Q waves) suggests severe transmural ischemia, is arrhythmogenic, and localizes the artery where there is spasm or a critical lesion (20, 21).

Dysrhythmias

Infrequent atrial or ventricular ectopic beats and short runs of supraventricular tachycardia commonly occur during exercise testing and do not appear to have diagnostic or prognostic significance for CAD. Similarly, the provocation or suppression of ventricular dysrhythmias during exercise testing does not necessarily signal the presence or absence of CAD, respectively (22). Threatening forms of ventricular ectopy are more likely to be asso-

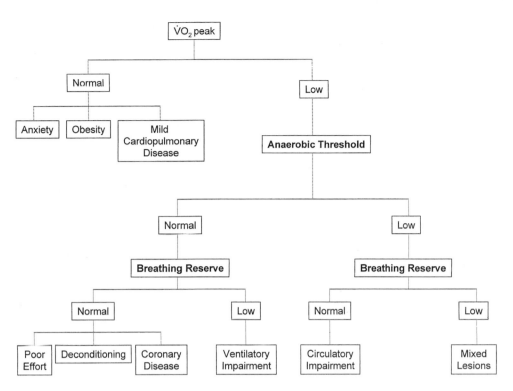

Figure 16.2. Flow chart for differential diagnosis of exertional dyspnea. (Adapted with permission from Wasserman K, Hansen JE, Sue DY, et al. Principles of Exercise Testing and Interpretation. Philadelphia: Lea & Febiger, 1987; Zavala DC. Manual on Exercise Testing: A Training Handbook. Iowa City: University of Iowa, 1985.)

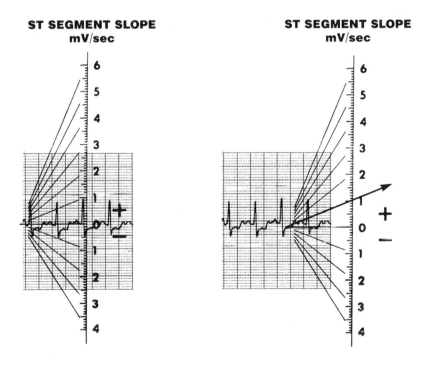

Figure 16.3. Calculation of the ST segment index by using a transparent overlay to determine the ST segment slope and depression. An abnormal ECG response with upsloping ST segment depression is shown.

ST depression = −2.0mm   ST slope = 1.0mV/sec

McHenry Index

ST depression = −2.0mm
ST slope   =   1.0mV/sec
SUM   =   −1.0 ST Index

ciated with significant CAD and a poor prognosis in the presence of ischemic ST segment depression (23).

HEMODYNAMIC RESPONSES

The evaluation of hemodynamic responses, specifically heart rate (HR) and blood pressure, has been shown to enhance the predictive value of exercise testing.

Heart Rate

A patient with a reduced HR response during exercise, in the absence of beta-blocker or calcium channel blocker therapy, is said to have chronotropic incompetence, which may be expressed as the peak heart rate attained; chronotropic index (ratio of heart rate reserve to metabolic reserve); or percent of age-predicted maximal heart rate achieved (24, 25). Traditionally this is identified by the failure of the exercise heart rate to rise to within two standard deviations (~ 20 beats/minute) of the age-predicted response to exercise, assuming the subject was highly motivated. This finding during exercise, even as an isolated anomaly, has been shown to predict the presence and angiographic severity of CAD and is associated with higher subsequent morbidity and mortality (25–27).

Systolic Blood Pressure

The normal systolic blood pressure response to incremental exercise is a progressive rise, typically 10 ± 2 mm Hg/MET, with a possible plateau at peak exercise. Exertional hypotension is defined as failure of the systolic blood pressure to rise, a drop below the pretest value (at standing rest), or a decrease of ≥ 20 mm Hg during exercise, after an initial rise. This abnormal response may be attributed to chronic ventricular dysfunction, exercise-induced myocardial ischemia causing left ventricular dysfunction, or papillary muscle dysfunction and mitral regurgitation. It is also associated with an increased risk of cardiac events during follow-up (28, 29).

Diastolic Blood Pressure

Diastolic blood pressure generally remains unchanged or decreases slightly during progressive exercise. Although an increase of more than 15 mm Hg during treadmill testing may be an indicator of severe CAD, it is more likely a marker for labile hypertension (30).

SYMPTOMS

It is important to note all symptoms that occur during and after the exercise test, especially substernal pressure that radiates across the chest to the left arm, jaw, back, or lower neck. Anginal symptoms can be rated by the patient on a scale of 1–4 ("perceptible but mild" to "severe"); however, ratings of >2 (moderate) are generally used as

end points for testing. Patients with angina during exercise, with or without concomitant ST segment depression, are at increased risk for subsequent coronary events (31).

STATIC AND ISODYNAMIC EXERTION

The myocardial demands imposed by static (isometric) or high-resistance effort may exceed those for low-resistance dynamic exercise. Because the pressor response to static exertion is proportionate to the relative intensity (percent of maximal voluntary contraction [MVC]), duration of effort, and muscle mass involved, a relatively mild static contraction in an isolated, weak muscle group may evoke an excessive pressor response despite relatively small increases in heart rate, somatic oxygen consumption, and cardiac output (32, 33).

Although static or combined static and dynamic (isodynamic) exercise has traditionally been discouraged in patients with CAD, it appears that these types of exertion may be less hazardous than once presumed, particularly in patients with normal or near-normal aerobic fitness and left ventricular function (34). Despite earlier reports that static exercise may precipitate arrhythmias, the appearance of new wall motion abnormalities and sudden cardiac death (rare), several studies now indicate that nonsustained isometric exercise, regardless of the percentage MVC used, generally fails to elicit angina pectoris, ischemic ST segment displacement, or threatening ventricular arrhythmias among clinically stable coronary patients (35–37). The rate–pressure product and estimated myocardial oxygen demands are lower during static than during maximal dynamic exercise, primarily because of a lower peak heart rate response (37). Increased subendocardial perfusion secondary to elevated diastolic blood pressure may also contribute to the lower incidence of ischemic ST segment depression and/or angina pectoris during static or isodynamic efforts. Furthermore, the myocardial oxygen supply–demand relationship appears to be favorably altered by superimposing static on dynamic effort, so that the magnitude of ST-segment depression is reduced at a given rate–pressure product (Fig. 16.4) (36, 38). These findings are changing the cautious attitude toward static and isodynamic exertion (and resistance training) for coronary patients, particularly in regard to vocational counseling and exercise prescription.

Since it is virtually impossible to participate in normal daily activities without engaging in some static efforts, realistic testing should include an evaluation of the physiological response to static forms of exercise, especially for patients at moderate to high risk. This applies to individuals involved in occupations with static requirements (carrying loads, operating a jackhammer, carpentry) as well as those involved in resistance training and selected recreational activities. Rather than arbitrarily prescribing such activities, the response to such predominantly static activities should be assessed and recommendations given

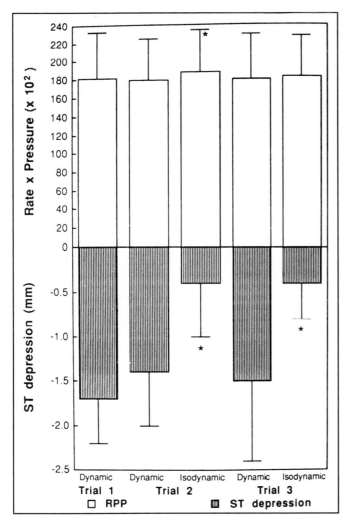

Figure 16.4. *Top,* Rate-pressure product (RPP). *Bottom,* Corresponding ST segment depression. Trial 1 is baseline dynamic exercise. Trials 2 and 3 are dynamic and isodynamic exercise. Values are mean ± SD. *P < 0.001 for differences between dynamic and isodynamic exercise trials. (Reprinted with permission from Bertagnoli K, Hanson P, Ward A. Attenuation of exercise-induced ST depression during combined isometric and dynamic exercise in coronary artery disease. Am J Cardiol 65:314–317, 1990.)

regarding minimizing adverse responses. For example, a shoulder strap for carrying weights, or luggage with wheels and an extendable handlebar can be recommended to minimize static efforts in selected patients.

PATIENTS WITH CHRONIC DISEASE

The electrocardiographic, cardiorespiratory, and hemodynamic responses to acute aerobic exercise may be markedly altered in patients with chronic disease. This section briefly reviews these anomalies with specific reference to patients with cardiopulmonary disease, hypertension, diabetes, obesity, and peripheral vascular disease.

Coronary Artery Disease

Typical circulatory data at rest and during maximal exercise in a healthy sedentary man and a patient with CAD are shown in Table 16.3. The 10-fold increase in oxygen consumption at maximal exercise ($\dot{V}O_{2max}$) in the sedentary man is contrasted to a 6-fold increase in the cardiac patient. The reduced oxygen transport capacity in the cardiac patient is primarily due to diminished cardiac output (stroke volume and/or heart rate) rather than a reduction in peripheral extraction of oxygen.

In some patients, a primary limitation appears to be decreased contractile force of the left ventricle due to residual myocardial ischemia or necrosis, causing a progressive decrease in ejection fraction and stroke volume with exercise. This may be manifested as exertional hypotension during progressive exercise (28). In others, cardiac output may be limited by the restriction in the rise of heart rate due to intrinsic disease of the sinoatrial or atrioventricular node, resulting in chronotropic impairment, or to the appearance of adverse signs and/or symptoms that preclude exercising at a higher work rate or intensity.

Pathophysiological evidence suggests that increased aerobic requirements imposed by progressive isotonic exercise may induce myocardial ischemia or electrical instability in patients with CAD. By increasing myocardial oxygen consumption and simultaneously shortening diastole and coronary perfusion time, exercise may evoke a tran-

Table 16.3. Hypothetical Circulatory Data at Rest and During Maximal Exercise for a Sedentary Man and a Patient With Heart Disease

Condition	Oxygen Consumption (L/min)	(mL/kg/min)	Cardiac Output (L/min)	Heart Rate (beats/min)	Stroke Volume (mL/beat)	Arteriovenous Oxygen Difference (mL/dL blood)
Sedentary man (70 kg)						
Rest	0.25	3.5[a]	6.1	70	87	4.0
Maximal exercise	2.50	35.0	17.7	190	93	14.0
Cardiac patient (70 kg)						
Rest	0.25	3.5[a]	6.1	82	74	4.0
Maximal exercise	1.50	21.5	10.4	165	66	13.6

[a] 3.5 mL/kg/min = 1 metabolic equivalent (MET); average resting metabolic rate expressed per unit body weight.

sient oxygen deficiency in subendocardial tissue that may be exacerbated by a decrease in venous return secondary to an abrupt cessation of exercise. Intracellular sodium–potassium imbalance, catecholamine excess, and increased circulating free fatty acids may also be dysrhythmogenic (Fig. 16.5). This scenario in the presence of documented or occult CAD may precipitate angina pectoris, ischemic ST segment depression, threatening ventricular dysrhythmias, or combinations thereof.

Pulmonary Disease

Patients with a ventilatory limitation to exercise become fatigued when limits of breathing reserve are reached, yet the cardiovascular system may remain largely unchallenged (1). Two reasons have been suggested for the premature exhaustion of breathing reserve (12, 14, 15). First, maximum ventilatory volume (MVV) is reduced by obstruction of airflow, restriction of lung volumes, or both. Second, ventilation–perfusion abnormalities increase physiological dead space, so that a higher minute ventilation ($\dot{V}_E$) at peak exercise is required to maintain gas exchange. In addition, arterial oxygen desaturation is often observed at peak exercise in patients with pulmonary disease but not in healthy subjects or patients with CAD.

Hypertension

Preliminary exercise testing is strongly recommended prior to vigorous exercise training in persons with a history of hypertension (above 140/90 mm Hg). It should be emphasized, however, that hypertensive patients frequently take diuretics, which by virtue of the potential association with hypokalemia, may cause spurious ST segment depression (39). Hypertensive patients may also demonstrate ECG evidence of left ventricular hypertrophy with or without strain, which confounds the interpretation of the exercise ECG with respect to myocardial ischemia (40). Thus, exercise induced ST segment depression should be interpreted with caution and additional studies obtained to differentiate true and false positive responses. Follow-up exercise testing with concomitant myocardial perfusion imaging may be particularly helpful in this regard.

Although those with hypertension generally exhibit above-normal systolic and diastolic blood pressure during exercise, most studies report no difference in the relative blood pressure increase between mildly hypertensive subjects and normotensive controls. In other words, it appears that blood pressure is simply reset and maintained at higher levels, whether the subject is at rest or performing static handgrip or treadmill exercise at varying percentages of maximum functional capacity Fig. 16.6 (41). Other patients with mild hypertension may normalize blood pressure during exercise relative to resting values. This phenomenon is presumably attributed to metabolic vasodilation, which transiently lowers an elevated resting peripheral resistance.

Several studies now suggest that an excessive blood pressure response to dynamic exercise in normotensive subjects may predict future hypertension (42, 43). This applies to an exaggerated systolic blood pressure rise (>220 mm Hg) and/or abnormal diastolic pressure (increase of more than 10 mm Hg or >90 mm Hg).

Figure 16.5. Physiological alterations accompanying acute exercise and recovery and their possible sequelae. CHD, coronary heart disease; HR, heart rate; $\dot{M}VO_2$, myocardial oxygen uptake; Na^+/K^+, sodium–potassium ion; SBP, systolic blood pressure.

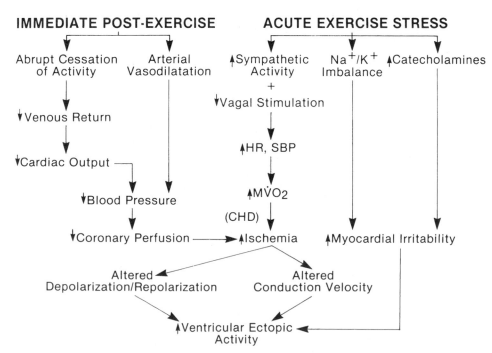

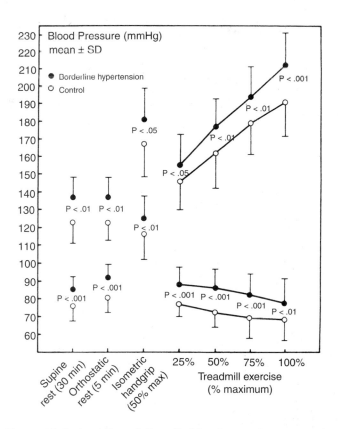

Figure 16.6. Systolic and diastolic blood pressure responses in normal and borderline hypertensive young men during supine rest, orthostatic stress, isometric exertion, and increasing percentages of maximum treadmill exercise capacity. (Reprinted with permission from Hanson P, Ward A, Painter P. Exercise training for special patient populations. J Cardiopulm Rehab 6:104–112, 1986.)

Diabetes

Before providing physical conditioning guidelines to diabetic patients, appropriate baseline studies should be performed to evaluate blood glucose and the potential for underlying CAD. Although treadmill or cycle ergometer testing may be used to assess the exercise ECG and acute cardiorespiratory response to progressive physical exertion, arm ergometry may be preferred in patients with peripheral neuropathy or peripheral vascular disease impairment of the lower extremities (44). The presence of autonomic neuropathy may result in chronotropic insufficiency, which may reduce functional capacity, as well as sensitivity of the exercise test.

Obesity

During treadmill testing, obese subjects often demonstrate a higher cardiac output, absolute oxygen consumption (L/minute), and minute ventilation at any given work rate (45). Systemic and pulmonary blood pressures and heart rate are also frequently higher in obese than in lean subjects during submaximal exercise (46). Because there is

little or no difference in maximal heart rate between overweight and lean subjects, the obese tend to perform a given work task at a higher percentage of maximal heart rate. Although obese persons may have a large absolute $\dot{V}O_{2max}$ by virtue of a large muscle mass, aerobic capacity is reduced when expressed relative to body weight (47). Other conditions that may limit exercise performance of obese patients include heat intolerance, hyperpnea, dyspnea, movement restriction, orthopaedic pain, local muscular weakness, balance problems, and anxiety (45).

Peripheral Vascular Disease

Patients with peripheral vascular disease (PVD) have discomfort, ischemic pain (claudication), or fatigue in the legs with walking. Like angina, claudication pain is attributed to a discrepancy between oxygen supply and demand in working muscle. This pain typically occurs in the calf, can be graded in severity from I–IV ("established but minimal" to "excruciating and unbearable") and disappears quickly with the cessation of walking. Accordingly, it is generally the limiting factor to performance in this patient population, since both circulatory and ventilatory systems may remain relatively unstressed at peak exercise or volitional fatigue.

Treadmill testing is the exercise modality of choice when patients with suspected PVD are being evaluated for diagnostic purposes (i.e., with Doppler studies) (48). On the other hand, when the assessment of CAD is the primary focus, arm ergometry may be preferred because many of these patients achieve suboptimal levels of cardiac stress during conventional treadmill or cycle ergometer testing (44).

► SUMMARY

Abnormal responses to exercise can be used to diagnose and classify persons undergoing exercise evaluation. Physiological changes that deviate from normal or that contrast markedly with normal response can be diagnostic of disease states leading to exercise intolerance. Categorizing functional status, the reason for the abnormal response, and the response itself may explain the intolerance and lead to identification of those disease states.

References

1. Neuberg GW, Friedman SH, Weiss MB, et al. Cardiopulmonary exercise testing: The clinical value of gas exchange data. Arch Intern Med 148:2221–2226, 1988.
2. Franklin BA. Diagnostic and functional exercise testing: Test selection and interpretation. J Cardiovasc Nurs 10:8–29, 1995.
3. Barthelémy JC, Roche F, Gaspoz JM, et al. Maximal blood lactate level acts as a major discriminant variable in exercise testing for coronary artery disease detection in men. Circulation 93:246–252, 1996.

4. Cannon RO III, Lesch M. The search for a better exercise test: A self-fulfilling prophecy? Circulation 93:205–207, 1996.

5. Laslett LJ, Amsterdam EA. Management of the asymptomatic patient with an abnormal ECG. JAMA 252:1744–1746, 1984.

6. Diamond GA, Forrester JS. Analysis of probability as an aid in the clinical diagnosis of coronary artery disease. N Engl J Med 300:1350–1358, 1979.

7. Froelicher VF, Quaglietti S. Handbook of Exercise Testing. Boston: Little, Brown, 1996:127–128.

8. Epstein SE. Implications of probability analysis on the strategy used for non-invasive detection of coronary artery disease. Am J Cardiol 46:491–499, 1980.

9. Buskirk E, Taylor HL. Maximal oxygen intake and its relation to body composition, with special reference to chronic physical activity and obesity. J Appl Physiol 2:72–78, 1957.

10. Mitchell JH, Blomqvist G. Maximal oxygen uptake. N Engl J Med 284:1018–1022, 1971.

11. Jones NL, Campbell EJM. Clinical Exercise Testing. Philadelphia: WB Saunders, 1981:2.

12. Weber KT, Janicki JS. Cardiopulmonary exercise testing for evaluation of chronic cardiac failure. Am J Cardiol 55(Suppl A):22A–31A, 1985.

13. Bruce RA, Kusumi F, Hosmer D. Maximal oxygen intake and nomographic assessment of functional aerobic impairment in cardiovascular disease. Am Heart J 85:546–562, 1973.

14. Wasserman K, Hansen JE, Sue DY, et al. Principles of Exercise Testing and Interpretation. Philadelphia: Lea & Febiger, 1987.

15. Zavala DC. Manual on Exercise Testing: A Training Handbook. Iowa City: University of Iowa Press, 1985.

16. McHenry PL, Phillips JF, Knoebel SB. Correlation of computer-quantitated treadmill exercise electrocardiogram with arteriographic location of coronary artery disease. Am J Cardiol 30:747–752, 1972.

17. Michaelides A, Ryan JM, VanFossen D, et al. Exercise-induced QRS prolongation in patients with coronary artery disease: A marker of myocardial ischemia. Am Heart J 126:1320–1325, 1993.

18. Chaitman BR, Waters DD, Théroux P, et al. ST-segment elevation and coronary spasm in response to exercise. Am J Cardiol 47:1350–1358, 1981.

19. Bruce RA, Fisher LD, Pettinger M, et al. ST segment elevation with exercise: A marker for poor ventricular function and poor prognosis. Circulation 77:897–905, 1988.

20. Chahine RA, Lowery MH, Bauerlein EJ. Interpretation of the exercise-induced ST-segment elevation. Am J Cardiol 72:100–101, 1993.

21. Yasue H, Omote S, Takizawa A, et al. Comparison of coronary arteriographic findings during angina pectoris associated with S-T elevation or depression. Am J Cardiol 47:539–546, 1981.

22. Califf RM, McKinnis RA, McNeer JF, et al. Prognostic value of ventricular arrhythmias associated with treadmill exercise testing in patients studied with cardiac catheterization for suspected ischemic heart disease. J Am Coll Cardiol 2:1060–1067, 1983.

23. Fuller T, Movahed A. Current review of exercise testing: Application and interpretation. Clin Cardiol 10:189–200, 1987.

24. Ellestad MH, Wan MK. Predictive implications of stress testing: Follow-up of 2700 subjects after maximum treadmill stress testing. Circulation 51:363–369, 1975.

25. Brener SJ, Pashkow FJ, Harvey SA, et al. Chronotropic response to exercise predicts angiographic severity in patients with suspected or stable coronary artery disease. Am J Cardiol 76:1228–1232, 1995.

26. Lauer MS, Okin PM, Larson MG, et al. Impaired heart rate response to graded exercise: Prognostic implications of chronotropic incompetence in the Framingham Heart Study. Circulation 93:1520–1526, 1996.

27. Ellestad MH. Chronotropic incompetence: The implications of heart rate response to exercise (compensatory parasympathetic hyperactivity?). Circulation 93:1485–1487, 1996.

28. Comess KA, Fenster PE. Clinical implications of the blood pressure response to exercise. Cardiology 68:233–244, 1981.

29. Irving JB, Bruce RA, De Rouen TA. Variations in and significance of systolic pressure during maximal exercise (treadmill) testing: Relation to severity of coronary artery disease and cardiac mortality. Am J Cardiol 39:841–848, 1977.

30. Sheps DS, Ernst JC, Briese FW, et al. Exercise-induced increase in diastolic pressure: Indicator of severe coronary artery disease. Am J Cardiol 43:708–712, 1979.

31. Cole JP, Ellestad MH. Significance of chest pain during treadmill exercise: Correlation with coronary events. Am J Cardiol 41:227–232, 1978.

32. Lind AR, McNichol GW. Muscular factors which determine the cardiovascular responses to sustained and rhythmic exercise. Can Med Assoc J 96:706–715, 1967.

33. Mitchell JH, Payne FC, Saltin B, et al. The role of muscle mass in the cardiovascular response to static contractions. J Physiol 309:45–54, 1980.

34. Fardy PS. Isometric exercise and the cardiovascular system. Physician Sportsmed 9:43–56, 1981.

35. DeBusk RF, Valdez R, Houston N, et al. Cardiovascular responses to dynamic and static effort soon after myocardial infarction: Application to occupational work assessment. Circulation 58:368–375, 1978.

36. DeBusk RF, Pitts W, Haskell W, et al. Comparison of cardiovascular responses to static-dynamic and dynamic effort alone in patients with ischemic heart disease. Circulation 59:977–984, 1979.

37. Ferguson RJ, Cote P, Bourassa MG, et al. Coronary blood flow during isometric and dynamic exercise in angina pectoris patients. J Cardiac Rehab 1:21–27, 1981.

38. Bertagnoli K, Hanson P, Ward A. Attenuation of exercise-induced ST depression during combined isometric and dynamic exercise in coronary artery disease. Am J Cardiol 65:314–317, 1990.

39. Georgopoulos AJ, Proudfit WL, Page IH. Effect of exercise on electrocardiogram of patients with low serum potassium. Circulation 23:567–572, 1961.

40. Schlant RC, Blomqvist CG, Brandenburg RO, et al. Guidelines for exercise testing. Circulation 74:653A–667A, 1986.

41. Hanson P, Ward A, Painter P. Exercise training for special patient populations. J Cardiopulm Rehab 6:104–112, 1986.

42. Wilson N, Meyer E. Early prediction of hypertension using exercise blood pressure. Prev Med 10:62–68, 1981.

43. Dlin R, Hanne N, Silverberg DS, et al. Follow-up of nor-motensive men with exaggerated blood pressure response to exercise. Am Heart J 106:316–320, 1983.

44. Franklin BA. Exercise testing, training and arm ergometry. Sports Med 2:100–119, 1985.

45. Foss ML. Lampman RM, Watt E, et al. Initial work tolerance of extremely obese patients. Arch Phys Med Rehab 56:63–67, 1975.

46. Alexander JK. Obesity and cardiac performance. Am J Cardiol 14:860–865, 1964.

47. Goodman C, Kenrick M. Physical fitness in relation to obesity. Obesity/Bariatric Med 4:12–15, 1975.

48. Berglund B, Eklund B. Reproducibility of treadmill exercise in patients with intermittent claudication. Clin Physiol 1:253–256, 1981.

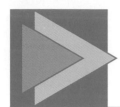

CHAPTER **17**

CARDIORESPIRATORY ADAPTATIONS TO EXERCISE

Barry A. Franklin and Jeffrey L. Roitman

Physical inactivity is now classified as a major contributing risk factor for heart disease, with an overall weight for preventive value similar to elevated blood cholesterol, cigarette smoking, and hypertension (1). Moreover, longitudinal studies have shown that higher levels of aerobic fitness are associated with a lower mortality from heart disease even after statistical adjustments for age, coronary risk factors, and family history of heart disease (Fig. 17.1) (2). These findings and other recent reports in persons with and without heart disease have confirmed an inverse association between aerobic capacity and cardiovascular mortality (3–8).

Endurance exercise training increases functional capacity and provides relief of symptoms in a majority of patients with coronary artery disease (CAD). This is particularly important since most patients with clinically manifest CAD have a subnormal functional capacity (50–70% age, gender-predicted) and some may be limited by symptoms at relatively low levels of exertion. Improvement in function appears to be mediated by increased central and/or peripheral oxygen transport and supply, while relief of angina pectoris may result from increased myocardial oxygen supply, decreased oxygen demand, or both.

This chapter reviews the cardiorespiratory adaptations to regular aerobic exercise in health and disease, with specific reference to alterations at submaximal and maximal exercise, gender differences and similarities, variables influencing exercise trainability, the role of training specificity, and responses in conditioned and unconditioned subjects.

SUBMAXIMAL AND MAXIMAL EXERCISE

Cardiovascular Changes

Cardiovascular changes induced by physical training during submaximal and maximal exercise are summarized in Table 17.1. Most exercise studies on healthy subjects demonstrate 20% ± 10% increases in aerobic capac-

ity ($\dot{V}O_{2max}$), with the greatest relative improvements among the most unfit (9). Because a fixed submaximal work rate has a relatively constant aerobic requirement, the physically trained individual works at a lower percentage of $\dot{V}O_{2max}$, with greater reserve after exercise training. Enhanced oxygen transport, particularly increased maximal stroke volume and cardiac output, has traditionally been regarded as the primary mechanism underlying the increase in $\dot{V}O_{2max}$ with training.

The effects of chronic exercise training on the autonomic nervous system act to reduce myocardial demands at rest and during exercise. Exercise bradycardia may be attributed to an intracardiac mechanism (an effect directly on the myocardium, e.g., increased stroke volume during submaximal work) or an extracardiac mechanism (e.g., alterations in trained skeletal muscle) or both. The result is reduced heart rate and systolic blood pressure at rest and at any fixed oxygen uptake or submaximal work rate.

The increased oxidative capacity of trained skeletal muscle appears to offer a distinct hemodynamic advantage. Lactic acid production and muscle blood flow are decreased at a fixed external work load, whereas submaximal cardiac output and oxygen uptake are unchanged or slightly reduced. As a result, there are compensatory increases in arteriovenous oxygen difference (a–vDO$_2$) at submaximal and maximal exercise (Table 17.1).

Recently, Hambrecht et al. reported improved coronary endothelial function after 4 weeks of training in patients with asymptomatic coronary artery disease. This may help to explain some of the cardioprotective effects of regular exercise. Patients may benefit via augmented coronary blood flow, increased myocardial perfusion and increased plaque stability, or combinations thereof (9a).

Respiratory Changes

Several respiratory adaptations result from physical conditioning regimens. Although ventilation generally does not limit exercise in apparently healthy individuals, in elite athletes the limits of ventilation may be reached at

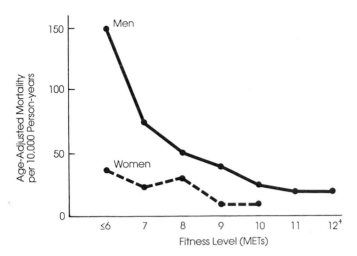

Figure 17.1. Age-adjusted all-cause mortality rates per 10,000 person–years of follow-up by physical fitness (METs) achieved during maximal treadmill exercise testing. (Adapted from Blair SN, Kohl HW III, Paffenbarger RS, et al. Physical fitness and all-cause mortality: a prospective study of healthy men and women. JAMA 262:2395–2401, 1989.)

$\dot{V}O_{2max}$ (10). Maximal minute ventilation is augmented by increased tidal volume and breathing frequency and is controlled by neural and chemical factors and by sensory mechanisms within the lungs and breathing muscles.

Table 17.1. Physiological Responses to Aerobic Conditioning in Untrained Individuals

Variable[a]	Unit of Measure	Response
$\dot{V}O_{2max}$	mL/kg/min	↑
Resting heart rate	beats/min	↓
Exercise heart rate (submax)	beats/minute	↓
Maximum heart rate	beats/min	↔ (or slight ↓)
A-vDO₂	ml O₂/100 mL blood	↑
Maximum minute ventilation	Liters/minute	↑
Stroke volume	mL/beat	↑
Cardiac output	Liters/min	↑
Blood volume (resting)	Liters	↑
Systolic blood pressure	mm Hg	↔ (or slight ↑)
Blood lactate	mL/100 mL blood	↑
Oxidative capacity skeletal muscle	multiple variables[b]	↑

[a] At maximum exercise unless otherwise specified.
[b] Represents increases in skeletal muscle mitochondrial number and size, capillary density, and/or oxidative enzymes.
↑, increase
↓, decrease
↔, no change

There is also increased ventilatory efficiency as substantiated by a reduced ventilatory equivalent for oxygen ($\dot{V}_E/\dot{V}O_2$) in trained as compared with untrained individuals. Ventilation increases linearly with $\dot{V}O_2$ up to about 50% $\dot{V}O_{2max}$, after which the increase is proportionately greater than the increase in work rate or $\dot{V}O_2$ (10, 11). Physically trained persons demonstrate larger lung volumes and diffusion capacity at rest and during exercise than their sedentary counterparts.

Ventilation is either unaffected or only modestly affected by cardiorespiratory training. Maximal ventilatory capacity may be increased by exercise training, but it is unclear that this provides any advantage other than increased buffering capacity for lactate. Submaximal ventilation is probably not affected, but it may be decreased in some circumstances because decreased production of lactate coincides with decreased need to buffer lactate and therefore decreased ventilation (11). Moreover, studies in subjects with and without heart disease have demonstrated increases in the ventilatory threshold after an exercise intervention, with associated decreases in blood lactate during submaximal work loads (12, 13).

GENDER-SPECIFIC IMPROVEMENT AND TRAINABILITY

The salutary effects of chronic endurance training in men are well documented. However, numerous studies now provide ample data on $\dot{V}O_{2max}$, cardiovascular hemodynamics, body composition, and serum lipids of middle-aged and older women, as well as changes with physical conditioning. The results demonstrate that women with and without CAD respond to aerobic training in much the same way as men when subjected to comparable programs in terms of frequency, intensity, and duration of exercise (Fig. 17.2) (14, 15). Improvement is negatively correlated with age, habitual physical activity, and initial $\dot{V}O_{2max}$ (which is generally lower in women than men) and positively correlated with conditioning frequency, intensity, and duration (16).

There are, however, large interindividual differences in the effects of physical conditioning independent of age, initial capacity, or conditioning program. These individual variations in response to aerobic exercise training may be due to childhood patterns of activity, state of conditioning at the initiation of the program, or degree of physiological aging. Body compositional differences in trainability may also play an important role with respect to the results of physical conditioning. Obese women demonstrate lower aerobic capacity (per-kilogram body weight), altered cardiovascular hemodynamics, and elevated serum lipids compared to leaner women (17). This initial varied profile may serve to modify the outcome of an aerobic conditioning program with respect to the magnitude of quantitative change.

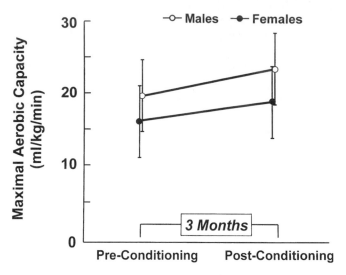

Figure 17.2. Aerobic capacity before and after physical conditioning in older (≥ 62 years) men and women with coronary heart disease. Maximal oxygen consumption increased by 19% and 17% in the men and women, respectively (both p < 0.001). (Adapted from Ades PA, Waldmann ML, Polk DM, et al. Referral patterns and exercise response in the rehabilitation of female coronary patients aged ≥ 62 years. Am J Cardiol 69:1422–1425, 1992.)

SPECIFICITY OF TRAINING

Decreased heart rate at rest and during fixed submaximal work rates, with an inherent reduction in myocardial aerobic requirements, is a well-documented adaptation to endurance exercise training. This response is believed to reflect intracardiac and/or extracardiac mechanisms. The former is attributed to enhanced stroke volume with a compensatory decrease in sympathetic stimulation and heart rate, the latter to alterations in the central nervous system, adaptations in trained muscles, or both (18, 19). Evidence supporting an extracardiac or peripheral mechanism includes an unchanged heart rate response or a considerably less marked bradycardia during exercise involving untrained muscles.

Numerous studies of normal subjects and cardiac patients have investigated the cardiorespiratory and metabolic adaptations of trained versus untrained muscle to physical conditioning. Results generally demonstrate little or no crossover of arm and leg training. After endurance training of one limb or set of limbs, several investigators report increased $\dot{V}O_{2max}$ and anaerobic (ventilatory) threshold or decreased heart rate (Fig. 17.3), blood lactate, pulmonary ventilation, ventilatory equivalent, blood pressure, and perceived exertion during submaximal exercise in trained but not untrained limbs (19, 20). These limb-specific training effects imply that a substantial portion of the conditioning response is attributed to extracardiac or peripheral factors such as alterations in blood flow and cellular and enzymatic adaptations in the trained limbs alone (21–23).

On the other hand, studies in both normal subjects and cardiac patients indicate some transfer effects (i.e., increased $\dot{V}O_{2max}$ or reduced submaximal exercise heart rate in untrained limbs), providing evidence for central circulatory adaptations to endurance training (24, 25). Although the conditions under which the crossover of arm and leg training may vary, some evidence suggests that the

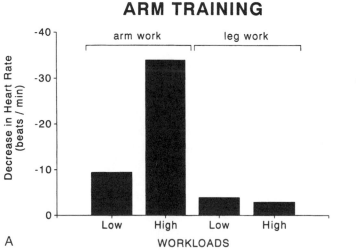

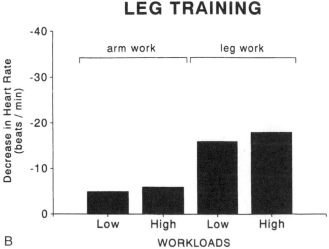

Figure 17.3. A. Arm training using an arm ergometer markedly decreased the heart rate response during arm exercise at low and high work loads, whereas the heart rate reduction during leg work was small. B. Similarly, leg training markedly decreased the heart rate during leg work, whereas the heart rate reduction during arm work was minimal. (Adapted from Clausen JP, Trap-Jensen J, Lassen NA. The effects of training on the heart rate during arm and leg exercise. Scand J Clin Lab Invest 26:295–301, 1970.)

initial fitness, as well as the intensity, frequency, and duration of training, may be important variables in determining the extent of cross-training benefits from arms to legs and vice versa (26).

The limited degree of cardiovascular and metabolic crossover from one set of limbs to another appears to discount the general practice of restricting aerobic conditioning to the lower extremities alone. Many recreational and occupational activities require sustained arm work to a greater extent than leg work. Consequently, individuals who rely on upper extremities for vocational or leisure-time pursuits should train arms as well as legs, with the expectation of improved cardiorespiratory, hemodynamic, and perceived exertion responses to both forms of effort. Specially designed arm ergometers or combined arm–leg ergometers are particularly beneficial for upper extremity training. Other equipment suitable for upper body training includes rowing machines, wall pulleys, vertical climbing devices, and cross-country skiing simulators.

Trainability of Arms Versus Legs

Arm training for persons with and without heart disease is now widely accepted as an integral component of a comprehensive physical conditioning program. Until recently, however, few data regarding the relative trainability of the upper extremities were available. Franklin et al. (27) reported the effects of a 6-week aerobic circuit training program on 13 post–myocardial infarction patients that involved alternating upper and lower extremity exercise devices for 15 minutes each at an intensity of 70–85% of peak heart rate. Postconditioning rate–pressure products during submaximal arm and leg ergometry were similarly decreased, while arm and leg $\dot{V}O_{2max}$ increased 13% and 11%, respectively (Fig. 17.4). These findings suggest that the upper extremities respond to aerobic exercise conditioning in the same qualitative and quantitative manner as the lower extremities.

CONDITIONED AND UNCONDITIONED RESPONSE

Adaptation to cardiorespiratory endurance exercise may be shown by contrasting responses to exercise in conditioned and unconditioned persons. The central effects (cardiorespiratory) of regular exercise (training) are manifested in several ways. The net outcome of increased ability to deliver oxygen to working muscle and to use nutrients at the cellular level is to increase $\dot{V}O_{2max}$. Changes in heart rate, stroke volume, $CaO_2 - C\bar{v}O_2$, cardiac output, blood lactate, and ventilation each contribute to increased $\dot{V}O_{2max}$ and to increased metabolic efficiency of the trained person. Table 17.1 summarizes the cardiorespiratory adaptations to exercise in conditioned and unconditioned persons.

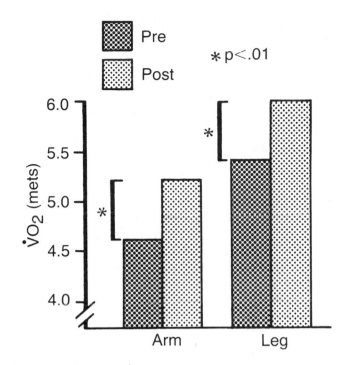

Figure 17.4. Mean $\dot{V}O_{2max}$ values, expressed as metabolic equivalents (METs; 1 MET = 3.5 mL/kg/min), during arm and leg exercise testing before and after training in men with previous myocardial infarction. (Adapted from Franklin BA, Vander L, Wrisley D, et al. Trainability of arms versus legs in men with previous myocardial infarction. Chest 105:262–264, 1994.)

Heart Rate

The heart rate response plays a critical role in the delivery of oxygen to working skeletal muscle. Heart rate increases during exercise to assist in augmenting cardiac output. The increase is initially caused primarily by neural influences, but as maximum exercise is approached, the increase is also influenced by neurohormonal and chemical factors. Resting heart rate is restrained by the vagus nerve (vagal tone), and vagal tone appears to be increased at rest, decreasing resting heart rate by approximately 10 to 15 beats/minute, whereas sympathoadrenergic drive (circulating catecholamines, particularly norepinephrine) is attenuated during exercise (18). Increased heart rate during exercise is influenced by mechanical receptors, sympathetic stimulation, and the release of vagal tone (11, 28, 29). Exercise in unconditioned persons causes a proportionately greater increase in heart rate at any fixed submaximal work rate than in conditioned persons.

Heart rate and stroke volume both contribute to cardiac output. In untrained persons, heart rate plays a more significant role because of the ability to induce relatively large changes in rate, as opposed to limited changes in stroke volume, which may be restricted by deconditioning. Heart rate, therefore, increases proportionately more during graded exercise and is higher at any given level of submaximal exercise in unconditioned persons (11, 30). Maximal heart rate is unchanged or slightly decreased (3 to 10 beats/minute) after aerobic conditioning (31). The latter is probably attributed to two training adaptations: cardiac hypertrophy via an increase in the size of the ventricular cavity and decreased sympathetic drive.

Stroke Volume

Stroke volume, the second factor used in determining cardiac output, increases during exercise secondary to increased venous return (Frank-Starling mechanism) and to increased contractile state (perhaps by neurohormonal influences) (11, 28, 32–35). The left ventricle is able to contract with greater force during exercise, in part because of increased end-diastolic volume and enhanced mechanical ability of myocardial fibers to produce force (36, 37). It is also likely that chronic cardiovascular exercise training strengthens myocardial tissue and enables more forceful contraction (11, 28, 38, 39). The result is augmented ejection of end-diastolic volume or increased ejection fraction.

Comparatively, cardiorespiratory training allows conditioned individuals to increase ejection fraction to a greater degree than their sedentary counterparts; hence stroke volume is higher in conditioned individuals at any fixed or relative submaximal work load (39). The increased stroke volume from training allows conditioned individuals to exercise at similar absolute and relative work loads at a lower heart rate, thus decreasing the myocardial oxygen demand of submaximal exercise (33, 35). The increase in ejection fraction is approximately 5–10% during maximal exercise.

Normal ventricular wall thickness and enlarged end-diastolic volume are consistently reported after endurance exercise training, with attendant increases in rest and exercise stroke volume (40). Cardiovascular morphological characteristics, including central blood volume and total hemoglobin, also increase with physical conditioning (41). Both of these variables are closely correlated with the $\dot{V}O_{2max}$.

Cardiac Output

Maximum cardiac output is significantly higher in trained than in untrained individuals, primarily because of the ability to increase stroke volume (28, 38, 39). Increased cardiac output during exercise is initially influenced by both heart rate and stroke volume, but stroke volume plateaus at approximately 40–60% $\dot{V}O_{2max}$, and increased heart rate is the sole contributor to increasing cardiac output thereafter. This is particularly evident in trained individuals with the ability to increase stroke volume significantly (39). It is generally accepted that cardiac output is essentially unchanged at any fixed submaximal workload before and after training and between conditioned and unconditioned individuals (38).

Arteriovenous Oxygen Difference

The final contributor to increased oxygen consumption during exercise is a-vDO$_2$. The difference between arterial and venous content of oxygen in blood reflects the ability of skeletal muscle tissue to extract oxygen (38, 42). Chronic training enhances the metabolic machinery within muscle, thereby enhancing the ability to use (i.e., extract) oxygen that is transported in circulating blood. Increased ability to deliver oxygen to working skeletal muscle and to remove and use it for generating energy is a hallmark of aerobic training.

Conditioned individuals have greater ability to use oxygen at the cellular level than unconditioned persons, but a-vDO$_2$ is similar in trained and untrained persons at submaximal levels of exercise until near $\dot{V}O_{2max}$ is reached. A-vDO$_2$ is greater at maximum exercise in trained than untrained persons.

Systolic Blood Pressure

Resting blood pressure is modulated by a number of factors, including cardiac output, general vasomotor tone (peripheral resistance), and arterial elasticity (28). Systolic blood pressure increases in a relatively linear fashion with cardiac output (and $\dot{V}O_2$) during exercise. Blood pressure can be expressed as follows:

$$BP \sim CO \times TPR$$

where BP = blood pressure
    CO = cardiac output
    TPR = total peripheral resistance

Primary control of blood pressure is exerted centrally by neural mechanisms affecting peripheral arterioles, which control peripheral resistance, and the arteriolar bed metabolites produced during exercise (38, 43). There is vasoconstriction in some areas during exercise (splanchnic areas, for example) and vasodilation in others (skeletal muscle and myocardium); the net effect is decreased vasomotor tone and peripheral resistance (28, 36). Systolic blood pressure increases during progressive exercise in healthy individuals because of increased cardiac output. Increased cardiac output maintains systolic blood pressure despite decreased peripheral resistance from arterial dilation (11). Diastolic blood pressure remains constant or may decrease slightly in both conditioned and unconditioned individuals.

At any fixed submaximal workload, conditioned individuals demonstrate comparable or lower systolic blood pressure than untrained individuals. Relative to $\dot{V}O_{2max}$ systolic blood pressure is lower in trained than untrained people.

Blood Lactate

Lactic acid (lactate) is a byproduct of anaerobic glycolysis. Though anaerobic threshold can be defined by many criteria, lactate threshold is commonly associated with the onset of significant anaerobic contribution to exercise metabolism. Blood lactate is buffered during exercise to

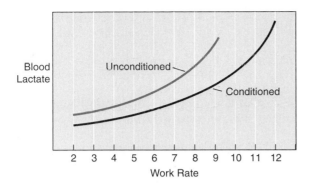

Figure 17.5. Blood lactate concentration during progressive exercise in conditioned versus unconditioned persons. The conditioned response typically exhibits lower lactate concentrations at any given work rate than unconditioned but has higher maximum lactate at $\dot{V}O_{2max}$.

maintain a tolerable acid-base balance. However, it begins to increase significantly when production exceeds buffering capacity of the blood. It is at this point that ventilation increases disproportionately and exercise begins to be perceived as more uncomfortable (10, 38).

Table 17.2. Factors Influencing the Training Response

VARIABLE(S)	COMMENT
Prolonged bed rest	Results in physiological deconditioning, including a significant reduction in $\dot{V}O_{2max}$
Intensity, frequency, and duration of training	Improvement in aerobic capacity generally demonstrates a positive correlation to these variables
Age, habitual physical activity, and initial $\dot{V}O_{2max}$	Improvement generally demonstrates an inverse relationship with these variables; however, recent studies suggest that older and younger adults demonstrate comparable exercise trainability
Adherence to the exercise prescription	Parallels the magnitude of improvement in cardiorespiratory function
Detraining	When physical conditioning is stopped or reduced, training-induced cardiorespiratory and metabolic adaptations are reversed to varying degrees over time
Coronary artery disease	Severity or progression of disease may present an obstacle to improvement
Left ventricular dysfunction[a]	Exercise training appears to be generally safe and effective in this population
Beta-blockade	Patients may derive considerable physiological benefit from exercise training in the presence of both cardioselective and nonselective beta-blockers, despite a reduced training heart rate
Calcium antagonists	No adverse effect on exercise trainability

[a] Ejection fraction $\leq 35\%$

Endurance exercise training improves oxidative capacity of skeletal muscle by stimulating increases in the size and number of skeletal muscle mitochondria, as well as increases in muscle myoglobin content, oxidative enzymes, and capillary density (44). Conditioned individuals have lower lactate at any fixed submaximal work rate, since they produce less and buffer more of the lactic acid produced (11, 38). However, at $\dot{V}O_{2max}$, lactic acid levels are significantly higher in conditioned individuals after training, since there is increased capacity to buffer and to tolerate lactate. At a fixed submaximal work rate, lactic acid is lower in trained than untrained individuals; thus, training increases lactate threshold (Fig. 17.5). Other variables affecting the training response are summarized (Table 17.2).

▶ SUMMARY

Exercise training induces many physiological changes that make a conditioned individual more efficient and better able to deliver and use oxygen and nutrients and resist fatigue. The conditioning effect also offers some protection against cardiovascular mortality and enhances ability to perform activities of daily living.

References
1. Fletcher GF, Balady G, Blair SN, et al. Statement on exercise: Benefits and recommendations for physical activity programs for all Americans. Circulation 94:857–862, 1996.
2. Blair SN, Kohl HW III, Paffenbarger RS, et al. Physical fitness and all-cause mortality: A prospective study of healthy men and women. JAMA 262:2395–2401, 1989.
3. Vanhees L. Fagard R. Thijs L, et al. Prognostic significance of peak exercise capacity in patients with coronary artery disease. J Am Coll Cardiol 23:358–363, 1994.
4. Blair SN, Kohl HW III, Barlow CE, et al. Changes in physical fitness and all-cause mortality: A prospective study of healthy and unhealthy men. JAMA 273:1093–1098, 1995.
5. Blair SN, Kampert JB, Kohl HW III, et al. Influences of cardiorespiratory fitness and other precursors on cardiovascular disease and all-cause mortality in men and women. JAMA 276:205–210, 1996.
6. Barlow CE, Kohl HW III, Gibbons LW, et al. Physical fitness, mortality and obesity. Int J Obes 19:S41–S44, 1995.
7. Paffenbarger RS, Hyde RT, Wing AL, et al. The association of changes in physical-activity level and other lifestyle characteristics with mortality among men. N Engl J Med 328:538–545, 1993.
8. Sandvik I, Erikssen J, Thaulow E, et al. Physical fitness as a predictor of mortality among healthy, middle-aged Norwegian men. N Engl J Med 328:533–537, 1993.
9. Pate RR, Pratt M, Blair SN, et al. Physical activity and public health: A recommendation from the Centers for Disease Control and Prevention and the American College of Sports Medicine. JAMA 273:402–407, 1995.
9a. Hambrecht R, Wolf A, Gielen S, et al. Effect of exercise on coronary entothelial function in patients with coronary artery disease. NEJM 342:454–460, 2000.

10. Beck KC, Johnson BD. Pulmonary adaptations to dynamic exercise. In: Durstine JL, ed. Resource Manual for Guidelines for Exercise Testing and Prescription. 2nd ed. Baltimore: Williams & Wilkins, 1993.

11. Durstine JL, Pate RR, Branch JD. Cardiorespiratory responses to acute exercise. In: Durstine JL, ed. Resource Manual for Guidelines for Exercise Testing and Prescription. 2nd ed. Baltimore: Williams & Wilkins, 1993.

12. Davis JA. Anaerobic threshold: Review of the concept and directions for future research. Med Sci Sports Exerc 17:6–21, 1985.

13. Sullivan MJ, Higginbotham MB, Cobb FR. Exercise training in patients with chronic heart failure delays ventilatory anaerobic threshold and improves submaximal exercise performance. Circulation 79:324–329, 1989.

14. Ades PA, Waldmann ML, Polk DM, et al. Referral patterns and exercise response in the rehabilitation of female coronary patients aged ≥62 years. Am J Cardiol 69:1422–1425, 1992.

15. Getchell LH, Moore JC. Physical training: Comparative responses of middle-aged adults. Arch Phys Med Rehab 56:250–254, 1975.

16. Franklin BA, Bonzheim K, Berg T. Gender differences in rehabilitation. In: Julian DG, Wenger NK, eds. Women and Heart Disease. London: Martin Dunitz, 1997:151–171.

17. Franklin B, Buskirk E, Hodgson J, et al. Effects of physical conditioning on cardiorespiratory function, body composition and serum lipids in relatively normal-weight and obese middle-aged women. Int J Obes 3:97–109, 1979.

18. Frick M, Elovainio R, Somer T. The mechanism of bradycardia evoked by physical training. Cariologia 51:46–54, 1967.

19. Clausen JP, Trap-Jensen J, Lassen NA. The effects of training on the heart rate during arm and leg exercise. Scand J Clin Lab Invest 26:295–301, 1970.

20. Rasmussen B, Klausen K, Clausen JP, et al. Pulmonary ventilation, blood gases, and blood pH after training of the arms or the legs. J Appl Physiol 38:250–256, 1975.

21. Davies CTM, Sargeant AJ. Effects of training on the physiological responses to one- and two-leg work. J Appl Physiol 38:377–381, 1975.

22. Henriksson J, Roitman JS. Time course of changes in human skeletal muscle succinate dehydrogenase and cytochrome oxidase activities and maximal oxygen uptake with physical activity and inactivity. Acta Physiol Scand 99:91–97, 1977.

23. Saltin B, Nazar K, Costill DL, et al. The nature of the training response: Peripheral and central adaptations to one-legged exercise. Acta Physiol Scand 96:289–305, 1976.

24. Clausen JP, Klausen K, Rasmussen B, et al. Central and peripheral circulatory changes after training of the arms or legs. Am J Physiol 225:675–682, 1973.

25. Thompson PD, Cullinane E, Lazarus B, et al. Effect of exercise training on the untrained limb exercise performance of men with angina pectoris. Am J Cardiol 48:844–850, 1981.

26. Lewis S, Thompson P, Areskog NH, et al. Transfer effects of endurance training to exercise with untrained limbs. Eur J Appl Physiol 44:25–34, 1980.

27. Franklin BA, Vander I, Wrisley D, et al. Trainability of arms versus legs in men with previous myocardial infarction. Chest 105:262–264, 1994.

28. Astrand PO, Rodahl K. Textbook of Work Physiology: Physiological Bases of Exercise. 4th ed. New York: McGraw-Hill, 1986.

29. Kenney WL. Parasympathetic control of resting heart rate: relationship to aerobic power. Med Sci Sports Exerc 17:451–455, 1985.

30. Rowell LB. Human cardiovascular adjustments to exercise and thermal stress. Physiol Rev 54:75–159, 1974.

31. Fox E, Bartels R, Billings C, et al. Intensity and distance of interval training programs and changes in aerobic power. Med Sci Sports 5(1):18–22, 1973.

32. Bevegard BS, Shepherd JT. Regulation of the circulation during exercise in man. Physiol Rev 47:178–213, 1967.

33. Longhurst JC, Kelly AR, Gonyea WJ, et al. Chronic training with static and dynamic exercise: Cardiovascular adaptation and response to exercise. Circ Res 48(6Pt2):1171–1178, 1981.

35. Levine BD, Lane LD, Buckey JC, et al. Left ventricular pressure-volume and Frank-Starling relations in endurance athletes: Implications for orthostatic tolerance and exercise performance. Circulation 84:1016, 1991.

36. Blomqvist CG, Saltin B. Cardiovascular adaptations to physical training. Ann Rev Physiol 45:169–189, 1983.

37. Perski A, Tzankoff SP, Engel BT. Central control of cardiovascular adjustments to exercise. J Appl Physiol 58:431–435, 1985.

38. Rerych, SK, Sholz PM, Sabiston DC, et al. Effects of exercise training on left ventricular function in normal subjects: A longitudinal study by radionuclide angiography. Am J Cardiol 45:244–252, 1980.

39. McArdle WD, Katch FI, Katch VL. Exercise Physiology: Energy, Nutrition and Human Performance. 3rd ed. Philadelphia: Lea & Febiger, 1991.

40. Smith ML, Mitchell JH. Cardiorespiratory adaptations to exercise training. In: Durstine JL, ed. Resource Manual for Guidelines for Exercise Testing and Prescription. 2nd ed. Baltimore: Williams & Wilkins, 1993.

41. Morganroth J, Maron B, Henry W, et al. Comparative left ventricular dimensions in trained athletes. Ann Intern Med 82:521–524, 1975.

42. Oscai L, Williams B, Hertig B. Effect of exercise on blood volume. J Appl Physiol 24:622–624, 1968.

43. Holoszy JO. Adaptations of skeletal muscle to endurance exercise. Med Sci Sports Exerc 7:155–164, 1975.

44. Rowell LB. General principles of vascular control. In: Human Circulation: Regulation During Physical Stress. New York: Oxford University Press, 1986.

45. Hermansen L, Wachtlova M. Capillary density of skeletal muscle in well-trained and untrained men. J Appl Physiol 30(6):860–863, 1971.

1.2.5, 1.2.6, 1.2.8, 1.2.11,   **2.2.0, 2.2.4, 2.2.7, 2.2.9,**   **4.8.6**
1.8.2, 1.8.3, 1.8.6, 1.8.15   **2.2.11, 2.2.18, 2.2.19,**
                      2.8.0.11

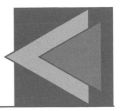

CHAPTER **18**

FACTORS AFFECTING THE ACUTE NEUROMUSCULAR RESPONSES TO RESISTANCE EXERCISE

William J. Kraemer and Jill A. Bush

Resistance training is repeated exposure to an acute exercise stimulus that is specific and characterized by various factors that define the physiological and biomechanical demands. Understanding the factors that affect acute resistance exercise stimuli is important in gaining insight into different resistance training protocols. Acute physiological changes are directly related to the configuration of external demands of resistance exercise and resistance exercise protocols must be specific to the physiological systems targeted.

PHYSIOLOGY OF RESISTANCE EXERCISE

Neuromuscular Activation

The stimulus for muscle activation comes from a high-level central control command signal originating from the premotor cortex and the motor cortex. The signal is relayed through a lower-level controller (brainstem and spinal cord) and transformed into a specific motor unit activation pattern. To perform a specific task, the required motor units meet specific demands for force production by activating associated muscle fibers (1, 2). Various feedback loops modify force production and provide communication to other physiological systems, such as the endocrine system. The high- and low-level commands can be modified by feedback from peripheral sensory or higher central command.

Motor Unit Activation

The functional unit of the neuromuscular system is the motor unit (3). It consists of the motor neuron and the muscle fibers it innervates. Motor units range in size from a few to several hundred muscle fibers. Muscle fibers from different motor units can be anatomically adjacent to each other, and therefore, a muscle fiber may be actively generating force while the adjacent fiber moves passively with no direct neural stimulation. When maximal force is required, all available motor units are activated. Another adaptive mechanism affected by heavy resistance training is the muscle force affected by different motor unit firing rates and/or frequencies.

Motor unit activation is also influenced by the size principle. This principle is based on the observed relationship between motor unit twitch force and recruitment threshold. Specifically, motor units are recruited in order according to recruitment thresholds and firing rates, resulting in a continuum of voluntary force. Thus, most muscles contain a range of motor units (type I and type II fibers), and force production can span wide levels. Maximal force production requires not only the recruitment of all motor units, including high-threshold motor units, but also recruitment at a sufficiently high firing rate. It has been hypothesized that untrained individuals cannot voluntarily recruit the highest-threshold motor units or maximally activate muscles. Furthermore, electrical stimulation has been shown to be more effective in eliciting gains in untrained muscle or injury rehabilitation scenarios, suggesting further inability to activate all available motor units. Thus, training adaptation develops the ability to recruit a greater percentage of motor units when required.

Few exceptions to the size principle have been identified; however, some advanced weight lifters and other athletes may not require the order of recruitment stipulated by the size principle. It may be possible to inhibit low-threshold motor units yet activate high-threshold ones to enhance rate of force development and power production. This hypothesis emerged from observations during rapid, stereotyped movements and voluntary eccentric muscle action in humans. The central nervous system can also limit force by engaging protective inhibitory mechanisms. Thus, training may result in changes in fiber recruitment order or reduced inhibition, which assists in the performance of certain types of muscle actions.

Muscle Fiber Types

Several nomenclatures have been used to classify skeletal muscle fibers, including color (red or white), contraction speed (fast or slow twitch), oxidative or glycolytic enzyme content (fast glycolytic, fast oxidative glycolytic, or oxidative), combination schemes (fast glycolytic), and

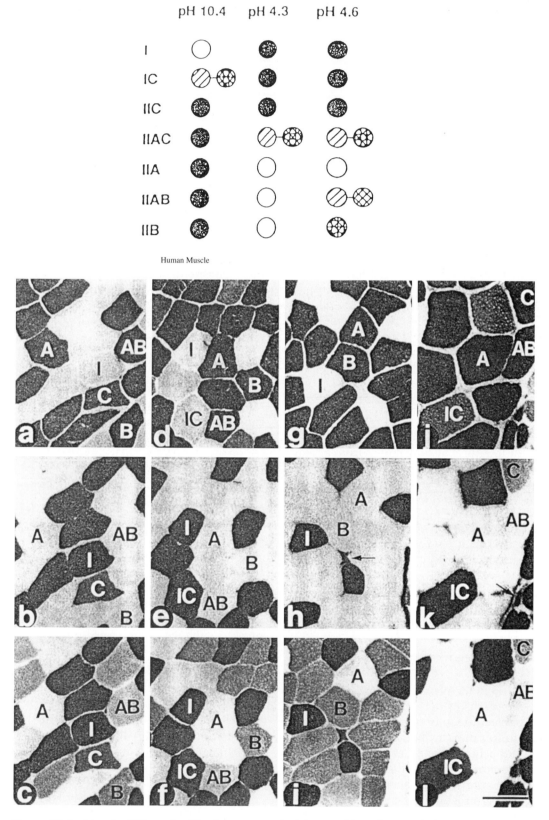

Figure 18.1. Myosin ATPase classification system. Staining profile and example fiber micrograph at 4.6 pH+. (Courtesy of Dr. Robert Staron, Ohio University, Athens, OH.)

myosin adenosine triphosphatase (ATPase) content (type I, IIa, IIb).

It is evident that exercise-induced changes in muscle have great plasticity (4–6). This is due in part to a complex yet readily adaptable group of contractile and regulatory proteins. Studies have focused on the myosin molecule and examination of fiber types. Fiber typing by myosin ATPase has been the most popular classification system (4–6). Figure 18.1 illustrates the continuum of human muscle fiber types from the most oxidative (type I) to the least oxidative (type IIB) fibers.

Three major types of polypeptide chains, including a heavy chain and two types of light chains, constitute the myosin molecule. The complexity of the system allows for different expression of isomyosin forms with different heavy and light chain compositions. The differential myosin expression is of interest because it is related to muscle function and adaptation. A link between the mATP-ase fiber type distribution and myosin heavy chain content in skeletal muscle has been investigated by examining relationships for entire biopsy samples or single fibers. The relative percentage of myosin heavy chain (MHC I, MHC IIa, MHC IIb) is highly correlated with the corresponding percentage of muscle fiber types (I, IIA, IIB) in both men and women (7).

Muscle Soreness

Muscle soreness may occur after an acute resistance training session. The exact mechanisms of muscle soreness remain speculative. Soreness is typically observed after excessively intense resistance training. It is most dramatic in relatively inexperienced or novice weight lifters. However, experienced weight lifters have soreness with novel exercise or excessive progression of intensity.

Several investigations demonstrate that eccentric exercise precipitates delayed-onset muscle soreness (DOMS). Eccentric contractions may damage the basic ultrastructure of the muscle cell. The focal point of the damage is the Z disk, a structural component that anchors the contractile protein actin.

The loss of structural integrity of the Z-disks may be the stimulus leading to the associated symptoms. The appearance of DOMS ranges from 24–48 hours after exercise and may last up to 10 days. Symptoms of DOMS include local muscular stiffness, tenderness, local edema, limited range of motion due to edema, and pain, which varies from low-grade ache to severe pain. Severity and location of discomfort specifically relate to the muscles used. The reason for increased soreness associated with eccentric training is unclear. However, one bout of eccentric exercise appears to result in protection from excessive soreness from another bout for up to 5–6 weeks in untrained or novice individuals. Thus, a slow progression in intensity is critical to limit soreness. It appears that excessive soreness develops from using resistance greater than the concentric 1 repetition maximum (RM).

PRINCIPLES OF RESISTANCE TRAINING PROGRAMS

The primary principles related to adaptation within the neuromuscular system during resistance training are specificity, progressive overload, and program variation.

Specificity

The principle of specificity states that resistance training should match the specific demands of the performance task. The concept of overload to enhance strength performance is a principle of progressive resistance training. Specificity comprises a number of concepts (8).

Speed of contraction relates to the speed of movement. Speed is important as an acute program variable, since it affects the safety of performing a specific movement (9). An intermediate training velocity is best if the aim is to increase strength at all velocities. Thus, for general strength, an intermediate training velocity is recommended through lifting and lowering the weight in a controlled manner. However, training at a fast velocity results in slightly greater gains in strength and power than training at a slow velocity. Thus, velocity-specific training is appropriate for athletes during selected periods.

Greater speed of movement requires proper equipment for safety. It has been shown that speed reps (i.e., loads of 30–45% of 1 RM) should not be performed when the weight is at the end of a limb (e.g., bench press, arm curls), since protective mechanisms decelerate the joint through activation of antagonist and inhibition of agonist muscles. If the goal is to develop an ability to accelerate through the range of motion, the mass must be released. Plyometric exercises, such as medicine ball throws; free-weight exercises in which the bar moves vertically; and sophisticated machines that catch the weight as it is released, are safest and most effective. In addition, different modes of resistance, such as isokinetic, pneumatic, or hydraulic machines, which do not accelerate through the range of motion, can be used to enhance speed. Appropriate exercises are required to train appropriate patterns of muscle activation (10).

Muscle group specificity requires that strength be developed through training of that muscle group. Increased elbow flexor and extensor strength requires exercises for both groups in a resistance program.

Metabolic specificity is also important in training. If the task requires high levels of muscular endurance, metabolic demands must be matched in training. Increased ability to perform anaerobic exercise requires reduced length of rest periods to stimulate anaerobic glycolysis and associated increased blood lactate. Likewise, increased aerobic capacity requires longer-duration, lower-intensity training.

Progressive Resistance

Adaptations from resistance training depend on the increased demands placed on the neuromuscular system (4,

8, 11). Progressive-resistance exercise refers to continual increases in stress on the muscle as training induces greater ability to produce and sustain force.

Ploutz et al. (12) demonstrated the importance of increasing resistance by using 1 RM for training. Strength increased by 14%, and cross-sectional area increased by 5% in trained left quadriceps, while strength increased by 7% and cross-sectional area did not change in untrained right quadriceps. This illustrates that neural factors mediate much of the improvement in 1-RM strength-induced adaptation. Also, in trained quadriceps, reduced muscle activation is required to lift a given resistance. Therefore, less muscle is activated as strength increases with training, unless resistance is also progressively increased.

Periodization

Variation in the volume and intensity of training, or periodization, is important for optimal strength gain (8, 10). Much of the early research focused on the concept that there is an optimal combination of sets and repetitions that induce increased strength. Such an optimal combination probably does not exist; instead, variations in resistance, number of sets, and number of repetitions is associated with greater strength gains. The most popular term for changing acute program variables is periodization. Periodization is planned variation in acute program variables.

Selye's general adaptation syndrome underlies the concept of periodization. This theory proposes three phases of adaptation during acute stress (i.e., resistance exercise): shock, adaptation, and staleness. The first stage, shock, occurs after the initiation of a novel stimulus (resistance exercise or new resistance), resulting in development of syndromes of maladaptation (e.g., soreness) and a resultant performance decrement. The second phase, adaptation, occurs during repeated training exposure to the stimulus and results in increased performance. In the third phase adaptation has occurred and the same stimulus does not produce further adaptation. Performance may reach a plateau in this phase, and for further adaptation to occur, a change in stimulus or rest must be imposed.

Programs that do not provide sufficient variation and rest result in a classic plateau of training or perhaps decreased performance (overtraining). Periodization can help avoid staleness and/or overtraining by allowing for adequate rest so that the exercise stimulus–response is maintained. Thus, variation in exercise stimulus is an important factor for consistent improvements in performance capacity.

The classic form of periodization breaks the training program into specific times. The longest period is the macrocycle, about a year. The macrocycle can be divided into mesocycles, generally 3–4 months each. A mesocycle may be further divided into a microcycle of approximately 2–6 weeks. Each training phase has a specific goal and is a planned part of the total program. This type of training was originally designed for track and field and weight lifting to assist competitors in peaking. Furthermore, only large muscle groups were normally periodized. Others have learned the benefits of such training and have adapted periodization for use in various sports and fitness activities. There are two models for periodization of training.

Classic Periodization Model

The goals of a program determine the number of training cycle phases, and it is thought that several cycles are better than one long cycle; therefore, the length of each phase typically ranges from 2–4 weeks. This example program contains only one set and repetition scheme; other schemes depend on the target training goal. Training frequency is typically 3 times per week. In this example the primary training goals are strength and power and associated muscle hypertrophy, which develops with such loadings.

GENERAL PRE-PREPARATION PHASE. At least 6–8 weeks is required for general conditioning to allow tolerance of strength training. Proper techniques should be emphasized with little or no resistance. Intensity allowing 12–15 repetitions, low volume (1 or 2 sets), and limited number of exercises is ideal for this phase. Exercises may be added as proper technique is demonstrated. Exercises for the large muscle groups are generally periodized, and small muscle groups are exercised at a slightly higher intensity (8–10 RM), but they can also be periodized. A length of 2–4 weeks is used for all of the following cycles.

PREPARATION PHASE. This is the first phase of a formal training cycle. The number of exercises and initial tolerance should be established in the previous cycle. The intensity allows 12–15 repetitions in 3–4 sets with a 1–2-minute rest between sets and exercises. This is a high-volume, low-intensity stimulus.

STRENGTH PHASE. Resistance work allows 3–5 repetitions in 2–3 sets with 2–2.5-minute rest periods between sets and exercises. Technique is emphasized along with progression of resistance.

POWER PHASE. This phase uses resistance allowing 1–4 repetitions at 30–60% of 1 RM in 5–6 sets with 3–4-minute rest periods between sets and exercises. The key is optimizing the rest for a maximal effort in all power exercise training. Again, technique is emphasized along with progression. Plyometric exercise or modalities such as isokinetics, pneumatics, and hydraulics can be added to the program for speed specificity at this point.

TRANSITION PHASE. The transition phase is used for active rest (i.e., performing endurance rather than resistance exercise). This phase can range from a few days to a couple of weeks, depending on the program and the amount of prior training.

Nonlinear Periodization Model

Nonlinear, or undulating, models for periodization are becoming more common. This model is nonlinear because it has larger resistance changes than those commonly used in linear models. The nonlinear model varies exercise within 1–2-week periods among light, moderate, heavy, and even very heavy resistance for appropriate exercises (e.g., core exercises). It begins with a general pre-preparation phase identical to that previously discussed. Then, for example, it uses 8–10 RM (moderate resistance) on the first training day of the week, 3–5 RM (heavy) on the next day, and 12–15 RM (light) on the third day for 12 weeks. The 12-week cycle is followed by a short active rest or transition phase and repeated. This model may be most appropriate for team and individual sports in which peaking is not primary because many competitions may take place in a season. A higher volume of training can be performed when light and moderate resistances are used and both training intensity and volume vary dramatically on a daily basis.

ACUTE PROGRAM VARIABLES

Several factors, termed acute program variables, affect configuration of resistance exercise stimuli. In 1983, Kraemer developed an approach for evaluating a single workout using five global variables as follows (8, 10):

- Choice of exercise
- Order of exercises
- Number of sets
- Rest periods
- Intensity of resistance

The acute program variables describe all possible single training sessions and determine acute physiological response to resistance exercise. A training session is designed by manipulating each variable and is specific to the combination effect of the acute program variables (8, 10, 13).

Choice of Exercise

The basis for choice of exercise relates to movement pattern and equipment (e.g., multijoint versus single joint, machine versus free weights, isokinetic versus constant external resistance, slow versus fast velocity). Furthermore, each time joint angle changes, the pattern of muscle tissue activation changes. Based on the needs analysis, exercises should stress both designated muscles and joint angles. Exercises can also be arbitrarily designated as **primary exercises** and **assistance exercises**. **Primary exercises** train prime movers in a particular movement and typically work major muscle groups (e.g., squat, bench press). **Assistance exercises** train smaller muscle groups and aid in the movement produced by the prime movers (e.g., triceps press, lat pull down, biceps curls).

Assistance exercises are often classified as single-joint or isolated movements.

Exercises can also be classified as **structural** or **isolation**. **Structural exercises** include whole-body lifts requiring coordinated action of multiple muscle groups. Power cleans, power snatches, dead lifts, and squats are examples of structural, whole-body, closed kinetic chain exercises. Exercises can also be classified as multijoint exercises, which use more than one joint in the movement. For example, the bench press, which involves movement of both the elbow and shoulder joints, is a multijoint exercise. Other examples of multijoint exercises are lat pull downs, military press, and leg press. **Isolation exercises** isolate a muscle group and are considered to be single-joint exercises. Bicep curls, sit-ups, knee extensions, and knee curls are good examples of isolated or single-joint exercises.

Order of Exercise

The order of exercises in resistance training programs typically consists of performing large-muscle prior to small-muscle exercises. It has been demonstrated that exercising the larger muscle groups first can achieve a higher intensity of exercise. Multijoint exercises (e.g., squats) are performed first, followed by exercises for smaller muscle groups (e.g., hamstring curls). Thus, order profiles focus on gaining a greater training effect for the large muscle groups by enhancing the amount of resistance that can be lifted.

Ordering of exercises also involves the sequence used in circuit weight-training protocols. For example, it is important to consider whether to perform a leg exercise followed by another leg exercise or to proceed to another muscle group. Inherent in this decision is the concept of pre-exhaustion. Pre-exhaustion is characterized by exercising smaller muscle groups prior to larger muscle groups. This method produces fatigue within the muscle group using isolation exercises prior to structural exercises. Arm-to-leg ordering allows for some recovery of arm muscles while legs are exercised. This is the most common order used in circuit weight training. Novice lifters are likely to be relatively intolerant of arm-to-arm or leg-to-leg exercise in circuit weight training because of their high blood lactate concentrations (10–14 mmol/L), especially with short rest periods (10 seconds) (14).

One final consideration for order of exercises is fitness level. The order of exercise can have a significant effect on the intensity level of a training session, and it is important to avoid excessive intensity for beginning lifters who may not be well conditioned.

Number of Sets

The number of sets is directly related to training results. For general fitness, the person does one set at the initiation of a training program and progresses to three or four sets. It has been suggested that multiple-set periodized systems (planned variation in sets, repetitions, and volume over a training period) are most effective for continued development of strength and local muscular endurance (8). Change in strength appears to be similar between one, two, and three sets of 10–12 RM during the first several weeks or months of training in untrained individuals when programs are not periodized. Thus, in a long-term training program, periodized multiple-set programs should be used.

Multiple sets of an exercise present a training stimulus during each set. Once initial fitness levels have been improved, multiple presentation of the stimulus is required to gain additional physiological benefit. Exercise volume (sets × repetitions × intensity) is vital to progression in each specific exercise, especially for those who have had several months of training (4, 5, 8). The interaction of sets and variation in training, or **periodized training**, may also help augment training adaptations.

Rest Periods

The length of the rest period between sets and exercises is often overlooked in exercise prescription. The rest period is a primary determinant of the overall intensity, and it influences the amount of resistance that can be used. It also significantly affects neuromuscular and metabolic demands. Rest periods determine how much of the adenosine triphosphate (ATP)–creatine phosphate (PC) (immediate) energy source is recovered and how high lactate concentrations increase in muscle and blood (14–17). Figures 18.2 and 18.3 show the effects of rest period length on blood lactate and growth hormone responses, respectively, in men and women.

The data indicate that for the same load (10-RM resistance) and total work, length of rest period dictates changes in the blood. In addition, heavier resistance does not always result in higher blood lactate concentrations; rather, the total amount of work performed and the duration of the force demands placed on the muscle actually determine blood lactate concentrations. For example, 10 RM allows more repetitions and longer sets, yet exercise remains at a relatively high percentage of the 1 RM (75–85% of 1 RM); therefore, higher lactate concentrations may result than from 1 or 2 RM exercises. Practically, it has been demonstrated that short rests are associated with greater psychological anxiety and fatigue. The psychological ramifications of using short rest periods should be carefully weighed when designing a training session. The anxiety appears to be due to dramatic metabolic demands of short-rest (1 minute or less) workouts (18).

Frequent use of high-intensity workouts with short rest periods and heavy resistance should be introduced slowly. Tolerance of increased muscle and blood lactate levels, and effective acid-base buffer mechanisms are re-

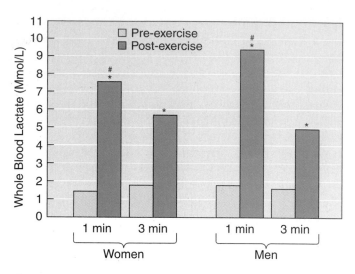

Figure 18.2. Pre-exercise to postexercise (peak value) response of blood lactate to short (1 minute) and long (3 minutes) rest period in men and women. *, P < 0.05 from corresponding pre-exercise value. #, corresponding 3-minute rest period. (Adapted with permission from Kraemer WJ, Fleck SJ, Dziados JE, et al. Changes in hormonal concentrations following different heavy resistance exercise protocols in women. J Appl Physiol 75:594–604, 1993; Kraemer WJ, Marchitelli L, McCurry D, et al. Hormonal and growth factor responses to heavy resistance exercise. J Appl Physiol 69:1442–1450, 1990.)

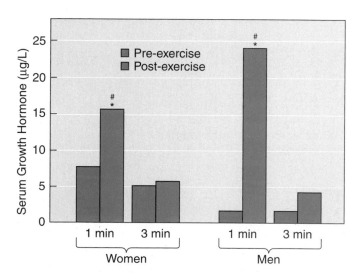

Figure 18.3. Pre-exercise to postexercise (peak value) response of growth hormone to short (1 minute) and long (3 minutes) rest period in men and women. *, P < 0.05 from corresponding pre-exercise value. #, corresponding 3-minute rest period. (Adapted with permission from Kraemer WJ, Fleck SJ, Dziados JE, et al. Changes in hormonal concentrations following different heavy resistance exercise protocols in women. J Appl Physiol 75:594–604, 1993; Kraemer WJ, Marchitelli L, McCurry D, et al. Hormonal and growth factor responses to heavy resistance exercise. J Appl Physiol 69:1442–1450, 1990.)

quired to offset associated adverse symptoms, such as nausea and dizziness must be developed (8, 14).

Short rest periods are also characteristic of circuit weight training, but resistances are typically moderate (40–60% of 1 RM) (8, 10). When rest periods are decreased to less than 1 minute, intensity is significantly reduced except in highly trained bodybuilders (7). Symptoms such as nausea and emesis do not indicate a quality workout; they are undesirable indications of having exceeded the ability to tolerate acid-base changes.

INTENSITY OF RESISTANCE

The amount of resistance used for a specific exercise is perhaps the most important variable in resistance training. It is probably the major stimulus related to changes in strength and local muscular endurance. The use of RM (the specific resistance that allows a specific number of repetitions) may be the easiest method to determine resistance. The RM continuum (Fig. 18.4) relates resistances to the broad training effects derived. It appears that RM resistances of six or fewer have the greatest effect on strength or maximal power output. RM resistances of 20 and above show the greatest effect on muscular endurance measures.

As resistances decrease from the strength stimulus zone, gains in strength diminish. The strength gains achieved above 25 RM resistances are small or nonexistent, and when they occur, they may be related to enhanced motor performance or learning effects. Pretraining status must be considered in evaluating strength improvement. The higher the pretraining level, the lower the percentage increase in the strength with training (8).

Another method of determining resistances uses a percentage of 1 RM (e.g., 70% of the 1 RM). This method requires that maximal strength in various lifts be evaluated regularly. If 1 RM is not assessed regularly, the percentage used in training decreases, and therefore training intensity is reduced.

Percentages of 1 RM are often used in training for competitive Olympic lifts, such as the clean and jerk, snatch, and pulls. Such lifts require coordinated movements and optimal power development to result in correct lifting technique. They cannot be performed at a "true" RM or to failure. Therefore, percent 1 RM allows correctly calculated resistances for such lifts. In addition, those in whom a Valsalva maneuver is contraindicated (e.g., cardiac patients) typically use a specific number of reps at a percent of 1 RM.

Interestingly, studies indicate that the relationship between percent of 1 RM and number of repetitions that can be performed with the resistance does not agree with the RM zones for optimal training (Fig. 18.4). This relationship varies with the amount of muscle mass required to perform the exercise (e.g., leg press requires more muscle recruitment than a leg extension). For example, using 80% of 1 RM typically results in the performance of more than 10 repetitions, especially for large muscle group exercises such as the leg press. Thus, number of repetitions must be carefully monitored to maintain resistance in the optimal training zone. Large muscle group exercises appear to require a higher percentage of 1 RM to maintain the strength RM zone (10 and under) (8).

Summary

A single resistance training session can be described by acute program variables. The configuration of these variables allows for a specific amount of exercise stimulus. Exercise sessions should be designed to meet training goals and to provide training variation. Because so many combinations are possible, a variety of sessions can be developed. Cognizance of the importance of each acute program variable is vital to understanding factors that affect acute physiological stress and ultimately the chronic adaptations to resistance training. Program variation is necessary to avoid overtraining. A reasonable guideline is to avoid increases in repetitions or volume of training of more than 2.5–5% at one time (8).

MUSCULAR STRENGTH AND ENDURANCE

The fitness characteristics of muscular performance typically targeted by a resistance training program include the following:

- Local muscular endurance, or the ability of a muscle or muscle group to perform repeated muscle actions against a submaximal resistance
- Muscle strength, or the ability of a muscle or muscle group to produce maximal force at a given velocity of movement

Within the concept of muscle strength, power should also be considered. Power is defined:

$$\frac{force \times distance}{time}$$

The ability to engage and produce force early in the activation pattern (rate of force production) is becoming

Theoretical Repetition Continuum

Loading Effects	Local Muscular Endurance	Power	Strength
Repetition Maximum	25 ←→ 12 ←→	10 ←→	5 ←→ 1

Figure 18.4. Theoretical repetition continuum for loading effects.

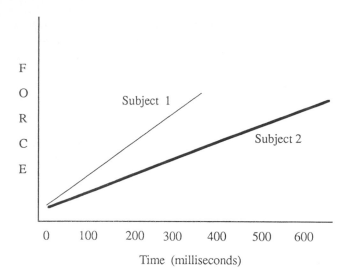

Figure 18.5. Typical force-time curve. Two individuals with equal maximal force capabilities but with different rates of force production are shown (Subject 1 high rate of force production).

recognized as an important feature of the acute functional ability of muscle (9, 10). This concept is shown in a typical force–time curve in Figure 18.5. Although maximum strength may be the same, the rate of force development to maximum is faster in some individuals than in others. The ability to engage the muscle rapidly seems to be important not only for sports performance but also for daily challenges, such as reacting to loss of balance, climbing stairs, and picking up a bag of groceries and putting it on a shelf (8).

ISOMETRICS

Isometrics, or static resistance training, occurs when contractions result in no apparent change in the length of the muscle and thus no movement. This type of resistance training is usually performed against an immovable object such as a wall or a weight machine loaded beyond maximal concentric strength. Isometrics is also performed when a weak muscle group contracts against a strong muscle group.

Isometric specificity is the result of isometric training. If isometric training is assessed isometrically, large strength gains are apparent; however, if progress is assessed using concentric or eccentric methods, little or no increase in strength may be demonstrated. Specificity in this case is related to recruitment of muscles and motor units specific to the activity. Increases in isometric strength are related to the frequency, duration, intensity, and number of exercises. Most studies using isometric training manipulate several variables simultaneously, making it difficult to evaluate any single factor. Some recommendations concerning isometric training are possible, however.

Increases in strength can be achieved with submaximal isometric muscle exercises. However, research supports the use of maximal voluntary muscle action (MVMA) as more effective for increasing strength (8). The majority of research has used MVMAs of 3–10 seconds' duration and a relatively small number of exercises per day. The length of time a muscle is activated is directly related to strength increase. Optimal gains in strength also result from fewer long-duration muscle actions or more short-duration exercises. The strength gain from isometric training occurs predominantly at the joint angle at which the isometric training is performed (joint angle specificity). There is, however, carryover of strength increase up to at least ±20° of the training angle. Isometric training is enhanced by visual feedback.

The safety of isometric training is well established. However, the Valsalva maneuver can occur, as in all resistance training, but should be discouraged, especially in those with cardiovascular disease because of the resulting exaggerated systolic and diastolic blood pressure response.

HEMODYNAMIC RESPONSES TO ACUTE RESISTANCE EXERCISE

Heart Rate and Blood Pressure

Heart rate and blood pressure increase during dynamic resistance exercise using machines, free weights, or isokinetics. Peak blood pressure response is higher during weight training in which a concentric and an eccentric phase occur than during isokinetic exercise (19). Blood pressure and heart rate may increase quite dramatically, with peak blood pressures of 320/250 mm Hg and heart rates of 170 beats per minute for a two-legged leg press at 95% of 1 RM to voluntary concentric failure with a Valsalva maneuver. Heart rate and blood pressure responses are also significant when the Valsalva maneuver is limited.

Peak blood pressure and heart rate normally occur during the last several repetitions of a set to voluntary concentric failure. Blood pressures are higher during sets at submaximal resistance to voluntary failure than at 1 RM. In dynamic resistance exercise, blood pressure but not heart rate rises during the concentric as compared to the eccentric portion of a repetition. In addition blood pressure increases with active muscle mass, but the increase is not linear (19).

Stroke Volume and Cardiac Output

Stroke volume (determined by electrical impedance) is not significantly elevated above resting during the **concentric** phase of resistance training exercise with or without a Valsalva maneuver. However, during the **eccentric** phase, stroke volume is significantly increased above rest (with or without a Valsalva maneuver) and is significantly greater than during the concentric phase of a repetition (19).

During both the concentric and eccentric phases of a repetition, cardiac output may be increased. Cardiac output during squat exercise may increase to approximately 20 L during the eccentric phase but be only 15 L during the concentric phase. However, during exercise involving smaller muscle mass (e.g., knee extension), cardiac output may be elevated above rest only during the eccentric phase. The differing response between eccentric and concentric phases may result in no overall change from rest in mean cardiac output and stroke volume during exercise involving a small muscle mass. Heart rate is not significantly different between the concentric and eccentric phases. Because stroke volume is significantly greater during the eccentric than the concentric phase of a repetition, the higher cardiac output during the eccentric phase is due to increased stroke volume.

CALORIC COST OF RESISTANCE EXERCISE

The caloric cost of resistance exercise can be increased both during and after exercise. The caloric costs of an acute exercise session have been studied in a variety of protocols from single exercises to multiple exercise circuits. The caloric cost ranges from 14–75 kcal/kg/day. It appears that the caloric cost of resistance exercise is related to the amount of muscle mass activated (choice of exercises), the length of the rest period, the intensity of the exercise, and the ability to tolerate higher volumes of total work (20).

► **SUMMARY**

The acute physiological stress of the neuromuscular system during resistance exercise is related to external demands. These demands are created by acute program variables that dictate the acute resistance exercise protocol. Careful consideration of these variables affecting the demands allows optimization of the exercise prescription for resistance exercise.

References
1. Edgerton VR, Roy RR, Gregor RJ, et al. Muscle fiber activation and recruitment. In: Knuttgen HG, Vogel JA, Poortmans S, eds. Biochemistry of Exercise. Champaign, IL: Human Kinetics, 1983:31–49.
2. Faulkner J, Claflin D, McCully K. Power output of fast and slow fibers from human skeletal muscles. In: Jones N, McCartney N, McComas A, eds. Human Muscle Power. Champaign, IL: Human Kinetics, 1986:81–90.
3. Noth J. Motor units. In: Komi PV, ed. Strength and Power in Sport. Oxford, UK: Blackwell Scientific, 1992:21–28.
4. Staron RS, Hikida RS. Histochemical, biochemical, and ultrastructural analyses of single human muscle fibers with special reference to the C fiber population. J Histochem Cytochem 40:563–568, 1992.
5. Staron RS, Karapondo DL, Kraemer WJ, et al. Skeletal muscle adaptations during the early phase of heavy-resistance training in men and women. J Appl Physiol 76:1247–1255, 1994.
6. Staron RS, Leonardi MJ, Karapondo DL, et al. Strength and skeletal muscle adaptations in heavy-resistance trained women after detraining and retraining. J Appl Physiol 70:631–640, 1991.
7. Fry AC, Allemeier CA, Staron RS. Correlation between percentage fiber type area and myosin heavy chain content in human skeletal muscle. Eur J Appl Physiol 68:246–251, 1994.
8. Fleck SJ, Kraemer WJ. Designing Resistance Training Programs. 2nd ed. Champaign, IL: Human Kinetics, 1997.
9. Newton RU, Kraemer WJ. Developing explosive muscular power: Implications for a mixed methods training strategy. J Strength Cond 16:20, 1994.
10. Kraemer WJ, Koziris LP. Muscle strength training: Techniques and considerations. Phys Ther Pract 2:54–68, 1992.
11. Sale DG. Neural adaptation to strength training. In: Komi P, ed. Strength and Power in Sports: The Encyclopaedia of Sports Medicine. Oxford, UK: Blackwell Scientific, 1992:249–265.
12. Ploutz LL, Tesch PA, Biro RL, et al. Effect of resistance training on muscle use during exercise. J Appl Physiol 76:1675–1681, 1994.
13. Kraemer WJ, Baechle TR. Development of a strength training program. In: Allman FL, Ryan AJ, eds. Sports Medicine. 2nd ed. Orlando: Academic, 1989:113–127.
14. Kraemer WJ, Noble BJ, Culver BW, et al. Physiologic responses to heavy-resistance exercise with very short rest periods. Int J Sports Med 8:247–252, 1987.
15. Kraemer WJ, Fleck SJ, Dziados JE, et al. Changes in hormonal concentrations following different heavy resistance exercise protocols in women. J Appl Physiol 75:594–604, 1993.
16. Kraemer WJ, Marchitelli L, McCurry D, et al. Hormonal and growth factor responses to heavy resistance exercise. J Appl Physiol 69:1442–1450, 1990.
17. Kraemer WJ, Gordon SE, Fleck SJ, et al. Endogenous anabolic hormonal and growth factor responses to heavy resistance exercise in males and females. Int J Sports Med 12:228–235, 1991.
18. Tharion WJ, Rausch TM, Harman EA, et al. Effects of different resistance exercise protocols on mood states. J Appl Sci Res 5:60–65, 1991.
19. Fleck SJ. Cardiovascular response to strength training. In: Komi P, ed. Strength and Power in Sports: The Encyclopaedia of Sports Medicine. Oxford, UK: Blackwell Scientific, 1992:305–315.
20. Stone MH. Weight gain and weight loss. In: Baechle TR, ed. Essentials of Strength Training and Conditioning. Champaign, IL: Human Kinetics, 1994:231–237.

1.2.5, 1.2.8

2.2.4, 2.2.7, 2.2.9, 2.2.18, 2.8.0.14

4.2.0.5

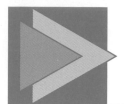

CHAPTER **19**

CHRONIC MUSCULOSKELETAL ADAPTATIONS TO RESISTANCE TRAINING

William J. Kraemer, Jeff S. Volek, and Steven J. Fleck

Both acute and chronic physiological changes occur with resistance exercise. An acute response usually results in an immediate change, whereas a chronic change is a function of the response to a repeated exercise stimulus. The term *adaptation* refers to the physiological process by which adaptation to physical training occurs. Ultimately, the adaptation to training determines whether resistance training is effective and whether a higher level of physiological function and/or performance is possible. Since resistance exercise protocols can be differentially configured to present a variety of demands, training adaptations appear to be specific to the type of protocol used. The specificity is related to the particular pattern of neuromuscular activation required to perform a resistance exercise. In turn, this neuromuscular stimulation activates a variety of other systems (e.g., endocrine, cardiovascular) that act to support the adaptive changes in the neuromuscular system. The sequence of adaptation events is initiated with the first exercise session and follows a time course specific to the individual and the type of protocol used.

Studies of chronic adaptations to resistance training have come primarily from training programs of less than 4 months' duration. Table 19.1 summarizes adaptations from heavy resistance training (i.e., resistances greater than 80% of 1 repetition maximum [RM]). This chapter discusses these adaptations, which are important to understanding program design for resistance training.

MUSCLE ENLARGEMENT

Hypertrophy

One of the most prominent adaptations to a properly designed and implemented strength training program is muscle growth. Increased muscle size has been primarily attributed to muscle fiber hypertrophy (increased size of individual fibers) (1). Only fibers activated during training are subject to this adaptation response. The mechanisms of muscle enlargement are unclear, but it is a multivariate phenomenon that affects the genetic machinery.

Initial increases in water content, changes in the type of muscle proteins, and eventual increases in contractile proteins are supported and signaled by a host of systematic trophic influences, from hormones to nutrition. Clearly, resistance exercise disrupts or damages certain muscle fibers, which later undergo repair and remodeling. This process may well involve many regulatory mechanisms (e.g., hormonal and metabolic) interacting with the training status as well as the availability of protein.

Increased muscle size is generally attributed to hypertrophy of existing muscle fibers. Muscle fiber hypertrophy is thought to occur through remodeling of protein within the cell, and increased size and number of myofibrils. Furthermore, increases in the number of contractile filaments (actin and myosin) and sarcomeres contribute to increased muscle fiber size and ultimately intact muscle. It has been suggested that the packing density of actin, but not myosin, increases as the contractile proteins are added to the outside of the myofibril without altering cross-bridge configuration. The contractile proteins and fluid (sarcoplasm) in muscle fibers turn over every 7–15 days (2). Resistance training influences this process by affecting the quality (i.e., the type of protein) and quantity (i.e., the absolute amount) of contractile proteins produced.

Changes in types of muscle protein, such as myosin heavy chains, begin with the initiation of heavy resistance training (3). As training continues, the quantity of contractile protein increases as the muscle fibers increase in cross-sectional area. It appears that more than eight sessions are required to increase contractile protein content in all muscle fibers to demonstrate significant muscle fiber hypertrophy. Ultimately, the amount of muscle fiber hypertrophy that occurs depends on the upper genetic limits of cell size. All fibers appear to hypertrophy, but not to the same extent. The amount of enlargement depends on the type of muscle fiber and the pattern of recruitment (4). It is believed that in type II muscle fibers the hypertrophy involves increased rate of protein synthesis, and in type I muscle fibers, decreased rate of degradation is responsible (2).

Table 19.1. Physiological Adaptations Associated With Chronic Resistance Training in Humans

VARIABLE	DIRECTIONAL CHANGE IN ADAPTATION
Performance	
Muscle strength and endurance	Increases
Aerobic power	No change
Maximal rate of force development	Increases
Vertical jump	Increases
Anaerobic power	Increases
Sprint speed	Improves
Muscle fibers	
Fiber size	Increases
Capillary volume density	No change or decreases
Mitochondrial volume density	Decreases
Myosin heavy chains	
Fast	Increases
Slow	No change or decreases
Enzyme activity	
Creatine phosphokinase	Increases
Myokinase	Increases
Phosphofructokinase	Increases
Metabolic energy stores	
Stored ATP	Increases
Stored creatine phosphate	Increases
Stored glycogen	Increases
Intramuscular triglycerides	May increase
Connective tissue	
Ligament strength	? (theoretically increases)
Tendon strength	? (theoretically increases)
Collagen content	? (theoretically increases)
Bone density	? (theoretically increases)
Body composition	
Percent body fat	Decreases
Fat-free mass	Increases
Neuroendocrine	
Growth hormone (acute exercise)	Increases
Growth hormone (chronic)	No change or decreases
Testosterone (acute and chronic)	Increases
Cortisol (acute)	Increases
Cortisol (chronic)	No change
Cardiovascular	
Heart rate	No change or decreases
Heart size	Increases
Blood pressure	Decreases
Max VO$_2$	No change
Serum lipids	
Total Cholesterol	Decreases
HDL	Increases
LDL	Decreases or no change
Triglycerides	Decreases
Neuromuscular	
Activation of synergistic muscles	Increases
Inhibition of antagonistic muscles	Increases
Neural protective mechanisms	Decreases
Motor neuron excitability	Increases

Hyperplasia

Although this hypothesis is controversial, it has been suggested that increased muscle size may also be due to muscle fiber hyperplasia (increased number of muscle fibers). Hyperplasia following resistance training has not been demonstrated in humans because of methodological difficulties (e.g., unavailability of whole muscle for examination), but it has been shown in response to various exercise protocols in both birds and mammals (1, 5). Hyperplasia was first implicated in adaptation to resistance training in laboratory animals. Critics of the hyperplasia hypothesis claim that methods of evaluation, damage to muscle samples, and degenerating muscle fibers account for the observed hyperplasia. Later studies, even while attempting to correct for such problems, continue to demonstrate increases in muscle fiber number. Though no clear evidence supports hyperplasia in humans, some findings indicate that it may occur.

One theory advanced to explain hyperplasia is activation of satellite cells (i.e., reserve cells outside the muscle fiber plasma membrane). Although activation of satellite cells and subsequent generation of new fibers are generally thought to occur in response to fiber injury or death, new muscle fibers may be formed as an adaptation to mild damage caused by intensive resistance training. While hyperplasia in humans may not be the primary adaptational response of muscle fibers, it may be an adaptation to resistance training that occurs when some fibers reach a theoretical upper limit in cell size. Intensive long-term training may make some type II muscle fibers primary candidates for such adaptation. If hyperplasia does occur, it probably accounts for only a small portion (5–10%) of the increase in muscle size.

MUSCLE FIBER TRANSFORMATION

Much plasticity exists with regard to changes in muscle with exercise, partly because of the complex yet readily adaptable group of myosin contractile and regulatory proteins. The majority of resistance exercise research has focused on the myosin molecule and examination of fiber types. Change in muscle adenosine triphosphatase (ATPase) also indicates associated change in the myosin heavy chain (MHC) content (6). A continuum of muscle fiber types exists, and transformation (e.g., type IIB to type IIA) within a particular subtype is a common adaptation to resistance training (7). Figure 19.1 illustrates the transformation that heavy resistance training produces in the muscle fiber subtypes. Using this classification scheme for evaluating changes in subtype, it is doubtful that in normal training conditions, muscle fibers transform from type II to type I. However, movement along the continuum within a fiber type clearly occurs (for reviews, see the suggested reading list).

It appears that as soon as a type IIB muscle fiber is stimulated, it begins a transformation toward the type IIA pro-

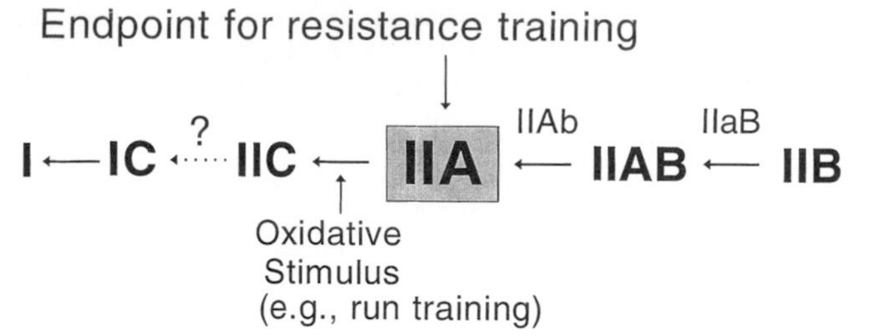

Endpoint for resistance training

Figure 19.1. The process of muscle fiber type transformation. Changes in myosin ATPase and myosin heavy chain proteins underlie this process.

file by changing the quality of proteins and expressing different types and amounts of mATPase. Thus, following resistance training, very few type IIB fibers remain. These alterations in the muscle fiber types are supported by MHC analyses with the replacement of MHC IIB with MHC IIA chains. Muscle fiber type conversions may occur very early during training, as early as four sessions. **Conversions of fast fiber types do not appear to be related to the rate of change of the cross-sectional area over either the short or long term.** In addition, some evidence indicates that women may undergo these conversions more quickly than men.

The shift from type IIB to type IIA reverses during detraining. Furthermore, it appears that when resistance training is restarted, the conversion from type IIB to type IIA is quicker relative to starting in an untrained state. Thus, type IIB fibers appear not to be a recruited pool of fibers that improve in oxidative ability when recruited for high threshold types of activities (i.e., heavy resistance exercise). In general, the proportion of type I muscle fibers and MHC I composition remain unchanged with resistance training. The extent that this muscle fiber remodeling contributes to muscle strength is unknown; however, gradual increases in number and size of myofibrils and perhaps the fast fiber type conversions of type IIB to IIA may contribute to force production. Thus, while nervous system alterations may be the most dramatic effects mediating strength and power changes early in training, many other changes that occur in the remodeling of muscle fibers may influence when hypertrophy reaches a critical threshold. Therefore, the quality of the protein type being generated because of the influence of resistance training is an important aspect of muscular development.

Information gained from studies examining simultaneous strength and aerobic training demonstrates that muscle fiber adaptations are not the same as the adaptive response produced by single-mode training (4). Thus, the mechanisms of adaptation to resistance exercise depend on the global exercise stimuli presented to the activated musculature. Such changes may begin to affect performance within 3 months of initiating training.

CONNECTIVE TISSUE

Physical activity also increases the size and strength of ligaments, tendons, and bone. To prevent injury, ligaments, tendons, and bones must adapt to support the greater forces generated by skeletal muscles. Bone tends to adapt more slowly (6–12 months for changes in bone density) than muscle (8). Both the attachment site of a ligament or tendon and the muscle–tendinous junction are frequent sites of injury. Research on laboratory animals demonstrates that with endurance training, the amount of force necessary to cause separation at these areas increases (9). It is probable that resistance training produces similar results.

The sheath of connective tissue that surrounds the entire muscle (epimysium), groups of muscle fibers (perimysium), and individual muscle fibers (endomysium) may also adapt to resistance training. These sheaths form the framework that supports an overload. Compensatory hypertrophy induced in the muscle of laboratory animals also causes an increase in the collagen content of the sheaths. Surprisingly, bodybuilders do not differ from age-matched control subjects in the relative amount of connective tissue in the biceps brachii. Thus, connective tissue sheaths appear to increase at the same rate as muscle tissue. Furthermore, resistance training has been demonstrated to increase the thickness of hyaline cartilage on the articular surfaces of bone. One major function of hyaline cartilage is to absorb shocks between the bony surfaces of a joint. Increasing the thickness of this cartilage may facilitate improved shock absorption.

ENZYMATIC ADAPTATIONS

The human body derives energy from three sources: the phosphagen, or adenosine triphosphate–creatine phosphate (ATP-PC) system, the glycolytic or lactic acid system, and the oxidative or aerobic system. Enzyme activity of the phosphagen energy source (creatine phosphokinase and myokinase) has been demonstrated to increase in humans as a result of isokinetic training, and in rats as a result of isometric training. Enzymatic changes associated with the phosphagen energy source appear to be linked to the duration of exercise bouts (i.e., no change with bouts shorter than 6 seconds). However, little or no change in creatine phosphokinase and myokinase has resulted from resistance training (10). Thus, the type of training program affects enzymatic adaptation. Neither of the glycolytic enzymes (phosphofructokinase and lactic dehydrogenase) appears to be affected by heavy resistance training (11, 12).

Increases in aerobic enzyme activity are reported with isokinetic and isometric training in humans and with isometric training in rats. These changes may also depend on the duration of individual exercise bouts. However, aerobic enzymes obtained from pooled samples of weight-trained muscle fibers do not demonstrate increased activity (10). Nevertheless, increases in oxidative enzymes have been demonstrated to be higher in type IIA fibers than in type IIB fibers. This may be because type IIB fibers are a nonrecruited population of type II muscle fibers that when activated, increase oxidative enzymes and begin to converge toward a type IIA fiber. Bodybuilders using training with high volume, short rest periods, and moderate resistance have higher citrate synthase activity in type II fibers than other types of lifters who train with heavier loads and longer rest periods (10). Again, the type of program may influence the magnitude of enzyme change. An enzyme associated with all three energy sources, myosin ATPase, undergoes minor changes in pooled muscle fibers (10). The fact that various types of myosin ATPase exist may suggest that interconversion of the type of myosin ATPase is more important than change in the absolute concentration.

ENERGY SUBSTRATES

The final source of energy for muscular activity is ATP that is ultimately derived from intramuscular phosphagens (phosphocreatine and ATP), carbohydrate (muscle glycogen and blood glucose), and lipids (plasma fatty acids and intramuscular triglycerides). In humans, it has been demonstrated that strength training increases resting intramuscular concentrations of phosphocreatine and ATP. However, this finding is not supported by other studies, even when significant amounts of muscle fiber hypertrophy occur (13). Recent evidence that creatine supplementation expands the total creatine content of muscle by about 20–30%, even in trained individuals, appears to support the concept that training induces only small changes even though stores can be improved by supplementation.

Five months of resistance training may increase intramuscular glycogen stores. However, muscle glycogen content does not change during resistance training (13). The aerobic energy system uses glycogen from hepatic and intramuscular sources, triglycerides from intramuscular and adipose tissue sources, and some protein to produce ATP; endurance training also enhances intramuscular storage and mobilization of triglycerides. Whether resistance training induces similar adaptations is equivocal, since increased triglyceride use has been observed in the triceps but not in the quadriceps after training. Thus, there may be differences in the response of different muscle groups with respect to triglyceride storage and mobilization.

Although dietary practices and type of program may affect triglyceride concentrations, it is possible that because most resistance training programs are anaerobic, intramuscular concentrations of triglycerides are minimally affected by resistance training. Storage and mobilization of energy within the body depend heavily on nutritional status and recent food consumption. Thus, both acute and chronic dietary intake influence adaptations associated with energy substrate availability and use.

Myoglobin content of muscle may decrease with resistance training (13). Thus, it has been postulated that long-term strength training may depress myoglobin content and therefore the ability of muscle fibers to extract oxygen. Again, the initial state of training and the specific type of program may influence the effect of resistance training on myoglobin content.

CAPILLARY SUPPLY AND MITOCHONDRIAL DENSITY

Oxidative metabolism is supported by capillary supply and the concentration of cellular mitochondria. Capillarization may be enhanced with resistance training of untrained subjects. Capillaries per unit area and per fiber are significantly increased in response to varying types of heavy resistance training (i.e., combinations of concentric and eccentric muscle actions). Olympic weight lifters and power lifters exhibit lower, and bodybuilders higher, capillary density than untrained men. In part, this may be due to the larger fibers exhibited by weight lifters and power lifters contributing to an area dilution. Thus, high-intensity, low-volume strength training (i.e., Olympic weight lifting or power lifting) actually decreases capillary density, whereas low-intensity, high-volume strength training (i.e., bodybuilding) increases capillary density. As with the selective hypertrophy of type II fibers, increased capillaries appears to be linked to the intensity and volume of resistance training. However, the time course of changes in capillary density appears to be slow, since studies have demonstrated that 6–12 weeks may not stimulate capillary growth beyond normal untrained levels (14).

Increased capillary density may facilitate performance of low-intensity weight training by increasing blood supply to active muscle. The short rest periods used by bodybuilders during training sessions result in large increases in blood lactate concentrations (1–2 mmol/L to more than 20 mmol/L). Increased capillary density may increase the ability to remove lactate and thereby improve the ability to tolerate training under highly acidic conditions. This theory is supported by the ability of bodybuilders to use heavier resistance under the same lactate conditions than power lifters, whose blood lactate concentrations in heavy resistance training are rarely above 4 mmol/L; therefore, the physiological stimulus to increase capillarization may not be as great in heavy resistance training (15).

Few studies have examined the effect of resistance training on mitochondrial density. Similar to capillaries per muscle fiber, mitochondrial density decreases with resistance training because of the dilution effects of muscle fiber hypertrophy. The observation of decreased mitochondrial density is consistent with the minimal demands for oxidative metabolism during most resistance training programs. The functional significance of this morphological alteration remains unclear.

NEURAL ADAPTATIONS

Following resistance training, the correlation between increases in strength and changes in whole muscle cross-sectional area, limb circumference, and muscle fiber cross-sectional area is low, indicating that other factors are responsible for gains in strength (3). This is true especially during the initial weeks of training. On the basis of this type of evidence, it has been concluded that neural factors profoundly influence muscular force production. Such neural factors are related to the following processes:

- Increased neural drive to muscle
- Increased synchronization of motor units
- Increased activation of the contractile apparatus
- Inhibition of protective mechanisms of the muscle (i.e., Golgi tendon organs)

Scientists have investigated the neural drive to muscle using integrated electromyogram (EMG) techniques (16–18). This technique measures electrical activity within muscles and nerves and indicates the amount of neural drive to a muscle (i.e., the number and amplitude of impulses). Evidence suggests that the amount of muscle required to be activated following resistance training is less than that required to perform the same exercise protocol prior to training. This reduction in the amount of muscle needed to move a given resistance post training demonstrates that unless resistance progressively increases, less muscle is activated as muscular strength increases.

Since less neural drive is required to produce a given submaximal force after training, either activation of muscle improves or muscle fibers develop a more efficient recruitment pattern. Since no improvement in activation of muscle after training has been demonstrated, some suggest that more efficient recruitment order may play an important role in increased force production in trained muscle. Furthermore, some evidence suggests that these neural adaptations are specific to certain muscle fibers and therefore may contribute to increased force output in some but not all muscles.

After the initial neural adaptations, muscle hypertrophy becomes the predominant factor in increased strength, especially for younger men. Sale (19) described this dynamic interplay of neural and hypertrophic factors. A significant increase in neural factor adaptation is observed over the time course used for most resistance training studies (e.g., 6–10 weeks). As training runs longer than 10 weeks, muscle hypertrophy eventually occurs and contributes more than neural adaptations to strength and power gain. Eventually muscle hypertrophy also reaches a plateau. Whole-muscle image systems (e.g., magnetic res-

onance imaging and computed tomography) have confirmed that fiber changes do not necessarily reflect the magnitude of change in whole muscle. Whole muscle must be frequently stimulated at several angles of movement to activate all available tissue over the cross-sectional area. Nevertheless, strength and power gains derived from the progressively and properly loaded and activated musculature appear to be bounded by a genetic upper limit of neuromuscular adaptation. Although neural adaptations account for much of the strength increase early in a resistance training program, strength and power improvement in advanced resistance trained athletes (i.e., Olympic weight lifters) may also be due to neural factors (18).

Morphological changes in the human nervous system with heavy resistance training are unclear. Evidence suggests that exercise increases the area of the neuromuscular junction (NMJ) and that this adaptation is differentially influenced by the intensity of exercise (19, 20). High-intensity endurance exercise appears to result in more dispersed, irregularly shaped synapses, while low-intensity training results in more compact, symmetrical synapses. High-intensity training also induces a greater total length of NMJ branching than does low-intensity exercise. Thus, it may be hypothesized that heavy resistance training produces morphological changes in the NMJ. These changes may have greater magnitude than adaptations to endurance training because of the differences in required quanta of neurotransmitter involved with the recruitment of high threshold motor units.

NEUROENDOCRINE ADAPTATIONS

The close association of hormones to the nervous system makes the neuroendocrine system potentially one of the most important physiological systems related to resistance training adaptations. Chronic adaptations in the neuroendocrine system are important in mediating many of the anabolic (tissue building) and catabolic (tissue breakdown) effects on muscle protein. The endocrine system also plays an important support function for adaptational mechanisms ultimately leading to enhanced muscular force production (21–24).

Hormones mediate changes primarily through metabolic or trophic effects on nerve and muscle cells. The alteration of metabolism (usually protein) and the molecular mechanisms associated with cell transport phenomena must be translated to enhanced synthesis, reduced degradation, or augmentation of the functional structure or secretory products leading to enhanced muscle mass and/or improved force production. Endocrine function is highly integrated with nutritional status, training status, and other external factors (e.g., stress, sleep, disease), which affect the remodeling and repair processes. Much of the work in the area of hormonal changes with resistance exercise has focused on the alteration of concentrations of hormones in circulating blood. Differential alterations in hormones have been observed to be a function of type of exercise protocol and associated physiological demands. The challenge is to link physiological response to chronic adaptation (e.g., muscle hypertrophy and strength).

The primary anabolic hormones are testosterone, growth hormone, and insulinlike growth factor I (IGF-I), while the primary catabolic hormones are cortisol and catecholamines. Resistance training increases resting and exercise-induced testosterone concentrations. The response of testosterone appears to be determined by the mode, intensity, and duration of the training program. In contrast, resistance training does not appear to alter resting concentrations of growth hormone; however, exercise-induced increases in growth hormone may be enhanced in trained individuals. There is less information available concerning the responses of IGF-I, cortisol, and catecholamines to resistance training. Some evidence indicates that a well-conditioned athlete has a less pronounced increase in cortisol during exercise than an unconditioned athlete (25).

Acute increases in circulating concentrations of hormones are differentially sensitive to manipulations of the acute program variables in a resistance training session. For example, the highest growth hormone concentrations (beta-endorphin and cortisol) are observed when short-rest (1 minute), 10-RM multiple sets (three sets) of exercises are performed. Testosterone appears responsive to high-intensity (5 RM), long rest (3 minutes) resistance exercise protocol and to a 10-RM, short-rest protocol (25). The following factors are important determinants of the hormonal response to resistance exercise:

- Amount of muscle mass recruited
- Intensity of the workout
- Amount of rest between sets and exercises
- Total volume of work
- Training level of the individual

The view of the endocrine system's response to resistance exercise has been somewhat limited to molecular forms that can be detected with an antibody-mediated assay (immunoreactive molecular forms), thus eliminating various molecular forms that are not immunoreactive (e.g., various forms of growth hormone). Finally, the understanding of receptors on the target tissue for various hormones is developing. It is now understood that the receptors can be differentially regulated in different fiber types in response to different types of exercise (20). These responses at the target level determine whether a hormonal message is realized at the level of individual cells.

CARDIOVASCULAR ADAPTATIONS

Cardiovascular adaptations, as with other adaptations to resistance training, are affected by training vol-
ume and intensity. Cardiovascular adaptations are due to the training stimulus on the cardiovascular system and thus are different from muscular adaptations to resistance training. In general, the differences are due to the large volume of blood pumped at a relatively low pressure during endurance exercise, and a relatively small volume of blood at a high pressure during resistance training.

Heart Rate and Blood Pressure

Strength-trained athletes have average or lower than average resting heart rates (26). Short-term resistance training studies result in either significant (5–12%) or no significant decrease in resting heart rate (27). Decreased resting heart rate due to physical training is attributed to a combination of decreased sympathetic and increased parasympathetic stimulation to the heart. Short-term training studies of men also demonstrate no change or slightly decreased resting systolic and diastolic blood pressures (26, 27). Decreased resting blood pressure is probably due to decreased body fat, decreased body salt, and alterations in the sympathetic drive to the heart. Rate–pressure product, an estimate of myocardial work and oxygen consumption, has been shown to decrease significantly as a result of resistance training. This indicates decreased myocardial oxygen consumption and is normally viewed as a positive adaptation to training. Despite evidence to the contrary, there is a common misconception that resistance training results in hypertension. Hypertension, when it occurs in resistance-trained athletes, is most likely related to essential hypertension, chronic overtraining, use of steroids, large increases in muscle mass, or increases in total body weight (27).

Stroke Volume

Highly resistance-trained men have normal or above normal absolute resting stroke volumes. However, relative to body surface area or lean body mass, resting stroke volume of highly resistance-trained men is not significantly different from normal. Greater than normal absolute stroke volume is due to a significantly greater left ventricular diastolic diameter, indicating increased ventricular filling and a normal ejection fraction. A long training period and/or a high training volume are probably required to increase absolute resting stroke volume (26).

Peak Oxygen Consumption

Heavy resistance training may induce small increases (5–10%) in peak oxygen consumption ($\dot{V}O_{2peak}$), in contrast to the 15–20% increases in $\dot{V}O_{2peak}$ that occur with traditional endurance training. Again, the volume of work appears to be critical for stimulating an adaptational response in aerobic power. For example, circuit weight training (e.g., 12–15 repetition sets at 40–60% of 1 RM) with short rest periods (15–30 seconds) has been shown to increase $\dot{V}O_{2peak}$ marginally (5–10%). The $\dot{V}O_{2peak}$ of competitive Olympic weight lifters, power lifters, and bodybuilders ranges from 41 to 55 mL/kg/min (22). The mechanism by which resistance training induces small increases in $\dot{V}O_{2peak}$ may be related to a true aerobic training effect. It is possible that certain training programs (e.g., circuit training and Olympic weight training) may reach a minimum threshold for improving $\dot{V}O_{2peak}$. Alternatively, increased cardiac output at peak aerobic workloads may explain the small improvements in $\dot{V}O_{2peak}$. Collectively this information indicates that a resistance training program designed to increase $\dot{V}O_{2peak}$ should consist of high volume with relatively short rest periods between sets and exercises.

Left Ventricular Mass

An increase in left ventricular mass can be associated with an increase in either wall thickness or chamber size. A thickened ventricular wall is an adaptation to intermittent elevated blood pressure during resistance training. Increased left ventricular chamber size or volume is an indication of volume overload on the heart and is a common adaptation observed in endurance athletes. Most studies on highly resistance-trained athletes and short-term training studies show absolute left ventricular mass and left ventricular and intraventricular septal wall thickness to be increased in both bodybuilders and weight lifters (26). However, only bodybuilders have a significantly greater than normal left ventricular end-diastolic dimension (i.e., both systolic or diastolic chamber dimensions). Thus, in bodybuilders, increased left ventricular mass is due to increases in both left ventricular wall thickness and chamber size, whereas in weight lifters, it is predominantly due to a thicker than normal wall. However, these differences are greatly reduced or nonexistent relative to body surface area or lean body mass. Factors related to increased left ventricular wall thickness include caliber of athlete, whether or not sets are carried to concentric failure, and size of muscle mass involved in the exercises.

Lipid Profile

The effect of resistance training on the lipid profile is controversial. Resistance-trained men demonstrate normal, higher than normal, and lower than normal high-density lipoprotein (HDL) cholesterol, low-density lipoprotein (LDL) cholesterol, total cholesterol, and ratio of total cholesterol to HDL cholesterol (22). Data on the lipid profile in strength-trained women are also mixed. The lipid profile of bodybuilders is similar to that of runners, while power lifters have lower HDL cholesterol and higher LDL cholesterol values than runners, when body fat, age, and steroid use (steroid use lowers HDL cholesterol concentrations) are considered. Other factors, such as nutrition and genetics, probably account for much of the variability in serum lipids. However, resistance train-

ing can improve this profile. High-volume programs with short rest periods between sets and exercises are probably most effective for positive effects on lipid profile.

BODY COMPOSITION

Body composition changes occur in short-term resistance training programs (6–24 weeks) (28). In general, strength training decreases body fat and increases body mass and fat-free mass in both men and women using dynamic, constant external resistance, variable resistance, and isokinetic training with programs involving a variety of combinations of exercises, sets, and repetitions. Because of the variation in the numbers of sets, repetitions, and exercises, and relatively small body composition changes, it is impossible to reach definitive conclusions regarding the optimal program for decreasing percent fat and increasing fat-free mass. The largest increases in fat-free mass are slightly greater than 3 kg (6.6 lb) in 10 weeks of training. This is equivalent to a fat-free mass increase of about 0.66 lb per week. Though some coaches desire huge gains in body mass for athletes during the off-season, this may not be possible if the added body mass is to be muscle mass.

▶ SUMMARY

Adaptations in resistance training focus on the development and maintenance of the neuromuscular units required for force production. Training neuromuscular units affects many other physiological systems (e.g., connective tissue, cardiovascular system, and the endocrine system). Training programs cause specific types of adaptation. Activation of specific patterns of motor units in training dictate which tissue and how other physiological systems are affected by exercise training. The time course of the development of the neuromuscular system appears to be predominated in the early phase by neural factors with associated changes in types of contractile protein. In the later phase, increased muscle protein and the contractile unit begin to contribute to the changes in performance capacity. A host of other factors can affect adaptations such as functional capabilities of the individual, age, nutritional status, and behavioral factors (e.g., sleep, health habits). Optimal adaptation appears to be related to the use of specific resistance training programs to meet individual training objectives.

References

1. MacDougal JD. Hypertrophy or hyperplasia. In: Komi P, ed. Strength and Power in Sports: The Encyclopaedia of Sports Medicine. Oxford, UK: Blackwell Scientific, 1992:230–238.
2. Goldspink C. Cellular and molecular aspects of adaptation in skeletal muscle. In: Komi P, ed. Strength and Power in Sports: The Encyclopaedia of Sports Medicine. Oxford, UK: Blackwell Scientific, 1992:211–229.

3. Staron RS, Karapondo DL, Kraemer WJ, et al. Skeletal muscle adaptations during the early phase of heavy-resistance training in men and women. J Appl Physiol 76:1247–1255, 1994.
4. Kraemer WJ, Patton J, Gordon SE, et al. Compatibility of high intensity strength and endurance training on hormonal and skeletal muscle adaptations. J Appl Physiol 78:976–989, 1995.
5. Antonio J, Gonyea WJ. Muscle fiber splitting in stretch-enlarged avian muscle. Med Sci Sports Exerc 26:973–977, 1994.
6. Fry AC, Allemeier CA, Staron RS. Correlation between percentage fiber type area and myosin heavy chain content in human skeletal muscle. Eur J Appl Physiol 68:246–251, 1994.
7. Staron RS. Correlation between myofibrillar ATPase activity and myosin heavy chain composition in single human muscle fibers. Histochem 96:21–24, 1991.
8. Conroy BP, Kraemer WJ, Maresh CM. Bone mineral density in elite junior weight lifters. Med Sci Sports Exerc 25:1103–1109, 1993.
9. Tipton CM, Matthes RD, Maynard JA, et al. The influence of physical activity on ligaments and tendons. Med Sci Sports 7:165–175, 1975.
10. Tesch PA. Short- and long-term histochemical and biochemical adaptations in muscle. In: Komi P, ed. Strength and Power in Sports: The Encyclopaedia of Sports Medicine. Oxford: Blackwell Scientific, 1992:239–248.
11. Komi PV, Karlsson J, Tesch P, et al. Effects of heavy resistance and explosive-type strength training methods and mechanical, functional and metabolic aspects of performance. In: Komi PV, ed. Exercise and Sports Biology: International Series on Sports Sciences. Champaign, IL: Human Kinetics, 1982:99–102.
12. Tesch PA, Komi PV, Häkkinen K. Enzymatic adaptations consequent to long-term strength training. Int J Sports Med 8(Suppl):66–69, 1987.
13. Tesch PA, Thorsson A, Colliander EB. Effects of eccentric and concentric resistance training on skeletal muscle substrates, enzyme activities and capillary supply. Acta Physiol Scand 140:575–580, 1990.
14. Tesch PA, Thorsson A, Kaiser P. Muscle capillary supply and fiber type characteristics in weight and power lifters. J Appl Physiol 56:35–38, 1984.
15. Kraemer WJ, Noble BJ, Clark MJ, et al. Physiological responses to heavy-resistance exercise with very short rest periods. Int J Sports Med 8:247–252, 1987.
16. Häkkinen K. Neuromuscular adaptation during strength training, again, detraining and immobilization. Crit Rev Phys Rehab Med 6:161–198, 1994.
17. Häkkinen K. Neuromuscular and hormonal adaptations during strength and power training: A review. J Sports Med 29:9–26, 1989.
18. Häkkinen K, Parkarinen A, Alen M, et al. Neuromuscular and hormonal adaptations in athletes to strength training in two years. J Appl Physiol 65:2406–2412, 1988.
19. Sale DG. Neural adaptation to strength training. In: Komi P, ed. Strength and Power in Sports: The Encyclopaedia of Sports Medicine. Oxford, UK: Blackwell Scientific, 1992:249–265.
20. Deschenes MR, Maresh CM, Armstrong LE, et al. Endurance and resistance exercise induce muscle fiber type specific responses in androgen binding capacity. J Steroid Biochem Molec Biol 50:175–179, 1994.
21. Deschenes MR, Maresh CM, Crivello JF, et al. The effects of exercise training of different intensities on neuromuscular junction morphology. J Neurocytol 22:603–615, 1993.
22. Kraemer WJ. Endocrine responses to resistance exercise. Med Sci Sports Exerc 20(Suppl):S152–S157, 1988.
23. Kraemer WJ. Endocrine responses and adaptations to strength training. In: Komi PV, ed. The Encyclopaedia of Sports Medicine: Strength and Power. Oxford, UK: Blackwell Scientific, 1992:291–304.
24. Kraemer WJ. Hormonal mechanisms related to the expression of muscular strength and power. In: Komi PV, ed. The Encyclopaedia of Sports Medicine: Strength and Power. Oxford, UK: Blackwell Scientific, 1992:64–76.
25. Deshenes MR, Kraemer WJ, Maresh CM, et al. Exercise-induced hormonal changes and their effects upon skeletal muscle tissue. Sports Med 12:80–93, 1991.
26. Fleck SJ. Cardiovascular adaptations to resistance training. Med Sci Sports Exerc 20:S146–S151, 1988.
27. Fleck SJ. Cardiovascular response to strength training. In: Komi PV, ed. The Encyclopaedia of Sports Medicine: Strength and Power in Sport. Oxford, UK: Blackwell Scientific, 1992:305–315.
28. Kraemer WJ, Fleck SJ. Designing Resistance Training Programs. 2nd ed. Champaign, IL: Human Kinetics, 1987:153–157.

Suggested Reading
Stone MH, Fleck SJ, Triplett NT, et al. Health- and performance-related potential of resistance training. Sports Med 11:210–231, 1991.
Komi PV, ed. Strength and Power in Sport: The Encyclopedia of Sports Medicine. Oxford, UK: Blackwell Scientific, 1992.

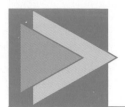

CHAPTER **20**

MECHANISMS OF MUSCULAR FATIGUE

Mark Davis and Robert Fitts

The etiology of muscle fatigue has interested exercise scientists for more than a century, yet definitive fatigue agents have yet to be identified. The problem is complex because muscle fatigue may result from deleterious alterations in the muscle (peripheral fatigue) and/or from changes in the neural input to the muscle (central fatigue). The latter may be mediated by central and/or peripheral changes. Furthermore, the nature and extent of muscle fatigue clearly depend on the type, duration, and intensity of exercise, the fiber type composition of the muscle, individual fitness level, and environmental factors. For example, fatigue experienced in high-intensity, short-duration exercise depends on factors differing from those precipitating fatigue in endurance activity. Similarly, fatigue during tasks involving heavily loaded contractions (e.g., weight lifting) probably differs from that produced during relatively unloaded movement (running and swimming). Finally, the often debilitating fatigue that accompanies viral or bacterial infections, recovery from injury or surgery, chronic fatigue syndrome, depression, sleep deprivation, and jet lag probably has little to do with the muscles themselves and likely involves factors within the central nervous system (CNS).

For the purpose of this review, muscle fatigue is defined as the loss of force or power output in response to voluntary effort leading to reduced performance. This definition illustrates the likelihood that both central and peripheral factors may be involved. Central fatigue is the progressive reduction in voluntary drive to motor neurons during exercise, whereas peripheral fatigue is the loss of force and power that is independent of neural drive. This chapter focuses primarily on muscle fatigue resulting from two general types of activity: short-duration, high-intensity and endurance exercise. However, it should be noted and remembered that muscle fatigue is a common phenomenon that confronts daily activities in ways that may be unrelated to athletic participation. This chapter includes a brief review of current theories and important supportive experimental results. Detailed discussions can be found in earlier reviews (1–5).

SHORT-DURATION, HIGH-INTENSITY EXERCISE

Fatigue during short-duration, high-intensity exercise may result from impairment anywhere along the chain of command from upper brain areas to contractile proteins (Fig. 20.1). Although the preponderance of evidence suggests that a dysfunction within the muscle itself is the most likely cause of fatigue under these circumstances, central deficits in motor drive may also occur.

Peripheral Mechanisms

It is clear that the primary sites of fatigue are within the muscle and do not generally involve peripheral nerves or the neuromuscular junction (NMJ). The observation that fatigued muscles generate the same tension whether stimulated directly or by the motor nerve argues against NMJ fatigue.

There are several possible sites within the excitation–contraction (E-C) coupling components of a muscle cell where alteration during heavy exercise may induce fatigue. With fatigue, the resting membrane potential is frequently altered and the action potential (AP) amplitude and duration are depressed and prolonged, respectively (6, 7). The membrane mechanism of muscle fatigue hypothesizes that K^+ efflux, Na^+ influx, and inhibition of the Na^+-K^+ pump cause cell depolarization, a reduced AP amplitude, and in some cells, complete inactivation (8). These may inhibit subsequent steps in E-C coupling, reduce propagation of the impulse into the T-tubules, and inhibit Ca^{2+} release, thus affecting the strength of contraction (4, 5).

Fatigued muscle frequently shows prolonged twitch duration and reduced peak rate of tension development (9). A prolonged twitch duration reflects a similar prolongation in the time course of the increase in intracellular levels of Ca^{2+} (Ca^{2+} transient), which suggests a reduced rate of release and/or re-uptake of Ca^{2+} by the sarcoplasmic reticulum (SR). Such changes may take place for any number of reasons. Several investigators have demonstrated that the amplitude of the Ca^{2+} transient decreases as fatigue develops (10, 11). Also, fatigue may result from a direct effect on the contractile proteins.

Central Fatigue

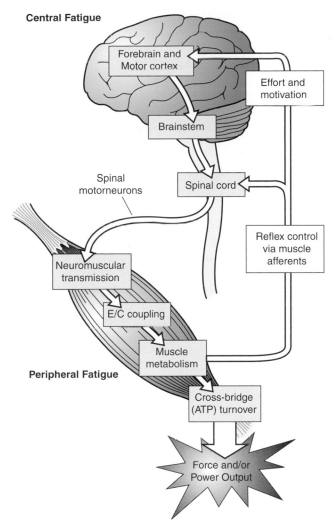

Figure 20.1. The chain of command for muscular contraction. Impairment along this pathway may be associated with fatigue.

High-intensity exercise involves an energy demand that exceeds maximal aerobic power and thus requires a high level of anaerobic metabolism. Consequently, the levels of high-energy phosphates, adenosine triphosphate (ATP), and creatine phosphate (CP) decrease, and levels of inorganic phosphate (Pi), ADP, lactate, and the H^+ ion increase as fatigue develops. All of these changes are possible fatigue-inducing agents, and each has been studied extensively (4, 5, 12).

Adequate tissue ATP levels must be maintained to avoid fatigue because this substrate supplies the immediate source of energy for force generation. ATP is required for the sodium–potassium pump to function. Additionally, ATP stabilizes the SR Ca^{2+} release channel and is a substrate of the SR ATPase, thus is required in the process of Ca^{2+} release and reuptake by the SR. A disturbance in any of these processes can lead to muscle fatigue; however, a cause and effect relationship between low cell ATP and muscle fatigue has not been demonstrated (13, 14).

CP levels decrease with contractile activity, and some suggest that low muscle CP levels may induce fatigue (15). The declines in CP concentration and tension during contractile activity, however, follow different time courses, making a causal relationship unlikely (13). The possibility exists that a critically low CP level may disrupt the ATP-CP shuttle system and slow the rate of adenosine diphosphate (ADP) rephosphorylation to ATP, which may lead to a critically low ATP at various subcellular sites, including the following:

The sarcolemma Na^+-K^+ pump
The SR Ca^{2+} release channel
The SR pump
The cross-bridges

However, this is not likely for these reasons:

1. Single cell analysis shows that the lowest postfatigue cell ATP concentrations are 100-fold higher than required for full cross-bridge activation (16).
2. Various levels of fatigue are generally associated with equal ATP and CP values.
3. The highest ATP use rate (and thus ATP synthesis) is observed in the exercise model producing the lowest force (17).
4. Cell ATP concentration rarely drops below 60–70% of the pre-exercise level even in cases of extensive fatigue (4).

Therefore, the evidence suggests that fatigue produced by other factors reduces the ATP use rate before ATP becomes limiting.

ADP, Pi, and H^+ ions increase during intense contractile activity and may cause fatigue by direct inhibition of hydrolysis of ATP (18–20). The hydrogen ion is a particularly interesting potential fatigue agent because it could produce fatigue at numerous sites. In addition to a direct inhibition of the cross-bridge actomyosin ATPase and ATP hydrolysis, a buildup in the intracellular H^+ (decreased intracellular pH [pHi]) may induce fatigue by any of the following:

1. Inhibiting phosphofructokinase and thus the glycolytic rate
2. Competitive inhibition of Ca^{2+} binding to troponin C, reducing cross-bridge activation
3. Inhibiting the SR ATPase reducing Ca^{2+} reuptake and subsequently Ca^{2+} release (21)

A major source of H^+ production during intense muscular activity is anaerobic production of lactic acid. Although lactic acid has long been implicated as a source of fatigue, the general consensus is that fatigue results from elevated H^+ (22).

Early work gave credence to the concept that elevated H^+ concentration inhibits glycolysis (22, 23). However, it was not until recently that a definitive relationship was found in both skeletal and cardiac muscle (24, 25). Decreasing pH (7.4 to 6.2) not only reduces maximal tension but also increases the threshold of free Ca^{2+} required for contraction (24, 25). Fast-twitch fibers are more sensitive to the acidotic depression of maximal tension than slow muscle fibers (25).

This is supported by the fact that elevated H^+ concentration, which inhibits the ATPase, can decrease the maximum speed of shortening (V_{max}) as well as Po during recovery (26, 27). Force recovers in two phases—a short, rapid phase (about 30 seconds) followed by a slower relatively prolonged phase of recovery (about 50 minutes) (14, 26). The rapid phase of force recovery is probably explained by reversal of a non-H^+-mediated alteration in E-C coupling. The second slower phase of recovery probably results in part from the removal of the excess intracellular H^+.

Changes in pH may also affect Ca^{2+} regulation by disturbing SR Ca^{2+} release and/or reuptake (27, 28). Changes in free H^+ may also effect the Ca^{2+} binding properties, which by itself would alter the Ca^{2+} transient and force output.

It has been suggested that an increased $H_2PO_4^-$ concentration can induce fatigue by inhibiting the cross-bridge transition from the low to the high force state (20, 29). The primary support for this hypothesis comes from the observation that high inorganic phosphate reduces peak force during the development of and recovery from fatigue as well as a close inverse relationship between inorganic phosphate and force in this state (16, 20).

Central Nervous System Mechanisms

The possible role of the central nervous system (CNS) in fatigue is usually addressed in studies involving the twitch interpolation technique (30). In these experiments, the maximum muscular force that a subject can elicit voluntarily is compared to that elicited by supramaximal electrical stimulation of the nerve or muscle itself. Many of these studies demonstrate that superimposing a supramaximal electrical stimulus does not usually increase maximal voluntary contractions of isolated muscle during fatiguing exercise in well-practiced and highly motivated subjects (2). These data are often used to conclude that reduced CNS drive is not a factor in muscular fatigue. However, many of these studies may have lacked the sensitivity to detect small reductions in central drive (30). Also in several examples this clearly was not the case (31–33). The preponderance of evidence suggests that sensory feedback can inhibit motor unit discharge rates at the level of the motor neuron in the spinal cord (34). This is known as the sensory feedback hypothesis. However, an important contribution from reduced central drive from upper brain regions cannot be excluded.

The possibility that specific brain mechanisms can reduce the magnitude of descending motor drive has received the least attention as a possible mediator of muscular fatigue even though willingness to maintain central motor drive (e.g., willingness to maintain a maximal effort) probably contributes to fatigue in most people during activities of daily life. It has been postulated that because failure to produce the necessary force during fatigue is usually preceded by increased perceived effort, the CNS processes are at least as likely to contribute to fatigue as are those that lie within the muscle (3).

Most evidence of central fatigue comes from studies often dismissed because of inadequate practice of the task or because the effect may represent alterations in "psychological factors" like attention, motivation, and perceptions of effort and pain. For example, it has been shown that force generation and electromyogram (EMG) activity during repeated maximal voluntary contractions may be enhanced by encouragement (35). Fatigue may also be more pronounced in subjects who are concentrating on performance rather than being distracted (36). The motivation issue has also been addressed in a series of studies in which rats were motivated to run on a treadmill by electrical stimulation of a reward system in the brain (37–39). Run time to fatigue is significantly longer in well-acclimated but untrained rats during pleasurable stimulation of brain versus electric shocks (38). The specific mechanisms of this effect have not been elucidated, but they are not likely to be due to cardiovascular or metabolic alterations.

Decreased motivation in conjunction with increased perceived exertion may also explain chronic debilitating fatigue affecting individuals with effort syndromes, such as chronic fatigue syndrome (CFS) (40–42). It has been demonstrated that isolated muscle function is normal in CFS patients but that the level of perceived exertion is much higher than expected (41). CFS patients appear to have normal muscle metabolism, muscle membrane function, and E-C coupling but fully activate skeletal muscle prior to exercise, which increases abnormally after 25 minutes of submaximal isometric exercise (40). It is likely, therefore, that the primary defect in CFS patients is an abnormality in the perception of effort translating into inability or unwillingness to reach and/or maintain the level of effort (central drive) necessary to achieve maximal performance during heavy work involving the whole body or large muscle groups. Therefore, it appears that there is a significant central component to muscle fatigue in CFS, although it is too early to determine the level of the defect within the CNS.

Only recently has direct evidence of reduced motor drive within the brain during fatiguing contractions become evident. The most convincing evidence comes from studies in humans using a new technique called transcranial magnetic stimulation (TMS) (43). Recent reports provide good evidence of inhibition of central motor drive following fatiguing exercise (44–47). The electrical stimulus reaching the muscle following magnetic stimulation of the motor cortex (motor-evoked potential) is suppressed following fatiguing exercise. Recently, a prolonged silent period following TMS has been demonstrated (46). These changes are not influenced by muscle afferent feedback and can result from altered voluntary drive to the motor cortex as well as intrinsic cortical processes (45, 46). The genesis of central fatigue may involve inadequate neural drive by the motor cortex at the highest levels of the brain.

ENDURANCE EXERCISE

Numerous factors have been linked to fatigue resulting from prolonged endurance activity, including depletion of muscle and liver glycogen, decreases in blood glucose, dehydration, and increases in body temperature. Undoubtedly each of these factors contributes to fatigue to a varying degree, the relative importance depending on environmental conditions and the nature of the activity. Mechanisms involving various neurotransmitters and neuromodulators have also recently been proposed to explain possible CNS involvement in fatigue during prolonged exercise. This section reviews some of these factors. In particular, carbohydrate depletion, alterations in SR function, and increased brain serotonin are discussed.

Glycogen Depletion

It has long been suggested that the rate of carbohydrate use depends on the intensity of work. This belief was based on the observation that the respiratory exchange ratio (RER) increases from rest to exercise. The early theories have been confirmed by direct measurements of glycogen use at different work intensities (12, 48). The rate of body carbohydrate usage depends not only on intensity but also on the state of fitness. At a fixed workload, trained individuals have a lower RER, deplete glycogen more slowly, and can work longer than untrained individuals (48). High-carbohydrate diets and ingestion of carbohydrate drinks during exercise can delay fatigue by increasing the availability and oxidation of carbohydrates (49). These observations support the hypothesis that depletion of carbohydrate stores causes muscular fatigue during endurance activity. However, the exact mechanism is not known. Low muscle glycogen concentration may reduce nicotinic acid dehydrogenase (NADH) production and electron transport, drain intermediates of the Krebs cycle, and/or reduce fat oxidation, the effects of which would be to inhibit ATP production and cause fatigue (5, 50).

It is also possible that central fatigue occurs in conjunction with carbohydrate depletion during prolonged exercise. Carbohydrate ingestion throughout exercise may attenuate the onset of negative CNS changes involving serotonin (discussed in more detail later in this chapter) (51). However, the effects of carbohydrate feedings on central fatigue mechanisms and the well-established beneficial effects on the contracting muscle are difficult to distinguish (49). It seems apparent that future efforts should focus on the mechanisms by which glycogen depletion causes fatigue.

Other Factors

Glycogen depletion is probably not an exclusive fatigue factor during endurance exercise. Other potential candidates include disruption of important intracellular organelles, such as the mitochondria, the SR, or the myofilaments (5). The role of mitochondrial damage in fatigue is controversial (5, 52).

The contractile proteins and in particular myofibril ATPase activity appear relatively resistant to change with endurance exercise (5, 9). Ca^{2+} uptake by the SR vesicles, however, is depressed in the slow- and fast-twitch red region of the vastus lateralis, which suggests uncoupling of the transport or a leaky membrane allowing Ca^{2+} flux back into the intracellular fluid. In addition to these functional changes, it has been demonstrated that exhaustive endurance exercise structurally damages the SR (5, 28). The exact nature of this change and its effect on muscle function has not been elucidated.

In one study, a prolonged swim produced a significant decrease in glycogen concentration in slow type I, fast type IIA, and fast type IIB fibers of muscles, but the type IIB fibers exhibited no fatigue and no change in any of the contractile or biochemical properties measured (9). The apparent explanation is that the type IIB (fast white glycolytic) fiber is recruited less frequently during endurance activity, but glycogen use is similar to other fiber types despite fewer total contractions. It is apparent that muscle fatigue during endurance activity is somehow related to the degree of muscle use and is not entirely dependent on glycogen depletion.

In some cases, fatigue is characterized by a period of prolonged recovery during which force may be depressed for days. This type of fatigue is frequently referred to as low-frequency fatigue (LFF) (53). Recent evidence suggests that it is caused by disruption of the E-C coupling process, perhaps because of excessive production of reactive oxygen species and/or prolonged exposure to high levels of intracellular Ca^{2+} (54, 55).

The long recovery period following LFF may be related to the time required for refolding of damaged proteins or the replacement of degraded proteins (54). Protein degradation could produce swelling and thus lead to muscle soreness. This possibility is supported by results of structural studies in which muscle soreness is related to changes in various intracellular organelles. The time course of recovery from muscle soreness (days) exceeds that observed for most forms of fatigue but correlates well with recovery from LFF and reflects the time required to synthesize new muscle proteins.

Of the many proposed causes of central fatigue during prolonged exercise, the role of brain serotonin has generated the most interest. Interesting new hypotheses implicate various neurotransmitters such as norepinephrine, dopamine, acetylcholine, and serotonin (2). However, a review of the mechanisms involved in the control of brain serotonin synthesis and turnover at rest and during exercise (Fig. 20.2), along with its well-known influence on depression, sleepiness, mood, and pain make it a particularly attractive candidate (2).

Evidence to support a role for brain serotonin in central fatigue during prolonged exercise is beginning to emerge. Concentrations of serotonin and 5-HIAA (a major metabolite) increase in several brain regions during prolonged exercise and peak at fatigue (56, 57). The administration of serotonin agonist and antagonist drugs decreases and increases, respectively, run times to fatigue in the absence of any apparent peripheral markers of muscle fatigue (56, 58, 59).

► **SUMMARY**

The studies and findings described in this chapter illustrate the complex nature of fatigue. Both central nervous system and muscle mechanisms are likely to contribute to fatigue. After short-duration, high-intensity exercise, recovery in force production usually occurs in two components that are probably caused by separate

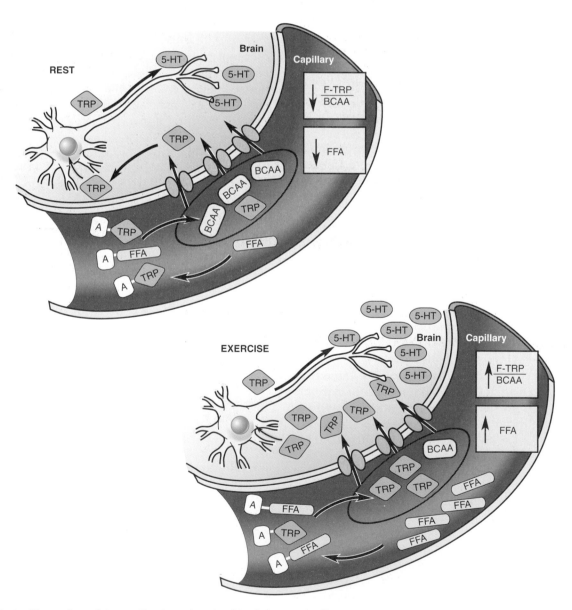

Figure 20.2. An illustration of the mechanisms involved in the control of brain serotonin synthesis and turnover at rest and during exercise. The well-known influence of these mechanisms on depression, sleepiness, mood, and pain make this a likely candidate for a center of fatigue.

mechanisms: (*a*) A rapidly reversible non–H$^+$-mediated perturbation, perhaps related to changes in E-C coupling, and (*b*) A slower change that is probably mediated by H$^+$ and Pi. The possible mechanisms of the deleterious effects of H$^+$ and Pi are described. Reduction in central motor drive occurring at the highest levels of the brain can also accompany fatigue, but this aspect is much less well studied and the mechanisms have not been elucidated.

In prolonged endurance exercise, the depletion of skeletal muscle carbohydrate stores frequently occurs, and it appears that muscle glycogen depletion is an important factor in fatigue. Additionally, minimal levels of muscle glycogen metabolism may be important in maintaining essential Krebs cycle intermediates. Undoubtedly, other factors are involved, however, because muscle glycogen depletion can exist without fatigue and vice versa. Disruption of muscle protein, particularly the E-C coupling complex, has been shown to be associated with LFF. This process may be mediated by elevated levels of reactive oxygen species (free radicals) and/or intracellular Ca^{2+}. Increased brain serotonin metabolism has also been implicated in central fatigue under these circumstances.

Practical Application

It is clear that exercise training reduces fatigue. The principles of specificity suggest that fatigue suppression applies to the specific intensities, durations, and modes of exercise regularly used in the training program, although some crossover effects may be possible. Training may somehow affect the basis of these components of fatigue. While the exact mechanisms may not be entirely clear, regular, specific exercise training reduces the onset and the effects of fatigue on the activities. In endurance exercise a number of factors are involved, including glycogen depletion which can be delayed by ingesting carbohydrates both before and during exercise. In this case, training may contribute by enhancing intracellular metabolic machinery, thus increasing cellular ability to use nutrients and produce energy. While other mechanisms also contribute to fatigue in endurance activity, the practical application of those mechanisms is at this point unclear.

References
1. Bigland-Ritchie B, Rice CL, Garland SJ, et al. Task-dependent factors in fatigue of human voluntary contractions. In: Gandevia SC, Enoka RM, McComas AJ, et al, eds. Fatigue: Neural and Muscular Mechanisms. New York: Plenum, 1995:361–380.
2. Davis JM, Bailey SP. Possible mechanisms of central nervous system fatigue during exercise. Med Sci Sports Exerc 29:45–57, 1997.
3. Enoka RM, Stuart DG. Neurobiology of muscle fatigue. J Appl Physiol 72:1631–1648, 1992.
4. Fitts RH. Cellular mechanisms of muscle fatigue. Physiol Rev 74:49, 1994.
5. Fitts RH. Cellular, molecular, and metabolic basis of muscle fatigue. In: Rowell LB, Shephard JT. eds. Handbook of Physiology: Section 12: Regulation and Integration of Multiple Systems. New York: Oxford University, 1996.
6. Lannergren J, Westerblad H. Force and membrane potential during and after fatiguing, continuous high-frequency stimulation of single Xenopus muscle fibers. Acta Physiol Scand 128:359, 1986.
7. Metzger JM, Fitts RH. Fatigue from high and low frequency muscle stimulation: Role of sarcolemma action potentials. Exp Neurol 93:320, 1986.
8. Sjogaard G. Role of exercise-induced potassium fluxes underlying muscle fatigue: A brief review. Can J Physiol Pharmacol 69:238, 1990.
9. Fitts RH, Courtright JB, Kim DM, et al. Muscle fatigue with prolonged exercise: Contractile and biochemical alterations. Am J Physiol 242:C65, 1982.
10. Allen DG, Lee JA, Westerblad H. Intracellular calcium and tension in isolated single muscle fibers from Xenopus. J Physiol 415:433, 1989.
11. Westerblad H, Allen DG. Changes of myoplasmic calcium concentration during fatigue in single mouse muscle fibers. J Gen Physiol 98:615, 1991.
12. Bergstrom J. Muscle electrolytes in man. Scand J Clin Lab Invest 14(Suppl 68), 1962.
13. Fitts RH, Holloszy JO. Lactate and contractile force in frog muscle during development of fatigue and recovery. Am J Physiol 231:430, 1976.
14. Fitts RH, Holloszy JO. Effects of fatigue and recovery on contractile properties of frog muscle. J Appl Physiol 45:899, 1978.
15. Sahlin K, Edstrom L, Sjoholm H. Force, relaxation and energy metabolism of rat soleus muscle during anaerobic contraction. Acta Physiol Scand 129:1, 1987.
16. Thompson LV, Fitts RH. Muscle fatigue in the frog semitendinosus: Role of high energy phosphates and P(I). Am J Physiol 263:C803, 1992.
17. Berstrom M, Hultman E. Energy cost and fatigue during intermittent electrical stimulation of human skeletal muscle. J Appl Physiol 65:1500, 1988.
18. Cooke R, Franko K, Luciana GB, et al. The inhibition of rabbit skeletal muscle contraction by hydrogen ions and phosphate. J Physiol 395:77, 1988.
19. Godt RE, Nosek TM. Changes of intracellular milieu with fatigue or hypoxia depress contraction of skinned rabbit skeletal and cardiac muscle. J Physiol 412:155, 1989.
20. Nosek TM, Fender KY, Godt RE. It is deprotonated inorganic phosphate that depresses force in skinned skeletal muscle fibers. Science 236:191, 1987.
21. Nakamura Y, Schwartz A. The influence of hydrogen ion concentration on calcium binding and release by skeletal muscle sarcoplasmic reticulum. J Gen Physiol 59:22, 1972.
22. Hill AV. The absolute value of the isometric heat coefficient T1/H in a muscle twitch, and the effect of stimulation and fatigue. Proc R Soc Lond B Biol Sci 103:163, 1928.
23. Sahlin K, Harris RC, Nylind B, et al. Lactate content and pH in muscle samples obtained after dynamic exercise. Plugers Arch 367:143, 1976.
24. Fabiato A, Fabiato F. Effects of pH on the myofilaments and the sarcoplasmic reticulum of skinned cells from cardiac and skeletal muscles. J Physiol 276:233, 1978.

25. Metzger JM, Moss RL. Greater hydrogen ion-induced depression of tension and velocity in skinned single fibres of rat fast rather than slow muscles. J Physiol 393:727, 1987.
26. Metzger JM, Fitts RH. Role of intracellular pH in muscle fatigue. J Appl Physiol 62:1392, 1987.
27. Thompson LV, Balog EM, Fitts RH. Muscle fatigue in frog semitendinosus: role of intracellular pH. Am J Physiol 263:C1507, 1992.
28. Byrd SK, McCutcheon LJ, Hodgson DR, et al. Altered sarcoplasmic reticulum function after high-intensity exercise. J Appl Physiol 67:2072, 1989.
29. Wilkie DR. Muscular fatigue: Effects of hydrogen ions and inorganic phosphate. Fed Proc 45:2921, 1986.
30. Allen GM, Gandevia SC, McKenzie DK. Reliability of measurements of muscle strength and voluntary activation using twitch interpolation. Muscle Nerve 18:593–600, 1995.
31. Bigland-Ritchie B, Furbush B, Woods II. Fatigue of intermittent submaximal voluntary contractions: Central and peripheral factors. J Appl Physiol 61:421–429, 1986.
32. Garner SH, Sutton JR, Burse RL, et al. Operation Everest II: Neuromuscular performance under conditions of extreme simulated altitude. J Appl Physiol 68:1167–1172, 1990.
33. Westing SH, Cresswell AG, Thorstensson A. Muscle activation during maximal voluntary eccentric and concentric knee extension. Eur J Appl Physiol 62:104–108, 1991.
34. Bigland-Ritchie B. EMG/Force relations and fatigue of human voluntary contractions. Exer Sports Sci Rev 9:75–117, 1981.
35. Rube N, Secher NH. Paradoxical influence of encouragement on muscle fatigue. Eur J Appl Physiol 46:1–7, 1981.
36. Asmussen E. Muscle fatigue. Med Sci Sports Exerc 11:313–321, 1979.
37. Burgess JM, Davis JM, Wilson SP, et al. Effects of intracranial self-stimulation on selected physiological parameters in rats. Am J Physiol 264:R149–R155, 1993.
38. Burgess ML, Davis JM, Borg TK, et al. Intracranial self-stimulation motivates treadmill running in rats. J Appl Physiol 71:1593–1597, 1991.
39. Burgess ML, Davis JM, Borg TK, et al. Exercise training alters cardiovascular and hormonal responses to intracranial self-stimulation. J Appl Physiol 75:863–869, 1993.
40. Kent-Braun SK, Weiner MW, Massie B, et al. Central basis of muscle fatigue in chronic fatigue syndrome. Neurology 43:125–131, 1993.
41. Lloyd AR, Gandevia SC, Hales JP. Muscle performance, voluntary activation, twitch properties and perceived effort in normal subjects and patients with the chronic fatigue syndrome. Brain 114:85–98, 1991.
42. Lloyd AR, Hales JP, Gandevia SC. Muscle strength, endurance and recovery in the post-infection fatigue syndrome. J Neurol Neurosurg Psych 51:1316–1322, 1988.
43. Gandevia SC. Insights into motor performance and muscle fatigue based on transcranial stimulation of the human motor cortex. Clin Exp Pharm Physiol 23:957–960, 1996.
44. Brasil-Neto JP, Pascual-Leone A, Valls-Sole J, et al. Post-exercise depression of motor evoked potentials: A measure of central nervous system fatigue. Exp Brain Res 93:181–184, 1993.
45. Gandevia S, Gabrielle MA, Butler JE, et al. Supraspinal factors in human muscle fatigue: Evidence for suboptimal output from the motor cortex. J Appl Physiol 490:520–536, 1996.
46. Taylor JL, Butler JE, Allen GM, et al. Changes in motor cortical excitability during human muscle fatigue. J Appl Physiol 490:519–528, 1996.
47. Zanette G, Bonato C, Polo A, et al. Long-lasting depression of motor-evoked potentials to transcranial magnetic stimulation following exercise. Exp Brain Res 107:80–86, 1995.
48. Saltin B, Karlsson J. Muscle glycogen utilization during work of different intensities. In: Pernow P, Saltin B, eds. Muscle Metabolism During Exercise. New York: Plenum, 1971.
49. Wagenmakers AJ, Bechers EJ, Brouns F, et al. Carbohydrate supplementation, glycogen depletion, and amino acid metabolism during exercise. Am J Physiol 260:E883–890, 1991.
50. Davis JM, Bailey SP, Woods JA, et al. Effects of carbohydrate feedings on plasma free-tryptophan and branched-chain amino acids during prolonged cycling. Eur J Appl Physiol 65:513–519, 1992.
51. Coggan AR, Coyle EF. Carbohydrate ingestion during prolonged exercise: Effects on metabolism and performance. In: Exercise and Sports Sciences Reviews. Baltimore: Williams & Wilkins, 1991:1–40.
52. Nimmo MA, Snow DH. Time course of ultrastructural changes in skeletal muscle after two types of exercise. J Appl Physiol 52:910, 1982.
53. Edwards RH, Hill DK, Jones DA, et al. Fatigue of long duration in human skeletal muscle after exercise. J Physiol 272:769, 1977.
54. Brotto MA, Nosek TM. Hydrogen peroxide disrupts calcium release from the sarcoplasmic reticulum of rat skeletal muscle fibers. J Appl Physiol 81:731, 1996.
55. Chin ER, Allen DG. The role of elevations in intracellular [calcium] in the development of low frequency fatigue in mouse single muscle fibers. J Physiol 491:813, 1996.
56. Bailey SP, Davis JM, Ahlborn EN. Neuroendocrine and substrate responses to altered brain 5-HT activity during prolonged exercise to fatigue. J Appl Physiol 74:3006–3012, 1993.
57. Meeusen R, Thorre K, Chaouloff F, et al. Effects of tryptophan and/or acute running on extracellular 5-HT and 5-HIAA levels in the hippocampus of food-deprived rats. Brain Res 740:245–252, 1996.
58. Bailey SP, Davis JM, Ahlborn EN. Brain serotonergic activity affects endurance performance in the rat. Intl J Sports Med 6:330–333, 1993.
59. Wilson WM, Maughan RJ. Evidence for a possible role of 5-hydroxytryptamine in the genesis of fatigue in man: Administration of paroxetine, a 5-HT re-uptake inhibitor, reduces the capacity to perform prolonged exercise. Exp Physiol 77:921–924, 1992.

1.2.7

2.2.2, 2.2.7, 2.2.16,
2.2.20

3.2.0

4.2.0.1

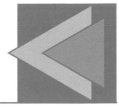

CHAPTER **21**

DETRAINING AND RETENTION OF ADAPTATIONS INDUCED BY ENDURANCE TRAINING

Edward F. Coyle

REVERSIBILITY OF ADAPTATIONS INDUCED BY TRAINING

The effects of regular exercise training show the remarkable ability of the human body to respond to the stimuli of regular exercise. After several weeks of training, the specific systems of the body (e.g., cardiovascular, muscular, nervous) that are stressed display physiological adaptations that improve tolerance for the type of exercise encountered in training. The level of adaptation and the magnitude of improvement in exercise tolerance are proportional to the potency of the physical training stimuli.

Although physical training promotes a variety of physiological adaptations, long periods of inactivity (i.e., detraining) are associated with a reversal of many adaptations. The reversibility concept holds that when physical training is stopped or reduced, the bodily systems readjust in accordance with the diminished physiological stimuli. The focus of this chapter is on the time course of loss of the adaptations to endurance training and the possibility that certain adaptations persist to some extent when training is stopped. Because endurance exercise training generally improves cardiovascular function and promotes metabolic adaptations within the exercising skeletal musculature, the reversibility of these specific adaptations is considered.

CARDIOVASCULAR DETRAINING

Maximal Oxygen Uptake

Endurance training induces increases in maximal oxygen uptake ($\dot{V}O_{2max}$), cardiac output, and stroke volume (1, 2). When sedentary people participate in a 6–10 week low-intensity training program, $\dot{V}O_{2max}$ increases by 6–10%, and it appears that $\dot{V}O_{2max}$ sometimes remains at this level for 2–3 weeks after cessation of low-intensity training (3, 4). However, more prolonged detraining (8–10 weeks) has been reported to result in a complete return of $\dot{V}O_{2max}$ to pretraining levels (5). Moderate endurance training increases $\dot{V}O_{2max}$ by 10–20%, yet

$\dot{V}O_{2max}$ may decline to pretraining levels when training is stopped (6–9). $\dot{V}O_{2max}$ values decline rapidly during the first month of inactivity, and a slower decline to untrained levels occurs during the second and third months of detraining (6–9). Therefore, the available evidence suggests that increases in $\dot{V}O_{2max}$ produced by endurance training involving exercise of low to moderate intensities and durations are totally reversed after several months of detraining and adoption of a totally sedentary lifestyle.

Whether years of intensive endurance training result in a more persistent maintenance of $\dot{V}O_{2max}$ after subsequent inactivity than do shorter periods of less intensive training has also been the subject of study. Present knowledge is limited to studies involving already-trained endurance athletes who cease training so that reversibility can be studied (10). Figure 21.1 illustrates the time course of the decline in $\dot{V}O_{2max}$ from one study and related variables (maximal stroke volume, heart rate, and arteriovenous oxygen difference [a-vDO$_2$]) when subjects become sedentary after training intensively for approximately 10 years.

The $\dot{V}O_{2max}$ value in trained subjects was relatively high (62 mL/minute^{-1} at 0 days without training), and it declined a total of 16% after 84 days of detraining. A rapid decline of 7% occurred in the first 12–21 days, with a further decline of 9% during the period from 21–84 days (10). The rapid early decline in $\dot{V}O_{2max}$ was associated with a reduction in maximal stroke volume and cardiac output measured during exercise in the upright position, despite an increase in heart rate (Fig. 21.1). Most of the decline in stroke volume occurred during the first 12 days of inactivity. Adaptive increases in maximal heart rate somewhat compensated for this loss of stroke volume. The decline in $\dot{V}O_{2max}$ during the 21–84-day period was associated with a decline in maximal difference a-vDO$_2$.

The 84 day period of detraining resulted in a stabilization of $\dot{V}O_{2max}$ and maximal stroke volume. Thus, the subjects appeared to have detrained for a sufficient length of time to display a complete readjustment of cardiovas-

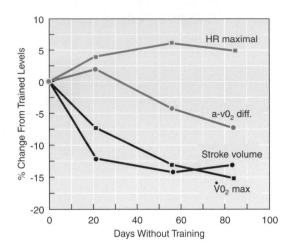

Figure 21.1. Effects of detraining on percent changes in stroke volume during exercise, maximal oxygen uptake $\dot{V}O_{2max}$), maximal heart rate (HR), and maximal arteriovenous oxygen difference (a-$\dot{V}O_{2diffmax}$). (Adapted with permission from Coyle EF et al. Time course of loss of adaptations after stopping prolonged intensive endurance training. J Appl Physiol, 57:1857–1864, 1984.)

Table 21.1. Responses When Highly Trained and After 3 Months of Detraining

		% OF SEDENTARY CONTROL		
		SEDENTARY CONTROL	TRAINED	DETRAINED 3 MONTHS
$\dot{V}O_{2max}$ (mL/kg/min) 43.3		143[a]	117[ab]	
Stroke Volume (mL)		128.0	120[a]	101[a]
a-$\dot{V}O_{2diffmax}$ (mL/100 mL)		12.6	122	116[ab]
Citrate synthase activity (mol/kg/hr)				
Whole muscle of both fiber types		4.1	243[a]	149[ab]
Type I fibers		4.8	140[a]	108[ab]
Type II fibers		2.6	246[a]	180[ab]
Capillary density (cap/mm^2)		318.0	146[a]	150[a]

Responses when trained and detrained are expressed as a percentage of sedentary control values observed in untrained subjects.
[a] Higher (p < 0.05) than sedentary control.
[b] Detrained lower than trained; p < 0.05.
Modified with permission from Coyle EF et al. Time course of loss adaptations after stopping prolonged intense endurance training. J Appl Physiol 57:1857–1864, 1984; Coyle EF, Martin WH, Bloomfield SA, et al. Effects of detraining on responses to submaximal exercise. J Appl Physiol 59:853–859, 1985; Costill DL et al. Metabolic characteristics of skeletal muscle during detraining from competitive swimming. Med Sci Sports Exerc 17:339–343, 1985.

cular response in accordance with a sedentary lifestyle. Maximal stroke volume during upright exercise in detrained subjects was virtually the same as that observed in people who had never engaged in endurance training (Table 21.1). The idea that this finding does not necessarily imply a loss of heart function is subsequently discussed. Although maximal cardiac output and stroke volume declined to untrained levels, $\dot{V}O_{2max}$ in the detrained subjects remained 17% above (i.e., 117% of) that of untrained individuals, primarily because of a persistent elevation of maximal a-vDO$_2$. The maintenance of $\dot{V}O_{2max}$ in detrained subjects was due to an augmented ability of exercising musculature to extract oxygen, which appeared to be related to the observation that these subjects displayed no loss of capillary density derived from training and only a partial loss of muscle mitochondria derived from training (Table 21.1).

Stroke Volume and Heart Size

Prolonged and intensive endurance training promotes increased heart mass, whereas detraining results in decreased heart mass (1, 11, 12). However, it is not clear whether training-induced increases in ventricular volume and myocardial wall thickness regress totally with inactivity. Athletes who become sedentary have larger hearts and higher $\dot{V}O_{2max}$ than those of people who have never trained (13).

One of the most striking effects of detraining in endurance-trained individuals is the rapid decline in stroke volume. To gain information regarding the cause of this large and rapid decline, Martin et al. (14) measured stroke volume during exercise in trained subjects in both the up-

right and supine positions and again after 21 and 56 days of inactivity (Fig. 21.2). Simultaneous measurements of the diameter of the left ventricle were obtained echocardiographically. The large decline in stroke volume during upright cycling was associated with parallel reductions in the diameter of the left ventricle at end-diastole (LVEDD). When the subjects exercised in the supine position, which usually augments ventricular filling because of increased venous return from elevated lower extremities, reduction in LVEDD was minimal. As a result, stroke volume during exercise in the supine position was maintained within a few percent of trained levels during the 56-day detraining period (Fig. 21.2). These observations indicate that cardiac filling is an important factor establishing stroke volume during exercise and that when it declines, perhaps as a result of reductions in blood volume, stroke volume also declines. Furthermore, it is possible that training-induced increases in stroke volume may be partially due to increased cardiac filling as a result of increased blood volume.

In studies of rats, it seems that endurance training programs promote significant increases in heart mass that are completely reversed after 3–7 weeks of detraining (12, 15). Endurance-trained athletes and professional soccer players also lose heart mass after 3–8 weeks of detraining; the loss is associated with reduced posterior and septal wall thickness of the left ventricle (11, 14, 16, 17). However, it appears that these reductions do not lower stroke

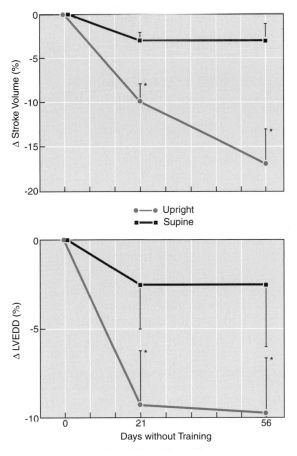

Figure 21.2. Percentage decline in exercise stroke volume (**A**) and LVEDD, measured by echocardiography (**B**) during exercise in upright and supine postures when trained and after 21 and 56 days of inactivity. *, responses in upright position are significantly ($p < 0.05$) lower than in supine position and lower than when trained (i.e., day 0). (Reprinted with permission from Martin WH, Coyle EF, Bloomfield SA, Ehsani AA: Effects of physical deconditioning after intensive training on left ventricular dimensions and stroke volume. J Am Coll Cardiol 7:982–989, 1986.)

volume during submaximal exercise when ventricular filling is high, such as when exercise is performed in the supine position (14).

Not all studies report a decline in left ventricular mass or $\dot{V}O_{2max}$ when endurance-trained subjects stop training. Cullinane et al. (18) found that 10 days of detraining in runners did not alter $\dot{V}O_{2max}$ or echocardiographically determined left ventricular mass. Furthermore, Pavlik et al. (19) reported that 60 days of detraining resulted in no reduction in LVEDD while at rest. Houmard et al. found $\dot{V}O_{2max}$ to decline 4% when a runner stopped training for 14 days; endurance performance declined 9% (20).

Blood Volume

It appears that rapid detraining-induced reduction of stroke volume during exercise in the upright position is

related to decreased blood volume (Fig. 21.3) (21). Intensive exercise training usually results in blood volume increasing by approximately 500 mL through the expansion of plasma volume (22, 23). This adaptation is gained after only a few bouts of exercise and is quickly reversed when training ceases (21–24). The decline in stroke volume and the increase in heart rate during submaximal exercise, which normally accompany several weeks of detraining, can be reversed, returning to near trained levels when the blood volume expands to a level similar to that of trained subjects (Fig. 21.3) (21).

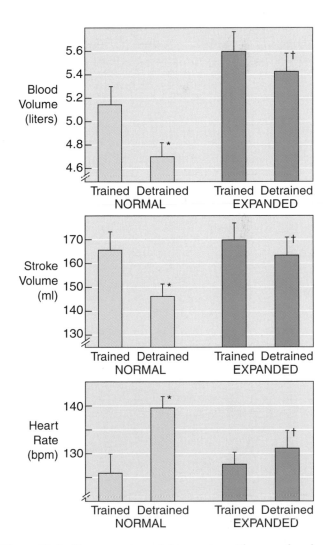

Figure 21.3. Responses to upright exercise with normal and expanded blood volume when trained and detrained. Significantly different from trained normal (*, $p < 0.05$). Detrained with expanded blood volume significantly different from detrained with normal blood volume (†, $p < 0.05$). (Reprinted with permission from Coyle EF, Hemmert MK, Coggan AR. Effects of detraining on cardiovascular responses to exercise: Role of blood volume. J Appl Physiol 60:95–99, 1986.)

Since stroke volume during exercise is maintained near trained levels when blood volume is high, the ability of the heart to fill with blood is not significantly altered by detraining. If ventricular mass does decrease, thinning of ventricular walls, not decreased LVEDD, may be responsible (14). Thus, decreased intrinsic cardiovascular function, at least during submaximal exercise, is apparently minimal after several weeks of inactivity in men who had been training intensively for several years (21). The large reduction in stroke volume during exercise in the upright position is largely a result of reduced blood volume, not deterioration of heart function (21).

HEART RATE DURING MAXIMAL AND SUBMAXIMAL EXERCISE

Maximal heart rate increases markedly with detraining, reflecting an attempt (cardiovascular compensation) to offset the large reductions in blood volume and stroke volume. Coyle et al. (10) observed 4% and 6% increases in maximal heart rate after 3 and 12 weeks of inactivity, respectively (figure 21.1). These results agree with the findings of others (18, 25). Heart rate also increases significantly during exercise at a given submaximal intensity over the course of detraining. For example, 12 days of in-

activity has been found to increase heart rate from 158 to 170 beats per minute, then to 184 beats per minute after 84 days of detraining (26).

DETRAINING AND MUSCLE METABOLISM

Enzymes of Energy Metabolism

Endurance exercise training induces enzymatic adaptations in exercising musculature that slows rates of glycogen use and lactate production and improves endurance during submaximal exercise (27). One of the more important alterations is an increase in the activity of mitochondrial enzymes, which results in increased ability to metabolize fuels in the presence of oxygen. Moderate endurance training (2–4 months' duration) increases mitochondrial enzyme activity by 20–40% from untrained levels (8, 28). When moderate training ceases and the stimuli for adaptation are removed, increases in mitochondrial activity are quickly and totally reversed. Mitochondrial activity returns to pretraining levels within 28–56 days after cessation of training (8, 10, 29–31).

Figure 21.4 illustrates the pattern of change in enzyme activity when individuals who trained intensively for 10 years ceased for 84 days (26, 30). Mitochondrial enzyme activity in trained subjects (i.e., citrate synthase, succinate

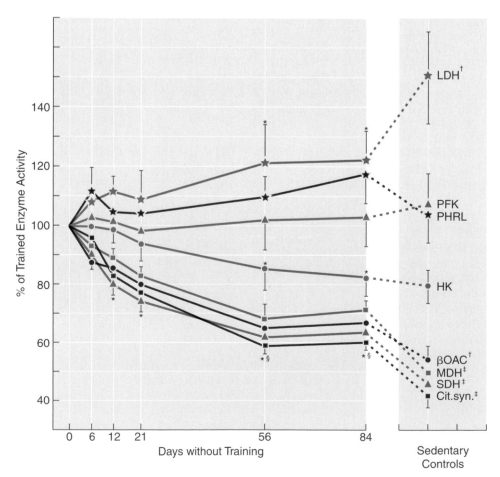

Figure 21.4. Enzyme activity during detraining period and comparison to sedentary control subjects. Values expressed as percentage of trained values. Cit. Syn., citrate synthase; SDH, succinate dehydrogenase; MDH, malate dehydrogenase; βOAC, beta-hydroxyacyl-CoA dehydrogenase; HK, hexokinase; LDH, total lactate dehydrogenase; PHRL, phosphorylase; PFK, phosphofructokinase; $*$, significantly different from trained ($p < 0.05$); §, significantly different from 21 days ($p < 0.01$); ‡, control significantly different from 84 days ($p < 0.05$); †, control significantly different from 84 days ($p < 0.001$). (Reprinted with permission from Coyle EF et al. Effects of detraining on responses to submaximal exercise. J Appl Physiol 59:853–859, 1985.)

dehydrogenase, malate dehydrogenase, and beta-hydrox-yacyl-CoA dehydrogenase), which is initially twofold higher than those in untrained persons (i.e., 243% of sedentary control in Table 21.1), decreases progressively during the first 56 days of detraining and then stabilizes at levels that are 50% higher than sedentary controls. Others have also subsequently reported that mitochondrial activity declines with detraining (29, 32). Figure 21.4 indicates that the half-life of decline is approximately 12 days (i.e., 50% decrease compared to trained in 12 days). Therefore, prolonged and intensive training, in contrast to training programs that last only a few months, appears to result in only a partial loss of mitochondrial enzyme activity; thus there is a persistent elevation of activity above untrained levels (i.e., detrained citrate synthase activity in whole muscle homogenates is 149% of sedentary control values) (Table 21.1). This elevation in whole-muscle citrate synthase activity occurred almost entirely because of a persistent 80% elevation above untrained levels in the mitochondrial enzyme activity in fast-twitch muscle fibers (30). The citrate synthase activity in slow-twitch fibers (type I) declined to levels of sedentary control. Although fast-twitch fiber (type II) activity declined (246–180% of sedentary control values), it stabilized at levels 80% higher than observed in the untrained sedentary control subjects (Table 21.1). The mechanism for this persistent elevation above sedentary levels in mitochondrial activity of fast-twitch fibers from detrained endurance athletes is unclear. One possibility is that these fast-twitch fibers were more readily recruited to contract during the daily activities of a sedentary lifestyle in these detrained persons. Another possibility is that some neuromuscular factors that stimulate mitochondrial synthesis (or reduce degradation) were better maintained. It is also possible that these individuals were atypical and predisposed to higher fast-twitch mitochondrial activity even before endurance training. However, this possibility seems unlikely, because high mitochondrial activity in fast-twitch muscle fibers of untrained people has not been observed (10, 30).

Muscle Capillarization

Endurance training promotes increased capillarization of the exercising musculature, which theoretically both prolongs the transit time of blood flow through the muscle and reduces diffusion distances, improving the availability of oxygen and nutrients to the muscle. It would also allow for better removal of metabolic waste products. Moderate endurance training of several months' duration increases muscle capillarization by 20–30% above pre-training levels (8, 33). However, it appears that 8 weeks of detraining can fully or partially reverse these increases in capillarization (8, 34). More prolonged and intensive training increases muscle capillary density by 40–50% from untrained levels (10, 33). It appears that this high degree of capillarization is maintained at trained levels for up to 3 months of detraining (Table 21.1) (10).

MUSCULAR ADAPTATIONS THAT PERSIST WITH DETRAINING

The detrained responses in the skeletal musculature of highly trained people, who regularly engaged in intensive exercise for several years, apparently differ from those who have trained for only a few months. No loss of increased muscle capillarization for at least 3 months occurs with cessation of prolonged intensive training, although such a loss does occur when moderate training is stopped. Cessation of moderate training results in a complete reversal of training-induced increases in mitochondrial enzyme activity, whereas only a partial decline, and therefore a persistent elevation of mitochondrial activity above untrained levels, occurs with cessation of exercise after prolonged intensive endurance training (10, 27, 30).

It is likely that the relatively high $\dot{V}O_{2max}$ observed in these detrained athletes is partially due to genetics. That is, untrained values are higher than normal, predisposing them to endurance athletics. However, it seems likely that some persistent muscular adaptation contributed to a relatively high a-vDO$_2$ and $\dot{V}O_{2max}$ (Table 21.1). It was also observed that these detrained subjects displayed the ability to exercise at a relatively high percentage of $\dot{V}O_{2max}$, before becoming fatigued or undergoing an increase in blood lactate concentration (26). Their blood lactate threshold occurred at 75% $\dot{V}O_{2max}$, which is considerably higher than observed in untrained people (63% $\dot{V}O_{2max}$) and not significantly lower than the percent $\dot{V}O_{2max}$ at blood lactate threshold when trained (79%). The ability to exercise at a high percentage of $\dot{V}O_{2max}$ in a detrained state reflects maintenance of muscular adaptations (i.e., high capillary density and mitochondria in fast-twitch muscle fibers).

REDUCED TRAINING RATHER THAN DETRAINING

Detraining is the total cessation of exercise training and therefore removal of the stimuli to maintain adaptations. Detraining produces more marked effects than reduced training, which may more effectively maintain cardiovascular and metabolic adaptations. Indeed, it has been demonstrated that $\dot{V}O_{2max}$ and heart size can be maintained at trained levels when training frequency is reduced from 6 to 1 or 2 days a week, provided that the intensity is sufficiently high (85–100% $\dot{V}O_{2max}$) (35, 36).

DETRAINING AND RETRAINING OF MUSCLE MITOCHONDRIA

While it seems logical that detrained subjects, who display only a partial loss of the adaptations to endurance training, should be able to retrain to former levels more rapidly than if they had never trained, that issue has not been directly studied in a controlled setting. Detrained former athletes seem to maintain for approximately 3

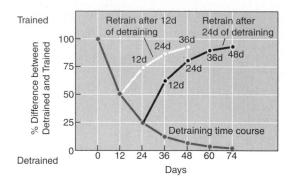

Figure 21.5. Theoretical time course of the decline in mitochondrial enzyme activity and endurance performance ability with detraining and the rate of increase when training is resumed after 12 days or 24 days of detraining.

months these morphological adaptations, such as heart size and muscle capillarization, which take years to develop. Detraining primarily causes reductions in blood volume and mitochondrial enzyme activity, and it appears that blood volume can be restored with several weeks of retraining (22, 23). Therefore, the limiting factor determining the time course of retraining seems likely to be the rate of increase in mitochondrial enzyme activity. The half-life of the decline in mitochondrial enzyme activity is approximately 12 days with detraining (Fig. 21.4). Therefore, if a person detrains for 12 days (i.e., a single half-time), approximately 50% of the improvements (above the detrained level) in mitochondrial enzyme activity will be lost. If after 12 days of detraining the person is able to resume full training, it will require approximately 36 days to achieve about 93% of the previous trained levels of mitochondrial activity (Fig. 21.5). Therefore, it is hypothesized that every 12 days of detraining requires three times the number of days retraining (i.e., 36 days) to approach fully trained levels. The theoretical decline after 24 days of detraining and the pattern of retraining is also displayed in Figure 21.5. The major point of this description is that a much longer period of retraining is required to restore the mitochondrial adaptations lost from a given period of detraining (total cessation of exercise). Since reduced training attenuates the loss, athletes should be encourage to perform some training if possible during the off season.

► SUMMARY

When physical training ceases (detraining), physiological systems readjust in accordance with the diminished physiological stimuli, and many training-induced adaptations are reversed to varying degrees. Available evidence suggests that the increased $\dot{V}O_{2max}$ produced by endurance training of low to moderate intensity and duration are totally reversed after several months of detrain-

ing. Detraining, after several years of intensive training, causes large reductions (5–15%) in stroke volume and $\dot{V}O_{2max}$ during the first 12–21 days of inactivity. These decreases do not indicate deterioration of heart function but instead largely result from reduced blood volume and venous return. $\dot{V}O_{2max}$ of endurance athletes continues to decline during the 21–56 days of detraining because of reductions in maximal a-vDO$_2$. These reductions are associated with a loss of mitochondrial enzyme activity within the trained musculature, which decreases with a half-life of approximately 12 days. Endurance athletes, however, do not regress to levels displayed by individuals who never participated in exercise training. Prolonged, intensive endurance training is associated with persistent elevation of mitochondrial enzyme activity, skeletal muscle capillarization, a-vDO$_2$, and $\dot{V}O_{2max}$.

References

1. Blomqvist CG, Saltin B. Cardiovascular adaptations to physical training. Annu Rev Physiol 45:169–189, 1983.
2. Rowell LB. Human cardiovascular adjustments to exercise and thermal stress. Physiol Rev, 54: 75–159, 1974.
3. Henriksson J, Reitman JS. Time course of changes in human skeletal muscle succinate dehydrogenase and cytochrome oxidase activities and maximal oxygen uptake with physical activity and inactivity. Acta Physiol Scand 99:91–97, 1977.
4. Moore RL, Thacker EM, Kelley GA, et al. Effect of training/detraining on submaximal exercise responses in humans. J Appl Physiol 63:1719–1724, 1987.
5. Orlander J, Kiessling KH, Karlsson J, Ekblom B. Low intensity training, inactivity and resumed training in sedentary men. Acta Physiol Scand 101:351–362, 1977.
6. Fringer MN, Stull GA. Changes in cardiorespiratory parameters during periods of training and detraining in young adult females. Med Sci Sports 6:20–25, 1974.
7. Fox EL, Bartels RL, Billings CE, et al. Frequency and duration of interval training programs and changes in aerobic power. J Appl Physiol 38:481–484, 1975.
8. Klausen K, Andersen LB, Pelle I. Adaptive changes in work capacity, skeletal muscle capillarization and enzyme levels during training and detraining. Acta Physiol Scand 113:9–16, 1981.
9. Drinkwater BL, Horvath SM. Detraining effects on young women. Med Sci Sports Exerc 4:91–95, 1972.
10. Coyle EF, Martin WH, Sinacore DR, et al. Time course of loss adaptations after stopping prolonged intense endurance training. J Appl Physiol 57:1857–1864, 1984.
11. Ehsani AA, Hagberg JM, Hickson RC. Rapid changes in left ventricular dimensions and mass in response to physical conditioning and deconditioning. Am J Cardiol 42:52–56, 1978.
12. Hickson RC, Hammons GT, Holloszy JO. Development and regression of exercise-induced cardiac hypertrophy in rats. Am J Physiol 236:H268–H272, 1979.
13. Saltin B, Grimby GG. Physiological analysis of middle-aged and old former athletes: Comparison with still active athletes of the same ages. Circulation 38:1104–1115, 1968.
14. Martin WH, Coyle EF, Bloomfield SA, Ehsani AA. Effects of physical deconditioning after intense training on left ven-

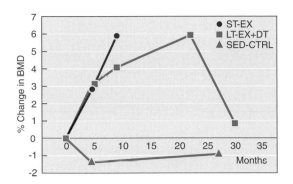

Figure 22.1. Gains in lumbar spine bone mineral density (BMD) with training for 9 months (ST-EX) and 22 months (LT-EX) and subsequent loss of BMD in exercisers remeasured after 8 months of sedentary living. ST-EX, short-term exercise; LT-EX, long-term exercise & detraining; SED-CTRL, sedentary control. (Adapted with permission from Dalsky G, Stocke KS, Ehsani AA, et al. Weight-bearing exercise training and lumbar bone mineral content in postmenopausal women. Ann Intern Med 108:824, 1988.)

cium balance and some weeks later, changes in bone mass. The external dimensions of bone in bed-rested adults do not change, but gradual loss of bone mineral content and organic matrix and some thinning of cancellous bone plates and cortical walls is eventually noted.

Calcium Balance

Maintaining normal bone mass requires a balance between resorption of existing bone and formation of new bone. Prolonged bed rest appears to disrupt this balance with either an absolute increase in resorption or a proportionately greater increase in resorption than formation when both activities are stimulated. Bone calcium released into general circulation by increased resorptive activity transiently increases serum calcium, allowing increased urinary excretion of calcium, which is mediated by the endocrine system, including parathyroid hormone (PTH) and other substances. This resorption-driven hypercalciuria is uniformly observed in bed-rested individuals, peaking at 60% above ambulatory values after 5–7 weeks of bed rest (8). A concomitant increase in fecal calcium also contributes to negative calcium balance, suggesting a reduction in intestinal calcium absorption. This has been verified with calcium balance studies in humans, in whom true calcium absorption by the gut decreases from 31% (while ambulatory) to 24% after bed rest (9).

Endocrine changes are not the primary events causing loss of bone mineral. That is, reduced mechanical usage produces a net increase in bone resorption by osteoclasts. The mobilization of bone calcium itself seems to drive certain endocrine responses to mediate increased calcium load. Intestinal calcium absorption is regulated by 1,25 dihydroxyvitamin D (1,25-D) and indirectly by PTH. In healthy men subjected to bed rest, no change or a decrease in serum PTH concurrent with a negative calcium balance has been observed; serum 1,25-D decreased or did not change (9–13). On the other hand, patients with acute spinal cord injury and functionally complete immobilization of affected limbs have consistently low PTH, low 1,25-D serum levels, and presumably reduced intestinal calcium absorption (14, 15).

Bone Mass

Negative calcium balance secondary to disuse eventually results in decreased bone mass. Krolner (16) first observed the deleterious effects of therapeutic bed rest combined with traction in lumbar disc disease patients, who had mean BMD loss of 0.9% per week in the lumbar spine. Healthy individuals, however, appear to have slower rates of bone loss (4% after 17 weeks) even with strict bed rest (17). Quantitative ultrasound measures of the calcaneus after 120 days of bed rest in healthy males revealed decreases of 0.07–0.11% per week using the speed of sound (SOS) as an indicator of bone loss (18). Figure 22.2 summarizes changes in bone mass with increasing durations of disuse.

Bony sites in weight-bearing lower limbs appear to be the most susceptible to bone loss secondary to disuse. Loss of BMD at the calcaneus (10%) is double that observed at the femoral neck (4%) and spine (4%) after 17 weeks of strict bed rest (Fig. 22.3) (17). By contrast, over the same period, no significant changes are noted in the radius of the forearm. The relative composition of bone is also likely to affect the rate of loss of bone at a particular anatomical site. Cancellous (trabecular) bone, with its greater surface area per volume, is particularly susceptible to increased activity of bone-resorbing osteoclasts during periods of reduced mechanical loading. For example, the proximal tibia (higher content of cancellous bone) is susceptible to more rapid bone loss with disuse than the cortical shaft (19–21). Loss of cortical bone occurs if duration of disuse is sufficient (13, 16). Cortical bone accounts for the major component of increased fragility of osteopenic bone (22).

Analyses of bone biopsy and changes in biochemical markers of bone formation and resorption from bed-rested subjects provide insight into tissue-level mechanisms for disuse bone loss. Biopsy data from healthy males subjected to 120 days of bed rest revealed no significant change in indices of cancellous bone mass and surprisingly subtle changes in bone cell activities (23, 24). By contrast, iliac biopsies from 11 healthy humans exposed to 12 weeks of bed rest disclosed a 250% increase in osteoclastic surface and a 39% decrease in osteoblastic surface, while the remaining structural and dynamic parameters remained unchanged (13). Changes in thickness and density of trabecular plates, with some indication of increased bone resorption, suggest that chronic unloading in healthy adults may exert effects primarily on bone

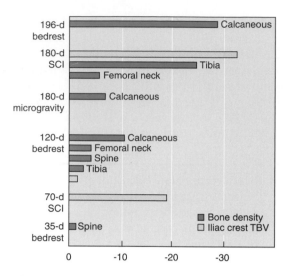

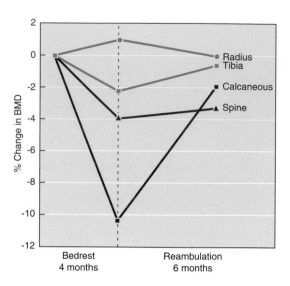

Figure 22.2. Decrements in trabecular bone volume (TBV) determined from iliac crest biopsies and bone mineral density at various sites observed after bed rest, exposure to microgravity, or spinal cord injury (SCI). (Adapted with permission from LeBlanc AD, Schneider VS, Evans HJ, et al. Bone mineral loss and recovery after 17 weeks of bed rest. J Bone Miner Res 5:843, 1990; Biering-Sorensen F, Bohr HH, Schaadt OP. Longitudinal study of bone mineral content in the lumbar spine, the forearm and the lower extremities after spinal cord injury. Eur J Clin Invest 20:330, 1990; Minaire P, Meunier P, Edouard C, et al. Quantitative histological data on disuse osteoporosis: Comparison with biological data. Calcif Tissue Res 17:57, 1974; Vico L, Chappard D, Alexandre C, et al. Effects of a 120-day period of bed-rest on bone mass and bone cell activities in man: Attempts at countermeasure. Bone Miner 2:383, 1987; LeBlanc A, Schneider V, Krebs J, et al. Spinal bone mineral after 5 weeks of bed rest. Calcif Tissue Int 41:259, 1987; Schneider VS, McDonald J. Skeletal calcium homeostasis and countermeasures to prevent disuse osteoporosis. Calcif Tissue Int 36:S151, 1984.)

Figure 22.3. Alterations in bone mineral density (BMD), expressed as percent change from baseline, during 4 months of bed rest and 6 months of reambulation in able-bodied young men. (Adapted with permission from LeBlanc AD, Schneider VS, Evans HJ, et al. Bone mineral loss and recovery after 17 weeks of bed rest. J Bone Miner Res 5:843, 1990.)

architecture, which may reduce bone strength independent of change in bone mass. These changes, after bed rest, may be quite different in lower limb bone (e.g., proximal tibia) as opposed to the non–weight-bearing iliac crest, where bone biopsies are typically taken.

Changes in biochemical markers of bone resorption or formation may better indicate more global changes in the skeleton with bed rest. Biochemical components of collagen fibril cross-links, released when bone matrix is resorbed, increase within 4 days of bed rest in healthy men (25). However, biochemical markers for bone formation do not increase during bed rest, suggesting an uncoupling of formation from resorption (13). Interestingly, some markers of bone resorption remain elevated for up to 6 weeks during renewed walking after a period of bed rest. This suggests that elevated resorption rates continue after activity resumes (12, 25, 26).

These changes in healthy men contrast with findings in patients with spinal cord injury (SCI), in whom iliac crest

cancellous bone volume decreases by 33% in the first 6 months after the injury (22). Maximal hypercalciuria observed in patients with acute SCI is 2–4 times greater than in healthy men at bed rest; disrupted calcium metabolism can persist for up to 12 months post injury (14). Factors unique to SCI (changes in bone blood flow or bone fluid pH) probably accentuate changes in bone cell activities noted in healthy men on bed rest. Bone mineral densities of the femoral neck, distal femur, and proximal tibia in individuals with long-standing SCI average 65%, 48%, and 45%, respectively, of healthy values (21, 27). Interestingly, BMD of the lumbar spine in persons with SCI remains within normal range (21, 27). Continued load bearing on the spine, or even impact force incurred during chair transfer, appears to provide sufficient mechanical stimulus to maintain bone mass in the spine.

REMOBILIZATION: CAN LOST BONE BE REGAINED?

Recovery of lost bone mass and reversal of presumed decreases in resistance to fracture require at least twice as long as the duration of disuse. Cancellous bone mass lost in dogs whose hind limbs were immobilized for 32 weeks was not fully regained after 28 weeks of remobilization (28). In young, healthy rats treadmill running during remobilization after 3 weeks of hind limb immobilization appeared to restore normal cancellous bone architecture (29). This effect should be confirmed in skeletally mature animals.

There are few data on recovery of bone mass after disuse in humans. Recovery is limited and very slow, although it varies among anatomical sites. A residual deficit in BMD of the calcaneus has been observed in astronauts 5 years after repeated exposures to microgravity (30). Loss of density at lumbar spine and femoral neck following 17 weeks of bed rest seems to be unaffected by 6 months of normal weight-bearing activity (Fig. 22.3) (17). BMD of the calcaneus and proximal tibia, however, appears to rebound adequately in this population. Significant tibial bone loss resulting from brief periods of non–weight bearing after hip joint surgery requires 1 to 1.5 years for recovery to baseline values (31). However, the residual deficit in BMD (−6% to −11%) noted in the lower limb of men 9 years after tibial shaft fracture and a 12% lower spine BMD imply that some BMD loss sustained after serious orthopaedic injuries may be permanent unless rehabilitation efforts are especially vigorous (32).

PRACTICAL IMPLICATIONS

It is doubtful that changes in bone mass of bed-rested subjects have any immediate effect on functional work capacity, as do decrements in muscle strength and endurance upon return to normal weight-bearing activity. A greater concern is increased risk of bone fracture, particularly after muscle strength is regained and resumed activity imposes higher forces on relatively weak osteopenic bone. There also is a possibility of increase in risk of clinically relevant osteoporosis later in life.

Each bony site has a critical bone density that constitutes a fracture threshold; that is, bone at a density below this threshold is susceptible to fracture with minimal trauma. It is also probable that during a period of bed rest, the age-related bone loss common to all adults over 40 years may be temporarily accelerated. The result would be an increased decline in bone mass over time and earlier arrival at fracture threshold at the bony site. Old individuals are particularly likely to undergo prolonged bed rest with illness or injury and to be close to a fracture threshold before a period of bed rest begins. The severe osteopenia in hip fracture, for example, almost certainly is worsened in prolonged immobilization during recovery (33).

Reduced BMD after bed rest significantly increases risk of bone fracture with even minor falls in older individuals. Concurrent decrements in muscle strength and balance after bed rest exacerbate the likelihood of falling once walking begins (34, 35). Hip fractures in elderly individuals can be life threatening, and mortality in the first year after hip fracture, usually from complications of prolonged immobility, is fairly common (36). For survivors, decreased mobility detracts significantly from functional capacity and general quality of life.

Exercise professionals must consider many practical implications of musculoskeletal changes with bed rest (Table 22.1). Clearly, the highest priority should be avoidance of prolonged immobility. Periods of bed rest

Table 22.1. Guidelines for Exercise Professionals Working with Severely Detrained or Bed-Rested Individuals

Emphasize strength training of back and lower limb postural muscle groups:
Back extensors
Quadriceps and associated hip extensors
Ankle extensors (soleus and gastrocnemius)
Use gradual, progressive overload starting at appropriately low intensities.
Incorporate training for postural stability and dynamic balance during walking, particularly if the client is elderly.
Be aware of increased risk of bone fracture even after muscle strength is normal, especially in osteopenia-prone individuals (estrogen-deficient women, elderly).

mandated by medical conditions should be as short as possible. Even short periods of weight bearing each day during a time of bed rest may help minimize disuse changes.

During remobilization, emphasis of training in muscle groups most significantly affected by relative disuse should be implemented using a conservative progressive overload program. Training to improve dynamic balance and postural stability should begin early in the remobilization period to reduce risk of falling, especially in the elderly. Given the slow time course of recovery of bone mass relative to muscle mass, awareness of the increased risk of fracture in remobilizing individuals after prolonged bed rest is important. The imbalance between muscle strength and bone strength is greatest when muscle strength has returned to normal and before bone mass is fully restored. These concerns are magnified in the frail elderly, who may enter a period of bed rest with little reserve of bone or muscle mass.

▶ SUMMARY

Training regimens can improve muscle strength and both static and dynamic balance. Aggressive use of these regimens, adapted in intensity and rate of progression, may make a major contribution to bone health by minimizing risk of fracture after a period of prolonged disuse or bed rest. Regular exercise training should be incorporated into the lifestyle thereafter so as to regain as much bone mass as possible, although it is unclear at present whether all lost bone can be replaced.

References
1. Bloomfield SA. Changes in musculoskeletal structure and function with prolonged bed rest. Med Sci Sports Exerc 29:197, 1997.
2. Uebelhart D, Demiaux-Domenech B, Roth M, et al. Bone metabolism in spinal cord injured individuals and in others who have prolonged immobilization: A review. Paraplegia 33:669, 1995.

3. Dalsky G, Stocke KS, Ehsani AA, et al. Weight-bearing exercise training and lumbar bone mineral content in postmenopausal women. Ann Intern Med 108:824, 1988.

4. Michel, BA, Lane NE, Bloch DA, et al. Effect of changes in weight-bearing exercise on lumbar bone mass after age fifty. Ann Med 23:397, 1991.

5. Vuori I, Heinonen A, Seivanen H, et al. Effects of unilateral strength training and detraining on bone mineral density and content in young women: A study of mechanical loading and deloading on human bones. Calcif Tissue Int 55:59–67, 1994.

6. Kiuchi A, Arai Y, Katsuta S. Detraining effects on bone mass in young male rats. Int J Sports Med 19:245, 1998.

7. Forwood MR, Burr DB. Physical activity and bone mass: Exercises in futility? Bone Miner 21:89, 1993.

8. Arnaud SB. Effects of inactivity on bone. In: Sandler H, Vernikos J, eds. Inactivity: Physiological Effects. Orlando, FL: Academic, 1986:56.

9. LeBlanc A, Schneider V, Spector E, et al. Calcium absorption, endogenous excretion, and endocrine changes during and after long-term bed rest. Bone 16:301S, 1995.

10. Ruml LA, Dubois SK, Roberts ML, et al. Prevention of hypercalciuria and stone-forming propensity during prolonged bedrest by alendronate. J Bone Miner Res 10:655, 1995.

11. Arnaud SB, Sherrard DJ, Maloney N, et al. Effects of 1-week head-down tilt bed rest on bone formation and the calcium endocrine system. Aviat Space Environ Med 63:14, 1992.

12. Van der Wiel HE, Lips P, Nauta J, et al. Biochemical parameters of bone turnover during ten days of bed rest and subsequent mobilization. Bone Miner 13:123, 1991.

13. Zerwekh JE, Ruml LA, Gottchalk F, et al. The effects of twelve weeks of bed rest on bone histology, biochemical markers of bone turnover, and calcium homeostasis in eleven normal subjects. J Bone Miner Res 13:1594, 1998.

14. Bergmann P, Heilporn A, Schoutens A, et al. Longitudinal study of calcium and bone metabolism in paraplegic patients. Paraplegia 15:147, 1977–1978.

15. Stewart AF, Adler M, Byers CM, et al. Calcium homeostasis in immobilization: An example of resorptive hypercalciuria. N Engl J Med 306:1136, 1982.

16. Krolner B, Toft B. Vertebral bone loss: An unheeded side effect of therapeutic bed rest. Clin Sci 64:537, 1983.

17. LeBlanc AD, Schneider VS, Evans HJ, et al. Bone mineral loss and recovery after 17 weeks of bed rest. J Bone Miner Res 5:843, 1990.

18. Laugier P, Novikov V, Elmann-Larsen B, et al. Quantitative ultrasound imaging of the calcaneous: Precision and variations during 120-day bed rest. Calcif Tissue Int 66:16, 2000.

19. LeBlanc A, Marsh C, Evans H, et al. Bone and muscle atrophy with suspension of the rat. J Appl Physiol 58:1669, 1985.

20. Young DR, Niklowitz WJ, Brown RJ, et al. Immobilization-associated osteoporosis in primates. Bone 7:109, 1986.

21. Biering-Sorensen F, Bohr HH, Schaadt OP. Longitudinal study of bone mineral content in the lumbar spine, the forearm and the lower extremities after spinal cord injury. Eur J Clin Invest 20:330–335, 1990.

22. Minaire P, Meunier P, Edouard C, et al. Quantitative histological data on disuse osteoporosis: Comparison with biological data. Calcif Tissue Res 17:57, 1974.

23. Vico L, Chappard D, Alexandre C, et al. Effects of a 120-day period of bed-rest on bone mass and bone cell activities in man: Attempts at countermeasure. Bone Miner 2:383, 1987.

24. Palle S, Vico L, Bourrin S, et al. Bone tissue response to four month antiorthostatic bedrest: A bone histomorphometric study. Calcif Tissue Int 51:189, 1992.

25. Lueken SA, Arnaud SB, Taylor AK, et al. Changes in markers of bone formation and resorption in a bed rest model of weightlessness. J Bone Miner Res 8:1433, 1993.

26. Uebelhart D, Bernard J, Hartmann DJ, et al. Modifications of bone and connective tissue after orthostatic bedrest. Osteoporos Int 11:59, 2000.

27. Bloomfield SA, Mysiw WJ, Jackson RD. Bone mass and endocrine adaptations to training in spinal cord injured individuals. Bone 19:61, 1996.

28. Jaworski ZF, Uhthoff HK. Reversibility of nontraumatic disuse osteoporosis during its active phase. Bone 7:431, 1986.

29. Bourrin S, Palle S, Genty C, et al. Physical exercise during remobilization restores a normal bone trabecular network after tail suspension-induced osteopenia in young rats. J Bone Miner Res 10:820, 1995.

30. Tilton FE, DeGioanni JJ, Schneider VS. Long-term follow-up of Skylab bone demineralization. Aviat Space Environ Med 51:1209, 1980.

31. Ito M, Matsumoto T, Enomoto H, et al. Effect of nonweight bearing on tibial bone density measured by QCT in patients with hip surgery. J Bone Miner Metab 17:45, 1999.

32. Kannus P, Jarvinen M, Seivanen H, et al. Osteoporosis in men with a history of tibial fracture. J Bone Miner Res 9:423–429, 1994.

33. Heaney RP. The natural history of vertebral osteoporosis: Is low bone mass an epiphenomenon? Bone 13:S23, 1992.

34. Dudley GA, Duvoisin MR, Convertino VA, Buchanan P. Alterations of the in vivo torque-velocity relationship of human skeletal muscle following 30 days exposure to simulated microgravity. Aviat Space Environ Med 60:659, 1989.

35. Dupui P, Montoya R, Costes-Salon MC, et al. Balance and gait analysis after 30 days-6 degrees bed rest: Influence of lower-body negative-pressure sessions. Aviat Space Environ Med 63:1004, 1992.

36. Cummings SR, Rubin SM, Black D. The future of hip fractures in the United States: Numbers, costs and potential effects of postmenopausal estrogen. Clin Orthop 252:163, 1990.

2.2.1, 2.2.4, 2.2.20   **3.2.0**   **4.2.0.1**

CHAPTER **23**

DECONDITIONING AND BED REST: MUSCULOSKELETAL RESPONSE

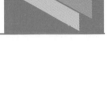

Gary A. Dudley and Lori L. Ploutz-Snyder

Reductions in physical activity are common occurrences that affect almost everyone and that are associated with physiological consequences. It is important to understand musculoskeletal adaptations to reduced physical activity so that functional ability can be predicted and appropriate exercise can be prescribed during disuse or rehabilitation. Decreased muscle activity can result from detraining, bed rest, casting, use of crutches, paralysis, aging, or even the microgravity of space flight. The effects of reduced muscular activity are not confined to diseased or disabled populations, but can also affect elite or weekend athletes.

The term **decreased muscle activity** refers to reductions in intensity and/or amount of total daily activity performed by a muscle or muscle group. Detraining (returning to a sedentary life style after training) does not evoke the same adaptive response as 1 month of bed rest in a sedentary person. The magnitude of the adaptive response to decreased activity depends on relative change in muscle use. For example, bed rest of previously sedentary individuals for 1 month causes greater skeletal muscle atrophy than does cessation of resistance training for the same period (1, 2). Muscle atrophy (reduction in muscle size) from disuse in this case is a normal response, not a maladaptation.

TYPES AND DEFINITIONS OF REDUCED USE (UNLOADING)

Detraining

Detraining is the process following the cessation of training in which adaptations to exercise are gradually reduced or lost (3–5). Detraining in athletes often occurs during the off-season, when normal training routines are interrupted. Detraining is most often observed in previously sedentary individuals who exercise for several weeks or months, then discontinue the practice.

Bed Rest

Periods of bed rest are commonly associated with disease processes, so it is difficult to determine the exact

cause of muscular adaptation. However, bed rest has been used as an experimental model of muscle unloading in healthy individuals to rule out underlying disease and yields similar results as casting or use of crutches (1, 6–10).

Casting

Skeletal muscle adaptations occur when a joint is immobilized by a cast. A unique feature to casting is that a joint is typically in a fixed position with the intent of immobilizing injured tissue, which also immobilizes muscle at a constant length. Muscles immobilized in a shortened position undergo more severe atrophy than muscles immobilized in a neutral or lengthened position (11, 12). Furthermore, after several weeks of casting, joint stiffness may be observed and must be considered when prescribing exercise for injured patients.

Crutches

The use of crutches may or may not be associated with casting. While a lower limb in a cast often necessitates crutches, minor injuries (sprains and strains) may not require casting but may require non–weight bearing. Human lower limb suspension is also used as an experimental technique to study adaptations to unloading (13–19).

Paralysis

Many diseases lead to partial or total paralysis. Spinal cord injuries are responsible for varying degrees of muscle paralysis, often in young and previously active individuals. While it is often difficult to discern how a disease process interacts with muscle disuse to produce functional changes, spinal cord injury is unique in that affected muscles may still be innervated, yet receive no input from higher nervous centers. Thus, muscles are innervated by intact motor neurons but are seldom activated except for spasm (20–27).

Space Flight

Though few individuals participate in space flight, studies of reduced muscle use have been inspired by lack of understanding of the effect of gravity on skeletal muscle. Astronauts adapt muscle function following space flight (28, 29). The mechanism or mechanisms responsible for compromised function and countermeasures or rehabilitation procedures are unknown.

Aging

Skeletal muscle size and strength decrease with increasing age (30, 31). The largest decrements in muscular strength occur after age 50. Decrements average 15% during the sixth and seventh decades of life and reach 30% per decade thereafter. Much of the reduction in strength is due to a reduction in muscle mass. There is controversy regarding whether these changes are inherent to the aging process, associated with increasingly sedentary lifestyle, and/or due to other disease processes.

CONSEQUENCES OF REDUCED USE (UNLOADING) ON SKELETAL MUSCLE

Morphological Consequences

Regardless of the method of unloading, the predominant adaptive response to decreased use is skeletal muscle atrophy (23, 24). Atrophy is the process whereby muscle size is reduced, almost exclusively because of reductions in the contractile proteins actin and myosin (30). Reduction in muscle size may occur through reduced cross-sectional area of individual fibers, a decrease in fiber number, or both. In unloading of a few weeks to a month, a decrease in fiber cross-sectional area is responsible. This is based on the finding that after 6 weeks of lower limb suspension, the decrease in average fiber cross-sectional area in vastus lateralis muscle (−14%) was comparable with the decrease in average cross-sectional area of the muscle (−15%) (18). In contrast, a reduction in fiber numbers due to functional denervation and fiber atrophy appears to contribute to the decreased muscle mass associated with aging (31).

For the first several weeks of disuse, atrophy is almost linearly related to duration and extent of unloading and differs among muscles depending on function (Fig. 23.1). Generally, atrophy is most severe in muscles that are involved in weight bearing and postural control; extensor muscles are typically more severely affected than flexor muscles (8, 18, 24). Likewise, it has recently been shown that the atrophic response of thigh adductor muscles to unloading is intermediate to that of extensor and flexor muscles (Table 23.1) (9, 18). Of particular concern are muscles of the thigh and calf. These are critical in normal walking and show marked atrophy in non–weight-bearing conditions (24). Generally, unloading the quadriceps femoris (knee extensor) muscle group causes reduced cross-sectional area of about 0.4% per day of unloading (Fig. 23.1).

The atrophic response to detraining appears to occur at least as slowly as the hypertrophic response to training

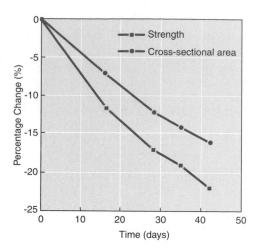

Figure 23.1. Time course of change in knee extensor strength and muscle cross-sectional area following unweighting using limb suspension. (Adapted with permission from Berg HE, Dudley GA, Haggmark T, et al. Effects of lower limb unloading on skeletal muscle mass and function in humans. J Appl Physiol 70:1882, 1991; Adams GR, Hather BM, Dudley GA. Effect of short-term unweighting on human skeletal muscle strength and size. Aviat Space Environ Med 65:1116, 1994; Hather BM, Adams GR, Tesch PA, et al. Skeletal muscle responses to lower limb suspension in humans. J Appl Physiol 72:1493, 1992; Ploutz-Snyder LL, Tesch PA, Crittenden DJ, et al. Effect of unweighting on skeletal muscle use during exercise. J Appl Physiol 79:168, 1995.)

(about 1% per week) (2–5). Thus, the atrophic response to resistance training cessation appears to be slower than to that of unloading in previously sedentary individuals. Therefore, with respect to muscle atrophy, detraining in exercising individuals is less deleterious than in bedridden, previously sedentary individuals. A short period of detraining may not be especially detrimental, but a patient on bed rest should attempt to walk as early as possible.

Table 23.1. Muscle Cross-Sectional Area Following 6 Weeks of Unloading

MUSCLE GROUP	% CHANGE IN SIZE
Knee extensor	16
Knee flexor	7
Knee adductors	9

Adapted with permission from Berg HE, Larsson L, Tesch PA, et al. Lower limb skeletal muscle function after 6 weeks of bed rest. J Appl Physiol 82:182–188, 1996.

In lower mammals, fiber type composition may influence the atrophic response to unloading; however, this has not been demonstrated in humans (24). Human skeletal muscle in general does not present the clear segmentation of fiber type found in lower mammals (32). Fast and slow fibers of human muscles show comparable atrophy after 4 to 6 weeks of bed rest (1). Fast fibers actually show greater atrophy 6 months after clinically complete spinal cord injury (SCI) (22). Likewise, soleus muscle, predominantly slow in humans, does not appear to exhibit greater atrophy after unloading than the gastrocnemius muscle (18, 24).

Fiber type composition of muscle, especially the relative area of muscle occupied by any given fiber type, has a marked effect on energy demands of contraction. Fast fibers evoke substantially greater energy demand per unit of contractile material than slow fibers and therefore require greater energy supply to sustain contraction. If a muscle becomes faster because of preferential slow-fiber atrophy with unloading, the result is increased energy demand per unit of force development and, all other factors being unchanged, increased relative fatigue. Muscle also becomes faster if slow fibers are transformed to fast fibers during unloading. Neither process appears to occur in humans during 4–6 weeks to 6 months of unloading (1, 9, 14, 16, 18, 22). Thus the energy demand of contraction is apparently not altered during several months of unloading in humans (27).

Fast subtypes, unlike fast versus slow fibers, appear to show transformation with several months of unloading or after detraining (2, 5, 22). Studies show that resistance training evokes a decrease in percent of type IIB fibers and a concomitant increase type IIA fibers in human skeletal muscle. When training is stopped, fiber type composition reverts to the composition that was evident prior to training (5). Consistent with these data, the proportion of type IIB fibers increases, while that of type IIA decreases several months after SCI (22). It appears that type IIB fibers in human muscle serve as the default expression of the fast myosin gene. These transformations would not be expected to markedly alter energy demand of contraction, unlike slow to fast fiber movement, because actomyosin adenosine triphosphatase (ATPase) activity is more different between slow and fast fibers than between fast subtypes (27).

The extent to which atrophy occurs depends in large part on the duration and extent of reduced use and the muscle in question. Most studies use several weeks' unloading. Patients with permanent paralysis, such as in SCI, exhibit marked atrophy (50% or more) of the most affected muscles, which reaches a nadir by approximately 6 months after injury (22–24). The fast-fiber composition of muscle is also high in patients years after injury, yet actomyosin ATPase activity is not elevated (21).

Skeletal muscle is one of the few multinucleated tissues in the human body. Recent research has investigated the influence of disuse on myonuclear number and myonuclear domain size (volume of cytoplasm per myonucleus). It has been hypothesized that dynamic modulation of myonuclear number provides a long-term adaptive response to both unloading and overloading of skeletal muscle. This has been widely studied in lower mammals and recently investigated in humans. Four months of bed rest resulted in no change in myonuclear number per millimeter of fiber length, but muscle fiber size was significantly reduced, resulting in smaller myonuclear domain sizes. Following bed rest, the correlation between fiber size and myonuclear number was decreased, suggesting that the muscle was in a more transitional state (33).

Following 6 weeks of unloading of the vastus lateralis muscle, the number of capillaries surrounding each fiber is unchanged, so capillaries per unit area of muscle (capillary density) actually increases (18). However, in moderate to severe denervation of human gastrocnemius muscle, capillaries per fiber is reduced in proportion to the degree of fiber atrophy, so capillary density is unchanged (34). This suggests that fiber atrophy exceeds capillary loss during initial weeks of unloading and that thereafter, loss of capillaries normalizes capillary density. In either case, it seems that unloading does not compromise the diffusional characteristics of the capillary–muscle milieu (22).

Metabolic Consequences

The influence of unloading on metabolic characteristics of human skeletal muscle has received less attention than atrophy and reduced strength. Homogenates of muscle biopsies show decreased concentrations of enzyme markers of aerobic oxidative capacity after unloading, while anaerobic enzymes of energy supply do not seem to change (1, 14). Reduced enzymes associated with aerobic capacity may reflect preferential loss of contractile protein with unloading; that is, aerobic oxidative enzyme content per fiber volume may not change and the anaerobic enzyme content may actually increase (26, 30). Nonetheless, fiber atrophy results in lower total mitochondrial content, so unloading compromises absolute muscular endurance (10, 14). This also suggests that relative muscular endurance is not significantly affected by unloading (14). However, preferential loss of contractile protein requires the remaining muscle to work against greater absolute load. This work is accomplished with reduced total capacity for aerobic–oxidative energy supply because mitochondrial content is lower.

Unlike short-term unloading, chronic but not acute SCI appears to reduce mitochondrial content, not only because of atrophy but also because there are fewer mitochondria per unit volume of contractile machinery (21, 22). This limited ability for aerobic–oxidative energy supply may in part account for the poor fatigue resistance evident after chronic but not acute SCI (20–23, 26).

Strength and Local Muscular Endurance

Unloading reduces muscular strength, regardless of the type of action or movement performed or the method of strength expression (6–10, 13–19, 35). Strength reduction is nearly linearly related to the duration of unloading and extent of muscle atrophy for the first few weeks (Fig. 23.1). Atrophy accounts for a large part but not all of decreased force production, suggesting that the ability to activate muscle is also compromised by unloading (discussed later). This is interesting because marked force during eccentric, isometric, and slow-speed concentric muscle contraction is believed to be controlled by some neural inhibitory mechanisms (36, 37). However, the relative decline in strength is comparable across speeds and types of muscle actions, so increased inhibition is not responsible for reduced voluntary activation, or if it is, the reduction is uniform across speeds and types of muscle actions (6, 9, 13, 17).

The lack of shape change in the speed–torque relationship with short-term unloading may suggest that muscle fiber type composition is not altered. However, as transformation to a faster muscle occurs with long-term extreme unloading, an increased ability to maintain force as speed increases during concentric actions should be evident (36). This finding has been reported after long-term space flight (28). However, 120 days of unloading of otherwise healthy individuals did not alter relative rise time during surface electrical stimulation of the triceps surae muscle group, suggesting that myofibrillar actomyosin ATPase activity is not altered by 3 months of disuse (35). Likewise, time to peak tension for a twitch of tibialis anterior muscle has been reported comparable between SCI patients and healthy controls, suggesting that long-term unloading does not markedly alter calcium kinetics (20). Comparable twitch mechanics in SCI patients and healthy controls may be interpreted to imply that fiber type composition of muscle and thereby myofibrillar actomyosin ATPase activity are not altered by SCI (26, 27). Martin et al. (21) report this finding in patients with chronic spinal cord injuries. Thus, a muscle appears faster in chronic SCI patients than controls yet is comparable with those of healthy individuals for myofibrillar actomyosin ATPase activity and mechanical function.

The magnitude of strength reduction is also specific to muscle group, with weight-bearing muscles most affected (Table 23.2). For knee extensors, decline in strength averages about 0.6% per day. In contrast, the first dorsal interosseus hand muscle is relatively resistant to adaptation after 3–5 weeks of immobilization (38).

Muscular endurance associated with disuse has not been widely studied. One recent report suggests that following 4 weeks of casting of the elbow flexors, endurance time was actually increased in female but not male subjects. Furthermore, the electromyography (EMG) activity during the endurance test was altered in the female subjects. The EMG was associated with intermittent motor unit activity instead of the continuous activity typically observed. This suggests that motor unit activation patterns are altered following disuse, at least in females (39). The ability to maintain force over repeat contractions is not altered within 6 months of SCI but is markedly compromised in chronic SCI patients (20, 22, 23).

Table 23.2. Muscle Strength Following 5 Weeks of Unweighting

MUSCLE GROUP	% CHANGE IN STRENGTH
Knee extensor	20
Knee flexor	8
Ankle extensor	26
Ankle flexor	10

Adapted with permission from Gogia PP, Schneider VS, LeBlanc AD, et al. Bed rest effect on extremity muscle torque in healthy men. Arch Phys Med Rehabil 69:1030, 1988; LeBlanc A, Gogia P, Schneider V, et al. Calf muscle area and strength changes after five weeks of horizontal bed rest. Am J Sports Med 16:624, 1988.

Neuromuscular Consequences

Decreased strength with reduced use has consistently been shown to be greater than that explained by muscle atrophy (19). An exception to this concept has been reported after short-term space flight. Muscle strength decreases in proportionately similar amounts, or perhaps less than fiber size, after 5 or 11 days of unloading (about 15% versus 20%) (28, 29). This implies increased ability to recruit muscle and/or greater specific tension (force per unit muscle size). Neither has been reported in studies of unloading at normal gravity (9, 10, 40). Thus, neuromuscular impairment may occur after unloading.

EMG studies demonstrate that maximal firing rate and maximal integrated EMG activity are decreased and periods of silent EMG activity appear during maximal voluntary contractions after unloading (41). The ability to recruit high-threshold motor units also seems to be compromised (10). The greater relative decline in strength than in size suggests that more muscle may be used to perform a given submaximal task. This has recently been reported using magnetic resonance imaging (MRI), supporting EMG analyses in which greater numbers of motor units are required to develop submaximal force (9, 15, 19, 42). It has also been reported that 4 weeks of leg casting leads to neuromuscular transmission defects such as end-plate dysfunction, resulting in neuromuscular jitter as evidenced by single-fiber EMG of the soleus (43).

The exercise professional should account for these neuromuscular adaptations to unloading in exercise prescriptions for subjects recovering from reduced muscular activity. Submaximal loads that were once easily borne require more absolute muscle involvement. Also, individuals may not have visible muscle atrophy but may be particularly weak because of irregularities in motor control.

VULNERABILITY TO MUSCLE DAMAGE

It has been demonstrated that unloading lower limb skeletal muscle for 5 weeks increases vulnerability to eccentric exercise-induced dysfunction and muscle injury (42). Following 5 weeks of unloading one lower limb, strength is reduced by 20%. Submaximal eccentric exercise performed by the already weakened limb results in further reductions in strength. There are no changes in strength in contralateral weight-bearing muscle. MRI obtained 3 days after eccentric exercise demonstrated muscle damage over the unloaded cross-sectional area, while none was evident in the contralateral weight-bearing limb.

These results have practical importance to the exercise professional. Dysfunction and injury during reloading may be sufficient to prolong recovery. In the previous study, 10 days after the eccentric exercise, strength remained reduced by 20% (before unloading). Low-intensity exercise should be used with care initially during renewal of walking to minimize muscle dysfunction and injury.

Increased vulnerability to exercise-induced muscle injury has also been reported in the elderly (30). Whether this is due to aging and/or low physical activity is not known, but when starting an exercise program for an elderly person, it is important to be cautious.

POSSIBLE COUNTERMEASURES

There are few data regarding efficacy of various countermeasures designed to prevent muscle atrophy and dysfunction or to enhance recovery during disuse. Endurance activity enhances fatigue resistance of skeletal muscle during unloading. Electrical stimulation of tibialis anterior muscle for 45 minutes to 2 hours/day in complete SCI patients evoked a marked increase in ability to maintain force during contraction. This response is attributed in part to increased muscle fiber aerobic–oxidative enzyme content (20, 21). Resistancelike exercise (high-force intermittent stimulation) in patients with SCI or ladder climbing in hindlimb-suspended rats has been shown to increase muscle size (25, 44), the former to near preinjury levels. One recent report using only four subjects suggests that wearing a Penguin antigravity suit for 10 hours/day and performing resistance exercise for 15 minutes each hour can prevent muscle atrophy associated with bed rest (33). However, this strategy is probably not practical for use in the bulk of the population.

Although it is not clear to what extent disuse is responsible for neuromuscular dysfunction in the elderly, it is clear that resistance exercise training can be used by individuals to increase strength and muscle mass (31). This may enhance performance of activities of daily living, decrease severity and occurrence of fall-related injury, and delay onset of disease.

Retraining

Short-term retraining after detraining appears to return muscle strength and size to those of the previously trained state (5). However, it appears that there is less deconditioning than expected during detraining and more rapid adaptation after resuming training than expected.

References
1. Hikida RS, Gollnick PD, Dudley GA, et al. Structural and metabolic characteristics of human skeletal muscle following 30 days of simulated microgravity. Aviat Space Environ Med 60:664, 1989.
2. Hather BM, Bruce M, Tesh PA, et al. Influence of eccentric actions on skeletal muscle adaptations to resistance training. Acta Physiol Scand 143:177, 1991.
3. Narici MV, Roi GS, Landoni L, et al. Changes in force, cross-sectional area and neural activation during strength training and detraining of the human quadriceps. Eur J Appl Physiol 59:310, 1989.
4. Houston ME, Froese EA, Valeriote P, et al. Muscle performance, morphology and metabolic capacity during strength training and detraining: A one leg model. Eur J Appl Physiol 51:25, 1983.
5. Staron RS, Leonardi MJ, Karapondo DL, et al. Strength and skeletal muscle adaptations in heavy-resistance-trained women after detraining and retraining. J Appl Physiol 70:631, 1991.
6. Dudley GA, Duvoisin MR, Convertino VA, et al. Alterations of the in vivo torque-velocity relationship of human skeletal muscle following 30 days exposure to simulated microgravity. Aviat Space Environ Med 60:659, 1989.
7. Gogia PP, Schneider VS, LeBlanc AD, et al. Bed rest effect on extremity muscle torque in healthy men. Arch Phys Med Rehabil 69:1030, 1988.
8. LeBlanc A, Gogia P, Schneider V, et al. Calf muscle area and strength changes after five weeks of horizontal bed rest. Am J Sports Med 16:624, 1988.
9. Berg HE, Larsson L, Tesch PA. Lower limb skeletal muscle function after 6 weeks of bedrest. J Appl Physiol 82:182–188, 1996.
10. Duchateau J. Bed rest induces neural and contractile adaptations in triceps surae. Med Sci Sports Exerc 27:1581, 1995.
11. Goldspink DF, Morton AJ, Loughna P, et al. The effect of hypokinesia and hypodynamia on protein turnover and the growth of four skeletal muscles of the rat. Pflugers Arch 407:333, 1986.
12. Pattullo MC, Cotter MA, Cameron NE, et al. Effects of lengthened immobilization on functional and histochemical properties of rabbit tibialis anterior muscle. Exp Physiol 77:433, 1992.
13. Berg HE, Dudley GA, Haggmark T, et al. Effects of lower limb unloading on skeletal muscle mass and function in humans. J Appl Physiol 70:1882, 1991.

14. Berg HE, Dudley GA, Hather BM, et al. Work capacity and metabolic and morphologic characteristics of the human quadriceps muscle in response to unloading. Clin Physiol 13:337, 1993.

15. Berg HE, Tesch PA. Changes in muscle function in response to 10 days of lower limb unloading in humans. Acta Physiol Scand 157:63–70, 1996.

16. Adams GR, Hather BM, Dudley GA. Effect of short-term unweighting on human skeletal muscle strength and size. Aviat Space Environ Med 65:1116, 1994.

17. Dudley GA, Duvoisin MR, Adams GR, et al. Adaptations to unilateral lower limb suspension in humans. Aviat Space Environ Med 63:678, 1992.

18. Hather BM, Adams GR, Tesch PA, et al. Skeletal muscle responses to lower limb suspension in humans. J Appl Physiol 72:1493, 1992.

19. Ploutz-Snyder LL, Tesch PA, Crittenden DJ, et al. Effect of unweighting on skeletal muscle use during exercise. J Appl Physiol 79:168, 1995.

20. Stein RB, T Gordon T, Jefferson J, et al. Optimal stimulation of paralyzed muscle after human spinal cord injury. J Appl Physiol 72:1393, 1992.

21. Martin TP, Stein RB, Hoeppner PH, et al. Influence of electrical stimulation on the morphological and metabolic properties of paralyzed muscle. J Appl Physiol 72:1401, 1992.

22. Castro MJ, Apple DF Jr, Staron RS, et al. Influence of complete spinal cord injury on skeletal muscle within six months of injury. J Appl Physiol 86:350–358, 1999

23. Hillegass EA, Dudley GA. Surface electrical stimulation of skeletal muscle after spinal cord injury. Spinal Cord 37:251–257, 1999.

24. Castro MJ, Apple DF Jr, Hillegass EA, Dudley GA. Influence of complete spinal cord injury on skeletal muscle morphology within six months of injury. Eur J Appl Physiol 80:373–378, 1999.

25. Dudley GA, Castro MJ, Rogers S, Apple DF Jr. A simple means of increasing muscle size after SCI: A pilot study. Eur J Appl Physiol 80:394–396, 1999.

26. Castro MJ, Apple DF Jr, Rogers S, Dudley GA. Influence of complete spinal cord injury on skeletal muscle mechanics within six months of injury. Eur J Appl Physiol 81:128–131, 2000.

27. Castro MJ, Apple DF Jr, Rogers S, Dudley GA. Muscle fiber-type specific Ca2+ actomyosin ATPase activity after complete spinal cord injury. Muscle Nerve 23:119–121, 2000.

28. Edgerton VR, Zhou MY, Ohira Y, et al. Human fiber size and enzymatic properties after 5 and 11 days of spaceflight. J Appl Physiol 78:1733, 1995.

29. LeBlanc A, Rowe R, Schneider V, et al. Regional muscle loss after short duration spaceflight. Aviat Space Environ Med 66:1151, 1995.

30. Manfredi TG, Fielding RA, O'Reilly KP, et al. Plasma creatine kinase activity and exercise-induced muscle damage in older men. Med Sci Sports Exerc 23:1028, 1991.

31. Tseng BS, Marsh DR, Hamilton MT, et al. Strength and aerobic training attenuate muscle wasting and improve resistance to the development of disability with aging. J Gerontol Series A 50A:113, 1995 (special issue).

32. Roy RR, Baldwin KM, Edgerton VR. The plasticity of skeletal muscle effects of neuromuscular activity. Exerc Sports Sci Rev 19:269, 1991.

33. Ohira Y, Yoshinaga T, Ohara M, et al. Myonuclear domain and myosin phenotype in human soleus after bed rest with or without loading. J Appl Physiol 87:1776–1785, 1999.

34. Carpenter S, Karpati G. Necrosis of capillaries in denervation atrophy of human skeletal muscle. Muscle Nerve 5:250, 1982.

35. Koryak Y. Contractile properties of the human triceps surae muscle during simulated weightlessness. Eur J Appl Physiol 70:344, 1995.

36. Harris RT, Dudley GA. Factors limiting force during slow, shortening actions of the quadriceps femoris muscle group in vivo. Acta Physiol Scand 152:63, 1994.

37. Westing SH, Seger H, Thorstensson A. Effects of electrical stimulation on eccentric and concentric torque-velocity relationships during knee extension in man. Acta Physiol Scand 140:17, 1990.

38. Fuglevand AJ, Bilodeau M, Enoka RM. Short-term immobilization has a minimal effect on the strength and fatigability of a human hand muscle. J Appl Physiol 78:847, 1995.

39. Semmler JG, Kutzscher DV, Enoka RM. Gender differences in the fatigability of human skeletal muscle. J Neurophysiol 82:3590–3593, 1999.

40. Kandarin SC, Boushel RC, Schulte LM. Elevated interstitial fluid volume in rat soleus muscles by hindlimb unweighting. J Appl Physiol 71:910, 1991.

41. Duchateau J, Hainaut K. Effects of immobilization on contractile properties, recruitment and firing rates of human motor units. J Physiol 422:55, 1990.

42. Ploutz-Snyder LL, Tesch PA, Hather BM, et al. Vulnerability to dysfunction and muscle injury after unloading. Arch Phys Med Rehabil 77:773–777, 1996.

43. Grana EA, Chiou-Tan F, Jaweed M. Endplate dysfunction in healthy muscle following a period of disuse. Muscle Nerve 19:989–993, 1996.

45. Herbert ME, Roy RR, Edgerton VR. Influence of one-week hindlimb suspension and intermittent high load exercise on rat muscles. Exp Neurol 102:190, 1988.

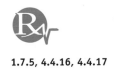

CHAPTER **24**

ENVIRONMENTAL CONSIDERATIONS: HEAT AND COLD

Thomas E. Bernard

The prevailing thermal environment can profoundly change the physiological response to exercise and increase the risk of an environment-related disorder. An understanding of the interrelationships between thermal environment and exercise allows better management of risk for heat or cold disorders during exercise.

The physiological response to heat and cold are different, and the disorders associated with these two stressors differ fundamentally. This chapter presents the interaction between the environment and exercise, disorders that may occur, and a plan for managing adverse environmental stress.

HEAT STRESS

Heat stress is the combination of environmental conditions, metabolic rate, and clothing that increases core temperature. The traditional approach to study and assessment of heat stress is to describe the balance that must be achieved between all sources of heat gain and heat loss (1–3). If a balance cannot be achieved, risk of excessive core temperature increases. A basic understanding of heat exchange is necessary to appreciate the interactions of environment, exercise, and clothing. The risk of a serious heat-related disorder is associated with the level of heat stress, and control of risk is based on maintaining health and managing exposure to heat stress.

Heat Balance

The major source of heat gain is internal heat generated by energy metabolism. Approximately 25% of metabolic energy expenditure is actually translated to mechanical work during locomotion (i.e., walking, biking); the remaining 75% is released as heat in contracting muscle (1). As metabolic rate increases to meet increasing demands of exercise, the rate of internal heat generation also increases. Rate of energy expenditure can be estimated using tables or equations (1, 4). An average man (73 kg) walking on a level surface at 1.6 m/second (3.5 mph) has a metabolic rate of about 350 watts (1).

Sweat Evaporative Cooling

The major avenue of heat loss is evaporation of sweat from the skin surface. Evaporative cooling by secreting water onto the skin surface through eccrine sweat glands is one response to heat stress. As water absorbs heat from the skin, it changes from liquid to vapor. Surrounding air carries the vapor away. Because the heat of vaporization is quite high, small amounts of sweat remove relatively large amounts of heat. Specifically, the evaporation of 0.5 L of sweat per hour is sufficient to remove the 350 watts of excess heat in the preceding walking example (2).

If sufficient volumes of sweat are produced quickly enough and evaporation is not impeded, thermal balance is maintained and core temperature does not rise. This scenario does not occur for several reasons. First, there are physiological limits to sweat evaporation. In the short term, it is not reasonable to expect a sustained sweat rate above 1 L/hour. In the long term (several hours), rate of evaporation may be reduced by dehydration (5).

The physiological limit to volume of sweat produced varies by state of acclimation, aerobic fitness, and genetically among individuals (2). Acclimation (also known as acclimatization) is a physiological adjustment that occurs naturally with repeated exposures to heat stress during exercise. Acclimation increases rate of sweating, shortens onset time, and conserves sodium. Resulting benefits include reduced cardiovascular strain and lower core temperature for the same level of heat stress. Most improvement occurs over the initial 3–5 days, with smaller additional improvements over the subsequent 2–7 days (1, 2). As a rule, 1 day of acclimation is lost for every 3 days away from exercise in heat stress, or in the case of illness, 1 day is lost per day of illness. Aerobic fitness is the single best indicator of ability to tolerate heat stress. On the other hand, about 1 in 20 people are heat intolerant for unknown reasons (6).

Second, the physical limits to rate of evaporative cooling are due to environmental conditions and clothing (1, 3, 7). The primary drive for evaporative cooling is the difference in water vapor pressures on the skin and in the air.

If the difference is small, rate of evaporative cooling decreases; if the difference is large, the evaporation rate can be sufficient to balance even high rates of metabolic heat. Water vapor pressure on the skin is relatively constant. The vapor pressure of water in air is the primary source of difference in environmental contribution to heat stress. It is for this reason that humidity is an important factor in heat stress. Air movement also modifies rate of evaporative cooling. If air movement is 2–3 m/second (4–6 mph), the maximum rate of evaporative cooling is achieved; higher speeds do not appreciably increase evaporative cooling (8).

Clothing

Clothing further restricts maximum rate of evaporative cooling. Clothing between skin and environment decreases cooling ability through evaporation of sweat (2, 7). Under some circumstances the effect of clothing is negligible. For example, if air is very dry (low humidity) or if metabolic rate is low, rate of sweat evaporation through clothing is sufficient to allow adequate cooling. The resistance of clothing to sweat evaporation depends on surface area covered, nature of the fabric, number of layers, and construction of the ensemble. The following are important to minimize the effect of clothing:

- The covered surface area should be as small as is reasonable.
- The fabric should be lightweight open weave or other material freely allowing water vapor to pass through.
- Trapped air spaces from multiple layers should be minimized.
- The construction should be loose, with openings to allow easy movement of air around and through the clothing.

At the other extreme is clothing that covers most of the body, is impermeable to water vapor (e.g., plastic or rubber rain clothing), and is tightly fitting around openings for arms, legs, and head. Little evaporative cooling can occur in a person wearing this type of clothing.

Convection and Radiation

Other factors that modify overall heat stress are convection and radiation. When the air temperature is greater than skin temperature (nominally 35°C or 95°F), heat is added by convection. Conversely, when air temperature is lower than 35°C, some heat is lost by convection. Rate of convection is enhanced by air movement and reduced by clothing insulation. Infrared radiation from the sun and warm or hot surfaces increase heat stress, while cool surfaces reduce heat stress. Clothing insulation reduces rate of heat flow (in either direction) by radiation. Convection and radiation combined usually account for less than 20% of either heat gain or heat loss during exercise.

Physiological Response

The physiological response to heat stress is reflected in body temperature, heart rate, and sweating. Metabolic heat raises temperature of working muscles, and circulating blood transports heat to the central organs, causing a rise in core temperature. Additional blood flow carries excess heat to the skin. To move heat from working muscles to the skin, cardiac output increases and blood flow is shunted from splanchnic and renal circulation (9).

HEAT-RELATED DISORDERS

The normal and acceptable response to heat stress includes elevated core temperature, increased heart rate, and water loss due to sweating. Left unchecked, however, these responses may lead to heat-related disorders and psychomotor and cognitive performance decrements. The disorders of particular importance during exercise are the following:

- Heat cramps
- Heat syncope
- Dehydration
- Heat exhaustion
- Heat stroke (1–3)

Table 24.1 lists these disorders and describes signs, symptoms, and first aid. It is important for exercise professionals to understand these features of heat disorders. Preventive measures are described next.

Heat Cramps and Syncope

Heat cramps are most likely to occur during or after sustained exercise with profuse sweating. Cramps usually appear in fatigued calf or abdominal muscles. Heat syncope may result from dehydration or excessive pooling of blood in peripheral vascular beds. The consequent hypotension may cause familiar blackout symptoms. Recovery is relatively quick, and most are generally aware of the occurrence. In addition to adequate hydration, risk of syncope can be reduced by avoiding prolonged standing or rapid transition to standing.

Dehydration and Heat Exhaustion

Dehydration and heat exhaustion are most likely to occur in the unacclimated and in those who do not drink enough or ignore early warning signs. In competitive sports, a 5% loss of body weight is not unusual (1, 2). Losses greater than 1.5% should be followed by a period of recovery and rehydration.

Heat Stroke

Heat stroke is a medical emergency, and the least suspicion that it may be present justifies an immediate and aggressive response. The risk of heat stroke is greatest among those who abuse alcohol or drugs, who are highly

Table 24.1. Heat-Related Disorders, Including Symptoms, Signs, and First Aid

Heat cramps
  Symptom
    Painful muscle cramps, especially in abdominal or fatigued muscles
  Sign
    Incapacitating pain in voluntary muscles
  First aid
    Rest in cool environment
    Drink salted water (0.5% salt solution)
    Massage muscles
Heat syncope
  Symptoms
    Blurred vision (gray out)
    Fainting (brief) (blackout)
  Sign
    Brief fainting or near fainting
    Normal temperature
  First aid
    Lie on back in cool environment
    Drink water
Dehydration
  Symptoms
    No early symptoms
    Fatigue, weakness
    Dry mouth
  Signs
    Loss of work capacity
    Increased response time
  First aid
    Fluid and salt replacement
Heat exhaustion
  Symptoms
    Fatigue
    Weakness
    Blurred vision
    Dizziness, headache
  Signs
    High pulse rate
    Profuse sweating
    Low blood pressure
    Insecure gait
    Pale face
    Collapse
    Body temperature normal to slightly increased
  First aid
    Lie flat on back in cool environment
    Drink water
    Loosen clothing
Heat stroke
  Symptoms
    Chills
    Restlessness
    Irritability
  Signs
    Red face
    Euphoria
    Shivering
    Disorientation
    Erratic behavior
    Collapse
    Unconsciousness
    Convulsions
    Body temperature >40°C (104°F)
  First aid
    Immediate, aggressive, effective cooling
    Transport to hospital

motivated and ignore symptoms of heat exhaustion, or who are heat intolerant (i.e., do not acclimate).

MANAGEMENT OF HEAT STRESS DURING EXERCISE

Exercise in a warm or hot environment always carries risk of heat disorder. Risk is increased if exercise is vigorous or clothing is improper or excessive. Managing risk depends on recognition of external factors and adjusting exercise intensity and/or duration appropriately. In addition, personal protective practices can minimize effects of heat stress. This section describes the ways to minimize risk of heat-related disorders during exercise.

External Factors

The wet-bulb–globe temperature (WBGT) is an environmental index originally developed for the military and widely accepted for use in occupational health and athletics (1–3). It is derived from measures of ambient temperature, relative humidity, and radiant heat. This index accounts for the impact of humidity on evaporative cooling (wet-bulb temperature, T_{WB}, WBT, or WB) as well as that of radiation and convection (globe temperature, T_g or GT). The dry-bulb (air) temperature (T_{air}, T_{db}, DB, or DBT) is also used for exercise in direct sunlight. Instruments for directly measuring the WBGT are commercially available. For exposures to direct sunlight:

$$\text{WBGT}_{out} = 0.7\, T_{wb} + 0.2\, T_g + 0.1\, T_{db}.$$

When the day is overcast or when the exercise is in the shade or indoors:

$$\text{WBGT}_{in} = 0.7\, T_{wb} + 0.3\, T_g.$$

If the instruments are not available, WBGT can be estimated (Table 24.2) from air temperature and any one of several measures of humidity, adjusting for direct sunlight. Dew point temperature (T_{dp}) is the best indicator of humidity for outside applications. Local news outlets often report dew point temperature. Because it remains relatively constant during the day if weather is stable, knowing the current value is less important than for the other indicators of humidity.

For indoor or outdoor environments, wet-bulb temperature can be easily measured by adapting a typical liquid-in-glass or electronic thermometer with a temperature-sensitive bulb. Alternatively, for indoor environments or if dew point is unknown, percent relative humidity (%rh) can be used. The value for %rh **must** be assessed at the same time and location as air temperature. If air temperature and either dew point temperature, wet bulb temperature, or relative humidity are known, Table 24.2 can be used to estimate WBGT. If exercise occurs in direct sunlight or on a partly cloudy day, 4°F is added to the value of WBGT to account for the effects of the sun. Adjustments for state of acclimation, metabolic

Table 24.2. Tables for Estimation of WBGT from Air Temperature and Either (1) Dew Point Temperature, (2) Wet Bulb Temperature, or (3) Relative Humidity. Estimated values must be increased by 4°F if exercise is in direct sunlight.

ESTIMATE OF WBGT (°F) FROM AIR TEMPERATURE (T_{air}) AND DEW POINT TEMPERATURE (T_{dp})

T_{dp} °F	60	65	70	75	80	85	90	95	100	105	110	T_{dp} °C
95	86	88	90	91	93	95	97	99	101	103	105	35
90	80	83	85	87	89	91	93	95	97	99	101	32
85	76	78	80	83	85	87	89	91	93	96	98	28
80	72	74	77	79	81	83	86	88	90	93	95	27
75	69	71	73	76	78	81	83	85	88	90	92	24
70	66	65	71	73	76	78	80	83	85	88	90	21
65	63	66	68	71	73	76	78	81	83	86	88	18
60	61	64	66	69	71	74	76	79	82	84	87	16
55	60	62	64	67	70	72	75	77	80	83	85	10
50	58	60	62	66	68	71	74	76	79	81	84	13
45	58	59	62	64	67	70	72	75	78	80	83	7
40	56	58	61	63	66	69	71	74	77	80	82	4
35	54	57	60	62	66	68	71	73	76	79	82	2
30	53	56	59	62	64	67	70	73	75	78	81	−1
	16	18	21	24	27	29	32	35	38	41	43	

T_{air} (°C)

For outdoor exercise, WBGT can be estimated from the current air temperature and the dew point temperature that has been recorded in the last few hours.

If the exercise occurs in direct sunlight, add 4°F to the estimated WBGT.

ESTIMATE OF WBGT (°F) FROM AIR TEMPERATURE (T_{air}) AND WET BULB TEMPERATURE (T_{wb})

T_{wb} °F	60	65	70	75	80	85	90	95	100	105	110	T_{wb} °C
94	84	86	87	88	90	91	93	94	96	97	99	34
92	82	84	85	87	88	90	91	93	94	96	97	33
90	81	83	84	86	87	89	90	92	93	95	96	32
88	80	81	83	84	86	87	89	90	92	93	95	31
86	78	80	81	83	84	86	87	89	90	92	93	30
84	77	78	80	81	83	84	86	87	89	90	92	29
82	75	77	78	80	81	83	84	86	87	89	90	28
80	74	76	77	79	80	82	83	85	86	88	89	27
78	73	74	76	77	79	80	82	83	85	86	88	26
76	71	73	74	76	77	79	80	82	83	85	86	24
74	70	71	73	74	76	77	79	80	82	83	85	23
72	68	70	71	73	74	76	77	79	80	82	83	22
70	67	69	70	72	73	75	76	78	79	81	82	21
64	66	67	69	70	72	73	75	76	78	79	81	20
	16	18	21	24	27	29	32	35	38	41	43	

T_{air} (°C)

For inside or outside, WBGT can be estimated from the air and wet bulb temperatures at the time and place of the exercise.

If the exercise occurs in direct sunlight, add 4°F to the estimated WBGT.

demands, and clothing are required (Table 24.3) (1, 3). Methods to reduce the level of heat stress include the following:

- Reduce exercise intensity (reduces metabolic rate).
- Reschedule exercise to cooler time of day or to cooler place.
- Reduce the amount of clothing.

Personal Protective Practices

Personal protective practices are steps an individual can take to minimize risk of heat disorder (3). Table 24.4 lists some common personal protective practices. Physiological monitoring is a useful method to assess heat. Oral temperature is a reasonably good measure under certain conditions. Oral temperature can be taken 10–15 minutes after fluid intake or strenuous exercise. Temperatures below 38°C (100.4°F) are considered safe. Temperatures above 38.5°C (101.3°F) indicate the need for immediate relief from exposure. Temperatures of 38–38.5°C suggest that relief is indicated. (Some clinical thermometers employ an infrared detector to estimate tympanic temperature; because hot environments and placement affect the outcome, use them with caution.)

Heart rate is an easily assessed index of heat strain. Recovery heart rate, assessed approximately 1 minute after discontinuing exercise, is a simple and useful method. If recovery heart rate is below 110 beats per minute (bpm), heat stress is not excessive; if the recovery heart rate is

Table 24.2. *Continued*

ESTIMATE OF WBGT (°F) FROM AIR TEMPERATURE (T_{air}) AND RELATIVE HUMIDITY (%)

RH%	60	65	70	75	80	85	90	95	100	105	110	RH%
95	60	65	70	75	80	85	90	95	100	105	110	95
90	60	64	69	74	79	85	90	95	100	105	110	90
85	59	64	68	73	78	83	89	95	100	105	110	85
80	59	63	68	72	77	82	88	93	99	105	110	80
75	58	62	67	71	76	81	86	92	98	103	110	75
70	58	62	66	71	76	80	85	90	96	102	108	70
65	57	61	68	70	74	79	84	88	94	100	105	65
60	57	60	66	69	73	78	83	87	93	98	103	60
55	56	60	64	68	72	77	81	86	91	96	101	55
50	55	59	63	67	71	75	80	84	89	94	99	50
45	55	58	62	66	70	74	79	83	88	92	97	45
40	54	58	62	65	69	73	77	82	88	90	95	40
35	54	57	61	64	68	72	76	80	84	89	93	35
30	53	57	60	64	67	71	76	79	83	87	91	30
25	53	56	59	63	66	70	73	77	81	85	89	25
20	52	55	58	62	65	69	72	76	79	83	87	20
15	51	54	58	61	64	67	71	74	76	81	85	15
10	51	54	57	60	63	68	69	73	76	79	82	10
	16	18	21	24	27	29	32	36	38	41	43	

T_{air} (°C)

For inside or outside, WBGT can be estimated from the air temperature and relative humdity at the time and place of exercise. Note: Relative humidity is very sensitive to air temperature.

If the exercise occurs in direct sunlight, add 4°F to the estimated WBGT.

above 110 bpm, relief is recommended (10, 11). The use of a heart rate monitor with an alarm for heart rate based on an acceptable limit in non–heat stress conditions (e.g., 75% of maximum heart rate) is another protective method (12).

If exercise involves cycles of exercise and recovery, oral temperature, recovery heart rate, or both may be used to assess length of the exercise and/or recovery period. Elevation of either temperature or heart rate indicates that exercise should be shortened or the recovery period extended.

COLD STRESS

Cold stress is the combination of environment, metabolic rate, and clothing that results in heat loss from the core as a whole or from local areas (2, 3, 13). Cold-related disorders include hypothermia and varying degrees of local tissue damage (1–3, 13). Again, control of cold stress is accomplished through managing risk factors.

Heat Balance

Like heat stress, cold stress is described as an imbalance between heat gained from metabolism and heat lost to the environment by convection, radiation, evaporation,

Table 24.3. Guidance Based on Estimated or Measured Values of Environmental WBGT Adjusted for Acclimation State, Metabolic Rate, and Clothing

Adjustments for external factors
   Step 1. Determine environmental WBGT.
   Step 2. If not acclimated (no recent heat stress exposure), add 3°F.
   Step 3. If the metabolic rate is light (e.g., walking), subtract 2°F.
         If the metabolic rate is heavy (e.g., sustained running), add 2°F.
   Step 4. If clothing is multiple layers, add 6°F.
         If clothing is impermeable to water, add 15°F.
Level of heat stress by WBGT and description
   <80°F: no appreciable heat stress
   80–85°F: low heat stress: implement personal protective practices
   86–88°F: moderate heat stress: increased risk; ensure adequate breaks; avoid strenuous exercise
   >88°F: high heat stress: significant risk; consider cancellation of exercise

Table 24.4. Personal Protective Practices to Reduce Risk of Heat Disorder

Seek relief from heat stress exposure with sensation of extreme discomfort, light-headedness, nausea, headache, loss of coordination, or weakness.
Main adequate hydration by drinking small amounts of water, sports drinks, diluted citrus-flavored drinks, diluted ice tea, and so on, at frequent intervals. A weight loss of 2% of body weight in 1 day is evidence of dehydration.
Maintain a healthy lifestyle through sound diet, adequate sleep, and avoiding drug abuse.
Avoid heat stress exposure and exercise during acute illness (e.g., fever, nausea, vomiting, diarrhea).
Seek medical advice if diagnosed with a chronic disease; disease or treatment may reduce heat tolerance.
Reduce expectations if no recent exercise in warm or hot environments.

and conduction (3). The problem, however, is net loss rather than net gain.

The sole source of heat gain during cold stress is metabolic heat released during muscular work along with basal biological processes. As exercise demands increase, rate of heat gain from metabolism increases. If the rate of metabolic heat decreases because of fatigue or changes in demand, a disorder is more likely (13).

Heat Loss

Heat is lost primarily by convection owing to the difference between skin and ambient temperature (2, 13, 14). The rate of convection increases with air movement from wind or motion through the air (e.g., cycling or running). Sitting or lying on a cold, solid surface may cause heat loss by conduction. Cyclic exercise and rest in which heat accumulates and the person sweats under clothing may be associated with heat loss through evaporation. Additional loss by radiant heat flow to colder surfaces is also possible.

Clothing

Proper clothing is the primary mechanism for achieving thermal balance during cold stress (13, 14). The amount of insulation that clothing affords is described in units called clo. A wool business suit has an insulating value of approximately 1 clo. Generally, each quarter-inch of clothing adds one clo of insulation. Figure 24.1 illustrates the relations among air temperature, metabolic rate, and clothing in maintaining thermal balance (14). The insulating quality of clothing decreases precipitously when it becomes wet.

Sometimes clothing is sufficient to protect from hypothermia, but exposed skin is still at risk for excessive local cooling. The major method of heat loss is convection, but conduction via contact with cold objects can also occur. Adequate heating from circulating blood may not be available because of reductions in peripheral blood flow (vasoconstriction) that naturally occur as a mechanism for heat conservation.

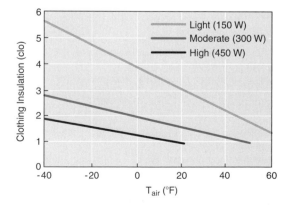

Figure 24.1. Relationship between air temperature and adequate clothing insulation for three levels of exercise.

COLD-RELATED DISORDERS

Normal physiological response to cold stress is directed toward heat conservation, decreasing peripheral circulation and increasing metabolic rate. These mechanisms, however, are not adequate for most cold stress, and behavioral thermal regulation is crucial for preventing cold-related disorders. Cold-related disorders can be systemic or local. Table 24.5 is a list of some common cold-related disorders along with symptoms, signs, and steps for first aid (1–3, 13).

Table 24.5. Cold-Related Disorders, Including Symptoms, Signs, and First Aid

Hypothermia
  Symptoms
    Chills
    Fatigue or drowsiness
    Pain in the extremities
  Signs
    Euphoria
    Slurred speech
    Slow, weak pulse
    Shivering
    Collapse and/or unconsciousness
    Body core temperature <35°C (95°F)
  First aid
    Move to warm area and remove wet clothing
    Modest external warming
    Drink warm carbohydrate-containing fluids
    Transport to hospital
Frostbite
  Symptoms
    Burning sensation at first
    Coldness, numbness, tingling
  Signs
    Skin color white or grayish yellow to reddish violet to black
    Blisters
    Response to touch depends on depth of freezing
  First aid
    Move to warm area and remove wet clothing
    External warming (e.g., warm water)
    Drink warm carbohydrate-containing fluids if conscious
    Treat as a burn; do not rub affected area
    Transport to hospital
Frost nip
  Symptoms
    Possible itching or pain
  Signs
    Skin turns white
  First aid
    Similar to frostbite
Trench foot
  Symptoms
    Severe pain
    Tingling, itching
  Signs
    Edema
    Blisters
    Response to touch depends on depth of cooling
  First aid
    Similar to frostbite

Table 24.6. Table for Determining Equivalent Chill Temperature in °F from Air Temperature and Air Motion

AIR SPEED		AIR TEMPERATURE (°F)												
		50	40	30	20	10	0	−10	−20	−30	−40	−50	−60	
MPH	M/S	EQUIVALENT CHILL TEMPERATURE (°F)												
0	0.0	50	40	30	20	10	0	−10	−20	−30	−40	−50	−60	
5	2.2	48	37	27	16	6	−5	−15	−26	−36	−47	−57	−68	
10	4.5	40	28	16	4	−9	−24	−33	−46	−58	−70	−83	−95	
15	6.7	36	22	9	−5	−18	−32	−45	58	−72	−85	−99	−112	
20	8.9	32	18	4	−10	−25	−39	−53	−67	82	−96	−110	−121	
25	11	30	16	0	−15	−29	−44	−59	−74	−88	−104	−118	−133	
30	13	28	13	−2	−18	−33	−48	−63	−79	−94	−109	−125	−140	
35	16	27	11	−4	−20	−35	−51	−67	−82	−98	−113	−129	−145	
>35	>16	26	10	−6	−21	−37	−53	−69	−85	−100	−116	−132	−148	

Little danger	**Increasing danger**	**Great danger**
If exposures with dry skin are less than 60 min. Caution: Avoid false sense of security.	Exposed flesh may freeze within 1 min.	Flesh may freeze within 30 sec.

Caution: Trench foot may occur anywhere on this chart.

Developed by the US Army Research Institute of Environmental Medicine, Natick, MA.

Systemic Cold

The systemic cold disorder is hypothermia. Mild cases are marked by shivering and cold sensation in extremities. Progression is associated with unstable cardiac function followed by central nervous system depression. Mild cases can be addressed by simple first aid, but moderate to severe hypothermia requires medical attention.

Local Disorders

Acute local disorders are associated with local tissue freezing (frostbite) or cooling (frost nip and trench foot). Frostbite can occur only when ambient temperature is < −1°C (30°F): it is marked by actual crystallization of water in tissue and subsequent destruction of cells. Because of the risk of further complication, significant cases of frostbite should be referred to medical personnel. Frost nip and trench foot are skin disorders resulting from extreme cooling of the skin and underlying tissue, but without actual freezing of water in the tissue. The distinguishing characteristic between frost nip and trench foot is the presence of damp clothing accelerating heat loss.

MANAGEMENT OF COLD STRESS DURING EXERCISE

Environmental conditions, especially air temperature and air speed, along with exercise demands are considered in management of cold stress. Ultimately, cold stress is managed through personal protective practices (3).

Evaluation of Cold Stress

Air temperature alone has utility for predicting degree of cold stress, but the role of air motion in facilitating loss of heat is also important. While cold stress indices are undergoing review, the equivalent chill temperature (ECT) is a useful way to account for both air temperature and motion. ECT translates a combination of air temperature and motion to an equivalent air temperature with no air motion. Table 24.6 is used to determine ECT. The table provides guidance with regard to overall risk of a cold-related disorder with an emphasis on exposed skin (1, 3). Table 24.7 provides guidelines for cold stress as a function of air temperature (T_{air}) and ECT. Generally, some risk may be present with exercise at air temperatures below 50°F.

Personal Protective Practices

Personal responsibility is key to successful management of cold stress. Table 24.8 provides minimal protective practices for risk management of cold-related disorders (3).

Table 24.7. Cold Stress Guidance Based on Air Temperature (T_{air}) and Equivalent Chill Temperature (ECT)

RISK	T_{air} (°F)	ECT (°F)
Decreases in manual dexterity	60	
Hypothermia (no special clothing)	50	50
Hypothermia (with special clothing)	Figure 24.1	
Frost nip		−22
Frostbite	30	
Prolonged contact with objects	30	
Incidental contact with objects	19	

Table 24.8. Personal Protective Practices to Reduce the Risk of Cold Disorders

Seek relief from cold stress exposure with sensation of extreme discomfort, especially extremities; fatigue or weakness; or loss of coordination.

Frequently drink warm, caffeine-free fluids containing carbohydrates.

Anticipate, wear, and adjust as necessary proper clothing.

Change wet clothing immediately, especially if the air temperature is <36°F.

Plan exercise to avoid fatigue at a location removed from a warm recovery station.

Maintain a healthy lifestyle through sound diet, adequate sleep, and avoiding drug abuse.

Seek medical advice for repeated or unusual intolerance to cold, such as repeated episodes of frost nip, apperances of welts, or severe shivering. Medical approval for exercise at ECT <−11°F is recommended.

Appropriate practices are recommended for exercise at air temperatures below 50°F.

► SUMMARY

Environmental stressors such as heat and cold can significantly affect exercise and can be dangerous if uncontrolled. Adequate preventive precautions for both heat and cold are possible and should be known by exercise professionals. Situations requiring medical attention are fairly common, and immediate referral of such problems is important.

References

1. McArdle D, Katch FI, Katch VL, eds. Exercise Physiology. 4th ed. Philadelphia: Lea & Febiger, 1996.
2. Pandolf B, Sawka MN, Gonzalez RG, eds. Human Performance Physiology and Environmental Medicine at Terrestrial Extremes. Carmel, IN: Cooper, 1986.
3. Bernard E. Thermal Stress. In: Plog BA, ed. Fundamentals in Industrial Hygiene. Itasca, IL: National Safety Council, 1996.
4. Eastman Kodak Company. Ergonomic Design for People at Work, vol 2. New York: Van Nostrand Reinhold, 1986.
5. International Organization for Standardization. Hot environments: Analytical determination and interpretation of thermal stress using calculation of required sweat rate. Geneva: ISO 7933, 1989.
6. Wyndham CH, Strydom NB, Benade JS, et al. Heat stroke risk in unacclimatized and acclimatized men of different maximum oxygen intakes working under hot humid conditions. Chamber of Mines Research Report 12/72. Johannesburg: Chamber of Mines of South Africa, 1972.
7. Parsons KC. Human Thermal Environments. Bristol, PA: Taylor & Francis, 1993.
8. Kamon E, Avellini BD. Wind speed limits to work under hot environments for clothed men. J Appl Physiol 46:340–349, 1979.
9. Rowell LB. Human Cardiovascular Control. Cary, NC: Oxford University, 1994.
10. Kenney WL, Humphrey RH, Bryant CX, et al., eds. ACSM's Guidelines for Exercise Testing and Prescription. 5th ed. Baltimore: Williams & Wilkins, 1995.
11. Bernard TE, Kenney WL. Heart rate recovery. American Industrial Hygiene Conference, 1988.
12. Humen DP, Boughner DR. Evaluation of commercially available heart rate monitors. Can Med Assoc J 131:585–589, 1984.
13. Holmer I. Cold Stress: 1.Guidelines for the practitioner. 2. The scientific basis (knowledge base) for the guide. Int J Indust Ergonom 14:139–159, 1994.
14. Holmer I. Assessment of cold stress in terms of required clothing insulation: IREQ. Int J Indust Ergonom 3:159–166, 1988.

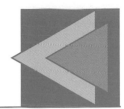

CHAPTER **25**

EXERCISE AND THE ENVIRONMENT: ALTITUDE AND AIR POLLUTION

George Havenith and Michael Holewijn

The condition of ambient air, which is inhaled into the lungs for respiratory gas exchange, has great importance for exercise capacity, physiological performance, and general health. This chapter discusses two main characteristics of ambient air: density, which changes with altitude, and contaminants, generally referred to as air pollution. It is necessary to be aware of hazards, since exposure to altitude and polluted air can have profound effects on physical performance and can cause serious illness even in well-trained individuals.

HIGH TERRESTRIAL ALTITUDE

Considerable evidence indicates that altitude training in preparation for competition at altitude is beneficial; therefore, many athletes spend considerable resources training at altitude. However, the value of this training for increasing performance at sea level is controversial. The lack of consensus may be attributed to differences in duration of exposure to altitude, elevations of training, initial fitness levels, and lack of a control group (1). Recent studies indicate that under specific conditions, intermittent altitude exposure may have some beneficial effects for sea level performance (2–4). In this section, physiological responses that occur at altitudes up to 3000 m (11,800 feet) are discussed. Above 3000 m, the negative effects of prolonged exposure to hypoxia outweigh any positive training effects (5).

Physiological Responses

The amount of oxygen bound to hemoglobin in red blood cells depends on the partial pressure of oxygen in the inspired air (P_IO_2). P_IO_2 decreases as a result of declines in barometric pressure with increasing altitude at constant oxygen percentage (Table 25.1). There is a fall in the arterial oxygen saturation (PaO_2) with the decline in P_IO_2 and, thus, in the amount of oxygen available. Acute exposure to reduced oxygen saturation triggers several compensatory mechanisms to increase oxygen transfer to tissue. Following these acute reactions acclimation occurs with more fundamental adaptations.

Acute Physiological Responses

One of the most significant physiological compensatory reactions during acute exposure above 1,200 m is increased pulmonary ventilation, or hypoxic ventilatory response, at rest and during exercise. Chemoreceptors in arterial blood vessels are stimulated, and signals are sent to the brain to increase ventilation. The increase in pulmonary ventilation is primarily associated with an increase in tidal volume, but with prolonged exposure or higher altitude, breathing frequency also increases. Hyperventilation substantially increases the arterial oxygen saturation. Increased ventilation also leads to washout of carbon dioxide in the blood. Therefore, uncompensated respiratory alkalosis (higher pH) may develop. This respiratory alkalosis can cause a left shift of the oxygen–hemoglobin dissociation curve, resulting in higher arterial oxygen saturation, a second compensatory mechanism (6). Finally, early in exposure to altitude, reduced oxygen pressure is compensated for by small increases in cardiac output. This is primarily because of an increased heart rate, since stroke volume is constant or even slightly reduced at rest and during submaximal and maximal exercise.

Despite acute responses that compensate for lower oxygen tension at altitude, arterial oxygen saturation is decreased (Fig. 25.1). The magnitude of desaturation is directly related to altitude and exercise intensity. The primary pulmonary factor leading to increasing desaturation with increasing exercise intensity is limited alveolar end capillary diffusion. The result is an almost linear decrease of maximal oxygen uptake at a ratio of 10% per 1000 m altitude above 1500 m (7). Since the oxygen uptake required by a fixed submaximal workload is not affected by altitude, the result is a higher relative exercise intensity for any given workload. Because of the nonlinear relationship between relative intensity (percent maximal oxygen uptake, or [$\dot{V}O_{2max}$]) and endurance time, the magnitude of the performance decrement at altitude is not constant but varies in proportion to the duration of the activity. Therefore, the longer the running distance, the larger the relative decrement (8).

Table 25.1. Barometric Pressure for a Standard Atmosphere and Inspired Partial Oxygen Pressure for Five Altitudes, Accounting for the Pressure of Water Vapor in the Lungs (47 mm Hg)

ALTITUDE (M)	BAROMETRIC PRESSURE (MM HG)	INSPIRED OXYGEN PRESSURE (P_IO_2)
0	760	149
1500	627	123
2000	596	115
2500	627	107
3000	522	100

Muscular strength and muscular endurance seem unaffected during acute exposure to altitude. However, subtle neuropsychological effects associated with acute mountain sickness can occur at altitudes of 3000 m within 6 hours of exposure. Above 4500 m the deterioration in most mental functions may be considerable, although variations between individuals are large (9). These neuropsychological effects may in turn affect muscular strength and endurance.

Long-Term Physiological Responses: Acclimation

With prolonged stay at altitude (days to weeks), acclimation occurs. This includes adjustments at the pulmonary, circulatory, and muscle tissue (cellular) level. Within 3–4 days, the increase in resting ventilatory rate at moderate altitude (3000 m) is stabilized at 40% above sea level values. The increase in exercise ventilation rate also stabilizes, but in a longer time frame, depending on exercise intensity and altitude. After acclimation, pulmonary ventilation during exercise can increase 100% over sea level controls. This increase becomes more pronounced as workloads increase (10).

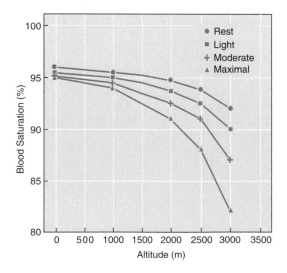

Figure 25.1. The effect of altitude and exercise levels on arterial oxygen saturation.

Red cell production increases (polycythemia) within 2 weeks, leading to a 4–12% increase in hemoglobin (11). Increased red blood cell production is the result of a substantial increase in erythropoietin (EPO) hormone concentration (11). Maximum levels of EPO (produced in the kidney) occur within the first few days, followed by a gradual fall to sea level concentration within a month. Hematocrit (ratio of red blood cells to total blood volume) and blood viscosity increase because of the polycythemia, but a substantial reduction of plasma volume during the first weeks at altitude (up to 15% at 3500 m) has the greatest early effect on hematocrit (6, 10).

With increasing acclimation to altitude, cardiac output at rest and during submaximal and maximal exercise is reduced because of decreased stroke volume. This process is complete within 2 weeks. The decrease in maximal stroke volume, which may be considered a negative side effect, is probably because of increased blood viscosity and lower filling pressure leading to a decreased venous return. Acclimation to altitude does not change heart rate during submaximal exercise (it remains elevated) (10). However, chronic hypoxia seems to lower maximal heart rate depending on altitude and duration of exposure (12).

It is unclear whether systemic oxygen transport is altered with acclimation by changes in the shape and position of the oxygen dissociation curve. The concentration of 2,3-diphosophoglycerate in red blood cells increases, shifting the dissociation curve to the right and facilitating unloading of oxygen from hemoglobin to tissue (10). This positive effect can be overwhelmed by the opposite effect, systemic alkalosis. The net effect of both mechanisms is unknown.

In skeletal muscle, capillary density, mitochondrial number, and tissue myoglobin concentration increase, so that in exercising muscle chronic hypoxic exposure results in an improved peripheral oxygen uptake. There is increased mobilization and use of free fatty acids, sparing muscle glycogen and increasing endurance time (13).

As a result of these physiological adaptations with acclimation, physical work capacity ($\dot{V}O_{2max}$ and endurance) at altitude improves and at moderate altitude may nearly reach sea level values with adequate acclimation time. Generally, about 2–3 weeks are needed to adapt to moderate altitude. Each 600-m increase requires an additional week. All of these adaptive changes are reversible on return to sea level, and within a month after ending exposure, adaptation is lost (6).

TRAINING AT ALTITUDE

Some coaches and athletes can provide "evidence from the practice" supporting the use of altitude training to enhance performance at sea level. Until recently, few well-controlled studies showing consistent improvement in sea level performance because of altitude training were available. Differences in type of athlete, altitude level, training, and testing method do not allow some of the improvements to be attributed solely to altitude residence (3). Furthermore, the measured performance indices (e.g., $\dot{V}O_{2max}$) can be inappropriate to reflect performance changes. It can be argued that the concept of $\dot{V}O_{2max}$ is not always relevant and sensitive enough to mirror performance changes (14). Recently some beneficial effects of altitude training for elite athletes who have reached a plateau have been suggested (4, 15, 16).

Altitude training can be performed by training at altitude, by using gas mixtures with lower partial oxygen pressure (Po_2) or by training in a hypobaric chamber. Each of these methods has advantages and disadvantages. Hypobaric chambers are sparsely available, and hypoxic gas mixtures interfere with high training intensities because of their flow and other equipment limitations; therefore, simulated altitude training has rarely been conducted except for research purposes.

Care should be taken to choose adequate altitude level, since the relationship between altitude and magnitude of physiological adaptation depends on the physiological variable in question. Adaptations aimed at changing oxygen transport are related to level of oxygen saturation. The most significant adaptations are seen when training is done at 2000–2500 m (3). The concept that "higher is better" may be compromised by severe side effects of exposure to high altitude. Altitudes above 4000 m are known to result in loss of body mass because of initial loss of water and subsequent loss of fat and muscle mass (5).

One of the major disadvantages that mitigates potential beneficial effects of altitude training is the necessary reduction in training workload. Because of the reduction in aerobic power, elite athletes may not reach and sustain normal training workloads at high altitudes (3, 17). In the initial days after arrival at altitude, training sessions of short duration (e.g., moderate to high intensity with prolonged rest intervals) can be performed at sea level intensities. Aerobic exercise in the first week of acclimation should be restricted to short durations, but within 2 weeks training workload can be increased, and maximal training performance can be achieved within 3–4 weeks of residence (18). Prolonged high-intensity exercise during initial exposure should be avoided to minimize exercise-induced decrease of EPO production, which delays polycythemia (11). Performance in activities with a large anaerobic component, which involve rapid body displacement, may actually be slightly improved because of decreased air resistance and weaker gravity. Special attention should be given to control of caloric and fluid intake. To meet the increased iron demand associated with polycythemia, supplemental oral iron intake in combination with vitamin C and vitamin E should be initiated 2–3 weeks before ascent and continued 2–4 weeks afterward (11).

Recently, alternatives for altitude training have been suggested. A primary reason for the absence of performance improvement in altitude training is reduced training intensity and volume. To avoid this, intermittent exposure or training in hypobaric chambers has been recommended. The time outside the chamber can be used to obtain a normal daily training volume. In this way it is possible to potentiate the effects of hypoxia (increases in hemoglobin, hematocrit, capillary density, and altered substrate use) without negative effects of prolonged living at high altitude (reduction of blood volume, loss of muscle and body mass, reduction of maximal heart rate) (1, 15). In five of six studies of subjects living at sea level and exercising at simulated altitude, enhanced performance at both sea level and altitude has been reported (2).

HIGH-ALTITUDE ILLNESS

Exposure to high altitude can lead to a number of illnesses that vary in seriousness. The speed of ascent and the absolute altitude are primary determinants of the incidence of altitude illness. Those exercising in or exposed to altitude (athletes and coaches) should anticipate the hazards and prepare through prevention and recognition of symptoms.

Acute Mountain Sickness

Acute mountain sickness (AMS) is characterized by severe headache and often accompanied by nausea, vomiting, decreased appetite, weariness, and sleep disturbances (19). AMS begins 6–12 hours after arrival, usually peaks on the second or third day, and disappears on the fourth or fifth day (20). AMS normally appears above 2500 m, and the frequency of AMS increases with altitude and rate of ascent. Generally, above 3000 m, 24 hours of acclimation should be acquired for every 300 m altitude gain (20). Although AMS is self-limiting, persistence of symptoms may require medical treatment. If AMS is not at least partially resolved within 2–3 days, descent is the only effective treatment. Supplemental oxygen and pharmacological treatment (acetazolamide, furosemide, analgesics) may be necessary for severe cases.

High-Altitude Pulmonary Edema

High-altitude pulmonary edema (HAPE) is considered a progression in the severity of AMS, associated with pulmonary edema (20). The onset may be subtle. Signs and symptoms include dyspnea, fatigue, chest pain, tachycardia, coughing, and cyanosis of lips and extremities. As HAPE progresses, affected individuals may cough frothy or blood-tinged sputum (19). This complication can be fatal if not treated promptly. Children and young adults are at higher risk of developing HAPE than adults, and immediate medical attention is necessary. Evacuation to lower altitude is essential. Individuals with a history of HAPE appear to be particularly susceptible to subsequent bouts upon return to altitude.

High-Altitude Cerebral Edema

High-altitude cerebral edema (HACE) may develop when the rate of ascent is too fast. The signs and symptoms of HACE include severe headache, fatigue, vomiting, nausea, ataxia, and changes of mental status (19). The incidence of HACE is low (1%), but HACE can be fatal if untreated. In cases of symptoms of cerebral edema, direct medical care with immediate evacuation to low altitude and supplemental oxygen is recommended (21).

Preventing Altitude Sickness

AMS is prevented by adjusting the amount and rate of ascent. Options include an interrupted ascent with time (days) to acclimate at successive altitudes before reaching final elevation or limiting daily gain in altitude to 300 m or less. Initially, unacclimated subjects should avoid vigorous exercise. Adequate hydration and a high-carbohydrate diet may aid prevention. Acetazolamide is the only drug for altitude sickness approved by the Food and Drug Administration (FDA). Since acetazolamide may affect exercise performance, it is contraindicated when training at altitude. Prophylactic administration of acetazolamide may be effective (19).

AIR POLLUTION

Air pollution can also affect exercise performance and health. Though nature contributes through ozone (O_3) from lightning, dust, and sulfuric oxides from volcano activity and other natural pollutants, the problem with polluted air is widespread since the start of the industrial revolution. Specific pollutants that affect human welfare reflect industrial development. Organizers of sporting events or exercisers are frequently confronted with problems related to exercising in polluted air. Both large sporting events and daily activity are performed in major cities, which are generally the sites with the highest pollution levels. Also, with indoor training and sports events, the infiltration of outdoor air pollution may be significant. Furthermore, the indoor environment may actually add to the problem with indoor air pollutants emitted by the occupants, activities, and building materials.

There are two major groups of pollutants: primary and secondary. Primary pollutants are directly attributable to a source of pollution, such as carbon monoxide (CO), sulfur oxides, nitrogen oxides, hydrocarbons, and particulates (dust, smoke, and soot). Secondary pollutants result from an interaction of the environment (sunlight, moisture, other pollutants) with primary pollutants. These include O_3, aldehydes, sulfuric acid (H_2SO_4), and peroxyacetyl nitrate (PAN). City air commonly contains both primary and secondary pollutants.

General Effector Mechanisms

The effect of pollutants is in part related to level of penetration. This "dosage" is determined by exposure time, concentration of pollutant in inspired air, ventilation rate, temperature and humidity of inspired air, and route of inspiration (the nose versus the mouth). Pollution primarily affects the respiratory tract. This tract provides a large surface area for contact by the pollutant. The mucous membranes of the nose effectively remove large particles and highly soluble gases (e.g., 99.9% of inhaled SO_2), preventing them from affecting deeper airways and lung tissue. However, smaller particles and agents with low solubility pass through this barrier easily. During exercise, when mouth breathing plays an important role, this air filtration is less efficient, and more pollutants reach the lungs, traverse the diffusion surface, and enter the blood and body tissues. Pollutants can have several effects during their course through the body, including the following:

- Irritation of the airways, which may lead to bronchoconstriction, hence increased airway resistance
- Reduction of alveolar diffusion capacity
- Reduction of oxygen transport capacity

Other effects of pollutants that can indirectly affect exercise performance are irritation of eyes (PAN and formaldehyde) and skin. Short-term effects of exposure to pollutants rather than long-term exposure is discussed in this chapter.

Outdoor Pollution

Geographical distribution of outdoor pollution is strongly related to industry and population density. Automobiles, trucks, buses, aircraft, industrial sources, and combustion of fossil fuels are major sources of CO, sulfur and nitrogen oxides, hydrocarbons, and particles. Areas with equal production of pollutants do not necessarily have equally polluted air, or smog, because climate and topography play major roles. River and mountain valleys generally have greater smog levels than hilltops and plains. High temperature and humidity typically promote photochemical smog with associated high O_3 levels. For example, in the Los Angeles area, such smog, trapped by summer winds toward the surrounding mountains, is a common phenomenon (22). Low temperature with a concomitant increase in fuel consumption for heating and high humidity (fog, rain) promote a different type of fog, in which high sulfur oxide concentrations combined with particulate matter are converted into sulfuric acid (acid rain) and sulfates. The most famous fog of this type is the London fog, which produced a large number of deaths in 1952 (4000 in a 4-day period) (23). Such fog can be persistent when temperature inversion occurs, a condition brought about by little wind and a layer of cool polluted air trapped beneath a layer of warmer air.

Specific Pollutants

Carbon monoxide

CO is the most common pollutant in urban areas. It plays a role in indoor events because of emissions from equipment (usually gas powered), but is more commonly associated with motor vehicle exhaust outdoors. The ambient concentration of CO tends to be highest during peak traffic flow and at low temperatures (Fig. 25.2) (23). The primary effect of CO is the formation of carboxyhemoglobin (COHb) because of its high affinity (> 200 times that of oxygen) for hemoglobin. Exposure to 100 parts per million (ppm) CO for 8 hours leads to more than 12% COHb. COHb is difficult to dissociate, and it impedes oxygen transport from lungs to cells (24). CO also reduces release of oxygen from hemoglobin in tissues because of a leftward shift in the lower end of the oxygen dissociation curve (25). COHb concentrations above 20% are required to produce these effects. However, during submaximal exercise, little effect has been observed. Such values are generally higher than those found in typically polluted air. At COHb concentrations below 20%, augmented heart rate, cardiac contractility, and cardiac output compensate for the COHb.

During maximal exercise, both exercise time and VO_{2max} are inversely related to CO concentration. The critical concentration for reduced $\dot{V}O_{2max}$ is near 4.3% COHb (approximately 100 ppm CO in inhaled air for 2 hours), which, considering that COHb concentration during prolonged exposure to heavy traffic can reach 5%, has practical importance (26). Individuals with coronary artery disease may be at risk during submaximal exercise. During exercise at COHb concentrations above 6%, arrhythmias have been observed, and concentrations of 2% COHb have been shown to decrease exercise time to the onset of angina. Smokers have higher baseline levels of COHb (> 4%). However, since the CO gradient between lungs and blood during ambient exposure is lower than for nonsmokers, the additional negative effect of CO from air pollution is less than for nonsmokers (22).

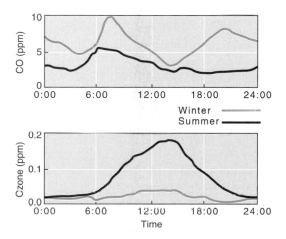

Figure 25.2. Daily and seasonal fluctuations in CO and ozone concentrations in the Los Angeles area. (Reprinted with permission from McCafferty W. Air Pollution and Athletic Performance. Springfield, IL: Charles C Thomas, 1981.)

Sulfur Oxides

Sulfur oxides, mainly in the form of sulfur dioxide (SO_2) or acid sulfides, have their main influence through irritation of the upper respiratory tract, which can cause reflex bronchoconstriction and increased airway resistance. Nose breathing strongly reduces this effect compared to mouth breathing, since nasal mucosa removes up to 99.9% of SO_2 before it reaches sensitive bronchial areas (27). Ambient air values of SO_2 do not normally reach concentrations that have important effects on lung function in normal, healthy subjects (28). In submaximal exercise, pulmonary function starts to be affected between 1 and 3 ppm; threshold values for maximal exercise are unknown. However, athletes in competition may be at risk because of extreme pulmonary ventilation and concomitant mouth breathing. Scrubbing in the upper respiratory tract may be less effective; thus, more pollutant is able to reach sensitive areas. People with reactive airway disease (asthma) are nearly five times as sensitive to SO_2 as those without. Sensitivity is exacerbated by cold and/or dry air (27).

Nitrogen Oxides

Of the nitrogen oxides, only nitrogen dioxide and nitric acid vapor have been studied in humans. Acute exposure to extreme concentrations of nitrogen dioxide (200–4000 ppm) can result in death. During submaximal exercise (below 50% $\dot{V}O_{2max}$) no effect has been observed for concentrations up to 1–2 ppm, which is rarely exceeded in the atmosphere. Effects of higher concentrations are unknown. Nitric acid inspiration up to a concentration of 500 $\mu g/m^3$ (0.18 ppm) has not been shown to cause any proximal airway or distal lung injury, nor has it been shown to increase airway resistance (29).

Particulate Matter: Aerosols, Soot, Dust, and Smoke

Particulate matter is solid or liquid particles in air. The physiological effect of minute particles in exercising humans has not been evaluated. Normally particulate inhalation is associated with bronchoconstriction. The penetration of particulates into the respiratory system is related to particle size (22). Particles smaller than 3 μm may reach alveoli, while those between 3 and 5 μm usually settle in areas of the upper respiratory tract. Particles larger than 5 μm are normally removed by coughing, sneezing, and ciliary action and do not reach the respiratory tract at all. Thus, particles smaller than 5 μm can be associated with bronchial inflammation, congestion, or ulceration. The shift from nose to mouth breathing during exercise increases the amount of particulates reaching the alveoli.

There are a large number of aerosols, and their effect on exercise performance is usually related to airway irritation. The most common aerosols are sulfates, which seem to have minimal adverse effects. Sulfuric acids have minimal adverse effects except when prolonged exposure occurs or there are large particles and/or high ambient relative humidity. Nitrate aerosols have minimal to no effect, and saturated and unsaturated aldehydes (e.g., formaldehyde, acrolein, and crotonaldehyde) have minimal effects other than irritation.

Ozone

The production of the secondary pollutant O_3 involves sunlight (UV) or electrical arcs, and therefore, concentration is highest during daytime (Fig. 25.2). In contrast to the O_3 in the upper atmosphere, O_3 at ground level can create a health risk. Most inhaled O_3 is absorbed by mucous membranes in the respiratory tract. The dose depends on inspiratory concentration, lung ventilation level, and duration of exposure. Symptoms related to O_3 exposure include throat irritation, cough, nausea, inability to take a deep breath, headaches, and substernal pain. Such symptoms predominate in asthmatics. O_3 poisoning has been reported in welders (secondary to electrical arcs) exposed to 9.2 ppm. Inhalation of 50 ppm O_3 for 30 minutes may be fatal.

During light to moderate submaximal exercise lasting several hours, exposures to 0.3–0.45 ppm O_3 have resulted in decrements in pulmonary function (reduced force vital capacity and forced expiratory volume) and increased subjective discomfort. However, no limitation of cardiorespiratory function has been observed. Adverse reactions have been observed at O_3 concentrations as low as 0.08 to 0.12 ppm after prolonged exposure (7 hours) (30). These concentrations are fairly common in ambient air. During heavy submaximal and perhaps maximal exercise, inspiration of 0.2–0.3 ppm O_3 may be limiting because of respiratory discomfort and associated changes in pulmonary function (shallow, rapid breathing) (25). Repeated exposure to O_3 (3–5 days) leads to desensitization, with a reduction in symptoms. Whether suppression of a natural defense mechanism is compatible with long-term health is questionable (23).

Peroxyacetyl Nitrate

The effects of the secondary pollutant PAN, formed from nitrogen oxides and organic compounds, have been studied for concentrations up to 0.27 ppm. Concentrations up to this level did not result in significant effects during either submaximal or maximal exercise. The threshold value is apparently higher but unknown. PAN concentration in the atmosphere rarely exceeds 0.1 ppm, however (28). Eye irritation can occur at concentrations lower than 0.27 ppm.

Indoor Pollution

Since many buildings where exercise and sports events are performed are ventilated with unfiltered outside air, the indoor air is also polluted. The choice of site for air intake can have a substantial effect on indoor air quality. Indoor air is also characterized by a wide spectrum of compounds occurring at low levels that emanate from building materials, furniture, carpeting, office equipment, human metabolism, and tobacco smoke. The major indoor substances of concern for human health are as follows:

- Soil gases: radon, gas from landfills, such as methane, CO_2, hydrogen sulfide, and volatile organic compounds from building materials
- Combustion products: CO and nitrogen dioxide leakage from garage spaces, cooking areas, heating appliances
- Tobacco smoke
- Formaldehyde from particle boards containing urea–formaldehyde resin-based adhesives or urea–formaldehyde foam insulation
- Metabolic gases from humans, animals

Most of these substances have long-term effects on health. Others, rather than being toxic hazards, present more of a nuisance odor.

Of the substances not previously described, short-term effects at realistic pollution levels are found from exposure only to formaldehyde, volatile organic compounds, and tobacco smoke. Formaldehyde is a colorless reactive gas with a pungent smell. Its effect on humans is irritation of the eyes and respiratory system, and it may affect exercise performance (31). Human response to volatile organic compounds in indoor air is acute or subacute inflammationlike reactions of skin or mucous membranes or subacute and weak stresslike reactions. The most commonly occurring and rapidly felt effects of tobacco smoke are irritation of mucous membranes of the eyes, nose, and throat. Circulating smoke in the environment is also an important source of CO for nonsmokers, producing a COHb concentration of up to 3% and resulting in irritation and discomfort in up to 20% of those exposed to 2 ppm (24, 31).

Interactions

Air commonly contains several pollutants, and the presence of more than one can result in interactions, which can make it additive, synergistic, or nullifying. Several combinations (CO and PAN, O_3 and SO_2, SO_2 and nitrogen dioxide) have been shown to produce additive effects, but additional research is needed. Furthermore, a pollutant and other environmental stressors, such as heat or cold and high altitude, can interact. Heat stress has generally been shown to be a more significant stressor than air pollution, and additive effects have been observed for heat stress and CO, PAN, and O_3 (26). Low relative humidity may facilitate adverse effects of O_3, whereas high relative humidity may facilitate adverse effects of SO_2 and nitrogen dioxide (23).

Humidity also plays an important role in the determination of indoor air quality. High humidity stimulates growth of bacteria, dust mites, molds, and other fungi, which may cause allergy and bad smells. Occasionally these organisms breed in and are distributed by poorly maintained humidifiers and air conditioning systems. High humidity also enhances the emission of chemicals from building materials. Conversely, low humidity causes dryness and facilitates irritation of skin and mucous membranes in some individuals. Indoor humidity levels of 30–70% without condensation in cold spots usually does not cause these types of problems (31). Breathing air colder than 0°C can result in reflex bronchoconstriction, especially in individuals with reactive airways. In addition, the combination of cold air and a pollutant, such as SO_2, may have a synergistic effect.

Interaction of pollutants with exercise at high altitudes has been studied only for CO. This combination is relatively common because of incomplete combustion of fuels at altitude. The combination of low Po_2 and competition between O_2 and CO for hemoglobin binding sites seems additive rather than synergistic and may impair performance (22). Smokers appear to be less affected by the combination of moderate altitude and low COHb levels (4%) (22).

Prevention

Avoidance of exposure is the primary method for preventing acute and long-term adverse effects of outdoor pollutants. Timing and selection of optimal location for exercise and moderating intensity and duration are key factors (26). Knowledge of daily and seasonal patterns and fluctuations (Fig. 25.2) is important when planning an event involving high-intensity exercise. Avoiding periods and areas with heavy traffic can minimize CO exposure. Summer and early autumn afternoons are unfavorable for O_3 exposure.

Information on air pollution can be acquired from local meteorological authorities, many of which provide a

pollutant standards index (PSI) developed by the Environmental Protection Agency. The PSI converts measured pollutant concentration to a number on a scale from 0–500. The critical number is 100, since this corresponds to the threshold established under the Clean Air Act (Table 25.2) (28). A PSI above 100 indicates pollution in an unhealthful range. PSI places maximum emphasis on acute health effects (24 hours or less), rather than chronic effects, making it useful for exercise planning. It does not incorporate interactions between pollutants. Table 25.3 has information on the PSI (28).

Table 25.2. National Ambient Air Quality Standards as Provided by the Environmental Protection Agency

POLLUTANTS	TIME PERIOD FOR AVERAGING	STANDARD LIMIT LEVEL
Carbon monoxide	8 hr	9 ppm
	1 hr	35 ppm
Ozone	1 hr	0.12 ppm
	8 hr	0.08 ppm
Nitrogen dioxide (NO$_2$)	AAM	0.053 ppm
Sulfur dioxide (SO$_2$)	AAM	80 µg/m^3
	24 hr	365 µg/m^3
Particulates (PM-2.5) (<2.5-micron diameter)	AAM	15 µg/m^3
	24 hr	65 µg/m^3
Particulates (PM-10) (<10-micron diameter)	AAM	50 µg/m^3
	24 hr	150 µg/m^3

AAM, annual arithmetic mean.
For pollutants with high hourly or daily fluctuations, longer duration averages and short-term peak level limits are provided. The numbers correspond to a pollution standards index (PSI) of 100.

Table 25.3. The PSI and Implications for Short-Term Health Effects

INDEX VALUE	PSI DESCRIPTOR	GENERAL HEALTH EFFECTS	CAUTIONARY STATEMENTS
Up to 50	Good	None for the general population.	None required.
51–100	Moderate	Few or none for the general population.	None required.
101–200	Unhealthful	Mild aggravation of symptoms among susceptible people, with irritation symptoms in the healthy population.	Persons with existing heart or respiratory ailments should reduce physical exertion and outdoor activity. General population should reduce vigorous outdoor activity.
201–300	Very unhealthful	Significant aggravation of symptoms and decreased exercise tolerance in persons with heart or lung disease; widespread symptoms in the healthy population.	Elderly and persons with heart or lung disease should stay indoors and reduce physical activity. General population should avoid vigorous outdoor activity.
>300	Hazardous	Early onset of certain diseases in addition to significant aggravation of symptoms and decreased exercise tolerance in healthy persons. At PSI levels above 400, premature death of ill and elderly persons may result. Healthy people have adverse symptoms that affect normal activity.	Elderly and persons with diseases should stay indoors and avoid physical exertion. At PSI levels above 400, general population should avoid outdoor activity. All people should remain indoors, keeping windows and doors closed, and minimize physical exertion.

PSI, pollution standards index.

The important factors for controlling exposure to indoor pollution include selecting an optimal location for air intake, using low-emission building materials, regularly cleaning and use of low-dust floor coverings, clean ventilation and air conditioning systems, and sufficiently high fresh-air ventilation rate. More specifically, exercise centers and fitness facilities require higher ventilation rates than offices and living quarters. A CO_2 concentration limit of 1000 ppm at an outdoor concentration of 350 ppm is often used as an indicator of adequate ventilation. At that level, 80% of the users are satisfied with air quality. A level of 650 ppm CO_2 is needed to increase satisfaction to 90% (31). Indoor exercise areas should maintain the lowest CO_2 concentration practically possible.

▶ **SUMMARY**

The environmental effects of altitude and air pollution can affect exercise and athletic performance. Physiological adaptation or maladaptation (in the case of altitude sickness or exposure to air pollution) is often a factor in fitness, exercise, and training programs. While some effects of altitude can be overcome with chronic adaptations to training at altitude, prevention of harmful effects of pollution is often a function of avoiding and/or minimizing exposure.

References

1. Favier R, Spielvogel H, Desplanches D, et al. Training in hypoxia vs. training in normoxia in high-altitude natives. J Appl Physiol 78:2286–2293, 1995.
2. Levine BD, Roach RC, Houston CS. Work and training at altitude. In: Sutton JR, Coates G, Houston CS, eds. Hypoxia and Mountain Medicine. Burlington, VT: Queen City Printers, 1992:192–201.
3. Levine BD, Stray-Gundersen J. A practical approach to altitude training. Int J Sports Med 13:S209–S212, 1992.
4. Rodriguez FA, Casa H, Casa M, et al. Intermittent hypobaric hypoxia stimulates erythropoiesis and improves aerobic capacity. Med Sci Sports Exerc 31:264–268, 1999.
5. Kayser B. Nutrition and energetics of exercise at altitude: Theory and possible practical implications. Sports Med 17:309–323, 1994.
6. Åstrand PO, Rodahl K. Textbook of Work Physiology: Physiological Bases of Exercise. Chicago: McGraw-Hill, 1986.
7. Buskirk ER. Decrease in physical working capacity at high altitude. In: Hegnauer AH, Natick MA, eds. Biomedicine of High Altitude. US Army Res Inst Environ Med 1969:204–222.
8. Fulco CS. Maximal and submaximal exercise performance at altitude. Aviat Space Environ Med 69:793–801, 1998.
9. Cudaback DD. Four-KM altitude effects on performance and health. Pub Astronom Soc Pac 96:463–477, 1984.
10. Young A, Young PA, Young AJ, et al. Human acclimatization to high terrestrial altitude. In: Pandolf KB, Swaka MN, Gonzalez RR, eds. Human Performance Physiology and Environmental Medicine at Terrestrial Extremes. Indianapolis: Benchmark, 1988:497–545.
11. Berglund B. High-altitude training: Aspects of hematological adaptation. Sport Med 14:289–303, 1992.
12. Savard GK, Areskog NH, Saltin B. Cardiovascular response to exercise in humans following acclimatization to extreme altitude. Acta Physiol Scand 154:499–509, 1995.
13. Bigard AX, Brunet A, Guezennec CY, Monod H. Skeletal muscle changes after endurance training at high altitude. J Appl Physiol 71:2114–2121, 1991.
14. Hopkins WG, Hawley JA, Burke LM. Design and analysis of research on sport performance enhancement. Med Sci Sports Exerc 31:472–485, 1999.
15. Fulco CS, Rock PB, Cymerman A. Improving athletic performance: Is altitude residence or altitude training helpful. Aviat Space Environ Med 71:162–171, 2000.
16. Baker A, Hopkins WG. Altitude training for sea level performance. In: Sportscience Training & Technology. Internet Society for Sportscience. http://www.sportsci.org/traintech/altitude/wgh.html
17. Levine BD, Stray-Gundersen J. Altitude training does not improve running performance more than equivalent training near sea level in trained runners. Med Sci Sports Exerc 24:1992.
18. Martin DE. The challenge of using altitude to improve performance. New Studies in Athletics. 9:51–57, 1994.
19. Malconian MK, Rock PB. Medical problems related to altitude. In: Pandolf KB, Swaka MN, Gonzalez RR, eds. Human Performance Physiology and Environmental Medicine at Terrestrial Extremes. Indianapolis: Benchmark, 1988.
20. Ward MP, Milledge JS, West JB. High Altitude Medicine and Physiology. New York: Chapman & Hall, 1989.
21. Hamilton AJ, Cymerman A, Black P. High altitude cerebral edema. Neurosurgery 19:841–849, 1986.
22. Haymes EM, Welss CL. Environment and Human Performance. Champaign, IL: Human Kinetics, 1986.
23. McCafferty W. Air pollution and athletic performance. Springfield, IL: Charles C Thomas, 1981.
24. Peterson JE, Stewart RD. Absorption and elimination of carbon monoxide by inactive young men. Arch Environ Health 21:165–171, 1970.
25. Folinsbee LJ. Air pollution and exercise. In: Welsh et al., eds. Current Therapy in Sports Medicine 1985–1986. Toronto: Mosby, 1985.
26. Cedaro R. Environmental factors and exercise performance: A review. II. Air pollution. Excel 8:161–166, 1992.
27. Anderson O. Dodging the deadly cocktail. Running Magazine Oct 1989:42–43.
28. Environmental Protection Agency. Public information provided on the World Wide Web server: http://www.epa.gov/1992.
29. Aris R, Christian D, Hearne PQ, et al. Effects of Nitric Acid Vapor Alone, and in Combination with Ozone, in Exercising, Healthy Subjects as Assessed by Bronchoalveolar and Proximal Lavage. Report ARB/R-94/552, San Francisco General Hospital. Center for Occupational and Environmental Health, 1994.
30. Horstman DH, Folinsbee LJ, Ives PJ, et al. Ozone concentration and pulmonary response relationships for 6.6-hour exposures with 5 hours of moderate exercise to 0.08, 0.10, and 0.12 ppm. Am Rev Respir Dis 142:1158–1163, 1990.
31. Bienfait D, Fanger PO, Fitzner K, et al. European Concerted Action Report 11: Guidelines for ventilation requirements in buildings. Office for Publications of the European Communities, Brussels, 1992.

SECTION FIVE

CORONARY ARTERY DISEASE

SECTION EDITOR: *Thomas P. LaFontaine, PhD, FACSM*

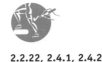

CHAPTER **26**

CORONARY ATHEROSCLEROSIS

Ray W. Squires

Coronary atherosclerosis (also called coronary artery disease) is the leading cause of death in all industrialized countries. Although coronary atherosclerosis was recognized in the 19th century, it has become more prevalent and better appreciated in the 20th century (1). Coronary atherosclerosis may result in the clinical syndromes of coronary heart disease (also called ischemic heart disease), angina pectoris, myocardial infarction, sudden cardiac death, and chronic heart failure. In the United States, each year approximately 1.5 million persons have myocardial infarction, and 500,000 deaths occur (2, 3). Each year more than 600,000 coronary artery bypass surgeries and more than 500,000 coronary angioplasties are performed. Although the rate of mortality from coronary heart disease has been declining in North America for the past 3 decades, the economic burden in direct costs of medical care and lost wages is staggering, exceeding $100 billion annually (4). Unfortunately, with economic improvement resulting in increased cigarette smoking, saturated fat intake, and less physical activity, it is also becoming an emerging epidemic in developing countries (5).

Coronary artery disease is not necessarily an inevitable consequence of a genetic predisposition and the aging process. Multiple powerful risk factors due to lifestyle choices are operative, as evidenced by the marked variation in the incidence of coronary heart disease around the world (6). This is powerfully illustrated by the observation that migrants, on leaving a geographical area of low incidence of cardiovascular mortality, assume the higher incidence of their new country (7).

Arteries undergo anatomical changes associated with aging, such as thickening of the intima, loss of elastic connective tissue, and an increase in diameter (8). These natural changes, which occur throughout the arterial tree, are called *arteriosclerosis*. In contrast, *atherosclerosis* (atherosis: soft, gruellike; sclerosis: hard, collagenous) is a pathological phenomenon resulting in potentially blood flow–obstructive lesions primarily in the coronary, carotid, iliac, and femoral arteries and the aorta (3). The disease is a multifactorial process and is incompletely understood at present. Several risk factors, characteristics that increase the probability of developing the disease, have been identified:

- Cigarette smoking
- Elevated blood concentration of low-density lipoprotein (LDL) cholesterol
- Low blood concentration of high-density lipoprotein (HDL) cholesterol
- Hypertension
- Sedentary lifestyle
- Obesity
- Diabetes mellitus and insulin resistance
- Genetic factors
- Psychological factors
- Male gender
- Advanced age

Risk factors may be causally related to the development of coronary atherosclerosis or merely associated with an increased chance of development of the disease. This chapter summarizes what is known about this.

THE NORMAL CORONARY ARTERY

Arteries are lined by a single layer of metabolically active cells, the *endothelium*, which serves as a barrier between the blood and the arterial wall (Fig. 26.1). The channel for the flow of blood within the artery is called the *lumen*. The endothelial cells are connected to each other at their borders and are attached to a basement membrane (9). The endothelial cells are selectively permeable, controlling the passage of substances from the blood into the arterial wall. Various receptors, such as for LDL and growth factors, are located on the endothelial cells. In addition, the endothelium is capable of producing several vasoactive substances, such as prostacyclin (a vasodilator and inhibitor of platelet aggregation), angiotensin-converting enzyme (important in vasoconstriction), and connective tissue molecules (9, 10). When in-

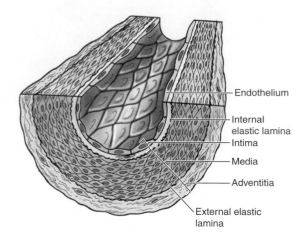

Figure 26.1. The normal coronary artery wall. (Reprinted with permission from Ross R, Glomset J. The pathogenesis of atherosclerosis. N Engl J Med 295:369, 1976.)

tact, the endothelium produces endothelial-derived relaxing factor (nitric oxide), which is released into both the lumen and arterial wall. This factor inactivates platelets, inhibits adhesion of cells from the blood to the arterial wall, and inhibits migration and proliferation of smooth muscle cells (11). These cells are also capable of manufacturing a form of platelet-derived growth factor, which stimulates the growth of connective tissue and smooth muscle cells. Endothelial cells can produce substances capable of dissolving blood clots, such as plasminogen, or factors that promote clotting, for example, von Willebrand factor (12). Under normal conditions, the endothelium protects against the development of atherosclerosis, but when deranged, it plays a critical role in the development of the disease.

Under the endothelial basement membrane is the *intima*, which consists of a thin layer of connective tissue with an occasional smooth muscle cell (Fig. 26.1). The intima is the area of the arterial wall where the lesions of atherosclerosis form (9).

The *media*, which contains most of the smooth muscle cells of the arterial wall in addition to elastic connective tissue, lies under the intima, between the internal and external elastic laminae (Fig. 26.1). The laminae consist of elastic connective tissue with occasional pores to allow passage of cells and other substances in either direction (9). Advanced atherosclerosis is characterized by proliferation of smooth muscle cells derived from the media. The smooth muscle cells maintain arterial tone (partial vasoconstriction) by their characteristic prolonged contractions. The vascular smooth muscle responds to various vasoactive stimuli, such as epinephrine and angiotensin II, which both cause vasoconstriction, and vasodilators, such as prostacyclin. Smooth muscle cells possess receptors for various substances, including LDL, insulin, and platelet-derived growth factor (13, 14). Smooth muscle cells in the arterial wall are capable of functioning as con-

tractile cells (as in maintenance of arterial tone) or when properly stimulated, as synthetic cells capable of the manufacture of collagen, elastin, and other connective tissue (15). When in the synthetic mode of action, these cells are sensitive to various growth-promoting factors, contribute to the formation of fibrous connective tissue, and directly contribute to the process of atherosclerosis.

The *adventitia*, the outermost layer of the arterial wall, consists of collagen, elastin, fibroblasts (cells capable of forming connective tissue), and a few smooth muscle cells (Fig. 26.1). This highly vascularized layer (its blood supply comes from small vessels called the vasa vasorum) provides the media and intima with oxygen and nutrients (9).

ATHEROGENESIS: RESPONSE TO INJURY

Over the past several decades, research has revealed much about the development and progression of atherosclerosis (*atherogenesis*), although our understanding of the disease is far from complete. The initial event is derangement or injury to the endothelium from substances in the blood. A subsequent *inflammatory response* results in proliferation (growth) of tissue within the arterial wall that may obstruct blood flow (9, 12). The process may begin in childhood and progress over many years before symptoms occur. The progression of the disease is not predictable or linear over time.

Injury to endothelial cells may result from multiple causes, such as the following (12, 16–21):

- Tobacco smoke and other chemical irritants from tobacco
- Hypertension and the resultant turbulent blood flow and increased shear stress
- Hypercholesterolemia, particularly oxidized LDL
- Glycated substances resulting from diabetes mellitus
- Vasoconstrictor substances
- Immune complexes
- Homocysteine
- Viral or bacterial infection (e.g., cytomegalovirus, *Chlamydia pneumoniae*, *Helicobacter pylori*)

Injury may result in *endothelial dysfunction*, potentially leading to the following abnormalities:

- Impaired vasodilation, increased propensity for vasospasm
- Increased permeability to lipoproteins and other bloodborne substances
- Increased adhesiveness of the endothelial cells leading to more platelet deposition and increased *thrombogenesis* along with increased adhesion of glycoproteins

LDL may alter the surface characteristics of endothelial cells, potentiating the adherence of cells and other substances to the arterial wall.

Platelets adhere to the injured endothelium (*platelet aggregation*), form small blood clots (*mural thrombi*), and release growth factors and vasoactive substances. Atherosclerosis thrives in a hyperthrombotic state. Platelets, after adhering to the endothelium, release thromboxane A2, a potent vasoconstrictor that may cause additional vascular injury (9, 12). A hyperthrombotic state may arise from a genetic trait or from excessive blood catecholamine concentration, for example because of smoking or psychosocial stress (22, 23). In addition, an impaired ability to dissolve intra-arterial thrombi (*fibrinolysis*) may result from smoking, a sedentary lifestyle, or elevated levels of lipoprotein(a), an atherogenic lipoprotein related to LDL (24).

Lipids from the blood, primarily carried by LDL, enter the arterial wall and may be taken up by endothelial or other cells, which augment the oxidized state of LDL, further increasing the ease of cell adherence to the endothelium. Monocytes from the blood may adhere to the endothelium, migrate into the intima, accumulate cholesterol, and be transformed into a distinctly different type of cell, the macrophage (9). Macrophages convert mildly oxidized LDL into highly oxidized LDL, which enters the cells more readily than the less oxidized form.

Growth factors, such as platelet-derived growth factor, enhance monocyte binding to the endothelium and increase the number of LDL receptors, inducing greater LDL binding and increased deposition of cholesterol in the arterial wall and in the macrophages (9, 13). Growth factors cause increased growth of certain tissues (*mitogenic effect*) and the migration of cells into the area of injury (*chemotactic effect*). In response to growth factors, *smooth muscle cells* and *fibroblasts* (a type of relatively undifferentiated connective tissue cell that can synthesize fibrous tissue) migrate from the media to the intima (9, 25). Some of these cells, in addition to macrophages, accumulate cholesterol, forming *foam cells* that release some of their cholesterol into the extracellular space, giving rise to *fatty streaks*, the earliest visually detectable (yellow macroscopic appearance) lesion of atherosclerosis (Fig. 26.2) (19, 26). With cholesterol lowering by diet or drug, fatty streaks may regress (lose bulk when cholesterol leaves the lesion and re-enters the blood). The *proliferation* (increase in cell numbers and cell size) of smooth muscle and fibrous connective tissue appears to be under the influence of several mitogenic (growth) factors in addition to platelet-derived growth factor from a variety of types of cells (e.g., injured endothelial cells, monocytes, vascular smooth muscle cells, fibroblasts), such as the following (12):

- Endothelial cell growth factor
- Fibroblast growth factor
- Smooth muscle cell–derived growth factor
- Low-density lipoprotein
- Angiotensin II

- Catecholamines
- Endothelin
- Thrombin

The proliferation of smooth muscle and fibrous tissues in the arterial wall results in part from the change to a "synthetic phenotype" of the cells, as mentioned previously.

T lymphocytes (immune system cells) are present in early fatty streaks (27). While their exact role in atherogenesis is uncertain, it appears that the immune system does have a role in the clinical syndromes resulting from the disease, discussed later in the chapter (28).

With continued accumulation of fibrous connective tissue, smooth muscle cells, cholesterol, and other cellular debris, the lesion progresses in size and appearance to a fibromuscular plaque (Fig. 26.2). The plaque is firm and pale gray, and it may contain a yellow cholesterol core called the atheroma.

The development of the early atherosclerotic plaque occurs with outward growth of the coronary artery, termed *remodeling* (28). Thus the **lumen size increases** to compensate for atherosclerotic plaque, whose obstructive bulk may constitute up to 40% of the vessel diameter without any reduction in inside vessel dimensions. However, if plaque bulk continues to increase over time, the vessel lumen diameter will be reduced and obstruction of blood flow may occur (9, 12). **The progression of the size of the lesions does not occur in a stable, linear manner over time** (12). **Some lesions appear to be relatively stable over many years; other plaque may progress wildly in size in a matter of months.**

Plaque rupture with subsequent thrombus formation has been established as a mechanism for rapid progression in plaque size. The *rupture*, or *fissuring*, of a plaque may result from local stress (from turbulent blood flow or vasoconstriction, for example) or chemical factors, exposing the contents of the inside of the lesion to the blood (12, 29). These sites may form *mural thrombi* of varying sizes. As fibrous organization of the thrombi occurs, the thrombi are incorporated into the plaque. The scenario of plaque rupture, thrombus formation, and incorporation into the arterial wall may repeatedly occur, giving a layered appearance to the lesion and resulting in considerable progression in size of the plaque. These highly complicated lesions, which include organized thrombus, are called *advanced atherosclerotic plaques* (Fig. 26.2).

Coronary atherosclerosis affects arteries in an extremely diffuse manner with occasional discrete, local areas of more pronounced narrowing of the vessel lumen that may produce obstruction of blood flow (30). Selective coronary angiography is the gold standard (best available technique) for determination of the severity of obstructive coronary atherosclerotic lesions. However, **based upon comparisons of angiographic and autopsy findings, with the exception of complete occlusion of**

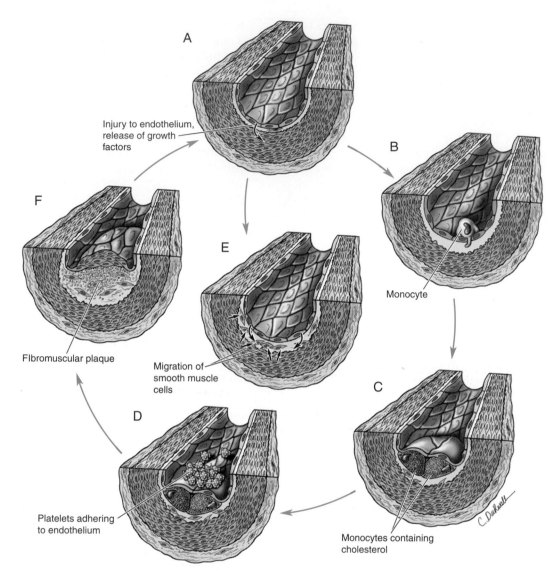

Figure 26.2. The atherosclerotic process: response to injury. **A.** Injury to endothelium with release of growth factors (*small arrow*). **B.** Monocytes attach to endothelium. **C.** Monocytes migrate to the intima, take up cholesterol, form fatty streaks. **D.** Platelets adhere to the endothelium and release growth factors. **F.** The result is a fibromuscular plaque. An alternative pathway is shown with arrows from A to E to F, with growth factor–mediated migration of smooth muscle cells from the media to the intima (**E**). (Reprinted with permission from Ross R. The pathogenesis of atherosclerosis: An update. N Engl J Med 314:496, 1986.)

the vessel (100% stenosis), the degree of stenosis is greatly underestimated by angiography because of the diffuse nature of the disease process (31). Standard coronary angiography provides a lumenogram only (an image of the size of the lumen of the vessel) and does not allow the angiographer to visualize the vessel wall where the atherosclerotic process occurs. New imaging techniques, such as intravascular ultrasound, improve the ability to assess the extent and severity of coronary atherosclerosis much more accurately than standard angiography (32).

Obstructive coronary atherosclerosis (disease severe enough to reduce blood flow) occurs most frequently in the first 4 to 5 cm of the epicardial coronary arteries, although flow-limiting lesions may occur anywhere in the coronary tree (27). Ostial lesions at the origins of the left main and main right coronary arteries may occur. Women tend to lag 5–20 years behind men in the extent and severity of coronary atherosclerosis (33). The exact reasons for the gender differences are not fully understood but are related to estrogen, since postmenopausal women have an accelerated course of coronary artery disease.

RISK FACTORS FOR ATHEROSCLEROSIS

Coronary risk factors are associated with an increased likelihood that coronary atherosclerosis will develop over time. Several such risk factors have been identified on the basis of epidemiological studies evaluating common characteristics of persons with the disease (6, 7). Some persons without traditional risk factors do develop coronary artery disease. However, persons without risk factors are much less likely to do so than those who have risk factors. Possible mechanisms of atherogenic effect for some risk factors have been identified, although a clear understanding of all possible actions of risk factors is still not a reality. Table 26.1 lists the major coronary risk factors that are described here.

Tobacco smoke exerts several atherogenic effects (19, 34–38):

- Endothelial damage
- Increased platelet adhesion to the injured endothelium
- Increased release of platelet-derived growth factor
- Carbon monoxide–induced arterial wall hypoxia and proinflammatory state
- Promotion of LDL oxidation
- Increased blood catecholamine concentrations via sympathetic nervous system stimulation
- Reduced blood HDL cholesterol concentration
- Increased thrombogenicity (formation of intra-arterial blood clots); increased fibrinogen levels
- Increased whole blood viscosity (secondary to polycythemia)
- Impaired endothelial-mediated vasodilation

Plasma lipoproteins play a crucial role in the development of atherosclerosis, and a basic understanding of their origins, structure, and functions is important for practitioners of cardiovascular rehabilitation. Data from epidemiological and experimental studies have resulted in the cholesterol–atherosclerosis hypothesis, although our understanding of the roles of blood lipids is not complete. Elevated levels of total and LDL cholesterol are strongly associated with the development of coronary artery disease, while high levels of HDL cholesterol are protective. Elevated triglycerides are also probably atherogenic. *Dyslipidemia* describes an adverse blood lipid profile. A substantial number of coronary events take place in patients who have moderate or even low levels of total or LDL cholesterol but who have low HDL cholesterol or elevated triglyceride concentrations (39). No threshold concentration for total or LDL cholesterol for atherogenesis has been determined. In addition to becoming incorporated into the atherosclerotic plaque directly, blood lipids may promote smooth muscle cell proliferation, enhance platelet reactivity and aggregation, and impair endothelial vasodilation (12, 40). The plasma lipoproteins are water-soluble complexes of lipids (cholesterol, triglycerides, phospholipids) and specific proteins (apolipoproteins) (41). They originate in the liver and/or intestine. Five classes have been described:

1. *Chylomicrons* are triglyceride-rich particles produced in the intestine after a fatty meal. They enter the circulation through the thoracic duct. After a half-life of a few minutes, they degrade into remnant particles by the enzyme lipoprotein lipase and are taken up by the liver. These postprandial triglyceride-rich lipoproteins and their remnants are potentially atherogenic (42).
2. *Very low density lipoprotein* (VLDL), secreted by the liver into the circulation, transports primarily triglyceride and a small amount of cholesterol (10–15% of total cholesterol). VLDL undergoes degradation in the blood by lipoprotein lipase to intermediate-density lipoprotein. Epidemiological data suggest that elevated VLDL (increased triglycerides) may be a risk factor for atherosclerosis. Elevated triglycerides result in heightened thrombogenicity.
3. *Intermediate-density lipoprotein* (IDL) is converted to LDL by the liver.
4. *LDL* transports most of the circulating cholesterol (60–70% of the total cholesterol). LDL's major apolipoprotein is apo B, which is believed to be highly atherogenic. In familial hypercholesterolemia, a genetic LDL receptor defect dramatically increases total cholesterol concentration and coronary risk (43). In the heterozygous form of the disease, which occurs in 1 in 500 persons, one defective and one normal LDL receptor gene are present, total cholesterol is approximately 350–400 mg/dL, and coronary artery disease usually becomes clinically apparent during the fourth or fifth decade of life. The homozygous form of the disorder is fortunately rare (1 in 1 million persons); it results in total cholesterol concentrations of more than 600 mg/dL, with myocardial infarction often occurring in childhood or adolescence. Additional genetic lipoprotein disorders are

Table 26.1. Established Risk Factors for the Development of Coronary Atherosclerosis

Cigarette smoking	High-fat diet
Dyslipidemia	Menopause
Hypertension	Family history
Sedentary lifestyle	Psychosocial distress
Diabetes mellitus/Insulin resistance	Abnormal blood clotting
Obesity	Elevated plasma homocysteine
Male gender	ACE DD genotype
Increased age	Elevated plasma C-reactive protein

discussed later. A particular type of LDL, *small dense LDL*, contains a greater complement of apo B than usual, is particularly susceptible to oxidation, and is believed to be very atherogenic. *Lipoprotein(a)* is LDL with apo B-100 linked to a specific protein called apo(a). This close relative of LDL is proatherogenic and prothrombic at concentrations of approximately 20 mg/dL or greater. Lipoprotein(a) is taken up by macrophages and interferes with clot lysis by inhibiting the conversion of plasminogen to plasmin (38).

5. *HDL* transports 20–30% of the total cholesterol. Apo A1 is the major apolipoprotein, and HDL cholesterol **is inversely related to the risk of developing coronary artery disease**. HDL probably mediates reverse cholesterol transport, the process by which cholesterol is removed from sites of deposit in the arterial wall and transported to the liver for excretion. This concept implies a dynamic situation of cholesterol entry and exit from the arterial wall, dependent on blood constituents. HDL also inhibits oxidation of LDL and prevents monocytes from adhering to the endothelium, from migrating into the arterial intimal layer, and from differentiating into macrophages (19, 44). With ultracentrifugation, HDL subfractions (HDL_2, HDL_3) may be identified, although these subfractions do not predict coronary atherosclerosis any better than HDL cholesterol.

Genetic lipoprotein disorders merit some discussion. As mentioned previously, *familial hypercholesterolemia* (the rare homozygous and the relatively common heterozygous forms) results in markedly elevated serum cholesterol concentrations and premature coronary artery disease (43). Extremely low levels of HDL cholesterol are seen in *familial hypoalphalipoproteinemia*, caused by a reduced synthesis of apo A1 (45). Individuals with this disease also develop premature coronary atherosclerosis. *Polygenic hypercholesterolemia* is a common abnormality that results from a relative deficiency of functioning LDL receptors, which leads to elevated HDL cholesterol in the setting of a high fat, high cholesterol diet (46). *Familial combined hyperlipidemia* results in elevations of both cholesterol and triglycerides. Approximately 10% of survivors of acute myocardial infarction have this disorder (42). *Familial defective apolipoprotein B-100* affects approximately 1 in 500 persons; it results in poor LDL receptor binding of cholesterol and elevated blood cholesterol concentrations (42).

In addition to genetic defects resulting in dyslipidemia, several secondary causes (adverse blood lipids as result of another disease process or condition) should be appreciated (19):

- Diabetes mellitus
- Hypothyroidism
- Obstructive liver disease
- Nephrotic syndrome
- Chronic renal failure
- Alcohol abuse
- Pregnancy

Correction or resolution of the secondary condition leads to normalization of the blood lipid profile.

Dietary intake of cholesterol and saturated fatty acids has been established as a critical determinant of plasma cholesterol concentrations in several diverse cultures (38). Epidemiological and experimental studies have demonstrated the effects of various levels of dietary fat and cholesterol on both blood lipid profiles and coronary event rates. For example, Table 26.2 compares the mean intakes of saturated fat in Japanese men living in Japan, Hawaii, and San Francisco and their associated death rate from coronary atherosclerosis. It is clear that the higher the dietary saturated fat intake, the greater the coronary death rate.

Hypertension exerts a direct effect on atherogenesis and worsens the prognosis of patients with documented coronary artery disease (47). Elevated blood pressure may cause arterial distension leading to remodeling of the arterial wall (medial thickening) (12). It may also result in endothelial dysfunction leading to increased endothelial permeability, increased platelet and monocyte adherence to the vessel wall, and smooth muscle proliferation (12, 47, 48). Hypertension also has adverse effects on the myocardium, such as left ventricular hypertrophy, increased wall stress, and myocardial oxygen requirements, which worsen the effects of reduced coronary blood flow secondary to coronary atherosclerosis.

Epidemiological investigations have demonstrated a direct relationship between a sedentary lifestyle and coronary artery disease morbidity and mortality (49, 50). Powell et al. (51) examined 47 such studies of habitual physical activity and coronary disease and reported a strong (relative risk 1.9 for a sedentary existence), consis-

Table 26.2. Dietary Intake of Saturated Fat in Japanese Men Living in Japan, Hawaii, and San Francisco Compared with Death Rates from Coronary Artery Disease

	JAPAN	HAWAII	SAN FRANCISCO
% Kcal from saturated fat	7%	12%	14%
Coronary death rate	1.0	1.7	2.8

Reprinted with permission from Tillotson JL, Kato H, Nichaman MZ, et al. Epidemiology of coronary heart disease and stroke in Japanese men living in Japan, Hawaii, and California: Methodology for comparison of diet. Am J Clin Nutr 26:177, 1973; Kagan A, Harris BR, Winkelstein W Jr., et al. Epidemiology studies of coronary heart disease and stroke in Japanese men living in Japan, Hawaii, and California: demographic, physical, dietary and biochemical characteristics. J Chronic Dis 27:345, 1974.

tent inverse relationship between regular exercise and coronary artery disease incidence.

Diabetes mellitus accelerates the development of atherosclerosis and increases the coronary death rate at least twofold (38, 52, 53). Elevated blood glucose (insulin resistance) results in increased platelet adhesiveness, dyslipidemia, abnormal blood coagulation, and impaired endothelium-dependent vasodilation. Elevated levels of various growth factors and glycated proteins found in diabetics result in proliferation of the fibromuscular component of atherosclerotic plaque (19). Diabetes is also associated with a high blood concentration of small dense LDL, which is especially susceptible to oxidation and highly atherogenic. Reaven (54) coined the term *syndrome X* to describe the common association of the following risk factors:

- Insulin resistance with elevated blood glucose levels
- Elevated triglycerides and low levels of HDL cholesterol
- Hypertension
- Central obesity (preponderance of fat accumulation at the waist as opposed to the hips)

Although only 2–6% of families in the general population have very strong family histories of early coronary heart disease (clinically apparent coronary disease at age 55 or earlier), they account for nearly 50% of early coronary deaths in the population (55). High-risk families share both genetic and environmental factors. Smoking, high-fat diet, sedentary lifestyle, depressed levels of HDL cholesterol, and elevated triglyceride concentrations cluster in families.

Men have a much higher incidence of coronary heart disease than do premenopausal women (38). The relative protection of women from coronary heart disease is thought to be related in part to the presence of estrogen. After menopause, women catch up with men in terms of coronary heart disease, and it is the leading killer of both women and men. In general, women lag behind men in terms of coronary risk by approximately 20 years. Estrogen replacement after menopause improves coronary risk factors and may decrease coronary risk, although this has not yet been demonstrated in prospective clinical trials (56).

Obesity is a major independent risk factor for the development of coronary artery disease and is related to other established risk factors, such as the following (19, 38, 57, 58):

- Dyslipidemia
- Insulin resistance and diabetes mellitus
- Hypertension and left ventricular hypertrophy
- Sedentary lifestyle
- Emotional distress
- Abnormal blood platelet function and impaired fibrinolysis

Abdominal (or central pattern) obesity, defined as a waist-to-hip ratio greater than 1.0 in men and 0.85 in women, is associated with a higher cardiovascular risk than leg and hip obesity (59, 60).

These psychosocial factors have been established as coronary risk factors: depression, anxiety, social isolation, low socioeconomic standing, life dissatisfaction, chronic life stress, and the coronary-prone behavior pattern (19, 38, 61). The coronary-prone behavior pattern, also known as the type A personality (high levels of ambition, aggressiveness, hostility, competitiveness, and time urgency), has been shown to be an especially powerful (relative risk 2.0) independent risk factor. Presumably the psychosocial factors exert their atherogenic potential through neuroendocrine activation mediated by the sympathetic nervous system.

Some specific markers of either abnormal blood clotting (increased thrombogenicity) or clot dissolution (impaired fibrinolysis) are risk factors for atherosclerosis when increased above normal levels (19, 42, 62):

- Fibrinogen
- von Willebrand factor
- Factor VIIa
- Platelet aggregation
- Tissue plasminogen activator (t-PA) antigen
- Plasminogen activator inhibitor-1
- Prothrombin
- Lipoprotein(a)

Three relatively newly identified coronary risk factors—elevated plasma homocysteine concentration, abnormalities in the gene that encodes angiotensin-converting enzyme (ACE), and C-reactive protein—warrant discussion. Homocysteine is an intermediary in the metabolism of the essential amino acid methionine (63, 64). Elevated plasma concentrations of homocysteine may result from genetic abnormalities, inadequate dietary intake of folic acid and other B vitamins, increasing age, male gender, and menopause. The precise level of plasma homocysteine considered atherogenic is unknown, but it appears that risk increases in direct proportion to the level of the substance in the blood, similar to the situation of blood cholesterol as a coronary risk factor. Elevated levels have been reported in up to 30% of patients with documented coronary artery disease. The upper limit of the normal range is approximately 17 μmol/L. Some patients with abnormal homocysteine metabolism have normal fasting plasma levels and require dietary loading with methionine to uncover the problem. Elevated blood concentrations of homocysteine are hypothesized to promote atherogenesis by causing direct damage to the endothelium, increasing the adhesiveness of platelets, and increasing the action of selected clotting factors. Treatment with folic acid and B vitamins lowers plasma homocysteine concentrations promptly.

Genes that influence the renin–angiotensin system are important for coronary artery disease because of the profound systemic vasoconstrictor effect of angiotensin II and because ACE-inhibiting drugs substantially reduce the risk of acute myocardial infarction. An abnormality (polymorphism) of the gene that encodes ACE (resulting in an ACE DD genotype) is associated with an increased risk of acute myocardial infarction in men, although it does not appear to be related to the development of coronary atherosclerosis (65). However, once coronary artery disease is present, gene polymorphism of ACE becomes a risk factor. Screening for this abnormality has not yet become clinically available.

Circulating levels of C-reactive protein are an independent coronary risk factor (66). The level of C-reactive protein reflects the amount of inflammation related to atherogenesis, but it is not clear whether it plays a direct role in the process. Clinical screening of this risk factor is not yet recommended.

NONATHEROSCLEROTIC CORONARY OBSTRUCTION

Most obstructive coronary artery disease is the result of atherosclerosis. Nonatherosclerotic coronary obstruction, although relatively uncommon, may result from the following (30):

- Coronary vasospasm (primary or cocaine induced)
- Embolism (thrombi from cardiac valves, calcium, tissue from tumors)
- Primary intracoronary thrombus
- Arteritis
- Spontaneous or traumatic coronary vessel dissection
- Congenital abnormalities of the coronary arteries (e.g., anomalous origin of the right or left main coronary)

CORONARY OBSTRUCTION AFTER CARDIAC INTERVENTIONS

The development of obstructive lesions in the coronary circulation after a revascularization procedure such as saphenous vein graft bypass surgery, percutaneous coronary intervention (coronary angioplasty, intracoronary stent, laser, atherectomy, rotablator), or cardiac transplantation is a major problem. Injury to saphenous vein grafts may occur at the time of harvesting from the legs, during operative handling, or with exposure to high-pressure flow of their new location in the circulation (arterialization of the vein). Injury may also arise from risk factors such as smoking or dyslipidemia or from other factors (67, 68). Atherosclerotic lesions may develop with intimal thickening, increased smooth muscle cell numbers and bulk, connective tissue accumulation, and lipid incorporation. At 5 years after surgery, up to 35% of vein grafts are occluded. Internal thoracic artery conduits are not nearly as prone to the development of graft atherosclerosis (69).

Angiographic *restenosis* rates of 45% at 6 months have been reported for percutaneous transluminal coronary angioplasty (PTCA) (70). Similar or higher restenosis rates are expected for laser angioplasty, atherectomy, and rotablator revascularization. The use of intracoronary stents with or without PTCA dramatically reduces the restenosis rate and is a major advance in revascularization (71). Restenosis is triggered by arterial injury at the time of catheter treatment. Typically, early thrombosis occurs with release of platelet- and macrophage-derived growth factors that stimulate migration and proliferation of smooth muscle cells, which reduces vessel lumen size. The lesions of restenosis are not lipid rich and are not typical atherosclerotic plaques.

After cardiac transplantation, *accelerated graft atherosclerosis* may result in clinically important reduction in coronary blood flow in less than a year. At 3 years after transplantation, approximately 40% of patients are affected (72). The initiating injury to the coronary endothelium is probably mediated by the immune system. The disease results in diffuse, severe, and progressive obstructive lesions. Intimal proliferation occurs with or without lipid deposition. This disease is not classic atherosclerosis.

CAN AGGRESSIVE RISK FACTOR MODIFICATION RETARD THE PROGRESSION OR CAUSE REGRESSION OF CORONARY ATHEROSCLEROSIS?

Progression of atherosclerosis in native coronary arteries and saphenous vein grafts is related to continued cigarette smoking, elevated blood cholesterol, hypertension, sedentary lifestyle, and an elevated fasting blood glucose concentration (73). Angiographic trials have been designed to determine the specific effects of aggressive blood lipid lowering and aerobic exercise training on the natural history of coronary atherosclerosis. Larger clinical trials have investigated the effects of lipid lowering on cardiovascular events and total mortality.

Lipid lowering by means of a very low fat diet, medication, or intestinal bypass surgery (to interfere with absorption of dietary fat and cholesterol) has been demonstrated in multiple trials to result in the following benefits (74):

- Less angiographic progression and more regression of coronary lesions
- Reduced rates of acute myocardial infarction
- Lower total and cardiac mortality

All types of interventions (diet, drugs, surgery) have resulted in similar favorable effects (75). In the Scandinavian Simvastatin Survival Study (4S), aggressive cholesterol lowering with drug treatment over 4 years in patients with coronary artery disease resulted in a 34% reduction in major coronary events and a 42% reduction in cardiac mortality compared with control conditions (76).

The magnitude of the improvement in clinical events has been far greater than the amount of angiographic improvement in all trials (75). In fact, the amount of angiographic improvement has been very modest in all trials (changes of 1–2% in stenosis severity). Furthermore, some untreated control group patients have shown angiographic regression of disease, while in some treated patients, in spite of marked HDL cholesterol lowering, the disease progresses (19).

The improvement in clinical outcomes for patients receiving cholesterol-lowering therapy may be due in part to regression of some lesions. Other more plausible explanations for the observed reductions in clinical events and mortality include the following (75, 77, 78):

- Stabilization of plaque resulting in less plaque rupture and thrombosis
- Improved endothelial function yielding less coronary vasoconstriction and more vasodilation
- Reduced rest and exercise in myocardial ischemia
- Less thrombogenesis

Among investigators, there is a consensus that early lipid-rich lesions are more likely to show angiographic improvement than are advanced plaques, with their considerable incorporation of thrombus and fibromuscular tissue. Lipid lowering is thought to stabilize potentially fracture-prone plaques, thereby reducing acute cardiac events (12). The amount of angiographic regression of disease is apparently not the most important factor in the impressive effects of lipid lowering on coronary artery disease outcomes.

Exercise training in sufficient amounts also appears to retard progression and increase regression of coronary atherosclerosis. A randomized, controlled trial demonstrated angiographic progression of disease in 45% of control subjects versus 10% of the treatment group. Regression of lesions was observed in 28% of treatment subjects compared with 6% of the controls (79).

It is clear that coronary atherosclerosis begins relatively early in life for many persons. Prevention of lesion development and its potentially lethal outcomes is of paramount importance (9, 12). Risk factor identification and modification in the children, grandchildren, and siblings of patients with established coronary artery disease should become a high priority. Moreover, intervention throughout the population to reduce tobacco use, decrease dietary saturated fat and total calorie intake, and increase habitual physical activity is necessary to stem the tide of this 20th century epidemic.

References

1. Report of the Working Group on Arteriosclerosis of the National Heart, Lung, and Blood Institute, vol 2. DHEW Publication (NIH) 82–2035. Washington: US Government Printing Office, 1981.
2. American Heart Association. 1998 Heart and Stroke Statistical Update. Dallas: AHA, 1998.
3. Gersh BJ, Clements IP. Acute myocardial infarction. A. Diagnosis and prognosis. In: Giuliani ER, Gersh BJ, McGoon DL, et al., eds. Mayo Clinic Practice of Cardiology. 3rd ed. St. Louis: Mosby, 1996.
4. Jones JH, Gotto AM. Prevention of coronary heart disease in 1994: Evidence for intervention. Heart Dis Stroke 3:290, 1994.
5. Reddy KS, Yusuf S. Emerging epidemic of cardiovascular disease in developing countries. Circulation 97:596, 1998.
6. Marmot MG. Epidemiologic basis for the prevention of coronary heart disease. Bull WHO 57:331, 1979.
7. Kannel WB. Cardiovascular disease: A multifactorial problem (insights from the Framingham study). In: Pollock ML, Schmidt DH, eds. Heart Disease and Rehabilitation. Boston: Houghton Mifflin Professional, 1979.
8. Lobstein JF. Cited in Li PL. Adaptation of veins to increased intravenous pressure, with special reference to the portal system and inferior vena cava. J Pathol Bacteriol 50:121, 1940.
9. Ross R. The pathogenesis of atherosclerosis. In: Braunwald E, ed. Heart Disease: A Textbook of Cardiovascular Medicine. 3rd ed. Philadelphia: Saunders, 1988.
10. Renkin EM. Multiple pathways of capillary permeability. Circ Res 41:735, 1977.
11. Schmieder RE, Schobel HP. Is endothelial dysfunction reversible? Am J Cardiol 76:117a, 1995.
12. Fuster V, Chesebro JH. Atherosclerosis: Pathogenesis, initiation, progression, acute coronary syndromes, and regression. In: Giuliani ER, Gersh BJ, McGoon DL, et al., eds. Mayo Clinic Practice of Cardiology. 3rd ed. St. Louis: Mosby, 1996.
13. Chait A, Ross R, Albers JJ, et al. Platelet-derived growth factor stimulates activity of low density lipoprotein receptors. Proc Natl Acad Sci U S A 77:4084, 1980.
14. Bowen-Pope DF, Seiffert RA, Ross R. The platelet-derived growth factor receptor. In: Boynton AL, Leffert HL, eds. Control of Animal Cell Proliferation: Recent Advances, vol 1. New York: Academic, 1985.
15. Campell GR, Campbell JH. Smooth muscle phenotypic changes in arterial wall homeostasis: Implications for the pathogenesis of atherosclerosis. Exp Mol Pathol 42:139, 1985.
16. Ross R, Glomset J. Atherosclerosis and the smooth muscle cell. Science 180:1332, 1973.
17. Clowers AW, Reidy MA, Clowers MM. Kinetics of cellular proliferation after arterial injury: 1. Smooth muscle growth in the absence of endothelium. Lab Invest 49:327, 1983.
18. Faggiotto A, Ross R, Harker L. Studies of hypercholesterolemia in the nonhuman primate: 1. Changes that lead to fatty streak formation. Arteriosclerosis 4:323, 1984.
19. Fuster V, Pearson TA. 27th Bethesda conference: Matching the intensity of risk factor management with the hazard for coronary disease events. J Am Coll Cardiol 27:957, 1996.

20. Mayer EL, Jacobsen DW, Robinson K. Homocysteine and coronary atherosclerosis. J Am Coll Cardiol 27:517, 1996.
21. Muhlestein JB, Hammond EH, Carlquist JF, et al. Increased incidence of chlamydia species within the coronary arteries of patients with symptomatic atherosclerotic versus other forms of cardiovascular disease. J Am Coll Cardiol 27:1555, 1996.
22. Rowsell HC, Hegardt B, Downie HB, et al. Adrenaline and experimental thrombosis. Br J Haematol 12:465, 1972.
23. Hampton JR, Gorlin R. Platelet studies in patients with coronary artery disease and in their relatives. Br Heart J 34:465, 1972.
24. Scott J. Thrombogenesis linked to atherogenesis at last? Nature 341:22, 1989.
25. Ross R, Glomset J, Karija B, et al. A platelet-dependent serum factor stimulates the proliferation of arterial smooth muscle cells in vitro. Proc Natl Acad Sci U S A 71:1207, 1974.
26. Stary HC. Evaluation of atherosclerotic plaques in the coronary arteries of young adults. Arteriosclerosis 3:471a, 1983.
27. Van Furth R. Current view on the mononuclear phagocyte system. Immunobiology 161:178, 1982.
28. Libby P. Molecular bases of the acute coronary syndromes. Circulation 91:2844, 1995.
29. Chesebro JH, Zoldelyi P, Fuster V. Plaque disruption and thrombosis in unstable angina pectoris. Am J Cardiol 68:9c, 1991.
30. Lie JT. Pathology of coronary artery disease. In: Giuliani ER, Fuster V, Gersh BJ, et al., eds. Cardiology: Fundamentals and Practice. 2nd ed. Chicago: Mosby–Year Book, 1991.
31. Arnett EN, Isner JM, Redwood DR, et al. Coronary artery narrowing in coronary heart disease: Comparison of cineangiography and necropsy findings. Ann Intern Med 91:350, 1979.
32. Higano ST, Nishimura RA. Intravascular ultrasound. In: Giuliani ER, Gersh BJ, McGoon DL, et al., eds. Mayo Clinic Practice of Cardiology. 3rd ed. St. Louis: Mosby, 1996.
33. Strong JP, McGill HC Jr. The natural history of coronary atherosclerosis. Ann J Pathol 40:37, 1962.
34. Brinson K. Effect of nicotine on human platelet aggregation. Atherosclerosis 20:137, 1974.
35. Astrup P. Some physiological and pathological effects of moderate carbon monoxide exposure. BMJ 4:447, 1972.
36. Mustard JF, Murphy EA. Effect of smoking on blood coagulation and platelet survival in man. BMJ 1:846, 1963.
37. Haft JI. Cardiovascular injury induced by sympathetic catecholamines. Prog Cardiovasc Dis 17:73, 1974.
38. Kottke TE, Weidman WH, Nguyen TT. Prevention of coronary heart disease. In: Giuliani ER, Gersh BJ, McGoon DL, et al., eds. Mayo Clinic Practice of Cardiology. 3rd ed. St. Louis: Mosby, 1996.
39. Kannel WB. Range of serum cholesterol values in the population developing coronary artery disease. Am J Cardiol 76:69c, 1995.
40. Anderson TJ, Meredith IT, Yeung AC, et al. The effect of cholesterol-lowering and antioxidant therapy on endothelium-dependent coronary vasomotion. N Engl J Med 332:428, 1995.
41. Lavie CJ, Gau GT, Squires RW, et al. Management of blood lipids in primary and secondary prevention of cardiovascular diseases. Mayo Clin Proc 63:605, 1988.
42. Genest J, Cohn JS. Clustering of cardiovascular risk factors: Targeting high-risk individuals. Am J Cardiol 76:8a, 1995.
43. Goldstein JL, Brown MS. Regulation of low-density lipoprotein receptors: Implications for pathogenesis and therapy of hypercholesterolemia and atherosclerosis. Circulation 76:504, 1987.
44. Navab M, Fogelman AM, Berliner JA, et al. Pathogenesis of atherosclerosis. Am J Cardiol 76:18c, 1995.
45. Scheidt S. Lipid regulation: A clinician's view of patient management. Am Heart J 112:437, 1986.
46. Brown MS, Goldstein JL. How LDL receptors influence cholesterol and atherosclerosis. Sci Am 251:58, November 1984.
47. Kannel WB, Cuppler LA, D'Agostino RB, et al. Hypertension, antihypertensive treatment, and sudden coronary death: The Framingham study. Hypertension 11(Suppl 2):45, 1988.
48. Leung DYM, Glagov S, Mathews MB. Cyclic stretching stimulates synthesis of matrix components by arterial smooth muscle cells in vitro. Science 191:475, 1976.
49. Paffenbarger RS, Hyde RT. Exercise in the prevention of coronary heart disease. Prev Med 13:3, 1984.
50. Leon AS, Connett J, Jacobs DR Jr, et al. Leisure-time physical activity levels and risk of coronary heart disease and death: The multiple risk factor intervention trial. JAMA 258:2388, 1987.
51. Powell KE, Thompson PD, Caspersen CJ, et al. Physical activity and the incidence of coronary heart disease. Annu Rev Public Health 8:253, 1987.
52. American Diabetes Association; National Heart, Lung, and Blood Institute; Juvenile Diabetes Foundation International; National Institute of Diabetes and Digestive and Kidney Diseases; American Heart Association. Diabetes mellitus: A major risk factor for cardiovascular disease (editorial). Circulation 100:1132, 1999.
53. Ginsberg HN, ed. A symposium: Implications of insulin resistance: Concerns beyond glucose. Am J Cardiol 84:1J, 1999.
54. Reaven GM. The role of insulin resistance in human disease. Diabetes 37:1595, 1988.
55. Williams RR, Hopkins PN, Hunt SC, et al. Population-based frequency of dyslipidemia syndromes in coronary-prone families in Utah. Arch Intern Med 150:582, 1990.
56. Stampfer MJ, Colditz GA. Estrogen replacement therapy and coronary heart disease: A quantitative assessment of the epidemiologic evidence. Prev Med 20:47, 1991.
57. Eckel RH, Krauss RM for AHA Nutrition Committee, American Heart Association. Call to action: Obesity as a major risk factor for coronary heart disease. Circulation 97: 2099, 1998.
58. Bray GA. Obesity and the heart. Mod Concepts Cardiovasc Dis 56:67, 1987.
59. Larsson B, Svardsudd K, Welin L, et al. Abdominal adipose tissue distribution, obesity, and risk of cardiovascular disease and death: 13 year follow up of participants in the study of men born in 1913. BMJ Clin Res 288:1401, 1984.
60. Vague J. The degree of masculine differentiation of obesity: A factor determining predisposition to diabetes, atherosclerosis, gout, and uric calculous disease. Am J Clin Nutr 2:20, 1956.

61. Rosenman RH, Brand RJ, Sholtz RI, et al. Multivariate prediction of coronary heart disease during 8.5 year follow-up in the western collaborative group study. Am J Cardiol 37:903, 1976.

62. Ma J, Hennekens CH, Ridker PM, Stampfer MJ. A prospective study of fibrinogen and risk of myocardial infarction in the physicians' health study. J Am Coll Cardiol 33: 1347, 1999.

63. Mayer EL, Jacobsen DW, Robinson K. Homocysteine and coronary atherosclerosis. J Am Coll Cardiol 27: 517, 1996.

64. Boushey CJ, Beresford SAA, Omenn GS, et al. A quantitative assessment of plasma homocysteine as a risk factor for vascular disease: Probable benefits of increasing folic acid intakes. JAMA 274:1049, 1995.

65. Ludwig E, Corneli PS, Anderson JL, et al. Angiotensin-converting enzyme gene polymorphism is associated with myocardial infarction but not with development of coronary stenosis. Circulation 91:2120, 1995.

66. Lagrand WK, Visser CA, Hermens WT, et al. C-reactive protein as a cardiovascular risk factor: More than an epiphenomenon? Circulation 100: 96, 1999.

67. Lie JT, Lawrie GM, Morris CG Jr, et al. Aorto-coronary bypass saphenous vein graft atherosclerosis: Anatomic study of 99 vein grafts from normal and hyperlipoproteinemic patients up to 75 months postoperatively. Am J Cardiol 40:906, 1977.

68. Fuster V, Fay WP, Chesebro JH. Antithrombotic agents in cardiac disease: Platelet inhibitors, anticoagulants, and thrombolytic agents. In: Giuliani ER, Gersh BJ, McGoon DL, et al., eds. Mayo Clinic Practice of Cardiology. 3rd ed. St. Louis: Mosby, 1996.

69. Lytle BW, Loop FD, Cosgrove DM, et al. Long-term (5 to 12 years) serial studies of internal mammary artery and saphenous vein coronary bypass grafts. J Thorac Cardiovasc Surg 89:248, 1985.

70. Garratt KN, Reeder GS, Holmes DS. Interventional cardiac therapy. In: Giuliani ER, Gersh BJ, McGoon DL, et al., eds. Mayo Clinic Practice of Cardiology. 3rd ed. St. Louis: Mosby, 1996.

71. Macaya C, Serruys PW, Ruygrok P, et al. Continued benefit of coronary stenting versus balloon angioplasty: One-year clinical follow-up of benestent trial. J Am Coll Cardiol 27:255, 1996.

72. Edwards BS, Rodeheffer RJ, McGregor CGA. Cardiac transplantation. In: Giuliani ER, Gersh BJ, McGoon DL, et al., eds Mayo Clinic Practice of Cardiology. 3rd ed. St. Louis: Mosby, 1996.

73. Squires RW, Gau GT, Miller TD, et al. Cardiac rehabilitation and cardiovascular health enhancement. In: Giuliani ER, Gersh BJ, McGoon DL, et al., eds. Mayo Clinic Practice of Cardiology. 3rd ed. St. Louis: Mosby, 1996.

74. Simoons ML, Vos J, Deckers JW, et al. Coronary artery disease: Prevention of progression and prevention of events. Eur Heart J 16:729, 1995.

75. Rossouw JE. Lipid-lowering interventions in angiographic trials. Am J Cardiol 76:86c, 1995.

76. Scandinavian Simvastatin Survival Study Group. Randomized trial of cholesterol lowering in 4,444 patients with coronary heart disease: The Scandinavian Simvastatin Survival Study (4S). Lancet 344:1383, 1994.

77. Gould KL, Ornish D, Scherwitz L, et al. Changes in myocardial perfusion abnormalities by positron emission tomography after long-term, intense risk factor modification. JAMA 274:894, 1995.

78. Seiler C, Suter TM, Hess OM. Exercise-induced vasomotion of angiographically normal and stenotic coronary arteries improves after cholesterol-lowering drug therapy with bezafibrate. J Am Coll Cardiol 26:1615, 1995.

79. Hambrecht R, Niebauer J, Marburger C, et al. Various intensities of leisure time physical activity in patients with coronary artery disease: Effects on cardiorespiratory fitness and progression of coronary atherosclerotic lesions. J Am Coll Cardiol 22:468, 1993.

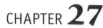

CHAPTER **27**

MANIFESTATIONS OF CORONARY ATHEROSCLEROSIS

Ray W. Squires

Coronary atherosclerosis may be present for decades without apparent clinical importance. In some patients, the disease makes itself known by the appearance of stable angina pectoris or by silent (symptomless) ischemia during stress testing. Unfortunately, in other patients the first manifestation is unstable angina, acute myocardial infarction, or sudden cardiac death. This chapter reviews the following topics related to the clinical appearance of coronary atherosclerosis:

1. Myocardial blood flow and metabolism
2. Myocardial ischemia
3. Stable coronary artery disease
4. Acute coronary syndromes, including myocardial infarction
5. Sudden cardiac death
6. Chronic heart failure

MYOCARDIAL BLOOD FLOW AND METABOLISM

Normal cardiac contractile function depends on the presence of adequate concentrations of high-energy phosphate supplies (primarily adenosine triphosphate, or ATP) in the myocardium. The heart is a highly aerobic organ with an extensive circulatory system and an abundance of mitochondria (1). The coronary arterial system is well developed and includes epicardial arteries (Fig. 27.1), which bifurcate into intramyocardial and endocardial branches (Fig. 27.2). At rest, coronary blood flow averages 60–90 mL/min/100 g of myocardium, and it may increase 5- to 6-fold during exercise (2). In normal conditions the heart produces ATP using the aerobic metabolic pathway; it is not adapted to anaerobic energy production. At rest, myocardial oxygen uptake is approximately 8–10 mL of oxygen per 100 g of tissue per minute. During intense exercise, the oxygen requirement may increase by 200–300% (3). Because the myocardium extracts nearly all of the oxygen from the arterial blood that flows through its capillary beds (70% extraction, much greater

than that of skeletal muscle at rest), coronary blood flow must be closely regulated to the needs of the myocardium for oxygen (4). With an increase in myocardial work, which increases oxygen demand (myocardial oxygen demand is determined by the heart rate, the contractile state of the left ventricle, the end-diastolic pressure, and the aortic pressure), coronary blood flow must increase to provide the necessary amount of oxygen (2).

Blood flow through any regional circulation, including the coronary system, is determined by the arterial blood pressure and the resistance to the flow of blood offered by the vasculature, primarily the arterioles, which can change caliber and dramatically alter the resistance to flow (4). Because of the high intramyocardial pressure generated during systole, which partially compresses the coronary arteries, increases vascular resistance, and inhibits forward flow, coronary blood flow to the left ventricle occurs primarily during diastole (Fig. 27.3). Control of coronary blood flow is primarily by local myocardial tissue metabolic factors, such as the vasodilators adenosine and prostacyclin, which are released during myocardial contraction (5, 6).

The autonomic nervous system also exerts some effect on myocardial blood flow (7). Sympathetic nervous system stimulation usually results in increased myocardial blood flow due to the augmentation of heart rate and contractility (increased myocardial oxygen requirement). However, alpha-receptor–mediated coronary vasoconstriction may occur with sympathetic stimulation if myocardial metabolism is not increased. Parasympathetic nervous system stimulation has been shown to result in coronary vasodilation.

A substantial reduction in vessel luminal (internal) diameter may occur before a decrease in blood flow can be measured distal to the narrowed coronary artery segment. When the plaque reduces the luminal cross-sectional area by 75% or more, blood flow through the artery when the person is at rest is reduced (termed a hemodynamically significant lesion) (2). Beyond this level of *critical stenosis*, further small decreases in cross-sectional area of the vessel result in large reductions in flow.

Anterior View

A

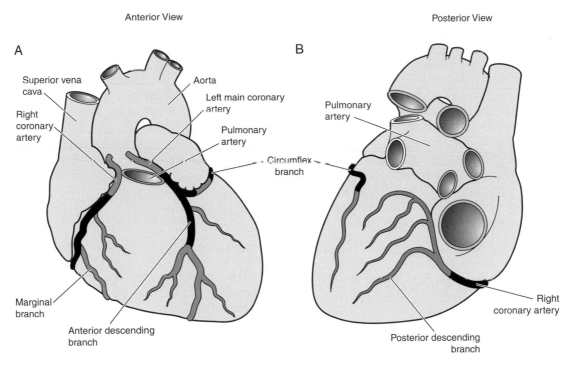

Superior vena cava

Aorta

Left main coronary artery

Right coronary artery

Pulmonary artery

Circumflex branch

Marginal branch

Anterior descending branch

Posterior View

B

Pulmonary artery

Right coronary artery

Posterior descending branch

Figure 27.1. The epicardial coronary arteries. **A.** Anterior view. Black segments are prime sites for the development of obstructive atherosclerotic plaques. Ao, aorta; IVC, inferior vena cava; SVC, superior vena cava; PA, pulmonary artery. (Reprinted with permission from Lie JT. Pathology of coronary artery disease. In: Giuliani ER, Fuster V, Gersh BJ, et al., eds. Cardiology: Fundamentals and Practice. St. Louis: Mosby–Year Book, 1991.)

The reduction in the cross-sectional area of the coronary artery may be caused by atherosclerotic plaque exclusively, by vasospasm of an artery without obstructive coronary atherosclerosis, by vasospasm superimposed over an atherosclerotic plaque, or by platelet aggregation leading to thrombus associated with a plaque rupture (discussed in detail later in the chapter) (8, 9).

Coronary vasospasm is defined as a temporary increase in epicardial coronary artery smooth muscle tone (contraction) that results in a reduced luminal cross-sectional area (10). Coronary vasospasm may result from a variety of factors:

- Local arterial wall abnormalities, including endothelial cell dysfunction, which result in an exaggerated response to vasoconstrictor agents such as thromboxane A2 and serotonin released from platelets
- Sympathetic nervous system activity stimulating alpha-adrenergic receptors in the artery, which leads to vasoconstriction (e.g., coronary vasoconstriction resulting from exposure to cold)

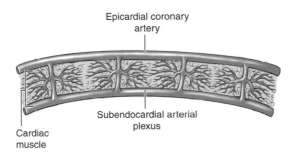

Epicardial coronary artery

Subendocardial arterial plexus

Cardiac muscle

Figure 27.2. Structure of the intramyocardial and subendocardial coronary arteries in relation to the epicardial arteries. (Reprinted with permission from Guyton AC. Textbook of Medical Physiology. 7th ed. Philadelphia: Saunders, 1986.)

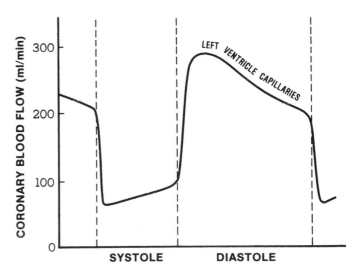

Figure 27.3. Coronary blood flow during systole and diastole. (Reprinted with permission from Guyton AC. Textbook of Medical Physiology. 7th ed. Philadelphia: Saunders, 1986.)

- Bloodborne substances such as epinephrine (which also stimulates the alpha-receptors)

Atherosclerotic arteries are deficient in the production and/or release of endothelium-derived relaxing factor (nitric oxide) and may exhibit an exaggerated vasoconstrictor response to bloodborne substances (11). They also have an impaired capacity to vasodilate.

Myocardial ischemia is a pathological condition in which blood flow to the myocardium is reduced below the amount needed to provide adequate amounts of oxygen to match the needs of the heart for ATP production (oxygen supply < demand) (2, 3). It results in oxygen deprivation accompanied by inadequate removal of metabolites. Three physiological abnormalities may result from ischemia:

1. Hypoxia (insufficient oxygen for the needs of aerobic energy metabolism)
2. Accumulation of toxic metabolites
3. Acidosis

Hypoxia inhibits aerobic metabolism, and the intracellular stores of ATP may become depleted. Toxic metabolites and acidosis likewise impair myocardial aerobic energy production. This results in a partial shift from the usual aerobic to the uncharacteristic anaerobic production of ATP, with metabolism of carbohydrate as the predominate fuel and a marked increase in the production of lactic acid. During ischemia the heart releases lactate into the venous blood rather than extracting lactic acid from arterial blood, as it does when ischemia is not present.

Ischemia may result in progressive abnormalities in cardiac function, the *ischemic cascade* (12). The first abnormality is stiffening of the left ventricle, which decreases the ability of the chamber to fill with blood during diastole (*diastolic dysfunction*). Second, systolic emptying of the left ventricle is impaired. Local areas of the heart that are ischemic may develop asynergic contraction patterns such as *hypokinesis* (reduced systolic contraction, decreased extent of myocyte shortening), *akinesis* (absent contraction, cessation of myocyte shortening), or *dyskinesis* (paradoxical aneurysmal bulging of the infarcted segment of myocardium during contraction) (13). In normal conditions, the ventricular myocytes shorten during systole and cause the chamber walls to thicken and move inward as contraction proceeds. During ischemia, altered systolic function, as demonstrated by the development of segmental wall motion contraction abnormalities, and a reduction in left ventricular ejection fraction and stroke volume may occur. Third, electrocardiographic changes associated with altered repolarization (ST segment depression or elevation, T wave inversion or pseudonormalization) may occur as a result of nonuniform repolarization through the ischemic and surrounding tissue. Ischemia may initiate serious ventricular arrhythmias (ventricular tachycardia and fibrillation). Finally, the patient may develop symptoms of *angina pectoris*.

Angina pectoris is transient referred cardiac pain resulting from myocardial ischemia (14). Some patients with ischemia, either mild or severe, do not develop pain or discomfort (*silent ischemia*). However, most patients do develop symptoms if the amount of ischemia is moderate to severe. The locations and sensations of angina pectoris are diverse. The pain is usually in the substernal region, jaw, neck, or arms, although it may occur in the epigastrium and interscapular regions. The characteristic pain is usually described as a feeling of pressure, heaviness, fullness, squeezing, burning, aching, choking, or boring. The pain may vary in intensity and may radiate. If the myocardial ischemia leads to an increase in left ventricular end-diastolic pressure and increased pulmonary vascular pressure, the patient may have dyspnea (*anginal equivalent*). *Typical angina* is usually provoked by exertion, emotion, exposure to cold or heat, meals, and sexual intercourse and is relieved by rest or nitroglycerin. *Atypical angina* refers to similar symptoms but with some characteristic that is apart from typical angina, such as no relation to exertion. *Stable angina* is reproducible and predictable in onset, severity, and means of relief. It is believed to be the result of a fixed stenosis of a coronary artery that limits blood flow in a consistent manner (15). *Unstable angina* is described as new onset of typical angina; increasing frequency, intensity, or duration of previously stable angina; or angina that occurs at rest or in the first few days after myocardial infarction (14). Unstable angina is believed to result from dynamic myocardial ischemia due to the development of transient partially or completely occlusive platelet thrombi (thrombi that develop and then dissolve) or periodic coronary vasospasm (*variant* or *Prinzmetal's angina*) mediated by local vasoconstrictors such as endothelin, which is produced by the injured endothelium (16).

With prolonged ischemia, myocyte necrosis (irreversible damage, myocardial infarction) occurs (12). If the episode of ischemia is relatively brief, the resultant contractile abnormalities of the ventricle (discussed earlier) are reversible. Brief postischemic left ventricular dysfunction is called *stunned myocardium* (17). More chronic but reversible left ventricular dysfunction is termed *hibernating myocardium*; it is the result of ongoing significant but not lethal (to myocytes) ischemia. In this condition, myocytes remain viable but exhibit depressed contractile function. This phenomenon appears to be a protective mechanism whereby myocytes reduce their oxygen demand when the oxygen supply is inadequate for normal function. Elimination of the chronic ischemia by revascularization results in a return of normal contractile function, which may occur rapidly or require as much as a year for resolution (18, 19).

STABLE CORONARY ARTERY DISEASE

Some patients with coronary artery disease have one or more hemodynamically significant lesions that remain anatomically stable over many years. These lesions limit coronary blood flow in a predictable and reproducible manner. Angina pectoris, if present, occurs consistently with various provocative stimuli. These lesions are thought to be advanced and fibrotic and to contain little lipid (15).

ACUTE CORONARY SYNDROMES INCLUDING MYOCARDIAL INFARCTION

The syndromes of **unstable angina, non–ST segment elevation myocardial infarction** (formerly termed non–Q wave myocardial infarction), **ST segment elevation myocardial infarction** (previously called Q wave myocardial infarction) and some instances of **sudden cardiac death** are related to atherosclerotic plaque rupture, vasoconstriction with subsequent occlusive thrombus formation (15, 20). The duration of thrombotic vessel occlusion is believed to be the critical determinant of the type of coronary event that occurs. Unstable angina is probably the result of plaque disruption followed by transient (<10 minutes) vessel occlusion (thrombus formation and/or vasospasm) followed by spontaneous thrombolysis (clot dissolution) and vasorelaxation. More severe plaque rupture, with thrombosis lasting approximately 60 minutes before lysis, is a postulated mechanism for non–ST segment elevation myocardial infarction. Disruption of a large amount of plaque with a fixed thrombus that occludes a coronary epicardial artery leads to ST segment elevation myocardial infarction. Ischemia resulting from any type of plaque disruption of thrombotic vessel occlusion may result in ventricular tachycardia or fibrillation and sudden cardiac death.

Why Do Some Plaques Rupture and Thrombose?

It appears that the strength and integrity of the fibrous cap overlying the lipid-rich core of the atherosclerotic plaque determines the stability of the lesion (21). Rupture-prone plaques tend to have thin fibrous caps, whereas stable plaques have thicker fibrous caps that protect the blood in the lumen from the thrombogenic core. These vulnerable plaques typically have a large amount of lipid in their core. Cytokines, protein mediators of inflammation, are present during various phases of atherogenesis. In particular, interferon-gamma from T cells inhibits collagen synthesis and thus weakens the fibrous cap. Interferon-gamma also inhibits smooth muscle cell proliferation, activates the program of cell death (apoptosis), and contributes to the relative scarcity of smooth muscle cells in rupture-prone lesions. The forces leading to plaque rupture may be hemodynamic stress, increased blood pressure and/or heart rate, local vasoconstriction,

nicotine, or immune complexes. Macrophages within the plaque may release proteases and tumor necrosis factor, which may erode the plaque from within. After plaque rupture, circulating platelets come in direct contact with the internal environment of the plaque, which provides a prothrombic state (16, 22).

Angiographic studies have demonstrated that rupture-prone plaques are not usually high-grade stenotic lesions. Typically, the lesions involved with rupture and thrombus formation are less than 50% occlusive (23). **Severe obstructive coronary atherosclerosis is not a prerequisite for the development of acute myocardial infarction.** This explains the finding that many patients who have an acute myocardial infarction do not provide a history of angina pectoris before their infarction. However, angiographically severe coronary atherosclerosis correlates with the likelihood to develop an acute coronary event, probably by serving as a marker of angiographically modest but rupture-prone lesions. Autopsy studies have shown that many patients have disrupted atherosclerotic plaques but no history of an acute coronary event. Thus, not all plaque ruptures lead to symptomatic events.

Acute Myocardial Infarction

Acute myocardial infarction is the necrosis (death) of cardiac myocytes resulting from prolonged myocardial ischemia caused by complete coronary artery occlusion lasting at least 60 minutes (24). The key event in differentiating reversible from irreversible (infarction) cell damage is disruption of the myocyte membrane. This appears to be the lethal event: the myocyte cannot recover if membrane disruption occurs and cytoplasmic contents (e.g., enzymes) spill into the circulation (24).

In a minority of cases it is possible to determine a precipitating event or trigger such as the following (25, 26):

- Physical exertion
- Emotional stress, anger
- Surgery associated with substantial loss of blood
- Circadian variation

Slightly more myocardial infarctions occur in the morning than at other times, suggesting a possible role for sympathetic nervous system activation in the onset of the event (24, 26).

The diagnosis of acute myocardial infarction is based on symptoms of myocardial ischemia that persist for at least 30 minutes, electrocardiographic (ECG) hallmarks, and evaluation of cardiac enzymes in the blood (evidence of myocyte necrosis). Echocardiographically determined regional wall motion abnormalities at rest and myocardial perfusion scanning may also be helpful in making the diagnosis (20, 24, 26).

Symptoms of acute myocardial infarction may include chest pain or other anginal pain, gastrointestinal upset, dyspnea, sweating, anxiety, or syncope or may be painless (*silent myocardial infarction*) in approximately 25% of patients (20, 26). Pain is often severe, but all intensities of discomfort are possible.

Myocardial infarctions may affect the entire thickness of the ventricle (*transmural infarction*) or only a portion of the wall of the ventricle (*subendocardial infarction*). Transmural infarction can be diagnosed from the ECG in the majority of cases (not in patients with pre-existing left bundle branch block, for example), but subendocardial infarction cannot be reliably diagnosed from the ECG (26). Transmural myocardial injury produces ST segment elevation on the ECG. During the acute phase of a transmural myocardial infarction, three zones of affected myocardium may be distinguished:

1. Central core of necrosis
2. Surrounding zone of ischemic injury
3. Peripheral area of ischemia

The necrotic core produces a *pathological Q wave* (about 30 ms wide and 0.2 mV in magnitude). The zone of ischemic injury results in *ST segment elevation*, and the peripheral ischemic zone produces an *inverted T wave* (20, 27). Figure 27.4 shows the evolution of the ECG changes of acute transmural myocardial infarction with hypera-

cute ST segment elevation—the most recognizable abnormality in the early hours of the infarction—the subsequent development of Q waves and T wave inversion, and the return of the ST segment to baseline. Over time, the scar tissue of the infarct may shrink, and the size of the Q wave may also diminish. Table 27.1 provides criteria for anatomical localization of myocardial infarctions by Q wave appearance. Myocardial infarction may involve more than one anatomical area simultaneously. Two or more infarctions, both acute and chronic, may coexist (27). Diagnosis of a Q wave myocardial infarction from the ECG is difficult or impossible in patients with left bundle branch block, left ventricular hypertrophy, or Wolff-Parkinson-White syndrome.

Categories of infarcts designated *Q wave* and *non–Q wave* have recently been replaced by the terms *ST segment elevation* and *non–ST segment elevation*, respectively (20). ST segment elevation infarcts are the result of an occluded epicardial coronary artery (usually with fibrin thrombus), with more myocardial damage and a worse prognosis than non–ST segment infarcts, which have less associated myocardial damage, partly because of spontaneous thrombolysis (clot dissolution) in approximately 75% of patients. These infarcts are associated with a platelet thrombus. Electrocardiographic signs include ST segment depression and/or T wave inversion.

Myocardial necrosis disrupts the myocyte membrane and releases some cytoplasmic contents into the blood. Cardiac enzymes and other substances released by the infarcted areas of the heart are useful in the diagnosis of acute infarction (20, 26). Creatine kinase (CK) catalyzes the hydrolysis of creatine phosphate, releasing energy for the resynthesis of ATP. This enzyme exists as three isoenzymes: BB, primarily in the brain and kidney; MM, in skeletal muscle; and MB, in the heart and in small amounts in skeletal muscle. An increase in the blood concentration of CK-MB is a specific early enzyme marker for

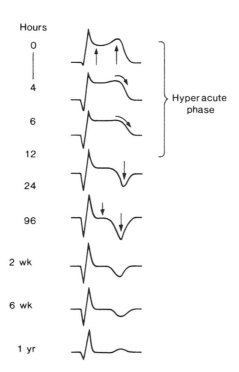

Figure 27.4. The evolution of electrocardiographic changes in Q wave myocardial infarction. (Reprinted with permission from Gau GT. Standard electrocardiography, vectorcardiography and signal-averaged electrocardiography. In: Giuliani ER, Fuster V, Gersh BJ, et al., eds. Cardiology: Fundamentals and Practice. St. Louis: Mosby–Year Book, 1991.)

Table 27.1. Criteria for Anatomical Localization of Myocardial Infarction by Q Wave Appearance

1. Inferior wall myocardial infarction (usually right coronary artery occlusion): Q wave (>40 ms duration, amplitude > 25% of the R wave) in leads II, III, aVf
2. Anterior wall myocardial infarction (left anterior descending coronary artery occlusion): Q wave in leads V1–V3 (anteroseptal), QS pattern in leads V1–V3 (anteroseptal), Q wave in leads V2–V4 (anterior), QS pattern in leads V2–V4 (anterior)
3. Lateral wall myocardial infarction (usually circumflex coronary artery occlusion): Q wave in leads V4–V6 or QS pattern in leads V4–V6
4. Posterior wall myocardial infarction (usually right coronary artery occlusion): prominent R wave in leads V1–V2 with positive T waves
5. High lateral wall myocardial infarction (usually circumflex coronary artery occlusion): Q wave in leads I and aVL or QS pattern in leads I and aVL

myocardial necrosis (28). CK-MB appears in the blood as early as 3 hours after the onset of myocardial infarction, peaks within 12–24 hours and returns to baseline by 48–72 hours. If a patient is seen in the hospital within the first 24 hours after the onset of the infarction, total CK and CK-MB measurements have an excellent sensitivity for detection of myocardial necrosis. If the patient presents more than 24 hours after the beginning of suspicious symptoms, the peak level of CK may have been missed, and measurement of other substances released from the damaged myocardium is necessary (26). Until recently, the enzyme lactate dehydrogenase was used as a late marker for myocardial necrosis (29). This has been replaced by cardiac troponin I, a specific myocardial contractile protein, which is released from necrotic myocardium beginning 3 to 6 hours after the onset of infarction (useful for early infarct detection) with peak values at 24–48 hours (20). It remains elevated for up to 10 days after infarction, hence is the preferred late marker for myocardial infarction. When both CK-MB and cardiac troponin I are measured and the results are concordant, the certainty of diagnosis is increased.

Additional cardiac imaging techniques may be helpful in the diagnosis of acute myocardial infarction (26). Echocardiography may disclose regional wall motion abnormalities of infarction and/or a subnormal left ventricular ejection fraction. Radionuclide imaging is helpful in identifying and quantifying the area of infarction.

Necrosis of myocytes, as with myocardial infarction, results in an inflammatory response with infiltration of neutrophils and macrophages (30). Since myocardial cells do not regenerate, infarct healing occurs via scar formation. Depending on the size of the infarction, completion of scar formation may take days to weeks. The scar cannot contract, as does normal myocardium. The greater the amount of infarcted myocardium, the larger the scar.

Treatment of Acute Myocardial Infarction

Treatment includes the following (31):

- Relief of symptoms
- Reperfusion of the infarct-related artery
- Hemodynamic monitoring and inotropic support with an intra-aortic balloon pump if required
- Risk factor modification for secondary prevention

Nitroglycerin, oxygen, and morphine are given to relieve the pain of infarction. Beta-blockers, aspirin, and heparin are routinely given. ACE inhibitors are given to patients with ST segment elevation myocardial infarctions, left bundle branch block, and/or left ventricular dysfunction.

Early reperfusion (restoring patency of the infarcted artery), ideally within 1 to 2 hours of the onset of symptoms, with either thrombolytic agents, such as tissue plasminogen activator or streptokinase, or immediate angio-

plasty without thrombolytics (primary angioplasty) may restore normal flow and reduce the size of the area of infarction (myocardial salvage). The speed of the application of reperfusion therapy after onset of symptoms is the critical factor in preventing a large area of necrosis. Reperfusion therapy applied more than 12 hours after the onset of infarction offers no benefit. Thrombolytic agents are given to patients with acute ST segment elevation myocardial infarcts (with fibrin thrombus amenable to thrombolysis). To prevent additional platelet aggregation at the infarct site, new drugs that bind to the platelet glycoprotein IIb-IIIa receptor (abciximab or eptifibatide) are now commonly given along with thrombolytic agents (32). These agents are also given in the setting of non–ST segment elevation myocardial infarction, with which thrombolytic agents are not used (platelet thrombus). In some instances, thrombolytic therapy may not result in complete resolution of symptoms and ECG abnormalities (failed thrombolysis), and subsequent angioplasty (rescue angioplasty) or emergency coronary artery bypass surgery may be performed. The use of intracoronary stents, metal support devices deployed in the coronary artery, is standard practice, with better short-term and long-term outcome than angioplasty alone.

Complications

Serious complications may arise from acute myocardial infarction. These complications may result in early or late mortality (24, 26). The most common complications are life-threatening ventricular arrhythmias (*ventricular tachycardia, ventricular fibrillation*). Additional possibly serious situations:

- *Rupture of the ventricular free wall* (occurs most commonly during the first week after infarction and affects 1–3% of infarcts)
- *Left ventricular aneurysm*
- *Rupture of the interventricular septum*
- *Extension* or *recurrence of infarction*
- *Severe left ventricular dysfunction* leading to *congestive heart failure* and *cardiogenic shock* (a downward cascade of cardiac pump failure resulting in further reduction in coronary blood flow because of hypotension and inadequate cardiac output; usually fatal)
- *Papillary muscle rupture* resulting in severe *mitral valve regurgitation*
- *Pericarditis* (Dressler's syndrome)

Contraction abnormalities of the ventricles are almost universal after myocardial infarction (24). Diastolic filling abnormalities are common; they indicate a stiff, noncompliant ventricle. Systolic contraction abnormalities (asynergic contraction) include hypokinesis, akinesis, and dyskinesis, as previously mentioned.

Myocardial infarction, particularly with anterior wall location or in other infarct locations with extensive myocardial necrosis, may over weeks to years produce progressive adverse changes in the geometry and contractile function of the ventricle (33). Left ventricular dilation involving both the infarcted myocardium (*infarct expansion*) and the adjacent uninfarcted tissue (*ventricular remodeling*) may occur. The process may result in progressive thinning of the ventricular wall, enlargement of the cardiac chambers, and congestive heart failure.

In-hospital mortality for conventionally treated patients after acute myocardial infarction is approximately 5–10% (26). Annual mortality thereafter averages 5%. However, the following clinical characteristics are associated with a higher (50% or greater) risk of reinfarction and death after hospital dismissal (34–37):

1. Left ventricular ejection fraction below 40% and congestive heart failure symptoms during hospitalization worsen the prognosis.
2. Patients with non–ST segment elevation myocardial infarction have lower hospital mortality than patients with ST segment elevation infarctions, but they are much more likely to have a recurrent infarction within 3 months of the initial event.
3. Patients who exhibit myocardial ischemia during low-intensity exercise are at an increased risk for a subsequent cardiac event.
4. Patients with poor exercise capacity as measured with graded exercise testing (<4 METs) are at high risk.
5. Psychosocial stress and social isolation are associated with an increase in the rate of recurrent cardiac events.
6. Complex ventricular arrhythmias portend an adverse prognosis.

SUDDEN CARDIAC DEATH

Death due to cardiovascular causes within approximately an hour of the onset of symptoms is *sudden cardiac death*. This phenomenon accounts for approximately 50% of cardiac deaths (38). Most sudden cardiac deaths are due to ventricular arrhythmias, usually ventricular tachycardia that degenerates into ventricular fibrillation. The pathophysiology of these lethal ventricular arrhythmias may be acute myocardial infarction, acute myocardial ischemia, chronic myocardial infarction (scar-mediated arrhythmia), or left ventricular hypertrophy or cardiomyopathy. Unfortunately, sudden cardiac death is the first manifestation of coronary artery disease for many patients.

Additional causes of sudden cardiac death are less common. Such causes include supraventricular tachycardia with an extremely fast ventricular rate, cardiac rupture (usually in the setting of acute myocardial infarction), pericardial effusion with cardiac tamponade (compression of the heart with subsequent rapid drop in cardiac output), and aortic rupture (38).

CHRONIC HEART FAILURE

Myocardial infarction and/or myocardial ischemia, if extensive in distribution in the heart, may lead to left ventricular dysfunction (chronic heart failure) (39). *Systolic dysfunction* results in poor contractile performance and is commonly diagnosed by a subnormal left ventricular ejection fraction (normal left ventricular ejection fraction is > 50%). *Diastolic dysfunction* is the condition in which the heart cannot accept blood and fill at a normal diastolic pressure. It results in inadequate left ventricular filling, slow filling, or abnormally high ventricular diastolic pressure. Systolic or diastolic dysfunction or both may result in a subnormal cardiac output.

The natural history of chronic heart failure usually includes a variable period with an asymptomatic stage of depressed left ventricular ejection fraction with cardiomegaly (*asymptomatic left ventricular dysfunction*). This progresses to a *minimally symptomatic stage* and finally to the *stage of congestive symptoms*. The rate of deterioration is highly variable (40). Common signs and symptoms in patients with heart failure:

- Fatigue, weakness
- Dyspnea, especially with exertion
- Reduced exercise capacity
- Orthopnea and/or paroxysmal nocturnal dyspnea

▶ SUMMARY

Obstructive plaque formation, lesion instability, and thrombosis can lead to a number of coronary syndromes, including stable or unstable angina pectoris, acute myocardial infarction (ST segment elevation or non–ST segment elevation), heart failure, or sudden cardiac death. The clinical conditions associated with these syndromes indicate that therapeutic modalities that are most appropriate should be administered immediately to increase the possibility of long-term survival.

References

1. Garratt KN, Morgan JP. Pathophysiology of myocardial ischemia and reperfusion. In: Giuliani ER, Fuster V, Gersh BJ, et al., eds. Cardiology: Fundamentals and Practice. St. Louis: Mosby–Year Book, 1991.
2. Braunwald E, Sobel BE. Coronary blood flow and myocardial ischemia. In: Braunwald, E. Textbook of Cardiovascular Medicine. 3rd ed. Philadelphia: Saunders, 1988.
3. Garratt KN, Morgan JP. Coronary circulation. In: Giuliani ER, Fuster V, Gersh BJ, et al., eds. Cardiology: Fundamentals and Practice. St. Louis: Mosby–Year Book, 1991.
4. Guyton AC. Textbook of Medical Physiology. 7th ed. Philadelphia: Saunders, 1986.
5. Rubio R, Wiedimeier VT, Berne RM. Relationship between coronary flow and adenosine production and release. J Mol Cardiol 6:561, 1974.

6. Schor K. Possible role of prostaglandins in the regulation of coronary blood flow. Basic Res Cardiol 76:239, 1981.

7. Bove AA, Santamore WP. Physiology of the coronary circulation. In: Giuliani ER, Fuster V, Gersh BJ, et al., eds. Cardiology: Fundamentals and Practice. St. Louis: Mosby–Year Book, 1991.

8. Maseri A. Myocardial ischemia in man: Current concepts, changing views and future investigation. Can J Cardiol Jul(Suppl A):225A, 1986.

9. Fuster V. Elucidation of the role of plaque instability and rupture in acute coronary events. Am J Cardiol 76:24C, 1995.

10. McGoon MD, Fuster V. Coronary artery spasm and vasotonicity. In: Giuliani ER, Fuster V, Gersh BJ, et al., eds. Cardiology: Fundamentals and Practice. St. Louis: Mosby–Year Book, 1991.

11. Griffith TM, Lewis MJ, Newby AC, et al. Endothelium-derived relaxing factor. J Am Coll Cardiol 12:797, 1988.

12. Hurst JW. Coronary heart disease: The overview of the clinician. In: Wenger NK. Hellerstein HK, eds. Rehabilitation of the Coronary Patient. 3rd ed. New York: Churchill Livingstone, 1992.

13. Squires RW, Williams WL. Coronary atherosclerosis and acute myocardial infarction. In: ACSM's Resource Manual for Guidelines for Exercise Testing and Prescription. 2nd ed. Philadelphia: Lea & Febiger, 1993.

14. Shub C. Angina pectoris and coronary heart disease. In: Giuliani ER, Fuster V, Gersh BJ, et al., eds. Cardiology: Fundamentals and Practice. St. Louis: Mosby–Year Book, 1991.

15. Fuster V, Chesebro JH. Atherosclerosis: Pathogenesis, initiation, progression, acute coronary syndromes, and regression. In: Giuliani ER, Gersh BJ, McGoon MD, et al., eds. Mayo Clinic Practice of Cardiology. 3rd ed. St. Louis: Mosby, 1996.

16. Assoian RK, Grotendorst GR, Miller DM, et al. Cellular transformation by coordinated action of three peptide growth factors from human platelets. Nature 309:804, 1984.

17. Ferrari R. Metabolic disturbances during myocardial ischemia and reperfusion. Am J Cardiol 76:17B, 1995.

18. Rahimtoola SH. From coronary artery disease to heart failure: Role of the hibernating myocardium. Am J Cardiol 75:16E, 1995.

19. Maseri A. Introduction to a symposium: From mitochondrial metabolism to coronary artery disease: New trends in the management of myocardial ischemia. Am J Cardiol 76:1B, 1995.

20. Wright RS, Santrach PJ, Kopecky SL. Diagnosis of acute myocardial infarction. In: Murphy JG, ed. Mayo Clinic Cardiology Review. 2nd ed. Philadelphia: Lippincott, 2000.

21. Libby P. Molecular bases of the acute coronary syndromes. Circulation 91:2844, 1995.

22. Frick RJ, Ostrach LH, Rooney PA, et al. Coronary thrombosis, ulcerated plaques and platelet/fibrin microemboli in patients dying with acute coronary disease: A large autopsy study. J Invest Cardiol 2:199, 1990.

23. Shah PK, Forrester JJ. Pathophysiology of acute coronary syndromes. Am J Cardiol 68:16C, 1991.

24. Pasternak RC, Braunwald E, Sobel BE. Acute myocardial infarction. In: Braunwald E, ed. Textbook of Cardiovascular Medicine. 3rd ed. Philadelphia: Saunders, 1988.

25. Mittleman MA, Maclure M, Sherwood JB, et al. Triggering of acute myocardial infarction by episodes of anger. Circulation 92:1720, 1995.

26. Gersh BJ, Clements IP. Acute myocardial infarction: Diagnosis and prognosis. In: Giuliani ER, Gersh BJ, McGoon MD, et al. Mayo Clinic Practice of Cardiology. 3rd ed. St. Louis: Mosby, 1996.

27. Gau GT. Standard electrocardiography, vectorcardiography and signal-averaged electrocardiography. In: Giuliani ER, Fuster V, Gersh BJ, et al., eds. Cardiology: Fundamentals and Practice. St. Louis: Mosby–Year Book, 1991.

28. Sobel BE, Shell WE. Serum enzyme determinations in the diagnosis and assessment of myocardial infarction. Circulation 45:471, 1972.

29. Agress CM, Kim JHC. Evaluation of enzyme tests in the diagnosis of heart disease. Am J Cardiol 6:641, 1960.

30. Edwards WD. Applied anatomy of the heart. In: Giuliani ER, Gersh BJ, McGoon MD, et al. Mayo Clinic Practice of Cardiology. 3rd ed. St. Louis: Mosby, 1996.

31. Murphy JG, Wright RS, Kopecky SL, Reeder GS. Management of acute myocardial infraction. In: Murphy JG, ed. Mayo Clinic Cardiology Review. 2nd ed. Philadelphia: Lippincott, 2000.

32. Wong SJ, Murphy JG. Thrombolytic trials for acute myocardial infarction. I. In: Murphy JG, ed. Mayo Clinic Cardiology Review. 2nd ed. Philadelphia: Lippincott, 2000.

33. Pfeffer MA, Braunwald E. Ventricular remodeling after myocardial infarction: Experimental observations and clinical implications. Circulation 81:1161, 1990.

34. Krone RJ. The role of risk stratification in the early management of a myocardial infarction. Ann Intern Med 116:223, 1992.

35. American College of Sports Medicine. ACSM's Guidelines for Exercise Testing and Prescription. 5th ed. Baltimore: Williams & Wilkins, 1995.

36. Frasure-Smith N, Lesperance F, Juneau M. Differentiated long-term impact of in-hospital symptoms of psychological stress after nonQ-wave and Q-wave acute myocardial infarction. Am J Cardiol 69:1128, 1992.

37. Case RB, Moss AJ, Case N, et al. Living alone after myocardial infarction: Impact on prognosis. JAMA 267:515, 1992.

38. Osborn MJ. Sudden cardiac death: Mechanisms, incidence, and prevention of sudden cardiac death. In: Giuliani ER, Gersh BJ, McGoon MD, et al., eds. Mayo Clinic Practice of Cardiology. 3rd ed. St. Louis: Mosby, 1996.

39. Karon B. Diagnosis and outpatient management of congestive heart failure. Mayo Clin Proc 70:1080, 1995.

40. Rodeheffer RJ, Gersh BJ. Dilated cardiomyopathy and the myocarditises. In: Giuliani ER, Gersh BJ, McGoon MD, et al., eds. Mayo Clinic Practice of Cardiology. 3rd ed. St. Louis: Mosby, 1996.

3.4.0   4.4.2, 4.4.3, 4.4.7, 4.6.3.0,   5.4.3, 5.6.0, 5.6.1
         4.6.4.5, 4.6.4.6, 4.6.4.5

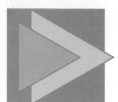

CHAPTER **28**

DIAGNOSIS OF CORONARY ARTERY DISEASE

Fredric J. Pashkow, Michael Lauer, and Sharon A. Harvey

The diagnosis of coronary artery disease (CAD) requires using a synergistic mix of traditional medical skills and cutting-edge technology (1). The judicious and appropriate use of tests in evaluating patients for CAD requires clinical judgment and knowledge of the indications, contraindications, sensitivity, specificity, predictive value, and limitations of each test (2). Tests can be used to confirm diagnosis, to define coronary anatomy, and to assess ventricular function and the extent of coronary involvement or amount of myocardial damage and thus to assess prognosis and the risk for future events. Typically, using cardiac tests in the diagnosis of CAD begins with the least costly and least invasive test. Abnormal or inconclusive findings lead the clinician to the next level. Each level of diagnostic testing increases diagnostic accuracy as well as expense. Also, as testing becomes more invasive, the risk increases.

PREDICTIVE ACCURACY OF DIAGNOSTIC TESTS

Calculation of predictive accuracy is based on the incidence of true and false findings. The following are important concepts in understanding the predictive accuracy of diagnostic testing:

1. In a *true-positive* test, the **patient has CAD** and the test findings are **abnormal**.
2. In a *true-negative* test, the **patient does not have CAD** and the test findings are **normal**.
3. In contrast, for a *false-positive* test, the **patient does not have CAD**, but the test findings are **abnormal**.
4. For a *false-negative* test, **the patient has CAD**, but the test findings are **normal**.

Effective test selection and interpretation of results requires a detailed understanding of the concepts of sensitivity, specificity, predictive accuracy, and relative risk. These values define how effectively a test identifies patients with and without CAD. The predictive ability of a test is significantly influenced by the prevalence of CAD in the population being tested.

If the population is skewed toward severity of disease, the test has higher sensitivity. For example, in the case of exercise testing, the test is more sensitive in individuals with triple-vessel CAD than in those with single-vessel CAD. Testing can also have low specificity if used in individuals who are likely to have false-positive results (e.g., exercise testing has relatively low specificity in women and those with mitral valve prolapse because of a higher prevalence of ST segment changes [false-positive findings] during exercise) (3).

Sensitivity

Sensitivity is the percentage of true-positive tests in patients with CAD. As the rate of false-negative tests increases, sensitivity decreases:

$$\text{Sensitivity} = [(\text{true-positive tests}) \div (\text{true-positive tests} + \text{false-negative tests})] \times 100$$

Specificity

Specificity is the percentage of negative tests in people who do not have CAD. As the rate of false-positive tests increases, specificity decreases:

$$\text{Specificity} = [(\text{true-negative tests}) \div (\text{true-negative tests} + \text{false-positive tests})] \times 100$$

Predictive Value

The predictive value of an abnormal test is the percentage of patients with an abnormal test who have CAD. It measures the accuracy of the test for identifying patients with disease and is a reflection of demonstrated sensitivity and specificity. Predictive value depends on the pretest likelihood of disease and prevalence of disease in the population being tested.

The equation to calculate predictive value for a **positive test**:

$$\text{Predictive value} = [(\text{true-positive tests}) \div (\text{true-positive tests} + \text{false-positive tests})] \times 100$$

The equation to calculate predictive value for a **negative test**:

Predictive value = [(true-negative tests) ÷ (true-negative tests + false-negative tests)] × 100

As with sensitivity and specificity, predictive value is improved when criteria other than electrocardiographic (ECG) findings are used to classify test findings as abnormal (e.g., hemodynamic and symptomatic responses).

Relative Risk

Relative risk, or risk ratio, indicates the chance of having disease if the test result is abnormal as opposed to the chance of having disease if the test result is normal.

Risk ratio = [true-positive tests ÷ all positive tests] ÷ [false-negative tests ÷ all negative tests]

PATIENT HISTORY

The patient's history is a fundamental and critical diagnostic tool. The evocation of a description of classical exertional angina provides diagnostic accuracy that is difficult to exceed with virtually any sophisticated diagnostic technology, particularly as emphasis on cost effectiveness increases (4, 5). Appraisal of ischemic symptoms, such as chest discomfort, is a key factor in differentiating CAD from other cardiovascular and noncardiac diagnoses and is an important guide for the selection of appropriate diagnostic testing (6). Bayes' theorem states that the probability of a hypothesis is variably modified as additional data are considered; that is, if the likelihood of CAD is low on the basis of coronary risk factors and history, an abnormal test result is likely to be a false-positive (7). Clinicians use assessment of pretest probability of having disease to determine whether additional testing will add incremental value for diagnosis.

THE 12-LEAD RESTING ELECTROCARDIOGRAM

The resting 12-lead ECG is a surface recording of cardiac electrical potentials. The resting 12-lead ECG can provide clinical information regarding the presence or absence of the following:

- Rhythm abnormalities
- Cardiac conduction disturbances
- Cardiac chamber enlargement
- Pre-excitation syndromes
- Ischemia
- Myocardial infarction (acute, recent, and old)
- Inflammation of the pericardium

Most of these findings may be a direct or indirect indication of suspected CAD. Identification of such abnormalities on the resting ECG, particularly if different from previous ECGs, should lead to additional diagnostic tests to establish the presence or absence of CAD.

In evaluating CAD, pathological Q waves (defined as > 0.04 seconds in duration), ST segment elevation, and the absence of R waves are characteristic and in certain situations diagnostic of CAD. When determined to be medically stable, such patients require additional functional testing or cardiac angiography to confirm the diagnosis and assess the severity of CAD. Abnormal ST segment depression can be ambiguous, particularly in the presence of hypertrophy, conduction delay, and certain drugs, such as digitalis. Such findings on the resting ECG render it uninterpretable for ischemia. Further diagnostic evaluation requires a stress imaging modality (i.e., radionuclide imaging or echocardiography) or coronary angiography.

THE EXERCISE ELECTROCARDIOGRAM

The value of exercise electrocardiographic testing is evolving, and our expectations are changing (2, 8, 9). Studies have demonstrated poor test accuracy for the diagnosis of CAD (10, 11). When used as a screening tool to evaluate asymptomatic people with at least one major risk factor or as a diagnostic test to evaluate patients with atypical angina, the exercise ECG can assist the clinician in making a preliminary diagnosis of CAD (12, 13). However, use of exercise testing as a screening tool in asymptomatic individuals with fewer than two risk factors may be more misleading than previously thought because of the relatively high rate of false-positive results (14). Therefore, use of the exercise ECG test in asymptomatic people requires awareness of the limitations of the test and an understanding of Bayesian principles.

Low prevalence of CAD (approximately 5% in asymptomatic men) results in a poor predictive value (about 23%) for a positive result but an excellent predictive value (about 99%) for a negative result (15). For practical purposes, this means that one must regard abnormal screening exercise ECGs in an asymptomatic population with skepticism, but negative results may be reassuring (16). Noninvasive diagnostic testing is being used to enhance clinical decision making in patients with intermediate pretest probability of having CAD (17).

The exercise ECG test is an accessible and cost-effective means of assessing cardiac function. Evaluation of hemodynamic and electrocardiographic responses to exercise permits prediction of the severity of underlying coronary disease and the patient's prognosis (18–20). Three features, all measurable during either exercise ECG or image-enhanced testing, determine the prognosis of CAD:

- The amount of myocardial ischemia
- The amount of left ventricular dysfunction
- The arrhythmic potential of the myocardial substrate

Studies suggest that certain parameters, measurable by the exercise test, provide reliable expectation for outcome after acute coronary events (21, 22). Since survival can be improved only in specific subsets of patients, it is important to carefully select a patient population in whom intervention with catheterization and subsequent revascularization can improve both quality and quantity of life (23, 24). This applies even to certain patients who have acute coronary syndrome, providing important prognostic information and improved outcomes.

There are significant differences in clinical, ECG, and hemodynamic measurements among patients with increasing coronary disease severity (25). Patients at high risk have more than 0.1 mV of ST segment depression at less than 7 metabolic equivalents (METs), while those at low risk do not have ST segment depression and are able to exceed 13 METs or achieve a heart rate greater than 160 bpm (26). In patients with known or strongly suspected CAD, an exaggerated exercise blood pressure response, defined as peak systolic pressure at least 210 mm Hg in men and at least 190 mm Hg in women, has been shown to be associated with relatively mild angiographic disease and a relatively good prognosis (27). Furthermore, impaired chronotropic response has been shown to be predictive of the presence and angiographic severity of CAD (28). In a study of healthy men, four exercise test variables were identified to be predictive of subsequent primary coronary events. They were exercise duration 6 minutes or less (i.e., < 6 to 7 METs), more than 0.1 mV ST segment depression during recovery, more than 10% heart rate impairment, and chest pain during maximal exertion.

Estimated functional capacity and thallium summary score are roughly equivalent predictors of cardiac mortality. In a large cohort of patients followed for 2 years, none of whom had prior invasive procedures, congestive heart failure, or valve disease, patients with fair or poor estimated exercise capacity were at markedly increased risk for CAD ($P < .0001$). In fact, 81% of the deaths occurred among these patients. The thallium scan, with results classified according to the total number of abnormal segments was also predictive of mortality ($P < .0001$). In multivariable analyses, including clinical, exercise, and thallium variables, estimated exercise capacity was the strongest predictor of death ($P < .0001$) (25). Exercise ECG alone, however, cannot reliably predict the location of angiographic CAD. Factors to consider in defining criteria for abnormal studies are summarized in Table 28.1.

Experience has clarified the significance of various findings and methodologies, such as logistic regression, applied in the interpretation of the exercise ECG. For example, it appears that the computer-generated ST/HR index (ST segment change divided by the difference between peak and resting heart rates) may be better than standard ST segment criteria with respect to diagnosis of CAD (29). In addition, unlike ST segment interpretation alone, the computerized ST/HR index seems to predict death independently of thallium perfusion defects. Important principles of exercise ECG interpretation are listed in Table 28.2.

Table 28.1. Criteria for Exercise ECG Interpretation, Abnormal Test

Diagnostic Test Criteria
  Horizontal or down-sloping ST segment depression ± 0.1 mV, persisting at least 1 minute post exercise
  ± 0.15 mV up-sloping ST, both inferior and lateral leads lasting beyond 1 minute recovery
  Typical pain, 0.1 mV up-sloping ST depression
  Elevation > 0.1 mV in any lead other than aVR
  ST/HR index ± 3.3 mV/bpm
  Any symptomatic drop in blood pressure, drop in systolic pressure below rest blood pressure, drop in heart rate during exercise
  Significant dysrhythmia, exercise-induced sustained SVT or VT
  Chronotropic index ≥0.8 or ≥10 bpm drop in heart rate during 1st minute of recovery

Nondiagnostic Test Criteria
  ST depression in the face of LVH, LBBB, WPW, nonspecific IVCD, digitalis therapy or other nonspecific ST-T wave abnormality
  Ventricular paced rhythm
  Failure to achieve 85% of age-predicted maximal heart rate (especially if due to submaximal effort)

Normal Test
  Exercise capacity normal for age
  ST segments exhibiting less than 0.1 mV of horizontal or down-sloping ST depression (beyond baseline) during exercise or recovery
  Systolic blood pressure increasing with each of the first 3 stages of exercise
  Achievement of 85% APMHR or <85% with normal BP, ST, and symptomatic response in a patient taking beta-blockers when the test is being performed for evaluation of medical therapy
  Use of "normal except for" to describe possibly important findings that do not meet the abnormal criteria

AMPHR, age-predicted maximal heart rate; LVH, left ventricular hypertrophy; LBBB, left bundle branch block; WPW, Wolff-Parkinson-White syndrome; IVCD, intraventricular conduction delay; SVT, supraventricular tachycardia; VT, ventricular tachycardia.

Sensitivity and Specificity

The exercise ECG is not sensitive when used alone for the diagnosis of CAD. However, the reliability and cost-effectiveness for monitoring progression of disease and determining therapeutic efficacy are not equaled by other diagnostic means (30).

The sensitivity and specificity of exercise-induced ST segment depression can be demonstrated by comparing the results of exercise testing and coronary angiography. The exercise threshold of 0.1 mV horizontal or down-sloping ST segment depression has a specificity for CAD of approximately 84%; that is, 84% of those without significant angiographic disease have normal exercise test findings. Studies have demonstrated an average 66% sensitivity of exercise testing for significant angiographic CAD (40% for one-vessel disease to 90% for three-vessel disease) (30). This level of sensitivity does, however, fail to detect disease in 34 of 100 who have CAD.

Sensitivity and specificity for each testing laboratory are related to the interpretive criteria used, the disease prevalence in the population, and the definition of significant angiographic CAD. The sensitivity of exercise test-

Table 28.2. Important Principles of Exercise ECG Interpretation

Ischemic ST depression normally occurs in the lateral leads (I, V4, V5)
Changes in both inferior and lateral leads suggests more significant CAD
Isolated inferior changes or changes in only one lead are often false-positives
ST changes that resolve within 1 minute of recovery are often false-positives
ST changes provoked in patients with an abnormal resting ECG are often false-positives
ST depression does not localize ischemia to an area of myocardium
ST depression without angina suggests milder CAD and lower risk
ST depression not interpretable in LBBB, previous CABG or PCI, Q wave myocardial infarction, LVH, digitalis, WPW, or ventricular pacing
ST elevation over Q wave areas indicates myocardial damage or aneurysm; over non–Q wave areas means local myocardial ischemia
Markers of poor prognosis and/or severe CAD:
  Exertional hypotension: a drop in SBP below pre-exercise value
  Angina that limits exercise
  Poor exercise capacity (<6 METs)
Down-sloping ST depression, especially in recovery
  ST depression starting at a low double product (<15,000)
  ST depression that persists into late recovery
  ST/HR index 3.3 mV/bpm
  Chronotropic index ≥10 bpm drop in heart rate during 1st minute of recovery

CABG, coronary artery bypass grafting; PCI, percutaneous coronary intervention; LVH, left ventricular hypertrophy; WPW, Wolff-Parkinson-White syndrome.

ing is improved when patients are exercised to maximal exertion, multiple lead systems are used, and test data other than ECG response, e.g., work capacity and chronotropic response, are included as criteria for an abnormal test. Sensitivity and specificity can also be manipulated by changing the criterion for an abnormal ST segment response. For example, an increase in the abnormal criterion for ST segment response from 0.1 mV to 0.15 mV will reduce the number of false-positives in women. Factors that lower sensitivity and specificity are summarized in Tables 28.3 and 28.4. The ability to diagnose CAD in

Table 28.3. Factors that Lower Diagnostic Sensitivity: False-Negatives

Failure to reach 85% of age-predicted maximal heart rate
Medications that decrease MVO_2 (e.g., beta-blockers)
Medications that increase myocardial oxygen supply
Equivocal tests that are called normal
Failure to use other test data in test interpretation (e.g., chronotropic response, symptoms, certain dysrhythmias)
Single-vessel disease
Good collateral circulation
Insufficient number of monitoring leads to detect ST changes
Increased criteria for abnormal ST depression (e.g., 0.15 mV rather than 0.1 mV)
Visual ST segment analysis

MVO_2, myocardial oxygen uptake.

Table 28.4. Factors that Lower Diagnostic Specificity: False-Positives

Categorization of up-sloping ST depression as abnormal
An abnormal resting ECG (e.g., LBBB, nonspecific ST-T abnormality)
Medications that produce ST-T changes (e.g., digoxin)
Cardiac hypertrophy or cardiomyopathy
Hypertension
Female gender
Mitral valve prolapse
Low prevalence of CAD in test population
Wolff-Parkinson-White syndrome
Pectus excavatum
Pre-exercise hyperventilation
Vasospasm
Hypokalemia and anemia
Technical or observer error

LBBB, left bundle branch block.

patients with confounding results is enhanced with the use of imaging.

Limitations

A major factor that affects the sensitivity of exercise ECG is the ability to obtain adequate workload and heart rate response. Patients who tolerate testing without complication should be encouraged to exercise to exhaustion. Some patients are not physiologically able to achieve 100% of age-predicted maximal heart rate (APMHR); others easily exceed this target. The practice of setting a mandatory termination point at 85% of APMHR precludes the opportunity to observe abnormalities occurring at higher workloads. Although the onset of ST changes at high workloads are less diagnostically significant than those occurring at lower levels, sensitivity improves, as does the opportunity for the documentation of ischemia by imaging techniques.

RADIONUCLIDE IMAGING

Radionuclide imaging in combination with exercise or pharmacological stress is a commonly applied means of coronary diagnosis (32). Use of radionuclide is indicated in follow-up of patients with abnormal ECG exercise test findings and in the diagnostic evaluation of women, patients taking digitalis, and those with abnormal resting ECG (i.e., left bundle branch block, left ventricular hypertrophy, Wolff-Parkinson-White syndrome, intraventricular conduction delay). It is also useful for the assessment of perfusion in patients with angiographically documented CAD and to study myocardial viability.

Perfusion Imaging

Thallium 201 (^{201}Th) injected at peak exercise is proportionally distributed within the myocardium in relation to regional myocardial blood flow and muscle viability. In normal myocardium, imaging following stress shows initial accumulation of the isotope, reflecting integrity of regional blood supply. In areas of decreased initial perfusion, peak isotopic concentrations are delayed and associated with slower washout. The presence of transient perfusion defects following exercise that fill in on the delayed images (obtained within 4–24 hours after exercise or at rest) is consistent with exercise-induced myocardial ischemia. Areas of scar characteristically show no uptake, either initially or during later redistribution. In addition to the uniformity of isotopic uptake, ventricular cavity size, myocardial wall thickness, and any pulmonary accumulation can be observed.

Planar ^{201}Th imaging provides average sensitivity and specificity of 83% and 88%, respectively. More recently, advances in radionuclide imaging, such as quantification of radionuclide data, tomographic imaging, and single photon emission computed tomography (SPECT) have enhanced sensitivity and specificity beyond that provided by planar imaging. A review of studies using SPECT analysis indicated overall sensitivity of 89% and specificity of 70% (33). Positron emission tomography (PET), a newer and significantly more costly image acquisition technology, appears to provide accuracy comparable with that of SPECT in diagnosing and predicting the severity of CAD. PET may be superior in obese patients or in those with equivocal thallium SPECT studies. Sensitivity and specificity for PET range from 78–100% and 87–97%, respectively (34).

Newer technetium 99m (^{99m}Tc) based radiopharmaceutical flow tracers, such as sestamibi, provide diagnostic benefits on the basis of their physical and biological attributes. ^{99m}Tc sestamibi has a shorter half-life than ^{201}Th. This allows administration of a larger dose, providing superior images. Also, the traditional stress–rest ^{201}Th scan can be replaced with a protocol in which the rest images are acquired before stress, reducing the time required for the study and allowing acquisition of ECG-gated functional images. Thus far, studies demonstrate similar sensitivity and specificity for ^{201}Th and ^{99m}Tc (34).

When diagnostic testing is needed in patients who are unable to exercise, potent selective coronary vasodilators, such as dipyridamole and adenosine, along with isotopes, such as ^{201}Th and ^{99m}Tc sestamibi or rubidium 82, are used with SPECT and PET (34). A typical hemodynamic response to these agents is decreased blood pressure due to vasodilation with a slight reflex increase in heart rate. These techniques have proven efficacy and are especially important for subjects who are incapable of exercise, are unable to achieve appropriate heart rates via exercise, or are in the early period after uncomplicated acute myocardial infarction and require a more definitive diagnostic study. Half of patients receiving dipyridamole and 80% of patients receiving adenosine have minor side effects. Mean sensitivity and specificity using dipyridamole SPECT imaging and either ^{201}Th or ^{99m}Tc sestamibi averages 90% and 70%, respectively, while use of adenosine averages 85% and 90%, respectively (35).

No test is clearly superior to all others in every clinical circumstance (34). Moreover, none have been shown to provide sensitivities and specificities consistently above 90% (32). Therefore, the use of radionuclide imaging for diagnostic purposes in populations with a lower prevalence of disease has only moderate value. However, for the assessment of patients with moderate pretest probability of disease or functional significance of CAD and for prognosis in patients with ischemic heart disease, the addition of these noninvasive imaging modalities to exercise testing is significant.

Ventriculography

Performing a multiple gated acquisition study (MUGA), or a first-pass study, during exercise can also aid the diagnosis of CAD. This allows assessment and comparison of resting and exercise cardiac function, including systolic and diastolic function, right and left ventricular ejection fraction, cardiac output, and regional wall motion.

An increase in left and right ventricular ejection fraction of 5% or more is a normal response to exercise. Failure to increase or a decrease in ejection fraction during exercise may indicate failing ventricular performance due to ischemia. This is confirmed by observing during exercise abnormal ECG changes and/or segmental wall motion abnormalities that would indicate compromised coronary flow. Abnormal left ventricular ejection fraction response to exercise is sensitive but not specific to CAD.

EXERCISE ECHOCARDIOGRAPHY

Exercise echocardiography combines surface echocardiography and exercise ECG testing (36). Echocardiographic images are viewed using side-by-side digital display of resting and exercise echocardiograms. Exercise echocardiographic images can be obtained during exercise using cycle ergometry or immediately after treadmill exercise. Acquisition of immediate postexercise images must be complete within 1–2 minutes of test termination. Both techniques require superior sonographic skill and experience.

Like radionuclide ventriculography, exercise echocardiography allows assessment of cardiac function, including wall motion abnormality, ejection fraction, and systolic and diastolic function. Exercise echocardiography significantly improves the sensitivity of stress testing (80% vs. 42%, $P < .0001$) even after exclusion of negative exercise ECGs with submaximal stress and all nondiagnostic exercise ECGs (87% vs. 63% for ECG, $P = .001$) (37). In a population with a high prevalence of symptomatic coronary disease (77%), a higher sensitivity (97% vs. 51% for ECG, $P < .0001$) has been observed (38). Specificity is also enhanced by exercise echocardiography. Specificity in normal tests is 93%, 82% after exclusion of nondiagnostic tests, compared to 77% for ECG (37).

Stress echocardiography is useful in women and in those with concurrent valvular or primary myocardial disease. Stress echo is less useful in patients with multiple myocardial infarctions, complex wall motion abnormality, or a poor imaging window (e.g., obese patients). Intravenous dobutamine, a beta-adrenergic stimulating agent, offers a pharmacological alternative for patients who are unable to exercise. Infusion of an incremental dose of dobutamine evokes a positive inotropic response, a less significant chronotropic response, and increased contractility. Unlike dipyridamole and adenosine, dobutamine closely parallels the exercise response by creating an oxygen supply and demand imbalance.

The most significant limitation in performing stress echocardiography is the learning curve associated with image acquisition and interpretation. High-quality images are required within 1–2 minutes of the termination of treadmill exercise. Interpretation of exercise echocardiographic images is still highly subjective, limited in part by current imaging technology and lack of algorithms for quantification and enhancement of data. Physicians require significant training before diagnostic reliability is achieved (39).

CORONARY ANGIOGRAPHY

Coronary arteriography entails the selective opacification of the coronary arteries during radiography. This produces a contrast image defining the internal diameter of a visualized artery. For many years, it was the gold standard for diagnosis of the presence and extent of coronary atherosclerosis, and it remains the most sensitive readily available test for this purpose. Findings at catheterization correlate well with clinical coronary events over an extended period (40). Arteriography does not provide extensive information about the wall of the artery or the structural content of the atherosclerotic plaque, nor does it address the presence of ischemia, the real bottom line of atherosclerotic disease.

Selective coronary angiography is generally combined with a contrast left ventriculogram. With the widespread availability of radionuclide and echocardiographic imaging, the left ventriculogram during catheterization is less important than in previous years. The measurement of left and right ventricular hemodynamics and pressures is rarely performed today. Echo Doppler is generally determined to be satisfactory for this purpose.

Coronary angiography is clearly indicated for patients with intractable or unstable angina to determine whether they are appropriate candidates for revascularization. Coronary arteriography may be indicated for patients with established disease who are stable, particularly those who demonstrate noninvasive indicators forecasting a poor prognosis. Randomized studies show improved survival rates following revascularization in patients with three-vessel CAD or its equivalent and in those with two-

vessel disease when the proximal portion of the left anterior descending coronary artery is critically obstructed (41, 42). In addition, patients with acute myocardial infarction and recurrent chest pain due to myocardial ischemia despite intensive medical therapy need coronary arteriography, as do those who have structural complications of acute infarction.

While angiography reflects only the luminal distortion of the atherosclerotic coronary plaque, intravascular ultrasound directly demonstrates the composition and structural anatomy of plaque invading the coronary arterial wall. However, the current major use of intravascular ultrasound is still mainly as a research tool and for specialized applications by the interventional cardiologist (43).

ELECTRON BEAM COMPUTED TOMOGRAPHY

Electron beam computed tomography (EBCT) allows noninvasive assessment of CAD. EBCT uses an electron beam that produces very fast scanning times and essentially eliminates the movement artifact that has been problematic in computed tomography. EBCT identifies calcified plaque in coronary atherosclerotic lesions. The amount of plaque is quantified using a scoring system to calculate total calcified plaque (44, 45).

EBCT appears to be a promising diagnostic tool that is being used with good sensitivity and relatively high specificity for the detection of CAD. The sensitivity and specificity in asymptomatic patients depend on the calcium score used as a cutoff point for a positive result. Current data show EBCT to be more sensitive and less specific than exercise testing (44, 45). EBCT may, in fact, be most useful and predictive when combined with other diagnostic tests, such as radionuclide stress testing. Finally, it appears that if EBCT results in a very low calcium score, the presence of significant atherosclerotic plaque is highly unlikely; conversely, if the calcium score is very high, the presence of calcified atherosclerotic plaque is highly likely. Thus, both positive and negative predictive value is good, but it also depends on the specific calcium cutoff score used for diagnosis (44, 45).

▶ SUMMARY

The diagnosis of CAD begins with careful consideration of the symptoms, signs, risk factor profile, and resting 12-lead ECG. The determination of pretest probability of having CAD assists in determining the need for additional diagnostic studies. People with a low pretest probability may not require further testing. Patients with low to intermediate probability may undergo exercise ECG testing for further risk stratification. Diagnosis of symptomatic patients with intermediate pretest probability frequently benefits from exercise ECG testing. The decision to use an imaging or nonimaging modality is based on multiple considerations. For detection of CAD, patients with high pretest probability receive little diagnostic advantage from noninvasive testing. Patients with a high pretest probability are most likely to be assessed with coronary angiography and may require subsequent noninvasive diagnostic procedures for localization of ischemia and determination of prognosis.

References

1. Pashkow FJ. Contemporary considerations in exercise ECG testing. Cleve Clin J Med 59:231–232, 1992.
2. American College of Sports Medicine. ACSM's Guidelines for Exercise Testing and Prescription. 6th ed. Philadelphia: Lippincott Williams & Wilkins, 335–336, 340–341, 2000.
3. Hanson P. Clinical Exercise Testing. In: ACSM Resource Manual for Guidelines for Exercise Testing and Prescription. Philadelphia: Lea & Febiger, 219–221, 1988.
4. Weiner D, Ryan T, McCabe C, et al. Correlations among history of angina, ST-segment response and prevalence of coronary artery disease in the Coronary Artery Surgery Study (CASS). N Engl J Med 301:230–235, 1979.
5. Patterson RE, Eng C, Horowitz SF, Gorlin R, Goldstein SR. Bayesian comparison of cost-effectiveness of different clinical approaches to diagnose coronary artery disease. J Am Coll Cardiol 4:278–289, 1984.
6. Hung J, Chaitman BR, Lam J, et al. A logistic regression analysis of multiple noninvasive tests for the prediction of the presence and extent of coronary artery disease in men. Am Heart J 110:460–469, 1985.
7. Morise AP, Duval RD. Comparison of three Bayesian methods to estimate posttest probability in patients undergoing exercise stress testing. Am J Cardiol 64:1117–1122, 1989.
8. Kligfield P. Rehabilitation of the exercise electrocardiogram. Ann Intern Med 128:1035–1037, 1998.
9. Froelicher VF, Lehmann KG, Thomas R, et al. The electrocardiographic exercise test in a population with reduced work-up bias: Diagnostic performance, computerized interpretation, and multivariable freedom. Ann Intern Med 128:965–974, 1998.
10. Gianrossi R, Detrano R, Mulvihill D, et al. Exercise-induced ST depression in the diagnosis of coronary artery disease: A meta-analysis. Circulation 80:87–98, 1989.
11. Detrano R, Gianrossi R, Froelicher V. The diagnostic accuracy of the exercise electrocardiogram: A meta-analysis of 22 years of research. Prog Cardiovasc Dis 32:173–206, 1989.
12. Sox H Jr, Littenberg B, Garber AM. The role of exercise testing in screening for coronary artery disease. Ann Intern Med 110:456–469, 1989 [see comments].
13. Pilote L, Pashkow FJ, Thomas JD, et al. Clinical yield and cost of exercise treadmill testing to screen for coronary artery disease in asymptomatic adults. Am J Cardiol 81:219–224, 1998.
14. Detrano R, Froelicher V. A logical approach to screening for coronary artery disease. Ann Intern Med 106:846–852, 1987.
15. Sheffield L. Exercise stress testing for coronary artery disease. In: Braunwald E, ed. Heart Disease: A Textbook of Cardiovascular Medicine. 3rd ed. Philadelphia: Saunders, 1988:223–241.
16. Patterson RE, Horowitz SF. Importance of epidemiology and biostatistics in deciding clinical strategies for using diagnostic tests: A simplified approach using examples from coronary artery disease. J Am Coll Cardiol 13:1653–1665, 1989.
17. Pashkow FJ. Role of routine exercise electrocardiographic testing. In: Marwick TH, ed. Cardiac Stress Testing and Imaging: A Clinician's Guide. New York: Churchill Livingstone, 1996:1–31.
18. Lauer MS, Mehta M, Pashkow FJ, et al. Association of chronotropic incompetence with echocardiographic ischemia and prognosis. J Am Coll Cardiol 32:1280–1286, 1998.
19. Cole CR, Blackstone EH, Pashkow FJ, et al. Association between mortality and recovery of heart rate immediately after exercise. N Engl J Med 341:1351–1357, 1999.
20. Lauer MS, Francis GS, Okin PM, et al. Impaired chronotropic response to exercise stress testing as a predictor of mortality. JAMA 281:524–529, 1999.
21. Froelicher V, Duarte G, Oakes D, et al. The prognostic value of the exercise test. Dis Mon 34:677–735, 1988.
22. DeBusk RF. Specialized testing after recent acute myocardial infarction. Ann Intern Med 110:470–481, 1989.
23. Weiner D, McCabe C, Ryan T. Identification of patients with left main and three vessel coronary disease with clinical and exercise test variables. Am J Cardiol 46:21–27, 1980.
24. Bogaty P, Dagenais GR, Cantin B, et al. Prognosis in patients with a strongly positive exercise electrocardiogram. Am J Cardiol 64:1284–1288, 1989.
25. Snader CE, Lauer MS, Pashkow FJ, et al. Importance of estimated functional capacity as a predictor of all-cause mortality among patients referred for exercise thallium SPECT: Report of 3400 patients from a single center. J Am Coll Cardiol 30:641–648, 1997.
26. McNeer J, Margolis J, Lee K. The role of the exercise test in the evaluation of patients for ischemic heart disease. Circulation 57:64–70, 1978.
27. Lauer M, Pashkow F, Harvey S, et al. Angiographic and prognostic implications of an exaggerated exercise systolic blood pressure response and rest systolic blood pressure in adults undergoing evaluation for suspected coronary artery disease. Am J Cardiol 26:1630–1636, 1995.
28. Brener S, Pashkow F, Harvey S, et al. Chronotropic response to exercise predicts angiographic severity in patients with suspected or stable coronary artery disease. Am J Cardiol 76:1228–1232, 1995.
29. Morise AP, Duval RD. Accuracy of ST/heart rate index in the diagnosis of coronary artery disease. Am J Cardiol 69:603–606, 1992.
30. Pashkow FJ, Harvey SA, Froelicher VF. Exercise electrocardiographic testing. In: Pashkow FJ, Dafoe WA, eds. Clinical Cardiac Rehabilitation: A Cardiologist's Guide. 2nd ed. Baltimore: Williams & Wilkins, 1999:65–101.
31. Detrano R, Gianrossi R, Mulvihill D, et al. Exercise-induced ST segment depression in the diagnosis of multivessel coronary disease: a meta-analysis. J Am Coll Cardiol 14:1501–1508, 1989.
32. Crawford MH. Overview: Diagnosis of ischemic heart disease by noninvasive techniques. Circulation 84:I50–I51, 1991.

33. Maddahi J, Rodrigues E, Berman DS, et al. State of the art myocardial perfusion imaging. In: Verani MS, ed. Nuclear cardiology: State of the art. Philadelphia: Saunders, 199–202, 1994.

34. Marwick T. Other noninvasive diagnostic tools: Tests of left ventricular function, perfusion and metabolism. In: Pashkow F, Dafoe W, eds. Clinical Cardiac Rehabilitation: A Cardiologist's Guide. 2nd ed. Baltimore: Williams & Wilkins, 1999:131–133.

35. Ritchie JL, Bateman TM, Bonow RO, et al. Guidelines for clinical use of cardiac radionuclide imaging: Report of the ACC/AHA Task Force on Assessment of Diagnostic and Therapeutic Cardiovascular Procedures. Circulation 82:2323–2345, 1995.

36. Ryan T, Feigenbaum H. Exercise echocardiography. Am J Cardiol 69:82H–89H, 1992.

37. Marwick TH, Nemec JJ, Pashkow FJ, et al. Accuracy and limitations of exercise echocardiography in a routine clinical setting. J Am Coll Cardiol 19:74–81, 1992.

38. Crouse LJ, Harbrecht JJ, Vacek JL, et al. Exercise echocardiography as a screening test for coronary artery disease and correlation with coronary arteriography. Am J Cardiol 67:1213–1218, 1991.

39. Orlandini A, Picano E, Lattanzi F, et al. Stress echocardiography and the human factor: The importance of being an expert. J Am Coll Cardiol 15:52a, 1990.

40. Ellis SG. Role of coronary angiography. In: Fuster V, Ross R, Topol EJ, eds. Atherosclerosis and Coronary Artery Disease, vol 2. Philadelphia: Lippincott-Raven, 1996:1433–1435.

41. Weiner DA, Ryan TJ, McCabe CH, et al. Value of exercise testing in determining the risk classification and the response to coronary artery bypass grafting in three-vessel coronary artery disease: A report from the Coronary Artery Surgery Study (CASS) registry. Am J Cardiol 60:262–266, 1987.

42. Ringqvist I, Fisher LD, Mock M, et al. Prognostic value of angiographic indices of coronary artery disease from the Coronary Artery Surgery Study (CASS). J Clin Invest 1983; 71:1854–1866.

43. DeFranco AC, Tuzcu EM, Brenner S, Nissen SE. Interventional applications of coronary intravascular ultrasound, angioscopy, and Doppler flow. In: Fuster V, Ross R, Topol EJ, eds. Atherosclerosis and Coronary Artery Disease, vol 2. Philadelphia: Lippincott-Raven, 1996:1451–1453.

44. O'Rourke RA, Brundage BH, Froelicher VF, et al. American College of Cardiology/American Heart Association Expert consensus document on electron-beam computed tomography for the diagnosis and prognosis of coronary artery disease. J Am Coll Cardiol 2000; 36:326–340.

45. Shavelle DM, Budoff MJ, LaMont DH, et al. Exercise testing and electron beam computed tomography in the evaluation of coronary artery disease. J Am Coll Cardiol 2000; 36:32–38.

Suggested Reading

Ellestad MH. Stress Testing: Principles and Practice. 4th ed. Philadelphia: Davis, 1996.

Fletcher GF, Balady G, Froelicher VF, et al. Exercise standards: A statement for healthcare professionals from the American Heart Association. Circulation 91:580–615, 1995.

Froelicher VF. Manual of Exercise Testing. 2nd ed. St Louis: Mosby, 1994.

Gibbons RJ, Balady GJ, Beasley JW, et al. ACC/AHA guidelines for exercise testing: Executive summary. Circulation 96:345–354, 1997.

Marwick T. Other noninvasive diagnostic tools: Tests of left ventricular function, perfusion and metabolism. In: Pashkow F, Dafoe W, eds. Clinical Cardiac Rehabilitation: A Cardiologist's Guide. 2nd ed. Baltimore: Williams & Wilkins, 1999:131–133.

Pashkow FJ, Harvey SA, Froelicher VF. Exercise electrocardiographic testing. In: Pashkow FJ, Dafoe WA, eds. Clinical Cardiac Rehabilitation: A Cardiologist's Guide. 2nd ed. Baltimore: Williams & Wilkins, 1999:65–101.

Ritchie JL, Bateman TM, Bonow RO, et al. Report of the ACC/AHA Task Force on Assessment of Diagnostic and Therapeutic Cardiovascular Procedures. Guidelines for Clinical Use of Cardiac Radionuclide Imaging. Am J Cardiol 25:521–547, 1995.

Roger VL, Pellikka PA, Oh JK, et al. Stress echocardiography: 1. Exercise echocardiography: Techniques, implementation, clinical applications, and correlations. Mayo Clin Proc 70(1):5–15, 1995.

1.4.0, 1.4.0.1, 1.4.0.2   2.4.1, 2.4.4   3.4.0   4.4.0, 4.4.3, 4.4.8, 4.4.9,   5.4.1, 5.4.3
                                                                        4.4.10

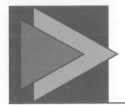

CHAPTER **29**

MEDICAL AND INVASIVE INTERVENTIONS IN THE MANAGEMENT OF CORONARY ARTERY DISEASE

L. Kent Smith, Sorin Brener, and Fredric J. Pashkow

Coronary heart disease is the major cause of morbidity and mortality in the United States. The prevalence is in excess of 12 million men and women in the United States. This includes 7 million myocardial infarction patients or survivors and an additional 6 million who have angina pectoris. By age 65 the prevalence of coronary artery disease in women reaches that of men, and it exceeds the men's prevalence in later years. Coronary heart disease produces nearly 500,000 deaths annually and is the largest single killer of American men and women. Annually, an estimated 1.1 million Americans will have either a new or recurrent coronary heart disease event, with 650,000 of these being an initial heart attack and 450,000 a recurrent heart attack. Approximately one-third of people who have a heart attack die. Sudden death accounts for 250,000 of these events. Of those who die of a coronary event, 85% are 65 years of age and older. Of sudden death patients, approximately 60% have no apparent previous symptom alerting them to seek medical evaluation. Because women have heart attacks when they are older, they are more likely to die within a year of the event (24% of men and 42% of women die within a year of having a documented myocardial infarction). Within the subsequent 6 years after surviving a heart attack, 21% of men and one-third of women have a recurrent myocardial infarction. Among infarct survivors, 21% of men and 30% of women have heart failure. In 1996, 1.2 million men and 930,000 women were hospitalized with coronary heart disease diagnoses, an increase in hospitalizations of 31% in men and 29% in women since 1979. Each year 350,000 new cases of angina pectoris are diagnosed (1).

RISK FACTOR MANAGEMENT

Well-established risk factors for coronary heart disease have been recognized for nearly a half-century. These risk factors include lipid disorders, cigarette smoking, elevation in systemic blood pressure, diabetes mellitus, and lack of physical activity. More recently, additional risk factors are being proposed. They include high levels of homocystine, lipoprotein(a), C-reactive protein and other markers of inflammation, certain markers of infection, fibrinogen, insulin resistance and small dense low-density lipoprotein (LDL). These emerging risk factors are not reviewed in this chapter. This chapter instead emphasizes risk factor management and its effect on reducing cardiovascular morbidity and mortality. Furthermore, this discussion pertains to patients with established coronary heart disease (secondary prevention) in contrast to managing of risk factors in patients who do not yet have manifest atherosclerotic cardiovascular disease (primary prevention). The following topics are addressed:

1. Lipid disorders
2. Cigarette smoking
3. Diabetes mellitus
4. Antiplatelet therapy and anticoagulation treatment
5. Role of angiotensin-converting enzyme inhibitors
6. Hormone replacement therapy

Management of Lipid Disorders

Four well-designed and well-executed large clinical trials have consistently demonstrated significant reduction in mortality in major cardiovascular events in patients with established coronary heart disease and management of lipid disorders with pharmacotherapy. In each of these studies, all double-blind, patients were assigned randomly to a placebo arm versus an active pharmacotherapy arm, and all patients were on a background lipid-lowering diet. Three studies used the beta-hydroxy-beta-methyglutaryl–coenzyme A (HMG-CoA) reductase inhibitor class of medications (one of the statin drugs). These drugs primarily reduce LDL cholesterol, although they have an additional benefit in raising HDL cholesterol. In each of these trials the active treatment arm resulted in significant reduction in cardiovascular events compared with the placebo arm. An additional trial using the fibric acid derivative gemfibrozil in male U.S. veterans was specifically designed to enroll patients with isolated low HDL cholesterol (mean HDL level 32 mg/dL). This study also documented reduction of cardiovascular events attributable to the increase in HDL cholesterol values in the active treatment arm versus placebo. These trials are summarized in Table 29.1 (2–5). The studies of simvastatin and pravastatin included elderly and women subjects in sufficiently large numbers to document significant reduction in clinical outcomes in patients over age 65 and in women as well as men (6–8).

One study has addressed the issue of lipid-lowering therapy in patients with coronary artery disease as compared to catheter-based coronary intervention (9). This clinical trial randomized 341 patients with stable coronary artery disease, ejection fraction greater than 40%, and baseline LDL cholesterol values at least 115 mg/dL. Following diagnostic coronary arteriography, patients with one- or two-vessel coronary artery disease and no left main coronary artery narrowing whose stenosis would qualify them for catheter-based treatment were randomly assigned to one of two groups. The first group received percutaneous revascularization, including coronary artery stenting (177 patients), to be followed by usual care. The second group received aggressive lipid-lowering treatment with atorvastatin 80 mg once daily and no coronary revascularization at the time of randomization (164 patients). The follow-up was 18 months. The revascularization subjects had an 18% reduction in LDL cholesterol and attained a mean level of 119 mg/dL. The aggressive lipid-lowering treatment group achieved a 46% reduction in LDL cholesterol level for a mean value of 77 mg/dL. The incidence of ischemic events at 18 months was 36% lower in the aggressive lipid treatment group than among the revascularization group (22 of the 164 aggressive lipid-lowering subjects compared to 37 events in the 177 initial revascularization group). The absolute event rate was 13% in the aggressive lipid-lowering group compared to 21% in the revascularization group (*P* = .045).

This study documented that aggressive lipid-lowering therapy is at least as effective as initial catheter-based intervention in patients with stable coronary artery disease. The potential annual economic impact on health care delivery in the United States of applying the strategies documented to be effective in this study is considerable. The number of annual catheter-based coronary interventions carried out in the United States exceeds 400,000 (1). The average cost of catheter-based coronary intervention is approximately $20,000. If one-quarter of the 400,000 intervention patients had aggressive lipid-lowering therapy and thus averted revascularization, the health care cost savings annually would approach $2 billion. Although the cost of managing 100,000 patients with aggressive lipid therapy, including medication costs and laboratory follow-up assessment, would approach $500 million annually, the net savings would be approximately $1.5 billion per year.

Smoking Cessation

According to the United States Surgeon General, cigarette smoking is the leading preventable cause of premature death in the United States, accounting for more than 400,000 deaths annually. Most of the excess mortality is from cardiovascular events, most specifically, coronary artery disease. For obvious ethical reasons, a planned randomized trial of smoking cessation compared to continued smoking has never occurred. However, 12 studies over the past 25 years have reported well-documented cohort studies comparing the outcomes regarding smoking cessation versus continued cigarette smoking in patients following myocardial infarction. Every study indicated mortality benefit favoring the smoking cessation cohort with all other risk factors statistically held even (10). The relative reduction in mortality ranged from 15–61%, and the absolute reduction was 1.2–27.5%. The odds ratio fa-

---

Table 29.1. Lipid Intervention

Trial	Intervention	# of Subjects	Reduction in LDL-C (%)	Increase in HDL-C (%)	Reduction in Cardiovascular Events (%)
CARE	Pravastatin[a]	4159	32	5	24
VA-HIT	Gemfibrozil[b]	2531	0	8	22
LIPID	Pravastatin[c]	9014	25	5	24
4S	Simvastatin[d]	4444	35	8	37

LDL-C, low-density lipoprotein cholesterol; HDL-C, high-density lipoprotein cholesterol.

[a] Sacks FM, Pfeffer MA, Moye LA, et al. The effect of pravastatin on coronary events after myocardial infarction in patients with average cholesterol levels. Cholesterol and Recurrent Events Trial investigators. N Engl J Med 335:1001–1009, 1996.

[b] Rubins HB, Robins SJ, Collins D, et al. Gemfibrozil for the secondary prevention of coronary heart disease in men with low levels of high-density lipoprotein cholesterol. N Engl J Med 341:410–418, 1999.

[c] Long-Term Intervention with Pravastatin in Ischaemic Disease (LIPID) Study Group. Prevention of cardiovascular events and death with pravastatin in patients with coronary heart disease and a broad range of initial cholesterol levels. N Engl J Med 339:1349–1357, 1998.

[d] Randomized trial of cholesterol lowering in 4444 patients with coronary heart disease: The Scandinavian Simvastatin Survival Study (4S). Lancet 344(8934):1383–1389, 1994.

voring cessation versus continued smoking was 0.54, which compares favorably with randomized controlled trials comparing other active therapies with placebo arms in the management of myocardial infarction (for instance, aspirin versus no aspirin: odds ratio, 0.77; beta-blocker versus placebo: odds ratio, 0.88). The strength and consistency of these findings underscore the significant beneficial role of smoking cessation in patients surviving myocardial infarction. Similar favorable outcomes have been reported for smoking cessation in cohort studies following coronary artery bypass surgery (11) and percutaneous coronary revascularization (12).

Diabetes Mellitus

Adult onset, or type 2, diabetes mellitus is a well-established risk factor for atherosclerotic cardiovascular disease. Approximately 11 million Americans have documented diabetes, with 625,000 new cases diagnosed each year in the United States (1). Diabetes is more common in women than men and is especially common among ethnic minorities. Two-thirds of diabetic patients die of cardiovascular disease (macrovascular disease), and 75% of hospitalizations of diabetic patients are due to macrovascular disease complications. The 7-year incidence of myocardial infarction in subjects with type II diabetes without history of prior myocardial infarction (20%) was practically the same as the 7-year incidence rate of repeat myocardial infarction in nondiabetic patients with a history of heart attack (19%). Therefore, diabetic subjects should be regarded as secondary prevention subjects with respect to aggressiveness of risk factor intervention and management. Furthermore, diabetic subjects who survive their myocardial infarction have a subsequent 7-year mortality of 45% (13). A major prospective study of 3867 newly diagnosed type II diabetics evaluated the effect of 10 years of intensive glycemic control (achieving hemoglobin A1c levels of 7% versus conventional therapy, with levels of 7.9%) (14). Disappointingly, no significant reduction in macrovascular disease end points was achieved. In contrast, the large randomized clinical trials of secondary prevention using HMG-CoA reductase intervention versus placebo documented highly significant beneficial outcome for the active-treatment arm. Specifically, in the simvastatin survival study, the relative reduction in major cardiovascular events favoring active treatment was 55% in diabetic patients (15). In another secondary prevention study involving myocardial infarction survivors, the diabetic cohort on active therapy with pravastatin resulted in a relative risk reduction of 25% compared to placebo (16).

Aspirin and Anticoagulation Management

The benefit of aspirin as contrasted with oral anticoagulation in patients with known coronary artery disease has been the subject of controversy, and the issue is characterized by different approaches in the United States and Europe. The principal approach in the United States has focused on aspirin, and the European approach has more often used oral anticoagulation with or without aspirin. A recent large meta-analysis of this issue has clarified the role of these two agents in managing patients with coronary artery disease (17). When compared with placebo, oral anticoagulation demonstrated superiority in reducing coronary mortality and stroke rates, but bleeding was significantly more common in the oral anticoagulation subjects. However, when oral anticoagulation therapy was compared with aspirin treatment in a blind trial, no significant difference in the rate of fatal and nonfatal heart attack or stroke was demonstrated. Once again, bleeding was more common in the anticoagulation subjects. Therefore, in patients without atrial fibrillation or known high risk of thromboembolic events (for example, patients with known intraventricular clot), aspirin alone appears sufficient to reduce cardiovascular morbidity and mortality in subjects with known coronary artery disease.

Angiotensin-Converting Enzyme Inhibitor Therapy

Angiotensin-converting enzyme inhibitors reduce activation of the renin–angiotensin system, with consequent benefits to the heart and vascular system. Their role in reducing mortality and myocardial infarction in heart failure patients has been well demonstrated for more than 20 years. However, the use of these agents for a general population of coronary artery disease subjects or patients with peripheral vascular disease or diabetes (but excluding those with ejection fraction under 40%) has only recently been evaluated (18). This large, randomized double-blind study (the HOPE trial) evaluated 9297 such high-risk patients aged 55 years and older. After a follow-up of 5 years, the absolute event rate of myocardial infarction, stroke, and cardiovascular death was 14% of the patients assigned to angiotensin-converting enzyme inhibition (ramipril 10 mg daily) compared to an event rate of 17.8% in the placebo subjects ($P < .001$). The relative risk in the active treatment arm compared to placebo arm was 0.74 for cardiovascular death, 0.8 for myocardial infarction, and 0.85 for revascularization. Furthermore, the relative risk of cardiac arrest was 0.63 and of heart failure, 0.77. This major study documents a broadened indication for the beneficial role of angiotensin-converting enzyme inhibitor treatment for patients with known cardiovascular disease and for high-risk patients who have preservation of left ventricular ejection fraction.

Hormone Replacement Therapy

Observational studies of postmenopausal women who were taking estrogen replacement therapy documented significant reduction in coronary heart disease event rates compared to women on no such hormone replacement therapy. A randomized trial rigidly evaluating the role of hormone replacement therapy has also recently been reported (19). A total of 2763 postmenopausal women with known coronary heart disease and with intact uterus were enrolled in this randomized, controlled trial (the HERS study). Women were randomly assigned to receive a combination of estrogen plus progestin or matching placebo and followed up for an average of 4.1 years. At the end of the trial, there were no significant differences between the groups regarding the primary end point of nonfatal myocardial infarction or coronary heart disease death. Furthermore, the secondary end point of coronary revascularization, unstable angina, heart failure, cardiac events, cerebral vascular events, and peripheral arterial disease showed no significant differences between the two groups. This study has led to a rethinking of the issue of hormone replacement therapy in women with established coronary heart disease.

STABLE ANGINA PECTORIS

More than 6 million Americans suffer from angina pectoris (3.9 million women and 2.3 million men). About 350,000 new diagnoses of angina pectoris occur annually, and angina pectoris was the prime reason for nearly 100,000 hospital admissions in 1996 (1). Angina pectoris is a symptom, and the original description by the physician William Heberden, initially published over 2 centuries ago, beautifully describes this clinical syndrome:

> A disorder of the breast marked with strong and peculiar symptoms . . . may make it not improperly be called angina pectoris. Those who are afflicted with it are seized with it while they are walking (more specifically if it be uphill, and soon after eating), with a painful and most disagreeable sensation in the breast, which seems as if it would extinguish life, if it were to increase or to continue; but the moment they stand still, all this uneasiness vanishes (20).

The painful sensation or symptom of cardiac ischemia arises from the afferent sensory fibers in the coronary vessels and myocardium. It indicates inadequate oxygenation of the myocardium (a disparity between demand and supply of oxygen in the myocardium). The development of ambulatory electrocardiographic monitoring has allowed for the detection of silent ischemia characterized by transient electrocardiographic ST segment depression (at least 1 mm persisting for at least 1 minute), which is common in patients with stable coronary artery disease and angina. A patient with angina pectoris of course requires objective evaluation to establish the diagnosis. Diagnostic tests are dealt with elsewhere in this text. The treatment of angina pectoris must address not only relief of the symptom but the issues that have brought coronary artery disease into play (i.e., management of the risk factors, previously discussed in this chapter). The medical management of angina pectoris as opposed to surgical intervention or catheter-based percutaneous intervention can be summarized as follows:

- In trials, daily aspirin reduced the clinical event rate compared to placebo.
- Nitroglycerin (sublingual or spray) for acute episodes or for daily use (oral form or transdermal patch) reduces left ventricular preload and afterload, thereby reducing oxygen consumption of the myocardium. Also, nitroglycerin dilates coronary arteries by relaxing smooth muscle.
- Beta-blocker medication to attenuate the catecholamine effects of increasing myocardial oxygen demand not only reduces the symptoms of angina but also has been shown to reduce mortality, particularly in patients who have survived myocardial infarction.
- The calcium channel blocker drugs significantly relax smooth muscle, produce peripheral arterial vasodilation, and reduce afterload. However, calcium channel blockers that raise the heart rate may have an adverse effect and should be avoided.

Nonpharmacological therapy, particularly emphasizing multidiscipline cardiac rehabilitation, should be part of the therapy for chronic stable angina pectoris. The value of interventional therapy is dealt with later in this chapter.

ACUTE CORONARY SYNDROMES

Acute coronary syndromes encompass clinical conditions intermediate between chronic stable angina pectoris and acute myocardial (Q wave) infarction. The underlying pathogenic mechanism is the rupture or fissure of an atheromatous coronary artery plaque. If plaque rupture does not completely disrupt blood flow in a major coronary artery (which would result in Q wave myocardial infarction), it is said to be unstable angina syndrome. The treatment of acute coronary syndromes has evolved greatly in recent years. The general supportive measures of pain relief (including the use of morphine or another opioid), application of oxygen, and the use of aspirin to inhibit platelet aggregation are standards of care. Unfractionated heparin and more recently low-molecular-weight heparin have demonstrated reduction in death and myocardial infarction. Low-molecular-weight heparin appears to be superior to standard unfractionated heparin (21). Several major clinical trials have established the beneficial effects of a new class of drugs, platelet glycoprotein IIb/IIIa antagonists (specific agents are abciximab, tirofiban, and Integrilin). International trials involving tens of thousands of patients with acute coronary syndromes have documented the benefit of this new class of drugs (administered acutely in the intravenous form) in reducing death and myocardial infarction. There is a relative reduction in risk of 34% and an absolute reduction of 1.3% (22). Early coronary revascularization also appears to add benefit (23, 24).

ACUTE MYOCARDIAL INFARCTION

Annually, slightly more than 1 million Americans have a new or recurrent attack of coronary artery disease (acute myocardial infarction or fatal coronary heart attack). Of these, approximately 650,000 are the initial event and 450,000 are recurrent episodes. Approximately one-third of patients having acute coronary events die. Of these deaths, approximately 250,000 are within an hour of the onset of symptoms, defined as sudden death (1). This has led to randomized trials evaluating the effect of prehospital use of thrombolytic therapy in patients having acute myocardial infarction. A recent meta-analysis of clinical trials documented that prehospital administration of thrombolytics advanced the initiation of this therapy by 45 minutes and saved 21 lives per 1000 patients treated (25). In the ideal setting, where cardiac catheterization laboratories are available to patients with acute myocardial infarction (ideally within 90 minutes of admission), angioplasty has been offered as an alternative to thrombolytic therapy and studied extensively in large clinical trials. A recent analysis of 10 randomized trials, carried out at centers where primary coronary angioplasty was efficiently conducted, documented a reduction in 30-day mortality favoring primary angioplasty (4.4%) compared with randomization to thrombolytic therapy (6.5%) (26). This benefit for primary angioplasty appears to persist for as long as 5 years of follow-up; mortality was 13% in the angioplasty group compared to 24% in the thrombolytic group. Also, reduction in nonfatal reinfarction from 22% to 6% was documented (27). In addition to these more aggressive and recent therapies for acute myocardial infarction, traditional treatment offers well-established benefit and is summarized as follows:

- **Aspirin.** Aspirin is a standard of care in the management of acute myocardial infarction and should be initiated as soon as the diagnosis is made or even suspected. The recommended dose is 160 mg to 325 mg daily.
- **Beta-blockade.** In the era of thrombolysis and primary angioplasty, the beneficial contribution of beta-blockade has been obscured. However, current recommendation for patients with acute myocardial infarction and good left ventricular function (ejection fraction 40% or higher) is to use beta-blockade orally. Patients who have hyperdynamic cardiovascular hemodynamics may benefit from intravenous beta-blockade.
- **Nitrate therapy.** The established beneficial role of nitroglycerin came from the prethrombolysis era, and recent large-scale trials of the benefit of nitroglycerine with thrombolysis are not positive. However, intravenous nitroglycerine is thought to be useful in reducing elevated systolic blood pressure in the setting of acute myocardial infarction and in patients with recurring angina pectoris.

- **Angiotensin-converting enzyme inhibitors.** Clinical trials demonstrate a consistent beneficial role for the use of angiotensin-converting enzyme inhibitors in patients with acute myocardial infarction and reduced left ventricular function. Early initiation (in the hospital) of angiotensin-converting enzyme inhibitors (unless not tolerated) offers proven benefit (28).
- **Calcium channel blockers.** Because clinical trials have not demonstrated benefit of calcium channel blockers in acute myocardial infarction, this therapy is not recommended.
- **Lipid management.** The well-established benefit of lipid-lowering therapy using the HMG-CoA reductase class of drugs (the statins) has been exceptionally well established in three large randomized controlled trials involving nearly 20,000 men and women. This class of drug should be made available to the patient during hospitalization for acute myocardial infarction and care taken to ensure continued use of this medication in the long term.

Recently controversy regarding the management of acute myocardial infarction in women as compared to men has arisen. Generally, women appear to receive less aggressive in-hospital management than men. A key issue relates to the possible adverse outcome of women compared to men resulting from this treatment difference. A large observational study using the Medicare database evaluated treatment differences and outcomes in men and women with acute myocardial infarction using the Medicare Cooperative Cardiovascular Project (29). Women were indeed documented to receive thrombolytic therapy and aspirin less often than men. However, the use of beta-blockers was equal, and women were more likely to receive angiotensin-converting enzyme inhibition treatment. Women were older than men, and 30-day mortality had to be adjusted to take the age difference into account. With such adjustment, 30-day mortality rates were no different between men and women in spite of the management differences.

INTERVENTION: PERCUTANEOUS CORONARY INTERVENTION VERSUS CORONARY ARTERY BYPASS GRAFT SURGERY

The American Heart Association's latest data document that 367,000 patients underwent coronary artery bypass surgery in 1996 in the United States. This was a 227% increase in this major surgery since 1979. The average cost of coronary artery bypass surgery was nearly $45,000. Also in 1996, 582,000 percutaneous transluminal coronary angiography (PTCA) took place at an average cost of $20,000 (1). The value of coronary angioplasty regarding quality of life has been assessed in the Randomized Interventional Treatment of Angina (RITA) trial comparing PTCA to continued medical treatment in patients with stable angina. At 3 years of follow-up in this 1018-patient study, the PTCA group had significantly greater improvement in quality of life scores pertaining to physical functioning, vitality, and general health at 1 year, but not at 3 years. The attenuation of the difference was attributed to 27% crossover of the initial medically assigned group to subsequent intervention (30). Continuing technical advances in percutaneous coronary intervention have occurred over the last 2 decades. Newer devices, especially stents, have come into widespread clinical use. The two national registries, a balloon angioplasty registry and a registry of newer coronary devices, allowed for a comparative study of clinical outcomes and mortality rates between the various devices. Perhaps surprisingly, this comparison "found no overall superiority to these newer devices in terms of patient survival or freedom from target lesion revascularization after adjustment for baseline risk profiles" (31). A recent comparison of longer versus shorter coronary stents found that the longer stent (> 25 mm) was associated with increased major procedural complications and with periprocedural non–Q wave myocardial infarction (32). A definitely beneficial addition to the management of patients undergoing percutaneous coronary revascularization has been the use of the new class of drug known as the platelet glycoprotein IIb/IIIa antagonist. The use of these agents in patients undergoing percutaneous coronary revascularization resulted in a relative reduction in the 30-day ratio for death or myocardial infarction of approximately 0.5 (33).

A recent report from the National Heart, Lung and Blood Institute provides interesting comparisons over the past decade between coronary artery bypass and catheter-based coronary intervention (34). This survey compared two periods, 1989 and 1997, regarding these two types of procedures in 17 large North American institutions. The findings can be highlighted as follows:

- The proportion of all procedures that were catheter based (versus surgery) increased from 52% to 62%.
- Patients with left main coronary disease who received catheter-based intervention increased from 2.2% to 5.7%.
- Catheter-based intervention in the setting of an acute myocardial infarction increased from 2.4% to 9.7% of all interventional procedures.
- The proportion of new devices other than balloons used in catheter-based procedures increased from 12% to 67%.
- For surgical patients, the prevalence of prior bypass surgery decreased from 13% to 7%.
- By 1997, 3% of surgical procedures were "minimally invasive."

With the advent of minimally invasive coronary artery bypass surgery, a comparison of this new approach with standard cardiopulmonary bypass graft surgery has been made. Although there has yet to be a randomized clinical trial comparing the two surgical approaches, a comparison has been provided from a single large university center (35). The comparisons can be highlighted as follows:

- Survival at 7 years was 80% in the beating-heart surgical group versus 79% in the cardiopulmonary bypass patient group (not significantly different).
- Of 107 patients from the beating-heart group, 21 (20%) needed subsequent angioplasty or a repeat coronary artery bypass procedure, compared with 8 (7%) of the 112 initial cardiopulmonary bypass patient group.

CORONARY ARTERY BYPASS SURGERY VERSUS PERCUTANEOUS CORONARY INTERVENTION

With the extensive use of interventional techniques in patients with coronary artery disease, the important issue of superiority of bypass surgery compared with catheter-based treatment is an issue of major importance both clinically and from the perspective of health care economics. Several studies of this issue provide useful information to health care providers, patients, and their families. The various studies are reviewed in the following paragraphs.

A registry regarding long-term outcomes of bypass surgery and angioplasty compared to medical therapy was carried out at the Duke University Medical Center from 1984 to 1990 (36). This registry covered outcomes for 9263 patients with a mean follow-up of 5.3 years. Of these patients, 2449 initially received medical therapy, 2924 underwent angioplasty, and bypass surgery was carried out in 3890 patients. (This was not a randomized trial.) After adjusting for patients' baseline differences that could affect prognosis, improved survival occurred in patients having undergone either angioplasty or bypass surgery compared to initial medical therapy alone. Furthermore, all patients with single-vessel coronary disease (except those with 90% or greater proximal left anterior descending coronary artery narrowing) benefited more from angioplasty than from bypass surgery. However, patients with three-vessel disease and those with two-vessel disease that included more than 95% proximal left anterior descending coronary artery narrowing benefited more from bypass surgery than from angioplasty. All other patients showed similar survival after either bypass surgery or angioplasty.

A randomized trial comparing bypass with percutaneous coronary intervention was carried out in Argentina on 127 patients with multivessel coronary artery disease. At 3 years' follow-up, freedom from the combined end point of death, myocardial infarction, angina, and repeat revascularization was significantly in favor of the bypass surgical group versus the angioplasty group (77% versus 47%, P < .001). However, there were no differences regarding either overall or cardiac mortality or frequency of myocardial infarction between the two groups. The benefit of bypass surgery resulted from freedom from angina (79% versus 57%) and far less need for additional interventional procedures (6.3% versus 37%). Also, the total medical costs at 3-year follow-up were greater in the bypass group than in the angioplasty group (37).

A large multicenter randomized trial has reported the long-term outcome of bypass surgery versus percutaneous coronary intervention (the RITA trial) (38). This study included patients with one-, two-, and three-vessel coronary artery disease and provided follow-up of a mean of 2.5 years in 1011 patients. All intended vessels were grafted in 97% of bypass patients. Successful angioplasty occurred in 87% of vessels. The number of deaths was not significantly different between the two groups (18 in the bypass patient group, 16 in the angioplasty group). Furthermore, there was no significant difference in the combined end point of death or myocardial infarction between the two groups (43 bypass patients compared to 50 angioplasty patients). However, within 2 years of randomization, 38% of the angioplasty patient group, compared to 11% of the bypass patient group, required revascularization, had a primary event, died, or had a myocardial infarction ($P < .001$). At 6 months' follow-up, 32% of the angioplasty group, compared to 11% of the bypass patients, had angina pectoris. At 1 month, functional status and employment status were lower in the bypass patient group, but thereafter no significant differences in the two groups persisted.

A randomized trial (single medical center) of bypass surgery versus angioplasty in patients with multivessel coronary artery disease has been reported from Emory University (39). This study, the EAST, randomized 194 patients to bypass surgery and 198 to initial coronary angioplasty. The primary end point (death, myocardial infarction, or large ischemic defect) was no different at 3 years. However, repeat revascularization was significantly greater in the initial angioplasty group. At follow-up of 8 years, survival was 83% in the surgical group compared to 79% in the angioplasty group ($P = 0.4$). The diabetic patients in this small study showed a trend toward better survival with bypass surgery that did not reach statistical significance.

A large multicenter randomized trial was carried out under the sponsorship of the National Heart, Lung and Blood Institute to compare long-term results in patients with multivessel coronary disease randomly assigned to initial revascularization by means of PTCA versus coronary artery bypass grafting. This study, known as BARI (40), examined 1829 patients. The end point of survival at 7-year follow-up favored the bypass surgical group (survival of 84.4% versus 80.9% in the angioplasty group; $P = .043$). This difference was the result of superior survival in patients with baseline treated diabetes mellitus, among whom 7-year survival was 76.4% in the bypass pa-

tient group compared to 55.7% in the angioplasty group ($P = .0011$). Among the 1476 nondiabetic treatment group, no survival difference occurred (86.4% bypass, 86.8% angioplasty groups). Subsequent revascularization was significantly greater in the initial angioplasty versus bypass patient group (59.7% versus 13.1%; $P < 0.001$) (41).

A substudy by the BARI investigators reported on medical care costs and quality of life in a subset of 934 patients (42). At 3 years' follow-up, functional status scores on the Duke Activity Status Index had improved more in the bypass than the angioplasty patients ($P < .05$). However, the angioplasty group returned to work on average 5 weeks sooner ($P < .001$) and had an initial mean cost considerably lower than the surgical patient group ($21,113 versus $32,347; $P < 0.001$). At 5 years, the cumulative medical cost for the angioplasty patient group averaged $56,224 versus $58,889 in the surgical group ($P = .047$).

▶ SUMMARY

Coronary heart disease is the major cause of morbidity and mortality in the United States, affecting more than 12 million people and causing in excess of 500,000 deaths each year. Aggressive treatment of the risk factors for coronary artery disease significantly affects morbidity and mortality. Invasive interventions in the treatment of acute coronary syndromes can be lifesaving and cost-effective.

References
1. American Heart Association. 1999 Heart and Stroke Statistical Update. Dallas, Tex.: American Heart Association, 1998.
2. Randomised trial of cholesterol lowering in 4444 patients with coronary heart disease: The Scandinavian Simvastatin Survival Study (4S). Lancet 344:1383–1389, 1994.
3. Sacks FM, Pfeffer MA, Moye LA, et al. The effect of pravastatin on coronary events after myocardial infarction in patients with average cholesterol levels. N Engl J Med 335:1001–1009, 1996.
4. Long-Term Intervention with Pravastatin in Ischaemic Disease (LIPID) Study Group. Prevention of cardiovascular events and death with pravastatin in patients with coronary heart disease and a broad range of initial cholesterol levels. N Engl J Med 339:1349–1357, 1998.
5. Rubins HB, Robins SJ, Collins D, et al. Gemfibrozil for the secondary prevention of coronary heart disease in men with low levels of high-density lipoprotein cholesterol. N Engl J Med 341:410–418, 1999.
6. Miettinen TA, Pyorala K, Olsson AG, et al. Cholesterol-lowering therapy in women and elderly patients with myocardial infarction or angina pectoris: Findings from the Scandinavian Simvastatin Survival Study (4S). Circ 96: 4211–4218, 1997.
7. Lewis SJ, Sacks FM, Mitchell JS, et al. Effect of pravastatin on cardiovascular events in women after myocardial infarction: The Cholesterol and Recurrent Events (CARE) trial. J Am Coll Cardiol 32:140–146, 1998.

8. Lewis SJ, Sacks FM, Mitchell JS, et al. Effect of pravastatin on cardiovascular events in older patients with myocardial infarction and cholesterol levels in the average range: Results of the Cholesterol and Recurrent Events (CARE) trial. Ann Intern Med 129:681–689, 1998.

9. Pitt B, Waters D, Brown WV, et al. Aggressive lipid-lowering therapy compared with angioplasty in stable coronary artery disease. N Engl J Med 341:70–76, 1999.

10. Wilson K, Gibson N, Willan A, Cook D. Effect of smoking cessation on mortality after myocardial infarction. Arch Intern Med 160:939–944, 2000.

11. Voors AA, Van Brussel BL, Plokker T, et al. Smoking and cardiac events after venous coronary bypass surgery. Circulation 93:42–47, 1996.

12. Hasdai D, Garrat KN, Grill DE, et al. Effect of smoking status on the long-term outcome after successful percutaneous coronary revascularization. N Engl J Med 336:755–761, 1997.

13. Haffner SM, Lehto S, Ronnemaa T, et al. Mortality from coronary heart disease in subjects with type 2 diabetes and in nondiabetic subjects with and without prior myocardial infarction. N Engl J Med 339(4):229–234, 1998.

14. UK Prospective Diabetes Study Group. Intensive blood-glucose control with sulphonylureas or insulin compared with conventional treatment and risk of complications in patients with type 2 diabetes (UKPDS 33). Lancet 352:837–853, 1998.

15. Pyorala K, Pedersen TR, Kjekshus J, et al. Cholesterol lowering with simvastatin improves prognosis of diabetic patients with coronary heart disease: A subgroup analysis of the Scandinavian Simvastatin Survival Study (4S). Diabetes Care 20:614–620, 1997.

16. Goldberg RB, Mellies MJ, Sacks FM, et al. Cardiovascular events and their reduction with pravastatin in diabetic and glucose-intolerant myocardial infarction survivors with average cholesterol levels: Subgroup analyses in the Cholesterol and Recurrent Events (CARE) trial. Circulation 98:2513–2519, 1998.

17. Anand SS, Yusuf S. Oral anticoagulant therapy in patients with coronary artery disease: A meta-analysis. JAMA 1282:2058–2067, 1999.

18. Yusuf S, Sleight P, Pogue J, et al. Effects of an angiotensin-converting-enzyme inhibitor, ramipril, on cardiovascular events in high-risk patients. N Engl J Med 342:145–153, 2000.

19. Hulley S, Grady D, Bush T, et al. Randomized trial of estrogen plus progestin for secondary prevention of coronary heart disease in postmenopausal women. JAMA 280:605–613, 1998.

20. Heberden W. Commentaries on the history and cure of diseases. In: Willius FA, Keys TE, eds. Classics of Cardiology. New York: Henry Schuman, Dover, 1941:I:221

21. Monrad ES. Role of low-molecular-weight heparins in the management of patients with unstable angina pectoris and non-Q wave acute myocardial infarction. Am J Cardiol 85(8A):2C–9C, 2000.

22. Boersma E, Akkerhuis KM, Theroux P, et al. Platelet glycoprotein IIb/IIIa receptor inhibition in non-ST-elevation acute coronary syndromes: Early benefit during medical treatment only, with additional protection during percutaneous coronary intervention. Circulation 100:2045–2048, 1999.

23. Kleiman NS, Lincoff AM, Flaker GC, et al. Early percutaneous coronary intervention, platelet inhibition with eptifibatide, and clinical outcomes in patients with acute coronary syndromes. Circulation 101:751–757, 2000.

24. Wallentin L, Lagerqvist B, Husted S, et al. Outcome at 1 year after an invasive compared with a noninvasive strategy in unstable coronary-artery disease. Lancet 356:9–16, 2000.

25. Morrison LJ, Verbeek PR, McDonald AC, et al. Mortality and prehospital thrombolysis for acute myocardial infarction. JAMA 283:2686–2692, 2000.

26. Weaver WD, Simes RJ, Betriu A, et al. Comparison of primary coronary angioplasty and intravenous thrombolytic therapy for acute myocardial infarction: A quantitative review. JAMA 278:2093–2098, 1997.

27. Zijlstra F, Hoorntje JCA, de Boer MJ, et al. Long-term benefit of primary angioplasty as compared with thrombolytic therapy for acute myocardial infarction. N Engl J Med 1999 Nov 4; 341(19):1413–1419, 1999.

28. Ball SG, Hall AS, Murray GD. Angiotensin-converting enzyme inhibitors after myocardial infarction: Indications and timing. J Am Coll Cardiol 25(7 Suppl):42S–46S, 1995.

29. Gan SC, Beaver SK, Houck PM, et al. Treatment of acute myocardial infarction and 30-day mortality among women and men. N Engl J Med 343:8–15, 2000.

30. Pocock SJ, Henderson RA, Clayton T, et al. Quality of life after coronary angioplasty or continued medical treatment for angina: Three-year follow-up in the RITA-2 trial. J Am Coll Cardiol 2000 Mar 15; 35(4):907–914.

31. King SB 3rd, Yeh W, Holubkov R, et al. Balloon angioplasty versus new device intervention: Clinical outcomes. J Am Coll Cardiol 31:558–566, 1998.

32. Kornowski R, Bhargava B, Fuchs S, et al. Procedural results and late clinical outcomes after percutaneous interventions using long (> or = 25 mm) versus short (< 20 mm) stents. J am Coll Cardiol 35:612–618, 2000.

33. Bhatt DL, Lincoff AM, Califf RM, et al. The benefit of abciximab in percutaneous coronary revascularization is not device-specific. Am J Cardiol 85:1060–1064, 2000.

34. Holubkov R, Detre KM, Sopko G, et al. Trends in Coronary Revascularization 1989 to 1997: The Bypass Angioplasty Revascularization Investigation (BARI) Survey of Procedures. Am J Cardiol 84:157–161, 1999.

35. Gundry SR, Romano MA, Shattuck OH, et al. Seven-year follow-up of coronary artery bypasses performed with and without cardiopulmonary bypass. J Thorac Cardiovasc Surg 115:1273–1277, 1998.

36. Jones RH, Kesler K, Phillips HR 3d, et al. Long-term survival benefits of coronary bypass grafting and percutaneous transluminal angioplasty in patients with coronary artery disease. J Thorac Cardiovasc Surg 111:1013–1025, 1996.

37. Rodriguez A, Mele E, Peyregne E, et al. Three-year follow-up of the Argentine Randomized Trial of Percutaneous Transluminal Coronary Angioplasty Versus Coronary Artery Bypass Surgery in Multivessel Disease. J Am Coll Cardiol 27:1178–1184, 1996.

38. Coronary angioplasty versus coronary artery bypass surgery: the Randomized Intervention Treatment of Angina (RITA) trial. Lancet 341:573–580, 1993.

39. King SB 3rd, Kosinski AS, Guyton RA, et al. Eight-year mortality in the Emory Angioplasty versus Surgery Trial. J Am Coll Cardiol 35:1116–1121, 2000.

40. BARI Investigators: Seven-year outcome in the Bypass An-

gioplasty Revascularization Investigation (BARI) by treatment and diabetic status. J Am Coll Cardiol 35:1122–1129, 2000.

41. Whitlow PL, Dimas AP, Bashore TM, et al. Relationship of extent of revascularization with angina at one year in the By- pass Angioplasty Revascularization Investigation (BARI). J Am Coll Cardiol 34:1750–1759, 1999.

42. Hlatky MA, Rogers WJ, Johnstone I, et al. Medical care costs and quality of life after randomization to coronary angioplasty or coronary bypass surgery. N Engl J Med 336:92–99, 1997.

1.4.0.1, 1.4.0.3   2.4.1, 2.4.2, 2.4.3   5.4.0, 5.4.2

CHAPTER **30**

COMPREHENSIVE CARDIOVASCULAR RISK REDUCTION IN PATIENTS WITH CORONARY ARTERY DISEASE

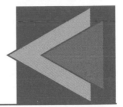

Thomas P. LaFontaine and Neil F. Gordon

Despite a 24.5% decline in the death rate from cardiovascular disease (CVD) during the past decade in the United States, CVD remains the leading cause of morbidity and mortality. In particular, coronary artery disease (CAD) causes approximately 1 million myocardial infarctions per year (1). More than 14 million Americans have established CAD (1). More than $50 billion is spent annually on the treatment of these individuals, and studies suggest that as few as 11% of patients achieve the target low-density lipoprotein (LDL) goal of 100 mg/dL (2). Evidence provides a strong rationale for long-term aggressive control of CAD risk factors as an essential strategy to do the following:

- Normalize coronary artery endothelial function
- Halt or reverse the progression of coronary atherosclerosis
- Prevent the instability, rupture, and thrombosis of atherosclerotic plaques
- Reduce mortality, recurrent hospitalization, and costs of medical care

This chapter provides a brief review of clinical data supporting aggressive CVD risk reduction in CAD patients, barriers to effective implementation of comprehensive cardiovascular risk reduction strategies, and recent expert guidelines for clinical practice.

PROGRESSION OR REGRESSION OF ATHEROSCLEROSIS

Atherosclerotic coronary artery occlusions are estimated to progress at a "natural" rate of 1.5% reduction in arterial diameter per year (3). Rate of progression is reported to be 3–6 times greater in grafted than ungrafted vessels (3). Recent arteriographic secondary prevention clinical trials have convincingly demonstrated that while progression of coronary atherosclerosis is common when CAD patients receive usual medical care, aggressive modification of risk factors may slow the rate of atherosclerosis progression, stabilize vulnerable plaques, and induce partial regression. This section summarizes key findings of these studies.

The National Heart, Blood and Lung Institute (NHLBI) Type II Coronary Intervention Study first suggested that lipid lowering using dietary therapy and cholestyramine could retard progression of atherosclerosis in patients with hyperlipidemia (4). In the Cholesterol Lowering Atherosclerosis Study (CLAS), 162 male patients who had had coronary artery bypass surgery were randomly assigned to diet therapy plus placebo or diet therapy plus colestipol and niacin (5). After 2 years, assessment of arteriographic change revealed significantly more regression in the drug-treated group than the placebo group (16.2% versus 2.4%). After 4 years of intervention, nonprogression of atherosclerosis occurred more often in the drug-treated group than the placebo group (52% versus 15%), as did regression (18% versus 6%) (6).

These initial trials prompted a series of arteriographic secondary prevention trials to evaluate the effect of CAD risk factor modification by pharmacological, lifestyle, and surgical strategies on the underlying atherosclerosis process (Tables 30.1–30.3). Differences in methodology preclude meaningful comparison of the amount of regression observed. However, analysis of arteriographic data from the study in which the greatest magnitude of regression occurred, namely the Lifestyle Heart Trial, provides insight into the degree to which the underlying process of atherosclerosis can be affected. In this study, the average stenosis regressed from 40% to 37.8% with 1 year of intensive lifestyle intervention and progressed from 42.7% to 46.1% with 1 year of usual medical care. When occlusions greater than 50% were analyzed, the average stenosis regressed from 61.1% to 55.8% in the intervention group and progressed from 61.7% to 64.4% in the usual care group (7). The 5-year results of the Lifestyle Heart Trial were recently reported to show continued progression of CAD in the control group and regression in the intensive lifestyle intervention group (8). Neibauer et al. (9) reported similar 6-year results. In this study and in earlier work this group reported that patients who expended

Table 30.1. Percentage of Patients with Progression or Regression of Atherosclerosis in Arteriographic Secondary Prevention Trials of Lifestyle Intervention Alone or with Drug Treatment

STUDY, YEAR (REFERENCE)	SUBJECTS	INTERVENTION	DURATION (YEARS)	PROGRESSION (% PATIENTS)		REGRESSION (% PATIENTS)	
				INTERVENTION GROUP	CONTROL GROUP	INTERVENTION GROUP	CONTROL GROUP
Lifestyle Heart Trial, 1990 (7)	Male: n = 36 Female: n = 5 Age 35–75 yr	Multiple lifestyle	1	18	53	82	42
STARS, 1992[a]	Male: n = 50 Female: n = 0 Age < 66 yr	Diet	3.25	15	46	38	4
	Male: n = 48 Female: n = 0 Age < 66 yr	Diet + cholestyramine	3.25	12	46	33	4
Heidelberg, 1992 (10)	Male: n = 113 Female: n = 0 Age 35–68 yr	Exercise + diet	1	23	48	32	17
Heidelberg, 1997 (9)	Male: n = 90 Female: n = 0 Age 35–68 yr	Exercise + diet	6	59	74	19	0
SCRIP, 1994 (14)	Male: n = 259 Female: n = 41 Age < 75 yr	Lifestyle + lipid-lowering drugs as needed	4	50	50	20	10
Omega-3, 1997[b]	(1997) Male: n = 134 Female: n = 28 Age < 75 yr	Omega-3 fatty acids	2	47	51	20	9

Design for all studies was randomized.
STARS, St. Thomas' Atherosclerosis Regression Study; SCRIP, Stanford Coronary Risk Intervention Project.
[a] Lancet 339:563–569, 1992.
[b] von Schacky C et al. Ann Intern Med 130:554–562, 1999.

about 1800 kcal/week (about 4 hours of aerobic exercise per week) demonstrated regression, while those who expended about 1240–1260 kcal/week showed progression of atherosclerotic plaques on quantitative angiography (9, 10).

Several important observations, including the following, have emerged from existing arteriographic secondary prevention clinical trials:

1. Progression of atherosclerosis can be expected when CAD patients receive usual medical care.
2. Nonprogression and regression of coronary atherosclerosis occur significantly more often in patients who aggressively modify CAD risk factors than in those receiving usual medical care.
3. The magnitude of regression is modest at best, usually on the order of 1–10% of the original stenosis.
4. The underlying atherosclerotic process can be favorably affected by single or multiple interventions and by pharmacological, lifestyle, or surgical modulation of CAD risk factors.
5. With continued adherence to therapeutic interventions, nonprogression or further regression may occur.

In addition, it is evident from these studies that effective interventions are well tolerated, safe, and acceptable to patients.

MYOCARDIAL PERFUSION AND CLINICAL EVENTS

Though modest changes in anatomical severity of coronary artery stenoses follow aggressive CAD risk factor modification, the precise value of such therapy may be questioned. More important than anatomical arteriographic improvement, however, is the effect of risk factor intervention on myocardial perfusion and clinical cardiac events.

According to the Poiseuille equation, resistance to flow is inversely proportional to the radius raised to the fourth power. Therefore, even minor reductions in stenosis can be expected to produce proportionately greater improvements in myocardial perfusion. In this respect, Schuler et al. (11) documented a reduction in exercise-induced myocardial ischemia, assessed by thallium scintigraphy, in patients with stable angina pectoris who participated in 12 months of exercise training combined with a low-fat diet. More recently, Gould et al. (12) evaluated changes in

Table 30.2. Percentage of Patients or Grafts with Progression or Regression of Atherosclerosis in Arteriographic Secondary Prevention Trials Involving Single-Drug or Ileal Bypass Surgery

STUDY, YEAR (REFERENCE)	SUBJECTS	INTERVENTION	DESIGN	DURATION (YEARS)	PROGRESSION (% PATIENTS OR GRAFTS)		REGRESSION (% PATIENTS OR GRAFTS)	
					INTERVENTION GROUP	CONTROL GROUP	INTERVENTION GROUP	CONTROL GROUP
NHLBI Type II Coronary Intervention Study, 1984 (4)	Male: n = 94 Female: n = 22 Age 21–55 yr	Cholestyramine	Randomized double blind	5	32	49	7	7
MARS, 1993[a]	Male: n = 247 Female: n = 23 Age 37–67 yr	Lovastatin	Randomized double blind	2	29	41	23	12
CCAIT, 1994[b]	Male: n = 269 Female: n = 62 Age 27–70 yr	Lovastatin	Randomized double blind	2	33	50	10	7
MAAS, 1994[c]	Male: n = 336 Female: n = 45 Age 30–67 yr	Simvastatin	Randomized double blind	4	3	4	4	4
REGRES, 1995[d]	Male: n = 885 Female: n = 0 Age < 70 yr	Pravastatin	Randomized double blind	2	22	28	8	5
POSCH, 1990[e]	Male: n = 760 Female: n = 78 Age 30–64 yr	Partial ileal bypass surgery	Randomized	9.7	55	85	6	4
Post CABG Trial, 1997[f]	Male: n = 1243 Female: n = 108 Age 21–74 yr	Lovastatin	Randomized double blind	4.3	27	39	NS	
					% grafts showing progression			
LCAS, 1999[g]	Male: n = 349 Female: n = 80 Age 35–75 yr	Fluvastatin	Randomized	2.5	29	36	14	7.6

[a] Ann Intern Med 119:969–976, 1993.
[b] Circulation 89:959–968, 1994.
[c] Lancet 344:633–638, 1994.
[d] Circulation 91:2528–2540, 1995.
[e] N Engl J Med 323:946–955, 1990.
[f] N Engl J Med 336:153–162, 1997.
[g] Am J Cardiol 80:278–286, 1997.
NHLBI, National Heart, Blood and Lung Institute; MARS, Monitored Atherosclerosis Regression Study; CCAIT, Canadian Coronary Atherosclerosis Intervention Trial; MAAS, Multicenter Anti-Atheroma Study; REGRESS, Regression Growth Evaluation Statin Study; POSCH, Program on the Surgical Control of the Hyperlipidemias; LCAS, Lipoprotein and Coronary Atherosclerosis Study. CABG, coronary artery bypass graft; NS, not significant.

size and severity of myocardial perfusion abnormalities by positron emission tomography in patients with CAD randomized to 5 years of intensive risk factor modification or to usual care as part of the Lifestyle Heart Trial. Risk factor modification consisted of a very low-fat, low-cholesterol vegetarian diet, smoking cessation, practice of stress management techniques for 82 minutes daily, and participation in mild to moderate aerobic exercise for more than 4 hours/week. The results showed that the size and severity of myocardial perfusion abnormalities at rest and after dipyridamole stress improve in patients undergoing intense risk factor modification, while patients treated with usual therapy demonstrated worsening perfusion abnormalities. The relative magnitude of change in size and severity of perfusion abnormalities was comparable with changes in stenoses.

Improvements in myocardial perfusion with aggressive risk factor modification are thought to be related to improved endothelial-mediated coronary artery and arteriolar vasomotor function (13–17). Animal and human studies document improvement in myocardial perfusion within weeks to months after vigorous cholesterol lowering by fat restriction and/or drugs, before anatomical regression (18–22). However, a recent well-controlled longer-term (6 months) study with a larger sample of patients with CAD and hypercholesterolemia suggested that cholesterol lowering of 40% on average with simvastatin did not improve endothelial function (23). Recent cross-sectional and longitudinal studies also have shown improved endothelial function following exercise training in elderly healthy persons, congestive heart failure patients, and patients with CAD (24–27).

Table 30.3. Percentage of Patients with Progression or Regression of Atherosclerosis in Arteriographic Secondary Prevention Trials Involving Multiple Drug Therapy

Study, Year (Reference)	Subjects	Intervention	Design	Duration (Years)	Progression (% Patients) Intervention Group	Control Group	Regression (% Patients) Intervention Group	Control Group
CLASS-I, 1987 (5, 6)	Male: n = 162 Female: n = 0 Age 40–59 yr	Colestipol + niacin	Randomized double blind	2.00	39	61	16	2
FATS, 1990[a]	Male: n = 82 Female: n = 0 Age < 63 yr	Colestipol + niacin	Randomized double blind	2.50	25	46	39	11
	Male: n = 84 Female: n = 0 Age < 63 yr	Colestipol + lovastatin	Randomized	2.50	21	46	32	11
SCOR, 1990[b]	Male: n = 31 Female: n = 41 Age 19–72 yr	Colestipol + niacin	Randomized double blind	2.17	20	41	33	13
CLASS-II, 1990	Male: n = 103 Female: n = 0 Age 40–59 yr	Colestipol + niacin + lovastatin	Randomized double blind	4	30	79	18	6
HARP, 1994[c]	Male: n = 70 Female: n = 9 Age 30–75 yr	Intensive drugs (1–4 lipid meds)	Randomized double blind	2.50	33	38	13	15
LCAS, 1999[d]	Male: n = 349 Female: n = 80 Age 35–75 yr	Fluvastatin + cholestyramine	Randomized double blind	2.50	29	51	17	11

[a] N Engl J Med 323:1289–1298, 1990.
[b] JAMA 264:3007–3012, 1990.
[c] Lancet 344:1182–1186, 1994.
[d] Am J Cardiol 80:278–286, 1997.
CLASS, Cholesterol-Lowering Atherosclerosis Study; FATS, Familial Atherosclerosis Treatment Study; SCOR, University of California, San Francisco, Arteriosclerosis Specialized Center of Research Intervention Trial; HARP, Harvard Atherosclerosis Reversibility Project; LCAS, Lipoprotein and Coronary Atherosclerosis.

These arteriographic secondary prevention trials were specifically designed to assess the effect of risk factor modification on atherosclerotic progression or regression. More recently, a significant reduction in major clinical cardiac events, including sudden cardiac death, nonfatal myocardial infarction, new-onset angina pectoris, and need for primary revascularization procedures, has been documented following single or multiple therapy interventions (Table 30.4).

Of the investigations performed to date, the Stanford Coronary Risk Intervention Project (SCRIP) perhaps has the greatest practical significance (28). SCRIP used aggressive modification of multiple risk factors via lifestyle intervention and medication. Moreover, SCRIP employed a physician-supervised nurse case manager model with consultation from other health professionals that could be implemented in other health care settings. SCRIP studied 300 men and women with arteriographically defined CAD. They were randomly assigned to usual care or multifactor risk reduction for the 4-year study period. Patients assigned to risk reduction were provided individualized programs including a low-fat, low-cholesterol diet, exercise, weight loss, smoking cessation, and medications to improve lipoprotein profiles. Intensive cardiovascular risk reduction resulted in significant improvements in various CAD risk factors, including LDL cholesterol and apolipoprotein B, high-density lipoprotein (HDL) cholesterol, plasma triglycerides, body weight, exercise capacity, and intake of dietary fat and cholesterol, compared with relatively small changes in the usual care group. Progression of atherosclerosis in the risk reduction group was 47% less than for the usual care group. In addition, there were 25 hospitalizations for clinical cardiac events in the risk reduction group versus 44 in the usual care group. Interestingly, during the final 3 years of the study, risk reduction patients were hospitalized for clinical cardiac events only 8 times compared with 35 times for the usual care patients.

Cholesterol lowering has caused some concern because the observed reduction of cardiac deaths appears to be offset by an increase in noncardiac mortality, particularly from cancer and violence. In the Scandinavian Simvastatin Survival Study (4S), a landmark secondary pre-

Table 30.4. Reduction in Clinical Cardiac Events with Risk Factor Modification in Secondary Prevention Trials

Study, Year (Reference)	Duration, Years	Cardiac Events	Intervention	Percent Reduction in Cardiac Events (P value)
DART, 1989[a]	2.00	All-cause, CAD death	200–400 g oily fish	29 ($p \leq .05$)
POSCH, 1990[b]	9.70	CAD death, MI, CABG	Partial ileal bypass surgery	49 ($p \leq .05$)
FATS, 1990[c]	2.50	CVD death, MI, revascularization	Colestipol + niacin	78 ($p \leq .05$)
			Colestipol + lovastatin	66 ($p \leq .05$)
STARS, 1992[d]	3.25	CVD death, MI, CABG, PTCA	Diet	($p \leq .05$)
			Diet + cholestyramine	89 ($p \leq .05$)
MARS, 1993[e]	2.00	CAD death, MI, CABG, PTCA, unstable angina	Lovastatin	28 (NS)
CCAIT, 1994[f]	2.00	CAD death, MI, unstable angina	Lovastatin	22 (NS)
SCRIP, 1994 (14)	4.00	CVD death, MI, CABG, primary PTCA	Multiple lifestyle, lipid meds as indicated	39 ($p \leq .05$)
MAAS, 1994[g]	4.00	CAD death, MI, CABG, PTCA	Simvastatin	24 (NS)
PLAC-II, 1994 (18)	3.00	CAD death, MI	Pravastatin	60*
HARP, 1994[h]	2.50	CAD death, MI, CHF, CABG, PTCA, unstable angina	Intensive meds (1–4 lipid meds)	33 (NS)
4S, 1994 (15)	5.40	CAD death, MI, resuscitated cardiac arrest	Simvastatin	34 ($p \leq .05$)
REGRESS, 1995[i]	2.00	CAD death, MI	Pravastatin	38*
PLAC-T, 1995 (18)	3.00	CAD death, MI	Pravastatin	53*
CARE, 1996 (19)	5.00	CAD death, MI	Pravastatin	24 ($p \leq .05$)
Singh et al., 1998[j]	1.00	CAD death, serious ventricular dysrhythmias	2 g omega-3 FFA	54 ($p \leq .05$) 30 ($p \leq .05$)
Post CABG, 1997[k]	4.30	Redo revascularization	Lovastatin	29 ($p \leq .05$)
Lifestyle Heart, 1998 (8)	5.00	CAD death, MI, CABG, hospitalizations	Multiple lifestyle	80 ($p \leq .05$)
LIPID, 1998[l]	6.10	CAD death, MI, stroke, all revascularizations	Pravastatin	19–29 ($p \leq .05$)
CARE, 1999[m] (revascularized patients)	5.00	CAD death, MI	Pravastatin	36 ($p \leq .05$)
VHA HDL Study[n]	5.10	CAD death, MI, stroke	Gemfibrozil	24 ($p \leq .05$)
Atorvastatin vs. PTCA Trial, 1999[o]	1.60	Any ischemia event	Lovastatin vs. PTCA	38 ($p \leq .05$)
Lyon Diet Heart Study, 1999[p]	3.86	CAD death, MI, other cardiopulmonary events	Mediterranean diet	68 ($p \leq .05$)
GISSI, 1999[q]	3.50	All-cause mortality, sudden death	850 mg omega-3 FFA	20 ($p \leq .05$) 45 ($p \leq .05$)
4S, 2000 (30)	7.40	All-cause death	Simvastatin	30 ($p \leq .05$)

* Statistical significance not provided. When data from these three trials are combined with data from Kuopio Atherosclerosis Prevention Study, $p \leq .05$ for reduction in CAD death and MI (51% reduction) (see reference 18).

** Differences in clinical events not significant after adjustment for interim analysis. See Tables 30.1, 30.2, 30.3.

[a] Lancet 2:757–761, 1989.
[b] N Engl J Med 323:946–955, 1990.
[c] N Engl J Med 323:1289–1298, 1990.
[d] Lancet 339:563–569, 1992.
[e] Ann Intern Med 119:969–976, 1993.
[f] Circulation 89:959–968, 1994.
[g] Lancet 344:633–638, 1994.
[h] Lancet 344:1182–1186, 1994.
[i] Circulation 91:2528–2540, 1995.
[j] Cardiovasc Drug Ther 11:485–491, 1997.
[k] N Engl J Med 336:153–162, 1997.
[l] N Engl J Med 339:1349–1357, 1998.
[m] J Am Coll Cardiol 34:106–112, 1999.
[n] N Engl J Med 341:410–418, 1999.
[o] N Engl J Med. 341:70–76, 1999.
[p] Circulation 99:779–785, 1999.
[q] Lancet 354:447–455, 1999.

DART, Diet and Reinfarction Trial; POSCH, Program on the Surgical Control of Hyperlipidemias; FATS, Familial Atherosclerosis Treatment Study; STARS, St. Thomas' Atherosclerosis Regression Study; MARS, Monitored Atherosclerosis Regression Study; CCAIT, Canadian Coronary Atherosclerosis Intervention Trial; SCRIP, Standford Coronary Risk Intervention Project; MAAS, Multicenter Anti-Atheroma Study; PLAC-I, Pravastatin Limitation of Atherosclerosis in the Coronary Arteries Trial; 4S, Scandinavian Simvastatin Survival Study; REGRESS, Regression Growth Evaluation Statin Study; PLAC-II, Pravastatin, Lipids, and Atherosclerosis in the Carotid Arteries Trial; LIPID, Long-Term Intervention with Pravastatin in Ischemic Heart Disease; CARE, Cholesterol and Recurrent Events Study; CAD, coronary artery disease; CVD, cardiovascular disease; MI, myocardial infarction; FFA, free fatty acids.

vention study, 4444 patients with angina pectoris or previous myocardial infarction and high serum cholesterol were randomized to double-blind treatment with simvastatin or placebo (29). Over the 5.4-year follow-up period, treatment resulted in a 42% reduction in cardiac deaths, a 37% reduction in risk of undergoing revascularization procedures, and a 30% reduction in all-cause mortality. This improvement in survival was achieved without an increase in non-CAD mortality. The benefit of simvastatin for CAD risk appeared to begin after about 1 year of therapy and increased steadily thereafter, a finding consistent with several angiographic studies (20). Recently, long-term observational results of the 4S study substantiated a 30% reduction in all-cause mortality in the group randomized to simvastatin compared to placebo (30).

Recent similar findings have been reported in the elderly, women, and patients with associated risk factors who were treated with diet, lovastatin, and cholestyramine following percutaneous coronary intervention or coronary artery bypass surgery (31–33). Aggressive lowering of LDL cholesterol to less than 100 mg/dL was associated with a 31% reduction per patient in grafts showing progression of atherosclerosis (32). It was concluded that these findings were consistent with the recommendation of the National Cholesterol Education program that the LDL cholesterol level should be reduced to less than 100 mg/dL in patients with documented CAD. These findings have been corroborated by the West of Scotland Coronary Prevention Study, the Pravastatin Atherosclerosis and MI Reduction Analysis, a combined analysis of clinical event data from four independent secondary prevention studies (Pravastatin Limitation of Atherosclerosis in the Coronary Arteries Trial [PLAC-I], Pravastatin, Lipids, and Atherosclerosis in the Carotid Arteries Trial [PLAC-II], Regression Growth Evaluation Statin Study [REGRESS], the Air Force Coronary Atherosclerosis Prevention Study/Texas Coronary Atherosclerosis Prevention study (AFCAPS/TEXCAPS), the Long-Term Intervention With Pravastatin in Ischemic Heart Disease [LIPID] Study, and the Cholesterol and Recurrent Events Study [CARE] Study (33–38).

Recent data from the Lipoprotein and Coronary Atherosclerosis Study (LCAS) of 429 CAD patients with mild to moderate elevations of LDL cholesterol (115–190 mg/dL) randomly assigned to placebo, fluvastatin 20 mg twice a day, or fluvastatin plus cholestyramine up to 12 g/day supported previous findings (39). In this trial, treatment with fluvastatin resulted in significantly less CAD progression ($p < .02$) and a nonsignificant reduction in clinical cardiac events (24–33% reduction).

MECHANISM OF REDUCTION IN CARDIAC EVENTS

Recent advances in understanding pathophysiology of atherosclerosis and acute cardiac syndromes are clarifying the paradoxical observation of a significant reduction in clinical cardiac events despite modest arteriographic

benefits following aggressive risk factor modification (40, 41).

1. Less severe atherosclerotic plaques may rapidly progress to severe stenoses or total coronary artery occlusions and may account for up to two-thirds of patients who develop unstable angina pectoris or acute myocardial infarction.
2. Rupture of a vulnerable plaque with resultant thrombus formation may be the most important mechanism underlying rapid progression.
3. Most ruptures occur at the periphery of the fibrous cap covering the lipid-rich core of the plaque, sites where the cap is usually thinnest and most heavily infiltrated by macrophage foam cells.
4. Vulnerability to plaque rupture depends on composition rather than size or volume. Although hard collagenous tissue usually constitutes the largest component, soft lipid-rich core and cap weakening (perhaps related to macrophages) predispose to plaque rupture and determine vulnerability.
5. The plaque components responsible for vulnerability (soft lipid and probably macrophages) appear to be more mobile, with greater potential to regress, than more voluminous collagenous components. Aggressive risk factor modification may stabilize plaques, leaving them less vulnerable though not necessarily less voluminous.
6. Aggressive risk factor modification may further stabilize plaques in the absence of atherosclerotic regression by normalizing endothelial function; endothelium can profoundly affect vascular tone by releasing contracting factors, such as endothelin-1, and relaxing factors, such as prostacyclin and endothelium-derived relaxing factor (EDRF, now known to be nitric oxide).

Possibilities other than plaque stabilization that are likely to contribute to reduced clinical cardiac events with aggressive risk factor modification include a favorable effect on thrombogenic propensity and on factors that trigger plaque rupture (e.g., reduced blood pressure and/or heart rate).

COST-EFFECTIVENESS

Health care costs in the United States exceed $1 trillion annually and consume 14% of gross domestic product. In 1994, approximately 850,000 coronary revascularizations, together with charges for hospitalization, medical personnel, health care facilities, and medications resulting from treatment of CAD, are estimated to have cost more than $50 billion. Strategies targeted at secondary prevention of CAD can be expected to reduce the economic toll. The public health approach to CAD prevention, targeting the entire population to modify risk factors, is the least expensive method of accomplishing this. To identify individuals with CAD and aggressively manage risk factors complements public health strategies but is more expensive. While the benefits of the clinical approach in reduced cardiac events is well documented, economic considerations dictate that such benefits be weighed against the costs to produce them.

Cost-effectiveness analysis is a method of considering the effectiveness and the cost of an intervention. In cost-effectiveness analysis, costs are expressed in monetary terms, whereas effectiveness is expressed as a health benefit (typically, years of life saved or quality-adjusted years of life saved). Cost-effectiveness analysis constitutes a useful method of expressing potential benefit from a particular investment. It has been proposed that if the cost per year of life saved (or quality-adjusted year of life saved) is less than $20,000, the intervention should be considered very cost-effective, whereas if it is greater than $75,000, the intervention should be considered very expensive (42).

Published cost-effectiveness analyses are available for a variety of strategies for modifying CAD risk factors, including smoking cessation, lipid management, blood pressure control, and cardiac rehabilitation exercise training (Table 30.5). Generally, these data support the cost-effectiveness of risk factor modification in CAD patients. The cost-effectiveness of aggressive modification of multiple risk factors (as compared to single risk factors) in patients with CAD has not been examined as rigorously or extensively as the clinical benefits. However, in view of the reduction (22–89%) in clinical cardiac events that can be expected with such approaches, there is little doubt that they are both clinically effective and cost-effective.

BARRIERS TO IMPLEMENTATION

There is overwhelming evidence as to the clinical benefits of aggressive risk factor modification in patients with established CAD. In fact, there are more published trials showing decreased cardiac events by aggressive risk factor modification than reports on decreased cardiac events by elective percutaneous transluminal coronary angioplasty or coronary artery bypass surgery in patients with stable CAD (18). Despite this, it is clear that long-term management of CAD patients is fragmented (and usually unsatisfactory) and that the proportion of patients receiving appropriate care is alarmingly low (Table 30.6) (42–45). The failure of the status of medical management of CAD to reflect recent advances in knowledge of risk factors and effective modification undoubtedly results in avoidable death, disability, and financial expenditure.

A variety of barriers to successful implementation of effective services for the secondary prevention of CAD have been identified (Table 30.7) (46). These include barriers at the level of the patient, physician, health care setting, community, and society. Strategies to overcome these barriers include the following:

1. Development of clinical practice guidelines for cardiovascular risk reduction
2. Implementation of model programs for cardiovascular risk reduction proven to be effective
3. Inclusion of risk factor management as a key indicator of quality of care in quality assurance programs
4. Adequate insurance reimbursement for effective risk reduction strategies
5. Requirement of expertise in risk factor management in training and accreditation programs

Table 30.5. Coronary Artery Disease Cost-Effectiveness Overview

INTERVENTION	CONDITION	PATIENTS	$/YLS OR $/QALY
Lovastatin (20 mg/dL)	Hyperlipidemia	CAD, chol ≤250 mg/dL, men 45–54 yr	Saves $ and lives
Enalapril	HF	Ejection fraction ≥0.35	Saves $ and lives
Nurse counseling manual	Smoking	Post myocardial infarction	250
Beta-blocker	Post myocardial infarction	High risk	3,600
Lovastatin (20 mg/dL)	Hyperlipidemia	CAD, chol ≤250 mg/dL, women 45–54 yr	4,700
PTCA	Chronic CAD	Severe angina, 1 vessel disease	8,700–10,200*
CABG	Chronic CAD	Severe angina, left main disease	9,200*
Cardiac rehabilitation	Post myocardial infarction	Depressed patients	9,200*
CABG	Chronic CAD	Mild angina, 3-vessel disease	18,200*
Beta-blocker	Post-myocardial infarction	Low risk	20,200
CABG	Chronic CAD	Severe angina, 2 vessel disease	42,500*
CABG	Chronic CAD	Severe angina, 1 vessel disease	72,900*
PTCA	Chronic CAD	Mild angina, 1 vessel disease	91,500*

* Dollars per quality-adjusted life years ($/QALY).
Other values in dollars per year of life saved ($/YLS).
CAD, coronary artery disease; chol, cholesterol; HF, heart failure; PTCA, percutaneous transluminal coronary angioplasty; CABG, coronary artery bypass grafting.
Values are in 1993 dollars.
Adapted with permission from Fuster V, Gotto AM, Libby P, et al. Task Force I. Pathogenesis of coronary disease: the biological role of risk factors. J Am Coll Cardiol 27:964–976, 1996.

Table 30.6. Estimates of Levels of Risk Factor Management in Patients Surviving Myocardial Infarction

Referral to cardiac rehabilitation program[a]	<5%
Smoking cessation counseling[b]	20
Lipid-lowering drug therapy[c]	25
Beta-blocker therapy[b]	40
ACE inhibitor therapy (reduced LV ejection fraction)[b]	60
Aspirin[b]	70

[a] Coronary Artery Surgery Study (CASS): a randomized trial of coronary artery bypass surgery. Quality of life in patients randomly assigned to treatment groups. Circulation 1983;68:951–960.
[b] Vogel RA. Risk factor intervention and coronary artery disease: clinical strategies. Coronary Artery Dis 1995;6:466–471.
[c] Pearson TA. Personal communication, September 1995.
ACE, angiotensin-converting enzyme; LV, left ventricular.
Reprinted with permission from Goldman L, Garber AM, Grover SA, et al. Task Force 6. Cost-effectiveness of assessment and management of risk factors. J Am Coll Cardiol 27:1020–1030, 1996.

It is clear that an appropriate level of care cannot be provided by health care personnel who do not understand the pathogenesis of atherosclerosis and the multiple factors that constitute safe and effective implementation of cardiovascular risk reduction (47). An American College of Cardiology task force has recently recommended use of **optimal medical management** rather than "secondary prevention" when referring to cardiovas-

Table 30.7. Barriers to Implementation of Preventive Services

Patient
  Lack of knowledge and motivation
  Lack of access to care
  Cultural factors
  Social factors
Physician
  Problem-based focus
  Feedback on prevention negative or neutral
  Time constraints
  Lack of incentives, including reimbursement
  Lack of training
  Poor knowledge of benefits
  Perceived ineffectiveness
  Lack of skills
  Lack of communication between specialist and generalist
  Lack of perceived legitimacy
Health care settings (e.g., hospitals, practices)
  Acute-care policy
  Lack of resources and facilities
  Lack of systems for preventive services
  Time and economic constraints
  Poor communication between specialty and primary care providers
  Lack of policies and standards
Community, society
  Lack of policies and standards
  Lack of reimbursement

Reprinted with permission from Goldman L, Garber AM, Grover SA, et al. Task Force 6. Cost-effectiveness of assessment and management of risk factors. J Am Coll Cardiol 27:1060–1070, 1996.

cular risk reduction in patients with established disease (46). Reasons for this:

1. In addition to lifestyle modification, comprehensive cardiovascular risk reduction includes appropriate use of cardioactive, vasoactive, lipid-lowering, and other drugs.
2. The qualifier "secondary" implies relative unimportance to patient and provider.
3. "Preventive" care services may not be compensated in insurance and managed care programs.

GUIDELINES FOR CLINICAL PRACTICE

Compelling scientific and clinical evidence supports aggressive management of risk factors as an integral part of optimal care of patients with established CAD (48, 49). The rationale for aggressive risk factor modification extends to patients with other types of documented atherosclerotic vascular disease, including transient ischemic attack, stroke, and aortic or peripheral vascular disease (46). A guide to comprehensive risk reduction has been developed by the American Heart Association and endorsed by the American College of Cardiology (48, 49).

Recent expert guidelines for comprehensive cardiovascular risk reduction emphasize individualization of risk factor management to the patient, the requirement for lifelong management of risk, and use of a team approach to ensure provision of optimal care (50–52). Physicians, nurses, exercise physiologists, dietitians, behavioral scientists, and other health professionals should collaborate in a structured fashion to manage risk reduction via follow-up techniques, including office or clinic visits, attendance of cardiac rehabilitation sessions, and mail and/or telephone contact.

Although the precise approach varies with a variety of factors, such as health care setting, patient population, and available resources, it is important to implement model programs for risk factor management that have been shown to be effective. Such approaches include the following fundamental components:

1. Initial evaluation and risk assessment.
2. Identification of specific goals for each CAD risk factor through risk stratification (53).
3. Formulation and implementation of an individualized treatment plan that includes lifestyle and pharmacological interventions for reaching specific goals.
4. Effective long-term follow-up to enhance compliance and revise the treatment plan as indicated.
5. Mechanism for outcomes-based long-term assessment of each patient.

The American Heart Association has urged that every effort be made throughout the spectrum of medical care to promote effective strategies for comprehensive cardiovascular risk reduction in all eligible patients (2).

ROLE OF CARDIAC REHABILITATION

Comprehensive cardiac rehabilitation combines prescriptive exercise training with risk factor modification (51). The goals of cardiac rehabilitation are to improve functional capacity, alleviate or lessen activity-related symptoms, reduce disability, and identify and modify CAD risk factors in an effort to reduce cardiovascular morbidity and mortality. A recent extensive review of existing scientific literature by the Agency for Health Care Policy and Research has substantiated the efficacy of traditional cardiac rehabilitation in reaching many of these goals (52). Moreover, it has been estimated that participation in cardiac rehabilitation by as few as 25–30% of eligible patients would translate into a savings of $31.4 million to $62.8 million in direct medical and nonmedical costs after 21 months (52).

Cardiac rehabilitation programs and health professionals are ideally positioned to assume a pivotal role in rendering comprehensive cardiovascular risk reduction. Primary target areas are lifestyle intervention, patient education, compliance, patient tracking and ongoing follow-up, and outcomes assessment. However, the extent to which traditional cardiac rehabilitation programs can successfully deliver key components of comprehensive cardiovascular risk reduction is limited by several fundamental deficiencies, including the following:

1. It is estimated that 11–38% of eligible patients participate in cardiac rehabilitation.
2. Most cardiac rehabilitation programs are 12 weeks in duration, with little structured follow-up; a lifelong approach is required if optimal results are to be achieved.
3. Cardiac rehabilitation services are generally not closely integrated with other aspects of medical care.

► SUMMARY

Increasing evidence supports aggressive risk factor modification in the medical treatment of CAD. Endothelial stabilization and decreased progression or even regression of atherosclerotic plaque lead to decreased mortality and morbidity in populations with and without CAD. This treatment is cost-effective and safe, and although barriers to this type of treatment exist, current programs and trained health care professionals are able to provide this type of care.

References

1. American Heart Association. Heart and Stroke Facts: 2000 Statistical Supplement. Dallas: American Heart Association, 2000.
2. Smith SC. Bridging the treatment gap. Am J Cardiol 85:3E–7E, 2000.
3. Superko HOUR, Krauss RM. Coronary artery disease regression: Convincing evidence for the benefit of aggressive lipoprotein management. Circulation 90:1056–1069, 1994.
4. Brensike JF, Levy RI, Kelsey SF, et al. Effects of therapy with cholestyramine on progression of coronary arteriosclerosis: Results of the NHLBI Type II Coronary Intervention Study. Circulation 69:313–324, 1984.
5. Blankenhorn DH, Nessim SA, Johnson RL, et al. Beneficial effects of combined colestipol-niacin therapy on coronary atherosclerosis and coronary venous bypass grafts. JAMA 257:3233–3240, 1987.
6. Cashin-Hemphill L, Mack WG, Pagoda JM, et al. Beneficial effects of colestipol-niacin on coronary atherosclerosis: A 4-year follow-up. JAMA 264:3013–3017, 1990.
7. Ornish D, Brown SE, Scherwitz LW, et al. Can lifestyle changes reverse coronary heart disease? The Lifestyle Heart Trial. Lancet 336:129–133, 1990.
8. Ornish D, Scherwitz LW, Billings, JH, et al. Intensive lifestyle changes for reversal of coronary heart disease. JAMA 280:2001–2007, 1998.
9. Niebauer J, Hambrecht R, Velich T, et al. Attenuated progression of coronary artery disease after 6 years of multifactorial risk intervention. Circulation 96:2534–2541, 1997.
10. Hambrecht R, Niebauer J, Marburger C, et al. Various intensities of exercise of leisure time physical activity in patients with coronary artery disease: Effects on cardiorespiratory fitness and progression of coronary artery disease. J Am Coll Cardiol 22:468–477, 1993.
11. Schuler G, Hambrecht R, Schlierf G, et al. Regular physical exercise and low-fat diet: Effects on progression of coronary artery disease. Circulation 86:1–11, 1992.
12. Gould KL, Ornish D, Scherwitz L, et al. Changes in myocardial perfusion abnormalities by positron emission tomography after long-term, intense risk factor modification. JAMA 274:894–901, 1995.
13. Celermajer DS, Sorensen KE, Bull C, et al. Endothelium-dependent dilation in the systemic arteries of asymptomatic subjects relates to coronary risk factors and their interaction. J Am Coll Cardiol 24:1468–1474, 1994
14. Treasure CB, Klein JL, Weintraub WS, et al. Beneficial effects of cholesterol-lowering therapy on the coronary endothelium in patients with coronary artery disease. N Engl J Med 332:481–487, 1995.
15. Andeson TJ, Meredith IT, Yeung AC, et al. The effect of cholesterol-lowering and antioxidant therapy on endothelium-dependent coronary vasomotion. N Engl J Med 332:488–493, 1995.
16. Kaufmann PA, Gnecchi-Ruscone T, Schafers KP, et al. Low density lipoprotein cholesterol and coronary microvascular dysfunction in hypercholesterolemia. J Am Coll Cardiol 36:103–109, 2000.
17. Benzuly KH, Padget RC, Kaul S, et al. Functional improvement precedes structural regression of atherosclerosis. Circulation 89:1810–1818, 1994.
18. Gould KL. Reversal of coronary atherosclerosis: Clinical promise as the basis for noninvasive management of coronary artery disease. Circulation 90:1558–1571, 1994.

19. Gould KL, Martucci JP, Goldberg DL, et al. Short-term cholesterol lowering decreases size and severity of perfusion abnormalities by positron emission tomography after dipyridamole in patients with coronary artery disease: A potential noninvasive marker of healing coronary endothelium. Circulation 89:1530–1538, 1994.

20. Cohen JD, Drury JH, Ostdiek J, et al. Benefits of lipid lowering on vascular reactivity in patients with coronary artery disease and average cholesterol levels: A mechanism for reducing clinical events? Am Heart J 139:734–738, 2000.

21. Yokoyama I, Momonura S, Ohtake T, et al. Improvement of impaired myocardial vasodilatation due to diffuse coronary atherosclerosis in hypercholesterolemics after lipid-lowering therapy. Circulation 100:117–122, 1999.

22. Dupuis J, Tardif JC, Cernacek P, et al. Cholesterol reduction rapidly improves endothelial function after acute coronary syndromes. Circulation 99:3227–3233, 1999.

23. Vita JA, Yeung AC, Winniford M, et al. Effect of cholesterol-lowering therapy on coronary endothelial vasomotor function in patients with coronary artery disease. Circulation 102:846–851, 2000.

24. Hornig B, Maier V, Drexter H. Physical training improves endothelial function in patients with chronic heart failure. Circulation 93:210–214, 1996.

25. Taddei S, Galetta F, Virdis A, et al. Physical activity prevents age-related impairment of nitric oxide availability in elderly athletes. Circulation 101:2896–2901, 2000.

26. Hambrecht R, Wolf A, Gielen S, et al. Effect of exercise on coronary endothelial function in patients with coronary artery disease. N Engl J Med 342:454–460, 2000.

27. Hambrecht R, Hilbrich L, Erbs S, et al. Correction of endothelial dysfunction in chronic heart failure: Additional effects of exercise training and oral L-arginine supplementation. J Am Coll Cardiol 35:706–713, 2000.

28. Haskell WL, Alderman EL, Fair JM, et al. Effects of intensive multiple risk factor reduction on coronary atherosclerosis and clinical cardiac events in men and women with coronary artery disease: The Stanford Coronary Risk Intervention Project (SCRIP). Circulation 89:975–990, 1994.

29. Scandinavian Simvastatin Survival Group. Randomized trial of cholesterol lowering in 4,444 patients with coronary heart disease: The Scandinavian Simvastatin Survival Study (4S). Lancet 344:1383–1389, 1994.

30. Pedersen TR, Wilhelmsen L, Faergeman O, et al. Follow-up study of patients randomized in the Scandinavian Simvastatin Survival Study (4S) of cholesterol lowering. Am J Cardiol 86:257–262, 2000.

31. Campeau L, Hunninghake DB, Knatterud GL, et al. Aggressive cholesterol lowering delays saphenous vein graft atherosclerosis in women, the elderly, and patients with associated risk factors: NHLBI Post Coronary Artery Bypass Graft Clinical Trial. Circulation 99:3241–3247, 1999.

32. Post Coronary Artery Bypass Graft Trial Investigators. The effect of aggressive lowering of low-density lipoprotein cholesterol levels and low-dose anticoagulation on obstructive changes in saphenous vein coronary artery bypass grafts. N Engl J Med 336:153–162, 1997.

33. Flaker GC, Warnica JW, Sacks FM. Pravastatin prevents clinical events in revascularized patients with average cholesterol concentrations. J Am Coll Cardiol 34:106–112, 1999.

34. Shepard J, Cobbe SM, Ford I, et al. Prevention of coronary heart disease with pravastatin in men with hypercholesterolemia. N Engl J Med 333:1301–1307, 1995.

35. West of Scotland Coronary Prevention Study Group. Baseline risk factors and their association with outcome in the West of Scotland Coronary Prevention Study. Am J Cardiol 79:756–762, 1997.

36. Byington RP, Jukema JW, Salonen JT. Reduction in cardiovascular events during pravastatin therapy: Pooled analysis of clinical events of the pravastatin atherosclerosis program. Circulation 92:2419–2425, 1995.

37. Sacks FM, Pfeffer MA, Moye LA, et al. The effect of pravastatin on coronary events after myocardial infarction in patients with average cholesterol levels. N Engl J Med 335:1001–1009, 1996.

38. Long-term Intervention With Pravastatin in Ischaemic Disease (LIPID) Study Group. Prevention of cardiovascular events and death with pravastatin in patients with coronary heart disease and a broad range of initial cholesterol levels. N Engl J Med 339:1349–1357, 1998.

39. Herd JA, Ballantyne CM, Farmer JA, et al. Effects of fluvastatin on coronary atherosclerosis in patients with mild to moderate cholesterol elevations: Lipoprotein and Coronary Atherosclerosis Study. Am J Cardiol 80:278–286, 1997.

40. Fuster V, Gotto AM, Libby P, et al. Task Force 1. Pathogenesis of coronary disease: The biological role of risk factors. J Am Coll Cardiol 27:964–976, 1996.

41. Falk E. Why do plaques rupture? Circulation 86(Suppl III):111-30–111-42, 1992.

42. Goldman L, Garber AM, Grover SA, et al. Task Force 6. Cost-effectiveness of assessment and management of risk factors. J Am Coll Cardiol 27:1020–1030, 1996.

43. Swan HJC, Brown J, Davidson MH, et al. ACC policy statement: Preventive cardiology and atherosclerotic disease. J Am Coll Cardiol 24:838, 1994.

44. Sueta CA, Chowdbury M, Bocuzzi SJ. Analysis of the degree of undertreatment of hyperlipidemia and congestive heart failure secondary to coronary artery disease. Am J Cardiol 83:1303–1307, 1999.

45. Bittner V, Olson M, Kelsey SF, et al. Effect of coronary angiography on use of lipid-lowering agents in women: A report from the Women's Ischemia Syndrome Evaluation (WISE) Study. Am J Cardiol 85:1083–1088, 2000.

46. Pearson TA, McBride PE, Houston-Miller N, et al. Task Force 8. Organization of preventive cardiology service. J Am Coll Cardiol 27:1039–1047, 1996.

47. Swan HJ, Gerch BJ, Graboys TB, et al. Task Force 7. Evaluation and management of risk factors for the individual patient (case management). J Am Coll Cardiol 27:1030–1039, 1996.

48. Smith SC, Blair SN, Criqui MH, et al. AHA consensus panel statement: Preventing heart attack and death in patients with coronary disease. Circulation 92:2–4, 1995.

49. Pearson TA, Fuster V. 27th Bethesda Conference. J Am Coll Cardiol 27:961–963, 1996 (executive summary).

50. Pearson T, Rapaport E, Cricqui M, et al. Optimal risk factor management in the patient after coronary revascularization. Circulation 90:3125–3133, 1994.

51. Balady GJ, Fletcher BJ, Froelicher ES, et al. AHA position statement: Cardiac rehabilitation programs: A statement for health care professionals from the American Heart Association. Circulation 90:1602–1610, 1994.

52. Wenger NK, Froelicher ES, Smith LK, et al. Cardiac rehabilitation. Clinical Practice Guidelines 17. Rockville, MD: U.S. Department of Health and Human Services, Public Health Service, Agency for Health Care Policy and Research and the National Heart, Lung and Blood Institute. AHCPR Publication 96–0672, October 1995.

53. Roitman JL, LaFontaine TP, Drimmer A. A new model for risk stratification and delivery of cardiovascular rehabilitation services in the long-term clinical management of patients with coronary artery disease. J Cardiopulmonary Rehab 18:113–123, 1998.

SECTION SIX
OTHER CHRONIC DISEASES

SECTION EDITOR: *Thomas P. LaFontaine, PhD, FACSM*

1.4.0, 1.4.0.1

2.4.6, 2.8.0, 2.8.0.9, 2.8.0.10

3.4.2, 3.4.3

4.4.0, 4.4.1, 4.4.14, 4.4.15, 4.8.0, 4.8.1, 4.8.1.9, 4.8.3.1–4.8.3.6, 4.8.6.1, 4.8.7, 4.8.8, 4.8.9

5.4.2, 5.8.0

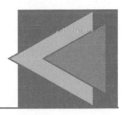

CHAPTER **31**

EXERCISE AND DIABETES MELLITUS

Barbara N. Campaigne

Exercise is an accepted adjunctive therapy in management of diabetes. One of the earliest indications of the effectiveness of exercise was the decreased sweetness of urine recorded in 600 B.C. by the Indian physician Shushruta. After the discovery of insulin in the early 1920s, the three cornerstones of diabetes care became insulin, diet, and exercise. Exercise appears to be beneficial in controlling blood glucose in non–insulin-dependent diabetes mellitus (NIDDM, or type II) and gestational diabetes mellitus (1, 2). Exercise can be made safe for individuals with insulin-dependent diabetes mellitus (IDDM, or type I) and may reduce the risk of cardiovascular disease (3–5).

This chapter describes exercise recommendations for managing patients with diabetes. Although background information is given individually for types I and II diabetes mellitus, issues relevant to both are discussed in greater detail. Both have distinct hereditary and environmental components, and they are separate diseases. Both cultural and geographical factors have roles in the cause of each disease. In type I diabetes, the primary abnormality is insulin deficiency, with insulin resistance as a secondary factor. In type II diabetes, a series of events caused by insulin resistance leads to stages of disease, including further insulin resistance and insulin and glucose abnormalities. Many complications are common to both type I and II diabetes. Chronic neurological and cardiovascular complications are brought about by long-term elevated levels of blood glucose and insulin. Short-term hypoglycemic and hyperglycemic responses result in acute complications. The complications of diabetes and use of exercise in a plan to manage blood glucose optimally are described. The major characteristics of type I and II diabetes are presented in Table 31.1.

TYPE I DIABETES MELLITUS

It is not well documented that exercise improves glycemic control in type I diabetes, perhaps because increased caloric consumption and/or decreased insulin treatment is used to prevent exercise-associated hypo-

glycemia. People with type I diabetes are prone to hypoglycemia; therefore, they tend to eat more to decrease the risk of hypoglycemia with exercise. The effects of eating more and the associated elevations in blood glucose negate the potential improvements in glycosylated hemoglobin (HbA1c) with exercise in type I patients. Regular exercise **does**, however, result in improvements in insulin sensitivity, glucose metabolism, and cardiovascular disease (CVD) risk factors. Exercise recommendations should be designed to assist individuals to exercise safely and to decrease their risk of CVD. Depending on duration and intensity, exercise is characterized by endocrine and neural responses. The balance of insulin, glucagon, and catecholamines (epinephrine and norepinephrine) largely controls the availability and use of metabolic fuel. Other factors that may significantly influence fuel metabolism during exercise in type I diabetes include the central nervous system, glycemic state, and general metabolic profile (6–8). Accordingly, this chapter focuses on diverse aspects of the physiological environment of diabetes that influence response to exercise and conversely, how acute exercise may affect the physiological environment. Table 31.2 gives the benefits of exercise for individuals with type I diabetes. Table 31.3 presents general recommendations for regular exercise in relatively healthy individuals with type I diabetes.

Blood Glucose Regulation

Because acute exercise results in increased glucose use, increased glucose production is necessary to maintain normal blood glucose levels. In the diabetic state, increased glucose production is sometimes compromised by presence of insulin and/or inability to increase glucose because of abnormal hormonal responses. Therefore, it is important to understand the effects of insulin on blood glucose when planning insulin use in conjunction with exercise. Figure 31.1 illustrates the powerful effects of circulating insulin on blood glucose in diabetes. If treatment with intravenous insulin infusion (insulin pump) brings about normal portal insulin levels, production of glucose

Table 31.1. Major Characteristics of Type I and Type II Diabetes

FACTOR	TYPE I	TYPE II
Age at onset	Usually early but may occur at any age	Usually over age 30 but may occur at any age
Type of onset	Usually abrupt	Insidious
Genetic susceptibility	HLA-related DR3, DR4, others	Frequent genetic background, not HLA-related
Environmental factors	Virus, toxins, autoimmune stimulation	Obesity, nutrition
Islet cell antibody	Present at onset	Not observed
Endogenous insulin	Minimal or absent	Stimulated response either adequate but delayed secretion or reduced but not absent; insulin resistance present
Nutritional status	Thin, catabolic state	Obese or normal
Symptoms	Thirst, polyuria, polyphagia, fatigue	Mild or frequently none
Ketosis	Prone; at onset or during insulin deficiency	Resistant except during infection or stress
Control of diabetes	Often difficult, with wide glucose fluctuation	Variable; helped by dietary adherence, weight loss, exercise
Dietary management	Essential	Essential; may suffice for glycemic control
Insulin	Required for all	Required for 20–30%
Oral hypoglycemics	Not effective	Effective
Vascular, neurological complications	Seen in most after 5 or more years of diabetes	Frequent

Adapted with permission from Shulman CR. Diabetes mellitus: definition, classification, and diagnosis. In: Galloway JA, Potvin JH, Shulman CR, eds. Diabetes Mellitus. 9th ed. Indianapolis: Lilly Research Laboratories, 1988.

Table 31.2. Benefits of Exercise for Type I Diabetes

Improved insulin sensitivity
Improved blood lipids and lipoproteins
Increased caloric expenditure resulting in reduction or maintenance of body weight, reduction in body fat, and preservation of lean body mass
Improved physical fitness
Improved flexibility and strength
Decreased blood pressure in hypertensives
Decreased risk of cardiovascular disease
Improved psychological well-being, including enhanced quality of life, improved self-esteem

Status of plasma insulin	Hepatic glucose production	Muscle glucose utilization	Blood glucose
Normal or slightly diminished	↑	↑	→
Markedly diminished	↑	↑	↑
Increased	↑	↑	↓

Figure 31.1. The influence of plasma insulin on blood glucose levels of individuals with IDDM. (Reprinted with permission from Campaigne BN, Lampman RL. *Exercise in the Clinical Management of Diabetes Mellitus.* Champaign, IL: Human Kinetics, 1994.)

Table 31.3. General Exercise Recommendations for Relatively Healthy Type I Diabetes

COMPONENT	RECOMMENDATION[a]
Type	[b]Aerobic: walking, jogging, cycling, stair climbing, cross-country skiing, etc. Strength (moderate-level resistance training): circuit programs using light weights with 10–15 repetitions
Intensity	60–90% maximum heart rate or 50–85%; $\dot{V}O_{2max}$
Duration	20–60 min plus 5–10-min warmup and cool-down periods
Frequency	Daily to ensure optimal blood glucose control
Timing	The timing of exercise is particularly important for those with IDDM. Both insulin therapy and blood glucose level at the time of exercise must be considered. Avoid exercise at time of peak insulin action.

[a] A bracelet or shoe tag identifying the individual as having diabetes and other relevant medical information should be worn at all times.
[b] Performed in ways that do not traumatize the feet.

equals that of glucose use and normal circulating glucose status can be maintained. In the case of insulin deficiency, glucose use may not take place with exercise. That circumstance, in combination with exercise-induced increase in liver glucose production, may bring about hyperglycemia. In the third scenario, if insulin absorption is enhanced with pre-exercise insulin (overinsulinization), as shown in Figure 31.1, glucose production may be inhibited. In conjunction with increased glucose use, too much insulin may lead to hypoglycemia.

Table 31.4 shows recommendations for adapting insulin in type I diabetes patients who exercise. In addition, other recommendations include avoiding intramuscular injection, perpendicular injection into a skinfold, and use of needles less than 8 mm in length.

Table 31.4. General Guidelines for Avoiding Hypoglycemia During and After Exercise

Blood glucose monitoring
1. Monitor blood glucose immediately before, during (if possible every 30 min) and 15 min after exercise.
2. Delay exercise if blood glucose is > 250 mg/dL and ketones are present in the urine or if > 300 mg/dL.[a]
3. Consume carbohydrates if blood glucose ≤ 100 mg/dL.
4. Learn individual glucose response to different types of exercise.
5. Avoid exercising late at night.

Insulin
1. Decrease insulin dose
   a. Intermediate-acting insulin: decrease by 30–35% on the day of exercise.
   b. Intermediate and short-acting insulin: omit dose of short-acting insulin that precedes exercise.
   c. Multiple doses of short-acting insulin: reduce dose prior to exercise by 30–35% and supplement carbohydrates.
   d. Continuous subcutaneous infusion: eliminate mealtime bolus or increment that precedes or immediately follows exercise.
2. Avoid exercising muscle underlying injections of short-acting insulin for 1 hr after injection.
3. Do not exercise at the time of peak insulin action (Table 31.5).

[a] ACSM guidelines state that 200–400 mg/dL requires medical supervision and that > 400 mg/dL contraindicates exercise. This guideline is taken from a recent ACSM position statement (Diabetes Mellitus and Exercise).
Adapted with permission from Vitug A, Schneider SH, Ruderman NB. Exercise and type I diabetes mellitus. Exerc Sport Sci Rev 16:285–304, 1988.

Table 31.5. Activity Characteristics of Insulin

	ONSET (HR)	PEAK (HR)	DURATION (HR)
Rapid acting			
Regular	0.5–1	2–4	6–8
Intermediate acting			
Lente or NPH	1–3	6–12	18–26
Long acting			
Ultralente or human	4–8	12–18	24–28

Onset, peak, and duration of action vary considerably and may depend on the individual patient, injection site, vascularity, and temperature.

Table 31.6. Benefits of Exercise for Type II Diabetes

Reduced blood glucose and glycosylated hemoglobin levels
Improved glucose tolerance
Improved insulin response to oral glucose stimulus
Improved peripheral and hepatic insulin sensitivity
Improved blood lipid and lipoprotein levels
Decreased blood pressure in hypertensives
Decreased risk of cardiovascular disease
Improved physical fitness
Increased caloric expenditure resulting in reduction or maintenance of body weight, reductions in body fat, and preservation of lean body mass
Improved psychological well-being, including enhanced quality of life and increased self-esteem
Improved flexibility and strength

Timing and Mode of Insulin Treatment

To optimize blood glucose control, most individuals with type I diabetes use subcutaneous injections consisting of a mixed-insulin split-dose regimen. This includes administration of a mixture of short-acting insulin and longer-acting (sustained release) insulin in morning and afternoon doses. Carbohydrate and caloric intake should be matched to insulin therapy. Optimal exercise times vary; general recommendations include avoiding exercise at peak time of insulin action or altering insulin dose to prevent peak effect at the time of exercise. It is recommended to exercise when insulin effects are low and blood glucose is rising. To prevent hypoglycemia when exercise is unplanned, a rapidly assimilated carbohydrate snack can be consumed prior to exercise. Exercising before insulin administration and breakfast may decrease need for short-acting insulin. Once an exercise routine is established, insulin dose and caloric intake can be adjusted. Table 31.5 gives a summary of action of various insulin preparations.

TYPE II DIABETES MELLITUS

The treatment of type II diabetes usually includes weight loss and oral hypoglycemic agents to help restore peripheral insulin receptor sensitivity and stimulate pancreatic insulin release. The benefits of regular exercise for individuals with type II diabetes have been clearly documented (1, 3, 5, 9, 10) (Table 31.6). Regular physical activity for individuals with type II diabetes is a recommendation of the American Diabetes Association (ADA) (4). Regular exercise improves daily blood glucose control and therefore causes a decrease in glycosylated hemoglobin. Exercise training improves insulin sensitivity and may be responsible for increased insulin receptor affinity (11). Reductions in blood pressure in individuals with hypertension and improvements in blood lipid profile resulting from regular exercise lower CVD risk. Lipid and lipoprotein changes include decreased triglycerides and very low density lipoprotein, and increased high-density lipoprotein (HDL). Decreases in systolic and diastolic blood pressure have been reported in mild to moderate hypertension and may be associated with effects of lowered insulin levels on renal sodium retention (1). An important effect of regular exercise for type II diabetes is weight loss in conjunction with dietary intervention and preservation of lean tissue (12).

Comparisons of rural and urban cultures provide evidence of lower prevalence of type II diabetes among active rural populations (13). Recent studies show that regular physical activity, even nonvigorous activity, is associated with a lowered risk of insulin resistance and type II diabetes (9, 10, 14, 15). Some data available from cross-sectional studies show that glucose intolerance and diabetes occur more often in sedentary than active individuals (16). These findings are independent of body mass and age. Physical activity has been recommended as an important approach to preventing type II diabetes in men and women (9, 17–19). In a prospective cohort of 70,102 women aged 40–65 years, Hu et al. (9) reported that women who exercised even moderately on a regular basis

had significantly lower risk of developing type II diabetes than women who did not exercise regularly. Statistical adjustment for age, body mass index, and other variables did not change the effects of exercise on diabetes risk. Thus, accumulating evidence indicates that physical activity does have a role in preventing type II diabetes. Table 31.7 presents recommendations for exercise in relatively healthy individuals with type II diabetes.

Diabetes Medication Other Than Insulin

Available evidence shows no effect of hypoglycemic agents on electrocardiograms, blood pressure, or heart rate. Because of other underlying medical conditions, individuals with diabetes may be treated with a variety of medications. If one is to prescribe safe and effective exercise, it is important to be aware of all medications and their effects on blood glucose. Table 31.8 shows the possible glucose-altering effects of various medications.

GESTATIONAL DIABETES

Three significant factors influence development of gestational diabetes mellitus (GDM): a genetic predisposition, a decrease in insulin action, and impaired beta-cell function (1). During pregnancy development of insulin

---

Table 31.7. General Exercise Recommendations for Relatively Healthy Persons With Type II Diabetes

COMPONENT	RECOMMENDATION
Type	Aerobic: walking, jogging, cycling, stair climbing, cross-country skiing, etc. Strength (moderate-level resistance training): circuit programs using light weights with 10–15 repetitions
Intensity	60–90% maximum heart rate or 50–85%; $\dot{V}O_{2max}$
Duration	20–60 min plus 5–10-min warmup and cool-down period
Frequency	3–5 times weekly, daily if taking insulin therapy

Modified with permission from Campaigne BN, Lampman RL. Exercise in the Clinical Management of Diabetes Mellitus. Champaign IL: Human Kinetics, 1994.

Table 31.8. Possible Glucose-Altering Effects of Common Medications

	MECHANISM OF ACTION		
	INSULIN SECRETION	GLUCOSE DISPOSAL	COMMENTS
Potentially increases blood glucose			
Diuretics (thiazides, chlorthalidone, furosemide, metolazone)	↓	↓	K^+ depletion, other effects
Beta-adrenergic antagonists (propranolol, nadolol, timolol)	0, ↓	0, ↓	More likely with noncardioselective agents
Ca^{2+} channel blockers (dihydropyridine derivatives)	0	0, ↓	Effect rarely significant
Glucocorticoids	↑	↓	Cause marked insulin resistance
Anabolic steroids	0	↓	Cause major lipid-altering effects
Growth hormone	↓	↓	A major insulin antagonist
Niacin	↑	↓	Particularly with high dosage
Cyclosporine	↑	↓	Often used with glucocorticoids
Potentially decreases blood glucose			
Alpha-adrenergic antagonists (prazosin, doxazosin, terazosin)	0, ↑	0, ↑	Rarely significant
ACE inhibitors	0	0, ↑	
Beta-adrenergic antagonists (propranolol, nadolol, timolol)			May prevent proper recovery from hypoglycemia
Salicylates	0, ↑	0	With high dosage
Alcohol	0, ↑	↑	May cause hyperglycemia with long-term use
Pentamidine	↑	0	May cause hyperglycemia with long-term use
Quinine	↑	0, ↑	May cause severe hypoglycemia

Modified with permission from Ganda OP. Patients on various drug therapies. In: Ruderman N, Devlin JT, eds. The Health Professional's Guide to Diabetes and Exercise. Alexandria, VA: American Diabetes Association, 1995:236.

resistance depends on several factors, including the following:

- The hormonal environment
- Genetic predisposition
- Age
- Excessive body weight
- Physical activity level

For those with GDM, glucose tolerance worsens during gestation. The effects of exercise on insulin secretion, insulin sensitivity, and glucose metabolism make it reasonable that regular exercise may prevent or treat GDM, although few data are available (20). Research indicates that exercise training improves glucose tolerance in women with GDM (21). Hyperglycemia, occurring with gestational diabetes, can be prevented by arm ergometry (22). In contrast, diet management alone produces no significant improvement in glucose control (21). These findings suggest that insulin administration may be avoided in some women with GDM by the safe application of regular exercise. Further research is needed in this area.

COMPLICATIONS OF DIABETES

Overview

Exercise is routinely recommended for patients with diabetes, but when secondary complications of diabetes occur, exercise is often neglected. Not only can inactivity affect the complications of diabetes, but also the complications can affect ability to tolerate exercise. The complications of diabetes combined with inactivity may lead to increased disability (22).

An understanding of diabetic complications is required for recommending clinically sound exercise for patients with diabetes. The screening process should reveal complications that would influence recommendations for exercise. Concerns for individuals with diabetes include autonomic and peripheral (sensory) neuropathy, retinopathy, and nephropathy. Most patients with diabetes develop some neuropathy after 2–3 years. Neuropathy is associated with poor glucose control, so individuals in poor control are most likely to develop neuropathy. Clinical manifestations of neuropathy include both sensory and motor deficits. Table 31.9 shows precautions for patients with specific complications.

Recommendations for Specific Complications

Autonomic Neuropathy

Exercise associated with change in position or high-intensity activity should be avoided because of the risk of hypotension, especially after vigorous activity. Exercise in hot or cold environments should be avoided because of the risk of dehydration and poor heat and cold tolerance.

Table 31.9. Special Precautions For Recommending Exercise for Patients With Complications of Diabetes

COMPLICATION	PRECAUTION
Retinopathy[a,b]	With proliferative and severe stages of retinopathy, avoid strenuous, high-intensity activities that involve breath holding (e.g., weight lifting and isometrics). Avoid activities that lower the head (e.g., yoga, gymnastics) or that risk jarring the head. Consult ophthalmologist for specific weight restrictions and limitations
Hypertension	Avoid heavy weight lifting or breath holding. Perform primarily dynamic exercise using large muscle groups, such as walking and cycling at a moderate intensity.
Autonomic neuropathy[b]	Likelihood of hypoglycemia and hypertension. Elevated resting heart rate and reduced maximal heart rate. Use of RPE recommended. Prone to dehydration and hypothermia.
Peripheral neuropathy	Avoid exercise that may cause trauma to the feet (e.g., prolonged hiking, jogging, or walking on uneven surfaces). Non–weight-bearing activities most appropriate (e.g., cycling and swimming). Swimming not recommended if active ulcers are present. Regular assessment of the feet recommended. Keep the feet clean and dry. Choose shoes carefully for proper fit. Avoid activities requiring a great deal of balance.
Nephropathy	Avoid exercise that raises blood pressure (e.g., weight lifting, high-intensity aerobic exercises) and breath holding.
All patients	Carry identification with diabetes information. Rehydrate carefully (drink fluids before, during, and after exercise). Avoid exercise in the heat of the day and in direct sunlight (wear hat and sunscreen when in sun).

[a] If patient has proliferative retinopathy and has recently undergone photocoagulation or surgical treatment or is not properly treated, exercise is contraindicated.
[b] Submaximal exercise testing is recommended for patients with proliferative retinopathy and autonomic neuropathy.
RPE, rate of perceived exertion.
Reprinted with permission from Campaigne BN, Lampman RL. Exercise in the Clinical Management of Diabetes Mellitus. Champaign, IL: Human Kinetics, 1994.

Such patients are prone to hypoglycemia and should be monitored carefully.

Additional recommendations:

1 Use of submaximal testing and rate of perceived exertion (RPE) to determine exercise intensity (avoidance of high-intensity activity)

2. Use of water activities or stationary cycling (maintain blood pressure)
3. Careful blood glucose monitoring
4. Avoidance of extreme environments

Peripheral Neuropathy

Complications of peripheral neuropathy include ulceration of the feet and decreased healing ability. Severe neuropathy can result in multiple fractures and dislocation of bones of the feet and ankle. Patients may or may not be aware of these problems because of loss of sensation in the periphery. Although exercise does not reverse peripheral neuropathy, it may prevent further deterioration of functional capacity associated with disuse. Range of motion activities for the major joints (ankle, knee, hip, trunk, shoulder, elbow, and wrist) should be performed daily to prevent or minimize contracture. Additional recommendations:

1. Use of RPE to determine exercise intensity
2. Use of non–weight-bearing activities (swimming, cycling, arm exercise)
3. Use of activities to improve balance
4. Use of proper foot care and footwear
5. Use of gentle, pain-free stretching

Retinopathy

Patients with **background retinopathy** do not require the same monitoring as those with proliferative retinopathy. Low-impact activities that do not significantly increase blood pressure (>180 mm Hg) are most suitable. Strenuous upper extremity exercise (e.g., arm ergometry) should be avoided because of the associated increased peripheral resistance, which raises the blood pressure. Exercise is contraindicated with recent retinal photocoagulation or eye surgery. Additional recommendations:

1. Use of heart rate and RPE based on blood pressure response to determine intensity
2. Maintenance of systolic blood pressure below 170 mm Hg during exercise
3. Avoidance of Valsalva maneuvers
4. Avoidance of heavy weight lifting, breath holding, high-intensity exercise

Table 31.10 has more detail on retinopathy.

Nephropathy

Renal patients often present with multisystem disease and should be fully evaluated before exercise is prescribed. Exercise should not be initiated until the patient has been stabilized on medication, dialysis when indicated, and diet. Fluid replacement is essential because of the effects of fluid balance changes on blood pressure. It is unclear whether exercise accelerates nephropathy; however, sustained elevations in blood pressure do accelerate diabetic nephropathy. It is prudent to avoid activities that involve sustained elevation in blood pressure. Additional recommendations:

1. Dynamic weight-bearing low-impact activities
2. Submaximal weight lifting or isometrics when blood pressure is controlled and left ventricular function is not significantly impaired
3. Avoidance of intensive aerobic activities and Valsalva maneuvers
4. Use of cushioned shoes (e.g., gel, air)
5. Special attention to maintain hydration

The importance and clinical significance of careful screening for underlying complications are evident. When complications are present, specific considerations and precautions should be considered.

Table 31.10. Considerations for Activity Limitation in Diabetic Retinopathy

LEVEL OF DR	ACCEPTABLE ACTIVITIES	DISCOURAGED ACTIVITIES	OCULAR AND ACTIVITY REEVALUATION
No DR	Dictated by medical status	Dictated by medical status	12 mo
Mild NPDR	Dictated by medical status	Dictated by medical status	6–12 mo
Moderate NPDR	Dictated by medical status	Activities that dramatically raise blood pressure: Power lifting, heavy Valsalva maneuvers	
Severe, very severe NPDR	Dictated by medical status	Limit systolic blood pressure, Valsalva maneuvers, active jarring: Boxing, heavy competitive sports	2–4 mo (may require laser surgery)
PDR	Low-impact cardiovascular conditioning: Swimming (not diving) Walking Low-impact aerobics Stationary cycling Endurance exercises	Strenuous activity, Valsalva maneuvers, pounding, jarring: Weight lifting, jogging, high-impact aerobics, racquet sports, strenuous trumpet playing	1–2 mo (may require laser surgery)

DR, diabetic retinopathy; NPDR, nonproliferative diabetic retinopathy; PDR, proliferative diabetic retinopathy.
Reprinted with permission from Aiello LM, Cavellerno J, Aiello LP, et al. Retinopathy. In: Ruderman N, Devlin JT, eds. The Health Professional's Guide to Diabetes and Exercise. Alexandria, VA: American Diabetes Association, 1995:163–174.

EXERCISE RECOMMENDATIONS AND SPECIAL CLINICAL CONSIDERATIONS

Contraindications to Exercise

Since it is not clear that exercise improves glycemic control in IDDM but that it does have specific health benefits, exercise programs should be designed to teach people with IDDM to exercise safely and decrease risk of CVD. The benefits of regular exercise in patients with type II diabetes are well established, but until recently, information for planning and carrying out individualized exercise prescriptions for patients with diabetes has not been readily available to exercise professionals.

Screening is required prior to recommending individual exercise programs. Glycemic control must be monitored closely, and frequent modifications in diet and insulin therapy may be necessary. Specific recommendations for type of exercise and precautions for patients with neuropathy, retinopathy, and nephropathy should be given. The specifics of exercise programs, including follow-up and risks and benefits, should be addressed to ensure the greatest chance of adherence. Table 31.11 gives specific recommendations for screening patients with diabetes for exercise programs. Absolute contraindications for vigorous exercise include the following:

1. Poor glycemic control (type I, > 250 mg/dL and presence of ketones in urine or type II, > 300 mg/dL without ketones)

2. Proliferative retinopathy
3. Microangiopathy
4. Severe neuropathy
5. Nephropathy
6. Evidence of underlying cardiovascular disease that has not been evaluated or referred from a cardiac rehabilitation program

Resistance Exercise

Recent research indicates that resistance exercise may be beneficial for patients with diabetes (23, 24). Eriksson et al. (24) evaluated the effects of circuit training on long-term glycemic control in a group of moderately obese, sedentary elderly subjects with type II diabetes. After 3 months of an individualized progressive resistance training program of moderate intensity and high volume performed twice a week, there was a significant improvement in HbA1c . There was a strong inverse relationship between HbA1c and muscle cross-sectional area after the exercise program. The inclusion of resistance exercise appropriate to the individual patient should be considered for both type I and type II diabetes. Blood pressure monitoring for those with underlying complications (i.e., retinopathy, nephropathy), as previously described, may be necessary. Young patients with newly diagnosed type I diabetes who have blood glucose stabilized and no other risk factors should be able to participate in resistance training safely. After appropriate screening, individuals with type II diabetes and those with type I of longer duration can participate in moderate resistance training.

Table 31.11. Recommended Screening Procedures Before Beginning Exercise in Patients With Diabetes

History and physical examination for those newly diagnosed or without up-to-date records
  Review all systems
  Identification of medical problems (e.g., asthma, arthritis, orthopaedic limitations)
Diabetes evaluation
  Glycosylated hemoglobin (HbA$_1$)
  Ophthalmoscopic examination (retinopathy)
  Neurological examination (neuropathy)
  Nephrological evaluation (microalbumin or protein in urine)
  Nutritional status evaluation (underweight, overweight)
Cardiovascular evaluation
  Blood pressure
  Peripheral pulses
  Bruits
  12-lead electrocardiogram
  Serum lipid profile (total cholesterol, triglycerides, HDL and LDL cholesterol)
  Exercise ECG in patients with known or suspected CAD (for IDDM, those over 30 years of age or diabetes of longer than 15 years' duration; for NIDDM, those over 35 years of age)

Modified with permission from Campaigne BN, Lampman RL. Exercise in the Clinical Management of Diabetes Mellitus. Champaign, IL: Human Kinetics, 1994.
HDL, high-density lipoprotein; LDL, low-density lipoprotein, CAD, coronary artery disease.

► SUMMARY

Regular physical activity is an important part of management for individuals with diabetes, particularly those with type II. Regular physical activity reduces risk of many diseases to which individuals with diabetes are predisposed, including hypertension, coronary heart disease, and obesity. A comprehensive approach to diabetes management, including diet, insulin, other medications, and exercise can facilitate optimal blood glucose and lipid levels, assist in weight management, and prevent exacerbation of underlying complications.

References
1. Horton ES. Exercise in the treatment of NIDDM: Applications for GDM? Diabetes 40 (Suppl 2):175–178, 1991.
2. Bung P, Atral R, Khodiguian N, et al. Exercise in gestational diabetes: An optional therapeutic approach? Diabetes 40(Suppl 2):182–185, 1991.
3. Campaigne BN, Lampman RL. Exercise in the Clinical Management of Diabetes Mellitus. Champaign, IL: Human Kinetics, 1994.
4. American Diabetes Association. Diabetes mellitus and exercise: Position statement. Diabetes Care 23 (Suppl 1):S50–S56, 2000.

5. Wallberg-Henriksson, H, Rincon J, Zierath JR. Exercise in the management of non-insulin-dependent diabetes mellitus. Sports Med 25(1):25–35, 1998.

6. Kjaer M, Secher NH, Bach FW, et al. Role of motor center activity for hormonal changes and substrate mobilization in humans. Am J Physiol 253:R687–R695, 1987.

7. Jenkins AB, Furler SM, Chisholm DJ, et al. Regulation of hepatic glucose output during exercise by circulating glucose and insulin in humans. Am J Physiol 250:R411–R417, 1986.

8. Katz A, Broberg S, Sahlin K, et al. Leg glucose uptake during maximal dynamic exercise in humans. Am J Physiol 251:E65–E70, 1986.

9. Hu FB, Sigal RJ, Rich-Edwards JW, et al. Walking compared with vigorous physical activity and risk of type II diabetes in women: A prospective study. JAMA 282:1433–1439, 1999.

10. Pan X, Li G, Hu Y, et al. Effects of diet and exercise in preventing NIDDM in people with impaired glucose tolerance: The Da Qing IGT and Diabetes Study. Diabetes Care 20:537–544,1997.

11. Denoria JT, Heishman M, Horton EL, et al. Enhanced peripheral and splanchnic insulin sensitivity in NIDDM after single bout of exercise. Diabetologia 365:434–439, 1987.

12. Lampman RM, Schteingart DE, Santinga JT, et al. The influence of physical training on glucose tolerance, insulin sensitivity, and lipid and lipoprotein concentrations in middle aged hypertriglyceridemic and carbohydrate intolerant men. Diabetologia 30:380–385, 1987.

13. Zimmet P, Dowse G, Finch C, et al. The epidemiology and natural history of NIDDM: Lessons from the South Pacific. Diabetic Metab Rev 6:1–124, 1990.

14. Torjensen PA, Birkeland KI, Anderssen SA, et al. Lifestyle changes may reverse development of the insulin resistance syndrome. Oslo diet and exercise study: A randomized trial. Diabetes Care 20:26–31, 1997.

15. Mayer-Davis EJ, D'Agostino R, Karter AJ, et al. Intensity and amount of physical activity in relation to insulin sensitivity: The insulin resistance atherosclerosis study. JAMA 279:669–674, 1998.

16. Dowse GK, Zimmet PZ, Gareeboo H, et al. Abdominal obesity and physical inactivity as risk factors for NIDDM and impaired glucose tolerance in Indians, Creoles, and Chinese Mauritians. Diabetes Care 14:271–282, 1991.

17. Helmrich SP, Raglund DR, Leung RW, et al. Physical activity and reduced occurrence of non-insulin dependent diabetes mellitus. N Engl J Med 325:147–152, 1991.

18. Manson JE, Rimm EB, Stampfer MJ, et al. Physical activity and incidence of non-insulin-dependent diabetes mellitus in women. Lancet 338:774–778, 1991.

19. Kriska AM, Blair SN, Pereira MA. The potential role of physical activity in the prevention of non-insulin dependent diabetes mellitus: Epidemiological evidence. Exerc Sport Sci Rev 22:121–143, 1994.

20. Jovanovic-Peterson L, Durak EP, Peterson CM. Randomized trial of diet versus diet plus cardiovascular conditioning on glucose levels in gestational diabetes. Am J Obstet Gynecol 161:415–419, 1989.

21. Jovanovic-Peterson L, Peterson CM. Dietary manipulation as a primary treatment strategy for pregnancies complicated by diabetes. J Am Coll Nutr 9:320–325, 1990.

22. Graham C, Lasko-McCarthey P. Exercise options for persons with diabetic complications. Diabetes Educator 16:212–220, 1990.

23. Rice B, Janssen I, Hudson R., Ross R. Effects of aerobic or resistance exercise and/or diet on glucose tolerance and plasma insulin levels in obese men. Diabetes Care 22:684–691, 1999.

24. Eriksson J, Taimela S, Eriksson K, et al. Resistance training in the treatment of non-insulin-dependent diabetes mellitus. Int J Sports Med 18:242–246, 1997.

Suggested Reading

American College of Sports Medicine. ACSM's Exercise Management for Persons with Chronic Disease and Disabilities. Champaign, IL: Human Kinetics, 1997.

American Diabetes Association. Diabetes mellitus and exercise: Position statement. Diabetes Care 23(Suppl 1):S50–S56.

Campaigne BN, Lampman RL. Exercise in the Clinical Management of Diabetes Mellitus. Champaign, IL: Human Kinetics, 1994.

Diabetes Mellitus and Exercise: A joint position statement of the American College of Sports Medicine and The American Diabetes Association. *Med Sci Sport Exerc* 29:1–5, 1997.

Report of the Expert Committee on the Diagnosis and Classification of Diabetes Mellitus. Diabetes Care 20:1183–1197, 1997.

Ruderman N, Devlin JT, eds. The Health Professionals Guide to Diabetes and Exercise. Alexandria, VA: American Diabetes Association, 1995.

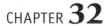

1.4.0.1, 1.4.0.2   2.4.4, 2.8.0, 2.8.0.9,   3.4.2, 3.4.3   4.4.1, 4.4.15, 4.8.1,
                      2.8.0.11   4.8.1.10

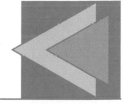

CHAPTER **32**

EXERCISE AND HYPERTENSION

Kerry J. Stewart

OVERVIEW OF HYPERTENSION

Approximately 50 million adults in the United States have systolic blood pressure (SBP) of at least 140 mm Hg and/or diastolic blood pressure (DBP) of at least 90 mm Hg (1). African Americans are more likely to have hypertension than whites, although specific reasons for this racial difference are not known. Hypertension is a primary risk factor for cardiovascular diseases such as stroke, congestive heart failure, angina, renal failure, and myocardial infarction at all ages and in both genders. While the highest risks are for stroke and congestive heart failure, coronary heart disease is the most common outcome of hypertension (2).

Epidemiological data suggest that the coronary disease risk in hypertensive patients is highest in those with a high ratio of total cholesterol to high-density lipoprotein (HDL) cholesterol, impaired glucose tolerance, high fibrinogen, electrocardiographic abnormalities, and cigarette smoking (2). The risk of stroke in hypertensive persons is highest in those with cardiovascular disease, diabetes, atrial fibrillation, left ventricular hypertrophy, and cigarette smoking. Because of the health risks of hypertension, treatment, including exercise, is necessary to improve outcomes. One advantage of exercise as a treatment for hypertension is its positive effect on multiple cardiac risk factors.

DEFINITION, CAUSES, EPIDEMIOLOGY, AND DIAGNOSIS

The 1997 Joint National Commission (JNC VI) on Detection, Evaluation, and Treatment of High Blood Pressure reclassified the risk categories for hypertension (Table 32.1) (3). Although stage 1 hypertension is the most prevalent form of high blood pressure, all stages are associated with increased risk of cardiovascular disease events and renal failure. A major change in the classification is the recognition that SBP below 120 mm Hg and DBP less than 80 are now considered optimal.

The Third National Health and Nutrition Examination Survey reported that two-thirds of those with hypertension were aware of their diagnosis, and 53% were taking prescribed medication (4). However, only 33% of Hispanics with hypertension were being treated, and 14% achieved control, in contrast to 25% and 24% of the non-Hispanic black and non-Hispanic white populations with hypertension, respectively (Fig. 32.1).

Increased blood pressure has a positive and continuous association with vascular events (5). Within the DBP range of 70–110 mm Hg, there is no threshold below which a lower blood pressure does not reduce the risk of stroke and coronary disease. Among individuals treated for hypertension, an average 15/6 mm Hg reduction in blood pressure reduced stroke by 34% and coronary heart disease by 19% over 4.7 years (6). The absolute benefits in older subjects were more than twice those seen in younger subjects. Hypertension may be a stronger independent risk factor for mortality from heart disease among elderly women than among elderly men (7).

PATHOPHYSIOLOGY AND IMPLICATIONS FOR EXERCISE TESTING AND TRAINING

Essential hypertension is the most common form of hypertension. It is characterized by an increased DBP and related general arteriolar vasoconstriction that increases the SBP. While there is no single cause of essential hypertension, blood pressure is mainly determined by the product of cardiac output and total peripheral resistance. Population factors closely associated with hypertension are obesity, high salt intake, low potassium intake, physical inactivity, heavy alcohol consumption, and psychosocial stress (8). Some studies suggest that accumulation of intra-abdominal visceral fat and hyperinsulinemia play a role in the pathogenesis of hypertension (9–11). For these reasons, lifestyle changes that favorably modify these factors are a substantial part of treatment for hypertension. Interactions between these lifestyle factors and

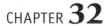

Table 32.1. Classification of Blood Pressure: Joint National Commission on Detection, Evaluation, and Treatment of Hypertension Recommendation

BLOOD PRESSURE CATEGORY	SYSTOLIC (MM HG)	DIASTOLIC (MM HG)
Optimal	<120	<80
Normal	120–129	80–84
High normal	130–139	85–89
Hypertension		
Stage 1	140–159	90–99
Stage 2	160–179	100–109
Stage 3	≥180	≥110

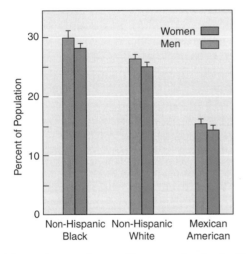

Figure 32.1. The prevalence of hypertension in the U.S. adult.

genetic endowment are also likely to contribute to the development of hypertension.

Hypertension imposes an afterload on the heart, resulting in increased left ventricular wall thickness (concentric hypertrophy) and reduced early diastolic filling (12–13). Aging also alters left ventricular mass and diastolic filling, and the combination of hypertension and advancing age markedly raises the risk of coronary disease and heart failure (14). The strong correlation of left ventricular mass with cardiovascular disease morbidity and mortality emphasizes the importance of classifying patients by this risk factor. In the Framingham study the predictive value of left ventricular mass on cardiovascular disease outcomes was independent of all other risk factors. Although several antihypertensive agents are capable of inducing regression of left ventricular hypertrophy, the long-term clinical benefits of reducing left ventricular mass have yet to be documented (15).

Some studies also suggest that hypertension and in particular the duration of hypertension promote the presence and extent of coronary calcium, itself a potential predictor of sudden coronary death (in parallel with the extent of peripheral atherosclerosis) (16). Hypertension is

also associated with subclinical changes in the brain (e.g., impaired cognitive function) and a thickening and stiffening of medium and small blood vessels. Hypertension may also lead to retinopathy and nephropathy.

ACUTE BLOOD PRESSURE RESPONSES TO EXERCISE

The typical blood pressure response to acute bouts of aerobic exercise is a gradual increase in SBP and a gradual decrease or no change in DBP. The expected peak blood pressure during maximal exercise is SBP of 180–210 and DBP of 60–85 mm Hg for most individuals. Age, gender, and body weight often cause variation in these responses. Along with resting blood pressure, excessive blood pressure responses to exercise may predict future hypertension. Recent exercise testing data from the Framingham study in subjects who were normotensive at baseline indicate the following:

- An exaggerated DBP response to exercise predicted risk of new-onset hypertension in normotensive men and women.
- An elevated recovery SBP predicted hypertension in men (17).

These findings may reflect subtle pathophysiological features in the preclinical stage of hypertension.

Exercise blood pressure may also predict coronary disease events. In apparently healthy men followed for an average of 16 years, exercise blood pressure at baseline was more strongly related to both morbidity and mortality from myocardial infarction than mildly elevated resting blood pressure (18). These results suggest that exercise blood pressure may distinguish between severe and less severe hypertension.

Another study compared cardiovascular responses to exercise in normotensive men at high risk for hypertension based on family history to those at low risk for hypertension (19). During exercise, high-risk men with exaggerated blood pressure responses (≥ 230/100 mm Hg) had blunted peripheral resistance. This suggests an impaired capacity for exercise-induced vasodilation as a mechanism for future hypertension.

POSSIBLE MECHANISMS BY WHICH EXERCISE MAY REDUCE HYPERTENSION

There are several possible hemodynamic mechanisms by which exercise may lower blood pressure. Lowering of both cardiac output and peripheral vascular resistance at rest and at any given level of work after exercise training is one hypothesis. Other possible exercise training–induced mechanisms are reduced serum catecholamines and reduced plasma renin activity (20).

Lack of a consistent association between exercise-induced changes in blood pressure with changes in body weight or composition suggest that anthropomorphic parameters may not be primary mechanisms in causing hypertension. Some studies have focused on body fat distribution. One study involving subjects with and without a parental history of hypertension showed that offspring of parents with hypertension had more central fat (9). However, there were no differences in fitness or physical activity based on parental hypertension, suggesting a role for central fat in the causation of primary hypertension.

Another study examined changes in blood pressure and fat distribution after a 12-week weight loss diet in obese hypertensive women (10). Subjects lost a mean of 9.4 ± 4.1 kg, and mean blood pressure fell from 112 ± 9 to 101 ± 12 mm Hg ($P < .001$). Change in blood pressure was not correlated with change in body weight or body mass index, but was correlated with a reduction in visceral fat area and ratio of visceral fat to subcutaneous fat. Thus, a decrease in visceral fat may reduce blood pressure in obese subjects. A contributing factor to the decrease in resting blood pressure as a result of exercise may be the decrease in central fat deposition (21–23).

MEDICAL THERAPY AND IMPLICATIONS FOR EXERCISE

Because the relationship between blood pressure and cardiovascular disease is continuous, the level of hypertension at which to initiate medical treatment is arbitrary. However, effective pharmacological and nonpharmacological management of hypertension can significantly reduce mortality for all patients (1).

Medical management of hypertension is often complicated by concomitant dyslipidemia, sedentary lifestyle, hyperinsulinemia, glucose intolerance, reduced arterial compliance, sympathetic overactivity, and obesity. These additional disorders compound the risk of hypertension. This cluster of risk factors (Table 32.2) has been called the metabolic cardiovascular syndrome, or hypertension syndrome (24, 25).

Age, race, sex, and the presence of other risk factors should be considered in determining treatment strategies. Subtle abnormalities in insulin resistance and hyperinsulinemia may cause systemic hypertension through multiple mechanisms (11). Insulin has a sodium-retaining effect on the kidney, augments catecholamine release, increases vascular sensitivity to vasoconstrictor substances, and decreases vascular sensitivity to vasodilator substances. In addition, insulin increases production of tissue growth factors and facilitates retention of cellular sodium and calcium. Insulin resistance, like hypertension, can be treated with regular aerobic exercise, weight reduction, high-fiber diet, and/or medications. To provide maximal protection against the cardiovascular complications, hypertension should be managed to reduce total cardiovascular risk burden (Table 32.3) (26).

Another consideration is that some antihypertensive

Table 32.2. Prevalence of Other Risk Factors in Patients With Hypertension

RISK FACTOR	PERCENT
Smoking	35
Hypercholesterolemia >240 mg/dL	40
HDL cholesterol <40 mg/dL	25
Obesity	40
Diabetes	15
Hyperinsulinemia	50
Sedentary lifestyle	>50

Adapted with permission from Kaplan NM. Management of hypertension. Dis Mon 38:769–838, 1992.

Table 32.3. Five Steps to Minimize the Total Cardiovascular Risk Burden

Carefully monitor the blood pressure in response to therapy
Assess concomitant cardiovascular risk factors
Institute lifestyle changes to control hypertension and other risk factors
Use antihypertensive drugs chosen to manage the individual patient's overall risk burden in a way that will lower blood pressure gradually while avoiding adverse reactions
Identify the goal of therapy: levels of blood pressure that are neither too high, to avoid increased risks of cerebral and renal damage, nor too low, to avoid increased risks of coronary ischemia.

Adapted with permission from Kaplan NM. Management of hypertension. Dis Mon 38:769–838, 1992.

agents adversely affect other risk factors, whereas exercise, diet, and weight loss improve multiple cardiac risk factors. The JNC VI recommendations regarding pharmacological agents provide a contemporary approach to hypertension control (3). The JNC VI recommends that a diuretic and/or a beta-blocker be used as initial therapy unless there are compelling or specific indications for another drug. One study (27) examined the use of the five major antihypertensive drug classes between 1982 and 1993. Diuretics accounted for 56% of all antihypertensive drugs in 1982 but only 27% in 1993. Use of beta-blockers and central agents also declined during this period, whereas the use of calcium antagonists and angiotensin-converting enzyme inhibitors increased. Although the use of newer agents has increased markedly, the large-scale clinical trials of antihypertensive drugs that have shown a reduction in morbidity and mortality from stroke and coronary disease used diuretics and beta-blockers (27, 28).

Patients' compliance with medication regimens is often a problem, particularly for active adults or individuals for whom exercise is encouraged (29). In many cases, exercise training may reduce or eliminate the need for antihypertensive medications in patients with mild or severe hypertension (30, 31).

AEROBIC EXERCISE AND THE TREATMENT OF HIGH BLOOD PRESSURE

Both the JNC VI and the ACSM (3, 32) recommend aerobic exercise to reduce blood pressure. The JNC VI treatment guidelines for hypertension are based on a risk stratification model that emphasizes diet, weight loss, and exercise. In this model, group A has no risk factors, no target organ disease (TOD), and no clinical cardiovascular disease (CCD); group B has at least one risk factor not including diabetes, but no TOD or CCD; and group C has TOD, CCD, and/or diabetes with or without other risk factors. Lifestyle modification, including diet, weight loss, and exercise, is recommended as initial therapy for individuals in groups A and B with high normal or stage 1 hypertension (Table 32.1). Individuals in group C at any level of hypertension, or anyone in any risk group with stage 2 or 3 hypertension should begin drug therapy along with lifestyle modification. Nevertheless, dietary and other nonpharmacological strategies have not been shown to reduce clinical events even when blood pressure is reduced (25).

In a study of adult men and women, subjects performing 4 months of aerobic exercise did not attain greater reductions in blood pressure than control subjects (33). A review from the same investigator concludes that although exercise and weight loss offer some promise as nonpharmacological treatments for hypertension, the available research is inconclusive, the mechanism is unknown, and further research is necessary to clarify the issue (34). However, several studies using moderate-intensity exercise show a fall in blood pressure by an average 7/7 mm Hg (35, 36). A meta-analysis of nine randomized controlled exercise trials of 245 subjects found decreases of approximately 7 ± 5 and 6 ± 2 mm Hg for resting SBP and DBP, respectively, in treatment groups (Fig. 32.2) (36).

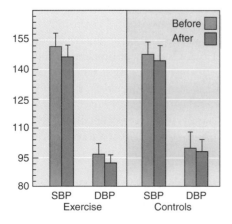

Figure 32.2. Blood pressure results from nine randomized studies of aerobic exercise in hypertension. SBP, systolic blood pressure; DBP, diastolic blood pressure

Another review summarized 47 studies concerned with endurance training in individuals with hypertension (37). More than 70% of the groups in these studies decreased resting blood pressure with exercise training, an average of 10.5/8.6 mm Hg from an initial level of 154/98 mm Hg. This review concluded that beneficial blood pressure responses associated with exercise are significantly more prevalent than negative or equivocal responses. Less consistent in the studies reviewed were reductions in ambulatory blood pressure with exercise training. A meta-analysis of seven studies that included 167 subjects engaged in aerobic exercise found a reduction of 2/3 mm Hg for average 24-hour blood pressure. In a recent 12-week study of exercise training in postmenopausal women with resting blood pressure of 130–159 over 85–99 mm Hg, resting blood pressure was reduced by 10/7 mm Hg. Walking blood pressure was unchanged, but reductions in blood pressure during submaximal exercise were significant. On average, subjects with stage 1 hypertension had a reduction in blood pressure into the high normal range, whereas subjects with high normal initial levels had a reduction in blood pressure into the normal range.

EXERCISE GUIDELINES

Aerobic Exercise

The ACSM recommends endurance exercise for mild hypertension (32). The recommended mode (large muscle activities), frequency (3–5 days/week), duration (20–60 minutes), and intensity (50–85% of maximal oxygen uptake) of the exercise recommended to achieve this effect are generally the same as those prescribed for healthy adults. For individuals with markedly elevated blood pressure, exercise training at somewhat lower intensities (40–70%) is recommended after initiation of pharmacological therapy.

The effectiveness of exercise training as a complement to pharmacological therapy was demonstrated in adult African American men with severe hypertension (SBP > 180 or DBP > 110) (31). After antihypertensive medications were administered in a stepped approach, subjects were divided into an exercise and sedentary group. Endurance exercise 3 days/week, 45 minutes/day at 75% of maximum heart rate for 16–32 weeks, was the training program. By week 16 the exercise group had lower SBP and DBP and reduced left ventricular mass. These effects persisted through 32 weeks, even after a reduction in antihypertensive medications. Thus, moderate aerobic exercise may reduce blood pressure, left ventricular hypertrophy, and the amount of antihypertensive medication required to control blood pressure.

Resistance Exercise

Acute bouts of resistance exercise increase SBP with an associated increase in DBP. Resistance exercise, however, increases the heart rate less than does aerobic exercise. In many instances, the myocardial oxygen demand (directly related to the heart rate × SBP, often called rate–pressure product) may be lower with resistance exercise than aerobic exercise performed at the same level of total body energy demand. This response was demonstrated in two studies of hypertensive men performing weight training and walking or jogging (29, 30). Heart rate during walking or jogging was higher than during weight training, while blood pressure was higher during weight training. The rate–pressure product was similar during weight training and walking or jogging. However, blood pressure responses to aerobic or resistive exercise are variable, and blood pressure at rest does not provide independent prognostic information about exercise responses. Therefore, exercise testing that includes assessment of blood pressure to resistance forms of exercise (e.g., hand grip, weight lifting, or isometrics) should be considered for subjects with hypertension.

While most studies have focused on endurance training, the benefits of resistance training for reducing blood pressure and improving cardiovascular health have been recognized in recent years. A recent position paper of the American Heart Association endorsed by the ACSM recommends mild to moderate resistance for improving muscular strength and endurance, preventing and managing a variety of chronic medical conditions, modifying coronary risk factors, and enhancing psychological well-being (39). Furthermore, resistance training attenuates the rate–pressure product when any given weight is lifted.

Several studies have investigated weight training as an intervention by itself or combined with aerobic exercise. A recent meta-analysis examined 11 studies (182 subjects) of progressive resistance training as the only intervention compared with randomized nonexercise control groups (138 subjects) (40). Across all designs and categories, resistance training decreased resting SBP by 2% and DBP by 4%. However, because only about 20% of the subjects in these studies could be classified as having at least mild hypertension, this analysis may be underestimating the benefits of resistance training among subjects with hypertension, who have the most to gain from lowering blood pressure.

In a study of men with mild hypertension, researchers examined the effects of circuit weight training combined with aerobic exercise in patients also randomly assigned to antihypertensive medications or placebo (29, 30). After 12 weeks of training, resting SBP and DBP fell by 13–14 mm Hg in all groups (Fig. 32.1). The most striking finding was that resting blood pressure fell equally between the drug and placebo groups, showing no added benefit of medications if subjects exercised regularly. All of these studies support the inclusion of resistance training as part of the exercise prescription for reducing blood pressure and improving cardiovascular health.

SCREENING AND TESTING

The Guide to Clinical Preventive Services states that blood pressure should be measured regularly in all persons aged 3 and above (41). The optimal interval for screening has not been determined but is left to clinical discretion. Current opinion is that blood pressure should be assessed every 2 years if a previous DBP and SBP were below 85 mm Hg and 140 mm Hg, respectively, or annually if the previous DBP was 85–89 mm Hg. Hypertension should not be diagnosed from a single measurement but should be confirmed from readings at each of three separate visits.

The ACSM does not recommend mass exercise testing specifically to determine blood pressure responses to exercise as a predictor of future hypertension (42). However, if exercise test results are available and the individual has a hypertensive response, the information does provide some indication of risk stratification and the necessity for further lifestyle counseling or treatment. Exercise testing before participation in moderate to vigorous exercise should be performed according to usual risk stratification guidelines. However, because hypertension often clusters with other cardiac risk factors, such as dyslipidemia, hyperinsulinemia, and obesity, many individuals with hypertension are likely to be candidates for exercise testing before exercise training.

► SUMMARY

Hypertension is a common and chronic problem, and adequate treatment is likely to reduce cardiovascular morbidity and mortality, particularly in the elderly. Physical activity has an important role in the treatment and prevention of hypertension.

Based on cross-sectional and experimental findings, regular physical activity and exercise training appear to lower blood pressure. Nevertheless, the specific mechanisms underlying this relationship are not entirely clear. Some major exercise-induced physiological changes from exercise that may account for the antihypertensive effects include decreased heart rate resulting from increased vagal tone and associated reductions in plasma norepinephrine and plasma renin levels. Although there are no consistent relationships between reduced body weight or improved body composition and decreased blood pressure, a growing body of evidence suggests that increased abdominal visceral fat, along with insulin and glucose intolerance, play a role in the pathogenesis of hypertension. These risk factors, which are also independent risk factors for coronary disease, can be improved substantially with physical activity.

Exercise prescription for hypertension should be based on medical history and risk factor status. Because resting blood pressure alone is often an inadequate prognostic indicator of hypertension risk, exercise testing may help to identify exaggerated blood pressure responses to exercise and latent ischemic heart disease. The exercise prescription should also be adapted to antihypertensive medications that may affect the exercise heart rate and blood pressure. Finally, although much of the exercise literature has focused on aerobic exercise for subjects with hypertension, there is ample evidence to recommend that resistance training be combined with aerobic exercise for controlling blood pressure and improving cardiovascular health.

References

1. Sutherland J, Castle C, Friedman R. Hypertension: Current management strategies. J Am Board Fam Pract 7:202–217, 1994.
2. Kannel WB. Potency of vascular risk factors as the basis for antihypertensive therapy. Eur Heart J 13:34–42, 1992.
3. The sixth report of the Joint National Committee on Detection, Evaluation, and Treatment of High Blood Pressure (JNC VI). Arch Intern Med 2413–2446, 1997.
4. Burt VL, Whelton P, Roccella EJ, et al. Prevalence of hypertension in the US adult population: Results from the Third National Health and Nutrition Examination Survey, 1988–1991. Hypertension 25:305–313, 1995.
5. MacMahon S, Peto R, Cutler J, et al. Blood pressure, stroke, and coronary heart disease: Part 1. Prolonged differences in blood pressure: Prospective observational studies corrected for the regression dilution bias. Lancet 335:765–774, 1990.
6. MacMahon S, Rodgers A. The effects of blood pressure reduction in older patients: An overview of five randomized controlled trials in elderly hypertensives. Clin Exp Hypertens 15:967–978, 1993.
7. Weijenberg MP, Feskens EJ, Bowles CH, Kromhout D. Serum total cholesterol and systolic blood pressure as risk factors for mortality from ischemic heart disease among elderly men and women. J Clin Epidemiol 47:197–205, 1994.
8. Perry IJ, Whincup PH, Shaper AG. Environmental factors in the development of essential hypertension. Br Med Bull 50:246–259, 1994.
9. de Visser DC, van Hooft IM, van Doornen LJ, et al. Anthropometric measures, fitness and habitual physical activity in offspring of hypertensive parents. Dutch Hypertension and Offspring Study. Am J Hypertens 7:242–248, 1994.
10. Kanai H, Tokunaga K, Fujioka S, et al. Decrease in intraabdominal visceral fat may reduce blood pressure in obese hypertensive women. Hypertension 27:125–129, 1996.
11. Mediratta S, Fozailoff A, Frishman W. Insulin resistance in systemic hypertension: Pharmacotherapeutic implications. J Clin Pharmacol 35:943–956, 1995.
12. Liebson PR, Grandits G, Prineas R, et al. Echocardiographic correlates of left ventricular structure among 844 mildly hypertensive men and women in the Treatment of Mild Hypertension Study (TOMHS). Circulation 87:476–486, 1993.
13. Missault LH, Duprez DA, Brandt AA, et al. Exercise performance and diastolic filling in essential hypertension. Blood Press 2:284–288, 1993.
14. Messerli FH, Ketelhut R. Left ventricular hypertrophy: A
15. Eselin JA, Carter BL. Hypertension and left ventricular hypertrophy: Is drug therapy beneficial? Pharmacotherapy 14:60–88, 1994.
16. Megnien JL, Simon A, Lemariey M, et al. Hypertension promotes coronary calcium deposit in asymptomatic men. Hypertension 27:949–954, 1996.
17. Singh JP, Larson MG, Manolio TA, et al. Blood pressure response during treadmill testing as a risk factor for new-onset hypertension: The Framingham heart study. Circulation 99:1831–1836, 1999.
18. Mundal R, Kjeldsen SE, Sandvik L, et al. Exercise blood pressure predicts mortality from myocardial infarction. Hypertension 27:324–329, 1996.
19. Wilson MF, Sung BH, Pincomb GA, Lovallo WR. Exaggerated pressure response to exercise in men at risk for systemic hypertension. Am J Cardiol 66:731–736, 1990.
20. Dubbert PM, Martin JE, Cushman WC, et al. Endurance exercise in mild hypertension: Effects on blood pressure and associated metabolic and quality of life variables. J Hum Hypertens 8:265–272, 1994.
21. Despres JP, Pouliot MC, Moorjani S, et al. Loss of abdominal fat and metabolic response to exercise training in obese women. Am J Physiol 261:E159–E167, 1991.
22. Schwartz RS, Shuman WP, Larson V, et al. The effect of intensive endurance exercise training on body fat distribution in young and older men. Metabolism 40:545–551, 1991.
23. Schwartz RS, Cain KC, Shuman WP, et al. Effect of intensive endurance training on lipoprotein profiles in young and older men. Metabolism 41:649–654, 1992.
24. Westheim A, Os I. Physical activity and the metabolic cardiovascular syndrome. J Cardiovasc Pharmacol 20:S49–S53, 1992.
25. Weber MA. Controversies in the diagnosis and treatment of hypertension: A personal review of JNC V. Am J Cardiol 72:3H–9H, 1993.
26. Kaplan NM. Management of hypertension. Dis Mon 38:769–838, 1992.
27. Manolio TA, Cutler JA, Furberg CD, et al. Trends in pharmacologic management of hypertension in the United States. Arch Intern Med 155:829–837, 1995.
28. Rutan GH, Cushman WC. Relative benefits of different antihypertensive drugs in the prevention of vascular complications. Curr Opin Nephrol Hypertens 4:240–244, 1995.
29. Stewart KJ, Effron MB, Valenti SA, Kelemen MH. Effects of diltiazem or propranolol during exercise training of hypertensive men. Med Sci Sports Exerc 22:171–177, 1990.
30. Kelemen MH, Effron MB, Valenti SA, Stewart KJ. Exercise training combined with antihypertensive drug therapy: Effects on lipids, blood pressure, and left ventricular mass. JAMA 263:2766–2771, 1990.
31. Kokkinos P, Narayan P, Colleran J, et al. Effects of regular exercise on blood pressure and left ventricular hypertrophy in African-American men with severe hypertension. N Engl J Med 333:1462–1467, 1995.
32. American College of Sports Medicine. Position Stand. Physical activity, physical fitness, and hypertension. Med Sci Sports Exerc 25:i–x, 1993.
33. Blumenthal JA, Siegel WC, Appelbaum M. Failure of exer-

pressure-independent cardiovascular risk factor. J Cardiovasc Pharmacol 22:S7–S13, 1993.

cise to reduce blood pressure in patients with mild hypertension: Results of a randomized controlled trial. JAMA 266:2098–2104, 1991.

34. Blumenthal JA, Thyrum ET, Gullette ED, et al. Do exercise and weight loss reduce blood pressure in patients with mild hypertension? N C Med J 56:92–95, 1995.

35. Arroll B, Beaglehole R. Does physical activity lower blood pressure: A critical review of the clinical trials. J Clin Epidemiol 45:439–447, 1992.

36. Kelley G, McClellan P. Antihypertensive effects of aerobic exercise: A brief meta-analytic review of randomized controlled trials. Am J Hypertens 7:115–119, 1994.

37. Hagberg JM. Physical Activity, Physical Fitness, and Blood Pressure. NIH Consensus Development Conference: Physical Activity and Cardiovascular Health. Bethesda, MD: National Institutes of Health, 1995:69–71.

38. Seals DR, Silverman HG, Reiling MJ, Davy KP. Effect of regular aerobic exercise on elevated blood pressure in postmenopausal women. Am J Cardiol 80:49–55, 1997.

39. Pollock ML, Franklin BA, Gary J, et al. Resistance exercise in individuals with and without cardiovascular disease: Benefits, rationale, safety, and prescription: An advisory from the Committee on Exercise, Rehabilitation, and Prevention, Council on Clinical Cardiology, American Heart Association. Circulation 101:828–833, 2000.

40. Kelley GA, Kelley KS. Progressive resistance exercise and resting blood pressure: A meta-analysis of randomized controlled trials. Hypertension 35:838–843, 2000.

41. U.S. Preventive Services Task Force Guide to Clinical Preventative Services. 2 ed. Baltimore: Williams & Wilkins, 1995.

42. ACSM's Guidelines for Exercise Testing and Prescription. 6th ed. Baltimore: Williams & Wilkins, 2000:207.

43. Kelley GA. Effects of aerobic exercise on ambulatory blood pressure: A meta-analysis. Sport Med Train Rehab 7:115–131, 1996.

Suggested Reading

The sixth report of the Joint National Committee on Detection, Evaluation, and Treatment of High Blood Pressure (JNC VI). Arch Intern Med 2413–2446, 1997.

American College of Sports Medicine. Position Stand. Physical activity, physical fitness, and hypertension. Med Sci Sports Exerc 25:i–x, 1993.

Pollock ML, Franklin BA, Gary J, et al. Resistance exercise in individuals with and without cardiovascular disease: Benefits, rationale, safety, and prescription: An advisory from the Committee on Exercise, Rehabilitation, and Prevention, Council on Clinical Cardiology, American Heart Association. Circulation 101:828–833, 2000.

CHAPTER **33**

EXERCISE IN THE MANAGEMENT OF PERIPHERAL ARTERIAL DISEASE

Judith G. Regensteiner and William R. Hiatt

Peripheral arterial disease (PAD) is a common manifestation of atherosclerosis. The prevalence of PAD increases with age, and the disease affects about 12% of the general population but up to 20% of older individuals (1, 2). Patients with PAD have similar cardiovascular risk factors to patients with coronary artery disease. In addition, since persons with PAD have systemic atherosclerosis, there is an associated increase in morbidity and mortality from other cardiovascular diseases (3).

PAD produces exercise-induced muscle aching or cramping (intermittent claudication) secondary to ischemia in the calf, thighs, or buttocks (Table 33.1). In patients with claudication, this symptom occurs only during walking, but in more severe forms of the disease, pain in the limb at rest, ischemic ulceration, gangrene, and ultimately the need for amputation may exist. There is a relatively stable natural history of symptoms of intermittent claudication such that the ability to walk may not worsen over intervals of up to several years (4). However, there is almost never spontaneous improvement in walking ability in the absence of intervention.

PAD has profound detrimental effects on functional status (5, 6). Clinically, PAD is an important cause of impaired functional ability because symptomatic patients are typically able to walk less than one to three blocks before rest is required. Peak oxygen consumption ($\dot{V}O_{2peak}$) ranges from 10–16 mL/kg/minutes equivalent to class C on the Weber scale of heart failure (7). Limited ability to walk leads to disability, which may prevent performance of personal, social, or occupational activities of daily living. For example, occupational activities that require walking short distances, shopping, and outdoor recreational activities may be limited. Thus, a major goal of therapy in PAD is to relieve symptoms of intermittent claudication and disability and to restore functional status.

Risk factors for PAD include diabetes mellitus, cigarette smoking, hypertension, hyperlipidemia (particularly disorders in the metabolism of triglycerides and high-density lipoprotein cholesterol), abnormalities of hemostatic function and hemorrheology, lipoprotein(a), and abnormalities of homocysteine metabolism (8–15). Aggressive treatment of risk factors may slow or stabilize the atherosclerotic disease process and may positively influence cardiac mortality, but does not for the most part improve exercise performance. In fact, of the risk factors, only smoking cessation has been shown to improve claudication symptoms (16). Helping patients to quit smoking and to normalize lipids is beneficial for preventing the progression of PAD.

AVAILABLE SURGICAL AND PHARMACOLOGIC TREATMENTS

Interventional Treatments

Surgery or angioplasty may be necessary for the relief of symptoms and/or limb preservation in patients with severe forms of the disease. In patients with claudication, interventional therapy is associated with improvements in ability to walk. However, there is higher morbidity and mortality, as well as higher costs for both surgery and angioplasty than for noninvasive treatments (17–21). In most cases, claudication can be treated with alternative methods.

Pharmacology

The only approved drug for treating intermittent claudication is pentoxifylline, a hemorheologic agent that decreases blood viscosity. This drug is associated with a 22% improvement over placebo in pain-free walking distance and 12% improvement in maximal walking distance (22). Thus, the clinical benefits are relatively modest. There is interest in the development of new drugs for claudication. Examples of drugs being tested include antiplatelet and anticoagulant drugs, hemorheologic drugs, novel vasodilators, prostaglandins, and drugs that alter muscle metabolism. Results of these studies are pending.

Table 33.1. Pathophysiology of Peripheral Arterial Disease

Acute	Muscle blood flow supply/demand mismatch
Chronic	Deconditioning and denervation + impaired oxidative metabolism
	Claudication during walking limits ability to carry out normal daily activities

Interventional and pharmacological therapies are used to treat claudication and improve walking ability. The development of new pharmacological therapies is growing, but it is unknown which agents will emerge as effective.

METHODS OF EVALUATION

Assessment Procedures

Programs using exercise rehabilitation or other therapies for claudication must have appropriate evaluations to assess hemodynamic and functional status of each patient before and after treatment. In this way, information about effectiveness can be provided to both the program director and the patient for purposes of feedback.

Screening

Prior to initiating an exercise rehabilitation program for a patient with PAD, cardiovascular screening should be performed because of the increased prevalence of coronary atherosclerosis in persons with PAD. Screening should include a history, physical examination, and resting and exercise electrocardiograms during the initial exercise test. If clinically significant coronary artery disease is present, the patient should be referred for treatment.

Hemodynamic Assessment

The peripheral circulation is commonly assessed by measuring resting and postexercise systolic blood pressures in the ankle and arm using Doppler ultrasound. At rest, the ratio of ankle to arm systolic blood pressure (ankle–brachial index [ABI]) is used to measure the severity of the underlying vascular disease (23). Using a large population of controls and diabetics, an abnormal ABI has been defined as less than 0.9 at rest and a 20% decrease after exercise (23).

Before the ABI is measured, patients should rest for 10–15 minutes. Blood pressure measurements in the dorsalis pedis, posterior tibial, and brachial arteries are duplicated for greater accuracy. These tests are practical because they are easy to perform, are well-tolerated by patients, require simple equipment, and are relatively inexpensive. The ABI measurements are important for assessing change in severity of PAD. However, the hemodynamic severity of vascular disease defined by ABI is not well correlated to treadmill exercise performance, and therefore, this measurement should not be used to test the functional effects of intervention (24).

Treadmill Testing in PAD

Treadmill testing on entry to an exercise rehabilitation program and after completion of the program is an objective means of assessing changes in performance. Importantly, in contrast to treadmill testing in healthy people, the protocol used in PAD patients must be much less strenuous, given the severe limitations. Slower speed and less rapidly increasing grade than other treadmill protocols are used. Claudication-free walking time or distance (initial claudication distance [ICD]) and maximal claudication-limited walking time or distance (absolute claudication distance [ACD]) are the most commonly used criteria to evaluate performance. Until recently, the most common type of treadmill protocol was a constant-load test conducted at 1.5–2 mph with a fixed grade of 8–12% (25). Despite the constant workload, most (but not all) persons reach maximum claudication pain, at which point walking is discontinued. Constant-load protocol tests are easy to administer and require simple equipment.

Graded treadmill protocols have been developed to test patients with PAD (24, 26). Two widely used graded protocols maintain a walking speed of 2 mph. One protocol increases grade 3.5% every 3 minutes, while the other uses 2% grade increments every 2 minutes (24, 26). All patients limited by claudication are reproducibly brought to maximal levels of discomfort using either protocol.

Measurement of Oxygen Consumption

Peak oxygen consumption ($\dot{V}O_{2peak}$) may be used to assess cardiopulmonary fitness in a PAD patient. The $\dot{V}O_{2peak}$ measurements are reproducible in the PAD population and can be modified with exercise training (24, 27, 28). However, obtaining $\dot{V}O_{2peak}$ measurements requires expensive equipment and specially trained personnel, and it is not available in most clinical settings.

Functional Status Measures

Laboratory-based tests, such as treadmill tests, and questionnaires, should be used to comprehensively evaluate functional status of PAD patients (Table 33.2). The Walking Impairment Questionnaire (WIQ) assesses defined walking distances, speeds, stair-climbing ability, and claudication severity in the PAD population (5, 6). The WIQ has been used to evaluate changes in walking ability resulting from an exercise training program and from peripheral bypass surgery (5, 6).

The Physical Activity Recall questionnaire provides a general measure of habitual physical activity in patients with PAD. This questionnaire has been modified from the original Stanford Physical Activity Recall for use in sedentary and diseased populations (6, 29). Energy expenditure in the home, at work, and during leisure time is measured (6).

Table 33.2. Questionnaires Used to Assess the Functional Status of Patients with Peripheral Arterial Disease

QUESTIONNAIRE	WALKING IMPAIRMENT QUESTIONNAIRE	PHYSICAL ACTIVITY RECALL	MEDICAL OUTCOMES STUDY (SF-36)
Domain(s) evaluated	Ability to walk distances, speeds, stair-climbing ability, claudication severity	Habitual physical activity level (work, housework, leisure)	Physical, role, social functioning, bodily pain, mental health, vitality, general health perception
Mode of administration	Interviewer	Interviewer	Self or interviewer
Time required for administration and scoring	6–8 minutes	6–8 minutes	5–7 minutes
Scoring	Four scores, 0–100% scale	One score MET/hr or kcal per week	Eight scores 0–100% scale
Validation	PAD population	PAD population Diabetes population Healthy sedentary adults	Numerous healthy and diseased populations (including PAD)

MET, metabolic equivalent; SF-36, short form 36.
For a complete review of the questionnaires, see Regensteiner JG, Hiatt WR. Exercise rehabilitation for patients with peripheral arterial disease. Exerc Sports Sci Rev 23:1–4, 1995.

The Medical Outcomes Study questionnaire evaluates physical, social, and role functioning and perception of general health and well-being. This questionnaire has been used to evaluate functional status in a number of disease states (including cardiac) as well as in healthy persons (30).

Questionnaires such as the ones discussed above are easily used to evaluate the effect of exercise rehabilitation on functional status in the PAD patient with claudication. The information provided is a valuable adjunct to laboratory-based measures. It is not recommended that the questionnaires replace treadmill testing in clinical trials given the valuable information obtained from more objective tests. However, when treadmill testing is not available, the questionnaires are useful in providing some outcome information.

EXERCISE REHABILITATION

A supervised exercise rehabilitation program has been shown to be highly effective in treating claudication (Table 33.3) (27, 28, 31–35). Repetitive programs, most often consisting of treadmill walking, are associated with improvements in both treadmill exercise performance and walking ability in patients with claudication. Therefore, for nearly 50 years exercise rehabilitation in varying forms has been recommended to improve walking ability in PAD.

Of the many exercise rehabilitation studies on PAD performed to date, relatively few have been randomized or controlled (27, 28, 31–35). However, all studies of exercise conditioning in persons with PAD report increased maximal claudication time and initial (pain-free) walking time during exercise. In randomized, controlled trials, it has been observed that both exercise performance (by treadmill) and functional status (by questionnaire) are improved after 12 weeks and 24 weeks (Table 33.4) (17,

Table 33.3. Improvements in Exercise Performance After Exercise Rehabilitation

Improved treadmill exercise performance
    Two- to threefold increase in walking distance
15–30% increase in oxygen consumption
Improved walking ability
    Increased speed, duration
    Less claudication pain
Improved perception of physical functioning
Increased level of habitual physical activity

27, 28, 31–36). Exercise performance prior to exercise conditioning is lower than that of normal, sedentary individuals. It is especially notable that VO_{2peak} is reduced in PAD by about 50% (27, 28). This finding reflects the extreme disability imposed by intermittent claudication.

Exercise Training-Specific Methods

Exercise rehabilitation should begin after entry screening and assessment of exercise performance and functional status, as described previously (5, 6, 27, 28). Exercise sessions should be held three times a week for 1 hour each for 3 months (Table 33.5). Telemetry monitoring can be used to evaluate heart rate response or may be required in the case of existent cardiovascular disease in addition to PAD. Warm-up should precede exercise, and cool-down should follow to minimize risk of injury (Table 33.5). The initial training load is determined from a symptom-limited maximal treadmill test, such that the intensity of the exercise causes claudication pain. In subsequent visits, the speed or grade is increased if the patient is able to walk 8–10 minutes or longer at the lower workload without moderate claudication pain.

The goal of the initial training session is for the patient

Table 33.4. Summary of Randomized Controlled Trials Evaluating the Efficacy of Exercise Rehabilitation for Patients With Peripheral Arterial Disease

Author	Group	N	Intervention	Treadmill Test	Duration of Program	Functional Assessment	Change in ICD	Change in ACD
Larsen and Lassen, 1966 (33)	T	7	Daily walks	Constant load	6 mo	No	106%[a]	183%[a]
	C	7	Placebo pill				−11%	−6%
Holm et al., 1973 (34)	T	6	Dynamic leg exercise	Constant load	4 mo	No	220%[a]	133%[a]
	C	6	Placebo pill				No change	No change
Dahllof et al., 1974 (31)	T	23	Dyanmic leg exercise	Constant load	6 mo	No	150%[a]	117%[a]
	C	11	Placebo pill				No change	No change
Dahllof et al., 1976 (32)	T	10	Dynamic leg exercise	Constant load	4 mo	No	170%[a]	135%[a]
	C	8	Placebo pill				120%[a]	75%[a]
Mannarino et al., 1991 (35)	T1	10	Dynamic leg exercise + daily walks	Constant load	6 mo	No	90%[a]	86%[a]
	T2	10	Exercise + antiplatelet				120%[a]	105%[a]
	T3	10	Antiplatelet				35%[a]	38%[a]
Lundgren et al., 1989 (36)	T1	25	Dynamic leg exercise	Constant load	6 mo	No	179%[a]	151%[a]
	T2	25	Surgery + dynamic leg exercise				698%[a]	263%[a]
	T3	25	Surgery				376%[a]	173%[a]
Creasy et al., 1990 (17)	T1	20	Exercise	Constant load	6 mo treatment (follow-up of 12 mo)	No	296%[a]	442%[a]
	T2	13	Angioplasty				21%	57%
Hiatt et al., 1990 (27)	T	10	Walking exercise	Graded	3 mo	Yes	165%[a]	123%[a]
	C	9	Nonexercising control				6%	20%[a]
Hiatt et al., 1994 (28)	T	10	Walking exercise	Graded	6 mo	Yes	209%[a]	128%[a]
	C	8	Nonexercising control		3 mo		−18%	−1%

T, treat; C, control; ICD, initial claudication distance; ACD, absolute claudication distance; functional assessment, use of questionnaire to evaluate community-based functional status. No change, a finding of no improvement is stated but the data are not given. For the Creasy study, the data given are for the 12 month follow-up time point.
[a] = P < 0.05 compared to baseline. Numbers in parentheses are reference numbers.

to spend 5 minutes of intermittent walking on the treadmill, exclusive of the warm-up and cool-down, with subsequent increases of 5 minutes each session until 35 minutes of treadmill walking in a 50-minute exercise session is accomplished. During exercise sessions, rest periods induced by claudication are interspersed between bouts of walking. The patient walks until mild to moderate claudication pain is perceived (3–4 on a 1-to-5 scale); at that point, the patient sits and rests until the pain abates. The patient resumes walking until a mild or moderate level of pain is reached again, followed by another rest period. This process is repeated until the 50-minute exercise period has elapsed. Generally, after some conditioning, walking constitutes about 35 minutes and rest periods total about 15 minutes of the 50-minute period (27, 28).

Resistive Training

The benefits of resistive training in PAD are less well known than those of walking. In one randomized controlled trial, 12 weeks of strength training alone was less effective than 12 weeks of supervised treadmill walking for improving walking ability (28). In addition, sequential use of strength training followed by aerobic exercise

Table 33.5. Specific Methods of Exercise Training

Warm-up period and cool-down period
(5 minutes each should precede and end the 1-hour session)
Training intensity
  Initial
    Set by results of peak treadmill
    Starting exercise work load brings on claudication pain
  Subsequent
    Speed or grade increased if patient walks > 8–10 minutes
      Grade increased first if speed ≥ 2 mph
      Speed increased first if < 2 mph
Duration
  Initial
    35 minutes (intermittent walking)
  Subsequent
    Add 5 minutes every session until 50 minutes (intermittent walking) is possible
  Total time
    3 months (36 sessions)
Frequency
  Three to five times per week[a]
Specificity of activity
  Treadmill walking is the recommended exercise

[a] ACSM Guidelines specify daily; literature supports the beneficial effects of 3 to 5 times per week.

or concomitant walking and strength training had no incremental effect on walking ability. Since in claudication the main deficit is ability to walk and given the principle of specificity of training, it is not surprising that walking results in greater benefit.

Assessment of Gait

Preliminary data suggest that gait is affected by PAD. Step length and steps per minute are lower in PAD patients than in controls (37). Changes in walking speed, step frequency, and other aspects of gait have not been measured in training studies, yet it is possible that inefficient gait may be a factor increasing the difficulty of walking. Rehabilitation physicians may be consulted if evaluation of gait abnormalities is desired.

Home-Based Walking Program

Home-based exercise programs have been evaluated for PAD patients (38). Results are variable but generally suggest that a hospital-based program has greater effectiveness. Clearly, where a home-based program is mandated, feedback and evaluation remain important.

Exercise Precautions and Special Considerations

For the most part, patients tolerate exercise training well. However, the potential for adverse events exists in any exercise program. There are two types of potential problems, cardiovascular and musculoskeletal. A cardiovascular problem is possible in PAD patients, since they have high prevalence of cardiac disease as well as PAD. To promote safety, all patients with clinical evidence of comorbid coronary disease are telemetry monitored during exercise sessions to evaluate heart rate and rhythm. Blood pressure is recorded before and after each training session. Thus far, in our experience in over 100 patients, no patient has experienced cardiovascular complication (serious arrhythmia, myocardial infarction, or stroke) during rehabilitation. Six patients have reported exacerbation of existing musculoskeletal problems (i.e., knee stiffness).

EXERCISE REHABILITATION: POTENTIAL MECHANISMS OF IMPROVEMENT

The mechanism or mechanisms by which an exercise rehabilitation program benefits persons with PAD remains incompletely delineated. Potential mechanisms for improvement include adaptations in peripheral blood flow or distribution of flow and changes in muscle metabolism.

Peripheral Blood Flow

Although various studies demonstrate increased peripheral blood flow with exercise training, more commonly, lack of increased peripheral blood flow has been observed (27, 32–36). Increased blood flow, when reported, is not correlated with changes in exercise performance. In addition to increased flow per se, other modifications of flow may occur and improve oxygen delivery to skeletal muscle. For example, decreased blood viscosity (39) or increased capillary density may alter exchange of oxygen and substrate at the capillary–muscle fiber interface.

Muscle Metabolism

In healthy subjects, exercise training is associated with improved oxidative metabolism of skeletal muscle (40). These changes are associated with improved extraction of oxygen and substrate during exercise. It has been postulated that chronic arterial insufficiency in PAD is associated with adaptive changes in the metabolic state of muscle (41). However, results have been variable. Increased oxidative enzyme activity in skeletal muscle is not always present in PAD (42). In addition, enzyme activities do not correlate with exercise performance, and one study demonstrated no change in citrate synthase after 12 weeks of rehabilitation (43).

In healthy individuals, carnitine is required for transport of long-chain fatty acyl groups into mitochondria. Under abnormal metabolic conditions, such as muscle ischemia, carnitine interacts with the cellular acyl–coenzyme A (CoA) pool to form acylcarnitines, which remove a variety of acyl groups derived from the corresponding acyl-CoA intermediates (44). In these circumstances, the formation of acylcarnitines reflects the underlying metabolic state of the cellular acyl-CoA pool and by removing potentially toxic acyl groups, may serve to maintain normal metabolism (45, 46).

Claudication pain during exercise is associated with (among other factors) an increased muscle concentration of acylcarnitines, reflecting the abnormal metabolic state of ischemic muscle (47). Exercise training reduces the plasma concentration of short-chain acylcarnitines. Furthermore, subjects who improved most from training also had the greatest reduction in plasma short-chain acylcarnitine concentration (27). It has recently been reported that training-induced changes in muscle carnitine metabolism are associated with improved functional status in the patient with claudication (43).

Changes in Walking Efficiency

It is possible that improvement in walking ability is related to a change in gait or pain threshold. The effects of exercise training on aspects of gait such as step length and steps per minute have not been assessed in PAD. However, it has been shown that oxygen consumption for a given constant workload decreases after exercise training (27). If the onset of claudication is due to mismatched oxygen delivery and oxygen demand, lower oxygen consumption per workload may be associated with an ability to walk longer after exercise training. This observation suggests that a change in the biomechanics of walking with training improves walking efficiency and decreases energy requirements of a given workload.

► **SUMMARY**

Intermittent claudication resulting from PAD impairs functional status. Reducing disability is therefore an important goal of treatment. To evaluate the efficacy of an intervention designed to improve functional status requires appropriate outcome measures. Such outcome measures include graded treadmill intervention (exercise rehabilitation). Importantly, exercise therapy has been shown to be effective and well tolerated. Patients improve both walking ability in the laboratory and functional status. Because of the effectiveness of this treatment, in addition to the low associated morbidity, exercise therapy is recommended as a major treatment option for persons with intermittent claudication due to PAD.

References

1. Criqui MH, Fronek A, Barret-Connor E, et al. The prevalence of peripheral arterial disease in a defined population. Circulation 71:510–515, 1985.
2. Hiatt WR, Marshall JA, Baxter J, et al. Diagnostic methods for peripheral arterial disease in the San Luis Valley Diabetes Study. J Clin Epidemiol 43:597–606, 1990.
3. Criqui MH, Coughlin SS, Fronek A. Noninvasively diagnosed peripheral arterial disease as a predictor of mortality: Results from a prospective study. Circulation 72:768–773, 1985.
4. Lassila R, Lepantalo M, Lindfors O. Peripheral arterial disease: Natural outcome. Acta Med Scand 220:295–301, 1986.
5. Regensteiner JG, Steiner JF, Panzer RJ, et al. Evaluation of walking impairment by questionnaire in patients with peripheral arterial disease. J Vasc Med Biol 2:142–152, 1990.
6. Regensteiner JG, Steiner JF, Hiatt WR. Exercise training improves functional status in patients with peripheral arterial disease. J Vasc Surg 1996:23;104–115.
7. Weber KT, Janicki JS. Cardiopulmonary Exercise Testing: Physiologic Principles and Clinical Applications. Philadelphia: Saunders, 1986.
8. Brand FN, Abbott RD, Kannel WB. Diabetes, intermittent claudication, and risk of cardiovascular events. Diabetes 38:504–509, 1989.
9. Coleridge-Smith PD, Thomas P, Scurr JH, et al. Causes of venous ulceration: A new hypothesis. BMJ 296:1726–1727, 1988.
10. Dormandy JA, Hoare E, Khattab AH, et al. Prognostic significance of rheological and biochemical findings in patients with intermittent claudication. BMJ 4:581–583, 1973.
11. Kannel WB, McGee DL. Diabetes and cardiovascular disease: The Framingham Study. JAMA 241:2035–2038, 1979.
12. Pomrehn P, Duncan B, Weissfeld L, et al. The association of dyslipoproteinemia with symptoms and signs of peripheral arterial disease: The lipids research clinics program prevalence study. Circulation 73 (Suppl I):1100–1107, 1986.
13. Kannel WB, McGee DL. Update on some epidemiologic features of intermittent claudication: The Framingham study. J Am Geriatr Soc 33:13–18, 1985.
14. Taylor LM, DeFrang RD, Harris EJ, et al. The association of elevated plasma homocyst(e)ine with progression of symptomatic peripheral arterial disease. J Vasc Surg 13:128–136, 1991.
15. Cantin B, Moorjani S, Dagenais GR, et al. Lipoprotein(a) distribution in a French Canadian population and its relation to intermittent claudication (The Quebec Cardiovascular Study). Am J Cardiol 75:1224–1228, 1995.
16. Quick CR, Cotton LT. The measured effect of stopping smoking on intermittent claudication. Br J Surg 69 (Suppl):S24–S26, 1982.
17. Creasy TS, McMillan PJ, Fletcher EW, et al. Is percutaneous transluminal angioplasty better than exercise for claudication? Preliminary results from a prospective randomized trial. Eur J Vasc Surg 4:135–140, 1990.
18. Regensteiner JG, Hargarten ME, Rutherford RB, et al. Functional benefits of peripheral vascular bypass surgery for patients with intermittent claudication. Angiology 44:1–10, 1993.
19. Doubilet P, Abrams HL. The cost of underutilization: Percutaneous transluminal angioplasty for peripheral vascular disease. N Engl J Med 310:95–102, 1984.
20. Jeans WD, Danton RM, Baird RN, et al. A comparison of the costs of vascular surgery and balloon dilatation in lower limb ischaemic disease. Br J Radiol 59:453–456, 1986.
21. Tunis SR, Bass EB, Steinberg EP. The use of angioplasty, bypass surgery, and amputation in the management of peripheral vascular disease. N Engl J Med 325:556–562, 1991.
22. Porter JM, Cutler BS, Lee BY, et al. Pentoxifylline efficacy in the treatment of intermittent claudication: Multicenter controlled double-blind trial with objective assessment of chronic occlusive arterial disease patients. Am Heart J 104:66–72, 1982.
23. Orchard TJ, Strandness DE, Cavanaugh PR, et al. Assessment of peripheral vascular disease in diabetes: Report and recommendations of an international workshop. Circulation 1993;88:819–828.
24. Hiatt WR, Nawaz D, Regensteiner JG, et al. The evaluation of exercise performance in patients with peripheral vascular disease. J Cardiopulm Rehab 12:525–532, 1988.
25. Patterson JA, Naughton J, Pietras RJ, et al. Treadmill exercise in assessment of the functional capacity of patients with cardiac disease. Am J Cardiol 30:757–762, 1972.
26. Gardner AW, Skinner JS, Cantwell BW, et al. Progressive vs single-stage treadmill tests for evaluation of claudication. Med Sci Sports Exerc 23:402–408, 1991.
27. Hiatt WR, Regensteiner JG, Hargarten ME, et al. Benefit of exercise conditioning for patients with peripheral arterial disease. Circulation 81:602–609, 1990.
28. Hiatt WR, Wolfel EE, Meier RH, et al. Superiority of treadmill walking exercise vs. strength training for patients with peripheral arterial disease: Implications for the mechanism of the training response. Circulation 90:1866–1874, 1994.
29. Sallis JF, Haskell WL, Wood PD, et al. Physical activity assessment methodology in the five-city project. Am J Epidemiol 121:91–106, 1985.

30. Tarlov AR, Ware JE, Greenfield S, et al. The medical outcomes study: An application of methods for monitoring the results of medical care. JAMA 262:925–930, 1989.
31. Dahllof A, Bjorntorp P, Holm J, et al. Metabolic activity of skeletal muscle in patients with peripheral arterial insufficiency: Effect of physical training. Eur J Clin Invest 4:9–15, 1974.
32. Dhallof A, Holm J, Schersten T, et al. Peripheral arterial insufficiency: Effect of physical training on walking tolerance, calf blood flow, and blood flow resistance. Scand I Rehab Med 8:19–26, 1976.
33. Larsen OA, Lassen NA. Effect of daily muscular exercise in patients with intermittent claudication. Lancet 2:1093–1096, 1966.
34. Holm J, Dahllof A, Bjorntorp P, et al. Enzyme studies in muscles of patients with intermittent claudication: Effect of training. Scand J Clin Lab Invest 31(Suppl 128):201–205, 1973.
35. Mannarino E, Pasqualini L, Innocente S, et al. Physical training and antiplatelet treatment in stage II peripheral arterial occlusive disease: Alone or combined? Angiology 42:513–521, 1991.
36. Lundgren F, Dahllof A, Lundholm K, et al. Intermittent claudication: Surgical reconstruction or physical training? A prospective randomized trial of treatment efficiency. Ann Surg 209:346–355, 1989.
37. Scherer SA, Bainbridge JS, Hiatt WR, Regensteiner JG. Gait characteristics of patients with claudication. Arch Phys Med Rehabil 79:529–531, 1999.
38. Regensteiner JG, Meyer T, Krupski W, et al. Comparison of home vs. hospital based rehabilitation for patients with peripheral arterial disease. Angiology 48:291–300, 1997.
39. Ernst EE, Matral A. Intermittent claudication, exercise, and blood rheology. Circulation 76:1110–1114, 1987.
40. Holloszy JO, Coyle, EF. Adaptations of skeletal muscle to endurance exercise and their metabolic consequences. J Appl Physiol 56:831–838, 1984.
41. Jansson E, Johansson J, Sylven C, et al. Calf muscle adaptation in intermittent claudication: Side-differences in muscle metabolic characteristics in patients with unilateral arterial disease. Clin Physiol 8:17–29, 1988.
42. Regensteiner JG, Wolfel EE, Brass EP, et al. Chronic changes in skeletal muscle histology and function in peripheral arterial disease. Circulation 87:413–421, 1993.
43. Hiatt WR, Regensteiner JG, Carry M, et al. Brass. Effect of exercise training on skeletal muscle histology and metabolism in peripheral arterial disease. J Appl Physiol 81:780–788, 1996.
44. Bieber LL, Emaus R, Valkner K, et al. Possible functions of short-chain and medium-chain carnitine acyltransferases. Fed Proc 41:2858–2862, 1982.
45. Brass EP, Hoppel CL. Relationship between acid-soluble carnitine and coenzyme A pools in vivo. Biochem J 190:495–504, 1980.
46. Brass EP, Fennessey PV, Miller LV. Inhibition of oxidative metabolism by propionic acid and its reversal by carnitine in isolated rat hepatocytes. Biochem J 236:131–136, 1986.
47. Hiatt WR, Wolfel EE, Regensteiner JG, et al. Skeletal muscle carnitine metabolism in patients with unilateral peripheral arterial disease. J Appl Physiol 73:346–353, 1992.

Suggested Reading

Ernst E, Fialka V. A review of the clinical effectiveness of exercise therapy for intermittent claudication. Arch Intern Med 153:2357–2360, 1993.
Gardner AW, Poehlman ET. Exercise rehabilitation programs for the treatment of claudication pain:A meta-analysis. JAMA 274:975–980, 1995.
Regensteiner JG, Hiatt WR. Exercise rehabilitation for patients with peripheral arterial disease. Exerc Sports Sci Rev 23:1–24, 1995.

1.1.0.1   2.4.7.   4.8.6, 4.8.6.1., 4.8.14.

CHAPTER **34**

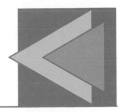

EXERCISE FOR SKELETAL HEALTH AND OSTEOPOROSIS PREVENTION

Janet M. Shaw, Kara A. Witzke, and Kerri M. Winters

Osteoporosis is a systemic skeletal disease characterized by low bone mass and microarchitectural deterioration of bone tissue leading to bone fragility and increased risk of fracture. It is estimated that more than 1.5 million osteoporotic fractures occur annually, which clearly establishes osteoporosis as a major public health care concern. Common fracture sites include the wrist, spine, and hip. Estimates of direct health care costs associated with these three types of fractures in white women over age 45 have been projected to be $45.2 billion over the next 10 years (1). Hip fractures will account for most of these expenses, and hip fractures have the most devastating personal consequences, such as loss of independence, prolonged immobility, and death due to multisystem failure. As with other chronic diseases, prevention of osteoporotic fractures is the focus of much research and debate (2). Preventive measures include altering lifestyle factors, such as nutrition and exercise, and administration of pharmacological agents (e.g., reproductive hormones, amino bisphosphonates, selective estrogen receptor modulators). This chapter provides a brief overview of skeletal physiology, presents research findings that help define the role of exercise in decreasing the risk of osteoporotic fractures, and suggests practical applications in developing an appropriate exercise prescription for skeletal health.

PURPOSE AND ORGANIZATION OF THE SKELETON

The skeleton has three primary purposes. The first is to support loads against gravity and to aid in locomotion by providing sites for muscular attachment. Second, bone provides a protective barrier for vital organs and bone marrow. Finally, the skeleton serves as a mineral reservoir that supports blood levels of calcium and phosphorus when needed.

The skeleton can be divided into appendicular (peripheral) and axial (central) components (see Figure 9.1). The appendicular skeleton comprises approximately 80% of total skeletal mass and consists primarily of cortical ("compact") bone. The concentric orientation of lamellae deposited around a central nutrient canal in cortical bone forms a dense tissue. Approximately 80–90% of the total volume of cortical bone is calcified. In contrast, the axial skeleton has a high percentage of trabecular ("spongy") bone, in which lamellae are arranged along a flat surface. Only 15–25% of trabecular bone volume is calcified; the remaining volume is occupied by bone marrow, fat, and blood vessels. Trabecular bone has a high ratio of surface area to volume and is close to hematopoietic activity of red marrow in the adult skeleton. Thus, trabecular bone is more metabolically active than cortical bone and consequently exhibits a greater rate of turnover.

BONE REMODELING

In the mature skeleton, bone is subjected to a dynamic process of breakdown and renewal termed *remodeling*. The purpose of remodeling is to maintain the mechanical integrity of the tissue by replacing fatigue-damaged older bone with new bone. Multinucleated osteoclasts erode portions of the bone surface, creating resorptive cavities. Within the cavity, osteoblasts secrete a collagen matrix that becomes mineralized. The events in a typical remodeling cycle are depicted in Figure 34.1. In normal conditions, remodeling is a coupled process, meaning that formation follows resorption. However, it is hypothesized that this process is inefficient in the adult skeleton and that small deficits in formation remain at the completion of one remodeling cycle. The accumulation of these formation deficits is thought to be partially responsible for age-related losses in bone mass. Thus, bone that undergoes the greatest number of remodeling cycles is at highest risk for age-related losses. Because of its high metabolic activity and the amount of surface area exposed, the relatively high rate of turnover in trabecular bone predisposes it to higher age-related loss than cortical bone and thus to fractures. In contrast to the mature skeleton, *modeling*, or new bone formation *not* preceded by resorption, is the dominant activity in growing bones. Modeling is the process by which bones gain mass as well as modifications in shape.

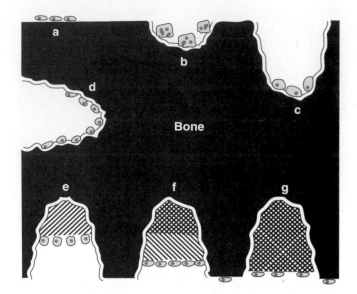

Figure 34.1. A. Resting trabecular surface. **B.** Multinucleated osteoclasts dig a cavity of approximately 20 μm. **C.** Completion of resorption to 60 μm by mononuclear phagocytes. **D.** Recruitment of osteoblast precursors to the base of the resorptive cavity. **E.** Secretion of new matrix by osteoblasts. **F.** Continued secretion of matrix with initiation of calcification. **G.** Completion of mineralization of new matrix. Bone has returned to a quiescent state, but a small deficit in bone mass persists. (Reprinted with permission from Marcus R. Normal and abnormal bone remodelling in man. Adv Intern Med 38:129–141, 1987.)

Reproductive hormones, calcium intake, and mechanical loading are three primary factors that regulate remodeling activity. When reproductive hormone status is compromised, such as in young, amenorrheic, or estrogen-depleted postmenopausal women, reductions in bone mineral density (BMD) are observed. Hypoestrogenism is characterized by increased resorption, which is typically reversed with hormone replacement therapy (HRT). Hence, HRT is an antiresorptive agent, as it arrests bone loss in most postmenopausal women. Other antiresorptive pharmaceutical therapies have recently become available. They include bisphosphonates such as alendronate (Fosamax), calcitonin, and a new class of drugs that act as selective estrogen receptor modulators (SERMs), such as raloxifene (Evista). The connection between bone metabolism and testosterone levels in men is less clear; however, in some cases, levels of testosterone in men have been weakly associated with BMD. Although their mechanism of action is poorly understood, androgens are generally thought to be important for skeletal health.

Remodeling activity increases when dietary calcium intake is insufficient. This effect, mediated by parathyroid hormone (PTH), provides an important means of maintaining adequate blood levels of calcium. Calcium intake during growth is essential to supply the raw materials necessary for optimal bone mineral accretion (see Table 3.3

for daily calcium requirements). On the other end of the spectrum, older individuals, particularly estrogen-depleted postmenopausal women, may have impaired intestinal absorption of calcium, and therefore calcium requirements are higher in this group. Recognizing the importance of calcium nutrition for bone health, the National Institutes for Health (NIH) Consensus Conference has put forth more aggressive guidelines for calcium intake than the recommended daily allowance (RDA) (3). For example, postmenopausal women who are estrogen-depleted are recommended to take 1500 mg of calcium per day, compared to the RDA of 800 mg per day. Calcium supplementation in these individuals may reduce the rate of bone loss and even reduce fracture risk. However, supplementation is less effective than hormone replacement for these purposes and appears unable to increase BMD (3). Hence, adequate calcium nutrition reduces the likelihood of hypersecretion of PTH and thus increased bone turnover. Attention to calcium intake is most important during growth and in older adults whose compensatory mechanisms for regulation of circulating calcium levels are less robust than among their younger adult counterparts.

Lastly, bone responds to alterations in mechanical forces, and the regulation of bone strength is a function of the loads to which the skeleton is subjected. In the absence of mechanical forces, such as during space flight and prolonged bed rest, urinary calcium excretion increases and BMD decreases (4, 5). This is likely to be a result of increased resorption and a reduction in new bone formation. Mechanical stimuli are important for maintaining bone mass and thus inducing a modeling response in mature bone. Mechanical force magnitude has been shown to be a more important stimulus for skeletal modeling than the number of force repetitions or load cycles (6). The rate at which peak force is delivered is emerging as another factor in determining the osteogenic potential of a loading regimen. This is supported by the number of studies that demonstrate increased BMD from impact exercise, in which forces on the skeleton are delivered very quickly (7–11). The absolute force magnitude and rate of force development that best promote skeletal health have yet to be defined, but both are important.

BONE MASS ASSESSMENT

Technological advances have enabled researchers to assess bone mass noninvasively with a high degree of precision at important fracture sites: the distal radius, proximal femur (hip), and lumbar spine. Dual-energy x-ray absorptiometry (DXA), the assessment technique used by many, quantifies mineral content per unit area of bone. The outcome variables include bone mineral content (BMC) in grams and BMD in grams per square centimeter. Bone mineral density is referred to as areal density, since it is expressed per unit area and therefore is not a true volumetric measure. In this chapter, BMD will be used synonymously with bone mass. It is highly correlated with bone strength, hence resistance to fracture (12, 13). Therefore, BMD is used as a primary outcome measure in research studies to determine the effectiveness of any particular intervention to reduce fracture risk. The U.S. Food and Drug Administration (FDA) has recently approved quantitative ultrasound (QUS) as a screening tool to determine which individuals will benefit most from a DXA scan. Measures from QUS scans, broadband ultrasound attenuation and ultrasound transmission velocity, have been correlated to the mechanical properties of bone and may provide information that is qualitatively different from that derived from DXA (14). A QUS scan is typically performed on the calcaneus (heel) or other peripheral site. Since many QUS devices are portable, the studies are low cost, the technology does not expose individuals to ionizing radiation, and QUS is being used extensively in health screenings across the country. However, while QUS fulfills a vital role in earmarking those who may be at increased risk, only a DXA scan or radiography (i.e., to detect fractures) can be used to make diagnoses of osteoporosis.

BONE MASS CHANGES WITH AGE

Changes in bone mass across the lifespan in girls and women are depicted in Figure 34.2. Periods of growth are dominated by modeling and rapid increases in bone mass. Peak bone mass is attained at the end of longitudinal growth, after which a plateau in BMD may be observed in the second and third decades of life. Age-related bone loss begins between the end of the second and the beginning of the fourth decade of life. The point at which losses begin probably varies in individuals as a function of factors such as sex (men may start losing bone mass later in life than women) and lifestyle (i.e., variations in exercise, diet, cigarette smoking, alcohol consumption,

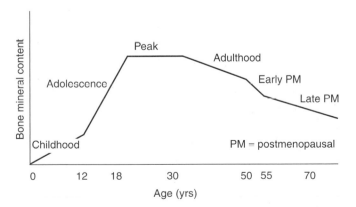

Figure 34.2. Model of bone mineral content changes with age in women. (Reprinted with permission from Snow-Harter, C.: Exercise, calcium and estrogen: Primary regulators of bone mass. Contemporary Nutrition 17(4), 1992.)

and parity). Age-related losses are most notable at sites with a high percentage of trabecular bone, occurring at a rate of 0.5–1% per year (15). This gradual rate of loss continues throughout the adult years but is interrupted by menopause in women. As a consequence of estrogen deficiency, women not taking HRT exhibit an accelerated rate of loss in the first 5–7 years of menopause (early PM) (16). Bone loss eventually returns to a slower rate once the woman has adapted to hormone deficiency (late PM).

Bone mass changes across the lifespan in boys and men are similar to those observed in girls and women with a few exceptions. Peak BMD is higher, the rate of loss in men may not be as great as in women, and losses may begin later in life (17). Testosterone levels decline with age; however, hormonal changes are not as uniform in men nor are they as strongly correlated with reductions in BMD as those observed with estrogen deficiency in postmenopausal women.

EXERCISE AND BONE MASS

Physical activity transmits mechanical loads to the skeleton via gravitational forces and muscular pull at the sites of attachment. Support for exercise as a preventive measure for osteoporosis was provided initially by the observation that physically active individuals and athletes typically have higher bone mass than sedentary controls. Within athletic groups, those involved in sports with unilateral activity, such as tennis, demonstrate higher BMD in the dominant (playing) arm than in the other arm (18). Further attempts to delineate the types of loading associated with the highest bone mass have resulted in more specific athletic group comparisons. Cross-sectional research demonstrates that individuals in activities that require very high muscle forces and impact loads (e.g., gymnastics) have higher bone mass than those in endurance training (e.g., distance running) (19). Furthermore, those who participate in activities characterized by substantial muscular involvement without gravitational forces or impact (e.g., swimming) have lower BMD than those engaged in activities with a weight-bearing component (20). This is not to de-emphasize the many benefits of water-based or other non–weight-bearing modes of exercise but rather to characterize the loading regimen of athletic groups with high BMD. Whether water-based exercise has detrimental effects on the skeleton has yet to be determined in controlled longitudinal trials. Finally, those who regularly engage in weight training typically have higher bone mass at the hip and spine than their non–weight training counterparts (21, 22). This is consistent with the studies on athletes, assuming that weight training affords higher than normal forces on the musculoskeletal system.

In addition to specific group comparisons, BMD has been correlated with parameters of fitness. Body composition, notably lean tissue mass and muscle strength, consistently correlate with bone mass in various age groups. Some associations between fat mass and BMD have been observed, although this relation is not well understood. Adiposity affords additional loading, albeit nonspecific, by increasing body weight. It is plausible that increased adiposity benefits the skeleton by increasing circulating levels of estrogens; however, the contribution of adrenal estrogens is probably small compared to that supplied by the ovaries. Muscle strength has been found to be an important determinant of BMD in children and in young and older adults, and this association appears to be site specific. For example, muscle strength of the hip abductors, which attach at the greater trochanter, has been shown to be a robust predictor of hip (femoral neck) BMD in both premenopausal and postmenopausal women (23). Recently, site-specific relationships between muscle strength and bone mass lost significance when the corresponding lean tissue mass was accounted for in correlational analyses (24, 25). Hence, lean tissue mass, a strong determinant of muscle strength, may be accounting for the relationship between muscle strength and bone mass.

Cross-sectional comparisons indicate that high BMD is typically observed in those with high lean tissue mass and high muscle strength and in those whose activities require high muscle forces and often involve significant impacts. The potential for selection bias warrants caution in the interpretation of these results, since causal attributions cannot be made from cross-sectional research. These data have been used, however, as the basis for designing longitudinal interventions to determine exercise training effects on bone mass.

LONGITUDINAL STUDIES AND PRINCIPLES OF TRAINING

Longitudinal data demonstrate equivocal findings in studies that induce mechanical loads through exercise. Results range from small (1–2%) increases in or maintenance (no change) of BMD to decrements in bone density. The improvements in BMD that have been observed are much smaller than would be expected from the cross-sectional literature. Any successful exercise program must

adhere to the principles of training to produce beneficial effects on a target tissue or system. Drinkwater (26) has emphasized the importance of including these training principles in exercise intervention programs for bone (Table 34.1). To date, many studies have neglected one or more of these principles, which may be the reason for minimal or no training effects on bone. Furthermore, training responses may depend on developmental stage, as young bone may be more responsive to additional loads than older bone.

Given the aforementioned cross-sectional research findings, weight training has been studied extensively as a means to increase bone mass. Most exercises on traditional weight machines, especially those for the lower body, are performed with the person seated, a position that reduces forces at the hip. This violates the principle of specificity and may partially explain why machine-based resistance training regimens have found increases in spine BMD but have had difficulty in achieving increases in hip BMD. The spine is sufficiently loaded when a person is seated. This notion is supported by the BMD patterns observed in those with spinal cord injury who are confined to a wheelchair. Specifically, spinal cord injury results in dramatically reduced hip BMD, but spine BMD in this population is similar to that of the able bodied (27). The use of free weights and/or machines that require standing have been shown to increase BMD at the hip in postmenopausal women (28, 29).

Appropriate overload in a program for improving bone mass must induce forces that are greater than those of the activities of daily living, in effect stimulating bone to respond and reorganize to meet the demands for increased loads. Optimal overload is difficult to define, given the scarcity of data on load quantification at specific skeletal sites, such as the hip and the spine, for various activities. Based upon the literature and preliminary laboratory studies, high skeletal loading intensity has been defined as ground reaction forces of greater than 4 times body weight, moderate intensity as 2–4 times body weight, and low intensity as ground reaction forces less than twice body weight (30). Thus, not all weight-bearing activities are likely to be osteogenic, given the range of intensities. Walking is an excellent mode of training for improving cardiovascular fitness, but its ability to produce a strong

Table 34.1. Principles of Training

SPECIFICITY	OVERLOAD	REVERSIBILITY	INITIAL VALUES	DIMINISHING RETURNS
Loading should occur at the bone site of interest because of a localized effect.	Loading to the bone must be significantly greater than that from daily activity.	In the adult skeleton, when loading is removed, the positive effect on bone is lost.	Individuals with low BMD have the most to gain from increased loading.	The biological ceiling of a person determines the extent of adaptation to the loading.

Adapted with permission from Drinkwater BL. C.H. McCloy research lecture: Does physical activity play a role in preventing osteoporosis? Res Q Exerc Sport 65:197–206, 1994.

enough signal for bone to adapt is questionable, especially in those who are able bodied and ambulatory. Limited information suggests that walking results in forces approximately equal to body weight at the lumbar spine. Walking alone has not been shown to be effective in arresting bone loss in postmenopausal women (31). Forces at the lumbar spine during weight training have been estimated to be 5–6 times body weight, but forces at the hip, which vary with the type of exercise, have not been quantified during weight training (32). Ground reaction forces of 10–12 times body weight have been observed in gymnastics training (33).

With respect to appropriate overload, gymnasts exhibit increased spine and hip BMD after 9 months of training (34). In this activity the forces on the skeleton not only are high but also develop fast because of the impact nature of the sport. Jumping mimics the forces exerted during gymnastics training. Increases in hip BMD of up to 4% have been observed in premenopausal women who performed 50 two-footed jumps from the floor, 3 days per week over 6 months (11). More recent reports have demonstrated similar response at the hip (2–3%) in addition to improvements in muscle strength, power, and balance with multicomponent programs (resistance training, step aerobics) that included jumping (8, 10). Jumping within the context of school-based interventions have also met with favor by increasing hip bone mass in prepubertal children (7, 35).

The principle of reversibility states that once the osteogenic stimulus is removed, the positive effects on bone will be lost. Improvements in spinal BMC were demonstrated in postmenopausal women with a program consisting of vigorous progressive exercises, including walking, jogging, stair climbing, and rowing (36). Those who discontinued participation in the exercise program had reversal in bone mass, which confirmed that the benefits of the training persist only as long as the stimulus is present. Reversibility has also been demonstrated in premenopausal women. Women who gained bone mass at the hip after a year of highly specific lower body resistance training plus impact exercise lost BMD after a 6-month detraining period during which no part of the specific training was maintained (8). In contrast, premenopausal women who continued to engage in voluntary, unsupervised aerobic and step training exercise 2 days per week for 10 months following a controlled 8-month intervention that took place 3 times per week maintained bone mass gains achieved during the original investigation (37). This indicates that the training stimulus was sufficient to maintain BMD despite reduced frequency and with a less structured format. Prospective bone mass increases in collegiate gymnasts during a training season are almost negated by declines observed in their off-season, when the impact loads are withdrawn (34). Young children are the only group likely to retain skeletal benefits associated with mechanical loading even after detraining.

Bone mineral increases at the hip observed with a jumping intervention in prepubertal children were maintained after 7 months of resuming preintervention activities (7; C.M. Snow, personal communication). A lack of reversibility response in young children supports the assertion that mechanical loading to increase peak bone mass may be a primary strategy to prevent osteoporosis.

Initial values play a role in the expected skeletal response to increased mechanical loads. Those with low initial values are most likely to demonstrate a response to exercise training. Once a training habit is established and maintained, further responses take longer to achieve, and the magnitude of change is less (diminishing returns). The time course for training responses to plateau is difficult to determine, given that most interventions have been conducted for only 6 months to a year. The ability of these training principles in formulating an exercise program to produce the desired response may depend on age. It has been proposed that young bone responds to increased mechanical stimuli more favorably than older bone. The aforementioned changes in gymnasts provide support for this idea, since the gymnasts demonstrated improvements despite having high initial BMD. Achieving a plateau where the magnitude of change is reduced would require continuous training without intervening summer sessions.

In addition to the principles of training, it is important to emphasize the time frame necessary to expect changes in bone mass and the likely magnitude of response. The time course of a trabecular remodeling cycle is approximately 3–4 months, and about 9 months to a year of follow-up is needed to detect significant changes in bone mass. In contrast to the muscular system, in which the magnitude of change is great (20–200%, depending on initial values) over a relatively short time (8–16 weeks), an increase in bone mass of more than 1% over 9 months is meaningful, especially given that average rates of loss are 0.5–1% per year and that DXA technology is precise. Furthermore, a 3–5% increase in BMD is associated with a 20–30% reduction in fractures (38). The magnitude of BMD change observed in young children and premenopausal women with impact exercise intervention is typically within 3–5%, which indicates the practical and clinical significance of these interventions.

SPECIAL CONSIDERATIONS

Amenorrheic and Postmenopausal Women

From puberty and into adulthood, the reproductive hormones assume a critical role in the maintenance of optimal bone health. This is especially evident in young women with menstrual cycle dysfunction and in early postmenopausal women (16, 35). These two groups have accelerated losses in bone mineral that are associated with hypoestrogenism. It has been proposed that reproductive hormones play a permissive role in the ability of mechanical loading to increase bone mass. It is improbable that additional loading from exercise can counteract the negative effects of hypoestrogenism observed in amenorrhea and early menopause. Low caloric intake and generally poor nutrition, low body weight and body fat, and high-volume physical training are likely contributing factors to exercise amenorrhea. However, bone mass of amenorrheic highly active women without eating disorders is still likely to be lower at most skeletal sites than that of menstruating women of similar body weight and training volume (39). The negative influence of amenorrhea on bone mass is well documented, and it is unlikely that bone losses with amenorrhea can be recovered with resumption of menses. Therefore, maintenance of normal reproductive endocrine function should be a high priority in young women. With respect to its effects on bone mass, exercise should be considered an adjunct to HRT in the early postmenopausal woman.

Exercise and Risk of Falling

Muscle strength, mass, and power decline with age, and it is well established that these factors are important for maintaining optimal function in older populations. Falls in older, nonclinical community-dwelling adults are associated with lower extremity muscular weakness, increases in reaction time, and postural instability. Most hip fractures and some vertebral fractures occur with a fall. Hence, fall risk, in addition to BMD, is a major consideration in the prevention of fractures in older adults. One intervention has successfully demonstrated improvements in muscle strength, muscle mass, bone mass, and dynamic balance in estrogen-depleted postmenopausal women (40). This regimen included dynamic resistance training at high relative intensity (80% of 1RM) two days per week on pneumatic machines. Earlier reports have confirmed via muscle biopsies that older men and women exhibit muscle hypertrophy in response to weight training and that older adults can tolerate well this type of program, using both free weights and machines.

Although falls are a leading cause of injury in older adults, most do not result in hip fracture. Close examination of falls reveals that the contact area and velocity at impact are important determinants of fracture (41). Falls to the side in which the impact is absorbed directly by the hip are most likely to result in fracture (42). Results of a recent intervention using a weighted vest and jumping exercises in postmenopausal women suggest potential for decreasing risk of falls to the side (43). Improvements in lower body muscle strength, power, and mass in addition to lateral postural stability were found after 9 months of training using weight-bearing exercises such as squats, lunges, rising from a chair, and jumping. The intervention encouraged development of the hip abductor muscles and leg extensor power, both of which were related to improvement in indices of lateral stability. One recent report

has demonstrated a reduction in total falls and injurious falls by 40% as a result of exercise intervention (44). This multicomponent intervention, which was conducted in community-dwelling individuals over 80 years of age, incorporated walking and resistance training and encouraged stair climbing in the context of daily activities. Very few studies have attempted to reduce falls and their injurious outcomes with exercise intervention, probably because of the large number of participants required for such research. From the data available, incorporation of functional activities that increase muscle strength, power, and mass and that also promote improvements in dynamic balance should be encouraged in older adults to prevent falls, especially those to the side, which are particularly likely to precipitate hip fractures.

PRACTICAL IMPLICATIONS

As an osteoporosis prevention strategy, exercise has four main applications: (*a*) to *increase* bone mass during and just after periods of growth, thus improving peak bone mass; (*b*) to *increase or maintain* bone mass in early to middle adulthood; (*c*) to *decrease* rates of bone loss in older adults; and (*d*) to reduce falls.

In light of the principles of training and available research, weight-bearing modes of exercise that emphasize high force magnitude and encourage development of the muscular system are recommended for skeletal health. Deciding on an exercise modality requires consideration of the age and/or physical limitations of the group or individual (Table 34.2). Certainly adolescents and younger individuals have more capacity to perform intensive activities, such as jumping, than do the frail elderly. Young and middle-aged adults can benefit from programs that include both impact and muscular development exercises, as this combination has been found effective for improving bone mass without consequent increases in joint injury (7, 8). Making 25–50 jumps in place at floor level 3 days per week has been well tolerated in healthy postmenopausal women without osteoporosis, and recent evidence suggests that older women who participate in long-term (5 years) weighted vest exercise with jumping maintain hip BMD (43, 45, 46). In addition to maintaining hip BMD, jumping exercise improves most women's muscle power, which is an important determinant of functional ability in elderly women (47). In addition, strength training in men and women in their 50s and 60s has produced similar absolute increases in muscular strength and power as in subjects in their 20s (48). In the frail elderly, many weight-bearing exercise modes, including high-intensity weight training and exercise with free weights, have met with success (49). In epidemiological research, the amount of walking and the overall caloric expenditure are higher in those who do not fracture, and thus, these general markers of habitual physical activity consistently emerge as factors that reduce the risk of hip

Table 34.2. **Activity Guidelines**

Children and adolescents	Activities involving jumping that mimic play are enjoyable and appear effective. 100 jumps from 24-inch boxes, 3 times/wk
Healthy premenopausal women	Lower body strength training in standing position with free weights: 2–3 sets at 6–10 RM (up to 80% of 1RM), 3 days/wk 50 two-footed jumps in place[a], 3 days/wk
Healthy nonosteoporotic postmenopausal women	Machine based or free weights as tolerated: 1–3 sets at 10–15 RM to begin, progress to 2–3 sets at 6–10 RM (up to 80% of 1RM), minimum of 2–3 days per week 50 two-footed jumps in place[a], 3 days/wk
Osteoporotic women	1–3 sets, 5–8 repetitions, of 4–6 weight-bearing lower body strength exercises using body weight as resistance, 2–3 days per week Additional resistance may be applied gradually and conservatively (up to 10 lb) with a weighted vest Therapy bands and rubber tubing may be used to facilitate range of motion exercises Avoid impact exercise, spinal flexion against resistance (e.g., keep back straight), high compressive forces on the spine, exercises that involve quick trunk rotation

[a] Jumps were performed in stocking feet (no shoes) on wooden floors within the context of the research, but this may go against risk management recommendations in many practical settings (10, 41).

fracture (50). Further research is needed to delineate the exercise mode that is most efficacious for reducing dangerous falls that result in hip fractures in the elderly.

Young bone is likely to respond more favorably to mechanical loading than old bone, and therefore, introduction of high mechanical loads during this stage of life may elicit the best skeletal response. Prepubertal children tolerate and even enjoy a high degree of mechanical loading. Children in the second grade jumped from 24-inch boxes up to 100 times 3 times per week. Bone mass at the hip was 5% higher in jumpers than in controls at the end of the 8-month intervention (7). Achieving optimal peak bone mass at the end of longitudinal growth will afford skeletal protection by delaying the point at which BMD is critically reduced, fractures are more likely, and preventive measures are few. Interestingly, premenopausal and postmenopausal women completing the same jumping intervention had different bone mass responses: the premenopausal women increased BMD at the hip, but the postmenopausal women exhibited no consistent pattern, despite having controlled for estrogen replacement status (45). Calcium intake and self-reported physical activity were important contributors to increases in spine bone mass in women in the third decade of life, a time at which

bone mass may level off (51). The premenopausal years may therefore be a fruitful time to increase bone mass, especially if progressive training regimens (i.e., impact exercise and/or free weight training) are used.

It is unlikely that dramatic increases in bone mass are attainable in the older skeleton. However, small improvements in or maintenance of bone mass can make a difference in the overall fracture risk profile. Resistance training that promotes functional ability may not elicit improvements in bone mass in all older persons, but the benefits of this training, such as reducing key indices of fall risk, are substantial. Weight training programs are therefore recommended for older adults, even for those who are frail. The frequency of training should be 2–3 times per week, with varying recommendations of the number of sets, repetitions, and intensity, depending on the characteristics of the target group (Table 34.2). Impact exercise should not be performed by those with osteoporosis and/or other conditions (i.e., osteoarthritis, urinary incontinence, severe dizziness) for whom the exercise may be contraindicated or otherwise objectionable. Other contraindicated activities for those with osteoporosis include exercises that place high compressive forces on the spine with trunk flexion as well as activities that result in quick trunk rotation. Standard screening practices should be followed, and older individuals with multiple risk factors for osteoporosis who have not been diagnosed should be treated conservatively.

References

1. Chrischilles C, Sherman T, Wallace R. Cost and health effects of osteoporotic fractures. Bone 15:377–386, 1994.
2. Salkeld G, Cameron ID, Cumming RG, et al. Quality of life related to fear of falling and hip fracture in older women: A time trade off study. BMJ 320:341–346, 2000.
3. Dawson-Hughes B. The role of calcium in the treatment of osteoporosis. In: Marcus R, Feldman D, Kelsey J, eds. Osteoporosis. San Diego: Academic, 1996.
4. Tipton CM, Hargens A. Physiological adaptations and countermeasures associated with long-duration spaceflights. Med Sci Sports Exerc 28:974–976, 1996.
5. Smith SM, Lane HW. Gravity and space flight: Effects on nutritional status. Curr Opin Clin Nutr Metab Care 2:335–338, 1999.
6. Rubin CT, Lanyon LE. Osteoregulatory nature of mechanical stimuli: Function as a determinant for adaptive remodeling in bone. J Orthop Res 5:300–310, 1987.
7. Fuchs RK, Snow CM. Jumping improves femoral neck bone mass in children. Med Sci Sports Exerc 31:S83, 1999.
8. Winters KM, Snow CM. Detraining reverses positive effects of exercise on the musculoskeletal system in premenopausal women. J Bone Miner Res 15:2495–2503, 2000.
9. Witzke KA, Snow CM. Effects of plyometric jump training on bone mass in adolescent girls. Med Sci Sports Exerc 32:1051–1057, 2000.
10. Heinonen A, Kannus P, Sievanen H, et al. Randomised controlled trial of effect of high-impact exercise on selected risk

factors for osteoporotic fractures. Lancet 348:1343–1347, 1996.

11. Bassey EJ, Ramsdale SJ. Increase in femoral bone density in young women following high-impact exercise. Osteoporosis Int 4:72–75, 1994.

12. Oden ZM, Selvitelli DM, Hayes WC, Myers ER. The effect of trabecular structure on DXA-based predictions of bovine bone failure. Calcif Tissue Int 63:67–73, 1998.

13. Bouxsein ML, Coan BS, Lee SC. Prediction of the strength of the elderly proximal femur by bone mineral density and quantitative ultrasound measurements of the heel and tibia. Bone 25:49–54, 1999.

14. Bouxsein, ML, Radloff, SE. Quantitative ultrasound of the calcaneus reflects the mechanical properties of calcaneal trabecular bone. J Bone Miner Res 12:839–846, 1997.

15. Marcus R, Kosek J, Pfefferbaum A, Horning S. Age-related loss of trabecular bone in premenopausal women: A biopsy study. Calcif Tissue Int 35:406–409, 1983.

16. Reeve J, Walton J, Russell LJ, et al. Determinants of the first decade of bone loss after menopause at spine, hip and radius. Q J Med 92:261–273,1999.

17. Orwoll ES, Klein RF. Osteoporosis in men. Endocrine Rev 16:87–116, 1995.

18. Kannus P, Haapasalo, Sievanen H, et al. The site-specific effects of long-term unilateral activity on bone mineral density and content. Bone 15:279–284, 1994.

19. Robinson TL, Snow-Harter C, Taaffe DR, et al. Gymnasts exhibit higher bone mass than runners despite similar prevalence of amenorrhea and oligomenorrhea. J Bone Miner Res 10:26–35, 1995.

20. Taaffe DR, Snow-Harter C, Connolly DA, et al. Differential effects of swimming versus weight-bearing activity on bone mineral status of eumenorrheic athletes. J Bone Miner Res 10:586–593, 1995.

21. Conroy BP, Kraemer WJ, Maresh CM, et al. Bone mineral density in elite junior Olympic weightlifters. Med Sci Sports Exerc 25:1103–1109, 1993.

22. Heinrich CH, Going SB, Pamenter RW, et al. Bone mineral content of cyclically menstruating female resistance and endurance trained athletes. Med Sci Sports Exerc 22:558–563, 1990.

23. Snow-Harter C, Robinson T, Shaw J, et al. Determinants of femoral neck mineral density in pre- and postmenopausal women. Med Sci Sports Exerc 25:Suppl S153, 1993.

24. Witzke KA, Snow CM. Lean body mass and leg power best predict bone mineral density in adolescent girls. Med Sci Sports Exerc 31:1558–1563, 1999.

25. Madsen KL, Adams WC, Van Loan MD. Effects of physical activity, body weight and composition, and muscular strength on bone density in young women. Med Sci Sports Exerc 30:114–120, 1998.

26. Drinkwater BL. C. H. McCloy research lecture: Does physical activity play a role in preventing osteoporosis? Res Q Exerc Sport 65:197–206, 1994.

27. Biering-Sorensen F, Bohr H, Schaadt O. Longitudinal study of bone mineral content in the lumbar spine, the forearm and the lower extremities after spinal cord injury. Eur J Clin Invest 20:330–335, 1990.

28. Lohman T, Going S, Pamenter R, et al. Effects of resistance training on regional and total bone mineral density in pre-

29. Kerr D, Morton A, Dick I, Prince R J. Exercise effects on bone mass in postmenopausal women are site-specific and load-dependent. J Bone Miner Res 11:218–225, 1996.

30. Hayes WC, Snow CM, McMahon TA. Toward a definition of impact loading in exercise studies of bone. Proc ASME Summer Bioengineering Conference, Sun River, OR, June 1997.

31. Cavanaugh DJ, Cann CE. Brisk walking does not stop bone loss in postmenopausal women. Bone 9:201–204, 1988.

32. Granhad H, Jonson R, Hansson T. The loads on the lumbar spine during extreme weight lifting. Spine 12:146–149, 1987.

33. Daly RM, Rich PA, Klein R, Bass S. Effects of high-impact exercise on ultrasonic and biochemical indices of skeletal status: A prospective study in young male gymnasts. J Bone Miner Res 14:1222–1230, 1999.

34. LaRiviere J, Snow-Harter C, Robinson TL. Bone mass changes in female competitive gymnasts over two training seasons. Med Sci Sports Exerc 27(Suppl):S68, 1995.

35. McKay HA, Petit MA, Schutz RW, et al. Augmented trochanteric bone mineral density after modified physical education classes: A randomized school-based exercise intervention study in prepubescent and early pubescent children. J Pediatr 136:156–162, 2000.

36. Dalsky GP, Stocke KS, Eshani AA. Weight-bearing exercise training and lumbar bone mineral content in postmenopausal women. Ann Intern Med 108:824–828, 1988.

37. Heinonen A, Kannus P, Sievanen H, et al. Good maintenance of high-impact activity-induced bone gain by voluntary, unsupervised exercises: An 8-month follow-up of a randomized controlled trial. J Bone Miner Res 14:125–128, 1999.

38. Black DM, Cummings SR, Genant HK, et al. Axial and appendicular bone density predict fractures in older women. J Bone Miner Res 7:633–638, 1992.

39. Rencken ML, Chestnut CH III, Drinkwater BL. Bone density at multiple skeletal sites in amenorrheic athletes. JAMA 276:238–240, 1996.

40. Nelson ME, Fiatarone MA, Morganti CM, et al. Effects of high-intensity strength training on multiple risk factors for osteoporotic fractures. JAMA 272:1909–1914, 1994.

41. Hayes WC, Myers ER, Morris JN, et al. Impact near the hip dominates fracture risk in elderly nursing home residents who fall. Calcif Tissue Int 52:192–198, 1993.

42. Greenspan SL, Myers ER, Maitland LA, et al. Fall severity and bone mineral density as risk factors for hip fracture in ambulatory elderly. JAMA 271:128–133, 1994.

43. Shaw JM, Snow C. Weighted vest exercise improves indices of fall risk in older women. J Gerontol A Biol Sci Med Sci 53:M53–M58, 1998.

44. Campbell AJ, Robertson MC, Gardner MM, et al. Randomised controlled trial of a general practice programme of home based exercise to prevent falls in elderly women. BMJ 315:1065–1069, 1997.

45. Bassey EJ, Rothwell MC, Littlewood JJ, Pye DW. Pre- and postmenopausal women have different bone mineral density responses to the same high-impact exercise. J Bone Miner Res 13:1805–1813, 1998.

46. Snow CM, Shaw JM, Winters KM, Witzke KA. Long-term ex-

ercise using weighted vests prevents hip bone loss in post-menopausal women. J Gerontol A Biol Sci Med Sci 55:M489–492, 2000.

47. Bassey EJ, Fiatarone MA, O'Neill EF, et al. Leg extensor power and functional performance in very old men and women. Clin Sci 82:321–327, 1992.

48. Jozsi AC, Campbell WW, Joseph L, et al. Changes in power with resistance training in older and younger men and women. J Gerontol A Biol Sci Med Sci 54:M591–596, 1999.

49. Brill PA, Probst JC, Greenhouse DL, et al. Clinical feasibility of a free-weight strength-training program for older adults. J Am Board Fam Pract 11:445–451, 1998.

50. Joakimsen RM, Magnus JH, Fonnebo V. Physical activity and predisposition for hip fractures: A review. Osteoporos Int 7:503–513, 1997.

51. Recker RR, Davies KM, Hinders SM, et al. Bone gain in young adult women. JAMA 268:2403–2408, 1992.

Suggested Reading

Drinkwater BL. C.H. McCloy research lecture: Does physical activity play a role in preventing osteoporosis? Res Q Exerc Sport 65:197–206, 1994.

Drinkwater BL. Exercise and bones: Lessons learned from female athletes. Am J Sports Med 24(6 Suppl):S33–S35, 1996.

ACSM Position Stand on Osteoporosis and Exercise. Med Sci Sports Exerc 27:I–vii, 1995.

Witzke, Kara A. Exercise and osteoporosis. In: Cotton R, ed. Clinical Exercise Specialist Manual: ACE's Source for Training Special Populations. San Diego: American Council on Exercise, 1999.

1.4.0.1, 1.4.0.2, 1.4.0.3

2.2.22, 2.4.1, 2.4.2, 2.4.3

3.4.0, 3.4.2

4.2.0.5, 4.4.15

5.2.0, 5.4.1, 5.4.2,

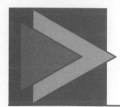

CHAPTER **35**

EXERCISE, NUTRITIONAL STRATEGIES, AND LIPOPROTEINS

Tom R. Thomas and Thomas P. LaFontaine

Cardiovascular disease (CVD) is the leading cause of death in the United States (1). One of the primary factors associated with CVD is atherosclerosis, an accumulation of cholesterol and smooth muscle cells in the arterial wall. This buildup can partially or totally occlude an artery and prevent adequate oxygen from reaching vital cells. Since fat and fatlike substances are found in atherosclerotic plaque, research has focused on the transportation system of fat and cholesterol in the blood as lipoproteins. Understanding this process may ultimately lead to the development of lifestyle prescriptions and drug therapies to prevent or reverse this disease.

OVERVIEW OF LIPOPROTEINS

Lipoproteins are large molecules that consist primarily of lipid and protein but that also contain various amounts of phospholipids, carbohydrate, and cholesterol. There are five general classes of lipoproteins, each having several subclasses. The largest lipoprotein is the chylomicron, which transports digested fat, primarily triglycerides (TG), to various tissues and to other lipoproteins after a meal (Fig. 35.1). Very low density lipoprotein (VLDL) receives much of its lipid content from chylomicrons, and VLDL is the major transporter of TG in the blood. Low-density lipoprotein (LDL) contains large amounts of esterified and nonesterified (free) cholesterol. It is the cholesterol associated with LDL that is thought to be taken up by the arterial wall, eventually to become a part of the atherosclerotic process (2). The cholesterol carried in the densest and smallest LDL subfraction, LDL_3, appears to have the highest association with atherosclerosis. Lipoprotein(a) [Lp(a)] shares many characteristics with LDL and has been linked to atherosclerosis, perhaps because it is susceptible to oxidation by free radicals. In addition, Lp(a) may be associated with cardiovascular disease by its ability to inhibit thrombolytic reactions in the blood. This effect would cause a greater tendency to form a thrombus (clot), which could get trapped in a narrowed artery. Cholesterol from LDL and peripheral tis-

sues can be transferred to high-density lipoprotein (HDL) and taken to the liver for degradation and excretion in feces. This reverse cholesterol transport process, or scavenger system, is believed to be helpful in preventing or reversing atherosclerosis. High-density lipoprotein also may hinder atherosclerosis by diminishing the oxidation of LDL cholesterol, by limiting LDL uptake by the scavenger system, and/or by serving as an oxidization substrate itself (3).

Although the lipid components of lipoproteins have received most of the attention from those studying cardiovascular disease, the proteins also are important in the prevention or cause of the disease. Apolipoprotein B (Apo B) has been shown to be associated with obstructive coronary artery disease (2). Apo B is the part of the LDL molecule that binds to the LDL receptor, which is responsible for clearing most of the cholesterol from blood. Apo B-100 is the primary protein of LDL, and Apo B-48, the primary protein of chylomicrons. Once taken up by the cell at the LDL receptor, some of the cholesterol is stored in the cell via the enzyme acyl-coenzyme A (CoA) acyltransferase. The increased cholesterol content reduces cellular synthesis of cholesterol by inhibiting the enzyme β-hydroxy-β-methyglutaryl (HMG) CoA reductase. In addition, the elevated cholesterol concentration causes a down-regulation of LDL receptors that decreases cellular uptake of cholesterol (4). Although all of these effects may be beneficial, uptake of cholesterol by either the LDL receptor or the unregulated scavenger system may allow free radical attack and cholesterol oxidation, one of the initiating steps in the atherosclerotic process (2).

Another important apoprotein is Apo A-I, the major protein of HDL. This protein activates lecithin cholesterol acyl transferase (LCAT), an enzyme that is important in attaching cholesterol to HDL for eventual deposition in the liver. Apo C-I and C-II, which are components of HDL and VLDL, also activate antiatherogenic enzymes LCAT and lipoprotein lipase (LPL), respectively. Apo E, found in VLDL, HDL, and chylomicrons, is another protein that interacts with the LDL receptor as well as another receptor in the liver for VLDL remnants (4).

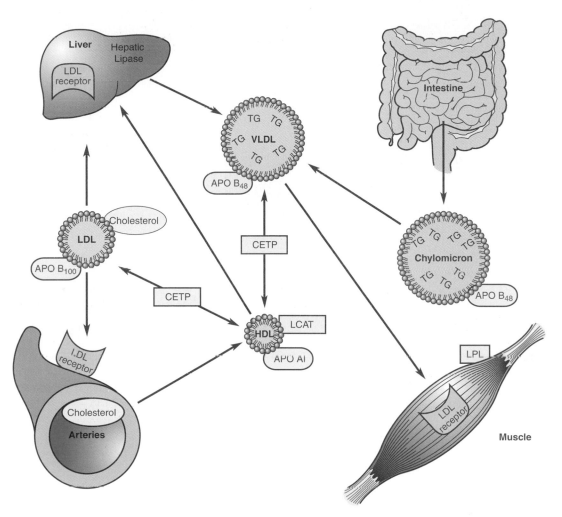

Figure 35.1. Interactions of lipoproteins. Many tissues play a role in lipoprotein synthesis, uptake, and degradation. Most of the transfer of particles between lipoproteins occurs in the blood. VLDL, very low density lipoprotein; LDL, low-density lipoprotein; HDL, high-density lipoprotein; apo, apolipoprotein; CETP, cholesterol ester transfer protein; LCAT, lecithin cholesterol acyltransferase; LPL, lipoprotein lipase; rec, receptor; TG, triglycerides.

The action of the lipoproteins is intimately tied to the activity of a variety of enzymes. Some of these enzymes are associated with atherogenesis. HMG-CoA reductase is the rate-limiting enzyme of cellular synthesis of cholesterol. Many drugs inhibit this enzyme and thus decrease blood cholesterol (e.g. simvastatin, pravastatin, atorvastatin). Another enzyme believed to be associated with atherogenesis is hepatic lipase, which is involved in the conversion of HDL_2 to HDL_3 in the liver (Fig. 35.1). HDL_2 appears to be the subfraction that is protective against cardiovascular disease. Hepatic lipase also reduces the cholesterol content of foam cells, and so its role in atherogenesis may be multifaceted.

More attention has been given to the antiatherogenic enzymes in the scientific literature. LCAT stimulates the attachment (esterification) of cholesterol to HDL (Fig. 35.1). This is a key step in the reverse cholesterol transport system. LCAT also is involved in the conversion of HDL_3 to HDL_2. Lipoprotein lipase (LPL), an enzyme located in the endothelium of capillaries, is involved in the conversion of chylomicrons and VLDL remnants to HDL and of HDL_3 to HDL_2 (Fig. 35.1). LPL degrades VLDL-TG, which allows the uptake of TG by cells for use as energy, for example in the working muscle. Other products of this reaction are called VLDL remnants. These proteins and lipids can be transferred to other lipoproteins or be transported to the liver, where they serve as precursors to lipoproteins, including HDL (4) (Fig. 35.2), especially during recovery from exercise. Triglyceride lipase (or hormone-sensitive lipase), which is found in adipose tissue and muscle, stimulates the degradation of TG to free fatty acids (FFA) and glycerol. The FFA can be used as energy, while the glycerol is released into the blood and can serve as a marker for fat mobilization. The use of FFA by muscle in turn stimulates LPL to degrade more VLDL-TG. Cholesterol ester transfer protein is believed to cause the

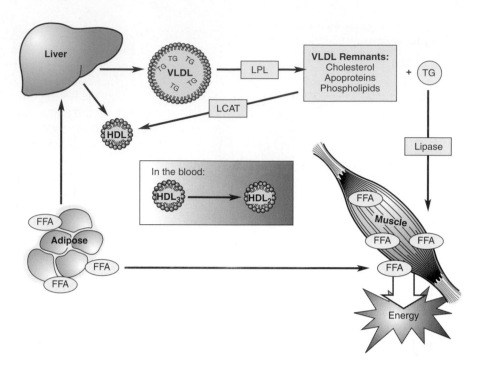

Figure 35.2. Proposed mechanism of exercise effect on HDL synthesis. The use of fat as energy by working muscles initiates a cascade of reactions that stimulate HDL production in the liver and HDL_2 conversion in blood. VLDL, very low density lipoprotein; HDL, high-density lipoprotein; FFA, free fatty acids; LCAT, lecithin cholesterol acyltransferase; TG, triglycerides.

transfer of triglycerides to HDL in exchange for cholesterol (Fig. 35.1). Since HDL would lose some of its free cholesterol, this transfer may decrease the capacity of HDL to promote the excretion of cholesterol.

Other enzymes important to the atherogenic process are those involved with cholesterol oxidation. Several reactions are involved in the generation of free radicals and their subsequent reaction with cell structures, especially those rich in unsaturated fat. Oxidative metabolism during exercise increases free radical production. This process may cause cholesterol to be more reactive with the arterial wall and form foam cells and/or cause endothelial injury. Both processes have been associated with atherosclerosis (2). Markers for cellular oxidation are called thiobarbituric acid-reactive substances. Fortunately, exercise training also increases antioxidant systems, including the enzymes superoxide dismutase and glutathione peroxidase, which inhibit free radical reactions within the cell. Another promising area of research involves antioxidant nutrients such as vitamin E, vitamin C, beta-carotene (a form of vitamin A), and selenium, which may help inhibit the oxidation of cholesterol by free radicals.

NORMAL AND RECOMMENDED VALUES FOR LIPIDS

Estimates are that nearly 95 million Americans over age 19 have a serum cholesterol level over 200 mg/dL (1).

In addition, 26.7 million Americans aged 19 and under have a cholesterol level over 170 mg/dL (1). One in five Americans over age 19 has a cholesterol level over 240 mg/dL, which is associated with a doubled risk of CVD compared to those with a blood cholesterol below 200 mg/dL (5).

In 1988, the National Institutes of Health established the National Cholesterol Education Program (NCEP) (6). The basis for the NCEP was twofold:

1. Cholesterol is an independent risk factor for the development of atherosclerosis.
2. Lowering cholesterol, particularly LDL cholesterol, results in a decreased rate of atherosclerotic events (e.g., heart attack, stroke, coronary artery bypass surgery).

Large population studies suggest that for every 1% reduction in cholesterol there is a 2–3% reduction in incidence of CVD events (5).

In 1993, the NCEP guidelines were updated (7). Table 35.1 summarizes target lipid values for adults over 19 years of age with and without documented atherosclerosis, and for youths 13–19 years of age (8). There is no consensus regarding target values for persons under age 13. However, it seems reasonable and prudent to strive for a cholesterol below 170 mg/dL in children under age 13. The NCEP II advises that both total cholesterol and HDL be assessed on initial screening.

Table 35.1. Target Lipid Levels in Adults over 19 Years of Age and Adolescents (7, 8)

Category	Total Cholesterol	LDL Cholesterol	HDL Cholesterol
Without documented CVD Age 20+	<200	<130	>35[a,b]
With documented CVD Age 20+	<200	<100	>35[a,b]
Age 13–19	<170	<100	No recommendation

All values are in milligrams per deciliter.
[a] It is the opinion of the authors that HDL should be > 45 in females with or without CVD.
[b] HDL > 60 mg/dL is considered a negative risk factor.

EXERCISE TRAINING AND LIPOPROTEINS

One of the most consistent benefits of a regular exercise program is the long-term effect that such a lifestyle has on the metabolism of lipoproteins. Many of the adaptations to exercise occur with a single vigorous or prolonged session of exercise. Decreased plasma TG is one of the most consistent effects of acute aerobic exercise. This decrease may be delayed for several hours after exercise, and TG may remain low for 24–48 hours (9). The cause is believed to be increased activity of LPL induced by exercise. If the VLDL-TG bond is broken, more TG can be taken up and used by muscle. Peak LPL activity appears to be delayed following aerobic exercise, perhaps because of the time necessary for protein synthesis and LPL gene expression (10, 11). This lag time appears to correspond to the time frame of the exercise-induced TG-lowering effect. The resulting increased availability of VLDL remnants may also stimulate the synthesis of HDL, which increases after a single exercise session. Cholesterol and LDL cholesterol may decrease in the 24 hours following a vigorous aerobic exercise bout, but this change is inconsistent and its physiological importance is unknown (12).

Another apparent beneficial effect of an aerobic exercise session is the transient effect on metabolism of fat ingested during a meal. It has been demonstrated that exercise prior to fat ingestion dramatically reduces the TG response to the meal, the so-called postprandial lipemia (13, 14). In addition, favorable HDL cholesterol changes occur when exercise precedes fat ingestion. The mechanism may be a stimulation of LPL by exercise, hence enhanced fat clearance following the meal. Thus, practically, if a person periodically ingests high-fat meals, exercising earlier in the day or even the day before may be advantageous from a health perspective. This may be one of the mechanisms by which chronic exercise may partially offset some of the ill effects of poor dietary habits.

Although many beneficial lipoprotein changes occur with a single exercise session, these adaptations are transient and do not become lasting unless exercise is regular over the long term. Data suggest that most of the beneficial lipoprotein changes are permanent if the exercise program continues for at least a year and is subsequently sustained (15–18). HDL cholesterol usually increases as a result of chronic exercise training. This increased plasma level is due to the increase in HDL_2 cholesterol (19), which is thought to be beneficial because of the potential for increasing cholesterol excretion by the liver. Total TG decreases with exercise training, and this reduction can be very large. The effects on total cholesterol are controversial. Except for HDL cholesterol, lipoproteins usually do not change substantially with exercise training unless accompanied by caloric restriction and weight loss (18, 20). However, a meta-analysis of studies of the effects of exercise on blood lipids suggests that modest beneficial changes do result from exercise training alone (21).

Changes in LDL subfractions also occur with aerobic exercise training. Cross-sectional studies indicate that endurance-trained individuals have higher levels of large LDL subfractions (LDL_1) and lower levels of small, dense LDL subfractions (LDL_3) than sedentary individuals (15). Other investigators have shown that overweight individuals who lost body weight through diet or exercise exhibited a decrease in dense LDL levels (18). Elevated LDL_3 levels, associated with increased plasma levels of TG, Apo B, and total cholesterol, have been observed in CVD patients (22).

Favorable enzyme changes have been associated with regular participation in aerobic exercise training. LPL, LCAT, and TG lipase increase, while hepatic lipase decreases. LDL receptors may be up-regulated after an aerobic training program. Lp(a) may resist exercise training, and cholesterol ester transfer protein has been shown either to decrease or to increase with exercise training (15, 23, 24). Antioxidant enzymes appear to increase, and cellular oxidation decreases with chronic aerobic exercise (25, 26).

The precise exercise intensity and duration necessary to induce beneficial lipoprotein changes are unknown, although it appears that the quantity of exercise is the major determining factor. That is, a person may exercise at a relatively low intensity (e.g., 60% of maximal heart rate) for a relatively long time (e.g., 60 minutes) or a higher intensity (e.g., 75% of maximal heart rate) for a shorter time (e.g., 30–40 minutes). Some lipoprotein changes require several months to become a lasting adaptation. After a training period of 8–16 weeks, the adaptations are rapidly reversed if exercise is discontinued. Among individuals who have participated in extended exercise training, the lipoprotein profile is more durable (27).

The effects of resistance training on lipoprotein metabolism are more equivocal. In a review of the topic, Hurley (28) noted that several studies demonstrated changes in lipoproteins similar to those found with aerobic training. In fact, some cardiovascular changes may follow resistance exercise training without increases in VO_{2max} (29). However, the investigators who observed lipoprotein changes used circuit resistance training that uses lower work rates and very brief rest periods; this type of resistance training more closely parallels the exercise intensity and cardiovascular effects of an aerobic exercise session. It is unknown whether traditional heavy resistance training influences lipoprotein metabolism. It is possible that such training is ineffective, since individuals involved in heavy resistance training over several years have lipoprotein profiles similar to those of untrained individuals. The exception may be bodybuilders, who appear to have better lipoprotein profiles than power lifters (28). It does not appear that heavy resistance training either augments or enhances the effects of aerobic training on lipoproteins, although LDL cholesterol levels may not be lowered as much if resistance training is part of the fitness program (30).

The mechanisms of the effects of exercise on lipoproteins have been examined, but no definitive conclusions have been reached. One commonly held hypotheses is illustrated in Figure 35.2. Exercise stimulates muscle oxidative processes, which increases the uptake of TG. The drop in blood fat stimulates the release from adipose tissue of FFA, which are carried in blood by the protein albumin. Some of this fat is carried to the heart and skeletal muscle, where it becomes an immediate source of energy for exercise. Some of the FFA is transported to liver, where it can be used to package VLDL released into the blood. By the action of LPL, the VLDL-TG can be broken down and the TG used as energy by muscle. The resulting VLDL remnants can be used to convert HDL_3 to HDL_2 in the blood or be transported to the liver to serve as precursors for HDL synthesis. Thus, the net result of increasing fat use by muscle would be elevated HDL levels. Ironically, much of this beneficial cascade of reactions may occur in recovery when fat use is very high (31). Therefore, even if carbohydrate is the primary energy source during the exercise, this series of events may occur in recovery from exercise when fat use is high. Some investigators speculate that the total energy expenditure is the key to lipoprotein changes rather than the specific use of fat. However, if this were true, anaerobic athletes undergoing vigorous training programs would have lipoprotein patterns similar to those of aerobic athletes. This generally is not the case (32). Finally, Despres and Lamarche (33) suggest that as long as the energy expenditure is sufficient, intensities of 50–80% should produce similar improvements in overall metabolic fitness, including blood lipids.

STRATEGIES TO IMPROVE BLOOD LIPIDS

Essentially there are three nonpharmacological strategies for improving blood lipids: diet, exercise training, and body weight and fat loss. This section discusses these strategies and summarizes guidelines for nonpharmacological management of blood lipids.

Dietary Therapy

Several dietary factors influence blood and tissue levels of lipoproteins. Connor and Connor (34) reported that after subjects consumed a cholesterol-free diet, there was a threshold dietary cholesterol intake of 100 mg/day before blood cholesterol began to rise. As cholesterol intake increased further, blood cholesterol reached a plateau (at 350–400 mg/day). There is a direct relationship between the level of dietary saturated fat intake and blood cholesterol, and reductions in saturated fat intake explain 50–60% of the change in blood cholesterol (35). Table 35.2 summarizes these findings.

Generally, studies show that the greater the dietary fat restriction, the more the blood cholesterol level falls (34, 36). However, there is wide interindividual variation in response to diet (37–39). A controlled study of 32 dyslipidemic middle-aged men and women reported a 5% increase to 40% decrease in blood cholesterol after 24 weeks of a daily diet of 26% fat, 4% saturated fat, and 45 mg cholesterol per 1000 kcal (38). Other studies of dyslipidemic subjects on a low-fat diet for 6 weeks showed similar results, perhaps secondary to genetic differences.

In 1984, the American Heart Association recommended a three-step approach to the dietary treatment of dyslipidemia (40). Table 35.3 summarizes this approach. In 1988, the NCEP I adopted the American Heart Association guidelines but conspicuously deleted step III (6). NCEP II did include recommendations to reduce saturated fat, total fat, and cholesterol further than step II if desired results were not obtained, particularly in patients with known atherosclerosis (7).

Some studies suggest that lowering fat and increasing carbohydrate intake may increase blood triglycerides and lower HDL cholesterol, particularly in patients with diabetes (41–43). However, in patients with coronary artery disease, a very low fat diet, exercise, and stress management resulted in regression of atherosclerosis in spite of a slight but not significant decrease in HDL cholesterol (36). The results of a recent controlled trial in patients with type II diabetes found that a hypocaloric low-fat diet (10% fat, 4% saturated fat) resulted in similar weight loss and changes in blood lipids, with slightly higher HDL cholesterol than in a hypocaloric, high-monounsaturated fat diet (44).

Finally, a recent trial illustrated the interaction of a low-fat diet and drug therapy of simvastatin (Zocor) 10 mg per day (45). Patients with coronary artery disease

Table 35.2. Predicted Blood Cholesterol Lowering Based on Dietary Fat, Saturated Fat, and Cholesterol Intake

	TOTAL FAT (% CALORIES)	SATURATED FAT (% CALORIES)	CHOLESTEROL (MG/DAY)	CHANGE IN BLOOD CHOLESTEROL (MG/DL)
Traditional diet	40	15	500	Baseline
Phase I diet	30–35	12–14	<350	−18
Phase II diet	25	8	200	−39
Phase III diet	<20	<5	<100	−53

Modified from Connor WE, Connor S. The dietary prevention and treatment of coronary heart disease. In: Connor WE, Bristow JD, eds. Coronary Heart Disease: Prevention, Complications, and Treatment. Philadelphia: Lippincott 1985:43–64.

Table 35.3. American Heart Association Dietary Therapy Recommendations for Treating Abnormal Lipids

STEP	FAT CALORIES (%)	SATURATED FAT CALORIES (%)	PROTEIN (%)	CARBOHYDRATES (%)	CHOLESTEROL (MG/DAY)
I	<30	10	15	55	300 or less
II	<25	8	15	60	200–250 or less
III	<20	<7	15	65	100–150 or less

Reprinted with permission from American Heart Association. Recommendations for treatment of hyperlipidemia in adults. Circulation 69:1065A–1084A, 1984.

randomized to an isocaloric diet containing less than 20% fat with or without simvastatin 10 mg showed a 29% increase in HDL cholesterol.

The following dietary factors also are known to influence blood lipids significantly:

- 2oz oat bran (11 g total fiber, 6 g soluble) may lower LDL by 3–7% (46).
- Replacing animal protein with 25 g soy protein may lower LDL by 13% (47).
- Omega-3 fatty acids may lower triglycerides 100 to 1200 mg/dL, and studies in patients with coronary artery disease show a reduction in sudden death, CVD mortality, and all-cause mortality following long-term treatment with omega-3 fatty acids (48–50).
- Some research suggests that replacing saturated and trans fatty acids with monounsaturated and omega-3 fatty acids found in nuts may improve lipoproteins (51, 52).

The importance of dietary fiber in improving blood lipids is well supported (53). Table 35.4 summarizes a suggested optimal diet for improving blood lipids.

Exercise Therapy

The primary effects of exercise on lipoproteins are decreased triglycerides and increased HDL. Forty-five minutes of aerobic exercise 4 or more days per week substantially lowers triglycerides. The minimal weekly caloric threshold to increase HDL appears to be 1000–1200. However, there is a dose–response relation between weekly calories expended and increase in HDL (16, 54).

Table 35.4. Optimal Diet for Improving Blood Lipids

DIETARY COMPONENT	RECOMMENDATION
Total calories	Adequate to support nutritional needs but low enough (not <1500 calories) to allow a 10% loss of weight if indicated
Total fat intake	No more than 20–25% of calories
Saturated fat intake	5–7% of calories or less
Polyunsaturated fat	5–7% of calories, focusing on omega-3s
Monounsaturated fat	10–15% of calories
Cholesterol intake	100–150 mg/day or less
Fiber intake	30–40 g/day
Soluble fiber intake	10–15 g/day
Protein	15% of calories (0.50–0.55 g/pound body weight in active persons) with an increase in vegetable and decrease in animal protein
Carbohydrate	65% of calories (55% complex)

Simultaneous weight loss may induce a greater increase in HDL (18, 20, 39). The lower the initial level of HDL, the greater the increase, and it often takes several months of consistent weekly caloric expenditure of more than 1000 kcal before it becomes apparent.

A recent study of 190 dyslipidemic men and women randomized to control, isocaloric diet (about 23% fat), exercise (1500–2000 kcal/week), or combined groups showed a significant 14% decrease in LDL cholesterol in the combined group compared to no change in the control and exercise groups, and a 7% decrease in the diet

Table 35.5. Target Exercise Guidelines for Improving Lipids

Type	Aerobic
Intensity (%VO$_{2max}$)	50–85
Frequency (days/wk)	3.5–7
Duration (min/session)	30–60
Minimum kilocalories/wk	1000–1200
Optimum kilocalories/wk	2000–3500
Time to goal	9–12 mo
Percent responding	90% for triglycerides; 70% for HDLs

These guidelines may have to be modified for sedentary, obese individuals and patients with chronic diseases such as diabetes, high blood pressure, and coronary heart disease. For more information on special populations, see ACSM Guidelines for Exercise Testing and Prescription. 6th ed. Philadelphia: Lippincott Williams & Wilkin, 2000.

group (55). There was a shift in the LDL cholesterol particle size in the exercise groups towards nonatherogenic, large, buoyant molecules. There also appears to be a positive interaction between lipid-lowering drug therapy and exercise (56). Table 35.5 summarizes recommendations for exercise to improve lipoproteins.

Weight Loss

The importance of weight loss in controlling serum lipids is underappreciated. A recent 18-year Danish study of men and women showed that weight gain was the most important predictor of increase in cholesterol (57). A 10-kg weight gain was associated with an 11.4 mg/dL and a 7.72 mg/dL increase in cholesterol in men and women, respectively. Considering that cross-cultural epidemiological studies suggest that for each 1 mg/dL increase in cholesterol there is a 2–3% increase in risk of coronary artery disease, this corresponds to a 23–34% increase in risk in men and women, respectively. Denke et al. (58, 59) also reported a significant relation between body mass index and cholesterol in 20- to 74-year-old men and women. Other work demonstrates that weight loss due to a low-fat hypocaloric diet and exercise may increase HDL cholesterol and lower LDL and VLDL cholesterol (18, 60).

One randomized trial showed a significantly ($P < .05$) greater decrease in triglycerides and LDL (18% and 7%, respectively) and increase in HDL (13%) in 44 men assigned to weight loss (10%) by diet compared to 49 men assigned to a vigorous exercise program with weight maintenance (triglycerides and LDL decreased 9% and 4%, respectively, and HDL increased by %) (61). Another study of 27 men and women aged 41 to 81 (LDL > 130 mg/dL) reported a 24.3% reduction in LDL cholesterol and no change in the ratio of total cholesterol to HDL cholesterol after consuming an ad libitum 15.1% fat diet that resulted in a 3.63 kg weight loss (39). In contrast, after consuming the diet without weight loss, there was a 17% reduction in LDL cholesterol but a 12.9% increase in the ratio of total cholesterol to HDL cholesterol.

Numerous studies suggest that weight loss through exercise and modest dietary restriction of total and fat calories is key to improving blood lipoproteins. In conclusion, the dietary guidelines in Table 35.4 and exercise guidelines in Table 35.5 should induce significant weight loss. For additional information, see Chapter 70.

▶ SUMMARY

The metabolism of lipoproteins is related to cardiovascular health and disease. Both the lipid and protein components of lipoprotein play a role in the prevention or cause of atherosclerosis. HDL$_2$, Apo A-I, and LCAT play significant roles in clearing cholesterol from the cells. Lipoprotein lipase and TG lipase are important in clearing fat from the blood and initiating a complex series of reactions that increase HDL. Elevated LDL cholesterol, Apo B-100, and hepatic lipase are associated with increased prevalence of atherosclerosis. Free radical–induced oxidation of LDL cholesterol is a relatively new theory of atherogenesis. The oxidation leads to an inflammatory process and the formation of foam cells and fatty streaks. Eventually plaque is formed and may rupture to form clots and cause a cardiovascular event.

To help reduce the prevalence of cardiovascular disease, the NCEP was developed with specific goals for blood lipid levels. The most notable of these goals is for all American adults to achieve plasma cholesterol levels below 200 mg/dL. The NCEP also proposed goals for LDL and HDL cholesterol. Various strategies have been used to reduce blood lipoproteins. The reduction of saturated fat in the diet has been one of the most successful strategies for lowering plasma cholesterol. Other dietary recommendations include ingestion of more complex carbohydrate and fish oils.

Exercise training of sufficient intensity, duration, and longevity will affect lipoprotein metabolism. The most predictable changes occur in plasma TG, HDL, and HDL$_2$ cholesterol. The effects on total and LDL cholesterol are less consistent and may be linked to weight loss. One of the primary factors related to the beneficial changes is the increased activities of LCAT and LPL. The antioxidant effect of exercise training also may be a major benefit, but the evidence for this is not consistent. Aerobic training appears to produce more consistent changes in lipoprotein than resistance training. However, circuit resistance training may be a useful method for producing some adaptations in the lipoprotein profile. The combination of exercise training and moderate caloric restriction may be the most effective means of altering blood lipids because of the effect of these combined strategies on weight loss.

References

1. American Heart Association. Heart and Stroke: 2000 Statistical Update. Dallas: American Heart Association, 2000.

2. Hensrud DD, Heimburger D C. Antioxidant status, fatty acids, and cardiovascular disease. Nutrition 10:170–175, 1994.

3. Parthasarathy S, Barnett J, Fong LG. High-density lipoprotein inhibits the oxidative modification of low-density lipoprotein. Biochim Biophys Acta 1044:275–283, 1990.

4. Mayes PA. Cholesterol synthesis, transport, and excretion. In: Murray RK, Granner DK, Mayes PA, Rodwell VW, eds. Harpers Biochemistry. Englewood Cliffs, NJ: Appleton & Lange, 1996:249–260.

5. Stamler J, Wentworth D, Neaton JD. Is the relationship between serum cholesterol and risk of premature death from coronary heart disease continuous and graded? Findings in 356,222 primary screenees of the Multiple Risk Factor Intervention Trial (MRFIT). JAMA 256:2823–2828, 1986.

6. National Cholesterol Education Program. Report of the Expert Panel on Population Strategies for Blood Cholesterol Reduction. Arch Intern Med 148:36–69, 1988.

7. Summary of the Second Report of the National Cholesterol Education Program (NCEP) Expert Panel on Detection, Evaluation, and Treatment of High Blood Cholesterol in Adults (Adult Treatment Panel II). JAMA 269:3015–3021, 1993.

8. National Cholesterol Education Program. Report of the Expert Panel on Blood Cholesterol Levels in Children and Adolescents. U.S. Department of Health and Human Services, Public Health Service, National Institutes of Health, National Heart, Lung and Blood Institute. NIH pub 91-2732, 1991.

9. Dufaux B, Order U, Muller R, W. Hollman W. Delayed effects of prolonged exercise on serum lipoproteins. Metabolism 35:105–109, 1986.

10. Kiens B, Richter EA. Utilization of skeletal muscle triacylglycerol during postexercise recovery in humans. Am J Physiol Endocrinol Metab 38: E332–E337, 1998.

11. Seip RL, Semenkovich CF. Skeletal muscle lipoprotein lipase: Molecular regulation and physiological effects in relation to exercise. Exerc Sports Sci Rev 26:191–218, 1998.

12. Kantor MA, Cullinane EM, Sady SP, et al. Exercise acutely increases high density lipoprotein-cholesterol and lipoprotein lipase activity in trained and untrained men. Metabolism 36:188–192, 1987.

13. Thomas TR, Fischer BA, Kist WB, et al. Effects of exercise and omega 3 fatty acids on postprandial lipemia. J Appl Physiol 88:2199–2204, 2000.

14. Zhang J., Thomas TR, and Ball SD. Effect of exercise timing on postprandial lipemia and HDL cholesterol subfractions. J Appl Physiol 85:1516–1522, 1998.

15. Berg A, Ifrey I, Baumstark MW, et al. Physical activity and lipoprotein lipid disorders. Sports Med 17:6–21, 1994.

16. Kokkinos PF, Fernhall B. Physical activity and high density lipoprotein cholesterol levels. Sports Med 28:307–314, 1999.

17. Williams PT, Krauss RM, Vranizan DM, Wood PD. Changes in lipoprotein subfractions during diet-induced and exercise-induced weight loss in moderately overweight men. Circulation 81:1293–1304, 1990.

18. Wood PD, Stefanick ML, Williams PT, Haskell WL. The effects on plasma lipids of a prudent weight-reducing diet with or without exercise in overweight men and women. N Engl J Med 325:461–466, 1991.

19. Despres JP, Pouliot MC, Moorjani S, et al. Loss of abdominal fat and metabolic response to exercise training in obese women. Am J Physiol 261:E159–E167, 1991.

20. Wood PD, Stefanick ML, Dreon DM, et al. Changes in plasma lipids and lipoproteins in overweight men during weight loss through dieting as compared with exercise. N Engl J Med 319:1173–1179, 1988.

21. Tran V, Weltman A, Glass GV, Mood DP. The effects of exercise on blood lipids and lipoproteins: A meta-analysis of studies. Med Sci Sports Exerc 15:393–402, 1983.

22. Austin MA, Hokanson JE. Epidemiology of triglycerides, small dense low-density lipoproteins, and lipoprotein(a) as risk factors for coronary heart disease. Med Clin North Am 78:99–115, 1994.

23. Gupta AK, Ross EA, Myers JN, Kashyap ML. Increased reverse cholesterol transport in athletes. Metabolism 42:684–690, 1993.

24. Seip RL, Moulin P, Cocke T, et al. Exercise training decreases plasma cholesteryl ester transfer protein. Arterioscler Thromb 13:1359–1367, 1993.

25. Alessio HM, Goldfarb AH. Lipid peroxidation and scavenger enzymes during exercise: Adaptive response to training. J Appl Physiol 64:1333–1336, 1988.

26. Ji LL. Exercise and oxidative stress: Role of cellular antioxidant systems. In: Holloszy HO, ed. Exercise and Sport Sciences Reviews. Baltimore: Williams & Wilkins, 1995:135–166.

27. Thompson CE, Thomas TR, Araujo J, et al. Response of HDL cholesterol, apoprotein A-I, and LCAT to exercise withdrawal. Atherosclerosis 54:65–73, 1985.

28. Hurley BF. Effects of resistive training on lipoprotein-lipid profiles: A comparison to aerobic exercise training. Med Sci Sports Exerc. 21:689–693, 1989.

29. Hurley BF, Hagberg JM, Goldberg AP, et al. Resistive training can reduce coronary risk factors without altering VO₂max or percent body fat. Med Sci Sports Exerc 20:150–154, 1988.

30. Kraemer WJ, Volek JS, Clark KL, et al. Influence of exercise training on physiological and performance changes with weight loss in men. Med Sci Exerc Sports 31:1320–1329, 1999.

31. Thomas TR. Prolonged recovery from eccentric versus concentric exercise. Can J Appl Physiol 19:441–450, 1994.

32. Thomas TR, Etheridge GL. The effect of track and field training on cardiovascular fitness. Phys Sportsmed 9:49–61, 1981.

33. Depres JP, Lamarche B. Low-intensity endurance exercise training, plasma lipoproteins and risk of coronary heart disease. J Intern Med 236:7–22, 1994.

34. Connor WE, Conner S. The dietary prevention and treatment of coronary heart disease. In: Connor WE, Bristow JD, eds. Coronary Heart Disease: Prevention, Complications, and Treatment. Philadelphia: Lippincott, 1985:43–64.

35. Messenick RP, Katan MB. Effect of dietary fatty acids on serum lipids and lipoproteins: A meta-analysis of 27 trials. Arterioscler Thromb 12:911–919, 1992.

36. Ornish DM, Brown SE, Scherwitz LW, et al. Can lifestyle changes reverse coronary artery disease? The Lifestyle Heart Trial. Lancet 336:129–133, 1990.

37. Denke MA, Grundy SM. Individual responses to a cholesterol-lowering diet in 50 men with moderate hypercholesterolemia. Arch Intern Med 154:317–322, 1994.

38. Schaefer EJ, Lichtenstein AH, Lamon-Fava, S, et al. Efficacy of a National Cholesterol Education Program step 2 diet in normolipidemic and hypercholesterolemic middle-aged and elderly men and women. Arterioscler Thromb Vasc Biol 15:1079–1085, 1995.

39. Schaefer EJ, Lichtenstein AH, Lamon-Fava S, et al. Body-weight and low-density lipoprotein cholesterol changes after consumption of a low-fat ad libitum diet. JAMA 274:1450–1455, 1995.

40. Gotto AM, Bierman EL, Connor WE, et al. Recommendations for treatment of hyperlipidemia in adults. Circulation 69:1065A–1084A, 1984.

41. Ginsberg H, Olefsky JM, Kimmerling G, et al. Induction of hypertriglyceridemia by a low fat diet. J Clin Endocrinol Metab 42:729–735, 1976.

42. Grundy SM, Nix D, Whelan MF, Franklin L. Comparison of three cholesterol-lowering diets in normolipidemic men. JAMA 256:2351–2355, 1986.

43. Tuswell AS. Food carbohydrates and plasma lipids: An update. Am J Clin Nutr 59(Suppl):710S–718S, 1994.

44. Heilbronn LK, Noakes M, Clifton PM. Effect of energy restriction, weight loss, and diet composition on plasma lipids and glucose in patients with type 2 diabetes. Diabetes Care 22:889–895, 1999.

45. Aquilani R, Tramarin R, Pedretti RFE, et al. Despite good compliance, very low fat diet alone does not achieve recommended cholesterol goals in outpatients with coronary heart disease. Eur Heart J 20:1020–1029, 1999.

46. Ripsin CM, Keenan JM, Jacobs DR, et al. Oat products and lipid lowering: A meta-analysis. JAMA 267:3317–3325, 1992.

47. Anderson JW, Johnstone BM, Cook-Newell ME. Meta-analysis of the effects of soy protein intake on serum lipids. N Engl J Med 333:276–282, 1995.

48. Davidson MH, Hurns JH, Subbaiah PV, et al. Marine oil capsule therapy for the treatment of hyperlipidemia. Arch Intern Med 151:1732–1740, 1991.

49. GISSI Prevenzione Investigators. Dietary supplementation with omega-3 polyunsaturated fatty acids and vitamin E in 11,324 patients with myocardial infarction: results of the GISSI-Prevenzione Trial. Lancet 354:447–455, 1999.

50. Singh RB, Niaz MA, Sharma JP, et al. Randomized, double-blind, placebo-controlled trial of fish oil and mustard oil in patients with suspected acute myocardial infarction. Indian Experiment of Infarct Survival 4. Cardiovasc Drug Ther 11:485–491, 1997.

51. Morgan WA, Clayshulte BJ. Pecans lower low-density lipoprotein cholesterol in people with normal lipid levels. J Am Diet Assoc 100:312–318, 2000.

52. Zambon D, Sabate J, Munoz S, et al. Substituting walnuts for monounsaturated fat improves the serum lipid profile of hypercholesterolemic men and women. Ann Intern Med 132:538–546, 2000.

53. Brow L, Rosner B, Willett WC, Sacks FM. Cholesterol-lowering effects of dietary fiber: A meta-analysis. Am J Clin Nutr 69:30–42, 1999.

54. Williams PT. Relationships of heart disease risk factors to exercise quantity and intensity. Arch Intern Med 158:237–245, 1998.

55. Stefanick ML, Mackey S, Sheehan M, et al. Effects of diet and exercise in men and postmenopausal women with low levels of HDL cholesterol and high levels of LDL cholesterol. N Engl J Med 339:12–20, 1998.

56. Wittke R. Effect of fluvastatin in combination with moderate endurance training on parameters of lipid metabolism. Sports Med 27:329–335, 1999.

57. Bakx JC, van den Hoogen JM, Deurenberg P, et al. Changes in total serum cholesterol levels over 18 years in a cohort of men and women: The Nijmegen Cohort Study. Prevent Med 30:138–145, 2000.

58. Denke MA, Sempos CT, Grundy SM. Excess bodyweight: An underrecognized contributor to high cholesterol levels in White American men. Arch Intern Med 153:1093–1103, 1993.

59. Denke MA, Sempos CT, Grundy SM. Excess bodyweight: An underrecognized contributor to dyslipidemia in White American women. Arch Intern Med 154:401–410, 1994.

60. Anderson SA, Haaland A, Hjermann I, et al. Oslo Diet and Exercise Study: A one-year randomized intervention trial: Effect on hemostatic variables and coronary risk factors. Nutr Metab Cardiovasc Dis 5:189–200, 1995.

61. Katzel LI, Bleecker ER, Colman EG, et al. Effects of weight loss vs aerobic exercise training on risk factors for coronary disease in healthy, obese, middle-aged, and older men. JAMA 274:1915–1921, 1995.

Suggested Reading

Drowtzky KL, Ainsworth BE, Durstine JL. Exercise, lipids, and lipoproteins in women. Clin Kinesiol 53:28–36, 1999.

Durstine JL, Haskell WL. Effects of exercise training on plasma lipids and lipoproteins. In: Holloszy JO, ed. Exercise and Sports Sciences Reviews. Baltimore: Williams & Wilkins, 1994:22:477–521.

Gotto AM. Lipid-regulating and antiatherosclerotic therapy: Current opinions and future approaches. Cleve Clin J Med 63:31–41, 1996.

Hamsten AG, Walldius A. Szamosi G, et al. Relationship of angiographically defined coronary disease to serum lipoproteins and apolipoproteins in young survivors of myocardial infarction. Circulation 73:1097–1110, 1986.

Keys A, Anderson JT, Grande F. Prediction of serum-cholesterol responses of man to changes in fats in the diet. Lancet 1:966, 1957.

Lipid Research Clinics Program. The Lipid Research Clinics Coronary Primary Prevention Trial results: II. The relationship of reduction in incidence of coronary heart disease to cholesterol lowering. JAMA 251:365–374, 1984.

Seip RL, Semenkovich CF. Skeletal muscle lipoprotein lipase: Molecular regulation and physiological effects in relation to exercise. In: Holloszy JO, ed. Exercise and Sports Sciences Reviews. Baltimore,: Williams & Wilkins, 1998:191–218.

Superko HR. Advances in lipoprotein metabolism: Applications in the Cardiac Rehabilitation Setting. In: Pashkow FJ, Dafoe WA, eds. Clinical Cardiac Rehabilitation: A Cardiologist Guide. 1st ed. Baltimore: Williams & Wilkins, 1993:196–226.

1.2.3

2.2.0, 2.2.2, 2.2.11,
2.2.15, 2.2.16, 2.4.5

3.4.3

4.2.0.5, 4.2.1.1, 4.2.3.2,
4.2.3.3

5.2.0

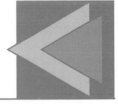

CHAPTER 36

PULMONARY ADAPTATIONS TO DYNAMIC EXERCISE

Kenneth C. Beck and Bruce D. Johnson

Key to Pulmonary Physiology Abbreviations

A-a D_{O2}	Alveolar–arterial oxygen difference
BTPS	Body temperature, ambient pressure, saturated with water vapor
EELV	End-expiratory lung volume
EILV	End-inspiratory lung volume
f_b	Breathing frequency
FEV_1	Forced expiratory volume in 1 second
Fio_2	Fractional concentration of oxygen in inspired gas
LT	Lactate threshold
MEFV	Maximal expiratory flow-volume (curve)
MIFV	Maximal inspiratory flow-volume (curve)
MVV	Maximal voluntary ventilation
$Paco_2$	Partial pressure of carbon dioxide in arterial blood
Pao_2	Partial pressure of oxygen in arterial blood
Pco_2	Partial pressure of carbon dioxide
Pio_2	Partial pressure of oxygen in inspired gas
P_{Emax}	Maximal expiratory pressure
Po_2	Partial pressure of oxygen
P_{pa}	Pulmonary artery pressure
P_{pw}	Pulmonary artery wedge pressure
$\dot{Q}$	Cardiac output (total pulmonary blood flow)
RER	Respiratory exchange ratio
STPD	Standard temperature and pressure, dry
T_E	Expiratory time
T_I	Inspiratory time
$\dot{V}_A$	Minute alveolar ventilation
$\dot{V}CO_2$	Carbon dioxide production
V_D	Dead space of the lungs
$\dot{V}_E$	Expired minute ventilation
$\dot{V}O_2$	Oxygen consumption
$\dot{V}O_{2max}$	Maximal oxygen consumption
V_I	Tidal volume
VT	Ventilatory threshold

Increasing levels of exercise require acute adaptations in the cardiorespiratory system to maintain homeostasis (1). As tissues increase $\dot{V}O_2$ and $\dot{V}CO_2$, cardiac output increases to deliver more oxygen to the tissues and transport more carbon dioxide away. Likewise, the ventilation must increase to meet the demand for oxygen and eliminate carbon dioxide. Without these adaptations, tissue hypoxia, hypercarbia, and acidosis compromise cellular function. This review focuses on adaptations in the pul-

monary system that meet increasing metabolic demands during exercise. The lungs, chest wall, and respiratory centers of the central nervous system meet this demand under most circumstances. However, while muscular and cardiovascular capacity chronically adapt to the demands of training, the capacity of the pulmonary system remains for the most part fixed. This chapter discusses normal pulmonary adaptations to exercise and definitions of the limits of the pulmonary response.

COUPLING OF INTERNAL TO EXTERNAL RESPIRATION

Internal respiration is the cellular exchange of oxygen and carbon dioxide. **External respiration** is the exchange of oxygen and carbon dioxide between organ systems, facilitated by the cardiac, circulatory, and pulmonary systems. Increased metabolic demand ($\dot{V}O_2$ and $\dot{V}CO_2$) raises the required level of cardiac output and pulmonary ventilation to maintain adequate tissue oxygenation and acid-base balance. The magnitudes of $\dot{V}O_2$ and $\dot{V}CO_2$ are related to the external workload.

As the tissues consume oxygen, they produce carbon dioxide at a rate dependent on the metabolic fuel being used and the amount of anaerobic metabolism. Carbon dioxide must be eliminated by the lungs to maintain the proper acid–base balance in the tissues. The ratio of $\dot{V}CO_2$ to $\dot{V}O_2$, the RER, steadily increases from about 0.7–0.8 at lower exercise intensities to 1 at moderate intensities and finally to 1.1–1.3 near maximum. This increase is due to a shift from predominantly fat metabolism to carbohydrate and finally to anaerobic metabolism. Although anaerobic metabolism (glycolytic pathways) neither consumes oxygen nor produces carbon dioxide, an increased anaerobic metabolism causes RER to rise secondary to buffering of lactic acid. Buffering releases carbon dioxide stored in blood and tissues through the combination of bicarbonate with hydrogen ions. The additional carbon dioxide excretion due to buffering can be substantial (2).

319

The Ventilatory (Anaerobic) Threshold

Pulmonary ventilation in a healthy person is generally adequate to support tissue oxygenation. Ventilatory demand increases linearly with $\dot{V}O_2$ as external work increases at low to moderate intensities. In the range of moderate to high intensities, the contribution of glycolytic pathways to total metabolism increases, which increases $\dot{V}CO_2$ by buffering action in the blood. Because of the need to eliminate carbon dioxide to maintain constant $Paco_2$, pulmonary ventilation increases out of proportion to the increased $\dot{V}O_2$. $\dot{V}CO_2$ therefore becomes proportionally greater than $\dot{V}O_2$. These relationships are demonstrated in Figure 36.1, which illustrates exercise-associated changes in minute ventilation (V_E), $\dot{V}O_2$, and $\dot{V}CO_2$ with increased work rate. Some of the increase may be related to hydrogen ion stimulation of peripheral chemoreceptors (3, 4).

The events shown in Figure 36.1 can be expressed mathematically. Within the lungs, mass balance relationships lead to the following equation which relates metabolic carbon dioxide production to minute ventilation at the alveolar level:

$$\dot{V}_A = \frac{0.863 \times \dot{V}CO_2}{Paco_2}$$

where $\dot{V}_A$ is converted to BTPS conditions and $\dot{V}CO_2$ is measured at the lungs and expressed in STPD conditions.

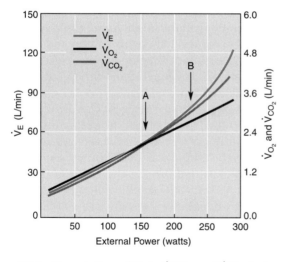

Figure 36.1. The relation of V_E to $\dot{V}CO_2$ and $\dot{V}O_2$ during progressive exercise. Note the parallel relation between V_E and $\dot{V}CO_2$ up to point B during the majority of exercise until the higher intensities (beyond point B). Below *arrow A*, metabolism is predominantly aerobic and RER is less than 1. Above *arrow A*, a significant portion of total metabolic rate becomes progressively dependent on glycolytic pathways. During anaerobic metabolism, additional carbon dioxide is transported to and eliminated by the lungs, and RER is above 1. Between *arrows A* and *B*, V_E keeps pace with increasing $\dot{V}CO_2$. At *arrow B*, minute ventilation begins to increase out of proportion to increases in $\dot{V}CO_2$.

The constant (0.863) is the factor required to transform fractional gas concentration to partial pressure and to express gas volumes at body temperature and pressure saturated with water vapor. V_A cannot be measured directly but is inferred from measurement of total minute ventilation at the mouth and the physiological dead space:

$$\dot{V}_A = \dot{V}_E \times (1 - V_D/V_T)$$

where V_E is converted to BTPS conditions and V_D/V_T is the ratio of physiological dead space to tidal volume (discussed later). Combining equations 1 and 2 gives the following:

$$\dot{V}_E = \frac{K \times \dot{V}CO_2}{Paco_2 \times (1 - V_D/V_T)}$$

This equation makes it apparent that V_E is proportional to $\dot{V}CO_2$ and inversely proportional to the $Paco_2$. In addition, increasing the V_D/V_T must result in an increase in V_E for $Paco_2$ to remain constant.

Use of the third equation and understanding cellular metabolism forms the basis for noninvasive methods to detect the so-called **anaerobic threshold**, which roughly corresponds to the point at which lactic acid begins to build up in the blood. Noninvasive detection of blood lactate acidosis relies on measurements of gas exchange ($\dot{V}O_2$, $\dot{V}CO_2$) and ventilation (V_E), referred to as the ventilatory threshold (VT). This distinguishes noninvasive determination from analysis of blood lactate, the lactate threshold (LT), and from the determination of anaerobic energy use at the cellular level, the anaerobic threshold. Though there is general agreement between VT and LT in most, but not all studies, a cause-and-effect relation between the two should not be inferred (5, 6).

There is no clear consensus in the literature for defining invasively determined LT from blood lactate versus $\dot{V}O_2$ curves. Some criteria are listed in Table 36.1. Despite the lack of consensus for determining LT, it is clear that there is a threshold exercise intensity in all healthy individuals above which exercise becomes increasingly difficult to sustain, probably because of a non–steady-state ac-

Table 36.1. Methods for Determining Lactate Threshold

CRITERION	(REFERENCES)
The $\dot{V}O_2$ or external power output at which blood lactate shows a "systematic" increase	(5, 12)
The $\dot{V}O_2$ or external power output at which blood lactate increases by 1 mM above value obtained at rest	
A clear change in slope of lactate plotted against either $\dot{V}O_2$ or external power output; includes log–log transformations to enhance the change in slope	(6)
The $\dot{V}O_2$ or external power output at which blood lactate exceeds a fixed value, such as 2 or 4 mM/L	(11)
The $\dot{V}O_2$ at which the slope of the lactate (mM/L) versus $\dot{V}O_2$ (L/min) curve equals 1	

cumulation of lactic acid (7, 8). This point occurs somewhere between 40% and 80% of maximal oxygen consumption, depending in part on fitness level (9). Use of methods to define this point from noninvasive criteria or invasively by one of the methods in Table 36.1 has demonstrated that $\dot{V}O_2$ at LT correlates better with exercise performance in predominantly aerobic tasks than maximum oxygen consumption ($\dot{V}O_{2max}$) (10, 11). Furthermore, exercise training raises $\dot{V}O_{2max}$ more effectively if training is performed at or just above LT (12).

Determination of the VT identifies the increase in $\dot{V}CO_2$ associated with buffering of lactic acid and the relative increase in V_E signaling the start of hyperventilation. In early studies, VT was determined from the point beyond which the RER exceeded 1. However, RER can be affected by hyperventilation, which transiently increases $\dot{V}CO_2$ measured at the mouth. A more sensitive method is to use the ventilatory equivalents for oxygen and carbon dioxide. To understand the utility of these two indices, the third equation can be rearranged:

$$\frac{\dot{V}_E}{\dot{V}CO_2} = \frac{K}{Pa_{CO_2} \times (1 - V_D/V_T)}$$

$$\frac{\dot{V}_E}{\dot{V}O_2} = \frac{K \times RER}{Pa_{CO_2} \times (1 - V_D/V_T)}$$

The ventilatory equivalents for carbon dioxide (top equation) normally decrease with increasing exercise intensity as V_D/V_T falls, reflecting improved gas exchange efficiency. Ventilatory equivalents for carbon dioxide increase near LT as ventilation is driven to the point that PA_{CO_2} and end-tidal P_{CO_2} begin to decrease. Similarly, ventilatory equivalents for oxygen decrease initially but begin to increase sooner than the increase in ventilatory equivalents for carbon dioxide because of increased RER. The commonly accepted definition of the VT using ventilatory equivalents is as follows: When following an exercise protocol with incrementally increasing exercise intensity, the VT is the $\dot{V}O_2$ at which these events occur:

- A rise in ventilatory equivalents for oxygen
- A steady or slowly falling ventilatory equivalents for carbon dioxide
- Constant or slowly rising end-tidal P_{CO_2} (13).

The final two criteria are included to avoid assigning VT to a point where simple hyperventilation is occurring, since hyperventilation can cause ventilatory equivalents for carbon dioxide to rise prematurely. In a normal response, the point at which the ventilatory equivalents for carbon dioxide rises and end-tidal P_{CO_2} begins to decline should occur later than the point at which ventilatory equivalents for oxygen rise, marking the beginning of relative hyperventilation and the end of isocapnic buffering.

To apply this method, data for V_E, $\dot{V}O_2$, $\dot{V}CO_2$, and end-tidal P_{CO_2} should be obtained at relatively short intervals using progressively increasing exercise intensity to volitional fatigue. No studies have addressed the "optimal" sampling interval for obtaining V_E, $\dot{V}O_2$, and $\dot{V}CO_2$. The interval should be long enough to smooth breath-to-breath variations but not so long that changes marking VT are obscured. An interval of 20–30 seconds is probably ideal. Thus, breath-by-breath data acquisition with 20–30 second averaging or a mixing chamber system with chamber size about 30–50% of the minute ventilation is sufficient.

A recent modification of the method for determining VT entails plotting the $\dot{V}CO_2$ against $\dot{V}O_2$ to locate a break point in the relationship (14). The break point identifies the $\dot{V}O_2$ at which the $\dot{V}CO_2$ rises disproportionately because of buffering.

Determination of VT is useful in many clinical and research settings. However, the identification of VT and the relation to blood lactate acidosis strongly depend on a normal breathing response to exercise. Some individuals do not have an identifiable VT by any method because of deviations in breathing pattern (carbon dioxide retention or hyperventilation).

The Ventilatory Response to Exercise

The mechanisms by which V_E is closely coupled to metabolism during exercise are unclear. During exercise, Pa_{CO_2} is maintained near resting levels until very heavy exercise, when it begins to decrease. An increase in V_E enough to decrease Pa_{CO_2} is thought to result from acidosis-stimulating chemoreceptors. Chemoreceptors are found in the brain and appear to be responsive to hydrogen ions and dissolved carbon dioxide primarily within the cerebrospinal fluid but are also influenced by local blood flow and metabolism (3). Also, peripheral chemoreceptors in the carotid bodies and aortic arch respond to decreased arterial pH and Pa_{O_2} and increased Pa_{CO_2}, serum K^+, and norepinephrine (15).

The mechanism that drives the increase in V_E to match increasing $\dot{V}O_2$ at lower levels of exercise is not known (3). Nerve centers (nuclei) in the brainstem that drive motor neurons of the respiratory muscles control the periodic nature of inspiration and expiration. These centers are probably influenced by afferent sensory inputs from the respiratory system and perhaps by working muscles (3). Lung stretch receptors may play a role in terminating a breath and in regulating end inspiratory lung volume. However, studies in heart–lung transplant patients devoid of stretch receptor feedback when tested at low levels of exercise demonstrate only small differences in breathing pattern from normal subjects. Lung irritant receptors are thought to lie between epithelial cells within the airways and appear to play a role during the bronchoconstriction of asthma in response to released histamine or bradykinin. Juxtacapillary receptors (J-receptors) in the alveolar walls respond to chemicals in the pulmonary circulation and to increases in interstitial fluid volume. Stimulation of these receptors causes rapid, shallow breathing. They may play a role in the dyspnea associated with congestive heart failure. They have also been implicated in the rapid, shallow breathing noted after heavy exercise (16). Additional receptors in the nose and upper airways respond to both mechanical and chemical stimulants. Respiratory muscles also contain muscle spindles, Golgi tendon organs, and nerve endings that may respond to length changes, rate of change, load, or metabolites produced with muscle fatigue.

BREATHING MECHANICS

The processes of increasing V_E through integration and recruitment of respiratory muscles and the alterations of airway diameter is known as breathing mechanics. The study of breathing mechanics includes the study of airway function, breathing pattern (respiratory rate and tidal volume), work of breathing, and the oxygen cost of doing the work.

Breathing Pattern

Light exercise is generally associated with increased depth, V_T, and f_b (Fig. 36.2). V_T and f_b increase until about 70–80% of peak exercise, after which increased frequency becomes the primary response (17). V_T usually levels off at 50–60% of vital capacity (18). Breathing frequency increases by a factor of one to three in most subjects, but in more fit athletes may be increased sixfold to sevenfold at high levels of V_E. In some subjects at extremely high ventilatory demands, V_T may decrease as f_b increases. Figure

36.2 shows average changes in breathing pattern with progressive exercise in a group of young, highly fit subjects and a group of older active individuals (19).

Increased V_T is due to both decreased EELV and increased EILV. Decreased EELV is thought to optimize inspiratory muscle length (for force development) and to help reduce the inspiratory work by allowing breathing at a lower average lung volume, therefore lowering average lung recoil pressure. In addition, the energy stored in the abdominal wall because of active expiration may provide some passive recoil at the initiation of the ensuing inspiration. In endurance athletes at high ventilatory demands (>150 L/minute), EELV may begin to increase, perhaps secondary to expiratory airflow limitation (17).

Increased f_b with exercise is associated with decreased inspiratory (T_I) and expiratory time (T_E). At moderate to high ventilatory demands, T_E decreases more than T_I (16). Because of the greater decrease in T_E, the increase in mean expiratory flow is greater than the increase in mean inspiratory flow.

Airflow and Pressure–Volume Responses

The MEFV curve produced by routine spirometry represents the maximal flow the lungs can sustain. Thus, the degree to which expiratory flows during exercise come close to the MEFV curve indicates the approach to a ventilatory limitation during exercise (discussed later). The MIFV curve represents the dynamic capacity of the inspiratory muscles, since the lungs do not limit inspiratory flows (Fig. 36.3).

Inspiratory pleural pressure generation gradually increases (becomes more negative) as ventilatory demand increases. Peak inspiratory pressure reaches only 50% of the dynamic capacity of the inspiratory muscles for pressure production (20). Peak expiratory pressures become positive only with heavy exercise and only near EELV. Thus, expiratory pressures for a given lung volume are well below the $P_{max,E}$ even in heavy exercise (17, 21).

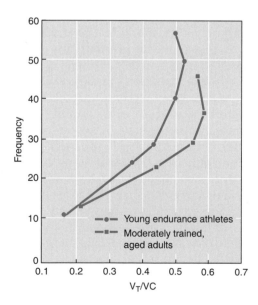

Figure 36.2. Frequency and tidal volume (V_T) relationship normalized for vital capacity (VC) during progressive exercise in young endurance athletes (*circles*) and moderately trained aged adults (*squares*). (Adapted with permission from Johnson BD, Badr MS, Dempsey JA. Impact of the aging pulmonary system on the response to exercise. Clin Chest Med 15:229, 1994.)

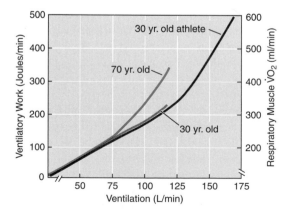

Figure 36.3. Ventilatory work and the oxygen cost of breathing during progressive exercise in 30-year-old untrained adults, 30-year-old athletes, and 70-year-old moderately fit older adults.

Airway Function and Pulmonary Resistance

The lungs are largely passive structures, and gas exchange occurs as respiratory muscles force lung expansion and contraction to move air in and out of alveoli. The muscles must work against the static recoil of the lungs and the resistance to movement of air in the pulmonary airways. Airway function is therefore an important parameter for normal lung function. It can be assessed in two ways: either through direct measurement of pulmonary resistance with assistance of an esophageal balloon or using MEFV curves.

The change in airway function during exercise is somewhat controversial. In normal individuals, airways are thought to dilate slightly during exercise, probably mediated by a change in vagus nerve activity. With asthma, airway function can show increased variability with changes in exercise intensity (22). After exercise, asthmatics can show marked deterioration in airway function, probably related to heat and water exchange in the airway during exercise.

The work that must be expended to move airflow can be estimated, and the oxygen cost of the work of breathing is thought to be less than 5% of the total $\dot{V}O_2$ at rest and during mild to moderate exercise. During heavy exercise in athletes, however, the work of breathing and the oxygen cost of the work can approach 15–20% of the $\dot{V}O_2$ (23). In pulmonary diseases, the oxygen cost of work that is related to increased airway resistance can also be substantial.

Nasal Breathing Versus Mouth Breathing

Though it varies, most people breathe through their nose at rest (24), although nasal airflow resistance is greater than mouth airflow resistance. The switch from primarily nasal breathing to oronasal breathing with exercise appears to occur at a V_E ranging from 22–44 L/min (24). The proportion of nasal to total ventilation has been found to vary between 26–64% during low-level activity and to decrease progressively to 25–30% during exercise at 90% of peak power (24).

Exercise has been shown to decrease nasal airflow resistance, presumably by dilation of the alai nasi muscles (22). Resistance to airflow can be decreased by 30% with the activation of these muscles (25). Despite this active dilation, airflow resistance is approximately 4 times greater through the nose than the mouth at rest and 9 times greater during exercise (24).

Indices of Ventilatory Constraint

Normal individuals who are not elite athletes generally do not have pulmonary limits to exercise. Pulmonary limitation can be defined in a number of ways. There is a mechanical limit to the amount of pressure the respiratory muscles can generate and the amount of inspiratory or expiratory flow the lungs can support. MVV is a crude index of maximal ventilation of the lungs and respiratory muscles. Calculated over 12–15 seconds, it may overestimate true maximal sustainable ventilation, but it represents an upper limit to the capacity of the pulmonary system. If an MVV is not measured, it can be estimated:

$$MVV = FEV_1 \times 37 \text{ (or 40)}$$

There are other methods for measuring mechanical limitation (4, 26).

Endurance athletes may approach both flow–volume and pressure-generating capacity near maximum exercise. As a result of increased lung volume at which peak inspiratory pressures occur, the demand for high flows (velocity of shortening), and the large pressures, peak inspiratory pressures approach a greater percent of the maximum available pressure (mean peak inspiratory pressure averaged 90% of the maximal available pressures) (17). An attempt to stimulate ventilation further by the addition of hypercapnic and hypoxic gases to inspired air near peak exercise results in little increase in ventilation (17). A likely explanation for this limitation is that despite the chemical stimulus to increase minute ventilation, the increased work, cost of breathing, and demand for blood flow competing with the locomotor muscles are too much for the system to effect a ventilatory response. The oxygen cost of breathing has been estimated to be on average 10–15% of total body $\dot{V}O_2$ in fit subjects. This requires a substantial percent of the available cardiac output to be diverted to respiratory muscles (17). Recent evidence suggests that the blood flow to respiratory muscles to support the work of breathing may steal blood flow from working muscles, which may affect performance (1).

GAS EXCHANGE

Adequate delivery of oxygen to and removal of carbon dioxide from working muscles depends on efficiency of gas exchange in the lungs. Oxygen delivery to the tissues is the product of blood oxygen content and cardiac output. When oxygen delivery is compromised, exercise may be limited by the ability to deliver oxygen to the tissues. Maintenance of partial pressure of oxygen in arterial blood (PaO_2) is critical to exercise performance and depends on the efficiency of gas exchange in the lungs. The lungs are efficient gas exchangers at rest and become more efficient at carbon dioxide removal during exercise. However, the efficiency of oxygenation deteriorates somewhat, requiring compensation through an enhanced ventilatory response (2).

Not all gas exchanging units of the lung (acini) have the same amount of ventilation (V_A) or perfusion ($\dot{Q}$), leading to inhomogeneity in ratios of V_A to $\dot{Q}$. A crude index of degree of $V_A/\dot{Q}$ mismatching is the V_D/V_T ratio, which is obtained by comparing $PaCO_2$ to mixed expired PCO_2 ($P_{\bar{E}CO_2}$, obtained by collecting expired air in a large bag or by digital integration of expiratory flow and P_{CO_2} signals):

$$\frac{V_D}{V_T} = \frac{Pa_{CO_2} - P\bar{E}_{CO_2}}{Pa_{CO_2}}$$

where Pa_{CO_2} is obtained from an arterial blood gas sample. The V_D/V_T ratio should decrease to less than 30% at maximal exercise (19, 27). However, the normal range for exercise V_D/V_T increases with age (19). It is tempting to substitute end-tidal P_{CO_2} ($P\bar{E}T_{CO_2}$) measurements for Pa_{CO_2} in the V_D/V_T equation. However, $P\bar{E}T_{CO_2}$ may not equate to Pa_{CO_2}, especially during exercise, so the noninvasive V_D/V_T should be used cautiously in diagnostic testing.

Oxygenation during exercise, as indicated by the Pa_{O_2}, is generally well maintained, though reduced oxygenation has been noted in elite athletes (4, 17). An example of arterial blood gases obtained during exercise in a highly fit group of young endurance athletes relative to average fit young subjects and fit older adults is shown in Figure 36.4. Data concerning the effect of age on arterial oxygenation near maximal exercise conflict. In one study, there was no age effect, though others suggest a deterioration in oxygenation with age (19, 27). However, there is a progressive decrease in $\dot{V}O_{2max}$ with age, and older athletes who can work at greater metabolic demands than sedentary individuals (near those achieved in the average fit young adult) may become hypoxemic for reasons similar to those that affect the elite young endurance athlete.

The A-a D_{O_2} is a useful index of gas exchange efficiency. The average Pa_{CO_2} is lowered by reduced Pi_{O_2} (e.g., at altitude) and by increased alveolar and Pa_{CO_2} (hypoventilation).

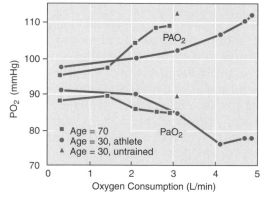

Figure 36.4. Alveolar and arterial partial pressures during incremental exercise in an average fit group of subjects (*diamonds*, peak exercise only, $\dot{V}O_{2max}$, = 42 ml/kg/min) relative to that found in a group of endurance athletes (*open circles*, n = 8, peak $\dot{V}O_{2max}$ = 73 ml/kg/min) and a group of relatively fit older adults (*circles*, n = 19, $\dot{V}O_{2max}$ = 42 ml/kg/min). (Reprinted with permission from Johnson BD, Badr MS, Dempsey JA. Impact of the aging pulmonary system on the response to exercise. Clin Chest Med 15:229, 1994.)

$$Pa_{CO_2} = Pi_{O_2} - Pa_{CO_2}\left[Fi_{O_2} - \frac{1 - Fi_{O_2}}{RER}\right]$$

Hypoxemia (reduced Pa_{O_2}) is caused by (2, 4, 28) the following:

- Decreased alveolar ventilation relative to carbon dioxide output, which increases Pa_{CO_2} (A-a D_{O_2} is normal)
- Diffusion limitation related to reduction in time the red blood cell is exposed to alveolar gas
- An increase in $\dot{V}_A/\dot{Q}$ mismatching
- Increased shunted blood
- Hypoxic environment (e.g., altitude)

PULMONARY HEMODYNAMICS

Pulmonary Circulation

The role of the pulmonary circulation is to provide for efficient gas exchange between mixed venous blood entering the pulmonary capillaries and alveolar air. This is achieved by an extremely thin interface between the capillaries and the alveoli and by a large network of capillary–alveolar interactions (discussed in the section on gas exchange). The perfusion of capillaries is thought to depend on body position (gravity) and the driving pressures through the pulmonary capillaries. Recent studies suggest inherent regional differences in vascular resistance dictating a gravity-independent anatomical distribution of blood flow (29). The driving pressure for pulmonary blood flow is determined by the difference between P_{pa} and the left atrial pressure or P_{pw}. The resting driving pressure through the pulmonary circulation is 7–8 mm Hg.

With moderate exercise ($\dot{V}O_2$ = 1.5–2.0 L/minute), the driving pressure increases to 11–12 mm Hg, which though small, probably increases the number of perfused capillaries and increases distention in already perfused capillaries. With heavy exercise ($\dot{V}O_2$ = 3–4 L/minute), the driving pressure may increase up to 10–15 mm Hg. Studies performed on older subjects note increased P_{pa} relative to younger individuals at a given $\dot{V}O_2$; however, the P_{pw} is also elevated, so that the driving pressures remain essentially unchanged (30). It is thought that in older adults, mild diastolic dysfunction may contribute to the elevated P_{pw}.

Bronchial Circulation

In addition to the pulmonary circulation, the lung has a vascular source provided by the bronchial circulation. This vascular supply originates from branches of the aorta, such as the intercostal, internal mammary, and subclavian arteries, and supplies the bronchi, branching with the airways as far as the terminal bronchioles (31). This circulation may play a role in temperature regulation and may be involved in lung fluid balance, as implied by its closeness to the lymphatic circulation. Some studies note marked increases in bronchial blood flow during exercise and during exposure to dry air (e.g., hyperventilation) (32). Under extremely adverse conditions, the bronchial circulation may play a role in gas exchange and in preventing pulmonary hypertension (31). Typically, however, it combines with thebesian vessels of the heart and contributes to a physiological venoarterial shunt (4, 31).

The bronchial circulation has been estimated to account for approximately 1–1.5% of total cardiac output at rest and during exercise. At the very high energy expenditures achieved by some endurance athletes, shunt would be expected to contribute proportionally more to increased widening in the A-a D_{O_2} because the mixed venous oxygen content is probably reduced to less than 5 mL oxygen per 100 mL blood. It is unlikely, however, that shunt accounts for all or even a major portion of the severe exercise-induced hypoxemia observed in some athletes, because mild hyperoxia during heavy exercise causes proportionate increases in alveolar and arterial P_{O_2} and Pa_{O_2} is normal, even in subjects who are the most hypoxemic (4).

AIRWAY FLUID BALANCE

The lumen side of the airway is a complex tissue composed of epithelial cells protected by the mucosal surface layer, secretory glands, nerves, smooth muscle, and cells of the immune system, including mast cells and macrophages. In disease states there may be more inflammatory cells populating the airway, including eosinophils and neutrophils. As with mast cells, the ionic milieu of the luminal surface may affect functioning of these cell types (33).

The amount of fluid present and the concentration of ions in the mucosa reflect a dynamic balance among fluid production by glandular structures, fluid transport from alveoli, fluid resorption by airway cells, and fluid evaporation (34). Most fluid evaporation probably occurs in the upper airway (oropharynx and nasopharynx) (35, 36). Although there are no studies in humans, animal research suggests that increased ventilation causes increased ionic concentration in the airway fluid layer of larger airways, presumably because of evaporative water loss (37). Modeling studies suggest that water loss also occurs in smaller airways (35, 36). The ionic milieu may be affected in important ways during exercise as evaporative water loss upsets the normal homeostatic balance. Both passive and active compensatory mechanisms activate to restore the ionic milieu. The passive compensations include increased fluid or ion fluxes across the airway secondary to changes in concentration gradients for ions or water as water evaporates from the airways. Active mechanisms include neural and humoral control of both glandular secretion and resorption mechanisms (34). Mechanical stresses associated with increased ventilation may cause increased production of mediators, such as nitric oxide and prostaglandins that influence airway fluid balance (34). The study of airway fluid balance in humans is in its infancy. Recent studies suggest that control of airway fluid balance may be different in normal persons from that of asthmatics (38).

► SUMMARY

As exercise intensity increases, oxygen consumption and carbon dioxide production by working muscles increase dramatically. The cardiorespiratory system is required to deliver oxygen to and transport carbon dioxide from these tissues in an attempt to maintain cellular homeostasis. The central nervous system responds by increasing neural ventilatory and cardiac drive, resulting in increased activity of cardiac and respiratory muscles. The lungs are largely passive, and the increased ventilatory and cardiac drives result in increasing blood and airflow and increased rate of transfer of oxygen and carbon dioxide across the gas-exchanging surfaces of the alveoli. However, limits to the degree to which increased airflow and blood flow can be supported can lead to pulmonary limitations to exercise either from mechanical ventilatory constraints or from compromised gas exchange. These limitations are generally not manifested in healthy individuals except in elite or older athletes.

References

1. Harms CA, Wetter TJ, McClaran SR, et al. Effects of respiratory muscle work on cardiac output and its distribution during maximal exercise. J Appl Physiol 85:609–618, 1998.
2. Dempsey JA, Wagner PD. Exercise-induced arterial hypoxemia. J Appl Physiol 87:1997–2006, 1999.
3. Forster HV. Exercise Hyperpnea: Where do we go from here? Exerc Sport Sci Rev 28:133–137, 2000.
4. Dempsey JA, Hanson PG, Henderson KS. Exercise-induced arterial hypoxemia in healthy human subjects at sea level. J Physiol 355:161, 1984.
5. Johnson BD, Weisman IM, Zeballos RJ, Beck KC. Emerging concepts in the evaluation of ventilatory limitation during exercise: The exercise tidal flow-volume loop. Chest 116:488–503, 1999.
6. Wasserman K et al. Gas exchange theory and the lactic acidosis (anaerobic) threshold. Circulation 81(Suppl 2):II14–II30, 1990.
7. Ribeiro JP et al. Metabolic and ventilatory responses to steady state exercise relative to lactate thresholds. Eur J Appl Physiol 55:215–221, 1986.
8. Roston WL et al. Oxygen uptake kinetics and lactate concentration during exercise in humans. Am Rev Resp Dis 135:1080–1084, 1987.
9. Normal values. In: Wasserman K et al., eds. Principles of Exercise Testing and Interpretation. Philadelphia: Lea & Febiger, 1987:72–86.
10. Kumagai S et al. Relationships of the anaerobic threshold with the 5 km, 10 km and 10 mile races. Eur J Appl Physiol 49:13–23, 1982.
11. Weltman A et al. Prediction of lactate threshold and fixed blood lactate concentrations from 3200-m running performance in male runners. Int J Sports Med 8:401–406, 1987.

12. Henritze J et al. Effects of training at and above the lactate threshold on the lactate threshold and maximal oxygen uptake. Eur J Physiol 54:84–88, 1985.
13. Wasserman K. The anaerobic threshold measurement to evaluate exercise performance. Am Rev Resp Dis 129(Suppl):S35–S40, 1984.
14. Beaver WL et al. A new method for detecting anaerobic threshold by gas exchange. J Appl Physiol 60:2020–2027, 1986.
15. Busse M, Maassen N, Konrad H. Relation between plasma K+ and ventilation during incremental exercise after glycogen depletion and repletion in man. J Physiol 443: 469–476, 1991.
16. Syabbalo NC, Krishnan B, Zintel T, et al. Differential ventilatory control during constant work rate and incremental exercise. Respir Physiol 97:175–187, 1994.
17. Johnson BD, Saupe KW, Dempsey JA. Mechanical constraints on exercise hyperpnea in endurance athletes. J Appl Physiol 73:874–886, 1992.
18. Blackie SP et al. Normal values and ranges for ventilation and breathing pattern at maximal exercise. Chest 100:136–142, 1991.
19. Johnson BD, Badr MS, Dempsey JA. Impact of the aging pulmonary system on the response to exercise. Clin Chest Med 15:229, 1994.
20. Leblanc P, Summers E, Inman MD, et al. Inspiratory muscles during exercise: a problem of supply and demand. J Appl Physiol 64:2482–2489, 1988.
21. Olafsson S, Hyatt RE. Ventilatory mechanics and expiratory flow limitation during exercise in normal subjects. J Clin Invest 48:564–573, 1969.
22. Syabbalo NC, Bundgaard A, Widdicombe JG. Effects of exercise on nasal airflow resistance in healthy subjects and in patients with asthma and rhinitis. Bull Eur Physiopathol Respir 21:507–513, 1985.
23. Aaron EA, Seow KC, Johnson BD, et al. Oxygen cost of exercise hyperpnea: implications for performance. J Appl Physiol 72:1818–1825, 1992.
24. Wheatley JR, Amis TC, Engel LA. Oronasal partitioning of ventilation during exercise. J Appl Physiol 71:546–551, 1991.
25. Strohl EP, O'Cain CF, Slutsky AS. Alae nasi activation and nasal resistance in healthy subjects. J Appl Physiol 52:1432–1437, 1982.
26. Johnson BD, Scanlon PD, Beck KC. Regulation of ventilatory capacity during exercise in asthmatics. J Appl Physiol 79:892–901, 1995.
27. Malmberg P, Hedenström H, Fridriksson HV. Reference values for gas exchange during exercise in healthy nonsmoking and smoking men. Bull Eur Physiopathol Respir 23:131, 1987.
28. Wagner PD. Ventilation-perfusion matching during exercise. Chest 101(Suppl):192S, 1992.
29. Beck KC, Rehder K. Factors determining pulmonary blood flow and gas distribution: New insights. Curr Opin Anaesthesiol 7:536–542, 1994.
30. Reeves JT, Dempsey JA, Grover RF. Pulmonary circulation during exercise. In: Weirand EK, Reeves JT, eds. Pulmonary Vascular Physiology and Pathophysiology. New York: Marcel Dekker, 1989:107–133.
31. Tobin CE. The bronchial arteries and their connections with other vessels in the human lung. Surg Gynecol Obstet 95:741–750, 1952.
32. Manohar M. Blood flow to the respiratory and limb muscles and to abdominal organs during maximal exertion in ponies. J Physiol 377:25–35, 1986.
33. Pearce FL, Flint KC, Leung KB, et al. Some studies on human pulmonary mast cells obtained by bronchoalveolar lavage and by enzymatic dissociation of whole lung tissue. Int Arch Allergy Appl Immunol 82:507–512, 1987.
34. Al-Bazzaz FJ. Regulation of salt and water transport across airway mucosa. Clin Chest Med 7:259–272, 1986.
35. Gilbert IA, Fouke JM, McFadden ER. Heat and water flux in the intrathoracic airways and exercise-induced asthma. J Appl Physiol 63:1681–1691, 1987.
36. Hanna LM, Scherer PW. A theoretical model of localized heat and water vapor transport in the human respiratory tract. J Biomech Eng 108:19–27, 1986.
37. Boucher RC, Stutts MJ, Bromberg PA, et al. Regional differences in airway surface liquid composition. J Appl Physiol 50:613–620, 1981.
38. Daviskas E, Anderson SD, Gonda I, et al. Changes in mucociliary clearance during and after isocapnic hyperventilation in asthmatic and healthy subjects. Eur Resp J 8:742–751, 1995.

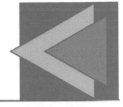

CHAPTER 37

PATHOPHYSIOLOGY OF LUNG DISEASE

Connie C. W. Hsia

Key to Pulmonary Physiology Abbreviations

A-a D_{O_2}	Alveolar–arterial oxygen difference
COPD	Chronic obstructive pulmonary disease
D_L	Lung diffusing capacity
$D_L/\dot{Q}$	Ratio of diffusion conductance of the alveolar tissue to perfusion of pulmonary vasculature
$D_L O_2$	Diffusing capacity of oxygen in the lungs
FEF_{25-75}	Forced expiratory flow at mid range (25–75%)
FEV_1	Forced expiratory volume in 1 second
PA_{O_2}	Partial pressure of oxygen in alveolar air
Pa_{CO_2}	Partial pressure of carbon dioxide in arterial blood
Pa_{O_2}	Partial pressure of oxygen in arterial blood
P_{CO_2}	Partial pressure of carbon dioxide
P_{O_2}	Partial pressure of oxygen
RV	Residual volume
RV/TLC	Ratio of residual volume to total lung capacity
TLC	Total lung capacity
$\dot{V}_A$	Minute alveolar ventilation
$\dot{V}_A/\dot{Q}$	Ratio of ventilation to perfusion (ventilation-cardiac output)

Diseases of the respiratory tract can be classified according to mechanisms of derangement:

- Obstructive airway disease
- Restrictive disease involving lung parenchyma, pleura, thorax, or respiratory muscles
- Pulmonary vascular disease
- Hypoventilation syndromes

This chapter reviews the general pathophysiological patterns of lung disease and the fundamental concepts of how lung disease limits aerobic capacity. It does not discuss exogenous causes of lung disease (infection, trauma, neoplasm, and congenital abnormalities).

NORMAL VENTILATORY MECHANICS

During inspiration the diaphragm contracts and descends while the rib cage moves upward and outward.

These actions generate negative pressure inside the thorax relative to pressure at the mouth, causing airflow into the lungs. During expiration the diaphragm relaxes and moves upward while the rib cage moves inward. At rest expiration requires no active muscular contraction. Lung tissue possesses intrinsic elasticity and a natural tendency to recoil inward, which forces air out of the lung. However, during exercise, expiration is aided by active contraction of the abdominal and thoracic expiratory muscles, which further pushes the abdominal contents upward and the rib cage inward. These muscular actions generate positive pressure inside the thorax, pushing air out of the lungs.

Large airways are supported by cartilage in the walls, and the dimensions are relatively unaffected by thoracic pressure changes. The amount of cartilage decreases as the size of the airway decreases, and the smallest branches have no cartilage. They are tethered to the surrounding alveolar mesh by radial traction and are influenced by intra-thoracic pressure changes. Negative intra-thoracic pressure increases lung volume, stretches the alveolar mesh, increases radial traction, and pulls airways open. Positive intrathoracic pressure reduces lung volume and radial traction; hence, airway caliber is larger during inspiration than expiration (Fig. 37.1). The potential energy stored in radial traction of airways and alveoli at a given lung volume is known as elastic recoil pressure; this pressure determines the diameter of small airways and resistance to flow. Elastic recoil pressure is greatest at high lung volumes and decreases as lung volume decreases.

During expiration a progressive loss of elastic recoil results in airway closure as lung volume decreases. The maximum expiratory flow that can be generated is related to intrathoracic pressure (determined by muscular effort at very high lung volumes and by chest wall and lung elastic recoil at lower lung volumes) and resistance of the airways (determined by airway diameter and geometry). Flow rates are reduced when there is neuromuscular weakness (polyneuropathy, polio), loss of elastic recoil (emphysema), or narrowing of airways (asthma, chronic

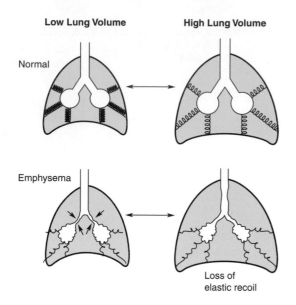

Figure 37.1. Small airways are tethered open by radial traction of lung tissue. Airway caliber depends on recoil of the lung, which is greater at a high lung volume; hence, airway caliber is also greater at a high lung volume. In diseases in which elastic recoil is lost, small airways are prone to dynamic collapse when pressure outside the airway becomes more positive, as during forced expiration.

bronchitis). Other sources provide a more detailed discussion of the mechanics of breathing (1, 2).

OBSTRUCTIVE AIRWAY DISEASES

Obstructive airway diseases result from a narrowing of airways. They can be caused by intraluminal, intramural, or extramural lesions. Airway narrowing within the lung increases resistance to air flow, resulting in uneven distribution of ventilation. Obstruction of extrathoracic airways causes a prominent reduction in inspiratory flow rates (3) (Fig. 37.2). Obstruction of intrathoracic airways causes a prominent expiratory flow limitation, shown by a disproportionate reduction in forced expiratory flow rates relative to lung volume, that is, low ratio of FEV_1 to forced vital capacity, or low FEF_{25-75}. The pattern of large, intrathoracic airway obstruction is distinct from obstruction distal to the trachea and mainstem bronchi.

In diffuse obstructive airway disease associated with a loss of lung elastic recoil, airways begin to close at an abnormally high lung volume above the resting end-expiratory volume, resulting in increased RV, or air trapping, at the end of a forced exhalation. TLC and the ratio of RV to TLC both increase in obstructive airway disease. Air trapping displaces the diaphragm downward, causing the muscle to lose its normal domelike configuration (Fig. 37.3). Flattening of the diaphragm places the muscle at a mechanical disadvantage, reduces the efficiency of contraction, and increases the oxygen cost of breathing. Air-

way involvement is usually not uniform; hence, regional distribution of ventilation becomes nonuniform, resulting in regional mismatch of $\dot{V}_A/\dot{Q}$, which impairs the efficiency of gas exchange between alveolar air and blood (4).

Chronic Obstructive Pulmonary Disease

COPD is a common disorder characterized by progressive expiratory flow obstruction, dyspnea on exertion, and some degree of reversible airway hyperreactivity (5). Symptoms develop insidiously over years to decades. Many such patients are chronic cigarette smokers. There are two main clinical and pathophysiological syndromes: chronic bronchitis and emphysema. A third syndrome, small airway disease, is sometimes designated separately to indicate obstruction of small airways. However, features of all three commonly overlap.

Chronic Bronchitis

Chronic bronchitis is characterized by a chronic cough and excessive sputum production. The histological hallmark of chronic bronchitis is enlargement and overabundance of mucous glands in the walls of large bronchi. The airway wall thickens, and the surface becomes irregular. Bronchial and peribronchial inflammation may reduce luminal diameter. These changes are exacerbated by bacterial colonization of the airway associated with episodes of acute bronchitis.

Narrowing of large bronchi produces a marked increase in air flow resistance, while intrathoracic pressure generated by muscular effort and lung elastic recoil is normal. Expiratory flow rates may improve after inhaled bronchodilator therapy but usually cannot be completely normalized. Lung units with high airway resistance receive little ventilation, while pulmonary blood flow either decreases or remains unchanged, and therefore, the lungs are underventilated and overperfused (i.e., low $\dot{V}_A/\dot{Q}$ ratio), which leads to arterial hypoxemia. Hypoxemia, a potent stimulus of smooth muscle constriction in pulmonary arterioles and venules, leads to increased pulmonary vascular resistance, pulmonary arterial hypertension, and right ventricular strain.

In chronic severe disease, secondary right heart failure (**cor pulmonale**) eventually develops. Hypoxemia stimulates the production of erythropoietin, resulting in excessive blood volume, hemoglobin concentration, and hematocrit (**secondary polycythemia**). Polycythemia may lead to high blood viscosity, increasing flow resistance in blood vessels and potentially compromising blood flow in small vessels of the brain and heart.

Typical patients with severe chronic bronchitis are known as **blue bloaters** because they exhibit a stocky habitus with central and peripheral cyanosis. Reduced airflow rate is associated with only mildly increased lung volumes and a relatively normal rate of oxygen transfer across the alveolar–capillary barrier (D_L). Secondary de-

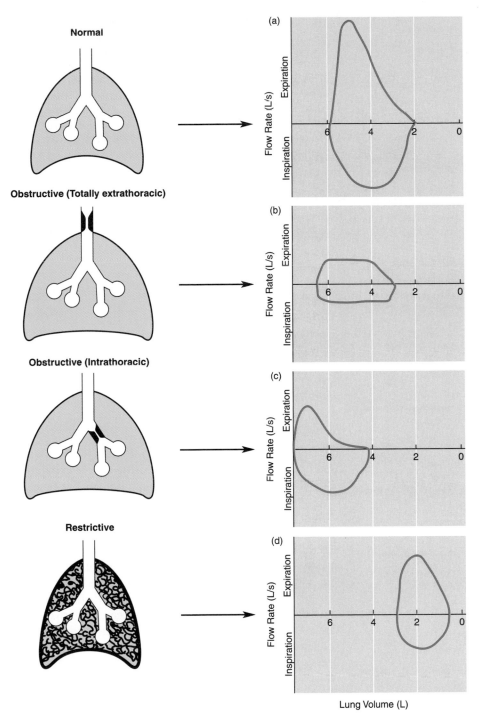

Figure 37.2. Maximal flow–volume curves in normal subject, extrathoracic airway obstruction, intrathoracic airway obstruction, and restrictive lung disease.

rangement in ventilatory control may develop, and patients with chronic bronchitis tend to maintain low minute ventilation, which may further decline during sleep, resulting in nocturnal hypoxemia. They may also develop daytime hypoxemia and carbon dioxide retention. The clinical progression of chronic bronchitis is shown in Figure 37.4.

Emphysema

Emphysema is technically a disease of the lung parenchyma secondarily affecting small airways (6). It includes abnormal permanent enlargement of air spaces accompanied by destruction of alveolar walls.

The biochemical basis of the disease is protease–antiprotease disequilibrium. Elastin is a major connective tissue component of the alveolar wall. Proteases promote degradation of elastin, and antiproteases inhibit degradation. Destruction of lung tissue results from either increased protease activity or deficient antiprotease activity. Smokers demonstrate significantly increased pulmonary proteolytic activities, possibly related to accumulation of inflammatory cells (neutrophils, macrophages) contain-

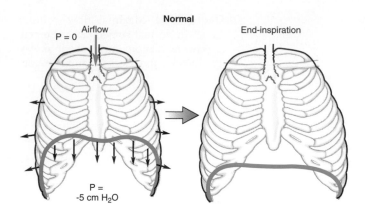

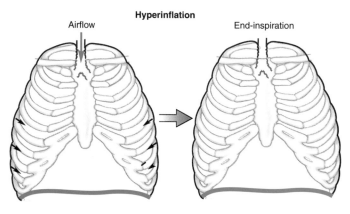

Figure 37.3. **Top.** Normally the diaphragm is dome shaped, with most of the muscle fibers nearly vertical. Diaphragm contraction causes muscle fibers to shorten and the dome to descend, simultaneously expanding the rib cage (*arrows*). These actions generate negative pressure inside the thorax, causing airflow into the lungs. **Bottom.** In lung hyperinflation caused by severe COPD, the diaphragm loses its dome shape. Upon contraction the diaphragm cannot descend normally, which can create a paradoxical inward movement of the lower ribcage (*arrows*).

Chronic cough and sputum production

↓

Expiratory airflow limitation
Progressive dyspnea on exertion

↓

Progressive $\dot{V}_A/\dot{Q}$ mismatch
↓arterial pO_2
↑arterial pCO_2

↓

Pulmonary hypertension
Right heart strain
Polycythemia

↓

Right heart failure

Figure 37.4. Progression of chronic bronchitis.

ing a high concentration of protease enzymes (7). On the other hand, those with a genetic deficiency of alpha-1-antitrypsin, a potent antiprotease, are prone to develop severe emphysema at an early age even if they never smoke.

The hallmark of emphysema is loss of lung elasticity and reduction of elastic recoil pressure due to accelerated alveolar destruction. Small airways lose radial traction to the surrounding alveolar walls and become easily collapsible during expiration because intrathoracic pressure

becomes more positive (Fig. 37.1). Patients with emphysema can expel a larger volume during a slow exhalation than during a maximal forced exhalation because intrathoracic pressure is less positive and airway compression is minimized during a slow exhalation.

Expiratory flow limitation in emphysema is unresponsive to bronchodilator therapy because the basis of obstruction is altered mechanical properties of the lung tissue. Patients can minimize air trapping and dyspnea by pursed-lip breathing, in which the lips are puckered during exhalation (8). Pursing the lips creates external resistance to flow and maintains a more positive intra-airway pressure during exhalation retarding small airway compression. Since loss of elastic recoil primarily affects airway resistance during forced expiration, airway resistance during quiet breathing may be relatively normal. However, even with normal airway resistance, the loss of elastic recoil as a driving force leads to a reduction in expiratory flow rate.

Distribution of ventilation is also not uniform in emphysema, and lung units that are not well ventilated tend to receive less perfusion because of destruction of the capillary bed. Some ventilation goes to lung units containing no capillaries; therefore dead space is increased. This physiological pattern is distinct from that seen in chronic bronchitis.

To overcome high physiological dead space, patients must chronically sustain high minute ventilation; therefore, typical patients with pure emphysema are known as

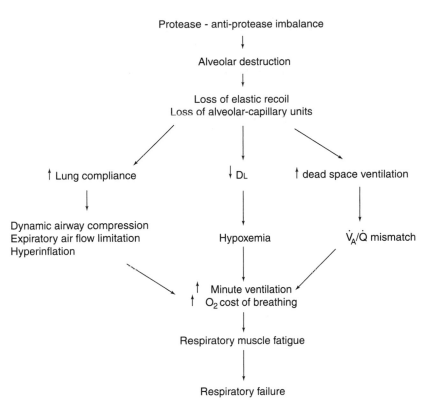

Figure 37.5. Progression of emphysema.

pink puffers. They are barrel-chested because of marked air trapping. There is little cough or sputum production. They are thin, with general muscle wasting attributed to malnutrition. Work of breathing is difficult, and a larger than normal fraction of oxygen supplied across the lung is required by respiratory muscles just to sustain ventilation, leaving an insufficient amount for other metabolic functions. In severe emphysema, excessive energy cost of breathing may divert oxygen away from the gut, leading to malnutrition. Malnutrition in turn impairs respiratory muscle strength and makes it more difficult to sustain the high ventilatory demands. In addition to reduced lung elasticity (i.e., high lung compliance), lung diffusing capacity is reduced by loss of alveolar–capillary units. Ventilatory control is normal.

In moderate emphysema PaO_2 and $PaCO_2$ are generally well maintained. With severe end-stage disease, respiratory muscle fatigue sets in and $PaCO_2$ rises, while PaO_2 drops. Progressive destruction of alveolar–capillary units leads to elevated pulmonary vascular resistance, right heart strain, and eventually right heart failure. Disease progression is outlined in Figure 37.5.

Small Airway Disease

Small airway disease is an early manifestation of the same pathological processes that eventually lead to chronic bronchitis and/or emphysema. Inflammation around small airways (< 2 mm in diameter) occurs in response to irritant exposure; it is associated with reduced FEF_{25-75}, while maximal expiratory flow rates at FEV_1 may be minimally affected. Cigarette smoking increases risk of small airway flow obstruction and loss of elastic recoil in a dose-dependent fashion. Objective abnormalities in small airway flow pattern can be demonstrated within 1–5 years of smoking; in early stages, such abnormalities are largely reversible with cessation of smoking. Subjective symptoms are usually mild in the absence of large airway or parenchymal involvement.

Management of COPD

The management of patients with these types of COPD generally includes the following strategies:

1. Identify and eliminate sources of bronchopulmonary inflammation (i.e., cigarette smoking, inhaled irritants, recurrent respiratory infections).
2. Identify and treat reversible airway narrowing with inhaled or oral bronchodilators and corticosteroids.
3. Prevent exacerbations by routine vaccination against infectious agents, such as pneumococcus and influenza; by adequate respiratory hygiene; and in selected patients, by prophylactic administration of antibiotics.
4. Establish individualized rehabilitation programs for stable patients.

Rehabilitation programs generally have some component of moderate physical and breathing exercises. Maximal oxygen uptake may improve if significant deconditioning is present. Selective respiratory muscle training can improve ventilatory capacity in patients with lung disease, and exercise performance may also improve in some patients (9). Neither cardiovascular nor selective respiratory muscle training significantly improves mechanical lung function or alveolar gas exchange. However, exercise training improves oxygen delivery and extraction; hence, overall efficiency of oxygen use is enhanced and endurance for submaximal exercise is improved (5).

Chronic home oxygen therapy is indicated for patients in respiratory failure whose PaO_2 remains below 55 mm Hg despite optimal medical therapy. The goal is to alleviate hypoxemia, minimize hypoxic pulmonary vasoconstriction, reduce pulmonary vascular resistance, and ultimately prevent right heart failure. The dose of oxygen must be determined individually. In the presence of chronic carbon dioxide retention, ventilatory response to carbon dioxide is blunted, and hypoxemia becomes the predominant stimulus to ventilation. Excessive oxygen administration can abolish the hypoxic ventilatory drive and lead to apnea.

Asthma

Asthma affects about 5% of the general population. It is characterized by increased airway reactivity to various stimuli, resulting in widespread reversible narrowing of airways (10, 11). The episodic nature and reversibility of the narrowing are important features. It is sometimes possible to identify specific agents that precipitate attacks (allergic asthma), such as pollens, dust mites, animal dander, drugs, foods, wine, fumes, and chemicals. Asthma attacks may also be induced by nonspecific stimuli, such as emotional stress, exercise, exposure to cold, or a viral respiratory infection. Often no precipitating factors can be identified (perennial asthma). Asthma may be associated with allergic rhinitis, nasal polyps, and aspirin sensitivity. There is a strong tendency for familial clustering.

The classical mechanism triggering an attack is coupling of an antigen to immunoglobulin-E antibodies on the surface of sensitized mast cells, leading to release of various biochemical mediators causing airway smooth muscle constriction (bronchospasm). The antigen–antibody interaction may also stimulate vagal neural reflexes directly to cause bronchoconstriction. Physical stimuli, such as cooling and fluid evaporation across airway epithelium during exercise or cold air exposure, may directly stimulate the release of chemical mediators (12).

Prolonged bronchospasm leads to secondary mucosal edema and mucus accumulation. These secondary processes must be aggressively prevented and treated, since they reduce the physiological response to bronchodilator therapy and further contribute to airflow obstruction, hyperinflation, and $\dot{V}_A/\dot{Q}$ mismatch.

The diagnosis is made by demonstrating airflow obstruction (reduced maximal expiratory flow rates, increased inspiratory and expiratory air flow resistance, ele-

vated RV, TLC, and RV/TLC) that is abolished by the administration of a bronchodilator or by a challenge test of inhaled methacholine, which causes bronchoconstriction in individuals with heightened airway reactivity (13). Patients with exercise-induced asthma may demonstrate normal airway function at rest, but bronchospasm may develop during or after exercise. This can be relieved by administration of an inhaled bronchodilator. Since exercise-induced asthma is thought to be related to physical stimuli directly causing mast cell degranulation, prophylactic use of an inhaled bronchodilator or a mast cell–stabilizing drug, such as cromolyn sodium, before exercise commonly prevents attacks.

During an acute asthmatic attack lung units distal to constricted bronchi are underventilated, and regions of low $\dot{V}_A/\dot{Q}$ ratio develop (14, 15). Patients typically hyperventilate initially, maintaining a normal PaO_2 while $PaCO_2$ drops. As the attack worsens, the distribution of $\dot{V}_A/\dot{Q}$ becomes more abnormal, and PaO_2 declines despite persistent hyperventilation. Severe or prolonged attacks unresponsive to therapy (i.e., status asthmaticus) may lead to respiratory failure with hypoxemia and hypercapnia.

Management of Asthma

Management of asthmatic patients generally includes the following strategies:

1. Identification and elimination of precipitating agents.
2. Preventing and minimizing attacks by teaching the patient to improve compliance with medication. Pharmacological prophylaxis can be achieved by use of inhaled corticosteroid preparations to reduce airway inflammation and inhaled cromolyn sodium to stabilize mast cells.
3. Establishing the best inhaled or oral bronchodilator therapy to achieve the maximal possible flow rates and maximal exercise tolerance.

RESTRICTIVE LUNG DISEASES

Restrictive lung diseases reduce lung volume by involving the thorax or the lung parenchyma; such diseases affect the rib cage and spine (kyphoscoliosis, ankylosing spondylitis, pectus excavatum), respiratory muscles and nerves (spinal cord injury, neuropathy, myopathy, diaphragm paralysis), pleura (effusion, pleuritis, fibrothorax, mesothelioma), or alveolar septum (interstitial fibrosis, alveolitis). Morbid obesity can also restrict the thorax and respiratory muscles. Restriction of the rib cage or pleura from any cause leads to low lung volume and reduced excursion of lung volume during exercise. Chronic restriction also leads to secondary atelectasis of some alveolar units. Functional surface of air–tissue interface decreases, eventually resulting in impaired gas exchange.

There are more than 200 causes of diffuse interstitial and alveolar lung disease, including the following (16):

- Infection (tuberculosis, fungus, virus)
- Neoplastic disease (lymphoma, metastatic cancer)
- Thromboembolism
- Toxic inhaled organic and inorganic substances (farmer's lung, bird fancier's disease, silicosis, asbestosis)
- Drugs (chemotherapeutic agents, amiodarone)
- Pulmonary edema
- Systemic immunological disease (rheumatoid arthritis, lupus erythematosus, sarcoidosis)
- Radiation injury
- Idiopathic interstitial lung disease (cause unknown)

The histological hallmark of many but not all types of restrictive lung disease is inflammation of the interstitium and alveolar tissue with varying degrees of fibrosis. These changes directly reduce lung compliance, leading to nonuniform distribution of ventilation, increased work of breathing, increased respiratory muscle oxygen demand, and increased airway size and expiratory flow rates.

A stiff lung requires more energy to stretch, and a greater transpulmonary pressure is required to achieve a given tidal volume. At the same time, maximal tidal volume is restricted. Hence, ventilation must be increased, primarily via faster breathing. This pattern of rapid, shallow breathing leads to alveolar hyperventilation and decreased Pa_{O_2}. Interstitial and alveolar inflammation eventually causes normal alveolar–capillary membrane to be replaced with fibrous tissue, leading to reduced rate of oxygen uptake by blood; therefore, both mechanical and gas exchange functions are impaired.

PULMONARY VASCULAR DISEASE

The most common pulmonary vascular disease is thromboembolism, in which a blood clot occludes a pulmonary blood vessel. A clot may originate within a pulmonary vessel (thrombus) or be dislodged from elsewhere in the venous system (embolus). Conditions that predispose to peripheral venous thrombosis include the following:

- Prolonged bed rest
- Postoperative convalescence
- Pregnancy
- Chronic cardiac or pulmonary disease
- Peripheral venous insufficiency
- Injury to a lower extremity
- Disorder of the clotting system

Occasionally a patient develops another form of embolus, such as an infected clot from intravenous drug abuse or indwelling vascular catheter, fat droplets following fracture of long bones, or amniotic fluid components following obstetrical procedures. The size of the embolus determines the site of occlusion and the functional consequences. A large embolus obstructing a main pulmonary artery may be immediately fatal; a smaller one obstructing a peripheral pulmonary arteriole may not cause symptoms. Since lung tissue is normally well supplied with oxygen from inspired air and from bronchial arterial circulation, pulmonary infarction (in which lung tissue distal to an embolus dies of ischemia) is uncommon. Usually, lung tissue remains perfused from the bronchial circulation. In time the embolus either is dissolved by endogenous fibrinolytic processes or exogenously administered drugs or organizes into a firm, adherent lump, after which distal perfusion is partially restored. In patients with pre-existing cardiopulmonary disease, the impact of an embolus is greatly exaggerated.

The obstruction of a pulmonary artery does not in itself cause hypoxemia. Ventilation reaching alveoli distal to the obstructed vessel is wasted, so dead space ventilation increases. Lung compliance is reduced, and local irritant receptors are activated, leading to tachypnea, hyperventilation, and a drop in Pa_{CO_2}. Secondary smooth muscle constriction develops in small airways, both in embolized lung units and adjacent normal units, causing redistribution of ventilation away from affected regions. Widespread airway constriction leads to distal atelectasis and shunting of blood through the underventilated lung units (17). These secondary processes are responsible for the arterial hypoxemia and high A-a D_{O_2} associated with pulmonary embolism.

Since total effective vascular bed available for gas exchange is reduced, there is also a reduction in lung diffusing capacity. In addition, a local inflammatory reaction may disrupt the integrity of alveolar–capillary membrane and cause fluid leakage into the interstitium to aggravate $\dot{V}_A/\dot{Q}$ mismatch and diffusion impairment. Pulmonary vascular resistance increases, and pulmonary arterial hypertension may develop. However, capacitance of the pulmonary vascular bed is sufficiently large that redistribution of pulmonary blood flow after an embolic event can often be accommodated without a rise in vascular pressure. In a normal subject almost 40% of the vascular bed must be occluded before there is any significant rise in resting pulmonary artery pressure (18). In less extensive occlusions, pulmonary artery pressure may be normal at rest, but rise abnormally during exercise. Right ventricular strain may result from an effort to maintain normal cardiac output against high pulmonary resistance.

Treatment consists of supportive measures (oxygen, fluids) and administration of anticoagulants (heparin and warfarin) to prevent further peripheral clot formation. Thrombolytic agents that promote dissolution of the clot are given to patients with massive pulmonary embolism who develop vascular collapse. In patients who are susceptible to recurrent embolization or already hemodynamically compromised, prophylactic insertion of a filter device into the inferior vena cava may trap dislodged clots from the lower extremities and prevent further episodes of embolism.

HYPOVENTILATION SYNDROMES

The neural drive to breathe may be blunted by opioids, diseases of the central nervous system (stroke, tumor, encephalitis), sleep apnea, or rarely, primary idiopathic disorders involving the respiratory control center. Sleep apnea syndromes are characterized by periodic cessation of breathing during sleep. Three pathophysiological patterns can be distinguished:

1. Obstructive apnea associated with oronasal blockage of air flow even though breathing efforts continue
2. Central apnea associated with cessation of respiratory muscle contraction
3. Mixed apnea associated with features of both obstructive and central apnea

Obstructive Sleep Apnea

The patency of the upper airway is normally maintained by contractions of muscles of the pharynx, tongue, and neck. In obstructive sleep apnea, these muscles lose tone during deep sleep, causing soft tissues of the posterior pharynx to collapse and obstruct air flow while the diaphragm and abdominal muscles continue to contract against the occluded airway. The highest incidence of obstructive sleep apnea is seen in obese middle-aged men. Many such patients have small nasal and oral passages, hypertrophied tonsils, or anatomical abnormalities of the jaw that predispose to upper airway obstruction.

Partial obstruction of the pharynx gives rise to snoring. Complete obstruction may lead to arterial hypoxemia and bradycardia. Eventually there is momentary arousal, muscular tone returns, the obstruction is abolished, and gas exchange and hemodynamics normalize. The same pattern repeats itself hundreds of times each night. Since patients cannot sleep restfully at night, they awake with a headache and may be somnolent during the day. In the early stages of disease, physiological function during waking hours is normal. With chronic sleep deprivation and nocturnal hypoxemia, a gradual change in personality and intellect may become apparent. Pulmonary and systemic arterial hypertension, secondary polycythemia, and a variety of cardiac arrhythmias may develop.

Diagnosis is made by the constellation of clinical symptoms and signs or documented by a sleep study demonstrating cessation of air flow accompanied by continued respiratory muscle effort (19). Treatment includes administration of continuous positive airway pressure via a tight face mask to prevent upper airway closure during sleep along with weight reduction. Both treatment measures require considerable motivation and persistence, so compliance is generally poor. Any anatomical abnormalities of the upper airway should be corrected, but surgical treatment by indiscriminately removing excessive soft tissue from the pharynx (uvulopalatopharyngoplasty) has mixed results and is not generally recommended.

Obesity Hypoventilation Syndrome

The most common form of central hypoventilation, also known as "Pickwickian Syndrome," occurs in association with morbid obesity. The causal relation between obesity and hypoventilation is incompletely understood. In addition to mechanical effects of morbid obesity (reduced chest wall compliance and restriction of lung volume) described previously, severe obesity is associated with impaired ability to augment ventilation in response to the usual stimuli, such as hypoxia or carbon dioxide inhalation. During deep sleep, patients develop periods of apnea, with cessation of both airflow and respiratory muscle effort. Secondary upper airway obstruction may develop because of the loss of pharyngeal muscle tone. Clinical manifestations are similar to those in patients with obstructive apnea. Weight reduction and careful administration of respiratory stimulants produce improvement in these abnormalities.

EXERCISE LIMITATION IN LUNG DISEASE

The following are general mechanisms by which lung disease limits exercise:
- Blunting of ventilatory response
- Mechanical limitation of airflow and respiratory muscle function
- Impairment of gas exchange by $\dot{V}_A/\dot{Q}$ mismatch, shunting, and diffusion limitation

Blunting of Ventilatory Response

In hypoventilation syndromes related to morbid obesity, neuromuscular disease, or respiratory depressant drugs, the respiratory center fails to respond appropriately to the normal metabolic and neural ventilatory stimuli during exercise (lactic acid and carbon dioxide accumulation and mechanoreceptor input from working muscles). Hypoxia is normally a secondary stimulus to ventilation, but it can assume greater importance in patients with significant lung disease who chronically retain carbon dioxide. Inadequate ventilatory response to carbon dioxide may be detected by a lower than normal relation between ventilation and inhaled carbon dioxide concentration (Fig. 37.6). Similarly, inadequate ventilatory response to hypoxia may be detected by lower than normal relation between ventilation and inhaled oxygen concentration (Fig. 37.6). With significant ventilatory suppression, carbon dioxide is not adequately eliminated from the blood; $Paco_2$ increases, causing a corresponding decline in Pao_2 and pH. The hypoxemia of hypoventilation is readily corrected by the administration of 100% oxygen.

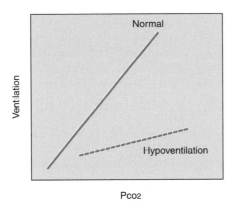

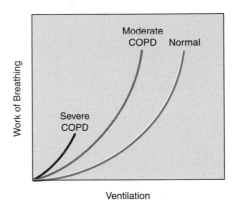

Figure 37.7. Work of respiratory muscles increases as ventilation increases. In moderate COPD the work of breathing is greater than normal at any given level of ventilation. In severe COPD with the onset of respiratory muscle fatigue, work of breathing is further increased; in addition, the maximum work that can be generated by respiratory muscle is diminished.

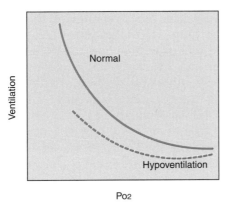

Figure 37.6. Ventilatory responses to high PCO_2 and low PO_2 are blunted in patients with hypoventilation syndromes.

Mechanical Ventilatory Limitation

Patients with obstructive lung disease and skeletal or neuromuscular disease of the thorax are primarily restricted by abnormal mechanics of breathing, manifested by derangement in the following:

- Respiratory pattern
- Maximal airflow rates
- Respiratory muscle energy balance upon exercise

At rest, ventilatory capacity assessed by maximal voluntary ventilation for 15 seconds and maximum sustained ventilation for 4 minutes are reduced. Dead space ventilation is increased and tidal volume is reduced; hence, the breathing pattern consists of rapid, shallow breaths at a high end-expiratory lung volume. This inefficient pattern results in a high energy cost of breathing. In patients with airflow obstruction, expiratory flow rate during exercise quickly reaches the limit and cannot be further increased. Bronchospasm may be induced or exaggerated on exercise. High transpulmonary pressure must be generated to overcome partial airway obstruction with each breath, further increasing respiratory muscle work and energy cost of breathing (Fig. 37.7).

Increased energy demand and oxygen cost of breathing may limit exercise by diverting a large fraction of the available oxygen from exercising locomotive muscles (20). If a significant fraction of total body oxygen supply is required by respiratory muscles to sustain ventilation, locomotive muscles must rely more heavily on anaerobic metabolism; muscle production of lactate increases, producing more carbon dioxide and further stimulating ventilation, which increases oxygen demand by respiratory muscles. The only way to mitigate the excessive rise in ventilatory oxygen demand is to blunt the ventilatory response to exercise, allowing $PaCO_2$ to rise. This response further compromises oxygen uptake. Furthermore, if right heart strain develops as a result of chronic lung disease, cardiac output and oxygen delivery are reduced, intensifying the competition for oxygen between respiratory and nonrespiratory muscle (21). Eventually exercise must be discontinued, either because locomotive muscles do not receive enough oxygen or because ventilatory capacity is exceeded.

Patients with neuromuscular or skeletal disease of the thorax are primarily limited by poor respiratory muscle strength and endurance. In neuromuscular disease, the mass of functioning respiratory muscle is diminished, indicated by low maximal inspiratory pressure. In addition, chronic thoracic disease may be associated with secondary atelectasis or fibrosis of the lung parenchyma, which reduces lung compliance, increases ventilatory work, and impairs gas exchange.

Gas Exchange Limitation

Impairment of gas exchange can be due to $\dot{V}_A/\dot{Q}$ mismatch, shunting, or diffusion limitation. Each is marked by incomplete oxygenation of blood leaving the lung, which results in arterial hypoxemia and abnormally high A-a D_{O2}. Abnormalities are accentuated during exercise.

$\dot{V}_A/\dot{Q}$ Mismatch

$\dot{V}_A/\dot{Q}$ mismatch occurs when ventilation and blood flow are not evenly distributed in different regions of the lung (4). In an ideal homogeneous lung, the $\dot{V}_A/\dot{Q}$ ratio should be 1.0; in regions with $\dot{V}_A/\dot{Q}$ mismatch, the ratio is either higher or lower than 1.0. Mismatch of $\dot{V}_A/\dot{Q}$ is the most common gas exchange derangement, although only low $\dot{V}_A/\dot{Q}$ ratios can cause hypoxemia. Mismatch may develop in any disease that disturbs the distribution of ventilation (chronic bronchitis, asthma) or the distribution of pulmonary blood flow (pulmonary hypertension, thromboembolism). $\dot{V}_A/\dot{Q}$ mismatch impairs efficiency of gas exchange because blood flow through low $\dot{V}_A/\dot{Q}$ regions remains hypoxic and blood flow through high $\dot{V}_A/\dot{Q}$ regions cannot be more than 100% saturated with oxygen; hence, the final mixture of blood leaving the lung still has a lower oxygen tension than mixed alveolar gas; that is, the A-a D_{O_2} is elevated.

Normal subjects commonly have a small degree of $\dot{V}_A/\dot{Q}$ mismatch. $\dot{V}_A/\dot{Q}$ mismatch is exaggerated in lung disease but may improve from rest to exercise. Anatomical distribution of $\dot{V}_A/\dot{Q}$ can be grossly assessed by ventilation and perfusion scans with inhaled or injected tracers, respectively. Hypoxemia related to lung regions characterized by low $\dot{V}_A/\dot{Q}$ ratio may be distinguished from hypoxemia due to shunt by application of 100% oxygen, which corrects the former but not the latter. Precise quantification of physiological distribution of $\dot{V}_A/\dot{Q}$ ratios requires invasive measurements such as the multiple inert gas elimination technique.

Shunting

Shunting develops when venous blood enters the arterial system without becoming fully oxygenated. Shunts, which are classified by anatomical location, can include the following:

- Intracardiac (right to left heart)
- Intrapulmonary
- Postpulmonary (venous return emptying directly into the left ventricle)

Intrapulmonary shunts can be viewed as an extreme form of $\dot{V}_A/\dot{Q}$ mismatch. Hypoxemia due to shunting worsens during exercise as blood flow through a shunted region increases and mixed venous P_{O_2} decreases; hypoxemia due to shunt cannot be corrected by the administration of 100% oxygen. Pa_{CO_2} is usually not increased if chemoreceptor control of ventilation is normal.

Diffusion Limitation

The rate of oxygen transfer from alveolar air to blood and combination with hemoglobin is D_L. The magnitude of D_L is determined by the alveolar–capillary surface available for gas exchange, oxygen-carrying capacity of blood, and pulmonary capillary blood volume. Normally, the $D_L O_2$ increases by 40–100% from rest to exercise. Increased D_L is the combined result of increased tidal volume, which opens partially collapsed alveoli and exposes more alveolar surface to inspired gas; increased pulmonary blood flow, which opens previously collapsed capillaries and increases capillary volume and surface for diffusion; and changes in red blood cell flow pattern so that the regional distribution of red blood cells within and among capillaries becomes more uniform.

Diffusion limitation develops when blood traverses and leaves the pulmonary capillary bed without fully equilibrating with PA_{O_2}, resulting in a low Pa_{O_2} and high A-a D_{O_2}. On average blood requires less than 1 second to traverse the lung. Upon exposure to oxygen, deoxygenated red cells require about 0.25 second to become fully oxygenated. Normally, red blood cells have sufficient time to equilibrate with alveolar oxygen before exiting the lung. The extent of oxygenation of blood flowing across the alveolar–capillary bed is determined by $D_L/\dot{Q}$ (22).

From rest to exercise $\dot{Q}$ increases faster than D_L; hence, $D_L/\dot{Q}$ progressively declines as exercise intensity increases. In the average subject during maximal exercise at sea level, maximal $\dot{Q}$ is relatively low and is reached before $D_L/\dot{Q}$ declines to a level that can cause a significant drop in arterial oxygen saturation. Therefore, in the average subject, maximal exercise at sea level is primarily limited by cardiovascular oxygen delivery, not by pulmonary diffusive oxygen uptake. Pulmonary diffusion impairment develops in two circumstances:

- When the increase in $\dot{Q}$ is so great that $D_L/\dot{Q}$ falls below a critical threshold for complete oxygenation of red cells
- When a significant portion of the alveolar–capillary membrane is destroyed or is ineffective for oxygen transfer, so that D_L cannot increase and the ratio of $D_L/\dot{Q}$ falls

The first condition may occur in elite athletes whose maximum $\dot{Q}$ is significantly increased through physical training. A lower ratio of $D_L/\dot{Q}$ at maximum exercise is achieved; hence, blood may not be fully oxygenated upon leaving the pulmonary capillary bed. In achieving maximum performance, the elite athlete may exhibit a significant drop in arterial oxygen saturation (23).

The second condition occurs in pulmonary fibrosis, emphysema, or pulmonary embolism. Because of the presence of large physiological reserves in D_L, more than 50% of total alveolar–capillary membrane must be destroyed before diffusion becomes the primary source of exercise limitation (24). Impaired diffusion may be detected by a reduction in D_L at a given cardiac output or by a failure of D_L to increase appropriately from rest to exercise (25–27). Since diffusion is a passive transport process, arterial hypoxemia due to a low D_L can be overcome by increasing the driving pressure, that is, increasing PA_{O_2} by the administration of 100% oxygen.

▶ **SUMMARY**

In a normal subject of average fitness, exercise capacity is usually limited by cardiovascular, not pulmonary, factors, because oxygen transport capacity of the lungs exceeds that of the heart. However, when capacity of the heart is enhanced to match that of the lungs, as in elite athletes, or when capacity of the lungs is reduced by disease, pulmonary factors may significantly limit exercise. In most patients with lung disease, a combination of mechanisms, including derangement of ventilatory control, lung and chest wall mechanics, and alveolar–capillary gas exchange, is responsible for exercise limitation. Progressive pulmonary disease eventually leads to increased ventilatory work, respiratory muscle fatigue, right heart strain, and impaired cardiac output. Understanding these mechanisms and the associated consequences lets the exercise professional rationally evaluate functional disability and appropriately direct therapy.

ACKNOWLEDGMENT

This work was supported by an American Heart Association Established Investigator Award.

References

1. Tisi GM. Pulmonary Physiology in Clinical Medicine. 2nd ed. Baltimore: Williams & Wilkins, 1985.
2. West JB. Respiratory Physiology: The Essentials. 3rd ed. Baltimore: Williams & Wilkins, 1985.
3. Kryger M, Bode F, Antic R, et al. Diagnosis of obstruction of the upper and central airways. Am J Med 61:85–93, 1976 (review).
4. West JB. Ventilation-perfusion relationships. Am Rev Respir Dis 116:919–943, 1977 (state of the art).
5. American Thoracic Society. Standards for the diagnosis and care of patients with chronic obstructive pulmonary disease. Am J Resp Crit Care Med 152:S77–S120, 1995.
6. Robins AG. Pathophysiology of emphysema. Clin Chest Med 4:413–420, 1983 (review).
7. Evans MD, Pryor WA. Cigarette smoking, emphysema, and damage to alpha 1-proteinase inhibitor. Am J Physiol 266(6 Pt 1):L593–611, 1995 (review). (Published errata appear in Am J Physiol 268(1 Pt 1):section L, 1995 and 268(6 Pt 3):section L, 1995.)
8. Faling LJ. Pulmonary rehabilitation: physical modalities. Clin Chest Med 7:599–618, 1986 (review).
9. Pardy RL, Rivington RN, Despas PJ, et al. The effects of inspiratory muscle training on exercise performance in chronic airflow limitation. Am Rev Respir Dis 123:426–433, 1981.
10. Tattersfield AE. The site of the defect in asthma. Neurohumoral, mediator or smooth muscle? Chest 91(6 Suppl):184S–189S, 1987 (review).
11. Hargreave FE, Dolovich J, O'Byrne PM, et al. The origin of airway hyperresponsiveness. J Allergy Clin Immunol 78(5 Pt 1):825–832, 1986 (review).
12. McFadden ER Jr. Exercise-induced asthma. Assessment of current etiologic concepts. Chest 91(6 Suppl):151S–157S, 1987 (review).
13. de Benedictis FM, Canny GJ, MacLusky IB, et al. Comparison of airway reactivity induced by cold air and methacholine challenges in asthmatic children. Pediatr Pulmonol 19:326–329, 1995.
14. Roca J, Ramis L, Rodriguez RR, et al. Serial relationships between ventilation-perfusion inequality and spirometry in acute severe asthma requiring hospitalization. Am Rev Respir Dis 137:1055–1061, 1988.
15. Ballester E, Reyes A, Roca J, et al. Ventilation-perfusion mismatching in acute severe asthma: Effects of salbutamol and 100% oxygen. Thorax 44:258–267, 1989. (Published erratum appears in Thorax 44:833, 1989.)
16. Reynolds HY, Matthay RA. Diffuse interstitial and alveolar inflammatory disease. In: George RB, Light RW, Matthay MA, et al., eds. Chest Medicine, Essentials of Pulmonary and Critical Care Medicine. Baltimore: Williams & Wilkins, 1990:209–248.
17. Kapitan KS, Buchbinder M, Wagner PD, et al. Mechanisms of hypoxemia in chronic thromboembolic pulmonary hypertension. Am Rev Respir Dis 139:1149–1154, 1989.
18. Moser KM, ed. Pulmonary Vascular Disease: Lung Biology in Health and Disease, vol. 14. New York: Marcel Dekker, 1979.
19. American Thoracic Society. Indications and standards for cardiopulmonary sleep studies. Am Rev Respir Dis 139:559–568, 1988.
20. Otis AB. The work of breathing. In: Fenn WO, Rahn H, eds. The Handbook of Physiology. Washington: American Physiological Society, 1964:463–476.
21. Hsia CC, Ramanathan M, Estrera AS. Recruitment of diffusing capacity with exercise in patients after pneumonectomy. Am Rev Respir Dis 145:811–816, 1992.
22. Piper J, Scheid P. Comparison of diffusion and perfusion limitations in alveolar gas exchange. Respir Physiol 51:287–290, 1983.
23. Dempsey JA. Exercise-induced arterial hypoxemia in healthy human subjects at sea level. J Physiol 355:161–175, 1984.
24. Johnson RL Jr. Exercise testing in lung disease. In: Sackner MA, ed. Diagnostic Techniques in Pulmonary Disease, Part I. New York: Marcel Dekker, 1980:473–501.
25. American Thoracic Society. Single breath carbon monoxide diffusing capacity (transfer factor): Recommendations for a standard technique. Am Rev Respir Dis 136:1299–1307, 1987.
26. Hsia CC, McBrayer DG, Ramanathan M. Reference values of pulmonary diffusing capacity during exercise by a rebreathing technique. Am J Resp Crit Care Med 152:658–665, 1995.
27. Hughes JM, Lockwood DN, Jones HA, et al. DLCO/$\dot{Q}$ and diffusion limitation at rest and on exercise in patients with interstitial fibrosis. Respir Physiol 83:155–166, 1991.

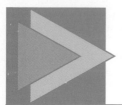

CHAPTER **38**

PULMONARY ASSESSMENT

Tony G. Babb

Key to Pulmonary Physiology Abbreviations

A-a D_{O2}	Alveolar–arterial oxygen difference
CPX	Cardiopulmonary exercise
DLco	Lung diffusing capacity of carbon monoxide
EELV	End-expiratory lung volume
EILV	End-inspiratory lung volume
FEV_1	Forced expiratory volume in 1 second
FRC	Functional residual capacity
FVC	Forced vital capacity
IC	Inspiratory capacity
MVV	Maximal voluntary ventilation
$Paco_2$	Partial pressure of carbon dioxide in arterial blood
Pao_2	Partial pressure of oxygen in arterial blood
$P\bar{e}co_2$	Partial pressure of expired carbon dioxide
P_{ETCO2}	Partial pressure of end tidal carbon dioxide
RPB	Rating of perceived breathlessness
SaO_2	Saturation of oxygen in arterial blood
TLC	Total lung capacity
$\dot{V}CO_2$	Carbon dioxide production
V_D/V_T	Ratio of ventilatory dead space to tidal volume
$\dot{V}_E$	Expired minute ventilation
$\dot{V}O_2$	Oxygen consumption
$\dot{V}O_{2max}$	Maximal oxygen consumption
VT	Ventilatory threshold

The purpose of cardiopulmonary exercise (CPX) testing in the pulmonary patient is to determine whether exercise tolerance is limited and to help identify and/or distinguish between various physiological factors contributing to the limitation. Distinguishing among these factors depends on recognition of normal and abnormal response patterns, including the following:

- $\dot{V}O_2$
- $\dot{V}CO_2$
- Pulmonary gas exchange
- $\dot{V}_E$
- Breathing pattern

- Metabolic demands
- Cardiovascular function
- Various combinations of these responses during incremental exercise
- Respiratory mechanics

Even in known pulmonary disease, the factors responsible for exercise limitation are not always apparent. Therefore, attention cannot be limited to the respiratory system during CPX testing in the pulmonary patient.

This discussion is divided into areas of assessment of pulmonary function and CPX testing for pulmonary patients. Although this material emphasizes assessment of known pulmonary disease, it is also applicable to CPX testing, especially in patients with unexplained shortness of breath upon exertion.

PRELIMINARY INFORMATION: PULMONARY FUNCTION TESTING

In the patient with known or suspected pulmonary disease, basic pulmonary function, including spirometry, lung volume, and diffusing capacity, should be assessed. Information on pulmonary function provides the basis for determining the type of pulmonary disease and the following:

1. Level of impairment (1, 2)
2. Type of exercise protocol that is appropriate
3. Possible causes of exercise-related limitations
4. Indications of exercise end points

Most patients with poor pulmonary function fall into one of three broad categories:

- Obstructive lung disease
- Restrictive lung disease
- Pulmonary vascular disease

The purpose of spirometry is to assess airway patency and the volume of air that can be moved in and out of the lungs in one breath (3). Spirometry includes measures of FVC, forced expiratory flow rates, such as FEV_1, the ratio of FEV_1 to FVC, and maximal flow–volume loops. MVV is sometimes included in pulmonary function assessment and is helpful in estimating maximal ventilatory capacity, but it can also be estimated from other measures of pulmonary function.

Lung volumes are commonly measured in pretest assessment; the procedures include measures of FRC, TLC, and residual volume. These assessments assist in evaluating the mechanical properties of the lungs and chest wall and inspiratory muscle strength. DLco indicates the rate at which carbon monoxide can enter the blood per driving pressure of the gas. When indicated, measurements of arterial blood gases, bronchoprovocation testing, and/or maximal inspiratory and expiratory pressures may also be helpful in the interpretation of pulmonary impairment.

TEST MODE

CPX testing generally begins at low work rates (even unloaded pedaling in patients with severe limitations) and continues with regular, progressive increases in work rate. The cycle ergometer is used most often for testing pulmonary patients for the following reasons:

1. Ease of use
2. Accuracy of work rate determination
3. Independence of body weight on determining work rate
4. Relative ease of the skill
5. Ease of performing invasive measurements during exercise
6. Ability to begin an incremental test at low work rates
7. Ability to make small adjustments in work rate
8. Availability of normal predictive values for cycle ergometry (4–6)

Although a treadmill may be used, it makes quantifying and incrementing work rate more difficult. In addition, many treadmills do not run slowly enough for pulmonary patients. Treadmill testing may be appropriate in patients who use it as a training mode.

Predicting End Points

The protocol for CPX testing should be individualized so that the test lasts 8–12 minutes. The maximum work rate can be predicted in a number of ways. Predicted $\dot{V}O_{2max}$ can be used as a target end point, but appropriate norms applicable to both patient population and mode of testing must be used (4–6). Comparing observed heart rate with predicted maximal heart rate may also be helpful for determining the relative intensity during each test stage and for targeting maximum exercise capacity.

Since respiratory function is likely to be the limiting factor in exercise for pulmonary patients, it may be help-

ful to estimate a mechanical ventilatory ceiling (7–9b). Using the method of Carter and others, with which FEV_1 × 37.5 estimates the maximal exercise $\dot{V}_E$, a patient with an FEV_1 of 1 L has an estimated mechanical ventilatory ceiling of 37.5 L (8). Using this as the estimated mechanical ventilatory ceiling and estimating the relation between $\dot{V}O_2$ and $\dot{V}_E$ ($\dot{V}_E = 29.28$), a 70-kg patient approaches the mechanical ventilatory ceiling at a $\dot{V}O_2$ of approximately 1184 mL/minute (about 80 W × [1184 − 3.5 × {weight in kilograms} / 2]/ 6) (10).

Although these are rough estimates, they may be useful for estimating mechanical ventilatory limitations for patients, which is helpful in selecting an individualized exercise protocol. Starting at 0 W with increments of 10 W, for example, may yield up to nine increments for data collection prior to the termination of the test because of mechanical ventilatory limitations. While a patient may obviously terminate for other respiratory or nonrespiratory reasons, this is also useful information. That is, that the test required termination before estimated mechanical ventilatory limitation indicates another reason for exercise limitation.

Variables

Assessment can determine the variables measured during CPX testing. Variables can be noninvasive or invasive, simple or complex. In general, all exercise tests in pulmonary patients require monitoring of the electrocardiogram, heart rate, blood pressure, SaO_2 by pulse oximetry, ratings of perceived exertion, ratings of perceived breathlessness, discomfort, symptoms, and/or fatigue. These measurements are required to assess safety of exercise and for safety of the CPX test. In addition, measurement of $\dot{V}O_2$, $\dot{V}CO_2$, anaerobic threshold, $\dot{V}_E$, and work rate establish physiological response, abnormal respiratory and/or cardiovascular function, acid–base status, ventilatory demand, neuromuscular function, and/or maximum exercise tolerance. Measurement of flow–volume characteristics helps to determine the mechanical ventilatory limitation, and arterial blood gas levels determine the effectiveness and efficiency of pulmonary gas exchange. With or without arterial blood gases, monitoring of P_{ETCO_2} yields valuable information regarding gas exchange (5, 9b).

Without proper presentation of results, the most sophisticated measurements offer little value to the exercise professional or the attending physician. It is important to present physiological responses so that each variable or combination of variables contributes to determining whether the patient is exercise limited and the factors most likely to be responsible. A standard general format is useful in this regard, as are normative data to compare responses. Further details on the display format of exercise test data and interpretation can be found in other sources (5, 6, 11).

MAXIMAL EXERCISE TOLERANCE

Although the primary objective of CPX testing is to determine the source of the limitation, other reasons for CPX testing in pulmonary patients include the following:

- Determining treatment strategies for improving respiratory mechanics or dyspnea
- Distinguishing other organ involvement
- Determining therapeutic strategy
- Determining appropriate exercise intensity
- Determining functional capacity after exercise training
- Determining whether changes in exercise tolerance are related to new causes

Recently, evaluation of candidates for lung transplant and lung volume reduction surgery are newer indications for CPX testing in pulmonary patients.

Predicted Maximum

The amount of exercise intolerance is determined by comparing predicted exercise capacity to measured exercise capacity. Predicted $\dot{V}O_{2max}$ or predicted maximal work rate can be used to quantify maximal exercise capacity. In Figure 38.1*A*, both of these variables are used (6).

Comparing $\dot{V}O_{2max}$ with predicted $\dot{V}O_{2max}$ requires caution, especially if 100% predicted $\dot{V}O_{2max}$ is obtained at a work rate significantly lower than predicted (i.e., normal cardiopulmonary functional capacity, but low exercise tolerance) (Fig. 38.1*B*). This result can be associated with obesity or increased work of breathing (increased ventilatory demand, airway resistance, or respiratory elastance) (6). However, in severely limited pulmonary pa-

tients $\dot{V}O_{2max}$ is not normally obtained. If predicted $\dot{V}O_{2max}$ is based on actual body weight, it may be overestimated in overweight patients, which produces an underestimate of cardiorespiratory capacity. Estimating relative peak $\dot{V}O_2$ (milliliters per kilogram per minute) is also useful for determining which activities of daily living are within the patient's capacity (12).

Maximal Effort

It is important to ensure that a "maximal" exercise test is obtained when determining whether exercise tolerance is normal (6). Maximal exercise is obtained if one or more of these conditions are met:

- Predicted $\dot{V}O_{2max}$ is reached.
- 90% or more of predicted maximal heart rate is obtained.
- A respiratory exchange ratio above 1.1 is achieved.
- $\dot{V}_E$ is near to or greater than MVV.
- Marked desaturation occurs.
- Blood lactate is above 8 mMol/L.
- The test is limited by discomfort or symptoms (e.g., dyspnea or termination of test because of electrocardiographic abnormality) (6).

However, attaining one of these criteria does not always indicate that it is the limiting factor (6). For example, $\dot{V}_E$ that matches or exceeds MVV does not necessarily indicate that ventilatory limitation is the primary cause of poor exercise tolerance. If lactic acidosis increases ventilatory demand, ventilatory limitation may be the reason to discontinue exercise, but cardiovascular disease may cause the limitation. In practice it may be difficult to make these distinctions.

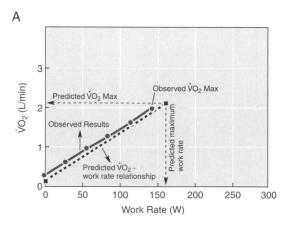

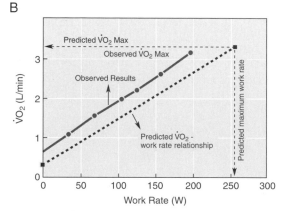

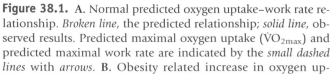

Figure 38.1. **A.** Normal predicted oxygen uptake–work rate relationship. *Broken line,* the predicted relationship; *solid line,* observed results. Predicted maximal oxygen uptake ($\dot{V}O_{2max}$) and predicted maximal work rate are indicated by the *small dashed lines* with *arrows.* **B.** Obesity related increase in oxygen up-

take–work rate relationship. *Dashed line* represents predicted relationship; *solid line* represents observed results. (Adapted with permission from Younes M, Kivinen G. Respiratory mechanics and breathing pattern during and following maximal exercise. J Appl Physiol 57:1773–1782, 1984.)

VENTILATORY LIMITATIONS

Mechanical Ventilatory Limitation

To determine possible causes of exercise limitation in pulmonary patients, it is important to determine the presence and extent of mechanical ventilatory limitations. Mechanical ventilatory limitation occurs when ventilatory requirement reaches or exceeds ventilatory capacity. There is no generally accepted objective method to quantify the magnitude of mechanical ventilatory limitation. However, certain measures do assist with this determination.

The $\dot{V}_E/MVV$ ratio is often used as an index of mechanical ventilatory limitation. $\dot{V}_E$ at maximal exercise (V_{Emax}) is expressed as a percentage of the MVV ($\dot{V}_E/MVV$). A ratio of 60–70% is normal, though the accepted range may vary with population (6, 13). Ventilatory limitation is not expected in individuals without pulmonary disease, but in patients with obstructive pulmonary disease, both MVV and ventilatory reserve are decreased. Reaching or exceeding the normal range for $\dot{V}_E/MVV$ may be an indication of a mechanical ventilatory limitation (6). However, patients with mild to moderate chronic obstructive pulmonary disease with a ratio of 60–70% may have significant mechanical ventilatory limitation, but only slightly reduced exercise capacity (14). Therefore, elevated $\dot{V}_E/MVV$ is helpful but not definitive. The difference between V_{Emax} and MVV, termed ventilatory reserve, may also be used as an index of mechanical ventilatory limitation. A reserve of 20–50% of the MVV is normal (5).

Tidal flow–volume loops measured at each increment of exercise or at maximal exercise can also reveal mechanical ventilatory limitation. The loops are compared to the maximal flow–volume loop measured at rest before exercise or immediately after exercise (7, 9b, 14). The postexercise maximal flow–volume loop should be used if there is suspected bronchodilation during exercise; otherwise, use of the pre-exercise loop may produce an overestimate of ventilatory limitation. Also, it is sometimes helpful to use the maximal flow–volume loop measured in a pressure-compensated volume displacement body plethysmograph (flow box), which corrects volume for the gas compression artifact. To compare the exercise tidal flow–volume loops to the maximal flow–volume loop, it is necessary to place the loops properly within the maximal flow–volume loop. Viewing the tidal flow–volume loops relative to the maximal flow–volume loop makes it easily apparent when the maximal flow–volume loop over a large percentage of tidal volume is reached (over 40–60% of tidal volume, expiratory flow meets maximal expiratory flow). However, by separate visual inspection of the flow–volume loops, it is difficult to quantify the magnitude of mechanical ventilatory limitation. Recently, techniques that more easily quantify mechanical ventilatory limitation have been developed, but they have not been validated for clinical use (7, 9b).

Calculations of dynamic lung volumes estimated during exercise from IC, EELV, and EILV can be used to assess mechanical ventilatory limitation. EELV and EILV, compared to resting lung volumes, indicate the degree of hyperinflation during exercise that occurs with tidal expiratory limitation (14). When EELV is at least as much as resting FRC and/or EILV is more than 90% of TLC, expiratory airflow limitation may be a factor in mechanical ventilatory limitation.

Ventilatory Response Limitations

The normal exercise response of $\dot{V}_E$ is linear up to approximately 50% of peak exercise. Beyond this, $\dot{V}_E$ becomes nonlinear with $\dot{V}O_2$ or work rate. It is important to determine whether $\dot{V}_E$ is appropriate or excessive for the external work rate during the linear portion of the relation. Increased ventilatory requirement increases ventilatory load on the respiratory system, which may already be limited. Increased demand also increases the likelihood of obtaining a ventilatory ceiling early in exertion. Identification of the cause of increased ventilatory demand (e.g., acidosis, hypoxemia, hyperventilation, dead space ventilation) is important because in some cases demand can be lowered therapeutically. If demand can be decreased, exercise function may be increased (6).

Comparison to norms or normal data collected in your own laboratory can help determine the appropriateness of $\dot{V}_E$ per work rate (5, 6, 10). Figure 38.2 illustrates $\dot{V}_E$ displayed for interpretation. The axes are expressed in relative units ($\dot{V}_E$ as a percentage of predicted MVV and $\dot{V}O_2$ as a percentage of predicted $\dot{V}O_{2max}$), making individual comparison easy (6). In addition, maximal and tidal flow–volume loops are shown. This type of representation may be helpful in determining whether $\dot{V}_E$ is within normal range.

Another method for determining whether ventilatory demand is elevated is to determine ventilatory equivalents for oxygen and carbon dioxide ($\dot{V}_E/\dot{V}O_2$ and $\dot{V}_E/\dot{V}CO_2$, respectively). Normal $\dot{V}_E/\dot{V}O_2$ ratio is 20–30 up to an intensity of approximately 50–60% $\dot{V}O_{2max}$, after which it increases (5, 15). Normal $\dot{V}_E/\dot{V}CO_2$ is 25–35; it does not increase significantly until near maximum. When ventilatory requirement is increased, these ratios may be near normal at rest, but they increase disproportionately during exercise. In other cases, the ratios may be elevated at rest and decrease during exercise, though remaining above normal. Ventilatory equivalents may be elevated at rest because of hyperventilation, which can be assessed by a respiratory exchange ratio near or exceeding 1. During exercise, ventilatory equivalents return to normal if the hyperventilation is secondary to anxiety or use of a mouthpiece.

The break point in the ventilatory response during exercise is the VT if it is determined from ventilatory variables. The VT may or may not be present in the pulmonary patient (16, 17). Absence of VT may be due to

Figure 38.2. A. Determination of mechanical ventilatory limitation from ratio of ventilation to percent predicted maximal voluntary ventilation ($\dot{V}_E$/%PMVV) plotted against oxygen uptake ($\dot{V}O_2$, percent predicted) and maximal and tidal flow–volume loops for individual with normal lung function. **B.** Mild to moderate chronic obstructive lung disease. **C.** Severe chronic obstructive lung disease. *Solid line,* observed results; *dotted line,* predicted relation. **Side panels.** Maximal flow–volume loop (large loop), tidal flow–volume loop at rest (smallest loop), and tidal flow–volume loop during maximal exercise (large loop inside maximal loop).

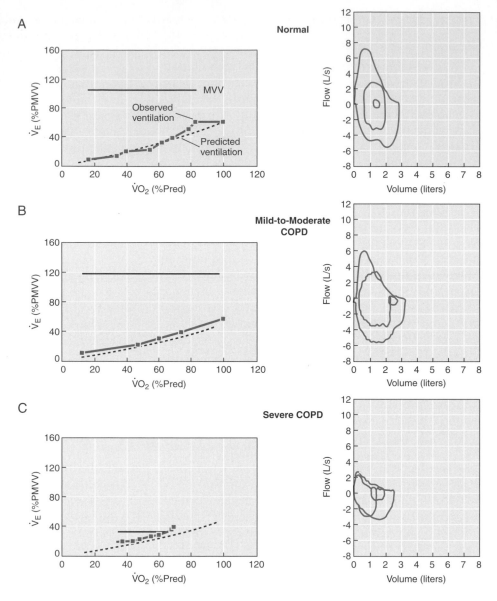

inability to exercise at an intensity sufficient to accumulate lactic acid or inability to hyperventilate. The most appropriate technique for determining VT in the pulmonary patient remains controversial (16–18).

It is important to know whether there is increased requirement for $\dot{V}O_E$ and whether mechanical ventilatory limitation is reached. In addition, it is important to distinguish between mechanical ventilatory limitation during exercise and exercise limited by ventilation.

Breathing Pattern

Pattern of breathing is important because of the association with V_D/V_T and economy of breathing. Increased $\dot{V}_E$ during low-level exercise occurs primarily by increased V_T. During heavy exercise, increased frequency of breathing contributes more to increased $\dot{V}_E$. V_T at maximum exercise is approximately 50–60% of vital capacity. Breathing frequency is generally 35–50 per minute and usually

less than 60 per minute (19). Variations in breathing pattern in combination with other exercise variables ($\dot{V}_E$ and gas exchange) can provide insight into the reason for the limitation (6, 20).

PULMONARY GAS EXCHANGE

Adequacy and efficiency of $\dot{V}_E$ are determined by pulmonary gas exchange. Any abnormality related to hypoventilation, the matching of $\dot{V}_E$ and perfusion in the lungs (maldistribution of $\dot{V}_E$ or perfusion), diffusion limitation in the lung, or right-to-left shunt alters gas exchange variables and indicates pulmonary disease. Hypoxemia can be caused by any of these four abnormalities. Hypercapnia can be caused by hypoventilation and ventilation–perfusion mismatch, and the presence of either one at rest or during exercise indicates inadequate gas exchange (21). Several reviews on CPX testing or gas exchange in pulmonary patients discuss these abnormalities in the context of disease (5, 6, 11, 21–23).

To assess gas exchange, such measures as SaO_2, P_{ETCO2}, diffusing capacity at rest, V_D/V_T using P_{ETCO2}, $P\bar{e}CO_2$, PaO_2, $PaCO_2$, and A-a D_{O2} (with calculation of V_D/V_T) are all useful. When using these variables, note rest abnormalities and exertional changes in the exercise test summary.

Saturation

SaO_2 can be determined noninvasively by pulse oximetry, which in most cases is adequate during exercise. SaO_2 is generally stable during exercise at a value similar to the resting SaO_2, which varies with age (24). Saturation below 90% indicates significant hypoxemia. Assessment of SaO_2 during exercise on room air, and if desaturation occurs, with supplemental oxygen, can determine the appropriate level of oxygen supplementation.

End-Tidal Carbon Dioxide

P_{ETCO2} is helpful in determining the adequacy of gas exchange (hypercapnia). Normal resting P_{ETCO2} is 36–42 mm Hg; it increases by 3–8 mm Hg during submaximal exercise, but it decreases during heavy exercise. While P_{ETCO2} is not always accurate when compared with $PaCO_2$, especially in pulmonary patients, the trend can be assessed with incremental exercise. If P_{ETCO2} changes, $PaCO_2$ is also likely to be changed. Inadequate gas exchange may be one reason (5).

Arterial Blood Gases

Sampling arterial blood gases during exercise may be important to assess the accuracy of a noninvasive measure such as SaO_2 or P_{ETCO2}. Multiple blood gas samples during incremental or constant load exercise are important for determining the adequacy of gas exchange. There is little change in PaO_2 during exercise (±10 mm Hg), but a significant decrease in PaO_2 (> 20 mm Hg) is associated with interstitial lung disease or pulmonary vascular disease. $PaCO_2$ is usually stable up to 50–60% of maximal exercise capacity (36–42 mm Hg), but decreases progressively thereafter.

Alveolar–Arterial Oxygen Difference

A greater A-a D_{O2} results from decreased SaO_2 (PaO_2), which indicates ventilation–perfusion mismatch, diffusion limitation, or right-to-left shunt. A-a D_{O2} is normally approximately 10 mm Hg (±5 mm Hg) at rest and increases to about 20 mm Hg (±10 mm Hg) during exercise (24). In some patients with ventilation–perfusion mismatch (pulmonary fibrosis or pulmonary vascular disease), PaO_2 decreases as exercise intensity increases. However, if PaO_2 decreases and A-a D_{O2} does not widen, desaturation usually indicates hypoventilation ($PaCO_2$

may increase as well), which may result from mechanical ventilatory limitation.

Dead Space Ventilation

When blood gases are measured, it is possible to calculate V_D/V_T, an indicator of physiological dead space (21, 24). V_D/V_T is normally about 40% at rest and progressively declines to about 20% during exercise. It decreases with age (30% at rest) (5). In the pulmonary patient, V_D/V_T increases at rest and may not decrease during exercise (22). This increases ventilatory demand in the pulmonary patient, who already has reduced ventilatory capacity. It is caused by ventilation–perfusion mismatch or by shallow breathing. It is important to determine the proportion of wasted $\dot{V}_E$ that must be overcome.

CARDIOVASCULAR RESPONSES TO EXERCISE

In most CPX testing, heart rate, electrocardiogram, and blood pressure should be monitored. Heart rate and oxygen uptake are strong indicators of cardiovascular function that may be limiting in known lung disease (11).

Maximum Heart Rate

Pulmonary patients, because of ventilatory limitations or leg discomfort, do not normally attain maximum heart rate. Maximum heart rate, expressed as a percent of predicted maximum, is lower in pulmonary patients than in age-matched individuals with normal pulmonary function (25). In contrast, $\dot{V}_E/MVV$ ratio is higher (at a lower exercise intensity) than in normals. Although heart rate is usually lower than normal at maximum exercise in severe pulmonary patients, it may be normal or near normal in patients with mild to moderate obstructive disease (26).

Relation of Oxygen Uptake to Work Rate

The $\dot{V}O_2$/work rate slope has been suggested as an indicator of cardiovascular status (11). In the absence of impaired cardiovascular status, the relation of heart rate to $\dot{V}O_2$ is usually normal in pulmonary patients (26).

Hemodynamics

Although hemodynamic measurements may be difficult to obtain during exercise, they may be useful, since changes may occur as a result of lung disease. Pulmonary patients usually have a normal cardiac output–$\dot{V}O_2$ relation during exercise, but discontinue exercise at a lower level of cardiac output and $\dot{V}O_2$ than normal individuals (27). Although cardiac output is normal, stroke volume is lower and heart rate is higher in pulmonary patients at the same $\dot{V}O_2$. Pulmonary artery pressure may be normal or slightly increased at rest, though during exercise it is usually inappropriately high for the level of cardiac output. Thus, pulmonary patients have increased vascular resistance given a normal cardiac output response (26, 27). This increases the incidence of right ventricular dysfunction during exercise in pulmonary patients; severity of this dysfunction depends upon the acuity of the pulmonary disease. Pulmonary hypertension may be present at rest and worsen with exercise secondary to airflow limitation and decreased arterial blood gases. A minority of pulmonary patients demonstrate left ventricular dysfunction during exercise, although it is unclear whether this is related to concomitant coronary artery disease (27). Hypoxemia, acidosis, bulging of the intraventricular septum in the left ventricular cavity, alterations in intrathoracic pressure, and the markedly negative swings in pleural pressure during exercise have been proposed to contribute to the possibility of left ventricular function during exercise in pulmonary patients (27).

SHORTNESS OF BREATH

It is important to note the influence of distress and discomfort during CPX testing. In the pulmonary patient, it is particularly important to note the effect shortness of breath or breathlessness on exercise tolerance (6). The complaint of breathlessness during exercise may be the primary reason pulmonary patients seek medical attention and may also be the factor most often responsible for discontinuing exercise. Pulmonary patients may also be limited by leg fatigue (25). Furthermore, rating of perceived breathlessness and leg fatigue at peak exercise are similar between pulmonary patients and normals, although pulmonary patients are limited by breathlessness more frequently and at a significantly lower exercise capacity (25). It is important to assess perception of breathlessness throughout exercise (28). There appears to be some desensitization to the rating of perceived breathlessness with regular exercise training in pulmonary patients (28). The Borg 0–10 scale and visual analog scale are commonly used to quantify breathlessness (25). These are valid, reliable, and responsive indicators (25, 28).

END OF TEST

Reasons for test termination are important to interpretation. The test summary should note the reason for termination, whether the test was a maximal test, whether the patient had distress or symptoms, who was responsible for stopping the test (i.e., patient, technician, or physician), and the maximum work load achieved.

SUMMARY OF INTERPRETATION

The interpretation of CPX testing should clearly indicate whether exercise tolerance was limited and name the factors most likely involved in the limitation. If the reasons for limitations are unclear, information from the CPX test may suggest appropriate clinical tests for follow-up. The interpretation of CPX testing is an art requiring

understanding of exercise physiology, integrative physiology, and clinical physiology.

References

1. American Thoracic Society. Evaluation of impairment/disability secondary to respiratory disorders. Am Rev Respir Dis 133:1205–1209, 1986.
2. American Thoracic Society. Lung function testing: Selection of reference values and interpretive strategies. Am Rev Respir Dis 144:1202–1218, 1991.
3. Enright PL, Hyatt RE. Office Spirometry: A Practical Guide to the Selection and Use of Spirometers. Philadelphia: Lea & Febiger, 1987:1–253.
4. Jones NL. Clinical Exercise Testing. Philadelphia: Saunders, 1988.
5. Wasserman K, Hansen JE, Sue DY, et al. Principles of Exercise Testing and Interpretation. Philadelphia: Lea & Febiger, 1987:261.
6. Younes M. Interpretation of clinical exercise testing in respiratory disease. Clin Chest Med 5:189–206, 1984.
7. Babb TG, Rodarte JR. Estimation of ventilatory capacity during submaximal exercise. J Appl Physiol 74:2016–2022, 1993.
8. Carter R, Peavler M, Zinkgraf S, et al. Predicting maximal exercise ventilation in patients with chronic obstructive pulmonary disease. Chest 92:253–259, 1987.
9a. Dillard TA, Piantadosi S, Rajagopal KR. Prediction of ventilation at maximal exercise in chronic air-flow obstruction. Am Rev Respir Dis 132:230–235, 1985.
9b. Johnson BD, Weisman IM, Zeballos RJ, Beck KC. Emerging concepts in the evaluation of ventilatory limitation during exercise: The exercise tidal flow–volume loop. Chest 116:488–503, 1999.
10. Levison H, Cherniack RM. Ventilatory cost of exercise in chronic obstructive pulmonary disease. J Appl Physiol 25:21–27, 1968.
11. Sue DY, Wasserman K. Impact of integrative cardiopulmonary exercise testing on clinical decision making. Chest 99:981–992, 1991 (review).
12. Becklake MR, Rodarte JR, Kalica AR, et al. Scientific issues in the assessment of respiratory impairment. Am Rev Respir Dis 137:1505–1510, 1988.
13. Dillard TA, Hnatiuk OW, McCumber TR. Maximum voluntary ventilation: Spirometric determinants in chronic obstructive pulmonary disease patients and normal subjects. Am Rev Respir Dis 147:870–875, 1993.
14. Babb TG, Viggiano R, Hurley B, et al. Effect of mild to moderate airflow limitation on exercise capacity. J Appl Physiol 70:223–230, 1991.
15. Ruppel GE. Manual of Pulmonary Function Testing. St. Louis: Stamathis, 1994:1–505.
16. Patessio A, Casaburi R, Carone M, et al. Comparison of gas exchange, lactate, and lactic acidosis thresholds in patients with chronic obstructive pulmonary disease. Am Rev Respir Dis 148:622–626, 1993.
17. Sue DY, Wasserman K, Moricca RB, et al. Metabolic acidosis during exercise in patients with chronic obstructive pulmonary disease: Use of the V-slope method for anaerobic threshold determination. Chest 94:931–938, 1988.
18. Belman MJ, Epstein LJ, Doornbos D, et al. Noninvasive de-

terminations of the anaerobic threshold: Reliability and validity in patients with COPD. Chest 102:1028–1034, 1992.

19. Blackie SP, Fairbarn MS, McElvaney MG, et al. Normal values and ranges for ventilation and breathing pattern at maximal exercise. Chest 100:136–142, 1991.

20. Gallagher CG, Younes M. Breathing pattern during and after maximal exercise in patients with chronic obstructive lung disease, interstitial lung disease, and cardiac disease, and in normal subjects. Am Rev Respir Dis 133:581–586, 1986.

21. West JB. Assessing pulmonary gas exchange. N Engl J Med 316:1336–1338, 1987 (editorial).

22. Jones NL, Berman LB. Gas exchange in chronic air-flow obstruction. Am Rev Respir Dis 129:S81–S83, 1984.

23. Wagner PD, Rodriguez-Roisin R. Clinical advances in pulmonary gas exchange. Am Rev Respir Dis 143:883–888, 1991.

24. Jones NL. Normal values for pulmonary gas exchange during exercise. Am Rev Respir Dis 129:S44–S46, 1984.

25. Killian KJ, Leblanc P, Martin DH, et al. Exercise capacity and ventilatory, circulatory, and symptom limitation in patients with chronic airflow limitation. Am Rev Respir Dis 146:935–940, 1992.

26. Gallagher CG. Exercise and chronic obstructive pulmonary disease. Med Clin North Am 74:619–641, 1990.

27. Macnee W. Pathophysiology of core pulmonale in chronic obstructive pulmonary disease: Part One. Am J Respir Crit Care Med 150:833–852, 1994.

28. Mahler DA, Horowitz MB. Perception of breathlessness during exercise in patients with respiratory disease. Med Sci Sports Exerc 26:1078–1081, 1994.

29. Johnson BD, Scanlon PD, Beck KC. Regulation of ventilatory capacity during exercise in asthmatics. J Appl Physiol 79:892–901, 1995.

Suggested Reading

Jones NL, Robertson DG, Kane JW. Difference between end-tidal and arterial P_{CO_2} in exercise. J Appl Physiol 47:954–960, 1979.

Macnee W. Pathophysiology of core pulmonale in chronic obstructive pulmonary disease: Part One. Am J Respir Crit Care Med 150:833–852, 1994.

Mahler DA, Horowitz MB. Perception of breathlessness during exercise in patients with respiratory disease. Med Sci Sports Exerc 26:1078–1081, 1994.

Marciniuk DD, Sridhar G, Clemens RE, et al. Lung volumes and expiratory flow limitation during exercise in interstitial lung disease. J Appl Physiol 77:963–973, 1994.

Younes M, Kivinen G. Respiratory mechanics and breathing pattern during and following maximal exercise. J Appl Physiol 57:1773–1782, 1984.

1.4.0

2.4.5, 2.8.0, 2.8.0.10

4.4.11, 4.4.12, 4.8.0,
4.8.1.6, 4.8.1.7, 4.8.4,
4.8.5, 4.8.6.1, 4.8.7,
4.8.10.7, 4.8.14

5.4.2, 5.8.0

CHAPTER **39**

SPECIAL CONSIDERATIONS FOR EXERCISE TRAINING

Richard Casaburi

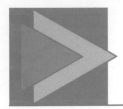

Key to Pulmonary Physiology Abbreviations

COPD	Chronic obstructive pulmonary disease
FEV_1	Forced expiratory volume in 1 second
$Paco_2$	Partial pressure of arterial carbon dioxide
Pao_2	Partial pressure of oxygen in arterial blood
$\dot{V}co_2$	Carbon dioxide production
V_D	Dead space of the lungs
V_D/V_T	Ratio of ventilatory dead space to tidal volume
$\dot{V}_E$	Level of ventilation
$\dot{V}o_2$	Oxygen consumption
V_T	Tidal volume

Before the 1950s, patients with chronic symptomatic lung disease were advised to avoid physical activity. For these patients, exercise elicits dyspnea, a sensation of uncomfortable shortness of breath. However, unlike some other unpleasant sensations (e.g. cardiac angina), dyspnea does not signal that tissue damage is taking place. Starting with the pioneering work of Barach et al. (1), a body of literature has been amassed indicating that patients with chronic lung disease benefit from physical activity.

The tendency of most patients with lung disease is to a gradual decrease in activity. By the time they seek medical attention, patients are often deconditioned and capable of only a low level of activity (2). For these patients, an organized exercise program is often greatly beneficial. Knowledge regarding exercise benefits and exercise prescription for chronic lung disease patients has accumulated rapidly in recent years. However, most research has concerned a single disease entity: COPD. This chapter focuses on exercise training in COPD; the final section presents what is known regarding other chronic lung diseases.

THE PULMONARY REHABILITATION MODEL

Though an exercise program can be prescribed as an isolated intervention, most commonly a coordinated program of pulmonary rehabilitation is prescribed. Table

39.1 lists the components usually included in such a program. A multidisciplinary team, often including a pulmonary physician; a nurse coordinator; physical, occupational, and respiratory therapists; a dietitian, and an exercise specialist, administers this therapy. Comprehensive pulmonary rehabilitation programs are not well standardized, but they generally run 6–8 weeks, with half-day sessions held three times per week. As exercise programs are acknowledged to have central importance, it is common to have 1–2 hours devoted to exercise in each rehabilitation session. As the benefits of rehabilitation have been shown to regress after the program is over, an organized maintenance program is useful. In particular, maintenance exercise sessions help to preserve the gains in exercise tolerance.

PSYCHOLOGICAL BENEFITS OF EXERCISE PROGRAMS

Two distinct strategies—psychological and physiological—for improving exercise tolerance in patients with lung disease have been defined. The psychological approach posits that patients can be desensitized to exertional dyspnea (3, 4). To date the most effective method to desensitize is a program of regular exercise. The desensitizing effects of exercise have been explained in several ways (4):

- Patients successfully participating in an exercise program gain positive feedback from mastering something perceived as being difficult.
- Progressive exercise in a supervised program with others having similar debilities calms unrealistic fears. This explanation is consistent with the generally inferior results obtained from home exercise programs (5).
- Dyspneic stimuli are perceived as less intense when attention is focused on stimuli that are not dyspneic. Thus, listening to music or exercising with a group of people distracts patients from respiratory sensations.

Psychological benefits of an exercise program can be substantial, though there are few established guidelines to

Table 39.1. Components of a Pulmonary Rehabilitation Program

Candidate assessment	Chest physical therapy
Education	Controlled breathing
Optimization of medical therapy	techniques
Psychosocial support	Nutritional therapy
Exercise training	Continuing care programs

define the most efficient program parameters to achieve such benefits. Intuitively, the setting, the exercise partners, and the experience and dedication of the rehabilitation staff are important. Precise frequency, duration, and intensity targets may be less important.

PHYSIOLOGICAL FACTORS LIMITING EXERCISE TOLERANCE IN COPD

Patients with COPD of moderate or greater severity are often *ventilatory limited* during exercise. Exercise terminates because pulmonary ventilation cannot be increased sufficiently to meet the physiological demand. A useful concept is the breathing reserve, defined as the difference between the maximal pulmonary ventilation that can be sustained and the peak ventilation achieved during a maximal exercise test. In COPD patients, but not in healthy individuals, breathing reserve is low because the ability to ventilate the lung is low and because the ventilatory requirement for a given level of exercise is high. Amelioration of either abnormality predictably improves exercise tolerance. COPD is associated with four physiological deficits that impair exercise tolerance:

1. *Impaired lung mechanics.* Airway resistance is high during expiration, which leads to high work of breathing. Furthermore, the airways tend to close as expiration proceeds and progressive hyperinflation ensues. This puts the respiratory muscles, especially the diaphragm, at a mechanical disadvantage. As a result, the respiratory muscles fatigue at low levels of exercise.
2. *Inefficient pulmonary gas exchange.* The factors dictating V_E required for a given level of exercise can be determined by consideration of the alveolar mass balance equation for carbon dioxide (6):

$$\dot{V}_E = \frac{k\,\dot{V}CO_2}{PaCO_2\,(1 - V_D/V_T)}$$

where V_D/V_T is the fraction of V_T that is not effective in expelling carbon dioxide from the lung, and k is a constant. In COPD, V_D/V_T is often high during exercise because emphysematous air spaces are ventilated, but poorly perfused. If the patient has clinically

significant hypoxemia with exercise (PaO_2 < approximately 60 torr), the carotid bodies are stimulated, resulting in an increased ventilatory drive and a lower $PaCO_2$. Some patients with severe COPD employ a compensatory technique that reduces the ventilatory requirement at a given level of exercise: They allow $PaCO_2$ to drift upward with exercise (carbon dioxide retention), allowing a lower level of ventilation, albeit at a cost of a lower arterial pH (7).

3. *Pulmonary vascular insufficiency.* In patients whose COPD involves extensive alveolar destruction, the pulmonary vasculature is destroyed as well. Instead of recruiting pulmonary capillaries during exercise, recruitment is limited and pulmonary artery pressure rises. This increases right heart work. If the right heart is unable to respond adequately, cardiac output and therefore oxygen delivery to the exercising muscle are inappropriately low. Whether this is an important mechanism of exercise intolerance in COPD is unclear. Most studies show that COPD patients do not have an abnormally low oxygen delivery to the exercising muscle for a given level of exercise (8).
4. *Abnormal skeletal muscle metabolism.* There is increasing evidence that an appreciable part of exercise intolerance in COPD patients can be traced to abnormalities in the exercising muscles (9). Several possible mechanisms of muscle dysfunction are present. COPD patients lead a sedentary life, so *deconditioning* is likely (2). It has been posited that *malnutrition* contributes to the muscle wasting (10). *Low levels of anabolic hormones* have been observed in ambulatory COPD patients (11). Both the growth hormone axis and the sex steroid axis seem to be abnormal. The resultant failure to provide anabolic stimuli to the muscle may well decrease muscle mass. Finally, it is plausible that a primary *skeletal muscle myopathy* is associated with chronic lung disease. Oral corticosteroid therapy (12) and perhaps chronic hypoxemia (9) may lead to maladaptive changes in muscle structure and function.

DESIGN OF ENDURANCE EXERCISE TRAINING PROGRAMS FOR COPD PATIENTS

Comprehensive reviews have reported the results of exercise programs for COPD patients (13, 14). It is clear that patients completing an exercise program feel that exercise tolerance has increased. On effort-dependent measures of exercise endurance, performance is generally better. It is clear that these benefits cannot be traced to improvements in lung function. However, until recently few studies featured a control group; the design of the exercise programs has varied widely; and the adequacy of the program has been difficult to evaluate (13). In particular, exercise has generally been performed on uncalibrated devices, and intensity was "increased as tolerated" during the program. Moreover, the outcome measures in most studies were effort dependent (e.g., timed walking tests). As a result, most of the published literature cannot be used to determine the parameters of an exercise program that are effective in improving the physiological ability to exercise.

However, several subsequent studies have confirmed that patients with COPD can indeed achieve a physiological training effect from a well-designed program of exercise training. Casaburi et al. (15) demonstrated that patients with predominantly moderate COPD respond to a program of high-intensity training with reduced levels of blood lactate and pulmonary ventilation at a given heavy work rate (Fig. 39.1). The same group demonstrated that a rigorous training program for patients with severe disease results in improved exercise tolerance and evidence of improved muscle function, including more rapid oxygen uptake kinetics following exercise onset (16). Maltais et al. (17) and Jobin et al. (18) have performed biopsies on the thigh muscle before and after a rigorous training program and demonstrated that aerobic enzyme concentrations and capillary density increase as a result of an endurance training program (Fig. 39.2).

Characteristics of an Effective Endurance Training Program

No detailed, well-controlled trials to ascertain the optimal characteristics of an exercise training program in patients with lung disease have been carried out. However, certain extrapolations from the responses of healthy subjects seem warranted. An aerobic training response can be expected only if training involves large muscle groups. Walking, cycling, stair climbing, and swimming, for example, are likely to be effective modalities. Upper extremity exercise involves a smaller muscle mass. However, upper extremity training may assist the patient in performing activities of daily living and also may improve the function of accessory muscles of respiration (14, 20). Training the muscles of respiration (e.g., by breathing against a resistance) may improve respiratory muscle strength, but usually does not improve exercise capacity (21).

It seems reasonable to advise that exercise programs for patients with lung disease feature sessions 3–5 times per week with at least 30 minutes per session, since these features are effective in healthy subjects. Programs should last at least 5 weeks and preferably longer. Once an aero-

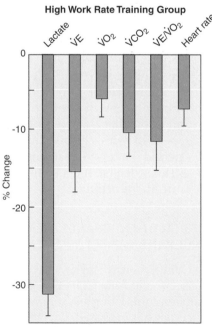

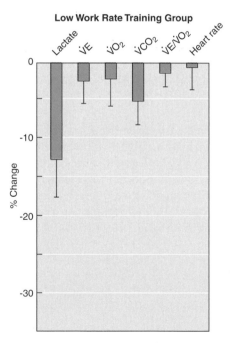

Figure 39.1. Changes in the physiological responses to an identical exercise task (a constant work rate test at a high exercise intensity) produced by two exercise training strategies in patients with COPD. The left panel shows the changes of responses in a group (N = 11) who trained at a high work rate; the right panel presents responses of a similar group (N = 8) who trained at a lower intensity but in a longer session, so that total work per session was identical irrespective Lof group assignment. Vertical bars are 1 SEM. Decreases in blood lactate, ventilation, oxygen uptake, carbon dioxide output, ventilatory equivalent for oxygen, and heart rate are observed for both training regimens, but decreases are appreciably greater for the high-work-rate group. (Reprinted with permission from Casaburi R, Patessio A, Ioli F, et al. Reduction in exercise lactic acidosis and ventilation as a result of exercise training in obstructive lung disease. Am Rev Respir Dis 143:9, 1991.)

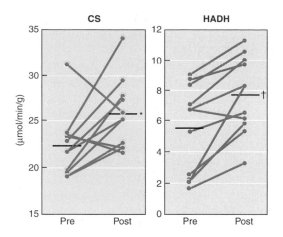

Figure 39.2. Eleven patients with severe COPD underwent a rigorous program of exercise training. Before and after training, patients underwent percutaneous biopsy of the vastus lateralis muscle. The activity of the oxidative enzymes citrate synthase (CS) and 3-hyroxyacyl-CoA dehydrogenase (HADH) increased significantly as a result of training (*P < .05; †P <.01). The activity of three glycolytic enzymes did not change significantly. These results show that skeletal muscle oxidative capacity of COPD patients improves after a rigorous exercise program. (Reproduced with permission from Maltais F, LeBlanc P, Simard C, et al. Skeletal muscle adaptation to endurance training in patients with chronic obstructive pulmonary disease. Am Respir Crit Care Med 154:442, 1996.)

bic training effect has been achieved, it is necessary to pursue a maintenance program or the benefits will be lost within a few weeks.

The Special Problem of Prescribing Intensity of Endurance Exercise

Intensity prescriptions suitable for healthy elderly subjects or even patients with other chronic diseases cannot be used for patients with chronic lung disease. Criteria based on heart rate or oxygen uptake are especially problematic. Since these patients are usually ventilatory limited, peak effort is associated with a heart rate and $\dot{V}O_2$ considerably less than predicted levels. Standard criteria that dictate an exercise intensity (e.g., 60% of *predicted* maximum heart rate) may well be above the peak exercise tolerance. On the other hand, basing the prescription on a similar percentage of the *observed* peak heart rate or $\dot{V}O_2$ sometimes leads to unreasonably low exercise intensity targets (e.g., below unloaded pedaling requirements). Calculating heart rate reserve is problematic, since resting heart rate is often high and varies considerably from day to day.

Casaburi et al. (22) proposed using the lactic acidosis threshold for a minimum training intensity target for COPD patients. However, an appreciable number of patients with severe COPD do not manifest elevated blood lactate levels at the highest work rate they can tolerate, yet

a rigorous exercise program has been shown to elicit a physiological training effect in these patients (16).

Ries and Archibald (23) and Punzal et al. (24) suggested a more practical approach. Patients with COPD have been found to tolerate high fractions of their peak exercise tolerance for prolonged periods, likely because levels of pulmonary ventilation mildly below the limiting ventilation are well tolerated. A reasonable procedure is to perform an incremental exercise test on a calibrated ergometer before initiating a training program. The target work rate can be selected as approximately 80% of the peak work rate observed in the incremental test. (Since the peak work rate varies with the rate of increase in work rate, it is important that an appropriately slow increase in work rate be used in the incremental test; the target should be an incremental phase lasting 8–12 minutes.) If exercise is not to be performed on a calibrated cycle ergometer, the heart rate associated with a work rate equal to 80% of the peak work rate during the incremental test can be used as the heart rate target. Several provisos accompany this approach. It is advisable to use the first few exercise sessions as low-intensity warm-up to ensure that disused muscles will not be inordinately sore. Once the high-intensity sessions begin, the rehabilitation therapist may have to adjust the intensity target up or down. Furthermore, it may be appropriate to allow the patient to break the exercise session into two or more portions for the first few sessions. As the exercise program proceeds and fitness improves, exercise intensity targets should be adjusted upward to maximize the training stimulus.

It is common practice in some rehabilitation programs to prescribe exercise intensity strictly on perceived exertion score. It seems unlikely that such a subjective criterion can reliably result in an stimulus sufficient to elicit a physiological training effect. If physiological benefits are the goal of the training program, perceived exertion should not be the sole yardstick for intensity.

Resistance Training

Resistance training has received little attention as a means to combat skeletal muscle dysfunction despite demonstrations that peripheral muscle weakness is common in COPD. Hamilton et al. (25) reported that strength scores of COPD patients averaged 81% of those in a control population. Bernard et al. (26) found that lower extremity voluntary strength measures (1-RM, or repetition maximum) for COPD patients averaged 73% of those in a matched control group, while thigh muscle cross-sectional size averaged 76% of that of the control group. The rationale for including resistance training is not only to provide a countermeasure against this loss of muscle strength and size but also to avoid a decrease in ability to perform daily functional activities, such as stair climbing and carrying objects. Loss of strength has been shown to be significantly related to use of health care resources in COPD (27). Decreased strength has also been linked to falls in the healthy elderly (28), which frequently lead to broken bones and substantial morbidity.

Resistance training has been shown to improve muscle function and performance of functional activities in patients with COPD, though this finding is based on only a few published studies. Simpson et al. (29) used an 8-week program of resistance training for three muscle groups and reported improvements of 16–40% in maximum voluntary strength versus no significant change in the control group. Bernard et al. (30) compared the results of aerobic exercise training to those of aerobic plus resistance training. In this 12-week intervention, thigh muscle cross-sectional area increased 8%; quadriceps muscle strength increased 20%; and pectoralis major strength increased 15% in the aerobic plus resistance training group. These increases were all significantly greater than those seen in the group receiving aerobic training only.

As with endurance training, there have been no studies to establish an optimal resistance training program for COPD patients. Extrapolations from programs used to develop strength, power, and endurance in healthy individuals (31) and the successful outcomes in COPD patients reported in the literature to date (29, 30) offer a template for program design. A synthesis of this information would suggest a training frequency of 2–3 days per week with 2–3 sets of 8–10 repetitions using loads progressing from 50–85% of a current 1-RM assessment. Studies using some combination of these guidelines have demonstrated substantial improvements in muscle strength and size (29, 30). Applying such principles in a maintenance pulmonary fitness program, significant changes have been documented in 1-RM of 12 people with COPD (average FEV_1 = 49% predicted, age 67 years) over 3 years (Storer et al., unpublished findings). These patients improved 1-RM leg press and chest press strength by 84% and 87%, respectively, in a twice-weekly resistance training program. The program used 1–3 sets of 1–2 exercises per muscle or muscle group (a total of 5–16 exercises) with loads beginning at 50–60% of the 1-RM and progressing to 8–10 repetitions maximum (8–10-RM) per set for each exercise. While much of the improvement was noted within the first year, average 1-RM strength continued to increase over the 3-year observation period. Recent resistance training guidelines for healthy individuals have suggested use of a single set of 8–12 repetitions to fatigue (32). While a single set of an exercise for each body part may be an ideal starting point for many people, principles of progression suggest that to maximize the response, 2 or perhaps 3 sets may be more advantageous as the patient progresses. Fewer rather than more repetitions seem to be better tolerated by the COPD patient, with 8–10 repetitions appearing optimal. As with endurance training, a gradual introduction to resistance exercise training, perhaps with 1 set of 8–10 repetitions using 50–60% of 1-RM for major muscle groups, avoids excessively sore muscles and allows the participant to establish a training base from which the exercise professional may advance the exercise program.

Other considerations in the formulation of a resistance training program for people with COPD include type of resistance used, the rest interval between sets or exercises, choice of exercises, and safety considerations. Many types of resistance are available; these include elastic resistance, machine weights, free weights, and body weight. Choice of equipment is often dictated by what is available. However, almost any form of resistance suffices so long as it can be graded in its application, is safe to use, and has some motivational appeal to the participant. The latter is often accomplished when the participant sees a known amount of weight move.

The ideal rest interval between sets is difficult to establish for the patient with COPD, primarily because of dyspnea and/or oxyhemoglobin desaturation. While a 1-minute rest interval between sets might be attempted, in practice, 2–3 minutes may be required. Choice of exercises may be dictated by the patient's goals (e.g., improving ability to climb stairs) or by contraindications, such as arthritic joints or osteoporosis (a particular problem in long-term corticosteroid therapy). A free weight squat, for example, is typically not appropriate in the COPD population.

Safety concerns in addition to those identified for endurance exercise training include the need to use biomechanically safe lifting technique. Also, periodic blood pressure measurements are needed to monitor the pressor response to the resistance exercise, and it may be necessary periodically to monitor oxygen saturation and level of dyspnea. While these training strategies have been shown to be safe and effective in improving muscle strength, size, and function in small groups of patients, they should be viewed as suggestions only; further research will be needed to establish firm resistance training guidelines for COPD patients.

SAFETY CONSIDERATIONS

Many patients with chronic lung disease are elderly and have high coexisting impairment of other organ systems. This is especially true of patients with COPD. Such patients require a systematic assessment before an exercise program can be safely undertaken. An evaluation by a physician, including a medical history, physical examination, basic blood tests (hematology and chemistry), chest radiography, and resting electrocardiogram should be on record. A recent pulmonary function test and arterial blood gas analysis offer objective evidence of disease severity. Patients should be in a stable phase of disease, and pharmacological therapy should be maximized. Since cigarette smoking is self-destructive behavior and may subvert the therapeutic environment of the group, most programs do not accept participants who have yet to stop smoking (though it is plausible that an exercise program may be a useful adjunct to smoking cessation efforts).

A cardiopulmonary exercise test (19) is useful for patients about to undertake an exercise program. Serial 12-lead electrocardiograms allow detection of cardiac arrhythmias or ischemia that might be contraindications to vigorous exercise. Pulse oximetry can be used to detect exercise-induced hypoxemia. If arterial oxygen saturation drops below approximately 90% or PaO_2 falls below 55 torr, supplemental oxygen via nasal cannula during exercise should be prescribed. Some authorities give supplemental oxygen to patients with lesser degrees of hypoxemia in the hope that exercise tolerance will improve and the training program will be more effective; however, this strategy has not been validated. Cardiopulmonary exercise testing can also be used to establish an exercise intensity prescription (discussed previously). Retesting after the exercise program can yield an objective measure of benefit.

TRAINING PROGRAM CONSIDERATIONS FOR PATIENTS WITH LUNG DISEASE OTHER THAN COPD

Often patients with chronic restrictive lung diseases, such as those with chest wall deformity, pneumoconiosis, or rheumatological lung disease, receive rehabilitative exercise training alongside the COPD majority. Though those with restrictive lung disease may well benefit from different training strategies, little work has been done to define optimal therapeutic programs for this diverse patient group (33). Other groups of patients with lung disease are generally treated in separate rehabilitative settings. Cystic fibrosis patients are generally young, and success with various exercise modalities has been reported, though secretion clearance and management of infections are continuing concerns (34). Asthmatics are often asymptomatic or minimally symptomatic between exacerbations; this provides an opportunity for a vigorous exercise program (35). The availability of lung and heart–lung transplantation and recently lung volume reduction surgery has led to the design of exercise programs for the preoperative and postoperative periods (2, 36). Occasionally, the exercise program is so effective that transplantation is no longer indicated. Finally, facilities have been established to care for patients dependent on mechanical ventilation. Exercise programs are a part of therapy designed to improve quality of life and decrease reliance on ventilatory support (37).

▶ SUMMARY

Pulmonary rehabilitation programs provide both psychological and physiological benefits for patients with chronic lung disease. Endurance training programs may require special design and different techniques for exercise prescription for pulmonary patients. Resistance training offers significant benefits to participants and should be an integral part of such programs. Appropriate screening and supervision of participants can enhance the safety of such programs.

References

1. Barach AL, Bickerman HA, Beck G. Advances in the treatment of non-tuberculous pulmonary disease. Bull N Y Acad Med 28:353, 1952.
2. Casaburi R. Deconditioning. In: Fishman AP, ed. Pulmonary Rehabilitation: Lung Biology in Health and Disease Series. New York: Marcel Dekker, 1996:213.
3. O'Donnell DE, McGuire M, Samis L, et al. The impact of exercise reconditioning on breathlessness in severe chronic airflow limitation. Am J Respir Crit Care Med 152:2005, 1995.
4. Haas F, Salazar-Schicchi J, Axen R. Desensitization to dyspnea in chronic obstructive pulmonary disease. In: Casaburi R, Petty TL, eds. Principles and Practice of Pulmonary Rehabilitation. Philadelphia: Saunders, 1993:24.
5. Puente-Maestu L, Sánz ML, Sánz P, et al. Comparison of effects of supervised versus self-monitored training programmes in patients with chronic obstructive pulmonary disease. Eur Respir J 15:517–526, 2000.
6. Casaburi R. Mechanisms of the reduced ventilatory requirement as a result of exercise training. Eur Respir Rev 4:42, 1995.
7. Barstow TJ, Casaburi R. Ventilatory control in lung disease. In: Casaburi R, Petty TL, eds. Principles and Practice of Pulmonary Rehabilitation. Philadelphia: Saunders, 1993:50.
8. Maltais F, Jobin J, Sullivan MJ, et al. Metabolic and hemodynamic responses of the lower limb during exercise in normal subjects and in COPD. J Appl Physiol 84:1573, 1998.
9. Casaburi R, Gosselink R, Decramer M, et al. Skeletal muscle dysfunction in obstructive pulmonary disease: A statement of the American Thoracic Society and European Respiratory Society. Am J Respir Crit Care Med 159 4 (part 2):S1–S40, 1999.
10. Schols AMWJ, Soeters PB, Dingemans AMC, et al. Prevalence and characteristics of nutritional depletion in patients with stable COPD eligible for pulmonary rehabilitation. Am Rev Respir Dis 147:1151, 1993.
11. Kamischke A, Kemper DE, Castel MA, et al. Testosterone levels in men with chronic obstructive lung disease with or without glucocorticoid therapy. Eur Respir J 11:41, 1998.
12. Decramer M, Lacquet LM, Fagard R, et al. Corticosteroids contribute to muscle weakness in chronic airflow obstruction. Am J Respir Crit Care Med 150:11, 1994.
13. Casaburi R. Exercise training in chronic obstructive lung disease. In: Casaburi R, Petty TL, eds. Principles and Practice of Pulmonary Rehabilitation. Philadelphia: Saunders, 1993:204.
14. Ries AL, Carlin BW, Carrieri-Kohlman V, et al. Pulmonary rehabilitation: Evidence based guidelines. Chest 112:1363, 1997.
15. Casaburi R, Patessio A, Ioli F, et al. Reduction in exercise lactic acidosis and ventilation as a result of exercise training in obstructive lung disease. Am Rev Respir Dis 143:9, 1991.

16. Casaburi R, Porszasz J, Burns MR, et al. Physiological benefits of exercise training in rehabilitation of severe COPD patients. Am J Respir Crit Care Med 155:1541, 1997.

17. Maltais F, LeBlanc P, Simard C, et al. Skeletal muscle adaptation to endurance training in patients with chronic obstructive pulmonary disease. Am Respir Crit Care Med 154:442, 1996.

18. Jobin J, Maltais F, Doyon JF, et al. Chronic obstructive pulmonary disease: Capillarity and fiber-type characteristics of skeletal muscle. J Cardiopulm Rehabil 18:432, 1998.

19. Wasserman K, Hansen JE, Sue DY, et al. Principles of Exercise Testing and Interpretation. 3rd ed. Philadelphia: Lippincott Williams & Wilkins, 1999.

20. Criner GJ, Celli BR. Effect of unsupported arm exercise on ventilatory muscle recruitment in patients with severe chronic airflow obstruction. Am Rev Respir Dis 138:856, 1988.

21. Smith K, Cook D, Guyatt GH, et al. Respiratory muscle training in chronic airflow limitation: A meta-analysis. Am Rev Respir Dis 145:533, 1992.

22. Casaburi R, Wasserman K, Patessio A, et al. A new perspective in pulmonary rehabilitation: Anaerobic threshold as a discriminant in training. Eur Resp J 2(Suppl):7:618s, 1989.

23. Ries AL, Archibald CJ. Endurance exercise training at maximal targets in patients with chronic obstructive pulmonary disease. J Cardiopulm Rehabil 7:594, 1987.

24. Punzal PA, Ries AL, Kaplan RM, et al. Maximum intensity exercise training in patients with chronic obstructive pulmonary disease. Chest 100:618, 1991.

25. Hamilton AL, Killian KJ, Summers E, et al. Muscle strength, symptom intensity, and exercise capacity in patients with cardiopulmonary disorders. Am J Respir Crit Care Med 152:2021, 1995.

26. Bernard S, LeBlanc P, Wittom F, et al. Peripheral muscle weakness in patients with chronic obstructive pulmonary disease. Am J Respir Crit Care Med 158:629, 1998.

27. Decramer M, Gosselink R, Troosters T, et al. Muscle weakness is related to utilization of health care resources in COPD patients. Eur Respir J 10:417, 1997.

28. Fiatarone MA, O'Neill EF, Doyle N, et al. The Boston FICSIT study: The effects of resistance training and nutritional supplementation on physical frailty in the oldest old. J Am Geriatr Soc 41:333, 1993.

29. Simpson K, Killian K, McCartney N, et al. Randomised controlled trial of weight lifting exercise in patients with chronic airflow limitation. Thorax 47:70, 1992.

30. Bernard S, Whittom F, LeBlanc P, et al. Aerobic and strength training in patients with chronic obstructive pulmonary disease. Am J Respir Crit Car Med 159:896, 1999.

31. Fleck SJ, Kraemer W. Designing Resistance Training Programs. 2nd ed. Champaign, IL: Human Kinetics, 1997.

32. Kenney WL, ed. ACSM's Guidelines for Exercise Testing and Prescription. 6th ed. Baltimore: Lippincott Williams & Wilkins, 2000.

33. Novitch RS, Thomas HM III. Rehabilitation of patients with chronic ventilatory limitation from nonobstructive lung diseases. In: Casaburi R, Petty TL, eds. Principles and Practice of Pulmonary Rehabilitation. Philadelphia: Saunders, 1993:416.

34. Orenstein DM, Noyes BE. Cystic fibrosis. In: Casaburi R, Petty TL, eds. Principles and Practice of Pulmonary Rehabilitation. Philadelphia: Saunders, 1993:439.

35. Clark CJ. The role of physical training in asthma. In: Casaburi R, Petty TL, eds. Principles and Practice of Pulmonary Rehabilitation. Philadelphia: Saunders, 1993:424.

36. Biggar DG, Malen JF, Trulock EP, et al. Pulmonary rehabilitation before and after lung transplantation. In: Casaburi R, Petty TL, eds. Principles and Practice of Pulmonary Rehabilitation. Philadelphia: Saunders, 1993:459.

37. Petty TL. The ventilator-dependent patient. In: Casaburi R, Petty TL, eds. Principles and Practice of Pulmonary Rehabilitation. Philadelphia: Saunders, 1993:468.

SECTION EIGHT

HEALTH AND FITNESS ASSESSMENT

SECTION EDITOR: Moira Kelsey, RN, MS

1.6.1, 1.6.2   2.6.0, 2.6.0.1, 2.6.0.2,   3.6.1   4.6.0, 4.6.0.1, 4.6.0.2,
                      2.6.0.3, 2.6.0.4   4.6.0.3

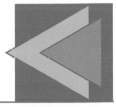

CHAPTER **40**

PREPARTICIPATION HEALTH APPRAISAL IN THE NONMEDICAL SETTING

Neil F. Gordon

It is clear that a physically active lifestyle provides partial protection against several major chronic diseases. In particular, there is now convincing evidence that regular exercise is beneficial in the primary prevention of coronary artery disease (CAD) and the reduction of mortality after myocardial infarction. Given the high prevalence of sedentary lifestyle and the fact that CAD remains the leading cause of death in Western industrialized countries, there is little doubt that considerable public health benefit would accrue if inactive individuals became more active.

The many health-related benefits of a physically active lifestyle are well documented. However, it is essential to realize that to be most effective, regular exercise must be combined with other positive lifestyle interventions and where applicable, with appropriate medical therapy. Furthermore, although exercise is extremely safe for most individuals, it is prudent to take certain precautions to optimize the benefit-to-risk ratio.

To ensure an optimal benefit-to-risk ratio, the exercise professional should incorporate some form of health appraisal before performing fitness testing or initiating an exercise program. The purpose of such an appraisal is to provide information relevant to the safety of fitness testing before beginning exercise training, to identify known diseases and risk factors for CAD and other preventable chronic diseases so that appropriate lifestyle interventions can be initiated, and to identify additional factors that require special consideration when developing an appropriate exercise prescription and programming that optimize adherence, minimize risks, and maximize benefits.

It is essential that the preparticipation health appraisal be both cost-effective and time-efficient so that unnecessary barriers to exercise can be avoided. The precise nature and extent of the appraisal should be determined by the age, sex, and perceived health status characteristics of the participants, as well as the available economic, personnel, and equipment resources. Health appraisals can range from a short questionnaire to interviews and sophisticated computerized evaluations.

This chapter presents information that may be incorporated into a health appraisal for the following:

- Safety of exercise
- Health behaviors and risk factors
- Other special considerations for exercise prescription and programming

SAFETY OF EXERCISE

Most prospective participants in exercise programs conducted in nonmedical settings are apparently healthy individuals whose goals are to enhance fitness and well-being, reduce weight, and reduce risk of chronic disease. For such individuals, the primary safety goal of a preparticipation health appraisal is to identify individuals who should receive further medical evaluation to determine whether there are contraindications to exercise testing or training, or whether referral to a medically supervised exercise program is necessary.

According to ACSM guidelines, asymptomatic, apparently healthy men under age 45 and women under age 55 with fewer than two CAD risk factors do not require medical evaluation by a physician before initiating a program of vigorous exercise training (i.e., exercise intensity $> 60\%$ $\dot{V}O_{2\,max}$) (1). It is also considered unnecessary for asymptomatic apparently healthy men and women, irrespective of age or CAD risk factor status, to have a medical evaluation by a physician before embarking on a program of moderate exercise training (i.e., exercise intensity 40–60% $\dot{V}O_{2\,max}$) (1). For such individuals, preparticipation screening can be accomplished using validated self-administered questionnaires, such as the Physical Activity Readiness Questionnaire (PAR-Q).

Although many questionnaires are available for pre-exercise screening, the PAR-Q is well developed and has a sensitivity of nearly 100% and specificity of approximately 80% for detecting medical contraindications to exercise (2). (When used in this context, **sensitivity** refers to the percent of persons with medical contraindications to

355

exercise who answer yes to one or more questions; **specificity** refers to the percent of persons without medical contraindications to exercise who answer no to all questions.) The PAR-Q is only one example of a pre-exercise screening questionnaire; limitations of this questionnaire are discussed later. The responsibility of adding to or modifying the pre-exercise screening tool lies with the director of the exercise program and should be determined primarily by the population served.

Despite the obvious ease of use and cost-effectiveness of the PAR-Q, its original format has several important limitations. These limitations, which should be kept in mind, include the following:

1. The less than desirable specificity for detecting contraindications to exercise
2. Limited sensitivity (approximately 35%) and specificity (approximately 80%) for predicting subsequent exercise electrocardiogram (ECG) abnormalities
3. Inability to screen out persons with two or more major CAD risk factors (who require a medical examination before participation in vigorous exercise)
4. Automatic referral for medical evaluation by a physician of asymptomatic, apparently healthy individuals over age 65, even if participation in moderate exercise is the goal
5. Inability to identify medications that may affect exercise safety
6. Inability to identify pregnant women, for whom special safety precautions may be required
7. From an overall health perspective, the absence of questions aimed at the identification of adverse health behaviors other than a sedentary lifestyle

Recognition of such limitations of the PAR-Q has led to several revisions of the questionnaire (1–3). The original and newest revision of the PAR-Q are shown in Table 40.1. The significance/clarification of each of the question in the new version of the PAR-Q is outlined in Table 40.2. This revised version enhances the specificity for detecting contraindications to exercise and thereby minimizes unnecessary medical referrals (3). It is important to note differences in phrasing of questions, so customized questionnaires may be developed within various settings that meet the needs of individual programs. Customized questionnaires can be developed to address the limited capability of the PAR-Q; to obtain information about risk factors, personal history, and health behaviors; and to obtain other information that may warrant special considerations.

PERSONAL HEALTH HISTORY AND CAD RISK FACTORS

In addition to readiness for and safety of exercise, it is important for exercise professionals to assess other aspects of personal health history and risk factors for chronic diseases, in particular CAD (which constitutes the leading cause of death in Western industrialized countries, including exertion-related sudden death). Because several risk factors for CAD (discussed elsewhere in this book) and other chronic diseases depend on behavior, health behaviors of participants should be assessed. The PAR-Q touches on several risk factors for CAD; however, it is designed to determine the safety of exercise, not the overall risk of CAD. The following includes additional information on aspects of the personal health history and risk factors that should be identified to clarify the risk of events during exercise, prioritize interventions, and encourage change in lifestyle to reduce disease risk. The information may also be important in developing or modifying the exercise program.

Table 40.1. Physical Activity Readiness Questionnaire: Matching Questions of Original and Revised Versions

ORIGINAL	REVISED
1. Has your doctor ever said you have heart trouble?	1. Has your doctor ever said that you have a heart condition and that you should only do physical activity recommended by a doctor?
2. Do you frequently have pains in your heart and chest?	2. Do you feel pain in your chest when you do physical activity?
3. Do you often feel faint or have spells of severe dizziness?	4. Do you lose your balance because of dizziness or do you ever lose consciousness?
4. Has a doctor ever said your blood pressure was too high?	6. Is your doctor currently prescribing drugs (for example, water pills) for your blood pressure or heart condition?
5. Has your doctor ever told you that you have a bone or joint problem such as arthritis that has been aggravated by exercise or might be made worse with exercise?	5. Do you have a bone or joint problem that could be made worse by a change in your physical activity?
6. Is there a good physical reason not mentioned here why you should not follow an activity program even if you wanted to?	7. Do you know of any other reason you should not do physical activity?
7. Are you over 65 and not accustomed to vigorous exercise?	(No matching question. Introductory comments state: If you are over 69 years of age, and you are not used to being very active, check with your doctor.)
(No matching question)	3. In the past month, have you had chest pain when you were not doing physical activity?

Table 40.2. Physical Activity Readiness Questionnaire (PAR-Q)

For most people, physical activity should not pose any problem or hazard. PAR-Q has been designed to identify the small number of adults for whom physical activity might be inappropriate and those who should have medical advice concerning the type of activity most suitable.

1. Has a doctor ever said that you have a heart condition and that you should only do physical activity recommended by a doctor?

    (**Significance/clarification:** Persons with known heart disease are at increased risk for cardiac complications during exercise. They should consult a physician and undergo exercise testing before starting an exercise program. The exercise prescription should be formulated in accordance with standard guidelines for cardiac patients. Medical supervision may be required during exercise training.)

2. Do you feel pain in your chest when you do physical activity?

3. In the past month, have you had chest pain when you were not doing physical activity?

    (**Significance/clarification:** A physician should be consulted to identify the cause of the chest pain, whether it occurs at rest or with exertion. If ischemic in origin, the condition should be stabilized before starting an exercise program. Exercise testing should be performed with the patient on his or her usual medication and the exercise prescription formulated in accordance with standard guidelines for cardiac patients. Medical supervision may be required during exercise training.)

4. Do you lose your balance because of dizziness or do you ever lose consciousness?

    (**Significance/clarification:** A physician should be consulted to establish the cause of these symptoms, which may be related to potentially life-threatening medical conditions. Exercise training should not be undertaken until serious cardiac disorders have been excluded.)

5. Do you have a bone or joint problem that could be made worse by a change in your physical activity?

    (**Significance/clarification:** Existing musculoskeletal disorders may be exacerbated by inappropriate exercise training. Persons with forms of arthritis known to be associated with a systemic component (for example, rheumatoid arthritis) may be at an increased risk for exercise-related medical complications. A physician should be consulted to determine whether any special precautions are required during exercise training.)

6. Is your doctor currently prescribing drugs (for example, water pills) for your blood pressure or heart condition?

    (**Significance/clarification:** See question 1. Medication effects should be considered when formulating the exercise prescription. The exercise prescription should be formulated in accordance with guidelines for the specific cardiovascular disease for which medications are being used. A physician should be consulted to determine whether the condition or factor requires special precautions during exercise training or contraindicates exercise training.)

7. Do you know of any other reason you should not do physical activity?

    (**Significance/clarification:** The exercise prescription may have to be modified in accordance with the specific reason provided. Depending on the specific reason, a physician may have to be consulted.)

If a person answers yes to any question, vigorous exercise or exercise testing may have to be postponed. Medical clearance may be necessary.

Personal History

A personal health history can be quite extensive and may require medically trained professionals for interpretations. As a part of an overall health risk appraisal, personal history should be tailored to emphasize specific factors that help categorize an individual in regard to several broad areas. The most important areas are those of **known diseases** and **manifestation of symptoms** (symptomatic or asymptomatic). Beyond this stratification is documentation concerning whether a symptom-free individual is at **high risk for the development of disease**. Some of this information is identified on the PAR-Q; however, in certain instances, more information may be beneficial.

Evidence of **known cardiovascular disease** or of **symptoms of cardiovascular disease**, such as angina pectoris, must be documented. Symptoms of peripheral vascular disease, particularly discomfort in one or both legs with walking, should also be determined and documented. A history of **respiratory disease** should be determined as well. Seasonal difficulties with breathing or breathing discomfort brought on by physical or emotional stress warrant particular attention.

Diabetes is an independent contributor to the risk of developing cardiovascular disease with the relative risk being higher in women than men (4). This excessive risk includes CAD, peripheral vascular disease, and congestive heart failure. Diabetes is a metabolic disease that requires specific diet and exercise therapy alone or in combination with prescribed medications (see Chapter 10 of *ACSM's Guidelines for Exercise Testing and Prescription*).

Obesity is a common problem, an independent risk factor for the development of CAD, and frequently a predecessor of type II diabetes (5). Body composition measurement is thoroughly discussed elsewhere in this book. The exercise professional must be able to identify the individual who is at risk for weight-related problems and appropriately intervene (or refer) for weight management.

Elevated blood pressure is associated with stroke, heart failure, and myocardial infarction. Exercise professionals are strongly encouraged to measure blood pressure during each patient visit (6). Blood pressure measurement and categorization of blood pressure elevations have been standardized. National guidelines for the follow-up and management of persons with high blood pressure are also available, and individuals with hypertension should be under medical care (6). Exercise training and dietary modifications are an important part of medical management of hypertension.

Abnormal blood lipid levels are known to be the basis of the atherosclerotic process. Serum total cholesterol and high-density lipoprotein (HDL) cholesterol should be measured in all adults 20 years of age and older (7). Triglyceride levels should be measured in patients with

CAD, diabetes, peripheral vascular disease, hypertension, chronic renal disease, and familial hyperlipidemic disorders. Individuals with abnormal lipid profiles are encouraged to modify diet to reduce, in particular, intake of saturated fat and cholesterol. These individuals should be identified and encouraged to maintain control of dietary fat and cholesterol intake in addition to participation in regular exercise.

Heart disease tends to be familial. The development of heart disease is independently associated with a positive **family history** (8). This history goes beyond measured risk factors such as cigarette smoking, excess weight, nutritional factors, and physical inactivity. Therefore, genetic predisposition to the development of CAD is important. The family history should identify any first-degree relatives (parents, siblings, and children). The risk of developing a myocardial infarction is particularly high when the family history documents myocardial infarction or sudden death before 55 years of age in a male first-degree relative or before 65 years of age in a female first-degree relative. Family history of other diseases, specifically diabetes mellitus and certain types of cancer, may be important in emphasizing dietary change in certain individuals.

Health Behaviors

There is a clear link between **dietary habits** and the development of several disease states. Most clear is a link between dietary saturated fat and cholesterol and the development of atherosclerosis. Diets high in cholesterol and saturated fat must be modified to decrease the risk of progressive atherosclerosis (9). Diets high in sodium can lead to persistent elevation of systemic blood pressure, or more important, worsening of heart failure. Diets deficient in complex carbohydrates and fiber have been linked with excessive rates of development of carcinomas of the gastrointestinal tract.

Ideally, diet appraisal should include documentation and analysis of usual dietary choices, specifically total caloric intake, saturated fat, cholesterol, sodium, and types of carbohydrates. Appraisal of dietary intake can range from a simple evaluation of dietary preferences to computer-scored instruments that analyze 24-hour dietary patterns, 3-day food records, and even 7-day food records.

Relating dietary analysis to objective measures of health (e.g., excessive calories in overweight individuals, excessive sodium and weight in hypertensive individuals) can be an excellent starting point for changing dietary patterns to improve health status.

Identification of past **exercise habits** assists the practitioner in developing appropriate prescriptions and programming with realistic goals, optimal adherence, and safety for the individual. The appraisal of exercise habits should include a history of vigorous physical activity, current physical activity habits (both leisure and vocational), and documentation of symptoms associated with activity, particularly chest discomfort, light-headedness, and/or disproportionate shortness of breath related to physical activity. Any muscle or joint discomfort associated with or aggravated by exercise should be identified.

Cigarette smoking is one of the best-established risk factors (10). The adverse impact of cigarette smoking is most dramatic in the areas of cardiovascular disease and lung cancer (the disease is attributable to smoking in 90% of persons with lung carcinoma). The rate of smoking in young women and adolescents is increasing. In addition to increased risk for developing CAD, risk of sudden death (defined as death within 1 hour in an apparently clinically stable or asymptomatic individual) occurs five times as commonly among pack-per-day smokers as among nonsmokers.

Such bleak statistics are counterbalanced by the encouraging and well-documented benefits of smoking cessation. Within 2 years of stopping cigarette smoking, the excess risk of cardiovascular disease drops dramatically. This decline in cardiovascular risk is a dose–response phenomenon; the heavier the prior habit, the more dramatic the benefits. The rate of progression of atherosclerosis is likely to decline in the ex-smoker as well. Every effort should be made to provide smoking participants with clear and persuasive information regarding risks associated with continuing smoking and benefits of cessation.

Table 40.3. Pathological Conditions Possibly Associated With Sudden Cardiac Death During Exercise

Conditions resulting in myocardial ischemia
    Atherosclerotic coronary artery disease
    Coronary artery spasm
    De novo coronary artery thrombus
    Myocardial bridging
    Hypoplastic coronary arteries
    Anomalous coronary arteries
Structural abnormalities
    Hypertrophic cardiomyopathy
    Idiopathic concentric left ventricular hypertrophy
    Right ventricular hypertrophy
    Mitral valve prolapse
    Other valvular heart disease
    Marfan's syndrome
    Congenital defects
Conduction abnormalities
    Wolff-Parkinson-White syndrome
    Lown-Ganong-Levine syndrome
    QT interval prolongation syndrome
Miscellaneous
    Heat stroke
    Myocarditis
    Sarcoidosis

Reprinted with permission from Sadaniantz A, Thompson PD. The problem of sudden death in athletes as illustrated by case studies. Sports Med 9:199, 1990; Kohl HW, Powell KE, Gordon NF, et al. Physical activity, physical fitness and sudden cardiac death. Epidemiol Rev 14:37, 1992.

The **type A behavior pattern** is believed to contribute to the overall risk of developing CAD (11). The original description and identification of type A behavior requires a difficult and elaborate technique of structured interview. Subsequent means of evaluating type A behavior are more objective and streamlined. One of these methods may be included as a component of an appraisal of health behavior. Identification of participants whose behavior pattern places them at high risk for myocardial infarction is important, and counseling should be provided to lower that risk.

OTHER FACTORS REQUIRING SPECIAL CONSIDERATION

The PAR-Q has been recommended as a minimum pre-exercise screening standard for entry into a low to moderate intensity physical activity program (1). Once an individual has been provided with medical clearance to participate in an exercise program (by virtue of either the PAR-Q or a more comprehensive health appraisal), it is important for the exercise professional to determine whether there are any additional health-related factors that require special consideration. Although a variety of risks are associated with exercise participation, the most important is precipitation of sudden cardiac death. Several studies clearly demonstrate that the transiently increased risk of cardiac arrest occurring during vigorous exercise results largely from the presence of preexisting cardiac abnormalities, in particular CAD (Table 40.3).

Other health-related conditions that may affect exercise prescription (or program) are discussed in Table 40.4. The significance and clarification in exercise prescription and programming are also presented in the table. The factors presented should be viewed as red flags, because they may indicate adaptation of type, frequency, intensity, du-

---

Table 40.4. Health-Related Factors That May Affect the Exercise Prescription

Factor: Alcohol and other substance abuse.
Implications/significance: Alcohol intake may elevate heart rate response to submaximal effort, impair exercise tolerance, promote dehydration, and increase risk of heart injury. Habit-forming drugs, such as cocaine, may accentuate risk of cardiac complications during exercise.

Factor: Cigarette smoking.
Implications/significance: Acute cigarette smoking may elevate heart rate, respiration, and blood pressure response to exercise, increase susceptibility toward ventricular arrhythmias, increase platelet aggregability (and risk of thrombosis), and predispose to coronary artery spasm. Chronically, cigarette smoking accentuates the risk of atherosclerosis.

Factor: Diet/nutrition.
Implications/significance: Dietary content, especially total fat, saturated fat, and cholesterol intake, affects serum lipids and lipoproteins and thus the risk for coronary artery disease. Individuals on a calorie-restricted diet should take care to consume adequate carbohydrates to replenish muscle glycogen stores that may be depleted during exercise. Resistance training may be of particular benefit for preservation of lean body mass and minimizing a decline in resting metabolic rate during dieting.

Factor: Diseases.
Implications/significance: Chronic diseases, such as coronary artery disease, diabetes mellitus, hypertension, cerebrovascular disease, AIDS, cancer, osteoporosis, renal disease, arthritis, and chronic obstructive pulmonary disease, require special consideration when devising an exercise prescription. For patients with such conditions, the exercise prescription should be individualized in accordance with standard guidelines.

Factor: Eating disorders, such as anorexia nervosa.
Implications/significance: Care should be taken to de-emphasize weight loss and possibly high-caloric expenditure exercise, where appropriate. To preserve lean body mass, resistance training should be emphasized.

Factor: Environmental considerations.
Implications/significance: The environment in which the individual exercise will occur must be considered when devising an exercise prescription; in particular, weather (heat, humidity, cold), altitude, and air pollution (carbon monoxide, ozone), should be factored into the design of the exercise prescription.

Factor: Family history.
Implications/significance: Family history of premature cardiovascular disease increases risk of such diseases in a given individual.

Factor: Medications.
Implications/significance: Certain medications may alter heart rate and/or blood pressure response to execise, evoke electrocardiographic abnormalities, and alter exercise capacity.

Factor: Obesity.
Implications/significance: Place emphasis on increasing caloric expenditure and minimizing risk of muscle soreness, orthopaedic injury, and other discomfort; initially, lower-intensity exercise of longer duration should be emphasized.

Factor: Past and present exercise history.
Implications/significance: Previous history of exercise experiences, specifically exertion-related orthopaedic injuries and reason for noncompliance, should be considered. Present exercise participation is important when decisions are made about the type, frequency, intensity, and duration at which exercise training should be initiated.

Factor: Personality, behavior pattern.
Implications/significance: May influence compliance with exercise guidelines and decisions regarding individual or group training.

Factor: Pregnancy and breastfeeding.
Implications/significance: Exercise should be prescribed in accordance with accepted guidelines for pregnant and lactating women. Women who already participate in a regular exercise program generally can continue during pregnancy. Other women are advised to obtain physician approval and begin exercising with low-impact or no-impact activities, such as walking and swimming.

Reprinted with permission from Sadaniantz A, Thompson PD. The problem of sudden death in athletes as illustrated by case studies. Sports Med 9:199, 1990; Kohl HW, Powell KE, Gordon NF, et al. Physical activity, physical fitness and sudden cardiac death. Epidemiol Rev 14:37, 1992.

ration, and/or progression of the exercise to make it most appropriate for the individual.

► SUMMARY

It is essential that the exercise professional obtain as much information as possible about a participant to optimize the benefit-to-risk ratio. A regular re-evaluation of health status and health behaviors via a health appraisal should be incorporated into long-term programs to update prescriptions and programming according to changing needs.

References

1. American College of Sports Medicine. Guidelines for Exercise Testing and Prescription, 6th ed. Baltimore: Lippincott Williams & Williams, 2000.
2. Shephard RJ, Thomas S, Weller I. The Canadian home fitness test: 1991 update. Sports Med 11:358, 1991.
3. Cardinal BJ, Esters J, Cardinal MK. Evaluation of the revised Physical Activity Readiness Questionnaire in older adults. Med Sci Sports Exer 28:468, 1996.
4. Kannel WB, McGee DL. Diabetes and cardiovascular disease: The Framingham study. JAMA 241:2035, 1979.
5. Kannel WB, et al. Obesity as an independent risk factor for cardiovascular disease; A 26-year follow-up of participants in the Framingham Heart Study. Circulation 67:968, 1983.
6. National High Blood Pressure Education Program. The sixth report of the Joint National Committee on Detection, Evaluation, and Treatment of High Blood Pressure (JNC VI). Arch Intern Med 157:2413–2446, 1997.
7. National Institutes of Health. Summary of the second report of the National Cholesterol Education Program (NCEP) Expert Panel on Detection, Evaluation, and Treatment of High Blood Cholesterol in Adults (Adult Treatment Panel II). JAMA 269:3015, 1993.
8. Snowden CB et al. Predicting coronary disease in siblings: a multivariate assessment: The Framingham Heart Study. Am J Epidemiol 115:217, 1982.
9. Forrester JS, Merz NB, Bush TL, et al. Task Force 4. Efficacy of Risk Factor Management. J Am Coll Cardiol 27:991, 1996.
10. Fielding JE. Smoking: Health effects and control. N Engl J Med 313:491, 1985.
11. Haynes SG, Feinleib M, Kannel WB. The relationship of psychosocial factors to coronary heart disease in the Framingham study III. Am J Epidemiol 111:37, 1980.

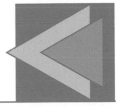

CHAPTER **41**

CARDIORESPIRATORY ASSESSMENT OF APPARENTLY HEALTHY POPULATIONS

Timothy R. McConnell

Several physiological responses to exercise are used to evaluate cardiorespiratory (CR) fitness, including oxygen consumption ($\dot{V}O_2$), heart rate, and blood pressure. Measuring these variables during exercise, particularly maximum exercise, increases the chance of detecting any coronary artery disease or pulmonary disease. Unfortunately, maximum exercise tests are impractical because they are expensive, require extensive clinical supervision, and subject individuals to levels of physical stress that may be unnecessary depending on the objectives of the test. Consequently, maximal testing is reserved for clinical assessments, athletic evaluation, and research. A submaximal exercise test costs less and carries a lower risk for the individual. Although less sensitive and specific for detecting disease or estimating maximal oxygen consumption ($\dot{V}O_{2max}$), correctly performed submaximal tests can provide a valid estimate of cardiorespiratory fitness.

PRETEST SCREENING

Pretest health screening is essential for risk stratification and for determining the type of test that should be performed and the need for an exercise test prior to exercise training (1). A thorough pretest health screening includes the following:

- Complete medical history
- Medical contraindications to exercise
- Symptoms suggesting cardiac or pulmonary disease
- Angina or other forms of discomfort at rest or during exercise
- Unusual shortness of breath at rest or during exercise
- Dizziness or light-headedness
- Orthopaedic complications that may prevent adequate effort or compromise the validity of test results
- Other unusual signs or symptoms that may preclude testing
- Risk factors for coronary heart disease
- History of major cardiorespiratory events
- Current medications
- Activity patterns

- Nutritional habits
- Reading and signing an informed consent form

Along with the appropriate informed consent, the Participant Activity Questionnaire has been recommended as a minimum standard for entry into a moderate-intensity exercise program (1). In addition, the American College of Sports Medicine and the American Heart Association have published a preparticipation screening questionnaire for health and fitness facilities (2). If any concerns are raised by the health screen appraisal or readiness questionnaire, a medical referral should be obtained before proceeding with the test.

SUBMAXIMAL EXERCISE TESTING

Heart rate varies linearly with $\dot{V}O_2$ to the point of maximum exertion; thus, $\dot{V}O_{2max}$ may be estimated using the relation between heart rate and $\dot{V}O_2$ without subjecting the individual to maximum levels of physical stress. During submaximal exercise testing, predetermined workloads are used to elicit a steady state of exertion (plateau of heart rate and $\dot{V}O_2$). The steady-state heart rate at each work level is displayed graphically and extrapolated to the $\dot{V}O_2$ at the age-predicted maximal heart rate (HR = 220 − age) (Fig. 41.1). A variety of protocols for different exercise modalities (i.e., treadmill, stationary cycle, and step increments) can be used as long as the $\dot{V}O_2$ requirements of each selected workload can be estimated with accuracy.

The objectives of CR fitness assessments in the apparently healthy population are as follows:

- Determine the level of CR fitness and establish fitness program goals and objectives.
- Develop a safe, effective exercise prescription for the improvement of CR fitness.
- Document improvements in CR fitness as a result of exercise training or other interventions.
- Motivate individuals to initiate an exercise program or comply with an established program.
- Provide information concerning health status.

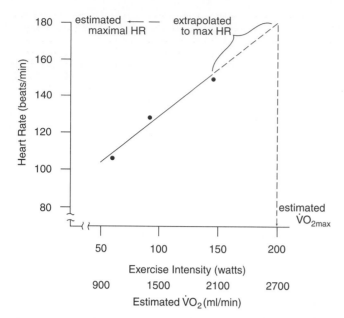

Figure 41.1. Heart rate (HR) obtained from at least two (more are preferable) submaximal exercise intensities may be extrapolated to the age-predicted maximal heart rate. A vertical line to the intensity scale estimates maximal exercise intensity from which an estimated $\dot{V}O_{2max}$ can be calculated. (Reprinted with permission from Franklin BA, ed. ACSM's Guidelines for Exercise Testing and Prescription. 6th ed. Philadelphia: Lippincott Williams & Wilkins, 2000:76.)

A few assumptions regarding testing are necessary to ensure the highest degree of accuracy when using submaximal exercise testing to estimate $\dot{V}O_{2max}$:

- Selected workloads are reproducible. A steady-state heart rate is obtained during each stage of the test. Usually, workload durations of 3 minutes or more are used to ensure steady state.
- The maximal heart rate for a given age is uniform (HR = 220 − age).
- Heart rate and $\dot{V}O_2$ have a linear relation over a wide range of values; thus, the slope of HR/$\dot{V}O_2$ regression can be extrapolated to an assumed maximum heart rate.
- Mechanical efficiency (i.e., $\dot{V}O_2$ at a given work rate) is consistent.

Although if done correctly, submaximal exercise tests provide valuable information concerning CR fitness, they have extremely limited diagnostic capabilities and should not be used as a replacement for clinical exercise tests or other clinical treatment or management modalities. Health care professionals should avoid detailed interpretation beyond the scope of the information obtained.

Considerations with Submaximal Exercise Testing

Considerations for selection of protocol and equipment include any physical or clinical limitations that may preclude certain types of exercise (i.e., age, weight, arthri-

tis, orthopaedic complications, individual comfort, level of fitness, type of exercise training that will be performed, and individual preference) (3–5). For example, some individuals may perform better on a non–weight-bearing modality (cycle versus treadmill), while others may not have the required range of motion in the hip or knee to pedal and may perform better walking. Deconditioned, weak, or elderly persons may have to start the test at a low work level and increase the workload in small increments. Also, field tests may not be appropriate for those who require strict supervision during testing, who do not understand the concept of pacing, or who cannot be expected to put forth a good effort. More consistent results may be obtained by testing in a controlled environment such as a laboratory setting. Creativity when selecting protocols may allow adaptations of commonly used protocols to accommodate athletes competing in specific sports (6, 7). Regardless of the type of exercise and protocol selected, the same type of exercise and protocol should be used for repeat testing if between-test comparisons are important.

Staffing

The staff administering the tests should be ACSM certified and academically trained in exercise science or at least have a basic knowledge of exercise physiology and exercise testing. Staff members should be able to do the following:

1. Establish rapport with the subject and make him or her feel comfortable.
2. Recognize normal acute and chronic responses to exercise.
3. Recognize abnormal signs and symptoms during exercise.
4. Provide basic life support measures competently.
5. Adhere to established procedures and protocols.
6. Clearly explain test results to the individual.

Budget

Financial considerations of exercise testing:

- Equipment costs
- Ratio of staff to patients
- Procedures for interpreting and reporting test results
- Space requirements
- Paper, forms, and other office supplies
- Other indirect costs

Table 41.1 provides a relative comparison of the costs of the various modalities used for submaximal exercise testing.

Individual Volumes

The volume of tests to be performed influences several administrative decisions. Although group testing has financial advantages, it may not be desirable for patient

Table 41.1. Cost Comparison of Submaximal Testing Modalities

Costs	Treadmill	Cycle	Step	Field
Equipment	+++	++	+	+
Staff needs	+++	+++	+	+
Interpretation	++	++	++	++
Space	+++	++	++	+
Paper, forms	++	++	++	++
Other indirect costs	+++	+++	++	+

+++, Greater expense; +, lesser expense

Table 41.2. Financial Considerations of Submaximal Testing

	Least Expensive	Most Expensive
Patient volumes	Group testing	One client at a time
Space	Field, track, or gym area	Allocated testing room
Equipment	Indoor or outdoor track	Treadmill
Staff	Multiple clients per staff	One-on-one testing

care and/or customer satisfaction. Group testing requires a staff-to-patient ratio that ensures safe and appropriate care as well as the accurate acquisition of data. For one-on-one testing it is important to allot a reasonable period for efficient and effective individual care that is also efficient in terms of staff use. Table 41.2 compares the relative cost of several options for submaximal testing.

Test Type

Procedural guidelines for several submaximal-testing protocols are provided in the *ACSM Guidelines for Exercise Testing and Prescription* (1).

Treadmill Tests

Treadmills are not commonly used for submaximal exercise testing because the equipment is expensive, the space requirement is high, and the test volume is limited. The prediction error for estimating $\dot{V}O_{2max}$ during treadmill exercise is higher (up to 17.5%) than with other modalities (8, 9). Reasons for the higher variation include unfamiliarity with the equipment, handrail support while walking, and the varying amount of time required to establish a steady state (10). Protocols should be based on the individual's exercise capacity and familiarity with treadmill walking or running. Work rate may be incremented in a more traditional step method or using more gradual and frequent small changes (ramping), which may be more comfortable for subjects and elicit lower perceptions of physical stress and anxiety (11).

Cycle Ergometer Tests

For the following reasons, cycle ergometers are the most commonly used modality for submaximal exercise testing:

- Low expense
- Portability
- Small space requirements
- Ease of use by both clients and providers
- Heart rate and $\dot{V}O_2$ responses highly reproducible at standardized workloads
- A low rate of prediction errors (coefficient of variation of less than 10%) (12, 13)

Frequently used cycle protocols include the YMCA protocol and the Astrand/Rhyming protocol. Both tests have norms and reliably predict $\dot{V}O_{2max}$ (12, 14). For well-trained cyclists, commonly used protocols may prove inadequate. Cycles with a high power output capacity and protocols employing faster pedaling rates may be necessary to elicit the desired range of physiological responses to ensure accuracy (15).

Stepping Protocols

With respect to equipment and staffing needs, stepping protocols are inexpensive because they allow testing of several subjects concurrently. Upon completion of the step test, the heart rate is counted for a fixed time. The use of a standard 8-inch step eliminates the need for different step heights and allows the test to be performed in any stairway.

The primary physiological assumption of the step test is that the rate of recovery indicates the level of CR endurance (16). The mean prediction error for step testing is 12%, and a 95% confidence interval of 16% has been demonstrated (17). Step tests are easily administered according to guidelines similar to those traditionally used by the YMCA (14).

Field Tests

The popularity of field tests for the cardiorespiratory assessment of healthy populations across age groups and those with a variety of disorders is increasing (18–20). Field tests offer the advantages of ease of administration, adaptability with regard to space needs, the possibility of concurrent testing of subjects, and reliable prediction of $\dot{V}O_{2max}$ (within 12%) (20). In walking or running tests, the participant is usually required to cover a fixed distance as quickly as possible or to walk as far as possible within a fixed time on the ground or treadmill (21, 22). For best results, participants should be told that test accuracy relies on their cooperation and willingness to give a good effort. The accuracy of the test may be improved with a pilot test or by having the participant perform the initial test at least twice and using the best score.

Cureton et al. (23) developed the following multiple regression equation for predicting peak oxygen consumption ($\dot{V}O_{2peak}$) from mile run or mile walk time for males and females:

$$\dot{V}O_{2peak} = -8.41(MRW) + 0.34(MRW)^2 + 0.21(age \times gender) - 0.84(BMI) + 108.94 \ (R = .72; SEE = 4.9 \ mL/kg/minute)$$

where MRW is mile run or walk time in minutes, age is in years, gender is 0 for females and 1 for males, BMI is body mass index in kilograms per square meter R is line of regression, and SEE is standard error of estimate.

Another commonly used field test is the Cooper 12-minute run/walk that requires the participant to walk or run as far as possible in 12 minutes. A single staff member can easily give this test on any measured area. The test results are used to estimate $\dot{V}O_{2max}$ as follows (24):

$$\dot{V}O_{2max} \ (mL/kg/minute) = 3.126 \times$$
$$(meters \ covered \ in \ 12 \ minutes) - 11.3$$

INDIVIDUAL MONITORING AND ABNORMAL RESPONSES

Submaximal exercise tests allow the exercise professional to obtain data about individuals at varying levels of fitness. For those at high risk and who require much supervision, individual testing in a laboratory may be more appropriate than field testing. During treadmill or cycle ergometer tests, heart rate, electrocardiogram, blood pressure, rate of perceived exertion, signs, and symptoms can be easily recorded. Vital signs should be assessed prior to the test, at each workload, and during recovery for a total of at least 4–8 minutes. Once the criterion heart rate or work rate has been obtained, the individuals should be given an adequate cool-down period. This may consist of slowing the pace of the treadmill, decreasing the resistance on an ergometer, or allowing subjects to walk freely. An adequate cool-down should last until the individual feels rested, ventilation and heart rate have slowed to near resting levels, and all symptoms resolve.

Field or group testing may be appropriate for low-risk individuals. During field testing, it may be possible to record only time or distance during the test and heart rate at test completion. Furthermore, it may be possible to monitor for signs of distress only visually. However, close supervision and monitoring are crucial, and participants should be carefully assessed prior to the test. Throughout the testing and recovery periods, supervisors should position themselves so that they can maintain visual contact with each participant.

Although individuals may be thoroughly screened prior to testing, evidence of occult disease may arise at any time during testing and recovery. For this reason, the following variables should be monitored throughout the test and recovery periods:

- Rating of perceived exertion (Table 41.3)
- Signs or symptoms of cardiac or pulmonary distress or signs of overexertion, including chest pain or other discomfort, shortness of breath, dizziness or light-headedness, or profuse sweating and nausea
- Heart rate and rhythm
- Blood pressure

Table 41.3. Original and Revised Scales for Ratings of Perceived Exertion

Original Scale			Category–Ratio Scale	
6		0.0	Nothing at all	No intensity
7	Very, very light	0.3		
8		0.5	Extremely weak	Just noticeable
9	Very light	0.7		
10		1.0	Very weak	
11	Fairly light	1.5		
12		2.0	Weak	Light
13	Somewhat hard	2.5		
14		3.0	Moderate	
15	Hard	4.0		
16		5.0	Strong	Heavy
17	Very hard	6.0		
18		7.0	Very strong	
19	Very, very hard	8.0		
20		9.0		
		10.0	Extremely strong	Strongest intensity
		11.0		
			Absolute maximum	Highest possible

TEST TERMINATION

Submaximal tests should be terminated according to ACSM or other accepted guidelines (Table 41.4). In the event of an abnormal response, the test should be terminated, the medical director of the facility and the individual's primary care physician notified, and all specified follow-up procedures performed. In the event of mechanical or electrical failure that may compromise the accuracy of the test results or monitoring capabilities, the test should be terminated until the problem is corrected.

Procedures and protocols for the most common emergencies that occur during exercise (e.g., angina, myocardial infarction, dysrhythmia, hypoglycemia, dizziness, and cardiac arrest) should be part of the institution's operations manual and clearly posted in the testing area, known by every staff member, and reviewed and practiced frequently. Make sure that all entrances are clear, staff members know their specific roles, and all telephone numbers and contact information are current and clearly posted. All professional exercise staff members should have the appropriate level of ACSM certification and a minimum of basic life support certification.

TEST INTERPRETATION

Regardless of the inclusive intent of performing a submaximal exercise test, it is human nature for those being tested to be curious as to how they did and how they compare to others. Results should be explained

Table 41.4. General Indications for Stopping an Exercise Test in Apparently Healthy Adults

Onset of angina or anginalike symptoms
Significant drop (20 mm Hg) in systolic blood pressure or a failure of the systolic blood pressure to rise with an increase in exercise intensity
Excessive rise in blood pressure: systolic pressure > 260 mm Hg or diastolic pressure > 115 mm Hg
Signs of poor perfusion: light-headedness, confusion, ataxia, pallor, cyanosis, nausea, or cold and clammy skin
Failure of heart rate to increase with increased exercise intensity
Noticeable change in heart rhythm
Subject requests to stop
Physical or verbal manifestations of severe fatigue
Failure of the testing equipment

Assuming that testing is nondiagnostic and is being performed without direct physician involvement or electrocardiographic monitoring.
Reprinted with permission from Franklin BA, ed. ACSM's Guidelines for Exercise Testing and Prescription. 6th ed. Lippincott Williams & Wilkins, 2000:80.

in an easily understandable format that may include percentile ranking regarding gender and age and whether the results were well above average (90%), above average (70%), average (50%), below average (30%), or well below average (10%) (25, 26). Not only will subjects realize how they compare to others, they will understand their improvement when they progress from one category to the next. Categories make more practical sense then the actual $\dot{V}O_{2max}$ value. Information concerning appropriate training intensities for fitness improvement may also be provided (27).

CONSIDERATIONS FOR ACCURACY

The ability to obtain valid and reproducible results is essential to ensure that any differences between pretreatment and posttreatment test results are due to exercise training rather than variations in testing procedures. Some inconsistencies that are inherent may increase variability:

- Submaximal heart rate is influenced by time of day, eating, smoking, and familiarization with test procedures (28).
- Prediction equations for estimating $\dot{V}O_{2max}$ may overestimate trained individuals and underestimate untrained individuals (29).
- The efficiency of motion during walking, running, and cycling varies.
- Cardiac output and $\dot{V}O_2$ have a test–retest variability of 3–4% (30)

Psychological factors, such as pretest anxiety, may influence the heart rate, especially at rates below 120 beats per minute and at low workloads. It is not unusual for the heart rate and/or blood pressure to be higher at rest than during the initial stages of exercise in these cases. Having the subject repeat the first test may improve reliability, particularly if the subject has never previously performed such a test (31).

Factors that can cause variation in the heart rate response to testing:

- Dehydration
- Prolonged heavy exercise prior to testing
- Environmental conditions (e.g., heat, humidity, ventilation)
- Fever
- Use of alcohol, tobacco, or caffeine 2 to 3 hours prior to testing

Because of these inherent inconsistencies, standard procedures for each test must be strictly followed to ensure the greatest accuracy and reproducibility possible:

- Standard testing protocol
- The same testing modality and protocol for repeat testing
- A constant pedal speed throughout cycle ergometry testing
- Cycle seat height properly adjusted, recorded, and standard for each test
- The time of day for repeat testing consistent
- All data collection procedures standardized and consistent
- Test conditions standard
- Subjects free of infection and in normal sinus rhythm
- Prior to the test, no intense or prolonged exercise for 24 hours, smoking for 2–3 hours, caffeine for 3 hours, or heavy meal for 3 hours
- Room temperature 18–20°C (64–68°F) with air movement provided

▶ SUMMARY

Cardiorespiratory endurance ($\dot{V}O_{2max}$) can be predicted accurately from submaximal exercise tests in individuals who do not require maximal testing. Test accuracy is enhanced by adhering to standardized protocols, selecting an appropriate test modality, and standardizing data collection methods, testing conditions, and procedures. Cardiorespiratory endurance is an important component of overall health status, since it indicates the capacity to perform routine activities of daily living, required occupational tasks, and recreational endeavors, thus, quality of life.

References

1. Franklin BA, ed. ACSM's Guidelines for Exercise Testing and Prescription. 6th ed. Philadelphia: Williams & Wilkins, 2000:22–29.

2. Balady GJ, Chaitman B, Driscoll D, et al. American College of Sports Medicine and American Heart Association Joint Position Statement: Recommendations for cardiovascular screening, staffing, and emergency policies at health/fitness facilities. Med Sci Sports Exerc 30:1009–1018, 1998.

3. O'Brien CP. Are current exercise test protocols appropriate for older patients? Coron Artery Dis 10:43–46, 1999.

4. McInnis KJ, Bader DS, Pierce GL, Balady GJ. Comparison of cardiopulmonary responses in obese women using ramp versus step treadmill protocols. Am J Cardiol 83:289–291, 1999.

5. Bader DS, Maguire TE, Balady GJ. Comparison of ramp versus step protocols for exercise testing in patients > or = 60 years of age. Am J Cardiol 83:11–14, 1999.

6. Dreger RW, Quinney HA. Development of a hockey-specific, skate-treadmill $\dot{V}O_{2max}$ protocol. Can J Appl Physiol 24:559–569, 1999.

7. Gibson AS, Lambert MI, Hawley JA, et al. Measurement of maximal oxygen uptake from two different laboratory protocols in runners and squash players. Med Sci Sports Exerc 31:1226–1229, 1999.

8. Ragg KE, Murray TF, Karbonit LM, Jump DA. Errors in predicting functional capacity from a treadmill exercise stress test. Am Heart J 100:581–583, 1980.

9. Haskell WL, Savin W, Oldridge N, Debusk R. Factors influencing estimated oxygen uptake during exercise testing soon after myocardial infarction. Am J Cardiol 50:299–304, 1982.

10. McConnell TR, Clark BA. Prediction of maximal oxygen consumption during handrail-supported treadmill exercise. J Cardiopulm Rehabil 7:324–331, 1987.

11. Will PM, Walter JD. Exercise testing: Improving performance with a ramped Bruce protocol. Am Heart J 138:1033–1037, 1999.

12. Astrand PO, Rhyming I. A nomogram for calculation of aerobic capacity (physical fitness) from pulse rate during submaximal work. J Appl Physiol 7:218–221, 1954.

13. deVries H, Klafs C. Predicting maximal oxygen intake from submaximal tests. J Sports Med 4:207, 1965.

14. Golding LA, Myers CR, Sinning WE, eds. The Y's Way to Physical Fitness. Rosemont, IL: YMCA of the USA, 1982:88–101.

15. Baron R, Bachl N, Petschnig R, et al. Measurement of maximal power output in isokinetic and non-isokinetic cycling. Int J Sports Med 20:532–537, 1999.

16. Blomqvist CG. Cardiovascular adaptations to physical training. Ann Rev Physiol 45:169–189, 1983.

17. Brouha L. The step test: A simple method of measuring physical fitness for muscular work in young men. Res Q Exerc Sport 14:31–35, 1943.

18. Draheim CC, Laurie NE, McCubbin JA, Perkins JL. Validity of a modified fitness test for adults with mental retardation. Med Sci Sports Exerc 31:1849–1854, 1999.

19. Oh-Park M, Zohman LR, Abrahams C. A simple walk test to guide exercise programming of the elderly. Am J Phys Med Rehabil 76:208–212, 1997.

20. Kline GM, Porcari JP, Hintermeister R, et al. Estimation of $\dot{V}O_{2max}$ from a one-mile track walk: gender, age, and body weight. Med Sci Sports Exerc 19:253–259, 1987.

21. Stevens D, Elpern E, Sharma K, et al. Comparison of hallway and treadmill six-minute walk tests. Am J Respir Critical Care Med 160:1540–1543, 1999.

22. Berthon P, Dabonneville M, Fellmann N, et al. Maximal aerobic velocity measured by the 5-minute running field test on two different fitness level groups. Arch Physiol Biochem 105:633–639, 1997.

23. Cureton KJ, Sloniger MA, O'Bannon JP, et al. A generalized equation for prediction of $\dot{V}O_{2peak}$ from 1-mile run/walk performance. Med Sci Sports Exerc 27:445–451, 1995.

24. Cooper K. A means of assessing maximal oxygen intake: Correlation between field testing and treadmill testing. JAMA 203:201–204, 1968.

25. Franklin BA, ed. ACSM's Guidelines for Exercise Testing and Prescription, 6th ed. Philadelphia: Williams & Wilkins, 2000:77.

26. Morris CK, Myers J, Froelicher VF, et al. Nomogram based on metabolic equivalents and age for assessing aerobic exercise capacity in men. J Am Coll Cardiol 22:175–182, 1993.

27. Dunbar CC, Glickman-Weiss EL, Burstyn DA, et al. A submaximal treadmill test for developing target ratings of perceived exertion for outpatient cardiac rehabilitation. Percept Motor Skills 87:755–759, 1998.

28. Taylor HL, Wang Y, Rowell L, Blomqvist G. The standardization and interpretation of submaximal and maximal tests of working capacity. Pediatrics 32:703–722, 1963.

29. Wyndham CH. Submaximal tests for estimating maximal oxygen intake. Can Med Assoc J 96:736–742, 1967.

30. Faulkner JA, Heigenhauser GF, Schork MA. The cardiac output-oxygen uptake relationship of men during graded bicycle ergometry. Med Sci Sports Exerc 9:148–154, 1977.

31. Capriotti PV, Sherman WM, Lamb DR. Reliability of power output during intermittent high-intensity cycling. Med Sci Sports Exerc 31:913–915, 1999.

1.2.3, 1.2.6

2.2.2, 2.2.11, 2.2.14,
2.6.0.1, 2.6.0.3,
2.6.0.4, 2.6.0.6,
2.6.0.7, 2.6.0.8

4.1.0.1, 4.1.0.2, 4.2.2.1, 4.2.3.1, 4.2.3.2, 4.2.3.3, 4.3.0.1,
4.4.0, 4.4.1, 4.4.2, 4.4.3, 4.4.4, 4.6.0.1, 4.6.1.2, 4.6.1.3,
4.6.1.5, 4.6.1.7, 4.6.2.1, 4.6.2.2, 4.6.2.3, 4.6.2.4, 4.6.2.5,
4.6.2.6, 4.6.2.7, 4.6.3.0, 4.6.4.5, 4.6.4.6

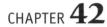

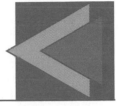

CHAPTER 42

CARDIORESPIRATORY ASSESSMENT OF HIGH-RISK OR DISEASED POPULATIONS

Peter H. Brubaker and Jonathan Myers

Of the many advances in the diagnosis of coronary artery disease (CAD), exercise testing remains an indispensable tool. When performed appropriately, exercise testing yields valuable diagnostic, prognostic, functional, and therapeutic information at a relatively low cost and with minimal risk. Data from several studies indicate that exercise testing is safe, even in high-risk patients, with no more than 1 death, 4 myocardial infarctions, and approximately 5 hospital admissions per 10,000 exercise tests (1). To minimize risk to the patient, the exercise professional must follow guidelines established by professional organizations, including the American College of Sports Medicine (ACSM), the American Association of Cardiovascular and Pulmonary Rehabilitation (AACVPR), and the American Heart Association (AHA) (2–4). This chapter describes these guidelines and other important considerations in test administration.

PRETEST CONSIDERATIONS

Prior to an exercise test, a complete medical history and a physical examination to identify contraindications for exercise testing are standard practice (2). The history includes past and current medical problems, symptoms, medications, and findings from previous physical examinations and laboratory tests. Physical activity patterns and vocational activity requirements must be assessed, as must any family history of cardiopulmonary and metabolic disorders. When any contraindications to exercise are identified, the patient should be referred to a primary physician for further medical management. Patients with precautions may be tested after careful evaluation of the risk–benefit ratio for the exercise test. Major CAD risk factors and signs and symptoms of cardiopulmonary disease are used to rate the risk to patients and to determine the appropriate level of medical supervision (2).

The patient should refrain from food, alcohol, caffeine, and tobacco for 3 hours before testing. Patients need to be well rested for the exercise test; therefore, they are also advised to avoid vigorous activity on the day of testing. Patients should continue any prescribed medical regimens unless instructed otherwise by a physician. For example, test sensitivity may increase in some individuals if patients taper their beta-blocker intake or discontinue antianginal medications for several days prior to testing. However, this practice is no longer recommended for routine testing (4).

The risks and possible discomforts associated with exercise testing should be explained to the patient as thoroughly as possible by an exercise professional prior to the test. Specific steps are taken to ensure the patient's safety during testing, such as demonstrating safe use of the treadmill. Steps to reduce anxiety, such as answering questions and describing expectations (e.g., reporting symptoms, level of exertion expected, test end points) are also advisable. Informed consent must be obtained, since it has important ethical and legal implications and ensures that the patient is aware of the purposes and risks associated with the test.

Appropriate and comfortable clothing ensure the patient's comfort during testing. Proper clothing also allows freedom of movement and proper placement of electrocardiogram (ECG) electrodes, as well as a blood pressure cuff. Properly fitting shoes with rubber soles are important to ensure good traction, particularly for treadmill testing.

EXERCISE TEST SELECTION

Selection of the specific exercise test is based on the purpose of the test, the health and fitness status of the client, and the most appropriate exercise modality and protocol. In many exercise laboratories, these issues are determined by the availability of equipment and by custom; however, each can have a profound effect on the response to the exercise test.

Modes

The purpose of exercise testing is to increase total body and myocardial oxygen demand at safe increments within a reasonable time. This requires dynamic exercise that uses major muscle groups, permitting a large increase in cardiac output, oxygen delivery, and gas exchange (Fig. 42.1). The modalities used for diagnostic testing include cycle ergometers, treadmills, arm ergometers, steps, and recently, chemical stressors.

Bicycle Ergometer

The bicycle ergometer and treadmill are the most commonly used exercise testing modalities. A bicycle is generally less expensive, occupies less space, and is less noisy. During cycling, upper body motion is decreased, facilitating the recording of blood pressure and ECG. However, the workload on simple, mechanically braked bicycle ergometers is not always accurate because it depends on pedaling speed, which may vary. This variation in work-

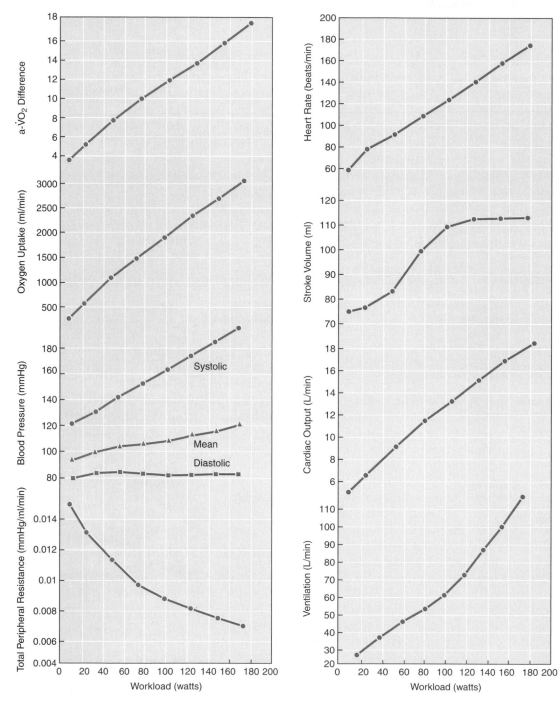

Figure 42.1. Response of basic hemodynamic and metabolic variables from rest to a moderately high level of exercise in the upright position. (Adapted with permission from Myers J. The physiology of exercise testing. Primary Care 21:415–437, 1994.)

load can be overcome by using electronically braked bicycle ergometers, which maintain a constant workload over a wide range of pedaling speeds. In either case, bicycle ergometer work is typically expressed in kilogram-meters per minute (kgm/minute), or watts.

Treadmill

The treadmill is used mainly in North America (5). It is more expensive than a cycle ergometer, relatively immobile, and noisier. Researchers comparing treadmill and bicycle ergometry report that maximal oxygen uptake is 10–20% higher (range, 6–25%) and maximal heart rate is 5–20% higher on the treadmill than the cycle ergometer (6–9). A slightly higher incidence of ST segment changes and angina has been reported during treadmill testing (7–9). Exercise-induced myocardial ischemia identified by thallium scintigraphy has been reported to be greater after treadmill testing than after cycle ergometry (8). Although most of the differences between the two modalities are minor, the treadmill may be preferred when the major goals of the test are to assess functional limits optimally and to identify ischemia.

Pharmacological Testing

Pharmacological stress, a relatively new consideration in exercise testing, has important applications for echocardiographic and nuclear techniques. Vasodilators, such as dipyridamole (Persantine) and adenosine, are commonly used to assess coronary perfusion in conjunction with a nuclear agent (thallium or sestamibi). These agents cause maximal coronary artery vasodilation in normal epicardial coronary arteries but not in stenotic segments. As a result, a coronary steal phenomenon occurs, with an increased flow to normal arteries and a decreased flow to stenotic arteries. Dipyridamole demonstrates similar or slightly better diagnostic accuracy than standard exercise testing (10, 11).

Dobutamine, a catecholamine that increases myocardial demand by increasing myocardial rate and force of contraction, is commonly used with echocardiography to identify myocardial ischemia. If the myocardial blood supply is limited by coronary artery stenoses, the increased myocardial demand provoked by the dobutamine infusion results in wall motion abnormalities (12).

Pharmacological stress techniques are advantageous for patients who are unable to exercise at an acceptable level, including patients with peripheral vascular disease or neurological or musculoskeletal disorders. The disadvantages of pharmacological stress testing include greater numbers of side effects (40–50%) and lack of a cardiovascular response (10%) (13, 14).

Protocols

It is most appropriate to select an exercise protocol based on the patient and the purpose of the exercise test. For example, a maximal, symptom-limited test using a relatively demanding protocol is not appropriate (or informative) for a severely limited patient. Similarly, a more gradual protocol may not be useful for an apparently healthy, active individual. Thus, the goals of testing help determine whether submaximal testing is appropriate and other specific protocol-related issues such as the mode of exercise, whether oxygen uptake is measured, and the need for a physician's supervision.

Submaximal Testing

Submaximal exercise testing is clinically appropriate for predischarge evaluations, especially for patients with acute myocardial infarction. Submaximal testing has been shown to be effective for risk stratification, activity recommendations, assessment of medical therapy, and to determine the need for further intervention (15). Submaximal testing is also appropriate for patients with a high risk of complex dysrhythmias. A submaximal predischarge test as well as a symptom-limited test have been shown to predict future events. The end points for submaximal testing are traditionally arbitrary but should always be based on sound clinical judgment. A heart rate limit of 140 beats per minute (bpm) and 7 METs (metabolic equivalents) are often used in patients younger than 40 years of age; 130 bpm and 5 METs are often used for patients over 40 years of age. The rating of perceived exertion (RPE) is an appropriate end point in patients taking beta-blockers; somewhat hard to hard exercise (13 to 15 on the Borg 6 to 20 scale) is a conservative end point for most patients. Maximal testing is more appropriate when conducted at least 1 month after acute myocardial infarction. It has been shown to be a safe and a useful tool for risk stratification.

A 1980 survey reported that approximately two-thirds of practitioners in North America use the Bruce protocol for exercise testing (5). Since that time, the use of more gradual, individualized protocols has been advocated (6, 7, 16–21). It is now appreciated that protocols with large, unequal work increments result in relatively inaccurate estimates of exercise capacity, particularly in patients with CAD. Recent investigations also demonstrate that excessive or rapid increments in rate of work can result in unreliable assessments of the effects of therapy and reduced accuracy of detecting CAD (20).

Thus, individualized protocols offer several advantages for cardiopulmonary assessment. Protocols that begin with a low-intensity warm-up phase followed by progressive, continuous exercise in which oxygen demand is elevated to its maximum level within 8–12 minutes are most efficacious. It is important to report exercise capacity in METs rather than treadmill time, so that measures of exercise capacity can be compared uniformly regardless of the protocol. Modifications of the Balke-Ware protocol are often used, employing a constant treadmill speed of 2 to 3.3 miles per hour and equal increments in grade (2.5% or 5%) every 2 minutes.

A ramp test can overcome some of the limitations of incremental protocols. A ramp protocol uses a constant and continuous increase in metabolic demand instead of the staging used in conventional tests. The uniform increase in work results in a steady rise in physiological responses and permits a more accurate estimation of oxygen uptake (7, 15). A Bruce ramp protocol has been developed to reduce problems associated with large increments in work (21).

A key issue emphasized in recent literature is individualization, a process designed to optimize the information yield and permit the use of tests that fall within the recommended range of 8–12 minutes to complete. This duration has been identified on the basis of convenience, evaluation of metabolic and hemodynamic responses, and optimally assessing the limits of the cardiorespiratory system, as well as for the ability to predict exercise capacity.

MEASUREMENT TECHNIQUES AND SEQUENCES

Electrocardiography

An electrocardiogram remains an integral part of cardiopulmonary assessment. Stress ECG must be performed correctly to ensure the patient's safety. Proper skin preparation and precise electrode placement are critical to obtaining an accurate ECG. Skin preparation decreases resistance at the skin–electrode interface and improves the signal-to-noise ratio. Hair should be removed from the general areas where the electrodes will be placed. Each placement site should be rubbed vigorously with alcohol to remove skin oil. The skin should then be abraded with abrasive pads, gels, or similar products to reduce resistance further. Finally, each electrode should be carefully placed in the proper location to ensure good contact with both the conducting gel and the adhesive surfaces of the electrode.

In clinical settings, the 12-lead Mason-Likar placement (Fig. 42.2) is generally used because it produces fewer artifacts and restricts movement less than standard limb placement. However, the Mason-Likar placement can alter the amplitude and axis of the ECG waveform (22). Because these shifts may be misinterpreted as diagnostic changes, a resting supine ECG should be recorded using standard limb lead placement. Furthermore, a change in body position from supine to standing can alter the ECG. Probably more than 90% of ST changes occur in lateral precordial leads. Miranda et al. (23) recently studied 178 men to evaluate the diagnostic value of ST depression in the inferior leads. The results indicated that the lateral leads had better sensitivity and specificity than the inferior leads and that ST depression isolated to the inferior leads frequently indicated a false-positive response.

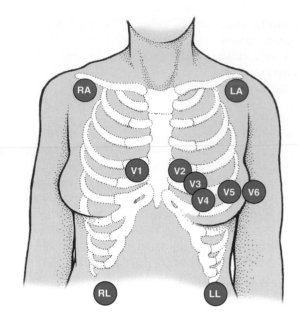

Figure 42.2. The Mason-Likar simulated 12-lead ECG electrode placement for exercise testing.

During the exercise test, at least 3 ECG leads representing lateral, inferior, and anterior views should be monitored continuously. A 12-lead ECG should be recorded in the latter part of each stage, more often if an abnormal reading or clinical symptoms are observed.

Serious dysrhythmias during exercise are indications to terminate the test. Serious dysrhythmias may be overt, as with ventricular tachycardia, or more subtle, as with unifocal premature ventricular contractions (PVCs) or supraventricular tachycardia. Second- or third-degree heart block and ventricular tachycardia (3 or more beats in succession) of any duration are reasons for immediate termination. If there is any doubt about the nature or origin of the dysrhythmia, the test should be terminated. Isolated PVCs, even when somewhat frequent, are not as ominous as previously thought. Recent studies demonstrate that PVCs during an exercise test are minimally prognostic (24). Therefore, PVCs should be interpreted within the context of the medical history along with observation of hemodynamic responses and/or associated symptoms.

Patients referred for exercise testing are likely to be taking medications that can have significant effects on the ECG and hemodynamic responses. The most common medications are beta-blockers and calcium channel blocking agents, which attenuate heart rate at rest and during exercise. Nitrates, which are commonly prescribed, can increase heart rate (2). In part because of the effects of these medications, age-predicted maximal heart rate should not be used as a test end point.

Blood Pressure

The systolic and diastolic blood pressures (SBP and DBP) are taken at rest and during exercise to ensure the patient's safety and to obtain important diagnostic and prognostic information. Properly trained personnel can obtain an accurate and reliable blood pressure using auscultatory techniques (25, 26). Blood pressure is measured at rest prior to the exercise test with the patient supine and standing to assess postural hypotension. Resting blood pressure may be elevated because of pretest anxiety. Persistent pretest hypertension is a precaution to exercise testing (2). However, anxiety-related elevations in blood pressure are fairly common. The blood pressure may decrease slightly during the initial stages of exercise; however, a fall in SBP below baseline carries a poor prognosis (27).

Systolic blood pressure and DBP should be assessed during the last minute of each stage of testing, more frequently if hypotension or hypertension is apparent. Normally, SBP increases with workload. Values exceeding 200 mm Hg are fairly common. However, when the SBP exceeds 250 mm Hg, the test should be terminated (2). The DBP normally stays the same or increases slightly during exercise. The fifth Korotkov sound is frequently heard to 0 mm Hg in some young, healthy individuals. When the DBP exceeds 115 mm Hg, the test should be terminated (2). If the SBP falls with increased workload, the blood pressure should immediately be taken again; if SBP decreases more than 10 mm Hg, the test should be terminated, particularly if symptoms are present.

Measuring Oxygen Consumption

Oxygen consumption ($\dot{V}O_2$) and other ventilatory variables provide important information about cardiopulmonary function. Measuring these variables requires careful attention to detail and a working knowledge of both the equipment and basic exercise physiology. Maximal oxygen consumption ($\dot{V}O_{2max}$) is the most common and generally the most useful measurement derived from gas exchange data during an exercise test. It defines the upper limits of cardiorespiratory function (i.e., the ability to increase heart rate, stroke volume, and oxygen extraction by active muscles). The clinical importance of an objective and accurate measurement of exercise capacity is underscored by studies on prognosis in patients with heart disease. In a review of the literature, exercise capacity was identified most frequently as a significant determinant of survival (28). In congestive heart failure, peak oxygen consumption ($\dot{V}O_{2peak}$) is one of the best predictors of survival and is widely used to determine the timing of cardiac transplantation. In one study of patients awaiting cardiac transplantation, a $\dot{V}O_{2peak}$ of at least 14 mL/kg/minute was associated with a 1-year survival of 94%; with a $\dot{V}O_{2peak}$ below 14 mL/kg/minute, the 1-year survival was 47% (29).

Although $\dot{V}O_{2peak}$ is most accurately determined by measuring expired gases directly, the technology to do so is not always available. Equations that can be used to predict $\dot{V}O_{2peak}$ for walking, running, arm and leg ergometry, and stair stepping have been described (2). These equations were developed from research that primarily used young, healthy subjects during steady-state exercise; therefore, using these formulas in other populations may result in significant errors in predicting $\dot{V}O_{2peak}$. Many factors, such as age, functional capacity, disease status, medications, and use of handrail support, can affect the accuracy of predicting $\dot{V}O_2$. Recently published equations can predict $\dot{V}O_{2peak}$ in clinical populations during treadmill testing with greater accuracy (30, 31).

Ventilatory and gas exchange variables should be monitored continuously during exercise, since they may be useful for determining maximum exertion and endpoints of testing. Symptoms, deconditioning, and/or unwillingness to tolerate fatigue may prevent the patient from reaching maximal levels; when these factors arise, it may be more appropriate to use $\dot{V}O_{2peak}$. Although breath-by-breath measurements of $\dot{V}O_2$ and other gas exchange parameters are now widely available on modern systems, they should be reserved for specific research applications. Peak exercise values based 30-second averages represent an acceptable balance between precision and variability, and are the most commonly used sample in the literature (20).

Subjective Assessments

Symptoms and perception of effort are assessed during exercise to help ensure the patient's safety and to optimize the diagnostic information yield. In order to make a valid assessment of subjective variables during exercise, the exercise professional must explain the scoring scale thoroughly prior to testing. For example, angina and dyspnea (the most common symptoms elicited during exercise testing) are each usually evaluated on a 4-point scale (2).

Patients should be encouraged to report all symptoms. In addition, they should be evaluated by the exercise professional at least once during each stage of the exercise test for the presence of cardiopulmonary symptoms, such as angina and dyspnea. Signs and symptoms can be reported while expired gases are being measured through the use of hand signals (Fig. 42.3) or by having the patient point at charts.

Typical Versus Atypical Angina

Distinguishing the precise features of anginal discomfort is important both diagnostically and prognostically. **Typical angina** is consistent in presentation and location, is brought on by physical or emotional stress, and is relieved by rest or nitroglycerin. **Atypical angina** refers to discomfort in an unusual location, with inconsistent precipitating factors, and of varying duration. It is usually unresponsive to nitroglycerin. Exercise-induced chest discomfort resembling typical angina confirms the presence of CAD better than any other test response. A combination of typical angina and an abnormal ST response is 98% predictive of significant CAD. Moderately severe angina

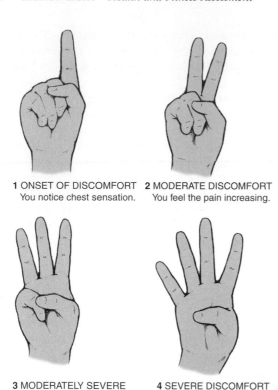

1 ONSET OF DISCOMFORT
You notice chest sensation.

2 MODERATE DISCOMFORT
You feel the pain increasing.

3 MODERATELY SEVERE
The discomfort would cause
you to rest or take nitroglycerin.

4 SEVERE DISCOMFORT

Figure 42.3. Rating scale for exertional chest discomfort. The scale is particularly useful when using gas exchange techniques, as chest discomfort can be expressed nonverbally using hand signals. A rating of 3 is the appropriate end point.

(grade III) or discomfort that would normally cause cessation of daily activities and/or administration of nitroglycerin are indications to terminate exercise (2, 4, 32).

Dyspnea

Dyspnea can be the predominant symptom in some patients with CAD, but it is more often associated with reduced left ventricular function or chronic obstructive pulmonary disease. In the former, it is usually accompanied by poor exercise capacity and can occur with an impaired SBP response. Dyspnea is appropriately quantified using a 4-point scale (2).

Rating of Perceived Exertion

The RPE, when properly assessed during exercise, can be used to identify the end point of maximum effort. The Borg perceived exertion scale provides reproducible measures of effort and is generally not affected by medications such as beta-blockers (2). An RPE should be obtained at least once during each stage of the exercise test.

TEST TERMINATION

The overall goal of the exercise test in individuals known or suspected of having cardiovascular disease is to obtain a near-maximum level of exertion to evaluate the cardiopulmonary response. Determining the end point of a clinical exercise test may be difficult, as it requires the integration of objective physiological data and termination criteria with subjective judgment based on clinical experience. Furthermore, patients may be unable or unwilling to exercise to an adequate level. A symptom-limited maximal test is generally useful when assessing cardiorespiratory responses in someone with known or suspected disease. Patients should be instructed to exercise to the point that they can no longer continue because of fatigue, dyspnea, or other symptoms. They should be informed that the test will be terminated if clinical evidence indicates distress. Patients should be encouraged to exercise as long as possible, but they should not be pushed beyond capacity. Furthermore, any patient's request to stop the test should be honored. When the exercise professional is unable to monitor responses fully, the test should be terminated immediately.

POSTTEST CONSIDERATIONS

The exercise test should include evaluation of the ECG, symptoms, and hemodynamic responses in recovery. Whether postexercise activities should be active or passive is controversial. For diagnostic purposes, the supine position may be the most valuable immediately after exercise because it increases venous return, thereby increasing ventricular volume, myocardial wall stress, and consequently, myocardial oxygen consumption. Several studies have shown that ST segment abnormalities are enhanced when a person is supine and that active recovery may attenuate these changes (33). ST segments observed 3–4 minutes into recovery may be helpful in detecting ischemia. Patients with symptom-limiting angina or dyspnea may be uncomfortable when supine and should be seated or semirecumbent during recovery. Passive recovery while standing should be avoided because of the possibility of complications associated with venous pooling. For a nondiagnostic test, such as when screening asymptomatic individuals, an active recovery at a low workload is more comfortable and less likely to be associated with a hypotensive response, and it may minimize the risk of dysrhythmia secondary to elevated catecholamines.

Regardless of the protocol, the recovery period should be monitored for at least 5 minutes. Blood pressure, ECG, and symptoms should be monitored and recorded at 1–2-minute intervals. The recovery period should be extended to resolve symptoms and abnormal hemodynamic or ECG responses.

It is important to avoid long, hot showers or baths immediately after recovery. Patients should be warned that fatigue and muscle soreness may occur and be instructed to avoid heavy exertion that day. Advise patients to report immediately to their physician any pain or discomfort the day after the test.

DATA INTERPRETATION

Most patients sent for exercise testing are referred for an evaluation of chest pain, most commonly to help make a diagnosis of CAD. Thus, the exercise test serves as a screen for further evaluation. Any screening test must be evaluated for its sensitivity and specificity. **Sensitivity** is the percentage of tests that correctly identify the condition, in this case, CAD. **Specificity** is the percentage of tests that correctly identify individuals without CAD. Sensitivity and specificity are inversely related, and they vary with the population tested, the definition of the disease, and the criteria used to define abnormality. For example, if the population being tested is at risk for severe forms of CAD (e.g., triple-vessel disease or left main coronary disease), the test will have a higher sensitivity. Alternatively, the specificity of the test will be higher in low-risk populations, such as a group of young, healthy subjects.

The diagnostic value of a test can be determined by its **predictive value. Positive predictive value** is the percentage of persons with an abnormal test who also have the disease. **Negative predictive value** is the percentage of persons with a normal test who do not have disease. The predictive value of a test cannot be determined directly from sensitivity and specificity; rather, it is strongly associated with the prevalence of disease in the population being tested. The calculations used to determine sensitivity, specificity, and predictive value are presented in Table 42.1.

False-Positive and False-Negative Responses

The factors that may be associated with a false-positive or false-negative response should be considered prior to the test. A **false-positive** test (an abnormal response in an individual without disease) decreases specificity, whereas a **false-negative** test (a normal response in an individual with disease) decreases sensitivity. When a false-positive or false-negative response is suspected, an alternative diagnostic procedure may be indicated, such as an exercise or pharmacological echocardiogram or radionuclide test.

Factors associated with false-positive and false-negative responses are listed in Table 42.2.

Prognosis

Exercise testing is valuable for determining the prognosis, or probability of a given outcome of disease, in patients with cardiovascular disease (34). Prognosis should be estimated because it provides information that can be useful for planning vocational and recreational activity and making important financial decisions. It is also useful for identifying additional interventions that may improve the outcome of therapy. An accurate estimation of risk can be obtaining by using any of a number of techniques to score exercise tests (15, 34).

Supplementary Diagnostic Tests

Radionuclide imaging complements the exercise ECG in known or suspected cases of CAD. It is particularly helpful with an equivocal exercise ECG or in patients who are likely to exhibit false-positive or false-negative responses. Nuclear imaging can be used to clarify the meaning of an abnormal ST segment response in asymptomatic individuals or the cause of chest discomfort. Patients with a positive exercise ECG and a positive radionuclide scan are 2.6 times more likely to have a subsequent event than patients with negative results (35).

Nuclear imaging of the coronary vessels is somewhat more sensitive and specific for CAD than the exercise ECG. The literature suggests that sensitivity and specificity of exercise thallium scintigraphy are 84% and 87%, respectively (35). This modality also permits localization of ischemia, which is not possible with an ECG, and permits differentiation between fixed defects (representing myocardial infarction) and reversible defects (representing ischemia).

Echocardiography is being used more often during exercise and pharmacological testing. The diagnostic accuracy of echocardiography depends primarily on the

Table 42.1. Terms Used to Demonstrate the Diagnostic Value of a Test

$$\text{Sensitivity} = \frac{TP}{TP + FN} \times 100$$

$$\text{Specificity} = \frac{TN}{TN + FP} \times 100$$

$$\text{Positive predictive value} = \frac{TP}{TP + FP} \times 100$$

$$\text{Negative predictive value} = \frac{TN}{TN + FN} \times 100$$

TP, true positives, or those with abnormal test results and with disease.
FN, false negatives, or those with normal test results and with disease.
FP, false positives, or those with abnormal test results and no disease.
TN, true negatives, or those with normal test results and no disease.

Table 42.2. Causes of False-Negative and False-Positive Tests

FALSE POSITIVE	FALSE NEGATIVE
Resting repolarization abnormalities	Failure to reach ischemic threshold secondary to medications
Cardiac hypertrophy	
Accelerated conduction defects	Monitoring an insufficient number of leads to detect ECG changes
Digitalis	
Nonischemic cardiomyopathy	
Hypokalemia	Angiographically significant disease compensated by collateral circulation
Vasoregulatory abnormalities	
Mitral valve prolapse	
Pericardial disease	Musculoskeletal limitations preceding cardiac abnormalities
Coronary spasm in absence of CAD	
Anemia	
Female gender	

methodology and the clinical experience of the interpreter. The sensitivity and specificity of this technique are both approximately 85% (36). These issues are addressed in more detail in Chapter 28.

► SUMMARY

The exercise test is useful in evaluating and managing patients with known or suspected CAD. The exercise test is a primary gatekeeper to more costly and invasive procedures, since it is the most accessible tool for evaluating medical therapy, quantifying exercise tolerance, helping to determine prognosis, and developing an exercise prescription. The exercise test is relatively inexpensive and safe. The most reliable information is obtained through careful attention to methodology and by interpretation of data by technicians who have a thorough understanding of the basic physiology of exercise, safety issues, experience interpreting ECGs and hemodynamic responses, and finally, familiarity with various professional guidelines.

References

1. Franklin BA, Gordon S, Timmins GC, O'Neill WW. Is direct physician supervision of exercise stress testing routinely necessary? Chest 111: 262–265, 1997.
2. American College of Sports Medicine. Guidelines for Exercise Testing and Exercise Prescription. 6th ed. Philadelphia: Lippincott Williams & Wilkins, 2000.
3. American Association of Cardiovascular and Pulmonary Rehabilitation. Guidelines for Cardiac Rehabilitation Programs. 3rd ed. Champaign: Human Kinetics, 1999.
4. Gibbons RJ, Balady GJ, Beasley JW, et al. ACC/AHA guidelines for exercise testing: A report of the American College of Cardiology/American Heart Association Task Force on Practice Guidelines (Committee on exercise testing). J Am Coll Cardiol 30:260–315, 1997.
5. Stuart RJ, Ellestad MH. National survey of exercise stress testing facilities. Chest 77:94–97, 1980
6. Buchfuhrer MJ, Hansen JE, Robinson TE, et al. Optimizing the exercise protocol for cardiopulmonary assessment. J Appl Physiol 55:1558–1564, 1983.
7. Myers J, Buchanan N, Walsh D, et al. Comparison of the ramp versus standard exercise protocols. J Am Coll Cardiol 17:1334–1342, 1991.
8. Hambrecht R, Schuler GC, Muth T, et al. Greater diagnostic sensitivity of treadmill versus cycle exercise testing of asymptomatic men with coronary artery disease. Am J Cardiol 70:141–146, 1992.
9. Wicks JR, Sutton JR, Oldridge NB, et al. Comparison of the electrocardiographic changes induced by maximum exercise testing with treadmill and cycle ergometer. Circulation 57:1066–1069, 1978.
10. Severi S, Picano E, Michelassi C, et al. Diagnostic and prognostic value of dipyridamole echocardiography in patients with suspected coronary artery disease: Comparison with exercise electrocardiography. Circulation 89:1160–1173, 1994.
11. Bolognese L, Sarasso G, Aralda D, et al. High dose dipyri-

damole echocardiography early after uncomplicated acute myocardial infarction: Correlation with exercise testing and coronary angiography. J Am Coll Cardiol 14:357–363, 1989.
12. Poldermans D, Fioretti PM, Forster T, et al. Dobutamine stress echocardiography for assessment of perioperative cardiac risk in patients undergoing major vascular surgery. Circulation 87:1505–1512, 1993.
13. Ranhosky A, Kempthorne-Rawson J. The safety of intravenous dipyridamole thallium myocardial perfusion imaging. Circulation 81:1205–1209, 1990.
14. Wilson RF, Laughlin DE, Ackell PH, et al. Transluminal, subselective measurement of coronary artery blood flow velocity and vasodilator reserve in man. Circulation 72:82–92, 1985.
15. Froelicher VF. Manual of Exercise Testing. St. Louis: Mosby, 1994.
16. Haskell W, Savin W, Oldrige N, et al. Factors influencing estimated oxygen uptake during exercise testing soon after myocardial infarction. Am J Cardiol 50:299–304, 1982.
17. Webster MWI, Sharpe DN. Exercise testing in angina pectoris: The importance of protocol design in clinical trials. Am Heart J 117:505–508, 1989.
18. Tamesis B, Stelken A, Byers S, et al. Comparison of the asymptomatic cardiac ischemia pilot versus Bruce and Cornell exercise protocols. Am J Cardiol 72:715–720, 1993.
19. Panza J, Quyyumi AA, Diodati JG, et al. Prediction of the frequency and duration of ambulatory myocardial ischemia in patients with stable coronary artery disease by determination of the ischemia threshold from exercise testing: Importance of the exercise protocol. J Am Coll Cardiol 17:657–663, 1991.
20. Myers J. Essentials of Cardiopulmonary Exercise Testing. Champaign, IL: Human Kinetics, 1996.
21. Kaminsky LA, Whaley MH. Evaluation of a new standardized ramp protocol: The BSU/Bruce Ramp Protocol. J Cardiopulm Rehab 18: 438–444, 1998.
22. Gamble P, McManus H, Jensen D, et al. A comparison of the standard 12-lead electrocardiogram to exercise electrode placement. Chest 85:616–622, 1984.
23. Miranda CP, Liu J, Kadar A, et al. Usefulness of exercise-induced ST-segment depression in the inferior leads during exercise testing as a marker for coronary artery disease. Am J Cardiol 69:303–307, 1992.
24. Yang JC, Wesley RC, Froelicher VF. Ventricular tachycardia during routine treadmill testing: Risk and prognosis. Arch Intern Med 151:349–353, 1991.
25. Bailey RH, Bauer JH. A review of common errors in the indirect measurement of blood pressure. Arch Intern Med 153:2741–2748, 1993.
26. Iyriboz Y, Hearon CM. Blood pressure measurement at rest and during exercise: controversies, guidelines, and procedures. J Cardiopulm Rehabil 12:277–287, 1992.
27. Mazzotta G, Scopinaro G, Falcidieno M, et al. Significance of abnormal blood pressure during exercise-induced myocardial dysfunction after recent acute myocardial infarction. Am J Cardiol 59:1256–1260, 1987.
28. Morris CK, Ueshima K, Kawaguchi T, et al. The prognostic value of exercise capacity: A review of the literature. Am Heart J 122:1423–1431, 1991.

29. Mancini DM, Eisen H, Kussmaul W, et al. Value of peak exercise oxygen consumption for optimal timing of cardiac transplantation in ambulatory patients with heart failure. Circulation 83:778–786, 1991.

30. Berry MJ, Brubaker PH, O'Toole ML, et al. Estimation of $\dot{V}O_2$ in older individuals with osteoarthritis of the knee and cardiovascular disease. Med Sci Sports Exerc 28:808–814, 1996.

31. Foster C, Crowe AJ, Daines E, et al. Predicting functional capacity during treadmill testing independent of exercise protocol. Med Sci Sports Exerc 28:752–756, 1996.

32. Myers JN. Perception of chest pain during exercise testing in patients with coronary artery disease. Med Sci Sports Exerc 26:1082–1086, 1994.

33. Lachterman B, Lehmann KG, Abrahamson D, et al. "Recovery only" ST segment depression and the predictive accuracy of the exercise test. Ann Intern Med 112:11–16, 1990.

34. Chang JA, Froelicher VF. Clinical and exercise test markers of prognosis in patients with stable coronary artery disease. Curr Prob Cardiol 19:533–588, 1994.

35. Kotler TS, Diamond GA. Exercise thallium-201 scintigraphy in the diagnosis and prognosis of coronary artery disease. Ann Intern Med 113:684–702, 1990.

Suggested Reading

Greco CA, Salustri A, Seccareccia F, et al. Prognostic value of dobutamine echocardiography early after uncomplicated acute myocardial infarction: A comparison with exercise electrocardiography. J Am Coll Cardiol 29:267–271, 1997.

1.8.6

2.2.19, 2.6.0.11,
2.6.0.14, 2.8.0.14

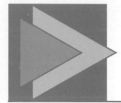

CHAPTER **43**

ASSESSMENT OF MUSCULAR STRENGTH AND ENDURANCE

James E. Graves, Michael L. Pollock, and Cedric X. Bryant

Muscular fitness is one of the primary components of physical health. It includes two basic physiological components: muscular strength and muscular endurance.

Muscular strength refers to the ability to generate force at a given speed (velocity) of movement (1). Muscular endurance refers to the ability to persist in physical activity or to resist muscular fatigue (2). Muscular strength and endurance are developed by placing an overload on the targeted muscle or muscle groups. Through adaptation, the muscle groups become stronger or better able to sustain muscular activity.

The process of overloading the muscular system is referred to as resistance training. **Resistance training,** in this chapter, refers to all types of strength or weight training, including free weights, isokinetic training, variable resistance, and static (isometric) training. Resistance training not only develops muscular strength and endurance, it also improves the ability of the muscles to recover from physical activity. In addition, properly performed resistance training can induce an increase in muscle mass, bone mineral density, and the strength and integrity of connective tissue (3).

Research demonstrates that physical fitness declines with age; however, many of the detrimental age-related changes in physiological function are due to decreased physical activity and can be attenuated or even reversed with proper exercise training. Just as aerobic training is required to develop and maintain cardiorespiratory fitness, resistance training is required to develop and maintain muscular fitness.

The importance of resistance training for maintaining muscle mass has been demonstrated in study of master athletes (4). The investigators measured the aerobic capacity and body composition of 24 master track athletes, 50 to 82 years of age, over a 10-year period. The results of the study demonstrate that cardiorespiratory fitness remains unchanged, but body fat increases during aerobic training. The change in body composition was attributed to reduced fat-free weight (i.e., muscle mass), specifically in the upper body, and not increased fat weight. Three athletes who supplemented aerobic training with either resistance training or cross-country skiing were able to maintain upper body muscle mass.

Recognizing the need for a well-rounded training program to develop and maintain muscular and cardiorespiratory fitness, the American College of Sports Medicine (ACSM) has revised its original position stand on "The Recommended Quantity and Quality of Exercise for Developing and Maintaining Fitness in Healthy Adults" to include resistance training (5). The ACSM recommends that resistance training of a moderate to high intensity, sufficient to develop and maintain muscle mass, become an integral part of fitness programs. One set of 8–12 repetitions consisting of 8–10 exercises with major muscle groups at least 2 days per week is the recommended minimum.

The adaptations that follow resistance training are benefits for middle-aged and older adults, especially postmenopausal women, who rapidly lose bone mineral density. Research has also demonstrated the following health benefits associated with resistance training:

- Modest improvements in cardiorespiratory fitness (6)
- Reductions in body fat (7)
- Modest reductions in blood pressure (8)
- Reduction in glucose-stimulated plasma insulin concentrations (9)
- Improvements in blood lipid–lipoprotein profiles (9)

These health benefits are most often associated with **circuit weight training,** a method of resistance training in which a series of exercises are performed in succession with a minimal amount of rest between exercises.

Muscular fitness is required for successful performance in most sports. Thus, resistance training is common among both recreational and professional athletes who wish to enhance athletic performance. Resistance training is also prescribed in rehabilitation programs designed to facilitate recovery from accidents and sport-related injuries. The effectiveness of resistance training exercises in clinical rehabilitation is well documented (10).

An important benefit associated with resistance training is a reduction in the risk of orthopaedic injury. Strong muscles and connective tissue support and help protect underlying joints. Inadequate levels of muscular strength can lead to serious musculoskeletal disorders, resulting in pain, discomfort, and loss of income due to disability and premature retirement. The overall strengthening of the musculoskeletal system (muscle, bone, and connective tissue) resulting from resistance training reduces the risk of elbow and shoulder injuries in tennis players and swimmers (11). Resistance training may have even greater importance for individuals participating in contact sports and for reducing the risk of injury due to accidents. Low back pain is a major health problem in all industrialized societies. Increasing muscular strength may reduce the risk of developing low back pain and minimize pain in patients with low back disorders (12, 13). Thus, the adaptations to resistance training increase the potential to enhance the quality of life. This chapter addresses methods of assessing muscular strength and endurance.

SPECIFICITY OF TRAINING

The increase in strength resulting from resistance training is specific to the following:

- The type of contraction used in training
- The range of motion (ROM) through which training occurs
- The velocity of contraction during training
- Whether exercises are performed unilaterally or bilaterally

These examples of specificity of training are at least partially attributed to neural adaptation; however, for specificity of contraction, and type and velocity of contraction, evidence suggests that resistance training also has specific effects on the contractile properties of the muscle. Each of these examples of specificity of resistance training will be discussed briefly.

There are two basic types of muscle activity: static and dynamic. In **static muscular activity**, the muscle attempts to shorten against a fixed or immovable resistance. There is no skeletal movement, and the muscle neither shortens nor lengthens forcibly. **Dynamic muscle action** involves movement, which may be concentric (i.e., the force produced by the muscle is sufficient to overcome resistance and muscle shortening occurs) or eccentric (i.e., the muscle exerts force, lengthens, and is overcome by the resistance).

Training a muscle group with dynamic actions (e.g., lifting weights) produces a relatively large increase in dynamic muscle strength but only small increases in isometric strength. Isometric training, on the other hand, improves isometric strength more than dynamic strength (14). Similar improvements in isometric strength at various positions through a ROM are noted following both isometric and dynamic training, when dynamic training involves slow, controlled repetitions (15). In addition to specificity in the isometric and dynamic modes of training, lifting weights improves weight-lifting strength to a greater extent than isokinetic (constant velocity), concentric muscular strength.

Increases in voluntary strength are specific to the ROM that is trained for both isometric and dynamic resistance training. A significant transfer of isometric strength within 20° of the training angle occurs following an isometric strength training program (16). At positions beyond 20° from the training angle, little transfer of isometric strength occurs. Thus, when isometric exercises are used to improve muscular strength, training should occur at multiple positions throughout the ROM. When training consists of dynamic muscle actions performed through a limited ROM, strength gains have been noted up to 50° away from the ROM used for training (17). However, improvements in the untrained ROM have been significantly less than those in the ROM in which training was conducted.

Strength training at slow speeds results in relatively large increases in the ability of the muscle to generate force at slow speeds but relatively small increases during contractions at faster speeds. The carryover of strength from high-speed training to slow-speed testing is also reduced (18). An intermediate training velocity is best for increasing strength at all velocities of movement. Thus, for individuals interested in general fitness, an intermediate training velocity is recommended (11).

REDUCED TRAINING

Muscle strength and muscle mass are decreased when resistance training is discontinued. Neither how much resistance training is required for long-term maintenance of muscular strength and endurance nor the exact effects of periodic reduction of either frequency or intensity on strength is known. Several studies indicate that if training intensity is maintained, training frequency can be reduced to as little as one day per week for up to 12 weeks without significant loss in strength (19, 20). It is important to note that the subjects in these studies were initially untrained and that the duration of training was 12–18 weeks. Whether highly trained athletes can similarly reduce training frequency or whether reduced training can be carried out for more than 12 weeks without loss of strength has not been determined. Available evidence suggests that an occasional missed session does not adversely affect muscular fitness. It is important not to discontinue training altogether.

MEASUREMENT DEVICES

The cable tensiometer is used to measure static strength by recording the tension applied to a steel cable. This instrument was originally designed to measure aircraft cable tension and was adapted and later refined to measure the strength of various muscle groups. One end of the cable is attached to a fixed object (e.g., a wall or the floor) and the other end is fitted with a device to which force can be applied. For the measurement to accurately reflect muscle force production, the cable must be in the plane of movement and must make a 90° angle at its point of attachment to the body or body part. The tensiometer, which is paced along the length of the cable, measures cable tension when the subject applies force to the cable.

Because the force-generating capacity varies through a ROM, establishing the proper angle of measurement is critical. A goniometer is used to set the joint angle for testing. The cable tensiometer strength test can accurately measure the static strength of virtually all major muscle groups. The device is highly reliable when used on normal subjects under standardized conditions. However, the cable and attachments often stretch during testing, making positional standardization difficult.

The dynamometer is used to measure static strength by recording the amount of force exerted. Two portable types of dynamometers are widely available, one for hand grip and one for back and leg strength. The most common type is the hand or grip dynamometer. Grip strength is measured as kilograms of force exerted by squeezing the hand dynamometer as hard as possible.

Dynamometers are popular for testing large numbers of people because they are easy to use and portable. Cumbersome setup procedures that often accompany other types of muscle performance measurements are not required. However, dynamometers can be used to measure only a few muscle groups, and their reliability is not well established. In addition, isolation of specific muscle groups is not accomplished, which makes standardization difficult.

Strain gauge devices can be employed to measure static and dynamic muscle force for a variety of muscle groups. Strain gauges are made of electroconductive material that is usually applied to the surfaces of finely machined metal parts. When a load from a muscle contraction is placed on the metal parts, the metal and the strain gauge attached to it deform. The deformation of the strain gauge changes the electrical resistance current passed through it. The change in voltage is related to the load and can be recorded on a strip chart, digital display, or volt meter. In most instances, strain gauges are used to measure static strain or compression by pushing or pulling on the device. Applications of strain gauges for dynamic strength measures, however, are commercially available (e.g., isokinetic machines). Strain gauge measurements are reliable, but they have the same limitations as the cable tensiometer.

One repetition maximum (1-RM) tests measure the greatest amount of weight that can be lifted one time for a specific weight-lifting exercise. The tests are usually limited to the amount of weight that can be lifted at the weakest position in the ROM and therefore do not assess muscle performance through a full ROM. Generally the test begins with an amount of weight that can be easily lifted. After a successful trial, a 2–3-minute rest period is allowed. The weight is increased by 5–10 pounds (or more, depending on the difficulty of the previous lift) and another trial is attempted. The 1-RM, the amount of weight for the last trial that can be successfully completed with good form, can usually be obtained in 4–6 trials. The 1-RM provides a measure of dynamic strength that can be applied to almost any weight lifting exercise. One-RM tests are commonly used because they are easy to administer and can often be performed with the same equipment used for training. They are highly reliable, although they do involve a skill factor, and subsequent tests may yield greater results due to practice. Thus, 1-RM tests may not be specific for muscle force production.

The application of computer technology and advancements in machine design have improved the accuracy and standardization of muscular strength testing. Electromechanical dynamometers have been developed for both static and dynamic measures of muscular strength, and some are capable of both static and dynamic strength measurements. Many electromechanical dynamometers employ a load cell to measure static strength. This method may be considered the electronic equivalent of the cable tensiometer. A major advantage of machines that use load cells, however, is the ease of making multiple measurements through a ROM. Cable tensiometer systems are usually cumbersome to adjust and therefore are usually used to provide a measure of static strength at only a single joint angle. Because strength varies through a ROM based on the biomechanical arrangement of the muscles and bony levers of the skeletal system, single joint angle measures do not provide an indication of how strength varies through the ROM. Multiple joint–angle isometric tests are often employed to quantify full ROM static strength. Multiple joint–angle isometric tests have been shown to be highly reliable for a variety of muscle groups.

Some electromechanical instruments have been designed to measure dynamic muscular strength at a preset movement speed. In theory, these constant-velocity (isokinetic) dynamometers are thought to measure the maximum force that can be applied throughout the constant-velocity movement. Because a period of acceleration is required to reach the preselected velocity of movement and a period of deceleration is required at the end of the movement, isokinetic dynamometers cannot measure force production through a full ROM. In addition, oscillation in observed forces, called torque overshoot, can limit the accuracy of these devices. Torque overshoot represents impact forces between the moving body part and the measurement device. Manufacturers have attempted with limited success to overcome these measurement errors by various software-controlled averaging systems called dampening mechanisms. While data averaging may be effective at presenting smooth force curves, it cannot eliminate potentially dangerous impact forces. Measurement error associated with the isokinetic dynamometer has been discussed in detail (21). Unfortunately, in spite of the shortcoming, isokinetic dynamometers are a common method of strength assessment in many clinical and research settings.

MEASUREMENT OF MUSCULAR STRENGTH

The primary function of skeletal muscle is to generate force. In most instances, forces generated by skeletal muscles are used to produce movement or for anatomical stabilization. The measurement of muscle force production is used for the following purposes:

- To assess muscular fitness
- To identify weakness
- To monitor progress in rehabilitation programs
- To measure the effectiveness of resistance training

The maximum amount of force that a muscle or group of muscles generates can be measured by a variety of methods, including a cable tensiometer, dynamometer, strain gauge device, 1-RM test, or computer-assisted force and work output determination. Each of these methods is briefly described.

Regardless of the method chosen to assess muscular strength, certain conditions are required for accurate and reliable measurement of muscle force output. Body position must be stabilized to allow only the desired movement. In the case of measuring muscle force generation during an isomeric contraction, the involved joint or joints at which movement would occur must be isolated. An example of the need for stabilization to isolate a specific group of muscles for functional assessment occurs during the measurement of lumbar extensor torque production. The lumbar extensors work in conjunction with the larger, more powerful gluteus and hamstring muscles to extend the trunk. If the pelvis is free to move during lumbar extension, the pelvis rotates as the gluteus and hamstring muscles contract. Pelvic rotation then contributes to the observed torque. Thus, pelvic stabilization is required to accurately assess isolated lumbar extensor function.

Muscle force production varies throughout the ROM. The most descriptive measures of muscle function account for this. The term *strength curve* describes a plot of the resultant force exerted versus an appropriate measure of the joint configuration. Because of acceleration at the initiation and deceleration at the termination of all move-

ments, and because dynamic strength is influenced by the speed of movement, dynamic strength tests are not appropriate for the quantification of muscle function through a ROM. In addition, if dynamic muscle actions are performed rapidly, kinetic forces that give an inaccurate measure of true force production may be recorded. Depending on the specific movement, these kinetic forces may be dangerous, especially for populations with orthopaedic problems, because of the impact that occurs upon rapid deceleration. Isometric tests can safely and accurately quantify muscle force production throughout the ROM if multiple joint angles are measured.

A final consideration required for the accurate assessment of muscle force production is whether the mass of the involved body part influences the measurement. For example, if the force generated by the quadriceps muscles during knee extension does not equal or exceed the mass of the lower leg, no measurable force is observed. Thus, the mass of the lower leg detracts from observed force production of the quadriceps muscles during knee extension testing. This mass must be accounted for to accurately quantify force. Although there is some controversy concerning the need for correction of the influence of gravitational forces during testing because most bodily actions are not corrected for gravity, the actual force generated by specific muscles in certain positions may be significantly influenced by body mass (22). Thus, although one cannot neglect the fact that in normal daily activities muscles are influenced by body mass, standardization of testing position and correction for gravitational forces are required for accurate quantification of muscle force production. The need for stabilization, positional standardization, compensation for gravitational influences, and measurement through a ROM have been recently discussed by Pollock et al. (12).

MEASUREMENT OF MUSCULAR ENDURANCE

Almost all of the devices for measuring strength can also be used for assessing muscular endurance. Tests of muscular endurance should be designed to evaluate the ability of muscle groups to produce submaximal force for repeated contractions. More specifically, the length of time a muscle contraction can be held or the number of repeated submaximal contractions a muscle group can make should be determined. Accordingly, similar to strength, muscular endurance can be assessed either statically or dynamically.

Measuring Muscle Endurance Statically

Two basic methods can be used to assess static muscular endurance. One method involves performing a maximal static contraction and sustaining that level of contraction for 60 seconds. The force being exerted by the muscle should be recorded at 10-second intervals. Accordingly, individuals who have a slower rate of decline in force production are exhibiting a greater level of muscle endurance for that specific muscle group than those whose level of recorded force falls faster. A second method for assessing static muscular endurance is to determine the length of time a given percentage of a maximum voluntary contraction can be sustained.

Measuring Muscle Endurance Dynamically

Several ways to determine dynamic muscular endurance exist. One way dynamic muscle endurance is assessed is to perform the maximum number of repetitions possible using a set weight, a given percentage of maximum strength (e.g., of 1-RM), or some set percentage of body weight. The endurance of a muscle group can be determined isokinetically through the performance of successive maximal repetitions. Isokinetic muscular endurance is measured as the number of repetitions completed before the torque production drops below 50% of the maximal torque value. Perhaps the most commonly used method for evaluating muscular endurance is calisthenics (e.g., situps, push-ups, pull-ups). During such tests, the maximum number of times one can lift the body weight is used as the measure of endurance. For persons of below average muscular fitness or above average body weight, however, calisthenics exercises often involve more of a measure of muscular strength than muscular endurance.

▶ SUMMARY

Resistance training is an important part of a fitness program and is recommended by the ACSM. Chronic resistance training stimulates many positive changes in physiology, and while much athletic competition requires strength, the benefits derived are particularly advantageous to adults, especially postmenopausal women. The measurement of muscular strength and endurance requires knowledge of the specificity of training and common measurement devices, and the advantages and disadvantages of each.

References

1. Knuttgen HG, Kraemer WJ. Terminology and measurement in exercise performance. J Appl Sport Sci Res 1:1–10, 1987.
2. Baumgartner TA. Jackson AS. Measurement for Evaluation in Physical Education and Exercise Science. Dubuque, IA: William C. Brown, 1987.
3. Stone MH. Connective tissue and bone response to strength training. In: Komi PV, ed. Strength and Power in Sport. Oxford: Blackwell Scientific, 1992:279–290.
4. Pollock ML, Foster C, Knapp D, et al. Effect of age and train-ing on aerobic capacity and body composition of master athletes. J Appl Physiol 62:725–731, 1987.
5. American College of Sports Medicine. Position stand: The recommended quantity and quality of exercise for developing and maintaining cardiorespiratory and muscular fitness in healthy adults. Med Sci Sports Exerc 22:265–274, 1990.
6. Fleck SJ. Cardiovascular adaptations to resistance training. Med Sci Sports Exerc 20:S146–151, 1988.
7. Wilmore JH. Alterations in strength, body composition, and anthropometric measurement consequence to a ten-week weight training program. Med Sci Sports Exerc 6:133–38, 1974.
8. Goldberg L. Elliot DL. Kuehl KS. A comparison of the cardiovascular effects of running and weight training. J Strength Condition Res 8(4):219–224, 1994.
9. Hurley BF, Hagberg JM, Goldberg AP, et al. Resistive training can reduce coronary risk factors without altering VO$_2$ max or percent body fat. Med Sci Sports Exerc 20(2):150–154, 1988.
10. Grimby G. Progressive resistance exercise for injury rehabilitation. Sports Med 2:309–315, 1985.
11. Fleck SJ, Kraemer WJ. Designing Resistance Training Programs. 2nd ed. Champaign, IL: Human Kinetics, 1997.
12. Pollock ML, Graves JE, Carpenter DM, et al. Muscle, In: Hockshuler SH, Colter HB, Colter RD, et al, eds. Rehabilitation of the Spine: Science and Practice. St. Louis: Mosby, 1993:263–284.
13. Risch SV, Norvell NK, Pollock ML, et al. Lumber strengthening in chronic low back pain patients. Spine 18:232–238, 1993.
14. Amusa LO, Obajuluwa VA. Static versus dynamic training programs for muscular strength using the knee-extensors in healthy young men. J Ortho Sports Phys Ther 8:243–247, 1986.
15. Graves JE, Pollock ML, Foster D, et al. Effect of training frequency and specificity on isometric lumbar extension strength. Spine 15:504–509, 1990.
16. Knapik JJ, Mawdsley RH, Ramos NU. Angular specificity and test mode specificity of isometric and isokinetic strength trading. J Orthop Sports Phys Ther 5:58–65, 1983.
17. Graves JE, Pollock ML, Jones AE, et al. Specificity of limited range of motion variable resistance training. Med Sci Sports Exerc 21:84–89, 1989.
18. Kanehisa H, Miyashita M. Specificity of velocity in strength training. Eur J Appl Physiol 52:104–106, 1983.
19. Graves JE, Pollock ML, Leggett SH, et al. Effect of reduced training frequency on muscular strength. Intl J Sports Med 9:316–319, 1988.
20. Tucci JT, Carpenter DM, Pollock ML, et al. Effect of reduced frequency of training and detraining on lumbar extension strength. Spine 17:1497–1501, 1992.
21. Winter DA, Wells RT, Orr GW. Errors in the use of isokinetic dynamometers. Eur J Appl Physiol 46:397–408, 1981.
22. Ford WJ, Bailey SD, Babich K, et al. Effect of hip position on gravity effect torque. Med Sci Sports Exerc 26:230–234, 1994.

1.1.0.1, 1.1.0.4,
1.1.1.1, 1.1.1.7, 1.2.5

2.1.0.1, 2.2.18,
2.3.0.2, 2.6.0.11,
2.6.0.14

4.1.0.4

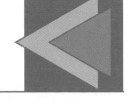

CHAPTER **44**

FLEXIBILITY AND RANGE OF MOTION

Elizabeth J. Protas

Joint flexibility is an important component of movement. The range of motion (ROM) of various joints is measured as a part of any evaluation of fitness or work capacity or clinical assessment of joint function. Consequently, ROM is measured in screening and intervention programs and listed among clinical outcomes and impairment ratings (1). In rehabilitation settings, ROM measures are used to do the following:

- Assess current status
- Describe any change in status
- Establish short-term and long-term treatment goals
- Explain performance
- Predict outcomes
- Motivate patients (2)

FACTORS THAT INFLUENCE RANGE OF MOTION

Joint ROM is the result of a combination of factors. The structure of the joint determines the degree of freedom of movement. For example, the elbow joint allows flexion and extension, but the articulation of its bony surfaces limits extension. In contrast, the shoulder allows movement in all planes; the loose fit between the head of the humerus and the acromion process offers less bony restriction to movement than in the elbow. Some movements are possible only when the joint is in a particular position. When bony surface areas are in maximum contact, the joint is in the close-packed position; that is, it is in a stable position and resists separation by distractive force (3). The knee in full extension is an example of the close-packed position. All other joint positions are loose packed. Spin, roll, and gliding motions occur in the loose-packed position.

The rigidity of ligaments helps stabilize and protect joints from excessive motion during dynamic movements. For example, the anterior cruciate ligament of the knee limits the movement of the tibia on the femoral heads. Intracapsular structures, such as articular cartilage

and synovial membranes, facilitate smoothness of movement while maintaining integrity of the joint. The extensibility of periarticular soft tissue, such as the joint capsule and surrounding muscle and tendon, also influence movement. One of the most common examples is the limitation imposed upon straight leg–raising by tight knee flexors (hamstrings). Some important functional ROMs are not limited to a single joint but result from a combination of movements by multiple joints. The ability to bend and pick up an object requires adequate ROM in trunk, hip, and shoulder; similarly, complete ROM in shoulder abduction requires both glenohumeral and scapulothoracic motion (4).

Table 44.1 shows the normative ROM of each of the major joints (5–7). These values vary with age; children generally have larger ROMs than adults, whereas adults more than 40 years of age have a gradual decline in ROM in many joints (Fig. 44.1) (8–10). Roach and Miles (11), using hip and knee ROM data from adults aged 25–74, in the United States, found evidence suggesting that the difference in ROM in younger and older age groups is small and not clinically significant (11). The exception is a 20% decrease in hip extension with age. Additionally, older African-American women exhibited significantly less hip flexion; this may be attributable to a larger body mass index. Range of motion may vary by gender in some joints, as girls tend to have greater hip joint ROM than boys. Women aged 60–84 tend to have a greater ROM than men in the shoulder and elbow and in medial hip rotation and ankle plantar flexion (8,9).

The published values for normal ROMs vary. For example, values for normal knee flexion vary from 130–150° and for hip flexion from 115–125°(11). Many sources do not categorize ROM by age, gender, or body type. Roach and Miles (11) suggest that a difference in active ROM of less than 10% of the expected norm may not be significant but may relate mainly to variability among individuals and measurement error. Even within the same individual, asymmetrical differences in ROM

381

Table 44.1. Range of Motion of the Major Joints

JOINT		MOTION	AVERAGE RANGES (DEGREES)
Spinal			
Cervical		Flexion	0–60
		Extension	0–75
		Lateral flexion	0–45
		Rotation	0–80
Thoracic		Flexion	0–50
		Rotation	0–30
Lumbar		Flexion	0–60
		Extension	0–25
		Lateral flexion	0–25
Upper extremity			
Shoulder		Flexion	0–180
		Extension	0–50
		Abduction	0–180
		Adduction	0–50
		Internal rotation	0–90
		External rotation	0–90
Elbow		Flexion	0–140
Forearm		Supination	0–80
		Pronation	0–80
Wrist		Flexion	0–60
		Extension	0–60
		Ulnar deviation	0–30
		Radial deviation	0–20
Thumb		Abduction	0–60
		Flexion	
		Carpal–metacarpal	0–15
		Metacarpal–phalangeal	0–50
		Interphalangeal	0–50
		Extension	
		Carpal–metacarpal	0–20
		Metacarpal–phalangeal	0–5
		Interphalangeal	0–20
Fingers		Flexion	
		Metacarpal–phalangeal	0–90
		Proximal interphalangeal	0–100
		Distal interphalangeal	0–80
		Extension	
		Metacarpal–phalangeal	0–45
Lower extremity			
Hip		Flexion	0–100
		Extension	0–30
		Abduction	0–40
		Adduction	0–20
		Internal rotation	0–40
		External rotation	0–50
Knee		Flexion	0–150
Ankle		Dorsiflexion	0–20
		Plantar flexion	0–40
Subtalar		Inversion	0–30
		Eversion	0–20

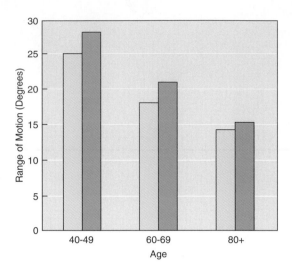

Figure 44.1. Changes in thoracic flexion with age for men and women. (Reprinted with permission from Olson S. Reliability and validity of trunk range of motion with age. Unpublished data, 1996.)

can occur as a result of joint use and/or limb dominance (Fig. 44.2).

NATURE OF MOVEMENTS IN MAJOR JOINTS

Movements occurring in the trunk and the upper and lower extremities are listed in Table 44.1. Flexion and extension occur in the sagittal plane. **Flexion** is an anterior movement for the head, trunk, upper extremity, and hip, but is a posterior movement for the knee, ankle (plantar flexion), and toes (12). **Extension** usually occurs in the direction opposite of flexion. **Hyperextension** refers to excessive movement in the direction of extension.

Abduction is movement away from the midline of the body; **adduction** is movement toward the midline in the coronal plane. Exceptions to this are the abduction and adduction of fingers and toes. The midline of the hand or foot rather than the body is the reference for these movements.

Rotation is movement in the transverse plane for the cervical and thoracic spine, pelvis (right and left rotation), shoulder, and hip (internal and external rotation). Some movements combine other motions, such as the subtalar and forefoot movements of inversion (supination, plantar flexion, and adduction) and eversion (pronation, abduction, and dorsiflexion).

The scapula has several additional motions as it moves on the thorax. **Scapular elevation** (shrugging) and **depression** (caudal movement) are upward and downward movements in the coronal plane. **Scapular protraction** is the position with shoulders slumped forward, whereas **retraction** is the position of the scapula in erect posture. Upward rotation of the scapula accompanies shoulder

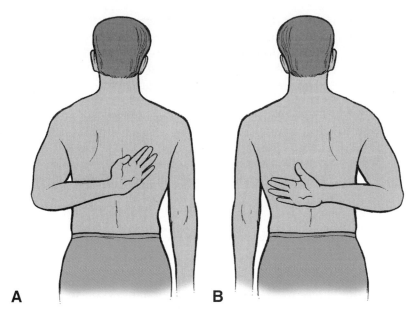

A   B

Figure 44.2 Difference in combined shoulder internal rotation and extension between left (**A**) and right (**B**) extremities. The individual is a right-handed water polo player. Muscle development on the right limits range of motion.

flexion, and downward rotation accompanies shoulder extension. Additional pelvic motions include the **anterior pelvic tilt**, which accompanies increased lumbar lordosis, and **posterior pelvic tilt**, which occurs with **bilateral** hip flexion and flattening of lumbar lordosis.

FLEXIBILITY EVALUATION

There are many methods for evaluating joint ROM. Visual estimates and/or measurements are made, often with a special instrument. Movement may be produced actively or passively. Differences in technique vary from the use of warm-up exercises prior to measurement to changing the starting position. Measurement technique may vary, depending upon the joint and motion. Differences in methodology suggest that accuracy and consistency can be achieved by following procedural principles. Furthermore, precision in assessment techniques enhances both accuracy and reliability.

Visual Estimate Versus Measured ROM

Visual estimates of ROM have been shown to be inaccurate for both extremity and spinal movements (1, 13). Gross or visual estimates of movement may, however, be useful for fitness screenings, group evaluations, and field testing, which are discussed later.

Active Versus Passive Movement

Although ROM measurements are commonly taken for both passive and active movements, it is more difficult to obtain an accurate measurement during passive ROM (13). Passive joint movement can exert variable forces that may alter the ROM. When the individual is unable to move an extremity actively, for example because of paral-

ysis or primary muscle disease, passive ROM can be measured reliably. Pandya et. al., (14) found high intratester reliability with repeated measurements of seven common passive upper and lower extremity ROMs in children with Duchenne muscular dystrophy. Passive goniometric measurement of ankle dorsiflexion in children with cerebral palsy has also been reliable (15).

Technique

Technique can have significant effect on accuracy. Improper identification of anatomical landmarks is a source of error in the trunk and extremities (1, 13). Use of surface markings and standardized bony landmarks increases reliability, as does the correct positioning of the individual and the proximal joint segment (1, 16). Using a standard position that stabilizes the proximal segment and allows full range of movement in the distal segment improves reliability (1, 13, 17). It is not clear whether a single measure or multiple measures of a single movement improves reliability. Measurement of a simple hinge joint movement (e.g., elbow flexion) is more accurate than the measurement of a complex movement (e.g., ankle inversion). Repeated trials of passive straight leg–raising can increase the ROM as a result of moving the limb to the extremes of the ROM (18). When possible, measurements should be taken starting with the limb in an anatomically neutral position to increase reliability; this is particularly important when edema or contracture is present. Placement and stabilization of the measuring device can affect measurement reliability (1).

Intratester Versus Intertester

Intratester reliability is greater than intertester reliability, regardless of the joint or method of measurement (1, 13).

Intratester reliability is also higher for upper extremity joints (19). Rothstein reported correlation coefficients of .86 to .99 for repeated measures of elbow and Knee ROM by the same tester using three different goniometers (20). The error of repeated measures for the same tester is usually up to 5 % between testers variability increases up to 10% (13). A single tester should conduct repeated measures on the same subject over time to reduce measurement error.

MEASUREMENT DEVICES

ROM is most often measured by goniometers, inclinometers, tape measures, and flexible rules. The selection of the device may depend upon the joint being measured.

Goniometers

Goniometers are the most commonly used measuring device for ROM because they are inexpensive and portable. The **universal goniometer** consists of two arms: a stationary arm that is stabilized on the proximal portion of the joint and a moving arm aligned with the distal portion of the joint, which is moved through the arc of motion during measurement. There are also dorsal and pendular goniometers (flexometers).

The reliability of goniometers is high if standard techniques are used. Rothstein compared three types of universal goniometer for elbow and knee ROM and found high interdevice reliablility ($r < 0.91$) (20). Goniometry may be inaccurate in spinal and complex movements (1).

Inclinometers

Inclinometers are handheld electronic or mechanical devices that use gravity to track the arc of motion during movement of the head, trunk or extremity. One type of inclinometer is a fluid-filled device, similar to a carpenter's level, attached to a compass. Good to excellent intratester and intertester reliability has been reported with inclinometers in the lumbers and cervical spines except during lumbar extension (21, 22). Both single and double inclinometer techniques have been described. Rondinelli et al. (23) report that a double inclinometer technique resulted in greater error (10.5°) than a single inclinometer technique (8.5°) when measuring lumbar flexion. Inclinometers are acceptable for measuring complex movements when standardized techniques are used.

Tape Measures

Tape measures can be used to measure spinal and finger movements. The skin distraction technique can be used to measure trunk flexion and lateral trunk flexion by comparing differences in position of two marks placed appropriately on the skin prior to and after movement (21). Variation for this were 10%. Tape measure techniques may be more reliable for lumbar flexion and lateral trunk flexion than inclinometry. Measurement of fingertip-to-floor distance using tape measure is unreliable (21).

Tape measures can also assess loss of ROM in the carpometacarpal and interphalangeal joints. These techniques are useful only if the individual cannot make a fist.

Flexible Rule

The flexible rule can be used to measure spinal movements. The tangent of an arc described by applying the rule to the contours of back during movement is the measure. Although the flexible rule is reliable, it is not widely used (1).

GROUP AND FIELD FLEXIBILITY SCREENING

Group or field assessment of flexibility is most appropriate when highly accurate measures of ROM are not required. Field testing is commonly used to observe postural alignment (malalignment may make an individual prone to injury). The most common field tests are shown in Figures 44.3–44.6. Tests that isolate trunk flexibility (Fig. 44.4C) from hamstring flexibility (Fig. 44.6D) are recommended because of the relationship to back injury. Figure 44.7 illustrates postural assessment.

FLEXIBILITY AND FITNESS

The relationship between level of fitness and flexibility is still being studied. It may be especially important in older adults, who usually exhibit a decline in movement capability. Walker et al. (q) found that physical activity, as measured by the Physical Activity Questionnaire, was not related to specific changes in ROM in men and women aged 60 to 80 years. Jette et al. (24), however, studied community-dwelling elders and found a relationship between decreased lower extremity ROM and functional impairments such as the ability to use public transportation or shop. There is limited evidence to support the assumption that flexibility is related to fitness level in older adults.

The relationship between flexibility and injury is another pertinent issue. Reid et al. (25) examined the correlation between lower extremity flexibility and hip and knee injuries in classical ballet dancers. Unbalanced flexibility, along with decreased ROM in hip adduction and internal rotation, was associated with increased incidence of lateral knee and anterior hip pain. Waddell et al. (26) found that reduced mobility in trunk flexion, lateral flexion and extension, and decreased straight leg–raising are frequently associated with chronic low back pain. However, decreased ROM is not always associated with injury. In a prospective study, men with increased lumbar mobility were more likely to have an acute episode of low back pain within 1 year of the flexibility examination (27).

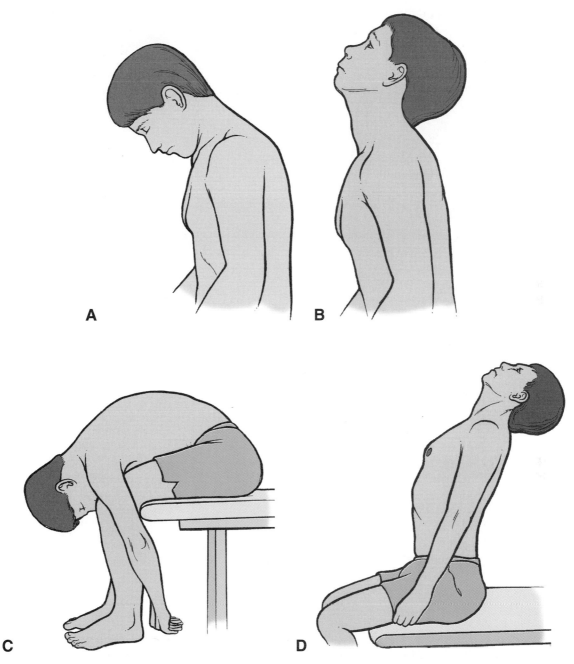

Figure 44.3. Neck and trunk flexibility screening. **A.** Cervical flexion. The chin should touch the chest. **B.** Cervical extension. The head should bend as far as possible posteriorly. **C.** Vertebral flexion. With the hips and knees bent, the trunk should touch the anterior thighs. **D.** Vertebral extension. Backward movement of the trunk as far posterior as possible without hip extension.

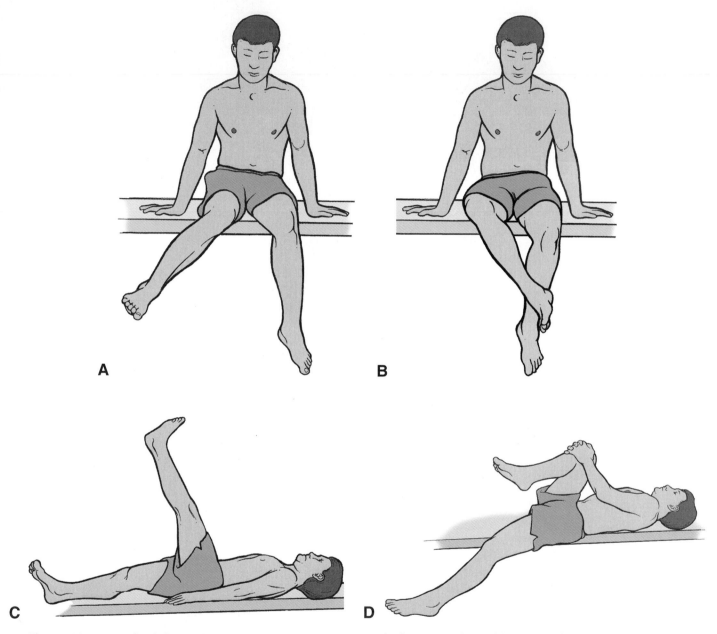

Figure 44.4. Hip flexibility screening. **A.** Internal rotation. With the hip and knee flexed, move the leg as far to the side as possible by rolling the thigh. **B.** External rotation. Move the leg as far as possible past the midline by rolling the thigh outward. **C.** Straight leg raising. Keep the contralateral lower extremity in full extension while lifting the other extermity without bending the knee. Note limited hamstring flexibility. **D.** Combined test of hip flexion on the right. Bring the bent hip and knee as close to the chest as possible with a Thomas test for hip extension on the left by allowing the limb to drop over the edge of the table into extension.

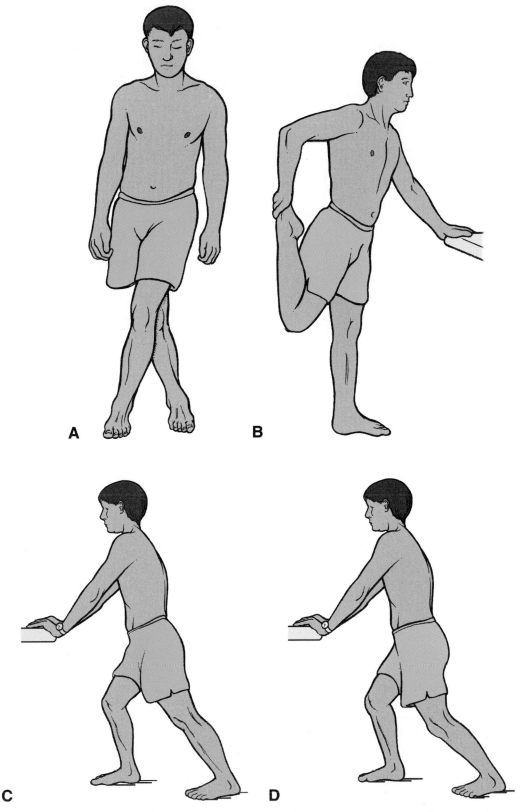

Figure 44.5. Lower extremity flexibility. **A.** Illiotibial band tightness. While standing, cross the lower extremity in front of the other limb and rotate the hip internally. **B.** Rectus femoris length. With full hip extension, the leg should almost touch the buttocks. **C.** Gastrocnemius ROM. With knee straight and limb placed as far posteriorly as possible, the heel remains flat on the floor. **D.** Soleus ROM. Same position as gastrocnemius except with bent knee. Heel remains on the floor.

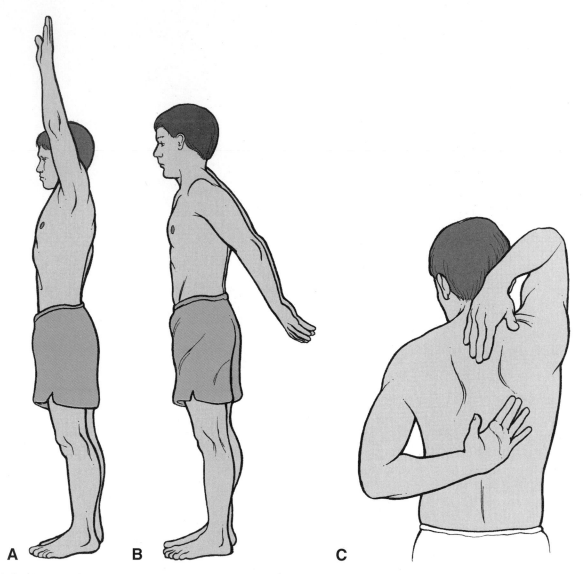

Figure 44.6. Shoulder flexibility **A.** Flexion, Reach forward and upward as far as possible; the humerus will be parallel to the ear. **B.** Extension. Reach as far backward as possible. **C.** Combined bilateral rotation and elbow flexion. Normally fingertips should almost touch.

Mobility is an important element in performing physical activities, but the ROM required may be specific to the activity. For example, a baseball player requires more dynamic shoulder flexibility than a soccer player. Flexibility assessment is often included in preseason evaluation as a means of preventing injuries, but the relationship between flexibility and injury remains unclear (28).

IDENTIFYING RISK FACTORS FOR ACTIVITY

Exercise professionals should be able to identify clients' conditions that require additional consultation before they begin an exercise program. An accurate and complete health history can elicit significant information. Persistent or recurrent joint pain may identify possibly arthritic joints. Medical consultation is advisable if pain, swelling, and /or heat in a joint or multiple joints is reported. A Change in physical activity is not recommended during an acute arthritic episode. Likewise, if these symptoms occur with activity and persist, the client should be referred to a physician to rule out joint injury, osteoarthritis and early rheumatoid arthritis.

Individuals sometimes report a trick knee or ankle, which suggests that the extremity may spontaneously collapse during weight-bearing activity. This is often accompanied by reports of an injury. It is important to determine whether a medical diagnosis was made.

An individual who reports either recent acute back pain or a history of chronic back pain should be referred to a physician. Back pain is one of the most common and

References
1. Lea RD. Current concepts review: range of motion measurements. J Bone Joint Surg 77A:78A, 1995.
2. Gilliam J, Barstow A. Assessment of joint range of motion. In : van Deusen K, Brunt D, D,eds. Assessment in Occupational and Physical Therapy. New York : Saunders, in press.
3. Soderberg GL, Kinesiology: Application to Pathological Motion. Baltimore: Williams & Wilkins, 1986:58.
4. Rowe CR. Joint measurement in disability evaluation. Clin Orthop 32:43, 1992.
5. American Academy of Orthopedic Surgeons Committee for the Study of Joint Morton. Joint motion: Method of measuring and recording. Chicago: American Academy of Orthopedic Surgeons, 1965.
6. Boone DC, Azen SP. Normal range of motion of joints in male subjects. J Bone Joint Surg 61A:756, 1979.
7. Greene WR, Heckman JD, eds. The Clinical Measurement of Joint Motion. Rosemont, IL: American Academy of Orthopedic Surgeons, 1994.
8. Svenningsen S, Terjesen T, Auflem M, et al. Hip motion related to age and sex. Acta Orthoped Scand 60:97, 1989.
9. Walker JM, Sue D, Miles-Elkousey N, et al. Active mobility of the extremities in older subjects. Phys Ther 64:919, 1984.
10. Olson S. Reliability and validity of trunk range of motion with age. Unpublished data, 1996.
11. Roach KE, Miles TP. Normal hip and knee active range of motion: The relationship to age. Phys Ther 71:656, 1991.
12. Kendall HO, Kendall FP, Wadsworth GF. Muscle: Testing and function. 2nd ed. Baltimore: Williams & Wilkins, 1971:21.
13. Gajdosik RL, Bohannon, RW. Clinical measurement of range of motion: Review of goniometry emphasizing reliability and validity. Phys Ther 67:1867, 1987.
14. Pandya, S, Florence J, King W, et al. Reliability of goniometric measurements in patients with Duchenne muscular dystrophy. Phys Ther 65:1339, 1985.
15. Tardieu C. de la Tour H, Bret MD, et al. Muscle hypoextensiblity in children with cerebral palsy: 1. Clinical and experimental observations. Arch Phys Med Rehabil 63:97, 1982.
16. Keeley I, Mayer TG, Cox R, et al. Quantification of lumbar function: 5. Reliability of range-of-motion measures in the sagittal plane and an in vivo torso rotation measurement technique. Spine 11:31, 1986.
17. Watkins MA, Riddle DL, Lamb RI, et al. Reliability of goniometric measurements and visual estimates of knee range of motion obtained in a clinical setting. Phys Ther 71:90, 1991.
18. Atha J, Wheatley DW. The mobilising effects of repeated measurement of hip flexion . Br J Sports Med 10:22, 1976.
19. Boone DC, Azen SP, Lin, CM, et al. Reliability of goniometric measurements. Phys Ther 58:1355, 1978.
20. Rothstein JM, Miller PJ, Roettger RF. Goniometric reliability in a clinical setting. Phys Ther 63:1611, 1983.
21. Merritt JL, McLean TJ, Erickson RP. Measurement of trunk flexibility in normal subjects: Reproducibility of three clinical methods. Mayo Clin Proc 61:192, 1986.
22. Youdas JW, Carey JR, Garrett, TR. Reliability of measurements of cervical spine range of motion: Comparison of three methods. Phys Ther 71:198, 1991.

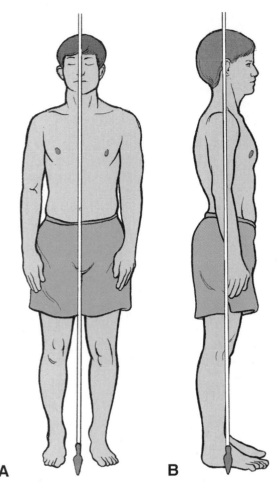

Figure 44.7. Postural assessment with a plumb line. **A.** Anterior. Observe for symmetry and knee position. **B.** Lateral. Observe alignment of head, shoulders, hips, knees, and ankles.

costly musculoskeletal problems in middle-aged adults. Although individuals with back pain are commonly able to participate in exercise programs, they should be referred to a physician and/or a physical therapist for an evaluation. Early intervention may reduce pain and decrease the likelihood that an acute problem will become chronic. This is consistent with the guide lines for management of acute back pain recently published by the Health Care Financing Administration (29). The chronicity of the problem impairs fitness by reducing activity during exacerbation of pain. An individualized exercise program for persons with chronic back pain, surpervised by a physical therapist, may improve function, decrease disability, and reduce pain (30).

Complaints of musculoskeletal pain persisting and/or increasing with exercise is a primary reason for seeking a medical consultation. Understanding the underlying cause of pain and the effect exercise are important considerations for the exercise professional in planning exercise programs.

23. Rondinelli R, Murphy J, Esler, A, et al. Estimation of normal lumbar flexion with surface inclinometry. Am J Phys Med Rehabil 71:219, 1992.

24. Jette AM, Branch LG, Berlin J. Musculoskeletal impairments and physical disablement among the aged. J Gerontol 45:M203, 1990.

25. Reid DC, Burnham RS, Saboe, LA, et al. Lower extremity flexibility patterns in classical ballet dancers and their correlation to lateral hip and knee injuries. Am J Sports Med 15:347, 1987.

26. Waddell G, Sommerville D, Henderson I, et al. Objective clinical evaluation of physical impairment in chronic low back pain. Spine 17:617, 1992.

27. Biering-Sorensen F. Physical measurements as risk indicators for low-back trouble over a one-year period. Spine 2:106, 1984.

28. Knapik JI, Bauman CL, Jones. BH, et al. Preseason strength and flexibility imbalances associated with athletic injuries in female collegiate athletes. Am J Sports Med 19:76, 1991.

29. Agency of Health Care Policy and Research. Clinical practice guidelines: Acute low back problems in adults. Washington: US Department of Health and Human Services, Public Health Service #14, 1995.

30. Beekman CE, Axtell L. Ambulation, activity level, and pain: Outcomes of a program for spinal pain. Phys Ther 65:1649, 1985.

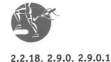
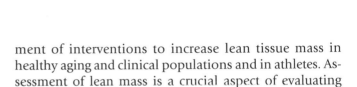

CHAPTER **45**

BODY COMPOSITION

Scott Going and Rebecca Davis

Body composition refers to the absolute and relative amounts of the body constituents. Body composition can be assessed on elemental (atomic), chemical, cellular, and tissue–system levels (1). It is possible to measure over 30 components of human body composition (2). Comprehensive descriptions of the technical aspects of most methods are available in several recent publications, although many methods are not applicable outside of the laboratory (3–5). Nevertheless, some familiarity with the principles underlying the more common laboratory methods is useful, since they provide the foundation for simpler field methods.

There are many reasons to assess body composition. The strong associations between obesity, especially excessive intra-abdominal (visceral) fat and increased risk of coronary artery disease, non–insulin-dependent diabetes, hypertension, and certain types of cancer, have received considerable attention in recent years. An excessively low level of fat is also detrimental, as evidenced by the physiological dysfunction of the chronically undernourished. In addition, assessment of body composition is useful to establish optimal weight for health and performance in athletes, to formulate dietary guidelines and exercise prescriptions for modifying body composition and evaluating efficacy, and to monitor changes in composition with growth, maturation, and aging to distinguish normal changes from disease states.

Although body fat is often the focus of assessment, lean tissue mass and its components (fluid, muscle, and bone) are at least as important. Low levels of lean mass and loss of lean tissue contribute to metabolic complications both directly and indirectly, through impaired functional capacity and reduced physical activity and energy expenditure, hence a greater risk of fat gain. Low bone mass and density are primary predictors of the risk of osteoporotic fracture. The muscle wasting (sarcopenia) that occurs with certain diseases and with aging not only decreases muscle strength and the capacity for even routine activities but is also a strong correlate of mortality. Recently there has been increased emphasis on the development of interventions to increase lean tissue mass in healthy aging and clinical populations and in athletes. Assessment of lean mass is a crucial aspect of evaluating progress toward that goal.

Exercise professionals generally use field techniques to assess body composition. Although the distinction between laboratory and field techniques is arbitrary, field techniques generally require less complex and more portable equipment, are less costly, and can be applied outside of controlled laboratory conditions. Anthropometric assessment using skinfolds and circumferences continues to be the most common approach, although newer techniques, such as bioelectric impedance analysis (BIA), are useful. There are literally hundreds of anthropometric and BIA equations for estimating body composition in various populations. As a result, one of the most difficult problems practitioners face is the selection of the most suitable method and equation.

To evaluate and choose the appropriate methods and equations for clients, exercise professionals must be familiar with the development of those methods. Validation procedures are followed when a new method or equation is developed. Cross-validation occurs when the method or equation is tested in another sample from the same or a different population. An understanding of these procedures requires a basic knowledge of criterion methods, the models, and the assumptions. Understanding the statistical criteria used to evaluate the outcomes of validation and cross-validation studies is also important. This discussion addresses these areas and provides practitioners with information needed to evaluate current and future methods so that the most accurate method may be selected.

HIERARCHY OF METHODOLOGY

Although more detailed taxonomies have been proposed, body composition methods can be categorized as being direct, indirect, or doubly indirect (6, 7). In vivo assessment is done using only indirect or doubly indirect

391

methods. Direct methods, such as dissection and chemical analysis of isolated tissues to whole cadavers, are not suitable for in vivo assessment. Nonetheless, they are central to in vivo assessment because they provide basic data that are the foundation from which indirect techniques are developed.

Indirect methods can be based on either property or component (2). Property-based methods are based on measurement of specific properties, such as body volume, decay properties of specific isotopes, or electrical resistance. The development of in vivo neutron activation analysis, for example, has made possible nondestructive chemical analysis by measuring the radiation given off during the decay of excited atoms (8). An example of a more common property-based method is the estimation of total body water (TBW) from tritium dilution (9).

Component-based methods depend on well-established models, usually ratios of measurable quantities to components that are assumed constant both within and between individuals. With component-based methods, the measured quantity is first assessed using a property-based method, and the component is estimated by application of the model. Thus, fat-free mass (FFM), a component of the two component models described later, can be estimated from body water by use of tritium dilution to measure TBW, which is converted to FFM according to the relation between TBW and FFM ($1.37 \times$ TBW = FFM).

Two types of mathematical functions are used to estimate composition with property- and component-based methods. The model approach, which depends on knowing the relation (ratio) between a particular constituent and the component of interest, is illustrated earlier. In the second approach, regression analysis is used with experimental data to derive an equation that relates a measured property or component to an unknown (estimated) component. Typically, the equation is developed by measuring the unknown component and the known component in the same subjects. Regression analysis is used to derive the equation relating the known component to the unknown component. Equations for estimating body fat from skinfold thickness or bioelectrical resistance are developed in this manner. Because they generally depend on a combination of methods used to estimate an unknown component, they are considered to be doubly indirect methods.

It is clear from the preceding discussion that a hierarchy of methods exists. Direct methods represent the most fundamental approach to assessment; property-based methods are one step removed; and component-based methods are two steps removed. Assessment methods are structured so that measurement errors or inaccurate assumptions are propagated from one level to the next. Thus, doubly indirect methods, farthest removed from direct methods, are most susceptible to inaccuracies unless precautions are taken to minimize errors.

MODELS

Many models have been proposed for characterizing the human body on various levels of analysis. A feature of all useful models is that the sum of the components closely approximates body weight. Molecular-level models are generally the most accessible and have been used in most validation studies of field methods. The usefulness of a model depends primarily on its validity for a given population and on the availability of the required technology. Simple models are accessible and require few measurements. However, simple models that combine constituents require more assumptions and are less generally applicable.

The TBW, total body potassium, and hydrodensitometry methods are three common laboratory methods for estimating fat and fat-free masses (8–10). Measurement errors and inaccuracies due to invalid assumptions are propagated from one step to the next and contribute to the total error in estimates of fat and FFM.

As noted earlier, the model is the conceptual basis from which the mathematical functions for estimating composition are derived. Thus, TBW and total body potassium can be converted to FFM according to their respective concentrations in the FFM determined through direct (chemical) analysis of human cadavers. In an analogous way, body density as determined by hydrodensitometry, can be converted to percent fat according to the relation between whole-body density and the proportions and densities of the components (10). Many equations can be derived. For example, the Siri equation ($f = 4.95 \div D_B - 4.5$), one of the most common two-component (2C) equations, was derived by use of the assumed densities for reference man from direct chemical analyses of cadavers (11, 12). It follows that equations reflect the models from which they are derived.

CRITERION REFERENCE METHODS

A criterion reference method is used to obtain accurate estimates of a body component or compartment against which regression equations are derived for estimating the same component or compartment from some measurable quantity. Reference methods are also used to derive the conversion constant that relates an unknown body component (e.g., FFM) to one of its constituents (e.g., TBW). It is essential that criterion estimates of composition be as accurate as possible, since error in the criterion measurement is propagated, hence contributes to the total error in the new equation.

According to the 2C model, laboratory methods, such as the TBW, total body potassium, and hydrodensitometry, are the most common reference methods. Each is based on an assumption of chemical constancy (i.e., that the composition and density of the FFM is similar and constant in everyone). This approach is accurate for all individuals for whom the model is valid. Model error is introduced when the actual composition of the individual is different from that assumed by the model. Higher-order models (3C and 4C models) require fewer assumptions about the composition of the FFM. For this reason, the higher-order models are valid for more people and should give more accurate results. However, their application requires more measurements, and the reduction in model error can be lost to increased technical error (measurement or method error) unless all measurements are made accurately.

The Siri equation generally gives accurate estimates of fat and FFM in young to middle-aged white men. In contrast, systematic differences among children, various racial and ethnic groups, athletes, and the elderly lead to errors in estimation of body fat and invalidate the Siri equation in these groups. The choice of an appropriate model depends on the component of FFM that is expected to vary the most. For example, young children have proportionally less mineral and more water than adults. Thus, a 4C model that adjusts for variability in both water and mineral is ideal, although good results can be achieved with a 3C model that adjusts for TBW. A 3C model that adjusts for differences in minerals is useful in African American men and women, the elderly, and many athletes, since racial, training, and age differences are due primarily to systematic variation in bone mineral mass and density. A more comprehensive review of the application of different models can be found elsewhere (2, 10).

When instruments are limited and 3C and 4C models are not possible, population-specific equations that are adjusted for systematic differences in the composition of the FFM can be used to improve accuracy. Population-specific equations appropriate for children and older adults, various racial and ethnic groups, and some clinical populations have been reviewed (3, 13, 14). Though inaccuracy is always a factor, adjusted equations are more valid and give more accurate estimates than general equations, since they are based on population-specific data.

METHOD SELECTION

Selection of an appropriate method is based on the relative precision, reliability, and accuracy of available methods, the availability of appropriate equations, and affordability (Table 45.1). Percent body fat and FFM can be estimated with field techniques with errors of more than 3% and more than 2.5–3 kg, respectively. Generally, they are adequate for screening and for following moderate changes in composition over time. When greater precision and accuracy are needed, laboratory techniques must be used.

Anthropometry

Weight-for-height indices and measurements of skinfold thicknesses, limb and trunk circumferences, and skeletal dimensions all have been used to estimate body composition. Generally, skinfolds give the most accurate estimates of percent fat and FFM, since they are direct measurements of subcutaneous fat. Circumferences are affected by both fat and muscle and do not provide accurate estimates of fatness in the general population. However, in obese persons, whose skinfold measurements can be difficult to obtain, circumferences can give useful estimates of fatness. Circumferences may also work well in athletic populations to estimate FFM, since athletes tend to vary more in muscularity than body fat.

Skinfolds and circumferences are also useful for assessing fat pattern and indirectly, distribution. The ratio of subscapular to triceps skinfolds, for example, has been used to reflect a central versus peripheral fat pattern, and the ratio of waist to hip circumferences (WHR) is a common index of upper versus lower body fat distribution. Epidemiological studies identify WHR as a predictor of chronic disease risk, and standards are available (Table 45.2). The assessment of fat pattern and distribution in combination with an estimate of total body fat is an important aspect of the assessment of disease risk.

The body mass index (BMI), a weight-for-height ratio widely used in epidemiological studies, is calculated as weight in kilograms divided by height in meters squared. Obesity standards (Table 45.3) based on BMI have been

Table 45.1. Ratings of the Validity and Objectivity of Body Composition Methods

METHOD	PRECISION	OBJECTIVITY	ACCURACY	VALID EQUATIONS	OVERALL
Body mass index	1	1	4, 5	4, 5	4
Near-infrared interactance	1	1, 2	4	4	3.5
Skinfolds	2	2, 3	2, 3	2, 3	2.5
Bioelectric impedance	2	2	2, 3	2, 3	2.5
Circumferences	2	2	2, 3	2, 4	3.0

1, excellent; 2, very good; 3, good; 4, fair; 5, unacceptable.
Precision is reliability within investigators; objectivity is reliability between investigators; accuracy refers to comparison with a criterion method; valid equations are cross-validated.

developed, and high BMI is associated with increased risk of chronic disease. Ironically, BMI is a poor predictor of percent body fat and often misclassifies individuals as obese if they have above average muscularity and skeletal mass rather than excess fat. In children and the elderly, for whom the ratio of muscle and bone to height is changing, BMI is especially misleading. Although the BMI may be useful when no other method is available, the results must be interpreted cautiously, and a follow-up examination with a more accurate method should be sought for persons for whom interventions are considered.

Excess fat in the abdomen, out of proportion to total body fat, is an independent predictor of risk factors and morbidity. Waist circumference is positively correlated with abdominal fat and is an acceptable measurement for indirectly assessing abdominal fat before and during weight loss. The sex-specific cut points given in Table 45.3 can be used in combination with BMI to identify in-

creased relative risk of the development of obesity-related risk factors in most adults with a BMI of 25–34.9 kg/m². These waist circumference cut points lose their incremental predictive power in people with a BMI above 35 kg/m² because these people exceed those cut points.

The reliability and validity of skinfolds and anthropometric methods are affected by the following:

- Skill of the measurer
- Type of caliper (due to pressure differences) or tape measure (if calibration is lost)
- Subject factors related to skinfold compressibility, edema, and variability in fat pattern and distribution
- The prediction equation used to estimate fatness

Failure to locate and measure the site properly is a major source of technical error in the skinfold method. To avoid these errors, technicians must be trained and certified by an expert, and all measurements should be made according to standard techniques (15). Equipment error can be controlled by regular calibration with Vernier calipers or a meter stick.

The skinfold method assumes that the distribution of subcutaneous and internal fat is the same for everyone to whom a particular equation is applied. Moreover, it is assumed that the sites in a particular equation adequately represent the subcutaneous fat pattern of the individual to whom it is applied. For example, an equation that includes only limb sites underestimates fatness in a person with predominantly truncal fat. Similarly, fatness is underestimated if an equation that includes only upper body sites is applied to a person with a predominantly lower body fat pattern. Equation error can be reduced by basing the selection of prediction equations on the age, sex, race, and level of physical activity in the population being assessed.

Table 45.2. Waist-To-Hip Circumference Ratio (WHR) Standard for Men and Women

	AGE	RISK			
		LOW	MODERATE	HIGH	VERY HIGH
Men	20–29	<0.83	0.83–0.88	0.89–0.94	>0.94
	30–39	<0.84	0.84–0.91	0.92–0.96	>0.96
	40–49	<0.88	0.88–0.95	0.96–1.00	>1.00
	50–59	<0.90	0.90–0.96	0.97–1.02	>1.02
	60–69	<0.91	0.91–0.98	0.99–1.03	>1.03
Women	20–29	<0.71	0.71–0.77	0.78–0.82	>0.82
	30–39	<0.72	0.72–0.78	0.79–0.84	>0.84
	40–49	<0.73	0.73–0.79	0.80–0.87	>0.87
	50–59	<0.74	0.74–0.81	0.82–0.88	>0.88
	60–69	<0.76	0.76–0.83	0.84–0.90	>0.90

(Reprinted with permission from Heyward VH, Stolarczyk LM. Applied Body Composition Assessment. Champaign, IL: Human Kinetics, 1996:82).

Table 45.3. Body Mass Index Standards and Risk of Disease

WEIGHT	BMI[b]	CLASS	DISEASE RISK[a]	
			MEN ≤ 102 CM (40 IN) WOMEN ≤ 88 CM (35 IN)	MEN >102 CM (40 IN) WOMEN >88 CM (35 IN)
Underweight	<18.5		—	—
Normal	18.5–24.9		—	—
Overweight	25.0–29.9		↑	↑↑
Obese	30.0–34.9	I	↑↑	↑↑↑
	35.0–39.9	II	↑↑↑	↑↑↑
Extremely obese	≥40.00	III	↑↑↑↑	↑↑↑↑

[a] Disease risk for NIDDM, hypertension, and CVD relative to normal weight and waist circumference.
[b] BMI is expressed in kilograms per square meter.
Adapted with permission from Expert Panel. Clinical Guidelines on the Identification, Evaluation, and Treatment of Overweight and Obesity in Adults. Bethesda, MD: National Institutes of Health, National Heart, Lung, and Blood Institute. U.S. Department of Health and Human Services, Public Health Service, 1998(22).

Bioelectrical Impedance Analysis

Bioelectrical impedance analysis (BIA) is a rapid, non-invasive, and relatively inexpensive method of estimating fat and FFM. Although the relative prediction accuracy is similar to that of the skinfold method, BIA may be preferable in some settings because it does not require a high degree of technical skill and is generally more comfortable, requires minimal cooperation, and intrudes less on privacy. Baumgartner (16) and Kushner (17) have published excellent overviews of BIA.

In the most common application of BIA, a single-frequency (50 kHz) low-level excitation current (500 μA) is used to measure whole body impedance. Unlike lower-frequency current, which flows through the extracellular fluid, higher frequencies penetrate the cell membranes and flow through both the intracellular and extracellular fluid. Given that the FFM contains large amounts of water (about 73%) and electrolytes, it is a good conductor, unlike fat, which is anhydrous and a poor conductor of electrical current. Thus, total body impedance at the constant frequency of 50 kHz primarily reflects the volumes of water (intracellular and extracellular fluid) and muscle compartments constituting the FFM.

As with anthropometry, the accuracy and precision of BIA are affected by the instruments used, subject factors, technical skill, and the prediction equation used to estimate FFM (17). Research indicates that whole-body resistance measured by different single frequency analyzers can differ as much as 36 ohms (18). To control this error, analyzers must be calibrated prior to measurement; the same instrument should be used when following changes in composition; and ideally the same brand of analyzer should be used as was used to develop the equation. Factors such as eating, drinking, and exercising must be controlled, since hydration status, fluid distribution, and temperature are sources of error in resistance measurements. Technician error is minor if standard procedures for electrode positioning and subject positioning are followed. Finally, as with skinfolds, equation error can be reduced by selecting prediction equations according to age, sex, race, and level of physical activity.

Recent research suggests that with multiple-frequency BIA (MFBIA), it may be possible to estimate extracellular and intracellular water compartments along with TBW (16). As a result, MFBIA may be less affected by hydration status and so better estimate FFM. Multiple-frequency BIA may also enhance the clinical application of BIA to assess changes and shifts between intracellular and extracellular fluid compartments associated with certain diseases.

EQUATION SELECTION

Prediction equations are either population specific or general. Population-specific equations are derived for use in a specific homogeneous population (e.g., prepubescent White boys or elderly African American women). Thus, they usually systematically underestimate or overestimate body composition if applied to individuals from other populations. In contrast, general equations can be applied to individuals who differ greatly in physical characteristics. General equations are developed from diverse, heterogeneous samples, and they account for differences in age, sex, race, ethnicity, and other characteristics by including these variables as predictors in the equation.

To develop prediction equations, it is necessary to select a representative sample of the specific population. The predictor variables (e.g., height and weight, age, race, skinfolds, or BIA) and the criterion estimates of body composition (percent fat or FFM) are measured in the same subjects, and the equation is developed using appropriate statistical methods. The usefulness of the equation depends on the strength of association between the variables and the accuracy with which the dependent variable is estimated. Useful equations give estimates of percent fat or FFM that are significantly correlated ($R \geq 0.8$) with criterion measurements. Moreover, the means and standard deviations of the estimated and criterion scores should be nearly equal, and the standard error of estimate (SEE) for predicting the criterion measurements from the estimated values should be approximately 2.5–3.5% for percent fat and 2.5–3.5 kg for FFM.

To select the most appropriate equation, it is important to evaluate the relative merit of the various methods and equations. The following questions should be considered (3):

1. *To whom is the equation applicable?* The answer lies in a careful examination of the characteristics of the population used to derive the equation. Factors such as age, race, sex, physical activity level, and amount of body fat must be examined carefully. Unless the equation has been shown to generalize to other groups, it should not be applied to groups with different characteristics.

2. *Was an appropriate reference method used to develop the equation?* Error in the reference measure is propagated and contributes to the total error in the equation. Multiple-component models require fewer assumptions and give more accurate reference measurements than methods based on the 2C model. Equations derived from reference measurements based on 3C and 4C models should be used in populations for whom the assumptions underlying the 2C model are not valid. Alternatively, population-specific conversion formulas should be used to derive reference estimates of FFM and percent fat.

3. *Was a representative sample of the population studied?* Large, randomly selected samples (100–400 subjects) are needed to ensure that the sample is representative. If random sampling is not possible and convenience samples are used, the procedure is acceptable as long as a sufficient number of subjects are studied. With an appropriate sample size, a more stable, valid, and generally applicable equation will be derived.

4. *How were the predictor variables measured?* When any equation is applied, it is important that the predictor variables be measured as the investigators who developed the equation measured them. Although it is recommended that standard procedures and sites be used, this is not always done, and errors are larger if the original procedures are not followed (5).

5. *Was the equation cross-validated in another sample of the population?* Because of investigator- and laboratory-specific procedural differences, equations that sometimes give accurate validation results may not be accurate when used in a different laboratory or by a different investigator, and the equation should be tested in other samples of the same population. Sometimes this is done by dividing the original sample into validation and cross-validation groups and testing in both groups. Although this approach is reasonable, it does not demonstrate whether the equation is reliable outside of the laboratory where it was developed. It is preferable to test the equation in samples in a different laboratory to determine its validity and generality. In addition, cross-validation studies in different populations are necessary to determine the accuracy in different groups.

6. *Does the equation give accurate estimates of composition?* In validation studies, the multiple correlation between the variables should be more than .80, and SEEs should range from 2.5–3.5% when estimating percent fat and 2.5–3.5 kg when estimating FFM. In addition, the prediction equation should yield a comparable average and distribution (range and standard deviation) of scores, and the total error should not be much larger than the SEE (13).

RECOMMENDED EQUATIONS

Heyward and Stolarczyk (3) recently made easier the task of equation selection. They reviewed the available equations and developed decision trees for selecting the most useful equations (Figs. 45.1 and 45.2). Decision trees can be used to find appropriate equations for African Americans, Whites, and Hispanics of both genders. The mathematical formulas for each equation are given in Tables 45.4 and 45.5. Equations for other minority groups (e.g., Asians and Native Americans) and athletes are also available (3); these equations do not meet all criteria previously outlined; however, they are the most useful to date.

BODY FAT STANDARDS

There are no accepted percent body fat standards for all ages. Most body composition studies use small groups, usually young adults. These studies demonstrate that body fat typically ranges from 10–20% for men and 20–30% for women. Based on these studies, recommendations of 15% for men and 25% for women have been made. These "standards" essentially are the average percent fat for young adults. Their usefulness in other groups has not been established.

National data for describing percent fat for the U.S. population are not available. However, there are skinfold data from the National Health and Nutrition Examination Survey (NHANES II) on a large (20,000) representative sample of U.S. men and women. Despite the limitations of skinfolds, these national data provide a better basis for developing standards than convenience samples. Conversion of the NHANES skinfold data (triceps and

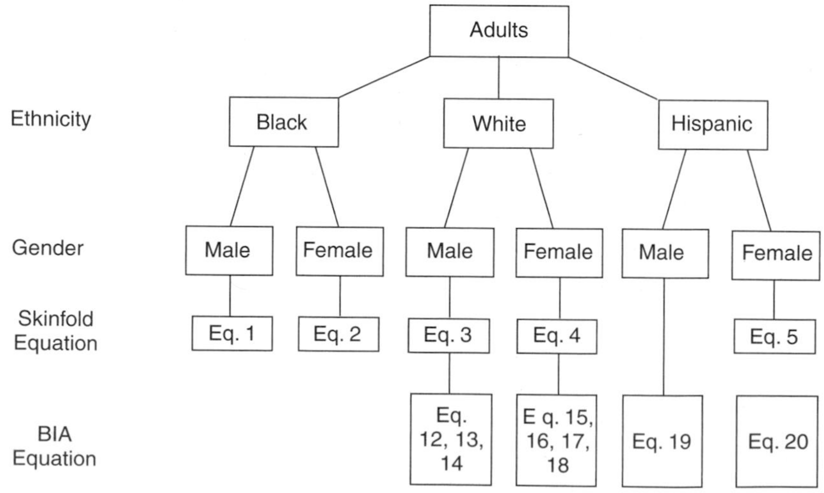

Figure 45.1. Skinfold and bioelectric impedance analysis (BIA) equation finder for adults. (Adapted with permission from Heyward VH, Stolarczyk LM. Applied Body Composition Assessment. Champaign, IL: Human Kinetics, 1996:165–168.)

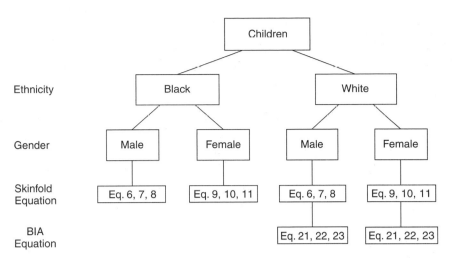

Figure 45.2. Skinfold and bioelectric impedance analysis (BIA) equation finder for children. (Adapted with permission from Heyward VH, Stolarczyk LM. Applied Body Composition Assessment. Champaign, IL: Human Kinetics, 1996:165–168.)

Table 45.4. Skinfold Prediction Equations

	ETHNICITY	GENDER	AGE	EQUATION	REFERENCE
1	Black	Men	18–61	Db (g/cc) = 1.1120 − 0.00043499 (Σ 7SKF chest, abdomen, thigh, triceps, subscapular, suprailiac, madaxillary) + 0.00000055 (Σ 7SKF)^2 − 0.00028826 (age).	19
2	Black	Women	18–55	Db (g/cc) = 1.0970 − 0.00046971 (Σ 7SKF chest, abdomen, thigh, triceps, subscapular, suprailiac, midaxillary) + 0.00000056 (Σ 7SKF)^2 − 0.00012828 (age).	20
3	White	Men	18–61	Db (g/cc) = 1.109380 − 0.0008267 (Σ 3SKF chest, abdomen, thigh) + 0.0000016 (Σ 3SKF)^2 − 0.0002574 (age).	19
4	White	Women	18–55	Db (g/cc) = 1.0994921 − 0.0009929 (Σ 3SKF triceps, suprailiac, thigh) + 0.0000023 (Σ 3SKF)^2 − 0.0001392 (age).	20
5	Hispanic	Women	20–40	Db (g/cc) = 1.0970 − 0.00046971 (Σ 3SKF chest, abdomen, thigh, triceps, subscapular, suprailiac, midaxillary) + 0.00000056 (Σ 7SKF)^2 − 0.00012828 (age).	20
6	Black & white	Boys	≤18	% BF = 0.735 (Σ 2SKF triceps, calf) + 1.0	23
7	Black & white	Boys (SKF > 35 mm)	≤18	%BF = 0.735 (Σ 2SKF triceps, subscapular) + 1.6	23
8	Black & white	Boys (SKF > 35 mm)	≤18	%BF = 0.783 (Σ 2SKF triceps, subscapular) − 0.008 (Σ 2SKF)^2 + 1*.	23
9	Black & White	Girls	≤18	% BF = 0.610 (2SKF triceps, calf) + 5.1	23
10	Black & white	Girls (SKF > 35 mm)	≤18	%BF = 0.546 (Σ 2SKF triceps, subscapular) + 9.7	23
11	Black & white	Girls (SKF > 35 mm)	≤18	%BF = 1.33 (Σ 2SKF triceps, subscapular) − 0.013 (Σ 2SKF)^2 − 2.5.	23

Db, body density; SKF, skinfolds; %BF, percent body fat.
* Intercept substitutions based on maturation and ethnicity for boys:

Age	Black	White
Prepubescent	−3.2	−1.7
Pubescent	−5.2	−3.4
Postpubescent	−6.8	−5.5

Adapted with permission from Heyward VH, Stolarczyk LM. Applied Bondy Composition Assessment. Champaign IL: Human Kinetics, 1996:173-185.

Table 45.5. Bioelectric Impedance Analysis Prediction Equations

	ETHNICITY	GENDER	AGE	EQUATION	REFERENCE
12	White	Men	18–29	FFM (kg) = 0.485 (HT²/r) + 0.338 (BW) + 5.32	13
13	White	Men (<20% BF)	17–62	FFM (kg) = 0.00066360 (HT²) − 0.02117 (R) + 0.62854 (BW) − 0.12380 (age + 9.33285)	24
14	White	Men (≥20% BF)	17–62	FFM (kg) = 0.00088580 (HT²) 0.02999 + 0.42688 (BW) 0.07002 (age) + 14.52435	24
15	White	Women	18–29	FFM (kg) = 0.476 (HT²/r) + 0.295 (BW) + 5.49	13
16	White	Women	30–49	FFM (kg) = 0.493 (HT²/r) + 0.141 (BW) + 11.59	13
17	White	Women	50-70	FFM (kg) = 0.474 (HT²/r) + 0.180 (BW) + 7.3	13
18	White	Women	22-74	FFM (kg) = 0.00151 (HT²) − 0.0344 (R) + 0.140 (BW) − 0.158 (age) + 20.387	25
19	Hispanic	Men	19-59	FFM (kg) = 13.74 + 0.34 (HT²/r) + 0.33 (BW) − 0.14 + (age) + 6.18	26
20	Hispanic	Women	20-40	FFM (kg) = 0.00151 (HT²) − 0.0344 (R) + 0.140 (BW) − 0.158 (age) + 20.387	25
21	White	Both	6–10	TBW (L) = 0.593 (HT²/r) + 0.65 (BW) + 0.04	17
22	White	Both	10–19	FFM (kg) = 0.61 (HT²/r) + 0.25 (BW) + 1.31	27
23	White	Both	8–15	FFM (kg) = 0.62 (HT²/r) + 0.21 (BW) + 0.10 (Σc) + 4.2	13

HT, height (cm); BW, body weight (kg); R, resistance (Ω); Σc, reactance (Ω); TBW, total body water (L).
To convert TBW to FFM, use the following hydration constants:
Boys   5–6 yr FFM (kg) = TBW/0.77   Girls   5–6 yr FFM (kg) TBW/0.78
       7–8 yr FFM (kg) = TBW/0.768   7–8 yr FFM (kg) = TBW/0.776
       9–10 yr FFM (kg) = TBW/0.762   9–10 yr FFM (kg) = TBW/0.77
Adapted with permission from Heyward VH, Stolarczyk LM. Applied Body Composition Assessment. Champaign IL: Human Kinetics, 1996:173–185.

subscapular skinfolds) to percent fat using published equations (19, 20) shows that the average (50th percentile) percent fat for 20–34-year-old men and women is 12% and 28%, respectively. The percent fat corresponding to the 15th (low) and 85th percentiles (high) is 5% and 22%, respectively, for young men and 22% and 39%, respectively, for young women. It is clear that the percent fat corresponding with the median, low, and high skinfold percentiles vary with age as well as sex. It is possible that standards should also vary with age, although typically the values for young adults are applied to all ages.

Using this approach, new percent fat health standards have been recently proposed (Fig. 45.3) (15). Some increase in percent fat with age was allowed. This was done in consideration of recent studies showing that lower body fat or reduced body fat in middle-aged women is associated with a lower bone mineral content, putting those women at risk for osteoporosis and bone fractures. Thus, the emphasis on lower percent fat to prevent heart disease, especially in women, must be balanced against the increased risk of bone fractures, especially if bone mineral content is already low.

Standards for active men and women have also been developed (Table 45.6). These standards are not necessarily associated with better health but may be associated with improved physical performance.

Recently, a unique approach to derive percent fat standards for children and adolescents has been reported (21). In this study, the authors sought to develop crite-

rion-referenced standards by assessing risk of high levels of blood pressure, total cholesterol, and low-density lipoprotein and low levels of high-density lipoprotein in girls and boys aged 6–18 years at different levels of body fatness. No excess risk was found until percent fat ex-

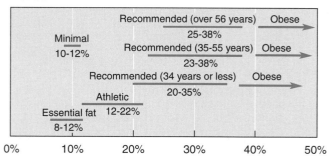

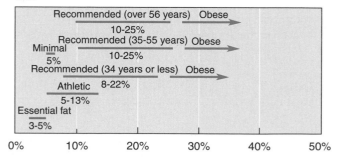

Figure 45.3. Percent fat standards for men and women.

Table 45.6. Percent Fat Standards for Active Men and Women

	Not Recommended	Recommended Body Fat Levels (%)		
		Low	Mid	Upper
Men				
young adult	< 5	5	10	15
middle adult	< 7	7	11	18
elderly	< 9	9	12	18
Women				
young adult	< 16	16	23	28
middle adult	< 20	20	27	33
elderly	< 20	20	27	33

Adapted with permission from Lohman TG, Houtkooper LB, Going SB. Body composition assessment: Body fat standards and methods in the field of exercise and sports medicine. ACSM Health Fitness J 1:30–35, 1997.

ceeded 25% in boys and 30% in girls. Age and race were not significant predictors of risk in this age group. Thus, 25% fat in boys and 30% fat in girls have been proposed as useful health standards for African Americans and Whites aged 6–18 years. A similar criterion-referenced approach would be useful in adults to determine whether risk varies with age and percent fat, or one standard is valid for all ages.

RESOURCES FOR BODY COMPOSITION ASSESSMENT

A number of excellent resources offer additional information on both laboratory and field methods for assessing body composition. Monographs by Lohman (13) and Roche et al. (5) provide comprehensive reviews of laboratory techniques. The proceedings from the ongoing international symposiums on in vivo body composition (28) are also excellent sources for current developments in measurement techniques. For information on field techniques, the monograph by Heyward and Stolarcyzk (3) is particularly helpful, as is the *Anthropometric Standardization Reference Manual* (4) from the Arlie conference, which describes recommended standard techniques for anthropometry. Videotapes, manuals, and software packages for training and standardizing procedures, and for simplifying calculations and reporting results are available from Human Kinetics Publishers, Champaign, Illinois. The recent evidence report, *Clinical Guidelines on the Identification, Evaluation, and Treatment of Overweight and Obesity in Adults* (29), is an important resource for practitioners involved in obesity prevention and treatment.

References

1. Wang ZM, Pierson RN, Heymsfield SB. The five level model: A new approach to organizing body composition research. Am J Clin Nutr 56:19–28, 1992.

2. Heymsfield SB, Wang ZM, Withers RT. Multicomponent molecular level models of body composition. In: Roche AF, Heymsfield SB, Lohman TG, eds. Human Body Composition. Champaign, IL: Human Kinetics, 1996:129–147.
3. Heyward VH, Stolarczyk LM. Applied Body Composition Assessment. Champaign, IL: Human Kinetics, 1996.
4. Lohman TG, Roche AF, Martorell R, eds. Anthropometric Standardization Reference Manual. Champaign, IL: Human Kinetics, 1988.
5. Roche AF, Heymsfield SB, Lohman TG, eds. Human Body Composition. Champaign, IL: Human Kinetics, 1996.
6. Wang ZM, Heshka S, Pierson RN, et al. Systematic organization of body composition methodology: An overview with emphasis on component-based methods. Am J Clin Nutr 61:457–465, 1995.
7. Heymsfield SB, Wang J, Lichtman S, et al. Body composition in elderly subjects: A critical appraisal of clinical methodology. Am J Clin Nutr 50:1167–1175, 1989.
8. Ellis KJ. Whole-body counting and neutron activation analysis. In: Roche AF, Heymsfield SB, Lohman TG, eds. Human Body Composition. Champaign, IL: Human Kinetics, 1996:45–61.
9. Schoeller DA. Hydrometry. In: Roche AF, Heymsfield SB, Lohman TG, eds. Human Body Composition. Champaign, IL: Human Kinetics, 1996:25–43.
10. Going SB. Densitometry. In: Roche AF, Heymsfield SB, Lohman TG, eds. Human Body Composition. Champaign, IL: Human Kinetics, 1996:3–23.
11. Brozek J, Grande F, Anderson JT, et al. Densitometric analysis of body composition: Revision of some quantitative assumptions. Ann N Y Acad Sci 110:113–140, 1963.
12. Siri WE. The gross composition of the body. Adv Biol Med Physiol 4:239–280, 1956.
13. Lohman TG. Advances in Body Composition Assessment. Champaign, IL: Human Kinetics, 1992.
14. Going SB, Williams DP, Lohman TG. Aging and body composition: Biological changes and methodological issues. Exerc Sport Sci Rev 23:411–458, 1995.
15. Lohman TG, Houtkooper LB, Going SB. Body composition assessment: Body fat standards and methods in the field of exercise and sports medicine. ACSM Health Fitness J 1:30–35, 1997.
16. Baumgartner RN. Electrical impedance and total body electrical conductivity. In: Roche AF, Heymsfield SB, Lohman TG, eds. Human Body Composition. Champaign, IL: Human Kinetics, 1996:79–107.
17. Kushner RF. Bioelectrical impedance analysis: A review of principles and applications. J Am Coll Nutr 11:199–209, 1992.
18. Graves JE, Pollock ML, Colvin AB, et al. Comparison of different bioelectrical impedance analyzers in the prediction of body composition. Am J Hum Biol 1:603–611, 1989.
19. Jackson AS, Pollock ML. Generalized equations for predicting body density of men. Br J Nutr 61:497–504, 1978.
20. Jackson AS, Pollock ML, Ward A. Generalized equations for predicting body density of women. Med Sci Sports Exerc 12:175–182, 1980.
21. Williams DP, Going SB, Lohman TG, et al. Body fatness and risk for elevated blood pressure, total cholesterol, and serum lipoprotein ratios in children and adolescents. Am J Public Health 82:358–363, 1992.
22. Department of Health and Human Services. Surgeon General's report on nutrition and health (DHHS Pub

88–50210). Washington: U.S. Government Printing Office, 1998.

23. Slaughter MH, Lohman TG, Boileau RA, et al. Skinfold equations for estimation of body fatness in children and youth. Human Biol 60:709–723, 1988.

24. Segal KR, Van Loan M, Fitzgerald PI, et al. Lean body mass estimation by bioelectrical impedance analysis: A four site cross-validation study. Am J Clin Nutr 47:7–14, 1988.

25. Gray DS, Bray GA, Bauer M, et al. Effect of obesity on bio-electric impedance. Am J Clin Nutr 50:255–260, 1989.

26. Rising R, Swinburn B, Larson K, et al. Body composition in Pima Indians: Validation of bioelectrical resistance. Am J Clin Nutr 53:594–598, 1991.

27. Houtkooper LB, Going SB, Lohman TG, et al. Bioelectrical impedance estimation of fat-free body mass in children and youth: a cross-validation study. J Appl Physiol 72:366–373, 1992.

28. Yasumura, S, Wang J, Pierson, RN, eds. In vivo body composition studies. Ann N Y Acad Sci 904, 1–631, 2000.

29. National Heart, Lung, and Blood Institute. Clinical Guidelines on the Identification, Evaluation, and Treatment of Overweight and Obesity in Adults: The Evidence Report. Bethesda, MD: National Institutes of Health, National Heart, Lung, and Blood Institute. U.S. Department of Health and Human Services, Public Health Service, 1998.

CHAPTER **46**

NUTRITION

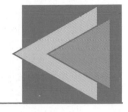

Donna Israel

Nutrition assessment is a broad-based method of determining the nutritional status and nutrient requirements of individuals. The assessment is designed to be completed by a registered dietitian (1). The American Dietetic Association defines nutrition assessment further as "the evaluation of nutrition needs of individuals based upon appropriate biochemical, anthropometric measurements, and laboratory data (2)." Thus, four types of data are evaluated in a nutrition assessment:

- Dietary
- Biochemical
- Anthropometric
- Physical

Information on which dietary data are based is typically subjective. It includes appetite, food habits, exercise habits, special diets, bowel function, and food allergies. In contrast, biochemical data are based on objective values, such as laboratory values for urine, blood, and other tissues, as are anthropometric data, which include height, weight, skinfold, and body circumferences. Physical data are based on an examination of the patient for clinical signs of nutrient deficiency or excess. Physical data can be obtained through observation of the skin, face, lips, nails, hair, teeth, eyes, and musculature. The musculoskeletal systems require functional assessments. Functional evaluations may be necessary in other systems also, to rule out impairment (2, 3).

The assessment often includes data from other health or clinical settings. It follows a model similar to the following:

- Identification and screening
- Planning
- Implementation
- Evaluation and monitoring

TOOLS FOR NUTRITION ASSESSMENT

Nutrition Screening

Nutrition screening is the "process of identifying characteristics known to be associated with nutrition problems. Its purpose is to pinpoint individuals who are malnourished or at nutritional risk" (2). The screening process should do the following:

- Work in any setting
- Complement the process of promoting early intervention
- Include data on risk factors and interpret them correctly to facilitate treatment
- Determine the need for nutrition assessment
- Be cost-effective

24-Hour Recall

The purpose of the 24-hour recall is to evaluate food choices within the past 24 hours. It is a method of estimating food intake that limits the risk of patient reporting food habits inaccurately. To enhance the accuracy of this tool, it should be based on a recent 24-hour period. The tool may be self-administered, but it is usually more accurate when a nutritionist uses it to interview the patient, asking open-ended questions designed to encourage the patient to report all foods and beverages consumed, usually in chronological order. This form of assessment is most appropriate when unhealthy eating habits are suspected or in an initial session.

Three-Day Diet Records

A 3-day diet record adds insight and accuracy to the assessment of eating patterns. The disadvantage of diet records is that patients often underestimate portion size. This can be overcome through proper instruction concerning estimating portion size. With a 3-day record, the patient may use food models, measure food, or even observe measuring cups and spoons to visualize portion size. Forms specifying time, location, food type (include brand name), portion size, method of preparation, and perhaps emotional state should be used. The patient is instructed to record each food and beverage consumed, including water, gum, and candy, over the course of the recording period (usually two weekdays and one weekend day). Three-day diet records are useful in tracking frequent eating patterns, analyzing diets for a deficiency or excess of nutrients, and as a teaching tool to demonstrate healthy alternatives to inappropriate food choices.

Diet History

A diet history is used to determine the patient's normal intake over time. Questions such as, "What do you typically eat for breakfast?" or "What do you usually eat first when you awaken?" are often included in the interview. Responses to these questions may be cross-checked with a food frequency from (Fig. 46.1), although such forms may not be appropriate when dietary patterns vary.

This tool differs somewhat from the food frequency method, described next, in that the diet history is used to determine overall intake and prevalence of certain foods in the diet rather than to identify food intake patterns. Unlike the food frequency method, the diet history method also requires significant interviewing skills to obtain accurate data.

Food Frequency Questionnaire

A food frequency questionnaire is useful for monitoring patterns of food intake. The questionnaire can be used to identify specific foods or types of foods that are consumed in excessive or insufficient amounts. Underestimation of portion size is a common problem with this tool, although food models and/or measuring devices may be used during the interview to indicate portion sizes as accurately as possible.

A French model recently challenged the reliability of information gained from the food frequency questionnaire (4). When used to assess the quality of food intake by French adults, the food frequency form revealed that the French diet failed to meet some of the U.S. Department of Agriculture (USDA) dietary guidelines (e.g., those summarized in the Food Pyramid and US Dietary Guidelines). However, a modified diet quality index (DQI), a dietary diversity (DD) score, and a dietary variety score (DVS) indicated that the French diet was more diverse than the standard American diet. This implies that the "French paradox"—the lower-than-expected mortality from coronary heart disease in a society where the diet is rich in fat, especially saturated fat—may be linked to overall diet quality rather than to specific foods.

Physical Examination

Clinical examination of a patient is an essential component of a thorough assessment. Even a gross examination of the eyes, hair, face, teeth, skin, nails, and lips can provide key information regarding the patient's nutritional status. Functional evaluation of the musculoskeletal, cardiovascular, and gastrointestinal systems can yield additional information.

ANTHROPOMETRIC DATA

Anthropometric data are based on measurements of the following:

- Height
- Weight
- Body mass index (BMI)
- Body composition
- Waist-to-hip ratio

These measurements are compared to norms that consider age, gender, body frame, and ethnicity. Anthropometry has many advantages. These measurements are usually less expensive and easier to obtain than clinical data. They are also safer for the patient because they can be obtained noninvasively. Anthropometric measurements may be obtained in the field as well as in clinical settings and can be taken by individuals with minimal training. However, field work presents a few disadvantages: 1) The measurements may be less accurate when taken by untrained or poorly trained individuals, and 2) measurements may be affected by the testing environment (2). The equipment used for assessment must be properly maintained and calibrated regularly for accurate results. To ensure the most accurate measures possible, the same person should assess the patient on each visit.

Height

It is usually more important to measure height in children than in adults. However, periodic measurements in adults (~ every 3 years) is recommended. Unfortunately, height is often self-reported by adults and thus may be inaccurate. An inaccurate measurement may make it difficult to assess body weight.

A stadiometer is often used to measure height. Height can be measured indirectly through knee height and arm span. Knee height is measured from the heel to the anterior surface of the thigh while the knee is flexed 90°. This may be useful for individuals with spinal deformities or for patients on bed rest or who are unable to stand (2). Knee height can be extrapolated to total height by means of a regression equation (5). **Arm span** may also be measured to estimate skeletal length. Arm span is the distance from the longest fingertip of one hand to the longest fingertip of the opposite hand when the arms are fully abducted at shoulder level (2).

Weight

Weight is most commonly measured using a platform balance scale. Weight without shoes, without objects in

FOOD INTAKE RECORD

Please indicate which foods you eat.

	Less than once a week	Not daily but at least once a week	Daily
Milk, yogurt			
Cheese			
Red meat			
Poultry			
Fish			
Eggs			
Mixed dishes			
Dried beans, legumes			
Peanut butter			
Nuts			
Breads, cereal			
Potatoes, pasta, rice			
Fruits, juices			
Vegetables			
Margarine, butter			
Cooking oil			
Sour cream, salad dressing			
Ice cream			
Cookies, cake, pie			
Candy			
Soft drink			
Coffee			
Tea, iced tea			
Alcohol			

Describe your usual daily eating pattern (include amount eaten).

Time	Meal	Food/method of preparation	Amount eaten	Calculations (for RD)
	Breakfast			
	Snack			
	Lunch			
	Dinner			
	Snack			

Medical Nutrition Therapy Across the Continuum of Care   ©1996, The American Dietetic Association

Figure 46.1. Food intake record.

pockets, and while wearing light clothing is standard. If a change in weight is crucial for a diagnosis or for selecting a treatment, it should be measured at least 2 hours after food or liquid intake and while wearing light clothing (2).

A weight history may help the health care professional determine patterns of nutrition and exercise behavior. Typical questions regarding weight history include high-est and lowest adult weight, preferred weight, usual weight, and weight change during the past 6–12 months (2).

The Metropolitan Life Insurance Company introduced normative tables for weight in 1959. Different norms have been introduced because of the increased weight in the general population, and the 1959 tables are no longer used (6, 7).

An alternative method for determining ideal body weight is presented in the following (8):

Women: ideal body weight
=100 lb for the first 5 feet + 5 lb for each inch over 5 feet

Men: ideal body weight
=106 lb for the first 5 feet + 6 lb for each inch over 5 feet

Body Mass Index

Body mass index (BMI) is a ratio of weight to height in adults that indicates body composition (9). BMI can be used to define the degree of adiposity without accounting for body frame size. It is calculated by the Quetelet equation (10):

$$BMI = Weight\ (kg)/[height\ (m)]^2$$

The BMI correlates the least with body height and the most with independent measures of body fatness in adults, including the elderly. A BMI score of 20 to 25 is associated with the lowest risk of excessive or deficient adipose tissue. Obesity is divided into three grades:

- Grade I = 25.0–29.9
- Grade II = 30–40
- Grade III = 40+

A BMI of at least 27 indicates obesity and increased health risk. Body mass index increases with age; therefore, age-specific guidelines for interpreting the BMI in the elderly have been recommended.

Body Composition

Percent body fat can be used to stratify the risk of cardiovascular disease in patients. The amount of body fat can be estimated by underwater weighing, skin-fold thickness measurements, circumferences, bioelectric impedance, and dual x-ray absorptiometry.

Waist-to-Hip Ratio

The waist-to-hip (W:H) ratio is used to estimate the risk of coronary artery disease (CAD). Values of > 0.8 for women and > 0.9 for men indicate an increased risk for cardiovascular disease and diabetes mellitus. A W:H value greater than 1.0 indicates a significantly increased risk of CAD. For lean and normal-weight individuals, the most accurate method of estimating the risk of CAD may be to combine the W:H ratio and BMI (11).

SUBJECTIVE GLOBAL ASSESSMENT

Subjective global assessment (SGA) includes a physical examination and medical evaluation. The medical evaluation assesses changes in weight and dietary intake; gastrointestinal(GI) symptoms, such as nausea, diarrhea, and vomiting; systemic function; metabolic demands; and environmental factors, such as stress and illness (2). The physical examination should include a measurement of subcutaneous fat to identify muscle wasting, edema, or ascites (2).

ADDITIONAL TOOLS FOR A COMPLETE ASSESSMENT

A complete medical history is the basis of a thorough and accurate nutrition assessment. The most pertinent components of that history are as follows:

1. Family history, including a history of diabetes mellitus, stroke, cancer, cardiovascular disease, hypertension, and GI or orthopaedic problems that may require nutrition intervention.
2. Personal medical history, including past and current illnesses and surgeries that may indicate nutritional status and intervention requirements.
3. Prescription medications, to rule out the possibility of drug–nutrient interactions, especially in elderly patients, who are 2 to 3 times more susceptible than younger patients (2) (Table 46.1). Common interactions include:
   - Reduced drug effectiveness because of the effects of food on gastric motility or pH
   - Nutrient deficiencies caused by appetite suppression or emesis (e.g., due to chemotherapy) or increased mineral loss
   - Nutrient excess caused by appetite stimulation (e.g., by steroids or tranquilizers)
   - Allergic reactions
4. Alcohol, smoking, and illicit drug use, which may alter caloric requirements and caloric intake, resulting in nutrient deficiencies.
5. Weight history, which may include patterns of change that indicate a positive or negative energy balance and may provide a reason for signs of nutrient deficiency or excess.
6. Exercise and activity, which may indicate total energy expenditure and can be used to estimate the basal metabolic rate (BMR). The BMR can be estimated by the Harris-Benedict equation and then multiplied by an activity factor (below) to yield caloric requirements.

Formula for calculation of BMR:

Men: BMR
= 66 + 13.8(weight in Kg) + 5(height in cm) − 6.8 (age)

Women: BMR
=655 + 9.6(weight in Kg) + 1.8(height in cm) −4.7(age)

Activity factors
- 1.2 Bed rest
- 1.3 Sedentary
- 1.4 Active
- 1.5 Very active

Table 46.1. Drug–Food Interactions

MEDICATION: BRAND NAME (GENERIC NAME) [FUNCTION]	NUTRITIONAL IMPLICATIONS
Cardiovascular agents	
Inderal (propranolol HCL) [beta-blocker]	Take with food to enhance absorption (may cause constipation, nausea)
Lanoxin (digoxin) [glycoside]	Take on an empty stomach (may cause anorexia, nausea)
Lasix (furosemide) [diuretic]	Take with food or milk (may cause nausea, diarrhea, potassium loss)
Procardia (nifedipine) [Ca^{2+} blocker]	Take with food or milk (may cause diarrhea, constipation)
Anti-infectives	
Amoxicillin [antibiotic]	Take tablet or liquid forms without regard to meals (may cause diarrhea, nausea, vomiting)
Ceclor (cefaclor) [antibiotic]	Take without regard to meals (may cause nausea, vomiting, diarrhea)
Erythromycin [antibiotic]	Take with meals (not milk) to prevent GI distress
Tetracycline [antibiotic]	Take on an empty stomach. Do not give with dairy products or medical nutritional products
Flagyl (metronidazole) [antifungal]	Take with food (may cause nausea, vomiting, diarrhea, GI distress)
Analgesics	
Tylenol (acetaminophen) [analgesic]	Take with food to prevent GI distress
Aspirin (acetylsalicylic acid) [analgesic]	Take with food to prevent GI distress
Motrin, Advil (ibuprofen) [analgesic]	Take with food to prevent GI distress
Codeine [analgesic, antitussive, narcotic]	Take with food or water to prevent GI distress
Antidepressants	
Tofranil (imipramine) [antidepressant]	Take with food to prevent GI distress (may cause diarrhea, nausea, vomiting)
Nardil (phenelzine) [MAOI antidepressant]	Avoid foods high in tyramine. Limit caffeine-containing foods and beverages.

7. Stress, which can increase metabolic and micronutrient requirements (1, 11–14).

LABORATORY DATA

The following laboratory data are often used in the nutritional assessment (15):

1. Blood nutrient levels
2. Urinary excretion rates for nutrients
3. Urinary nutrient metabolite levels
4. Abnormal metabolic byproducts in blood
5. Changes in blood components or enzyme activities related to nutrient intake
6. Response to a loading, saturation, or isotopic test

Pertinent laboratory data include albumin, creatinine, cholesterol (blood lipids), triglycerides, glucose, white blood cell (WBC) count, transferrin, hemoglobin, hematocrit, potassium, sodium, chloride, calcium, phosphorus, and carbon dioxide content. Diagnoses are not usually made on the basis of laboratory values alone.

ASSESSMENT THROUGHOUT THE LIFE CYCLE

Protocols for nutrition assessments taken during a specific stage of life should address risk factors common to that age group (16–26). Several of these are discussed next.

Pediatric Population

One of the best indicators of nutritional status in children may be physical growth. Length or stature and weight are commonly used to assess growth. Physical examination of the teeth, gums, and tongue is also helpful in determining the nutritional status of children (2). However, the fact that their eating habits may be affected by a myriad of factors—including flavor acceptance and the physiological development of taste, as well as habits, ethnicity, social interaction, food availability and convenience, family economic status, emotions, the physical appearance of food, current or prior nutritional status—must be taken into consideration in the development of nutrition interventions (11, 12).

Anthropometric measures commonly used in children include the weight-for-height index, height-for-age index, weight-for-age index, head circumference, mid-upper-arm circumference, and triceps skinfold thickness. These indexes can be plotted on standardized forms. The mid-upper-arm circumference and triceps skinfold thickness can help identify wasting, since these measures correlate with lean body mass (27, 28). The triceps skinfold can help determine whether excessive weight is due to excessive fat or excessive lean tissue (e.g., muscle hypertrophy in athletes); however, this measurement is not the most reliable measure of body composition (2).

Assessments of children should also consider activity level. The Harris-Benedict equation can be used to estimate children's caloric requirements (18).

Adolescent Population

The patient is considered an adolescent on reaching puberty. Up to 20% of adult height and 50% of weight may be gained during this period. Both body fat and lean muscle mass increase. Girls generally gain more body fat than boys, and boys usually gain more lean tissue (29). It is important to use age-specific norms in assessing adolescents (16).

Nutrient needs increase significantly during adolescence to accommodate rapid growth. Adolescents are likely not to obtain adequate amounts of vitamins and minerals because of their sudden increase in requirements and generally poor food choices. Nutritional assessment should include an evaluation of the patient's nutritional environment—including parental, peer, school, cultural, personal, and lifestyle factors—as well as attitude toward food and nutrition in general (29). Growth rate and exercise habits should be considered when determining the nutritional requirements of adolescents. The development of body image concerns during adolescence may lead to a desire to change the growth rate or body proportions with further dietary manipulation and often has a negative consequence. Consequently, a variety of eating disorders may develop during this period (30, 31). Use of tobacco, alcohol, marijuana, and other drugs can also affect nutritional status.

Adult Population

When the epiphyseal plates close about age 18, adolescents may be considered adults for the purposes of nutrition assessment. Weight is particularly useful in assessing the nutritional status of adults. Height and weight should both be measured, as adults commonly overestimate height and underestimate weight. Weight loss reflects an acute inability to meet nutritional requirements and may indicate a nutritional risk factor or illness (29). The use of the Metropolitan Life Insurance table and/or the BMI can help determine appropriate body weight (7, 9). The previously mentioned methods of assessing body composition may also be used to determine nutritional status. Assessments for adults should consider activity and exercise levels. The Harris-Benedict equation can be used to estimate caloric requirements.

Elderly Population

Aging is marked by a progressive loss of lean body mass and increased body fat, and is accompanied by changes in most physiological systems (29). Lean body mass in the healthy elderly is 30–40% less than in young adults. This represents the loss of both muscular and visceral protein and leads to functional and metabolic changes. Basal metabolic rate and therefore energy requirements decrease by 20% between ages 30 and 90, mainly because of decreased lean body mass (29). The Harris-Benedict equation can be used to estimate caloric requirements in this population.

Nutrition assessment of older adults should take into consideration the activity level and the possibility of chronic disease. Physical activity helps maintain bone and muscle mass and functional capacity in this population, and also helps maintain a normal metabolic rate. When caloric requirements fall below 1800 calories a day in the elderly, inadequate amounts of protein, calcium, iron, and vitamins may be consumed (19). For this reason, the metabolic rate should be maintained to ensure an adequate nutritional status (29). Most older adults maintain eating habits that they established at younger ages (29). This may present a challenge to the dietitian, who may have to assist in altering their eating habits to meet current needs.

Causes of malnutrition in the elderly include ignorance of appropriate nutrition, financial restrictions, physical disabilities that interfere with the purchase and preparation of food, social isolation, mental disorders, loss of vision, chewing and swallowing difficulties, and changes in taste acuity. Other causes of malnutrition include malabsorption, anorexia, alcohol abuse, and long-term use of certain therapeutic drugs (29).

Approximately 5% of persons aged 65 years and older are institutionalized. Nutrition care of institutionalized elderly is directed at meeting their physiological and psychological needs. The nutrition assessment of elderly patients should consider the current nutritional status, as well as recent illnesses, surgeries, and changes in appetite, bowel function, and weight. Excellent sources of information regarding the clinical nutrition assessment of elderly individuals with chronic disease are available (13, 19, 32, 33).

▶ SUMMARY

Nutritional assessment is an important tool for evaluating health behavior. In the hands of a good interviewer, this assessment can be used to identify specific factors, such as lifestyle, taste, cultural background, disease, economic status, and ability to process food, that affect food intake and to use the information to help the patient achieve a positive behavior change (34).

Five of the leading causes of death in the United States are related to food practices; therefore, changes in these practices may have a significant effect on the health of the nation. By combining expertise in food and nutrition with a strong background in medical care and behavior modification techniques, medical nutrition therapy provided by a registered dietitian can help prevent or delay the development of disease.

References

1. Posthauer RD et al. Identifying patients at risk: ADA's definitions for nutrition screening and nutrition assessment. J Am Diet Assoc 94:838–839, 1994.
2. Simko MD, Cowell C, Gilbride JA. Nutrition Assessment: A Comprehensive Guide for Planning Intervention. Gaithersburg, MD: Apsen, 1995.
3. Detsky AS. Is this patient malnourished? JAMA 27:54–57, 1994.
4. Drewnowski A et al. Diet quality and dietary diversity in France: Implications for the French paradox. J Am Diet Assoc 96:663–669, 1996.
5. Chumlea WC, Roche AF, Mukherjee D. Nutritional Assessment of the Elderly Through Anthropometry. Columbus: Ross Laboratories, 1987.
6. Metropolitan Life Insurance Company. New weight standards for men and women. Stat Bull 40:1–4, 1959.

7. Metropolitan Life Foundation. 1983 Metropolitan height and weight tables. Stat Bull 64:2–9, 1983.

8. Dikovics A. Nutritional Assessment: Case Study Methods. Philadelphia: George F. Stickley, 1987.

9. Fidanza F. Nutritional Status Assessment: A Manual for Population Studies. New York: Chapman & Hall, 1991.

10. Kuskowska-Wolk A, Bergstrom R, Bostrom G. Relationship between questionnaire data and medical records of height, weight, and body mass index. Int J Obes 16:1–9, 1992.

11. Snetselaar LG. Nutrition counseling Skills: Assessment, Treatment, and Evaluation. Gaithersburg, MD: Aspen, 1989.

12. Israel DA, Moores S, eds. Beyond Nutrition Counseling. Chicago: American Dietetic Association, 1996.

13. American Dieteic Association. Medical Nutrition Therapy Across the Continuum of Care: Patient Protocols. Smyrna, GA: Morrision Health Care, 1996.

14. Gates G. Clinical reasoning: An essential component of dietetic practice. Top Clin Nutr 7(3):74–80, 1992.

15. King JW, Faulkner WR, eds. Critical Reviews in Clinical Laboratory Science. Cleveland: CRC, 1973.

16. American Dietetic Association Public Health Nutrition Dietetic Practice Group. Quality assurance criteria for nutritional care of prenatal women and adolescents. Atlanta: US Dept of Agriculture, Public Health Service, Centers for Disease Control and Prevention, Division of Nutrition, 1993.

17. Dietetics in Developmental and Psychiatric Disorders Dietetic Practice Group. Clinical Criteria and Indicators for Nutrition Services in Developmental Disabilities, Psychiatric Disorders, and Substance Abuse. Chicago: American Dietetic Association, 1993.

18. Dietitians in Pediatric Practice Dietetic Practice Group. Quality Assurance Criteria for Pediatric Nutrition Conditions. Chicago: American Dietetic Association, 1988.

19. Dwyer JT. Screening Older Americans' Nutritional Health: Current Practices and Future Possibilities. Washington: Nutrition Screening Initiative, 1991.

20. Franz MJ. Practice guidelines for nutrition care by dietetics practitioners for outpaients with non-insulin-dependent diabetes mellitus: Consensus statement. J Am Diet Assoc 92:1136, 1992.

21. Gerwick C, ed. Consultant Dietitians in Health Care Facilities Dietetic Practice Group. Nutrition Care in Nursing Facilities. Chigaco: American Dietetic Association, 1992.

22. Minimum Data Set (MDS) Manual. Natick, MA: Eliot, 1993.

23. Nutrition Services Payment Systems Committee. Reimbursement and Insurance Coverage for Nutrition Services. Chicago: American Dietetic Association, 1991.

24. Queen P, Caldwell M, Balogun L. Clinical indicators for oncology, cardiovascular and surgical patients: Report of the ADA Council on practice quality management committee. J Am Diet Assoc 93:338, 1993.

25. Wilkins K, Schiro K, eds. Renal Dietitians Dietetic Practice Group. Suggested Guidelines for Nutrition Care of Renal Patients. 2nd ed. Chicago: American Dietetic Association, 1992.

26. Winkler M, Lysen L, eds. Dietitians in Nutrition Support Dietetic Practice Group. Suggested Guidelines for Nutrition and Metabolic Management of Adult Patients Receiving Nutrition Support. Chicago: American Dietetic Association, 1993.

27. Trowbridge FL, Hiney CD, Robertson AD. Arm muscle indicators and creatinine excretion in children. Am J Clin Nutr 36:691–696, 1982.

28. Chen LC et al. Anthropometric assessment of energy-protein malnutrition and subsequent risk of mortality among preschool aged children. Am J Clin Nutr 33:1836–1845, 1980.

29. Mahan KL, Arlin M. Krause's Food Nutrition and Diet Therapy. 8th ed. Philapdelphia: Saunders, 1995.

30. American Diatetic Association. Nutrition intervention in the treatment of anorexia nervosa, bulimia nervosa, and binge eating. J Am Diet Assoc 94:902–907, 1994.

31. Berg F. Health risks of weight loss. Hennings, SD: Health Weight Journal, 1994.

32. Dietitian's Patient Education Manual. Gaithersburg, MD: Aspen Publishers, 1995.

33. Shils ME, Young VR. Modern Nutrition in Health and Disease. 8th ed. Philadelphia: Lea & Febiger, 1993.

34. Helm KK, Klawitter B, eds. Nutrition Therapy: Advanced Counseling skills. Lake Dallas, TX: Helm Seminars, 1995.

2.2.10

4.1.0.2

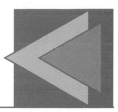

CHAPTER **47**

BASIC PRINCIPLES OF ELECTROCARDIOGRAPHY

John A. Larry and Stephen F. Schaal

Electrocardiography (ECG) is the study of the electrical events that occur in the heart. Despite the development of newer modalities that assist clinicians in evaluating cardiac disorders, the ECG has remained an invaluable diagnostic tool. By careful assessment of the ECG tracing, one may obtain information about the heart rate and rhythm, any chamber enlargement and conduction derangements, evidence of acute or previous myocardial infarctions, myocardial ischemia, drug and metabolic effects, and much more. The monitoring of the ECG during exercise is a valuable means of evaluating patients with chest pain.

Although much information can be obtained from ECG, it has limitations. A patient may have ECG abnormalities and have no underlying heart disease or exhibit a normal ECG in the setting of significant cardiac disease. It is therefore important to interpret the ECG in the context of the history and physical examination findings. This chapter provides an introductory discussion of ECG.

ACTION POTENTIALS

Electrical events occur because of the movement of ions across the membrane of the cell. In the resting phase, cardiac myocytes have a greater number of negatively charged ions within the cell, which results in a voltage difference across the cell membrane. This difference is called the transmembrane potential and is approximately -80 to -90mV. When the cell is stimulated, channels in the cell membrane open and allow positively charged sodium ions to enter the cell, causing depolarization (Fig. 47.1). The changes in membrane potential over time can be depicted as in Figure 47.2, a diagram of the action potential. Depolarization occurs during phase 0 of the action potential. The depolarization of one cell leads to the depolarization of neighbor-

ing cells; in this fashion an impulse (phase 1) is propagated through the heart. Once a cell depolarizes, it cannot depolarize again until repolarization has occurred. The time during which the cell cannot depolarize is termed the refractory period. Repolarization, the restoration of transmembrane potential, occurs during phases 2 and 3 of the action potential. Phase 4 is a quiescent phase for most cardiac cells. However, in certain cells, such as those at the sinus node, ions travel across the membrane during phase 4, resulting in a gradual decrease of the membrane potential. Once the voltage reaches a threshold level, depolarization occurs. Cells that possess this property of automaticity include the sinus node, atrioventricular (AV) node, and His-Purkinje fibers. The sinus node possesses the most rapid phase 4 depolarization causing it to depolarize first and thereby function as the pacemaker of the heart. The rate of phase 4 depolarization may be delayed by certain classes of medications, namely beta-blockers and some calcium channel antagonists, resulting in a slowing of the heart rate. Exercise, via enhanced sympathetic nervous system stimulation and elevated circulating catecholamines, increases the phase 4 depolarization rate, elevating the heart rate.

ECG measures the summation of the action potentials of the cardiac cells. The P wave is the summation of atrial action potentials, which the QRS complex is an aggregation of depolarization of the ventricular cells. Each depolarization can be thought of as a vector, a force with both direction and magnitude. Placing recording leads at different locations on the chest wall allows a variety of views of these electrical forces to be obtained. If the recording lead is parallel with the vector of depolarization, the maximum voltage is recorded. Conversely, if the recording lead is perpendicular to the vector, less displacement of the recording electrode takes place. By definition, electrical depolarization moving toward a positive lead produces an upright deflection on the ECG.

ELECTROCARDIOGRAPHIC LEADS

The standard ECG records the cardiac impulse using 12 leads. **Bipolar limb leads**, which were introduced by Einthoven, record the changes in voltage potentials occurring in the frontal plane. Lead I records the differences in potential between the left arm and the right arm, lead II between the left leg and the right arm, and lead III between the left leg and left arm. By definition, the right arm is the negative pole and the left arm is the positive pole for lead I; the right arm is negative and the left leg is positive for lead II; and the left arm is negative and the left leg is positive for lead III. Figure 47.3 depicts the locations and directions of the standard limb leads and illustrates

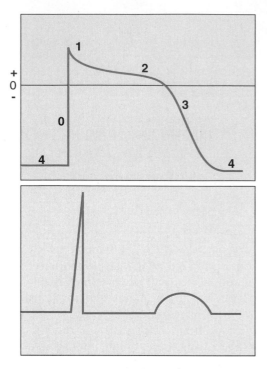

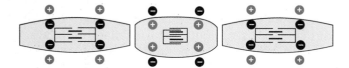

Figure 47.1. When the cell is stimulated, channels in the cell membrane open and allow positively charged sodium ions to enter the cell, causing depolarization. Repolarization is the restoration of transmembrane potential.

Figure 47.2. Changes in membrane potential over time.

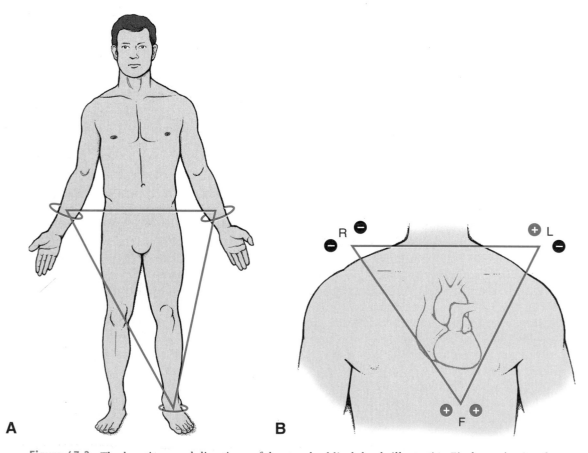

Figure 47.3. The locations and directions of the standard limb leads illustrating Einthoven's triangle.

Einthoven's triangle. Einthoven's law states that the sum of the complexes in leads I and III is equal to the complex in lead II.

$$Lead\ I\ +\ lead\ III\ =\ lead\ II$$

This rule is helpful in detecting situations of lead malposition or transposition.

The **unipolar limb leads** are created by connecting all three limb electrodes through a resistance of 5000 ohms to form a central terminal that for practical purposes is considered to have a zero potential (Fig. 47.4). The central terminal can be connected to an exploring electrode (designated by the letter V), where the potential difference recorded is dominated by local events. Potentials are recorded from the right arm (R), the left arm (L), and the left leg (F). Since this recorded voltage is quite low, the central terminal is disconnected from the location of the exploring electrode, augmenting the location of the exploring electrode augmenting the voltage recorded. These leads consequently are named aVR, aVL, and aVF.

Figure 47.5 depicts the location and direction of each lead in the frontal plane. Each lead has a positive and a negative pole. Leads I and aVL are considered the high lateral leads, while II, III, and aVF are the inferior or diaphragmatic leads. The positive directions of the limb

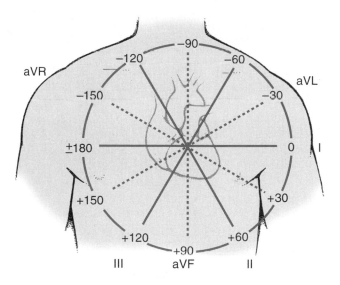

Figure 47.5. The hexaxial reference systems, depicting location and direction of each frontal plane lead.

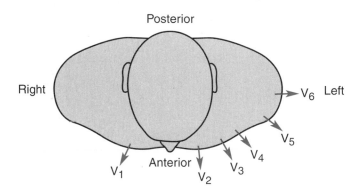

Figure 47.6. The exploring electrode is placed at various locations on the chest wall to allow evaluation of the anteroseptal, anterior, and anterolateral walls of the left ventricle. The positive direction of these leads are shown here.

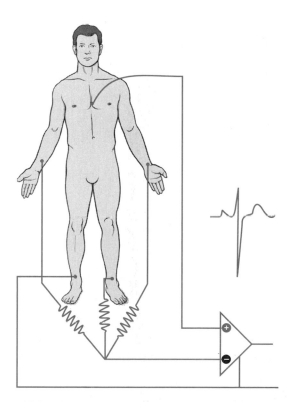

Figure 47.4. The unipolar limb leads are created by connecting all three limb electrodes through a resistance of 5000 ohms to form a central terminal that for practical purposes is considered to have zero potential.

leads are illustrated in Figure 47.5. Leads V1 through V6 are the precordial leads; they record electrical potentials in the transverse plane of the body. The exploring electrode is placed at various locations on the chest wall, which allows evaluation of the anteroseptal, anterior, and anterolateral walls of the left ventricle. The positive direction of these leads are shown in Figure 47.6.

PERFORMANCE OF AN ECG

The location of the recording leads is important, since minor variations in lead placement can significantly affect the ECG recording. The limb electrodes are attached to the appropriate wrists and ankles. The electrode attached to the right leg serves as a ground. Important landmarks on the chest wall are vital to correct precordial lead placement. These include the following:

1. The sternal angle (i.e., the junction between the manubrium and the sternum, at the level of the second rib)
2. The midclavicular line, halfway between the sternoclavicular and acromioclavicular joints
3. The anterior axillary line, an imaginary vertical line down the anterior fold of the axilla
4. The midaxillary line, an imaginary vertical line down the midportion of the axilla.

The standard placement of the unipolar precordial leads is depicted in Figure 47.7. The patient should be supine to achieve proper lead placement. Lead V1 is placed in the fourth intercostal space to the right of the sternum. Lead V2 is placed to the left of the sternum, also in the fourth intercostal space. Lead V4 should lie in the midclavicular line in the fifth intercostal space, with lead V3 halfway between leads V2 and V4. Leads V5 and V6 are aligned with the anterior axillary line and midaxillary line respectively at the level of lead V4.

The apposition of the ECG leads to the patient is quite important to ensure a technically good tracing and mini-mize artifacts. In some cases it may be necessary to shave the chest. Relative quiet is necessary to minimize skeletal muscle twitching and reduce the likelihood of recording artifact. The skin where the leads will be placed can be cleaned with alcohol and in some cases abraded gently with fine sandpaper or gauze after the alcohol evaporates to remove the top layer of skin. This improves the electrical conductance between the patient and the recording electrode.

The standard ECG paper is designed with horizontal and vertical lines at 1-mm intervals. At each 5-mm interval, the line on the grid is accentuated. The ECG is recorded at a speed of 25 mm/second and such that a 5-mm distance represents 0.2 seconds (200 msec). A 1-mm interval (each small box) is equivalent to 0.04 seconds or 40 msec. A 1-second interval is defined by 5 bold lines or large boxes.

The ECG is calibrated so that 1 mV recorded is represented by 10 mm of vertical deflection on the grid. In only rare instances, when the voltage is not totally recorded on the paper or too great to be displayed without merging with the lead above, should this be altered. All modern ECG recorders display a calibration signal. The vertical height is the standardization of a 1-mV signal. The calibration signal, 0.2 seconds in duration, documents the paper speed. A 5-mm width of the calibration signal confirms a paper speed of 25 mm/second.

Different ECG recorders display the standard 12 leads in varying formats. In the most common format, three leads are recorded simultaneously. The initial group consists of leads, I,II, and III, followed by leads aVR, aVL, and aVF, then V1, V2, and V3, and finally V4, V5, and V6. In addition to recording a 12-lead ECG, a rhythm strip can be recorded. A rhythm strip, a recording of a single lead or three leads simultaneously—usually leads V1, II, and V5— may be useful when a rhythm is unclear on the standard 12-lead ECG.

► SUMMARY

Proper technique is vital to obtain a high quality 12-lead ECG recording. The patient must be supine, the leads correctly placed with good contact to the chest wall and limbs, and the correct standardization of settings on the recorder must be employed. The standard 12-lead ECG comprises the standard limb leads (I, II, and III), the augmented limb leads (aVR, aVL, and aVF), and the precordial leads (V1 through V6). These leads record the summation of the electrical forces or vectors that are generated by depolarization of the myocardial cells.

Suggested Reading

Braunwald E. Heart Disease: A Textbook of Cardiovascular Medicine. 5th ed. Philadelphia: Saunders, 1997.

Wagner GS. Marriott's Practical Electrocardiography. 9th ed. Baltimore: Williams & Wilkins, 1994.

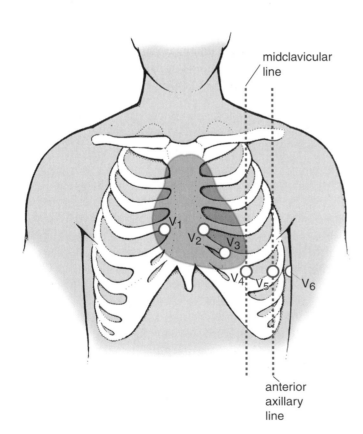

Figure 47.7. The standard placement of the unipolar precordial leads.

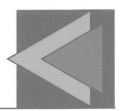

CHAPTER **48**

NORMAL ELECTROCARDIOGRAMS

John A. Larry and Stephen F. Schaal

ANATOMY OF THE CONDUCTION SYSTEM

The anatomy of the conduction system is depicted in Figure 48.1. The impulse that drives electrical depolarization of the heart originates in the sinoatrial (SA), or sinus node. This area is located in the right atrium near the superior vena cava. The wave of activity initially spreads in a radial fashion through the right atrium and subsequently the left atrium. The impulse reaches the atrioventricular (AV) node, an ovoid structure that lies at the base of the intra-atrial septum. The impulse takes approximately 100 ms to traverse the AV node and depolarize the bundle of His. In the normal heart, the AV node and the His bundle are the only point of connection between the atria and ventricles. The bundle of His extends through the fibrous skeleton of the heart into the superior portion of the intraventricular septum and divides into right and left bundles. The right bundle is quite discrete and travels down the right side of the interventricular septum and through the moderator band, beyond which it branches into the right ventricle. The left bundle divides into anterior and posterior divisions; in reality, these divisions are more complex and diffuse as they fan out into the left ventricle. The bundle branches terminate in Purkinje fibers (specialized cells that spread the electrical activity rapidly through the myocardium). The depolarization wave stimulates myocardial cells to contract by initiating a series of events referred to as excitation–contraction coupling.

ELECTROCARDIOGRAM NOMENCLATURE: THE NORMAL DEPOLARIZATION AND REPOLARIZATION SEQUENCE

A normal rhythm strip is depicted in Figure 48.2. The correlation between the electrical events and their electrocardiogram (ECG) manifestations is illustrated in Table 48.1. The electrical activity recorded during atrial depolarization is the P wave. Following the inscription of the P wave, the impulse travels through the AV node, the His bundle, and the Purkinje system. These structures are electrically silent on the surface ECG and are depolarized during the PR interval. The delay of the impulse through the AV node permits optimal contribution of atrial contraction to ventricular filling.

Depolarization of the myocardial cells of the ventricles generates the QRS complex. By definition, the initial downstroke of the QRS complex is designated the Q wave. The initial upstroke is termed the R wave. Depending on the lead and the underlying cardiac disease, the initial deflection from the baseline may be a Q wave or an R wave. The negative deflection that follows the R wave is an S wave.

The ST segment and the T wave are the surface correlates of repolarization of the cardiac myocytes (phases 2 and 3 of the action potential). The ST segment begins at the J point, the point separating the termination of the QRS complex from the ST segment. The J point is important because criteria established to evaluate ST segment changes during exercise testing (indicative of myocardial ischemia) use the J point as a reference. The T wave represents the completion of repolarization. During or shortly after repolarization, the myocardial cells will not depolarize again if presented with another stimulus. This period is called the refractory period.

Certain patients exhibit a U wave. The exact cause of this wave is not clearly defined, but investigators have suggested it may represent repolarization of the papillary muscles, Purkinje fibers, or special cells in the ventricle known as M cells.

VECTORS RESPONSIBLE FOR THE NORMAL ECG

The P wave exhibits certain characteristics when the depolarization originates in the sinus node. Because the sinus node is in the right superior portion of the right atrium, the initial atrial depolarization wave is directed leftward, inferiorly, and anteriorly. This results in an upright P wave in leads I, II, and aVL and an initial upright

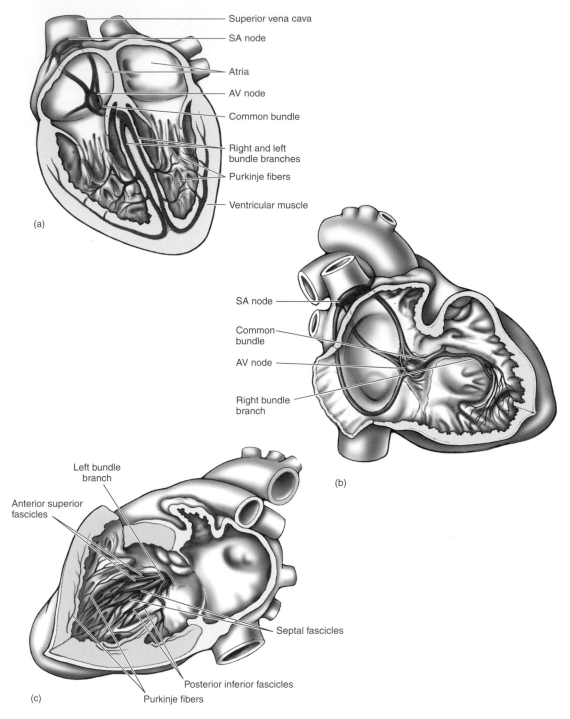

Superior vena cava

SA node

Atria

AV node

Common bundle

Right and left bundle branches

Purkinje fibers

Ventricular muscle

(a)

SA node

Common bundle

AV node

Right bundle branch

(b)

Left bundle branch

Anterior superior fascicles

Septal fascicles

Posterior inferior fascicles

Purkinje fibers

(c)

Figure 48.1. The anatomy of the conduction system.

deflection in lead VI (Fig. 48.3). Depolarization vectors moving toward the positive pole of a lead result in an upright deflection (see Chapter 46). As the impulse spreads to the left atrium, the mean vector of depolarization rotates posteriorly (the left atrium is posterior to the right atrium), causing the P wave in lead VI to become inverted. Consequently, a biphasic P wave is recorded in lead V1 in sinus rhythm with upright P waves in leads I, II, aVL, V5,

and V6. Other leads may exhibit some variability in P-wave morphology.

The vectors that generate the normal QRS complex are more complex than those responsible for the P wave. After the AV node and the bundle of His are depolarized, the impulse traverses the left and right bundle branches. The left bundle branch gives off branches to the septum first; thus the left side of the septum depolarizes earliest. Con-

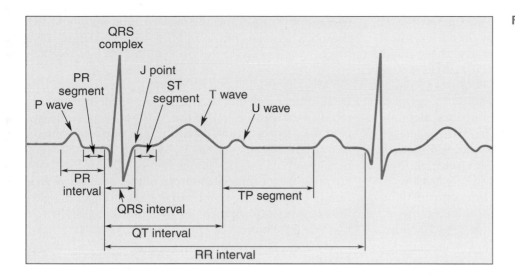

Figure 48.2. A normal rhythm strip.

Table 48.1. Normal Sequence of Depolarization and the ECG Correlation

Sinoatrial node	Silent
Atrial depolarization	P wave
Atrioventricular node	PR interval
His bundle	PR interval
Purkinje fibers	PR interval
Ventricular muscle depolarization	QRS complex
Ventricular isoelectric period	ST segment
Ventricular muscle repolarization	T wave

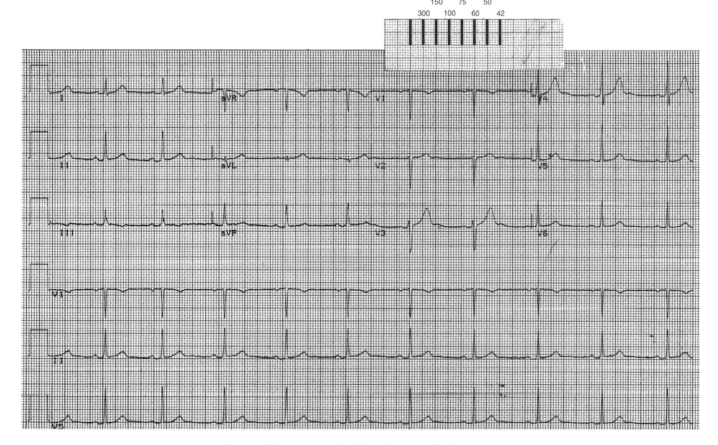

Figure 48.3. A normal EKG and 3-lead rhythm strip.

sequently, the impulse travels across the intraventricular septum from left to right, causing an initial vector directed superiorly, rightward, and anteriorly. This yields an initial force on the ECG depicted as small upright R waves in leads V1 and V2, and small, narrow Q waves may be noted in leads I, II, III, aVL, aVF, V5, and V6 (Fig. 48.3). Subsequently, the impulse travels through the right and left ventricles nearly simultaneously. Since the left ventricle has a much greater mass than the right ventricle, the electrical activity generated by the left ventricle overwhelms that of the right ventricle. This generates a vector directed leftward, posteriorly, and inferiorly. This inscribes an upright R wave in leads I, II, aVL, and the precordial leads; variable morphology in lead III; and a downgoing complex in lead aVR.

Repolarization is the regeneration of the membrane potential of the cardiac cells. The repolarization of the atrium occurs during depolarization of the ventricle and is therefore not seen on the ECG. Ventricular muscle repolarization generates the T wave. The ventricle depolarizes from endocardium to epicardium but repolarizes from epicardium to endocardium, producing a T wave vector that generally follows the QRS vector. Consequently, the T wave is typically upright when the QRS is upright and usually deflected downward when the QRS is downward (Fig. 48.3).

BASIC INTERPRETATION STRATEGY

Many recording systems provide a computer interpretation of the ECG, but they can be inaccurate and should not be relied upon as a final diagnostic tool. A systematic approach is necessary when interpreting ECGs.

Initial Assessment

Before beginning to interpret the ECG, it is necessary to check the name of the patient and the date and time the ECG was performed. It is useless to render an interpretation of the wrong patient; attributing findings to the wrong patient may have serious consequences. Once you are certain the tracing is the correct one, check the calibration signal to determine that the paper speed is 25 mm/second and that the amplitude of the signal is such that 1 mV is represented by 10 mm. The calibration signal displays 1 mV for 0.2 second. Consistency with Einthoven's law should be ensured (see Chapter 46).

Rate

The first step is to determine the ventricular rate in beats per minute (bpm). There are several methods to achieve this. One strategy is to mark off a 6-second period (30 heavy lines on the ECG grid), count the number of QRS complexes in that interval, and multiply by 10. This method is not efficient, but can be useful and should be used when the heart rate is irregular. A second method used when the rhythm is regular requires dividing 60,000

(the number of milliseconds in one minute) by the milliseconds between QRS complexes. This calculation yields bpm.

$$bpm = \frac{60,000 \ ms/minute}{ms/beat}$$

In addition, applying this principle for derivation of a rapid approach to estimate the heart rate is possible. If a complex occurs at every heavy line (i.e., one beat every 0.2 second) the rate is 300 bpm. If a complex occurs every second large box, the rate is one-half of 300, or 150 bpm. Frequent use of this method can allow rapid quantification of the heart rate by identifying the number of heavy lines between QRS complexes. In Figure 48.3, the ventricular rate is 80 bpm. A normal heart rate is 60–100 bpm.

Rhythm

The second step, evaluation of the rhythm, is performed after the ventricular rate is ascertained. To assess the rhythm, one must identify the P waves and QRS complexes and determine the relationship between them. In the example of normal sinus rhythm (Fig. 48.3), a single P wave is responsible for generating a single QRS complex. Furthermore, the P wave exhibits a normal vector. The P wave is upright in leads I, II, V5, and V6 and is biphasic in lead V1, with an initial upright deflection. These two criteria are required for a rhythm to be considered a normal sinus rhythm. The common arrhythmias are reviewed in Chapter 49.

Axis

The QRS axis in the frontal plane is simply the direction of the mean QRS vector. Determination of the axis requires knowledge of the vectors of each normal lead, as depicted in Figure 47.5. In young people, the axis may be nearly vertical (near +90°), but as people age, the axis moves gradually leftward and becomes more horizontal. Authors disagree mildly about the normal ranges for the QRS axis. The axis can be considered normal if it falls between −30° and ≤+100°. An axis between −30° and −90° is considered left axis deviation (Fig. 48.4). The pathological process causing left axis deviation is usually block of the left anterior division or divisions of the left bundle branch. An axis of +100° to 180° is termed right axis deviation. Tables 48.2 and 48.3 list the most common causes of right and left axis deviation. Axes falling between −90° and +180° may result from extreme left or right axis deviation and are quite uncommon.

Plotting the mean voltage of deflection for leads I, II, and III on a grid and drawing a line from the origin through the intersection of the three lines is an accurate method to determine the mean QRS axis. However, this method is time consuming. An alternative method can reliably and quickly approximate the mean axis. First, estimate the QRS axis by determining which of the four quadrants (created by the intersection of leads I and aVF) contains the maximum QRS positive voltage. This can be

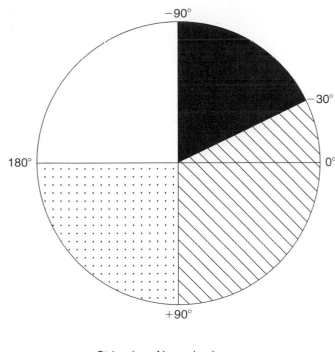

Striped — Normal axis
Solid — Left axis deviation
Dotted — Right axis deviation
White — Extreme right or
left axis deviation

Figure 48.4. Schematic depicting the ranges of normal axis, left axis deviation, right axis deviation, and extreme right or left axis deviation.

Table 48.2. Abnormalities Associated With Left Axis Deviation

Left anterior fascicular block
Left ventricular enlargement
Inferior myocardial infarction
Hypertensive heart disease
Cardiomyopathy
Congenital heart disease
Wolff-Parkinson-White syndrome

Adapted with permission from Marriott HL. Practical electrocardiography. 8th ed, 1988.

Table 48.3. Abnormalities Associated With Right Axis Deviation

Right ventricular enlargement
Left posterior fascicular block
Congenital heart disease
Mechanical shifts (i.e., emphysema, pneumothorax)
Dextrocardia
Wolff-Parkinson-White syndrome
Normal variant

Adapted with permission from Wagner GS. Marriott's Practical Electrocardiography. 9th ed. Baltimore: Williams & Wilkins, 1994.

quickly accomplished by looking at the QRS complex in leads I and aVF. If the predominant deflection of the QRS is positive in both, the axis must lie between 0° and +90°. If the complex is mainly upright in lead I but downward in lead aVF, the axis falls between 0° and −90°. Axes between +90° and +180° produce a downward complex in lead I and an upright complex in aVF. Once you have determined the quadrant in which the axis lies, find the limb lead that most nearly approximates a complex with equal upward and downward deflections. This is often called the isoelectric lead. A perpendicular line from this lead into the quadrant previously determined approximates the mean QRS axis. In Figure 48.4, the QRS complex is predominantly upright in lead I and mainly downward in lead aVF. Lead aVR is the most isoelectric lead, placing the axis at −60°, consistent with left axis deviation.

Intervals

The next step in the assessment of the ECG is the measurement of intervals. Figure 48.2 depicts the intervals measured on the ECG. The PR interval extends from the beginning of the P wave to the initial QRS deflection. This may be a Q wave or an R wave, depending on the morphology of the complex. This interval represents the time for the impulse to travel from the sinus node to the ventricles. Prolongation may reflect conduction abnormalities in the atrium, AV node, or His–Purkinje system. A normal PR interval in adults ranges from 120 to 200 ms. Each small box represents 40 ms. The normal PR interval may vary, depending on the relative contributions of the sympathetic and parasympathetic nervous systems and the effect of medications on conduction through the AV node. A PR interval greater than 200 ms is termed first-degree AV block, whereas a PR interval less than 120 ms is labeled a short PR syndrome.

The QRS interval may be measured in any limb lead. The QRS interval begins at the initial deviation from the baseline, either a Q wave or an R wave, and terminates at the end of the QRS, which may be an R wave or an S wave. A normal QRS interval is less than 100 ms. Common causes of prolongation of this interval include conduction defects such as bundle branch block, myocardial disease, and metabolic, electrolyte, and drug effects on the ventricular myocardium.

The QT interval encompasses both depolarization and repolarization of the ventricular muscle. It is measured from the onset of the QRS complex to the end of the T wave (Fig. 48.2). The QT interval is usually corrected for the ventricular rate by Bazett's formula:

$$QTc = \frac{measured\ QT\ interval}{square\ root\ of\ the\ R\text{-}R\ interval\ (ms)}$$

A normal corrected QT interval is less than 440 ms. This interval may be prolonged by certain medications, such as antiarrhythmic agents (quinidine, procainamide,

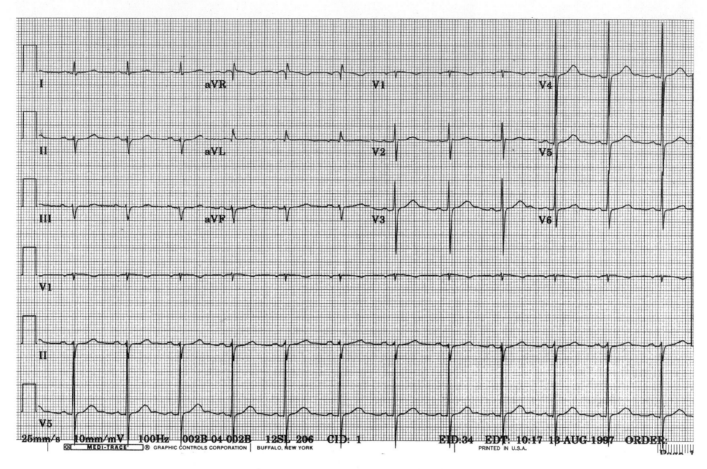

Figure 48.5. This ECG depicts an axis of −60° (left axis deviation).

disopyramide, sotalol, amiodarone), tricyclic antidepressants, electrolyte disorders (hypokalemia, hypocalcemia), ischemia, or myocardial disease. Congenital QT prolongation is associated with an increased risk of sudden cardiac death from a type of polymorphic ventricular tachycardia known as torsades de pointes.

Wave Form Analysis

The wave forms must be critically assessed in terms of their orientation, amplitude, contour, and position. The initial wave to interpret is the P wave. Knowledge of the basic vectors allows one to distinguish normal from abnormal. The initial vector is directed leftward, inferiorly, and anteriorly as the right atrium is depolarized, followed by a leftward, inferior, and posterior vector generated by left atrial depolarization. The mean P wave axis in the frontal plane is between 0° and 90°, meaning that the P wave must be upright in lead II if it originates from the sinus node. In addition to being upright in lead II, the P wave is upright in leads I, aVL, and V3–V6 and is biphasic (initially upright then downgoing) in lead V1. The other leads exhibit variable P-wave morphology. The amplitude of a normal P wave is usually less than 3 mm in lead II.

Next, note the QRS complexes and scan for any pathological Q waves. Small, narrow (<30 ms) Q waves in leads I, aVL, II, III, and aVF reflect the normal vector loop and do not indicate previous myocardial infarction. The progression of the height of the R wave should increase across the precordial leads, with the transition zone (the lead where the R wave becomes greater than the S wave) usually occurring at lead V4. The increase in height of the R wave from V1 to V6 reflects closer proximity to the left ventricle, which has greater mass than the right ventricle.

The ST segments should be evaluated in each lead. Typically, the ST segment should be isoelectric (on the baseline) at the level of the PR or TP segment. ST segment depression or elevation may be abnormal. Many entities may affect the ST segment such as conduction system abnormalities, ischemia, ventricular hypertrophy, medications such as digitalis, and electrolyte and metabolic disorders.

T wave evaluation primarily involves ascertaining the T wave vector. In general, the T wave is directed toward the QRS complex. Abnormally flattened or inverted T Waves (due to alteration of the T wave vector) may be caused by ischemia, infarction, hypertrophy, electrolyte disorders, hyperventilation, medications, and noncardiac illness.

► SUMMARY

A summary of the objective findings should be presented as the interpretation. The final interpretation must integrate the features into a common theme that includes consideration of the history and diagnosis. As in any area, repetition is the key to proficiency. Many hundreds of ECGs must be evaluated to achieve comfort with the numerous abnormalities and normal variants. Reading tracings in an organized fashion will allow the most accurate and concise interpretation.

Suggested Reading

Braunwald E. Heart Disease: A Textbook of Cardiovascular Medicine. 5th ed. Philadelphia: Saunders, 1997.

Wagner GS. Marriott's Practical Electrocardiography. 9th ed. Baltimore: Williams & Wilkins, 1994.

4.11.0.9, 4.11.2,   5.11.0, 5.11.1, 5.11.3
4.11.2.1, 4.11.2.2

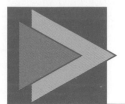

CHAPTER **49**

ISCHEMIA AND INFARCTION

John A. Larry and Stephen F. Schaal

One of the most prevalent uses of electrocardiography is the identification of patients with myocardial infarction or myocardial ischemia. Monitoring the electrocardiogram (ECG) during exercise testing is a commonly used technique to assess whether myocardial ischemia is the cause of chest discomfort.

MYOCARDIAL INFARCTION

Myocardial infarction results when blood flow to a region of heart muscle is interrupted by total occlusion of a coronary artery. ECG changes occur as a result of the impairment of flow to the myocardium. The initial manifestation is elevation of the ST segment and peaking of the T waves. The ST segment change is termed an injury current. The ST segments exhibit an upward convex shape as shown in Figure 49.1, an example of anterior myocardial injury. Within hours or days, the T waves invert and the ST segment gradually returns to baseline. Pathological Q waves or loss of R waves may develop in the involved leads, depending on the location and extent of myocardial damage. These may develop soon after the occlusion or take several days to evolve. Q waves or loss of R waves are caused by the loss of electrical activity that normally results from the depolarization of that region of myocardium. Myocardial infarctions that do not develop Q waves are termed non–Q wave infarcts. Patients with a non–Q wave infarct have a better short-term, but a worse long-term prognosis than patients with Q wave infarcts.

The age of the infarct may be determined in relative terms. When ST elevation or hyperacute T waves are identified, acute injury is present. When Q waves are present, the ST segments have returned to baseline, and the T waves remain inverted, the infarct is recent, between 2 weeks and 1 year old. These are often read as infarcts of indeterminate age. When the only manifestation is the presence of Q waves and no ST or T wave changes are present, the infarct is considered to be remote.

The ECG leads that exhibit changes permit determination of the region of myocardial infarction (Table 49.1). Figure 49.2 is an ECG from a patient with acute inferior

wall injury. Note the ST segment elevation in leads II, III, and aVF. Inspection of Figure 49.3 shows loss of R wave in the precordial leads consistent with an anterior wall myocardial infarction. The ST changes have resolved, but T wave inversions persist in leads V6, I, and aVL, suggesting that this is a recent but not acute infarction.

A common difficulty is differentiation of pathological Q waves from those resulting from the normal depolarization sequence of the myocardium. The location, depth, and width of the Q waves may be useful in this determinaton. As previously stated, the normal vector loop of depolarization results in small Q waves in leads I, II, III, aVL, aVF, V5, and V6. These deflections are typically quite small in amplitude and narrow in width (less than 30 ms). Significant Q waves are typically greater than 30 ms, often at least one-third the height of the R wave, and occur in contiguous leads that reflect a particular region of the heart.

Myocardial infarction is not the only entity affecting ST segments. Causes of ST segment elevation other than myocardial injury are common. Pericardial inflammation present in **acute pericarditis** (Figure 49.4) causes generalized ST segment elevation (all ECG leads), whereas acute injury due to an occluded coronary artery affects contiguous leads. In general, the ST segment typically has an upward concave appearance in pericarditis, whereas the appearance is convex upward in the setting of myocardial injury.

Benign repolarization variants (also called early repolarization) are another common cause of ST segment elevation. These variants are most commonly seen in young African-American men, but may be seen in other patients as well. Elevation of the J point from the baseline is present. The ST segments are elevated, but exhibit a concave upward appearance; this helps in the differentiation from myocardial injury (Figure 49.5).

Bundle branch blocks (see Figs. 50.21 and 50.22) also exert influence on the ST segment. In the left bundle, the ST vector is directed away from the QRS vector, resulting in elevated ST segments in the right precordial leads (see Fig. 50.22).

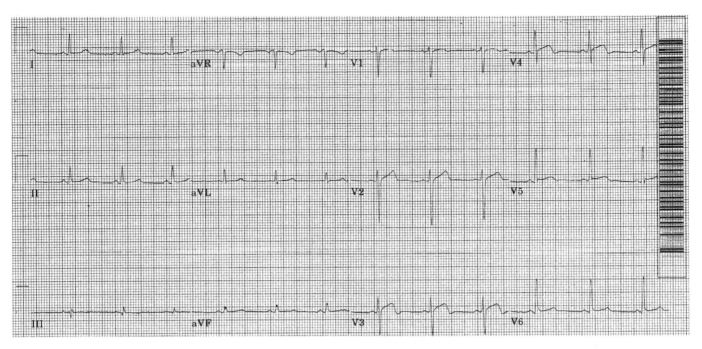

Figure 49.1. Acute anterolateral injury.

Table 49.1. Locations of Myocardial Infarction and Ischemia

LOCATION	LEADS AFFECTED
Anteroseptal	V1, V2
Anterior	V1–V4
Extensive anterior	V1–V6, I, aVL
Anterolateral	V3–V6, I, aVL
High lateral	I, aVL
Inferior	II, III, aVF
Posterior	V1, V2 (ST depression, tall R waves noted)

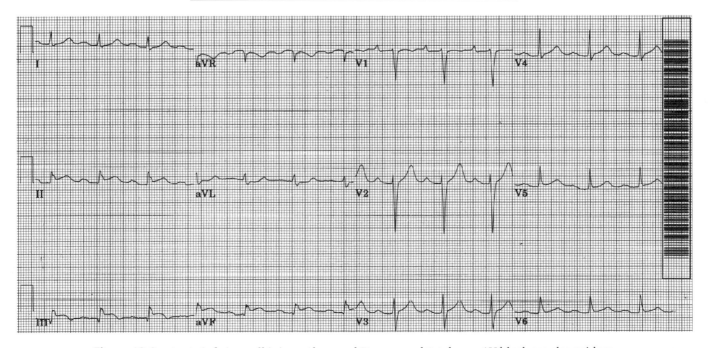

Figure 49.2. Acute inferior wall injury. Abnormal P waves and 1st degree AV block are also evident.

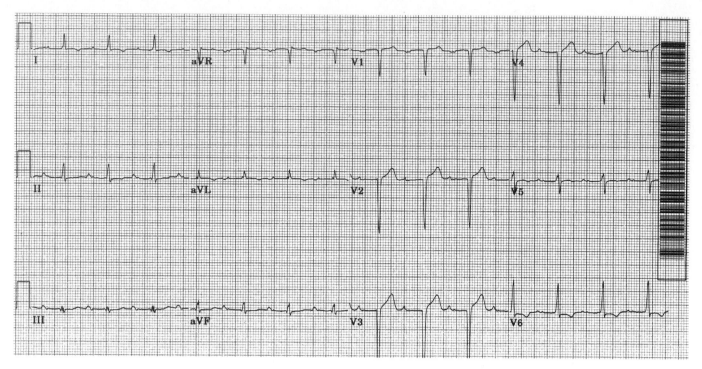

Figure 49.3.   Recent anterior wall myocardial infarction with left anterior fasicular block.

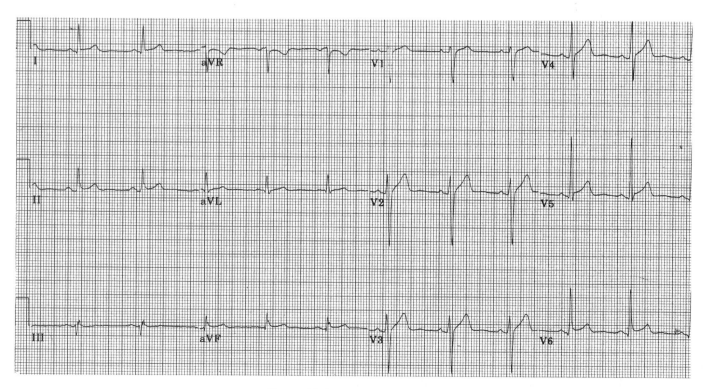

Figure 49.4.   Acute pericarditis.

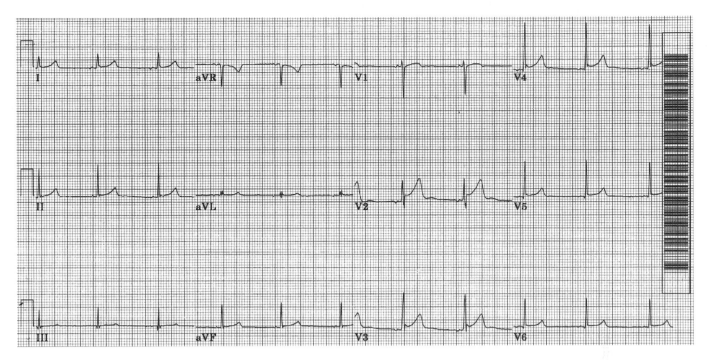

Figure 49.5. Benign repolarization variant.

Persistent ST segment elevation after an infarction may suggest **ventricular aneurysm** formation. This typically involves the anterior wall of the left ventricle and occurs after large infarcts. The presence of Q waves in the involved leads in a patient post-myocardial infarction suggests this diagnosis.

MYOCARDIAL ISCHEMIA

When the supply of blood flow is inadequate to meet the demands of the myocardium, myocardial ischemia results. The patient often has chest pain with exertion. ECG changes include ST segment depression and/or inversion of the T waves (Figure 49.6). Alteration in the ST segments

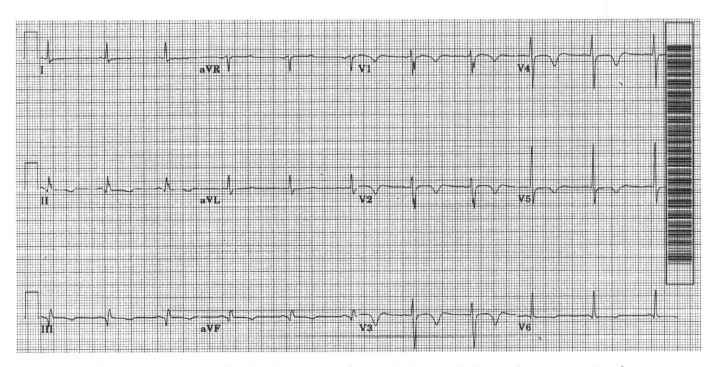

Figure 49.6. 54-year-old male with previous inferior wall MI now with T wave changes suggestive of anterolateral ischemia.

and T waves is in most cases nonspecific, as numerous factors may contribute to similar appearing ST segment and T wave changes. Symmetrically inverted T waves suggest ischemia, while other disorders typically cause asymmetrical inversion. Although many ECGs are interpreted as nonspecific ST and T wave changes, some of these changes may actually be the result of myocardial ischemia. The location of the ischemia may be determined by noting which leads exhibit the ST segment or T wave changes, as seen in Table 49.1.

EXERCISE ECG TESTING

Monitoring the ECG during exercise testing affords the opportunity to detect **arrhythmias** and to ascertain ischemic changes. Arrhythmias, discussed in Chaper 50, may be provoked during or after exercise. It is important for individuals performing exercise testing to be comfortable with the interpretation of these rhythm disorders and the advanced cardiac life support (ACLS) protocols to treat them.

The lead placement for an exercise ECG deviates slightly from the standard 12-lead ECG. The leads typically placed on the right and left wrists are moved proximally to the upper chest near the shoulders. The lower extremity leads are moved to the lower abdomen. These recording sites reduce the motion artifact that occurs with movement of the extremities during exercise.

A history and examination are necessary to rule out contraindications to exercise testing. ECG monitoring is continuous throughout the test and during the recovery. After exercise is initiated, a 12-lead ECG is recorded according to protocol and during any symptoms or change in heart rhythm. Monitoring should continue for 4 to 6 minutes during recovery or until changes on the ECG have resolved. Ischemia may induce several changes on the ECG; the most common change is ST segment depression. When baseline ST abnormalities exist, the test becomes less specific. In addition to the magnitude of change, the character of the ST depression is important. Up-sloping ST depression has less specificity for significant coronary disease than does horizontal or down-sloping ST depression. Several clinical and electrocardiographic criteria exist for termination of the exercise test.

Because the subendocardial area of the left ventricular apex region is most often rendered ischemic during exercise, the ST segment shifts in V4, V5, and V6 are the most sensitive for detection of ischemia.

▶ SUMMARY

ECG is useful in determining the presence of acute or remote infarctions and may detect resting ischemia. Combining exercise testing with ECG recording is a useful strategy to evaluate patients for exertional angina.

Suggested Reading

Braunwald E. Heart Disease: A Textbook of Cardiovascular Medicine. 5th ed Philadelphia: Saunders, 1997.

Wagner GS. Marriott's Practical Electrocardiography. 9th ed. Baltimore: Williams & Wilkins, 1994.

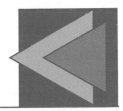

CHAPTER **50**

DYSRHYTHMIAS

John A. Larry and Stephen F. Schaal

The sinus node is typically responsible for initiating depolarization of the myocardium. The impulse generated then travels through the atria, atrioventricular (AV) node, His–bundle branch–Purkinje system, and finally the ventricular myocardium. However, in patients with structural heart disease, as well as those with normal hearts, deviations from the normal depolarization sequence occur. These abnormalities in heart rhythm are called arrhythmias (or dysrhythmias). Arrhythmias may be fast (tachyarrhythmia) or slow (bradyarrhythmia). This chapter examines the most common arrhythmias and the mechanisms responsible for their generation.

PREMATURE COMPLEXES

It is fairly common for patients to exhibit either premature atrial complexes (PACs) or premature ventricular complexes (PVCs), especially during exercise testing when catecholamine levels are increased. PACs occur when a site in the atrium other than the sinus node depolarizes prematurely (Fig. 50.1). The resulting impulse traverses the AV node, bundle of His, bundle branches, and Purkinje system and in the absence of bundle branch block or myocardial disease, generates a narrow QRS complex.

Occasionally the premature atrial complex occurs early enough that a portion of the conduction system may be refractory. If the impulse finds the AV node not recovered, the impulse extinguishes at that point, and no QRS complex results. These are *blocked PACs.* The block at the AV node is physiological if the PAC occurs quite early. If the AV node conducts the impulse but one of the bundle branches is refractory, the QRS complex exhibits features of a bundle branch block (discussed later in this chapter), a phenomenon termed *bundle branch aberration.* If one of the fascicles of the left bundle is refractory when the premature beat arrives, the QRS complex may exhibit features of left anterior fascicular or left posterior fascicular

block aberration. A normal sinus beat alternating with a premature atrial contraction is atrial bigeminy.

PVCs occur when a site in the ventricle fires before the next wave of depolarization from the sinus node reaches the ventricle (Fig. 50.2). These QRS complexes have bizarre, wide morphologies. Unlike PACs, these beats may not reset the periodicity of the sinus node; that is, the next sinus beat is often two cycle lengths from the beat prior to the PVC. A pattern of a sinus beat alternating with a PVC is ventricular bigeminy, and every third beat, ventricular trigeminy. PACs and PVCs may occur in patients with normal hearts during rest or exercise, or they may be markers of underlying cardiac disease.

MECHANISMS OF TACHYARRHYTHMIAS

Electrophysiological mechanisms responsible for the generation of most cardiac arrhythmias have been identified as circus re-entry, enhanced automaticity, and triggered activity. The substrate for re-entry requires two pathways for current to travel. The first pathway depolarizes rapidly and recovers slowly, while the second depolarizes slowly, but recovers rapidly (Fig. 50.3). Re-entry occurs when an area of altered conduction exists and unidirectional block occurs. If an impulse arrives prematurely at a time when the slow pathway has recovered, but the fast pathway is refractory (not recovered from the previous depolarization), the impulse conducts over the slow pathway. If conduction over the slow pathway reaches the fast pathway when recovered, the impulse may travel retrograde over the fast pathway. If the slow pathway has recovered, depolarization of the slow path occurs, and a re-entrant loop is established.

Enhanced automaticity is another mechanism responsible for the generation of arrhythmias. In this situation, an increased rate of phase 4 depolarization (see Figure 47.2) of a myocardial cell occurs, thereby reaching the threshold potential more rapidly than usual. The cell

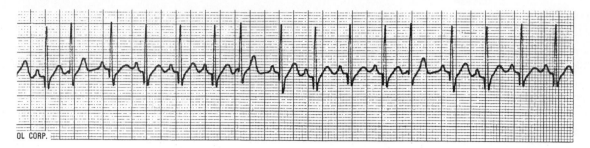

Figure 50.1. Sinus tachycardia with frequent PACs.

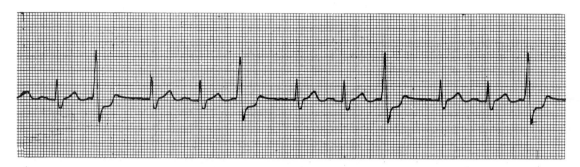

Figure 50.2. Normal sinus rhythm with PVCs.

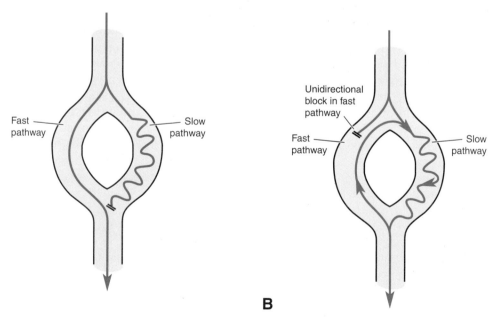

A   **B**

Figure 50.3. Substrate for re-entrant arrhythmias. **A.** Normal depolarization wave arrives, finding both fast and slow pathways recovered from previous depolarization. Impulse travels via fast pathway to distal conducting tissue. **B.** A premature beat blocks in the fast pathway but is able to travel over the slow pathway, which has a short refractory period. The impulse travels to the distal conducting tissue and also retrograde over the fast pathway, which by this time has recovered. If the slow pathway is recovered, a reentrant loop is generated, resulting in tachycardia.

depolarizes, and the impulse generated depolarizes the remainder of the myocardium.

A third mechanism of arrhythmias is called triggered activity, which exhibits features of both re-entry and automaticity. Myocardial cells may exhibit after-depolarization or increases in the membrane potential that occur during the repolarization phase of the action potential. These depolarizations can be characterized as early, occurring during phase 3, and late, occurring after phase 3. If the magnitude of these after-depolarizations is great enough, depolarization may be triggered. Early after-depolarizations are related to conditions that prolong the action potential, such as antiarrhythmic agents (type IA and III drugs), and electrolyte disorders, such as hypokalemia and hypomagenesemia. Generally, the tachycardia develops after a pause. Delayed after-depolarizations occur in the setting of myocardial ischemia, digitalis toxicity, and congenital long QT syndromes. These after-depolarizations are tachycardia dependent and high catecholamine states contribute to the development of the tachycardia.

Circus re-entry, enhanced automaticity, and triggered activity may occur in any portion of the myocardium or specialized conducting tissue. The atrial myocardium, ventricular myocardium, sinoatrial (SA) node, atrioventricular (AV) node, and the His–Purkinje system all may be susceptible to variations in conduction. The location of the abnormality and the underlying cardiac substrate govern the type of arrhythmia and its properties.

TYPES OF TACHYARRHYTHMIAS
Sinus Tachycardia

Sinus tachycardia (Fig. 50.4) is the result of enhancement of the rate of firing of the sinus node. The sinus node is under the control of the parasympathetic and sympathetic nervous systems and will therefore accelerate or decelerate depending on the physiological requirements. Sinus tachycardia results when increased activity of the sympathetic nervous system is present. These include situations such as fear, exercise, fever, hypovolemia, bleeding, thyrotoxicosis, hypoxia, or other acute illness. Decreased stroke volume in severe left ventricular dysfunction may also result in sinus tachycardia, since the sympathetic nervous system is activated in an attempt to preserve adequate cardiac output.

Three key features of sinus tachycardia are important. First, patients typically exhibit a gradual increase in heart rate (i.e., sudden acceleration from 80 beats per minute to 150 beats per minute does not occur). Second, although exceptions occur, the sinus rate typically does not exceed the maximum rate as calculated by this formula: **Maximum heart rate = 220 − the age.** Finally, the P wave vector must be normal.

Atrial Fibrillation

Atrial fibrillation (Fig. 50.5), a relatively common arrhythmia, is the result of multiple re-entrant waves of electrical activity in the atria. These depolarization waves do not result in organized atrial contraction, and the appearance of the atria has been described as a bag of worms when in fibrillation. The AV node is stimulated at frequent and irregular intervals by the very rapid atrial activity, resulting in an irregular ventricular rate (R-R response). The rate of the ventricular response is governed by the AV node's refractory period. The hallmarks of atrial fibrillation are the absence of organized P wave activity and an irregular ventricular response. This rhythm has important consequences for the patient: the absence of a properly timed atrial contraction results in decline of the cardiac output (as much as 20% in those with relatively normal ventricles). In patients with cardiac disease, the cardiac

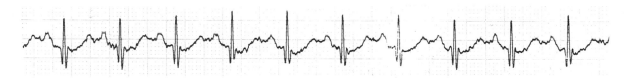

Figure 50.4. Sinus tachycardia.

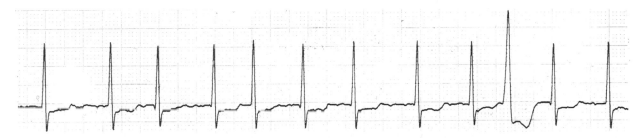

Figure 50.5. Atrial fibrillation with rapid ventricular response. The wide QRS complex likely represents aberrant ventricular conduction, although a PVC cannot be excluded.

output may decline by up to 40%. Atrial fibrillation may compromise ability to perform physical activities.

In addition, patients with atrial fibrillation are at increased risk for developing atrial thrombus that may embolize to the brain, kidneys, a peripheral artery, etc. The incidence of embolic stroke in patients with atrial fibrillation is fivefold the incidence among age-matched patients in normal sinus rhythm.

Treatment of atrial fibrillation focuses initially on decreasing the ventricular response with agents such as digitalis, calcium channel blockers (specifically diltiazem and verapamil), and beta-blockers, which prolong the refractory period of the AV node. Anticoagulation is necessary prior to the restoration of normal sinus rhythm, which is usually attempted with type IA, IC, or III antiarrythmic agents, namely quinidine, propafenone, sotalol, or amiodarone. Electrical cardioversion is required if the rhythm does not convert to normal sinus rhythm with the use of an antiarrhythmic drug.

Most patients with atrial fibrillation have underlying cardiac disease. A list of the common causes is presented in Table 50.1. Rarely, a patient has lone atrial fibrillation, in which the arrhythmia exists in the absence of structural heart disease or other definable trigger. Because of the presence of underlying cardiac disease, even when sinus rhythm has been restored, almost 50% of patients have reverted to atrial fibrillation 1 year later.

Atrial Flutter

Atrial flutter (Fig. 50.6) classically results from a macro–re-entrant circuit in the atria, generating flutter waves at a rate of 250–350 atrial depolarizations per minute. The atrial waves are typically best seen in the inferior leads (II, III, aVF) and lead V1. As in atrial fibrillation, the ventricular rate depends on the refractory period of the AV node, and the QRS complexes may be regular or irregular depending on whether a fixed or variable relationship exists between the atria and ventricles. The classic appearance of this rhythm is the sawtooth shape of the flutter waves in the inferior leads at a rates of 250–350 per minute. In the absence of medications or disease of the AV node, 2:1 block exists, so that one of every two atrial flutter waves is conducted to the ventricle. Consequently, whenever a ventricular rate near 150 beats per minute is detected, the tracing must be scrutinized for atrial flutter waves. The same underlying causes listed in Table 50.1 for atrial fibrillation apply to atrial flutter. In general, this rhythm may not persist for extended periods but often converts to sinus rhythm or more commonly degenerates into atrial fibrillation.

Patients with hypoxemia, hypokalemia, and other metabolic abnormalities, as occasionally seen in chronic obstructive lung disease or congestive heart failure, may exhibit a rhythm known as **multifocal atrial tachycardia** (Fig. 50.7). This rhythm is likely due to multiple sites within the atrium functioning as the pacemaker of the heart, thereby generating multiple P wave morphologies. The AV node is stimulated at variable intervals by the atrial impulses, leading to irregular, narrow QRS complexes. Recognition of this rhythm depends on defining at least three different P wave morphologies in the same lead with an irregular and usually rapid ventricular response.

Atrioventricular Nodal Re-entrant Tachycardia

Atrioventricular nodal reentrant tachycardia (AVNRT) is a narrow complex tachycardia that occurs when a patient has two functional pathways in the AV node region. The pathways exhibit the classic characteristics that promote re-entry: a fast pathway that depolarizes rapidly but recovers slowly and a slow pathway that depolarizes slowly but recovers quickly. The initiation of this rhythm is usually a premature atrial contraction timed so that it finds the fast pathway refractory and the slow pathway recovered. The PAC blocks in the fast pathway and conducts down the slow pathway. After the slow pathway depolarizes, the fast pathway has recovered, allowing the impulse to conduct in a retrograde fashion to the atria and again arrive at the slow pathway. This results in a re-entrant loop of depolarization traveling down the slow pathway

---

Table 50.1. Cardiac and Noncardiac Conditions Predisposing to Atrial Dysrhythmias

Hypertensive heart disease
Valvular heart disease
Ischemic heart disease
Cardiomyopathy
Congenital heart disease
Conduction system disease
Pericarditis
Thyrotoxicosis
Pulmonary embolus
Hypoxia
Holiday heart syndrome
Sepsis

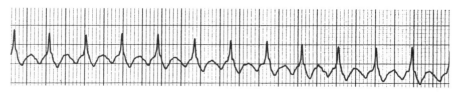

Figure 50.6. Atrial flutter with 2:1 AV conduction. Note the "sawtooth" pattern of the atrial flutter waves.

and up the fast pathway. The atria and ventricles are depolarized nearly simultaneously. The P waves are typically inverted in the inferior leads (the atria are depolarized in a retrograde fashion from the AV node with the vector going superiorly) and may occur shortly after the QRS complex or even simultaneously with the QRS complex, so that the P wave cannot be visualized on the surface ECG (Fig. 50.8).

Atrioventricular Re-entrant Tachycardia

Atrioventricular re-entrant tachycardia (AVRT) occurs in the setting of the substrate of an accessory pathway (AP). The AP is a muscle bridge of connection between the atria and ventricles. The onset of the tachycardia occurs when a PAC conducts over the AV node and returns to the atrium via retrograde conduction over the AP. Alternatively, depolarization from a PVC may travel retrograde over the accessory pathway, stimulating the atrium, and return antegrade down the AV node. The P waves are typically at some interval after the QRS complex, usually greater than 100 ms (Fig. 50.9).

Atrial Tachycardia

Atrial tachycardia (Fig. 50.10) may be the result of rapid firing of an automatic or triggered atrial focus or re-entry within the atrium. The ventricular rate depends on the atrial rate and the refractory period of the AV node. The P wave has altered morphology (exhibits a different vector from sinus rhythm), and the PR interval is often short.

Ventricular Tachycardia

Ventricular tachycardia (Figs. 50.11 and 50.12) is typically seen in patients with underlying heart disease, most

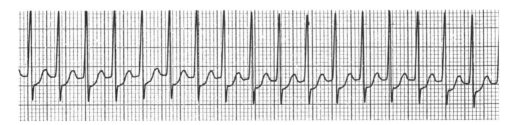

Figure 50.7. Multifocal atrial tachycardia.

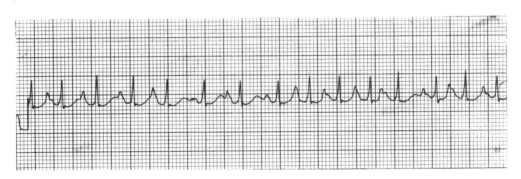

Figure 50.8. AV nodal re-entrant tachycardia. The P wave is buried in the QRS complex.

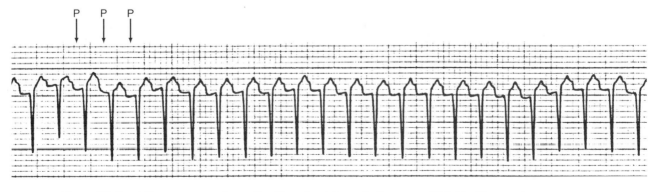

Figure 50.9. AV re-entrant tachycardia. Note the retrograde P waves within the T wave.

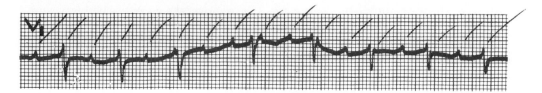

Figure 50.10. Atrial tachycardia with variable AV block. Markers label the atrial activity.

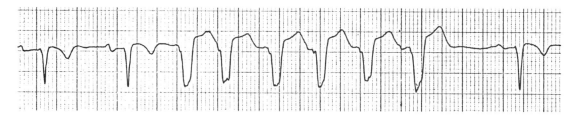

Figure 50.11. Normal sinus rhythm with a run of nonsustained ventricular tachycardia.

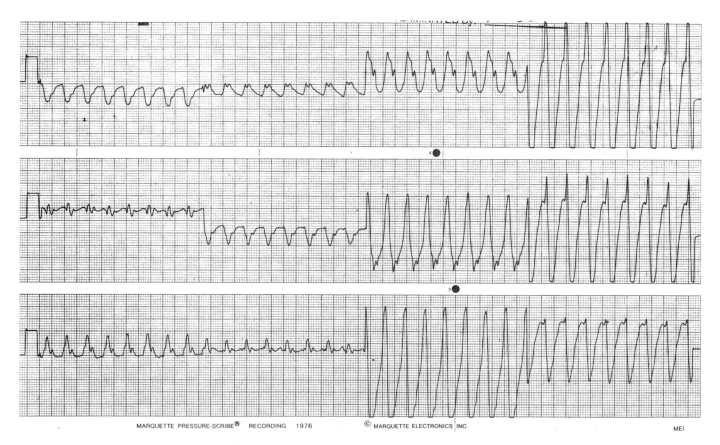

MARQUETTE PRESSURE-SCRIBE® RECORDING 1976   © MARQUETTE ELECTRONICS INC.   MEI

Figure 50.12. Sustained ventricular tachycardia.

commonly coronary artery disease with previous myocardial infarction or cardiomyopathy. Three or more consecutive ventricular beats at 100 beats per minute defines ventricular tachycardia. Nonsustained ventricular tachycardia is a run of tachycardia lasting less than 30 seconds. Sustained ventricular tachycardia is tachycardia lasting longer than 30 seconds or terminated because of hemodynamic consequences prior to 30 seconds. Ventricular tachycardia is usually recognized by the presence of a wide QRS complex (120 ms or greater), AV dissociation (the P waves and QRS complexes have no relationship), and a QRS complex that does not have the morphology of typical bundle branch block. Re-entry is the most common mechanism of ventricular tachycardia; however, abnormal automaticity or triggered activity due to afterdepolarizations may be responsible. Depending on the cardiac and hemodynamic status of the patient and the rate of the tachycardia, the patient may have normal blood pressure with minimal to no symptoms or be in cardiac arrest requiring immediate cardioversion.

Torsade de Pointes

Torsade de pointes is a type of ventricular tachycardia named because the morphology of the ventricular tachycardia exhibits a twisting of the points. An example of this rhythm is shown in Fig. 50.13.

Ventricular Fibrillation

Ventricular fibrillation (Fig. 50.14) is a life-threatening rhythm that must be treated with immediate electrical defibrillation per advanced cardiac life support protocol.

BRADYARRHYTHMIAS AND DISORDERS OF THE CONDUCTION SYSTEM

Sinus Node Dysfunction

Sinus bradycardia (Fig. 50.15) occurs when the impulse originates from the sinus node at a rate less than 60 beats per minute. This may be seen in individuals who are well trained and exhibit high parasympathetic (vagal) tone, in patients who are receiving drugs that slow the heart rate (e.g., beta-blockers), or in individuals who have disease of the sinus node (sick sinus syndrome).

Sinus pauses may be due to high vagal tone or disease of the sinus node. If the pause interval is a multiple of the intrinsic sinus rate, one may suspect **sinus exit block**. In this instance, the sinus node fires but the impulse does not conduct through the perisinus nodal tissue, and the atrium is not depolarized. **Sinus arrhythmia**, a variation of the rate of firing of the sinus node, is commonly seen in younger persons and does not reflect disease of the sinus node.

If the sinus node fails and none of the atrial cell take over the pacemaker role, the AV junction (His bundle region) may assume the role of pacemaker, resulting in a **junctional rhythm** (Fig. 50.16). This rhythm is typified by narrow QRS complexes at regular intervals; the P waves often are generated by retrograde atrial conduction. P waves may occur during or after the transcription of the QRS complex. Typically the AV junction has a much slower phase 4 depolarization than the sinus node. Therefore, the normal junctional rate ranges between 40 to 60 beats per minute. Occasionally, the rate is more than 60 beats per minute; the rhythm is called **junctional tachycardia** or **accelerated junctional rhythm**.

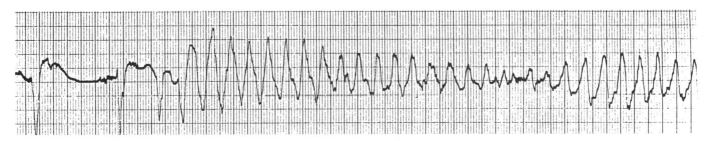

Figure 50.13. Torsade de pointes.

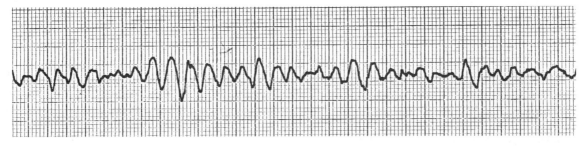

Figure 50.14. Ventricular fibrillation (coarse).

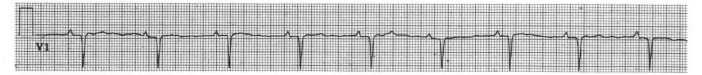

Figure 50.15. Sinus bradycardia.

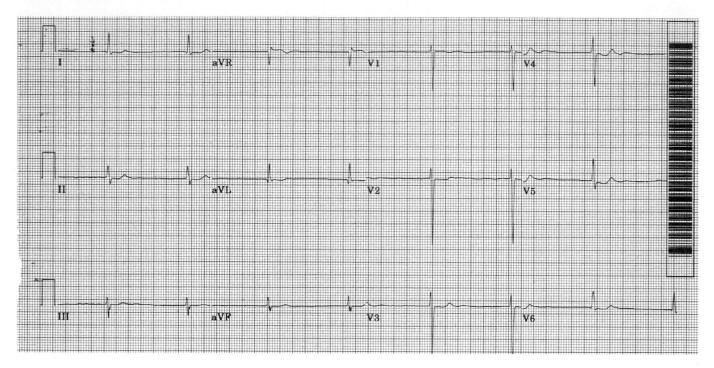

Figure 50.16. Junctional rhythm.

Disorders of the AV node and His–Purkinje system

AV nodal disease may be due to a number of causes: infarction, ischemia, primary conduction system disease, and medication effect are the most common. The types of AV block are classified as follows:

- **First-degree AV block** is simply prolongation of the PR interval (see Fig. 48.3). This may be the result of intra-atrial or interatrial conduction delay, delayed conduction through the AV node, impaired conduction through the His-Purkinje system, or a combination of these.
- **Second-degree AV block** may be divided into two types: *Mobitz type I* and *Mobitz type II*. In type I, also known as Wenckebach, the disease process is usually in the AV node. In Mobitz type I, the PR interval progressively lengthens with each beat until a P wave is not conducted to the ventricles (Fig. 50.17). In type II block, the disease usually is below the AV node in the His bundle–bundle branch region. The PR interval is fixed until a P wave is not conducted to the ventricles (Fig. 50.18). Type II block is often associated with a wide QRS complex. A rhythm disorder that may cause confusion is called *2:1 AV block* (Fig. 50.19). The con-

fusion arises with the semantics used to describe *arrhythmias*. Constant 2:1 AV block may indicate second-degree type I or second-degree type II. Although the width of the QRS complex may be helpful, it is impossible to distinguish whether a progressively prolonging PR interval with a dropped beat or a fixed PR interval with every other beat dropped is present unless the onset or offset of 2:1 AV block is recorded. Further confusion results in the setting in which atrial flutter is present with 2:1 AV block. In this setting, no disease of the AV nodal–His bundle system exists; the refractory period of the normal AV node prevents the atrial impulses from reaching the ventricle in a one-to-one relationship. Therefore depending on the clinical setting, 2:1 AV block may indicate disease below the AV node, disease in the AV node, or no disease.

- **Third-degree** or **complete heart block** occurs when the atrial activity is unable to traverse the AV junction to generate a QRS complex (Fig. 50.20). The atrial rate is faster than the ventricular rate, and the P waves have no influence on the QRS complexes. Depending on the site of origin of the QRS complexes, the QRS complexes may be narrow or wide.

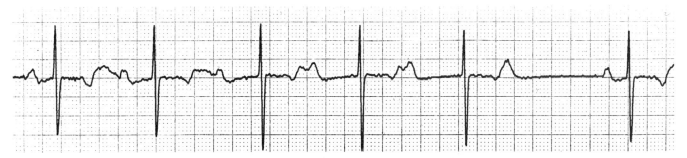

Figure 50.17. Second-degree Type I AV block (Wenckebach).

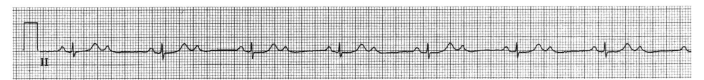

Figure 50.18. Second-degree AV block, type II.

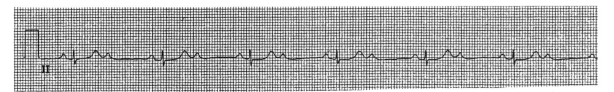

Figure 50.19. 2:1 AV block.

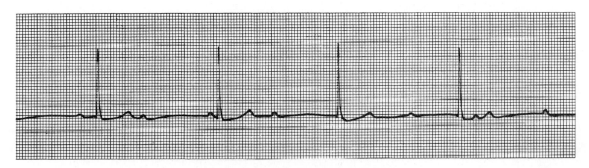

Figure 50.20. Complete heart block.

DISORDERS OF THE BUNDLE BRANCHES AND FASICLES

Bundle Branch Blocks

When one of the bundle branches is diseased, the QRS complex is wide (greater then 120 ms). Wide QRS complexes may result from disease in the bundle branches, abnormalities of the ventricular myocardium, or the effects of drugs, electrolyte, or metabolic disorders on the ventricular myocardium. Depending on the morphology of the QRS complex, these may be characterized as right bundle branch block, left bundle branch block, or nonspecific interventricular conduction defects.

In **right bundle branch block** (Fig. 50.21), activation of the left ventricle occurs prior to that of the right ventricle. The initial force due to left-to-right activation of the septum is normal. Consequently, the small Q waves seen in the inferior and lateral leads and the small R waves seen in leads V1 and V2 are unchanged. After the septum is depolarized, the impulse travels through the mass of the left ventricle, generating the initial portion of the QRS complex. After the left ventricle has been partially depolarized, the right ventricle depolarizes, resulting in a terminal vector that is directed anteriorly and rightward. This results in a triphasic impulse in lead V1, often described as a rabbit ears configuration or an RSR complex. The abnormal depolarization results in abnormal repolarization with ST and T wave vectors directed away from the QRS complex in leads V1,V2, and sometimes V3. Right bundle branch block does not prohibit electrocardiographic interpretation of ST changes in leads other than V1,V2, and V3 during an exercise test.

In **left bundle branch block** (Fig. 50.22), the initial force travels across the septum from right to left, altering the initial QRS deflection. This results in an initial negative deflection in lead VI and an initial upright deflection in lead V6. As the remainder of the left ventricle is depolarized, the QRS vector continues to be toward V6. The depolarization of the right ventricle is mainly obscured by that of the left ventricle; therefore, little effect of right ventricle depolarization on the vector forces is noted. The repolarization pattern is altered in left bundle branch block, with the ST and T vector directed rightward and anteriorly. Consequently, the electrocardiogram may not be used to ascertain ischemic changes during an exercise study.

A QRS greater than 120 ms without the morphology of right or left bundle branch block is best termed a nonspecific intraventricular conduction delay.

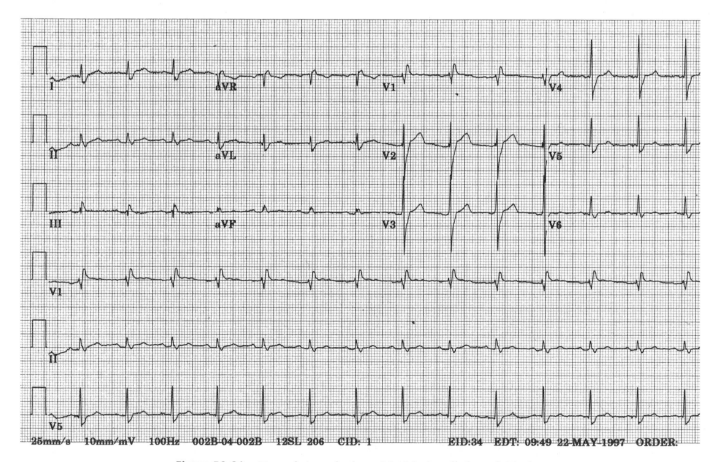

Figure 50.21. Normal sinus rhythm with right bundle branch block.

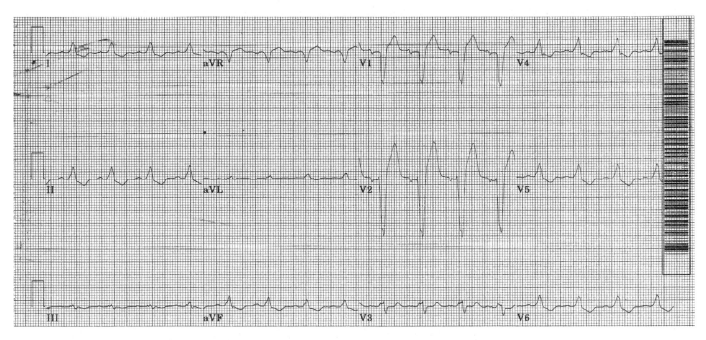

Figure 50.22. Normal sinus rhythm with left bundle branch block.

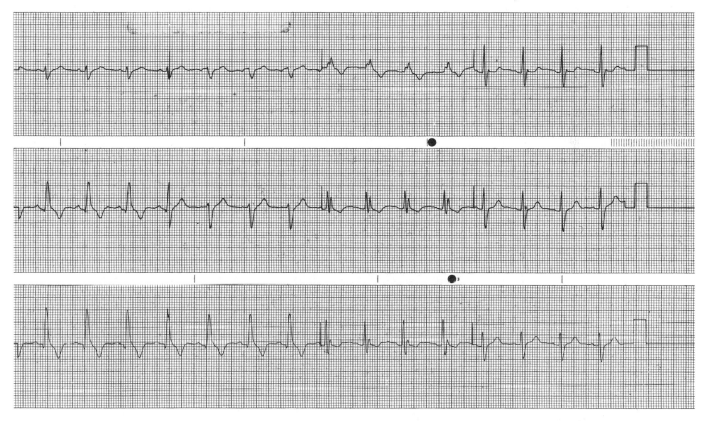

Figure 50.23. Normal sinus rhythm with right bundle branch block and left posterior fascicular block.

Fascicular Blocks

Disease in the fasicles of the left bundle branch results in minimal prolongation of the QRS complex. Fascicular block (hemiblocks) are recognized by their effects on the frontal plane axis. **Left anterior fascicular block** (see Fig. 47.4) causes significant left axis deviation (greater than − 30°), resulting in small Q waves in lead I and aVL and small R waves in leads II, III, and aVF. **Left posterior**

fascicular block (Fig. 50.23) produces right axis deviation, (usually 90–110°) with small Q waves in leads II, III, and aVF and a small R waves in leads I and aVL. Unlike left bundle branch, these entities have no adverse effect on the ability to interpret electrocardiographic changes during an exercise test.

► **SUMMARY**

Many derangements in the normal depolarization sequence may occur. Three mechanisms for arrhythmia genesis have been described. By careful interpretation of the relationship between the P waves and QRS complexes and the effect on other aspects of the ECG (i.e., axis, intervals, complex width and P wave and QRS vectors) one may readily ascertain the causes of tachyarrhythmias, bradyarrhythmias, and atrioventricular and interventricular conduction defects.

Suggested Reading

Braunwald E. Heart Disease: A Textbook of Cardiovascular Medicine. 5th ed Philadelphia: Saunders, 1997.

Wagner GS. Marriott's Practical Electrocardiography. 9th ed. Baltimore: Williams & Wilkins, 1994.

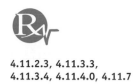

CHAPTER **51**

OTHER ABNORMAL ELECTROCARDIOGRAMS

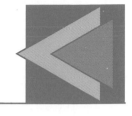

John A. Larry and Stephen F. Schaal

Many common pathologies of the heart cause changes in the electrocardiogram (ECG). These include hypertrophic patterns, ECG changes mediated by pharmacological agents or by electrolyte disorders, and conduction defects, which often require pacemakers for correction and treatment. Some of the more common ECG patterns associated with them are discussed below.

VENTRICULAR HYPERTROPHY

While echocardiography remains the gold standard, ECG can determine chamber enlargement with a reasonable degree of accuracy. Various criteria have different degrees of sensitivity and specificity. There follows a discussion of the most commonly used criteria that have reasonable sensitivity and specificity for determining ventricular hypertrophy.

Left Ventricular Hypertrophy

Left ventricular hypertrophy (LVH) or enlargement (Fig. 51.1), as detected by ECG, is associated with two mechanisms: hypertrophy of the walls and dilation of the chamber. LVH is an important ECG finding, as it has been associated with increased morbidity and mortality. The terms enlargement and hypertrophy are often used interchangeably, although some experts do distinguish these entities. The best known criteria for determining LVH are the **Estes criteria** (Table 51.1). This is a weighted scoring system in which points are assigned for certain characteristics. Increased voltage is the result of a greater mass of myocardium, which must be depolarized. Repolarization changes that develop with LVH classically are described as a strain pattern. The ST segments are depressed, but exhibit an upward convexity and blend into a biphasic or inverted T wave. This pattern is most commonly seen in the inferior and lateral leads. Often, left atrial enlargement can be found in association with LVH. The QRS width may increase, and the time from the R wave to the S wave, the **intrinisicoid deflection**, also may increase. The tracing in Figure 51.1 would receive 11 points by the Estes scoring.

The **Scott criteria** (Table 51.2), another commonly used method for ECG analysis, are simpler to use. The voltage changes caused by the left ventricular enlargement are measured and used as an index for left ventricular enlargement. Consideration of the secondary changes in repolarization or in left atrial size are not used in the Scott criteria.

The presence of LVH on the baseline tracing may result in an indeterminate or false positive stress ECG. Because of this, evaluation for chest pain requires supplemental radionuclide imaging to confirm or exclude ischemia.

Right Ventricular Hypertrophy

Right ventricular hypertrophy (RVH) or enlargement (Figure 51.2) is much less common than LVH. The major causes are pulmonary disease, valvular disease (particularly mitral and tricuspid), and congenital heart disease. A variety of ECG types of RVH have been described, but are beyond the scope of this chapter. Table 51.3 lists some of the electrocardiographic manifestations of RVH.

Left Atrial Enlargement

Left atrial enlargement (Fig. 51.1) may be inferred from changes in P-wave morphology. The P-wave changes of broadening and notching, when present, are usually best seen in lead II. A more sensitive finding is enlargement of the negative component of the P wave in lead V1. As previously noted, the negative deflection in lead V1 reflects left atrial depolarization, a posteriorly directed vector. In left atrial enlargement, the negative component in lead V1 is greater than one small box on the grid, that is, greater than 0.04 seconds in duration and 1 mm in amplitude.

Right Atrial Enlargement

Right atrial enlargement also produces changes in P-wave morphology. Tall, peaked P waves (>3 mm) may be seen in lead II and the right sided chest leads. However, this criterion is less sensitive for right atrial enlargement than are the criteria for left atrial enlargement.

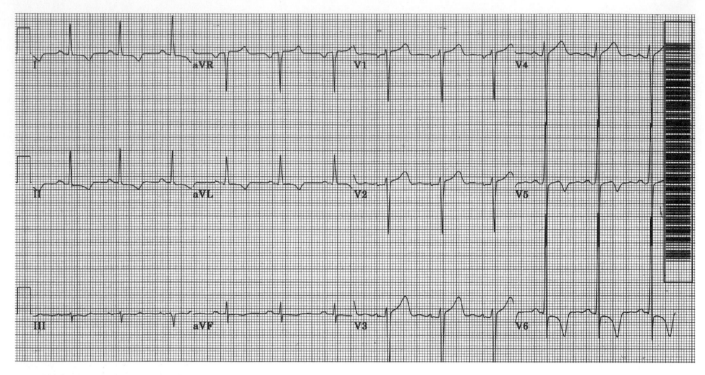

Figure 51.1. Left ventricular hypertrophy and left atrial enlargement.

Table 51.1. Estes ECG Criteria for the Determination of Left Ventricular Enlargement

	POINTS
1. Any of the following	
R or S in limb lead ≥ 20 mm	
S wave in V1, V2, V3 ≥ 25 mm	
R wave in V4, V5, V6 ≥ 25 mm	3
2. Any ST shift	3
Typical strain ST-T changes:	1
3. LAD > 15 degrees	2
4. QRS interval > 0.09 sec	1
5. Intrisicoid deflection > 0.04 sec	1
6. P-terminal force in V1 > 0.04	3
Total (LVH > 5 points. probable LVH > 4 points)	13

Adapted with permission from Wagner GS. Marriott's Electro-cardiography. 9th ed. Baltimore: Williams & Wilkins, 1994.

Table 51.2. Scott ECG Criteria for the Determination of Left Ventricular Hypertrophy

Any one listed below
S in V1 or V2 + R in V5 or V6 ≥ 35 mm
R in V5 or V6 ≥ 26 mm
R + S in any V lead ≥ 45 mm
R in I + S in III ≥ than 25 mm
R in aVL ≥ 7.5 mm
R in aVF ≥ 20 mm
S in aVR ≥ 14 mm

Adapted with permission from Wagner GS. Marriott's Practical Electro-cardiography. 9th ed. Baltimore: Williams & Wilkins, 1994.

COMMONLY USED MEDICATIONS THAT AFFECT THE ELECTROCARDIOGRAM

Digitalis

Digitalis is often used to treat patients with congestive heart failure or atrial arrhythmias. In addition to its effect of prolonging the refractory period of the atrioventricular (AV) node, digitalis effects the ST segment and T wave. Figure 51.3 demonstrates these changes. The ST segment appears scooped out and depressed. These changes typi-cally occur in the inferior and lateral leads. Digitalis may cause false-positive stress ECG findings, and additional imaging modalities may be required to increase the speci-ficity of the study.

Quinidine

Quinidine is a commonly used antiarrhythmic agent that is predominantly used to maintain sinus rhythm in patients with a history of atrial fibrillation. Historically, it has been used to treat ventricular arrhythmias, although recently it has been replaced with other agents and im-plantable defibrillators. Quinidine prolongs the QT inter-val on the ECG. Other agents in its class, **procainamide** and **disopyramide**, have a similar effect. Some of the an-

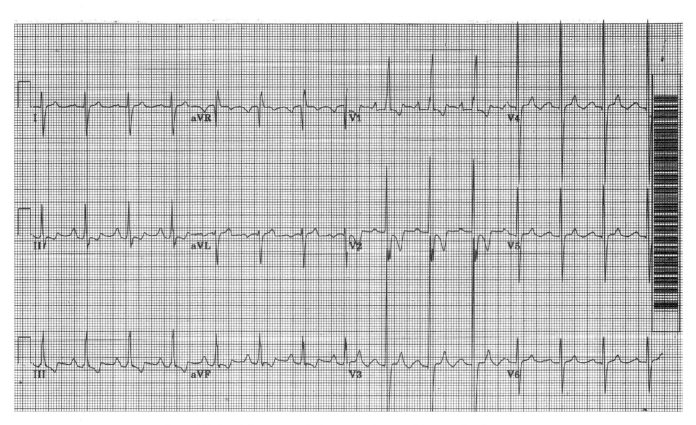

Figure 51.2. Right ventricular hypertrophy and right atrial enlargement.

Table 51.3. Electrocardiographic Manifestations of Right Ventricular Hypertrophy

Right axis deviation
R wave in V1 >than 7 mm
R in V1 + S in V5 or V6> 10 mm
R:S ratio in V1 >1.0
S:R in V6 >1.0
Right intraventricular conduction defect
Right ventricular strain pattern in V1, V2, or II, III, and aVF

Adapted with permission from Wagner GS. Marriott's Electrocardiography. 9th ed. Baltimore: Williams & Wilkins, 1994.

tidepressant agents, particularly the **tricyclic antidepressants**, may also prolong the QT interval. Significant prolongation of the QT interval predisposes the patient to torsades de pointes, which can be fatal.

ELECTROLYTE DISORDERS

Hyperkalemia is associated with a variety of ECG changes, depending on the serum potassium. Initially the T waves peak (Fig. 51.4), followed by prolongation of the QRS interval (not illustrated). Subsequently, the PR interval prolongs and finally the P waves disappear. At ex-

tremely high levels of potassium the rhythm has the appearance of a sine wave.

Hypokalemia may cause diminution of the T wave voltage, prolongation of the QT interval, and rarely, ST segment depression. Prominent U waves may develop, although these can also be seen in the absence of potassium abnormalities. **Hypercalcemia** results in shortening of the Q-T interval, while **hypocalcemia** prolongs the Q-T interval.

WOLFF-PARKINSON-WHITE SYNDROME

Typically, the AV node is the only connection between the atria and the ventricles. In Wolff-Parkinson-White syndrome there is an additional myocardial bridging connection, termed an accessory pathway, between the atria and ventricles. When the patient is in normal sinus rhythm, a short PR interval and a slurred QRS upstroke, termed a delta wave, are present (Fig. 51.5). While patients with an accessory pathway may be asymptomatic, they are predisposed to three types of tachycardias: orthodromic AV re-entrant tachycardia, antidromic AV re-entrant tachycardia, and atrial fibrillation. When the reentrant loop travels antegrade over the AV node and retrograde over the accessory pathway, the tachycardia is referred to as **orthodromic** AV re-entrant tachycardia

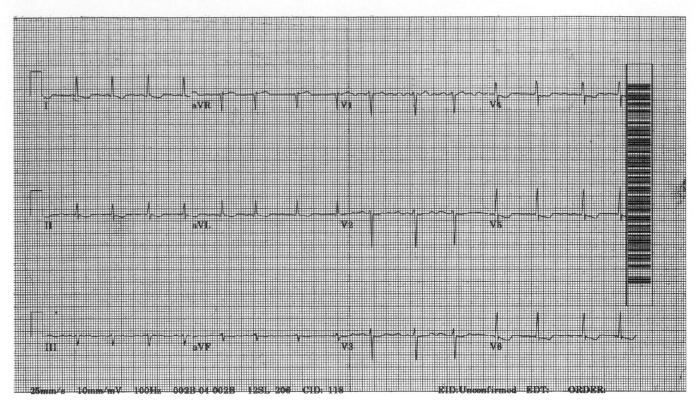

Figure 51.3. ST depression caused by digitalis. The rhythm is atrial fibrillation.

Figure 51.4. Peaked T waves seen in hyper-kalemia.

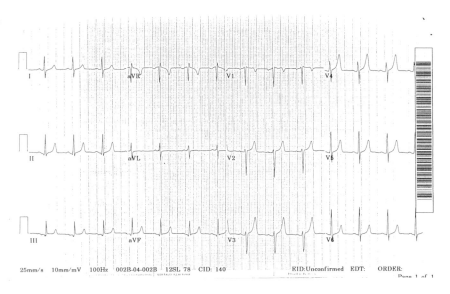

(Fig. 51.6). This tachycardia has a narrow QRS complex. The alternative situation, when the impulse travels ante-grade over the accessory pathway and retrograde through the AV node, results in a wide complex tachycardia called **antidromic** AV re-entrant tachycardia. Atrial fibrillation in patients with Wolff-Parkinson-White syndrome may result in very rapid ventricular rates with hemodynamic instability. These arrhythmias can be provoked during ex-ercise testing; therefore, it is important to note the acces-

sory pathway prior to testing and be alert for the develop-ment of a tachyarrhythmia.

PACEMAKERS

A variety of pacemakers are available, and a compre-hensive review is beyond the scope of this text. Nonethe-less, many patients undergoing treadmill testing or enter-ing cardiac rehabilitation programs have pacemakers.

100Hz

Vent. rate(BPM) 96
PR interval(ms) 143
QRS duration(ms) 106

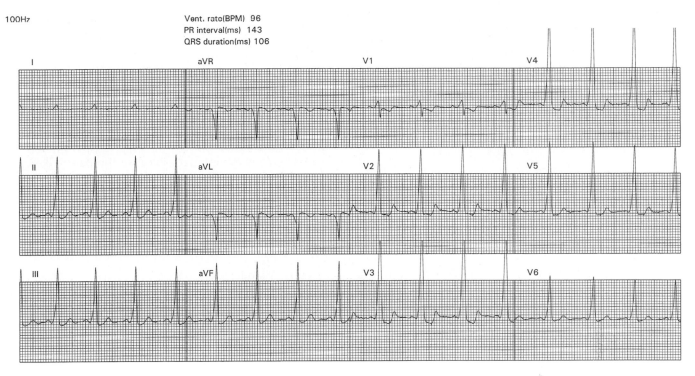

Figure 51.5. Wolff-Parkinson-White syndrome.

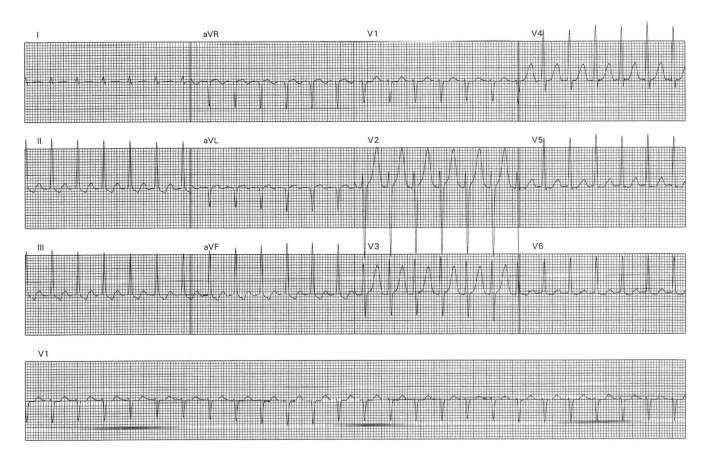

Figure 51.6. Orthodromic AV re-entrant tachycardia.

Table 51.4. Standardized Pacemaker Code

1st letter: paced chamber
 A = atria
 V = ventricle
 D = dual chamber
2nd letter: sensing chamber
 A = atria
 V = ventricle
 D = dual chamber
3rd letter: mode of pacemaker
 I = inhibit
 T = trigger
 D = both inhibit and trigger
4th letter: rate modulation present
 R = rate responsive

Pacemakers are inserted for patients with bradycardia due to disease of the conduction system. The most common reasons for pacing are sinus node dysfunction and AV block.

Pacemakers are described by a standard code adopted by both Europe and the United States. Table 51.4 shows the standard pacemaker code and describes the designation for each position in the code.

The simplest type of pacemaker is a VVI (Fig. 51.7). In this mode a single pacing wire in the right ventricle senses any impulses in the ventricle. If the rate is set at 60 beats per minute, the pacemaker senses for ventricular depolarization for the 1-second interval between depolarization of the sinoatrial node. If no impulses are detected during the predetermined interval, the pacemaker delivers an impulse to the right ventricle, resulting in ventricular depolarization. The timing interval is reset and the pacemaker begins to sense for ventricular impulses during the next interval. If an impulse is detected, the pacemaker is inhibited from firing, the timing interval is reset, and ventricular sensing is restarted. Because the pacemaker is in the right ventricle, the paced complexes have a wide morphology similar to left bundle branch block. Normally a pace artifact, or spike, is noted before the QRS complex. Because of the abnormal sequence of depolarization in pacing, abnormal repolarization causes ST and T changes. This prevents interpretation of ST and T changes during an exercise study.

The most common pacemaker in use today is a DDD pacemaker (Fig. 51.8). This pacemaker has two leads, one in the right atrium and one in the right ventricle. This permits the maintenance of atrial and ventricular synchrony. Proper timing of atrial contraction to augment diastolic filling is more physiological. Depending on the underlying conduction disease and the programmed characteristics of the pacemaker, four conditions may appear on the ECG. These are depicted in Table 51.5. As many of the new pacemakers are rate responsive (DDDR), it is possi-

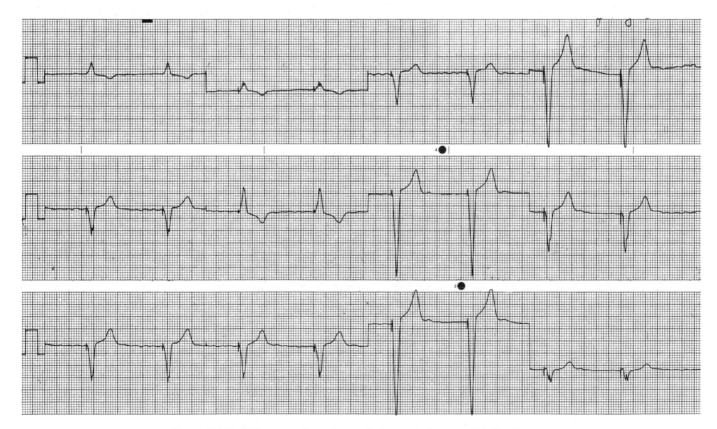

Figure 51.7. VVI pacemaker. The underlying rhythm is atrial fibrillation.

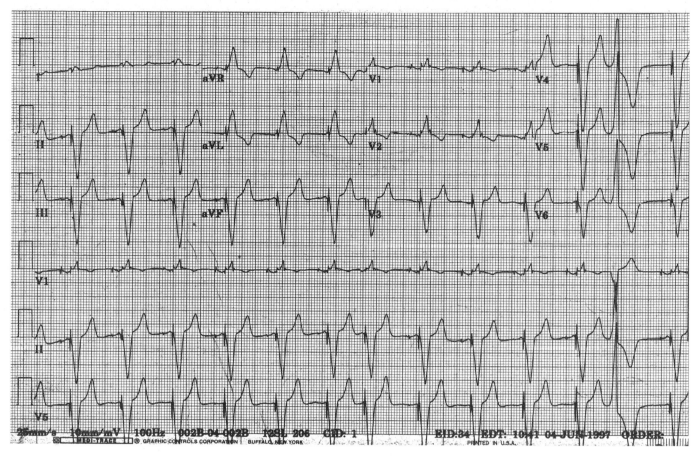

Figure 51.8. DDD pacemaker with pacing spikes present before the P waves and QRS complexes.

Table 51.5. Complexes Seen in DDD Pacing

Native P wave	Native QRS
Paced P wave	Native QRS
Native P wave	Paced QRS
Paced P wave	Paced QRS

ble to see an increase in the paced atrial rate with exercise.

Rate-responsive pacemakers use one of several strategies to detect the need for increased cardiac output. The most common sensor is a gyroscope in the generator that senses movement of the upper body. Depending on the rate of vibrations sensed, the pacer increases its rate based on a predetermined algorithm to the maximum programmed rate. A second sensor commonly used measures the respiratory rate and relative tidal volume to calculate minute ventilation. When the minute ventilation increases, so does the rate of the pacer.

► **SUMMARY**

Many cardiac and noncardiac phenomena can exert effects on the ECG. Some of the more common situations have been highlighted. Pacemakers are becoming more common as our population ages, and one should not be surprised by the ECG findings in these patients. Competence in ECG interpretation requires repetition in reading tracings. We hope to have provided a framework of understanding through which basic electrophysiological principles govern the approach to ECG interpretation. The ECG remains an invaluable diagnostic tool; the better skilled the interpreter, the more information can be derived about patients and their cardiac condition.

Suggested Reading

Braunwald E. Heart Disease: A Textbook of Cardiovascular Medicine. 5th ed. Philadelphia: Saunders, 1997.

Wagner GS. Marriott's Practical Electrocardiography. 9th ed. Baltimore: Williams & Wilkins, 1994.

SECTION TEN

EXERCISE PROGRAMMING

SECTION EDITOR: *Michael Wegner, PhD, FACSM*

1.2.0, 1.2.5, 1.2.10,
1.8.0, 1.8.3, 1.8.5,
1.8.8, 1.8.9

2.2.0, 2.2.19, 2.8.0.3,
2.8.0.11

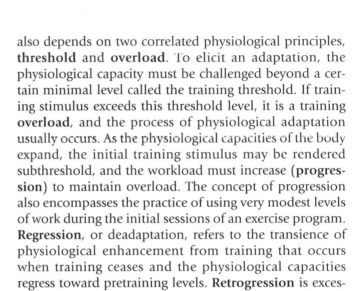

CHAPTER **52**

CARDIORESPIRATORY ENDURANCE

Robert G. Holly and James D. Shaffrath

Physical activity is defined as any bodily movement produced by skeletal muscles that results in energy expenditure. Exercise is defined as planned, structured, and repetitive bodily movement done to improve or maintain one or more components of physical fitness. The focus of this chapter is exercise planning or programming to increase cardiorespiratory (CR) fitness; however, some of the health benefits associated with less structured but regular moderate-intensity physical activity are also discussed (1, 2).

Cardiorespiratory activities are those that cause an increase in the transport and uptake of oxygen by skeletal muscle. These activities, appropriately performed on a regular basis, increase CR fitness and lead to numerous health benefits (1, 2). However, CR exercise and activity performed inappropriately or by those for whom it is contraindicated may result in serious complications. Thus, it is important to understand both the principles of exercise programming and the actual approach to CR conditioning to safely meet the goals of the individual.

PRINCIPLES

This section discusses the following topics:

- Principles of exercise adaptation
- Medical clearance and supervision
- Types of fitness
- Goal setting
- Components of an exercise session

Principles of Exercise Adaptation

A basic assumption in exercise programming is that something useful or beneficial occurs as a result of repeated bouts of exercise. This assumption is predicated on a number of physiological principles. The most central of these is the **principle of adaptation**, which states that if a specific physiological capacity is taxed by a physical training stimulus within a certain range and on a regular basis, this physiological capacity usually expands. Adaptation also depends on two correlated physiological principles, **threshold** and **overload**. To elicit an adaptation, the physiological capacity must be challenged beyond a certain minimal level called the training threshold. If training stimulus exceeds this threshold level, it is a training **overload**, and the process of physiological adaptation usually occurs. As the physiological capacities of the body expand, the initial training stimulus may be rendered subthreshold, and the workload must increase (**progression**) to maintain overload. The concept of progression also encompasses the practice of using very modest levels of work during the initial sessions of an exercise program. **Regression**, or deadaptation, refers to the transience of physiological enhancement from training that occurs when training ceases and the physiological capacities regress toward pretraining levels. **Retrogression** is excessive taxing of physiological capacities leading to their diminution. Retrogression can refer to either acute or chronic periods of excessive overload. That is, either a single bout or chronic bouts of excessive overload can cause retrogression. These principles are illustrated in Figure 52.1.

A final principle of central importance in exercise programming is the concept of **specificity**. Specific physiological capacities expand only if they are stressed in the course of an exercise program. For example, swimmers have an 11% increase in swim ergometry performance over the course of a training season but show no change in run time to exhaustion on a treadmill (3). Each of these principles guides the design of an exercise program.

Medical Clearance and Supervision

Exercise training may not be appropriate for everyone. Patients whose adaptive reserves are severely limited by disease processes may be unable to adapt to or benefit from exercise. In this small subpopulation of people with severe or unstable cardiac, respiratory, metabolic, systemic, or musculoskeletal disease, exercise programming may be fatal, injurious, or simply not beneficial, depending on the clinical status and condition of the individual.

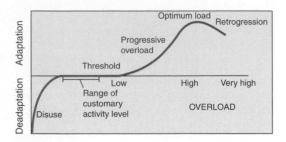

Figure 52.1. Adaptive effects of decreased (disuse) and increased (overload) levels of physical activity relative to usual activity levels. See text for explanation of terms. (Reprinted with permission from Adams WC. *Foundations of Physical Education, Exercise, and Sport Sciences.* Philadelphia: Lea & Febiger, 1991.)

The *ACSM Guidelines for Exercise Testing and Prescription* (4) lists contraindications to both exercise training and testing. Medical clearance to rule out these conditions prior to beginning an exercise program is warranted for those with known disease or suggestive symptoms.

For individuals without known contraindications to exercise training, various levels of screening and supervision relative to health and fitness status, goals, and personal preferences are appropriate. These topics are covered in detail in the *ACSM Guidelines* and are discussed only briefly here (4). The recommended level of screening prior to beginning or increasing an exercise program depends on the risk of the individual and the intensity of the planned physical activity (4). For individuals planning to engage in low- to moderate-intensity activities, the Physical Activities Readiness Questionnaire (PAR-Q) should be considered the minimal level of screening (5). A yes answer to any question indicates the necessity of a physician's referral before the person begins or increases physical activity. The PAR-Q can be found in the *ACSM Guidelines* along with specific recommendations for screening (4).

Supervised exercise programs are recommended for those with low functional capacity (<8 METs) or poor health status (4). Beyond health and functional status, whether a person exercises under supervision depends primarily on goals and personal preference.

Types of Fitness

For most people the question is not whether or in what setting they will benefit from exercise but rather which of the benefits are desired outcomes. The principle of specificity implies that fitness is a diverse and varied group of related adaptations that may be differentially developed. Physical fitness has been defined as a set of attributes that people have or achieve that relates to the ability to perform physical activity (1). The components of physical fitness that lead to increased vigor in daily life and help protect against degenerative diseases associated with physical

inactivity are called the health-related aspects of fitness (4). They are CR endurance, muscular strength and endurance, flexibility, and body composition.

Cardiorespiratory, or aerobic, fitness refers to the constellation of improvements that enhance $\dot{V}O_{2max}$ and/or aerobic work capacity. Clearly, CR conditioning is the primary focus of exercise programs for endurance athletes. It is also a primary goal in cardiac rehabilitation programs, since such training can enhance peripheral oxygen delivery, and thus helps compensate for an impaired myocardium (6). Finally, this type of conditioning is also most strongly associated with health benefits in the general population (2, 4, 6–10).

Goal Setting

One of the first considerations in designing an exercise program is to determine the expected outcomes. Goal setting is an essential preliminary step in a successful program. The goals of an exercise program provide a focus for its detailed structure. In general, goals should realistically attempt to meet the medical, emotional, and functional needs of the exerciser within the context of limitations of time, interest, and physical ability.

The first step in goal setting is to clarify stated goals or objectives. Occasionally the stated goal reflects incomplete knowledge or unrealistic expectations about the effects of exercise training ("I want to lose 50 pounds without restricting my eating habits"). In such cases, further education about the effects of training combined with clarification of priorities and values should result in more practical goals. There may be conflicts between the emotional and medical or functional needs ("I want to run a 400-meter dash to show that I'm over my heart attack"). Although the actual activities proposed may be unattainable or contraindicated, the exercise professional must recognize, respect, and attempt to address the emotional realities of the situation. Once the objectives have been clarified, the next step is to assess resources for meeting these goals. Medical or physical limitations may define the scope of activities in the exercise program. Exploring past successes and failures with physical activity is often useful for identifying specific modes of exercise that may be enjoyable. Personal preferences for group or individual exercise should be considered. Facilities and equipment needed for various modes of exercise should be evaluated for convenience and affordability. Finally, a realistic appraisal of the time available for an exercise program can be made through examination of a personal calendar or datebook.

Before a new exercise program is implemented, a means of evaluating effectiveness in meeting established goals should be considered. If the primary goal is to feel better, evaluation may be as simple as assessing perception of well-being after 1 to 2 months of regular exercise. In many cases, especially when more concrete performance or physiological goals are stated, goal-specific assessment is valuable. For most exercise programs, subjective evaluations or simple pre–post physiological evaluation of the goals is sufficient.

Record keeping is a powerful tool for meeting exercise goals that should be used in the implementation of a new exercise program. Most programs for health maintenance or recreation do not require this degree of vigilance for success; however, record-keeping may be invaluable in programs for patients with major medical problems that cause restriction of activity, for individuals who are restarting exercise after years of inactivity, for exercisers for whom weight management is a major goal, and for performance-oriented athletes.

To be useful, a record of physical activity should include day, date, time of day, type of exercise, an estimate of the external work or work rate (e.g., miles, watts, METs) and the physiological response (heart rate or rate of perceived exertion [RPE]). Symptoms or problems, such as specific physical complaints ("left knee sore again") or general symptoms ("couldn't catch breath for first 10 minutes") should be recorded. A carefully kept exercise record can provide early warning of impending overuse injuries and overtraining as well as powerful feedback about improvement or patterns of avoidance. In addition, the vagaries of human impulse and appetite are such that any person attempting to include dietary portion control or caloric restriction as a goal is likely to benefit from keeping a record, by kilocalories, weight, or volume, of all food consumed.

In summary, exercise programming is a purposeful activity. Identifying the goals of each participant clarifies and directs the development of a specific activity plan that addresses these goals while acknowledging the limitations of the exerciser. Evaluation of the effects and outcomes is part of this process. Certain groups may benefit further from keeping a record of their exercise (and dietary) activities.

Components of an Exercise Session

The three basic components to any exercise conditioning session are warm-up, conditioning stimulus, and cool-down. An appropriate warm-up can improve performance and decrease risk of ischemic and dysrhythmic events (11, 12). Cool-down has these benefits as well as helping to clear metabolic waste from skeletal muscle (11). Warmup and cool-down are periods of metabolic and CR adjustment from rest to exercise and exercise to rest, respectively. Thus, the most appropriate types of warm-up and cool-down are activities similar to the conditioning stimulus activities, performed at approximately 50% of the stimulus intensity (11). Older individuals and those who have or are at increased risk for ischemic heart disease benefit from longer periods of warm-up and cool-down that may further decrease their risk of ischemic or dysrhythmic events (12). Warmup and cool-down may take 5–15 minutes, depending on the age and risk of the

individual and the time allotted for flexibility exercises. Stretching to increase flexibility is appropriate at these times but should not substitute for activity that alters metabolism. The conditioning stimulus may contain a period of aerobic conditioning, muscle conditioning, or both. It may be as short as 20 minutes or longer than an hour, depending on the exercises selected (4, 7).

CARDIORESPIRATORY CONDITIONING

This section discusses the following topics:

- Benefits of CR activities and fitness
- Conditioning for health versus fitness
- FITTE factors (see page 452) for increasing fitness
- Prescribing and determining exercise intensity
- Progression and maintenance
- Modifications for sport and activity-specific conditioning

Benefits of CR Activities and Fitness

The benefits of physical activity and fitness relative to health have been exhaustively reviewed and are summarized in Table 52.1 (2, 4, 6, 9, 10, 13). Both CR conditioning and enhanced physical fitness decrease fatigue in

Table 52.1. Benefits of Increasing Cardiorespiratory Activities and/or Improved Cardiorespiratory Fitness

Decreased fatigue in daily activities
Improved work, recreational, and sports performance
Improved cardiorespiratory function
   Increased maximal oxygen uptake
   Increased maximal cardiac output and stroke volume
   Increased capillary density in skeletal muscle
   Increased mitochondrial density
   Increased lactate threshold
   Lower heart rate and blood pressure at a fixed submaximal work rate
   Lower myocardial oxygen demand at a fixed submaximal work rate
   Lower minute ventilation at a fixed submaximal work rate
Decreased risk of the following:
   Mortality from all causes
   Coronary artery disease
   Cancer (colon, perhaps breast and prostate)
   Hypertension
   Non–insulin-dependent diabetes mellitus
   Osteoporosis
   Anxiety
   Depression
Improved blood lipid profile
   Decreased triglycerides
   Increased high density lipoprotein cholesterol
   Decreased postprandial lipemia
Improved immune function
Improved glucose tolerance and insulin sensitivity
Improved body composition
Enhanced sense of well-being

Many of the health benefits accrue from physical activities that may have relatively little effect on increasing cardiorespiratory fitness (2, 8–10).

daily activities, improve sports performance, and are associated with decreased all-cause, cardiovascular, and cancer mortality (14–17).

Conditioning for Health Versus Fitness

While there are unresolved issues concerning the amount of CR exercise necessary to achieve a specific response, in recent years it has become apparent that the level of physical activity necessary to achieve the majority of health benefits is less than that needed to attain a high level of CR fitness (Fig. 52.2) (2, 8–10, 14–16, 18). For example, Blair et al. (16) recently demonstrated that activity sufficient to cause only a small improvement in CR fitness may have significant health benefits. Such research, combined with the low physical activity level of the U.S. population, has stimulated recommendations for levels of activity less than previously suggested for the general public (2, 8, 18). A recent joint statement from the Centers for Disease Control and Prevention (CDC) and the American College of Sports Medicine (ACSM) concludes that "every US adult should accumulate 30 minutes or more of moderate-intensity physical activity on most, preferably all, days of the week" (2). Consistent with this recommendation is the report of the Surgeon General (10), which recommends moderate exercise energy expenditures, roughly 1000 kcal/week or 150 kcal/day. This recommendation differs from previous exercise recommendations by acknowledging the health benefits of moderate-intensity activities, by recognizing that benefits accrue from intermittent regular activity as well as regular continuous exercise, and by stressing the efficacy and safety of higher-frequency activities when intensity is moderate and activities are nonimpact. An example of activity meeting the CDC–ACSM criteria would be brisk walking over uneven ground at 3–4 mph (3–6 METs), 3 times a day for 10–15 minutes each session, 5–7 days of the week. Using stairs instead of elevators is an additional means of engaging in intermittent moderate exercise.

Reports of additional specific health benefits elicited by higher-intensity exercise do not contradict this recom-

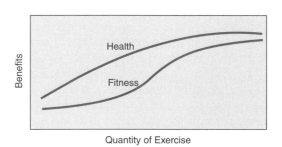

Figure 52.2. Theoretical representation of the relation between the quantity of exercise and expected health and fitness benefits. A level of exercise that has little effect on increasing fitness may yield substantial health benefits. (Courtesy of William L. Haskell, Stanford University School of Medicine, division of Cardiovascular Medicine.)

mendation (17). Thus, the CDC–ACSM recommendation complements but does not replace recommendations based on the scientific evidence supporting the type of exercise needed to improve CR fitness (7). As suggested in Figure 52.2, the health benefits of physical activity and exercise run along a continuum of intensity. Higher levels of exertion are likely to yield specific (18) and, as noted in the Surgeon General's report (10), greater health and fitness benefits.

FITTE Factors for Increasing CR Fitness

Exercise programming for fitness emphasizes focused training periods of at least 20–30 minutes, high levels of exercise intensity, and for those pursuing goals in specific activities or sports, a commitment to the principle of specificity. As such, the ACSM position stand remains a useful and accurate document for those whose goals focus on achieving a higher level of CR fitness (7).

The total training stimulus provided by an exercise program can be quantified by frequency (usually days per week), intensity, duration, and type of exercise. Coupled with the nonquantitative but crucial adherence factor of enjoyment, these factors form the acronym FITTE. The minimum levels of the FITTE factors recommended by the ACSM to achieve an increase in CR fitness (4, 7):

- Frequency: 3–5 days a week
- Intensity: 65–90% of maximal heart rate (HR_{max}), or 50–85% of maximal oxygen uptake reserve ($\dot{V}O_{2R}$) or HR_{max} reserve (HRR), where $\dot{V}O_{2R}$ and HRR are calculated from the difference between resting heart rate and HR_{max} and oxygen uptake ($\dot{V}O_2$) at rest and maximal oxygen uptake ($\dot{V}O_{2max}$), respectively. To estimate training intensity, a percentage of this value is added to the resting heart rate or resting $\dot{V}O_2$ and is expressed as a percentage of HRR or maximal oxygen uptake reserve ($\dot{V}O_{2R}$ [19]). For very unfit individuals, lower-intensity values of 40–49% of $\dot{V}O_{2R}$ or HRR or 55–64% of HR_{max} may apply.
- Time: 20–60 or more minutes per session, continuous or intermittent activity
- Type: Aerobic (run, brisk walk, bike, swim, cross-country ski, dance)
- Enjoyment: Preferably enjoyable aerobic activities

The art of exercise programming is to create a program that fits the unique needs of the individual and the performance demands of the specific sport or activity. A major part of this individualization is accomplished through differential emphasis of the interrelated FITTE factors. Different programs seeking to improve CR fitness begin at the lower end of the ranges for each of the quantifiable FITTE factors and diverge as they focus more precisely on goals and functional demands of the selected activities. For example, an exercise program for health benefits is focused on frequent and enjoyable activity with broad latitude in the levels of exercise intensity, duration, and type (F i t t E).

Generally, there is an inverse relation between the intensity and duration in a single session; that is, as intensity increases, duration decreases and vice versa. It is for this reason that larger caloric expenditures can be practically achieved in exercise sessions of low to moderate intensity and longer duration. The total volume of work is described by frequency, intensity, and time and may be expressed in kilocalories per week. Thus, for weight management, frequent, enjoyable exercise periods of low to moderate intensity and relatively long duration (F i T t E) result in the largest weekly caloric expenditures. Finally, the athlete in competition seeks to perform an event at the highest possible intensity. Thus, for the athlete, it is intensity and type of activity which are most emphasized (f I t T e). The remainder of this chapter further details how the FITTE factors are tailored to the individual needs of those in specific activities.

Prescribing and Determining Exercise Intensity

Health benefits and caloric expenditure accrue even at low levels of intensity; therefore, precise specification of intensity may not be necessary for an effective exercise program. If the goal is simply recreation or health, an adequate prescription of intensity might be "hard enough to increase breathing but not hard enough to make you breathless or exhausted." A rigidly quantitative cookbook approach to the prescription of intensity can be a recipe for disaster. Without proper application of the principles of training and careful personal observation, no specific prescription of intensity is likely to result in optimal training.

Paradoxically, the groups most likely to benefit from a precise determination of exercise intensity are patients and athletes (20). Cardiac, pulmonary, and other patients with chronic disease who develop signs of exertional intolerance such as ischemia or hypoxemia at specific physiological workloads need a reasonably exact determination of intensity. This topic is discussed in the *ACSM Guidelines* (4). Endurance athletes, however, attempt to maintain a maximal overload stimulus without crossing over into retrogression. Answering two questions can help determine the optimal range of training intensity for the development of CR fitness:

1. What is the optimal range of training intensities for a particular individual?
2. How can this range of intensities best be determined in the course of training?

The threshold level for training intensity to initiate an adaptation in CR fitness is approximately 50% of $\dot{V}O_{2R}$, or 65% of maximal heart rate (7). Relatively unfit individuals may achieve significant training effects at intensities as low as 40% of $\dot{V}O_{2R}$, while those at higher levels of aerobic fitness may require intensities greater than 60% of $\dot{V}O_{2R}$. Training intensities above 50% of $\dot{V}O_{2R}$ generally facilitate greater improvement in aerobic capacity, whereas training very far above the lactate threshold (LT) results in smaller gains as exercise tolerance is compromised and an increased risk of cardiovascular events, orthopaedic injury, and lower compliance exists (7). For this reason, ACSM recommends programs emphasizing low to moderate intensity for most adults, with an upper limit of 85% of $\dot{V}O_{2R}$ (4, 7). Competitive athletes may require intensities above these levels to attain performance goals.

Therefore, the ideal intensity for an individual may range from 40–85% of $\dot{V}O_{2R}$. This range may even be applied in a single training session in some cases. For example, sports such as soccer and lacrosse feature a pattern of continuous, moderate aerobic activity punctuated by frequent surges of intensity up to and beyond $\dot{V}O_{2max}$. For these athletes, the optimal range of training intensities should include the range and pattern of intensity demands encountered in competition.

Intensity during training can be determined in a number of distinct and complementary ways. The goal is to guide efforts so that work occurs within the range most conducive to developing CR endurance (50–85% of $\dot{V}O_{2R}$). Quantitative laboratory measurements such as $\dot{V}O_{2max}$ or serum lactate level can precisely describe certain levels of intensity but usually are connected to more readily available field measures of intensity, such as heart rate or RPE. The quantification of external work rate (such as speed of running or watts in cycle ergometry) complements the more usual measurements of the physiological response such as heart rate, lactate level, or RPE. Comparing such markers of internal and external work intensity can provide unique and valuable information, and both should be included in a system for monitoring progress. A decline in physiological response (e.g., heart rate) to a fixed rate of external work (e.g., 160 watts of cycle ergometry) suggests a classic training effect. If, however, physiological responses to a fixed external work rate become elevated, this suggests retrogression (overtraining), incipient illness, environmental stress, or some other diversion of the physiological resources (21–24).

While laboratory methods can precisely identify $\dot{V}O_{2max}$ or LT, these are not necessary for successful intensity prescription and ultimately must be referenced to techniques that can be employed by athletes during training. The most common means of determining exercise intensity in the field are based on either training heart rate range or non–heart rate methods of assessing intensity. Non–heart rate methods are most appropriate for the recreational exerciser, those working at low intensity to expend calories, exercisers without major medical problems, and the experienced exerciser with a well-developed internal sense of work intensity. One such method is to estimate intensity of physical activity by using metabolic calculations or tables listing the metabolic cost of various activities at different levels of intensity (4,

25). A second method quantifies internal perception of intensity using a scale such as the Borg RPE scale (26). Activities eliciting perceived work intensities of 13–16, corresponding to perceptions of somewhat hard through hard, correlate well with intensities of 50–85% of $\dot{V}O_{2R}$ (7). Perceptions of work as light (RPE of 11–12) are appropriate as initial exercise intensities for unconditioned subjects.

A final non–heart rate method of estimating work intensity is the so-called talk test. Exercising at or above LT and ventilatory threshold generally does not allow complete conversational sentences without pausing for breath. Thus, inability to complete simple sentences is a semiquantitative test of ceiling intensity used by many apparently healthy adults in recreational programs. Combining them with determinations of intensity based on heart rate further enhances the use of these methods.

Heart rate is a useful means of prescribing exercise intensity, since it increases linearly with oxygen consumption and intensity, is easily assessed, and can be cross-referenced with other objective and subjective indices of intensity. Heart rate methods are particularly useful for beginning exercisers, those with intensity-related medical problems such as angina, and competitive athletes. Two basic techniques are used to establish a training heart rate range. The first is to connect a specific heart rate with some other intensity-related marker, such as a measured oxygen consumption at 75% $\dot{V}O_{2max}$, an RPE of 12, or the onset of clinical events. In cardiac patients, it is common to identify the heart rate at which signs or symptoms of exertional intolerance (such as angina or ST depression) occur and use a training heart rate that is at least 10 beats per minute lower, depending on the setting in which the patient exercises and the severity of work intolerance. A second technique is to assign a range of training heart rates based on a percentage of the maximal heart rate. These methods are described in detail in the *ACSM Guidelines* (4).

In general, the recommended intensity range of 50–85% of $\dot{V}O_{2R}$ corresponds to 65–90% of HR_{max}. The HR_{max} estimated from equations such as 220 − age has a standard deviation of plus or minus 10–12 beats per minute (4). Therefore, in a group of 40-year-olds, all with a predicted HR_{max} of 180 beats per minute, the actual HR_{max} will be less than 168 or greater than 192 beats per minute in about one-third of the subjects. This emphasizes the importance of actually measuring HR_{max} (if safe and appropriate) whenever a precise estimate of intensity is required. The HR_{max} can also be assessed in young, healthy individuals by determining the pulse immediately after a field test such as a 12-minute or 1.5-mile run to exhaustion (i.e., runs performed with true maximal effort).

During exercise, heart rate is usually quantified by counting a radial or carotid pulse. Assessing the carotid pulse requires gentle pressure at or below the level of the laryngeal cartilage to avoid disturbing carotid barorecep-

tors and possible atherosclerotic lesions, which frequently occur at the carotid bifurcation beneath the angle of the mandible. Simultaneous palpation of carotid arteries bilaterally should be avoided. During cardiac emergencies, assessment of the pulse at the carotid is preferable to peripheral pulses because of concerns regarding cerebral perfusion.

Counting a Pulse Rate

To obtain a pulse rate, the following can be done:

1. Locate a pulse with the index and long fingers of one hand.
2. Count the number of pulsations in a given period.
3. For the highest precision, if timing is initiated simultaneously with a pulsation, this first pulsation is counted as zero. If a second person is keeping time or if there is lag between the initiation of timing and the first pulsation that is felt, the first pulse is counted as one.
4. To determine the pulse rate, multiply the number of pulse beats by the number of counting intervals in 1 minute.
   10 seconds = 6 intervals (multiply pulse beats by 6)
   15 seconds = 4 intervals
   20 seconds = 3 intervals
   30 seconds = 2 intervals

The margin of error may be one pulse count within the counting period, which can lead to substantial errors in heart rate (in beats per minute) when short counting periods are used. Longer pulse counts afford greater accuracy and provide more time for detection of some dysrhythmias. However, the heart rate of fit persons can decrease quite rapidly following exercise, possibly making long counts less accurate than short ones.

Locally telemetered heart rate monitors (heart watches) are commonly available and can be a useful aid in training, particularly for athletes and others desiring frequent, immediate feedback regarding exercise heart rate. However, the only advantages such monitors have over manual pulse counts are the ability to assess heart rate without interrupting exercise and the capacity for data storage. These devices do not perform any of the functions of a medical electrocardiographic monitor. Manual pulse counts have the advantages of detecting some forms of dysrhythmia and being constantly available to any person who carries a timepiece. Thus, it may be preferable to continue to use manual pulse counts in clinical or older populations.

It is important to recognize that the prescription of exercise intensity via heart rate is not rigidly quantitative. Exercise heart rate may be influenced by a number of factors other than work intensity, and the presence of such factors may uncouple the connection between a given intensity-related event (such as the LT or a 5-minute-per-mile pace) and a specific heart rate. These factors include environmental conditions that influence heat dissipation, such as temperature, airflow, and humidity; the degree of rest or overtraining of the athlete; altitude; illness; and the timing and amount of specific cardiovascular medications. Environmental effects that impair the dissipation of heat are particularly important. At the same absolute level of work intensity, heart rates may be 10–20 beats per minute higher during exercise in heat or in the absence of airflow (21–24).

This discussion makes it apparent that cookbook approaches to prescribing exercise intensity are inappropriate. In three 40-year-old individuals, using the equation 220 − age to predict HR_{max} and a 75% training HR level will result in a training heart rate of 135 beats per minute. This may be detrimental to an individual with coronary disease, too low for a fit individual who is an experienced exerciser, and too high for an individual with hypertension who is taking beta-blocking medication, which may inhibit increases in heart rate. A flexible and thoughtful approach to assessing and assigning exercise intensity provides the most likely recipe for success.

Selecting Appropriate Modes of Exercise

It is important that the type or mode of exercise be appropriate to individual goals and limitations. Apparently healthy adults seeking recreation or health benefits from exercise may engage in a wide range of physical activities, their choices guided by personal preferences, which may change. For the athlete or competitive recreational exerciser, the mode of training is usually tightly connected to the performance activity.

An important distinction among modes of training for those who are obese or have musculoskeletal problems is the distinction between high- and low-impact activities. Activities such as cycling, swimming, water aerobics, rowing, and low-impact aerobics avoid the impact of body mass against the ground and may be better tolerated by those who are overweight or have orthopaedic limitations. Some activities that are technically low impact, such as cross-country skiing and roller-blading, have a high fall potential and so may not be appropriate for those with orthopaedic problems. They may, however, be useful for younger athletes recovering from impact-related overuse injuries. It is particularly important among the FITTE factors that the type or types of exercise selected be suitable and enjoyable to the participant.

Progression and Maintenance

The FITTE factors must change over the course of an exercise program to match progress. Just as an exercise session progresses through a warm-up stage to the conditioning stimulus, over a broader scale of weeks and months, a training program progresses through several discrete stages. Most training programs feature three stages: initiation, improvement, and maintenance.

Initiation Stage

The initial stage of training allows time to begin the adaptive process. Typically, this is accomplished by working at lower intensity and shorter duration and with careful attention to signs of intolerance, particularly musculoskeletal or cardiopulmonary. The initial stage is the time to develop the habit of exercise. A relatively high frequency of exercise (3 alternate days per week up to 5–6 sessions per week) may assist this process, as long as other FITTE factors are maintained at low levels.

Suitable initial intensities may range from 40% of $\dot{V}O_{2R}$ (RPE of 11–12) for beginners to more than 50% of $\dot{V}O_{2R}$ for individuals with higher aerobic capacities or experienced exercisers returning from time off regular exercise. Appropriate initial levels of duration range from 12–15 to 40 minutes per session. Older, obese, or profoundly sedentary individuals may start with as little as 12–15 minutes or less of continuous exercise. In such situations, especially if the factor limiting duration is stable angina or claudication, intermittent exercise or multiple daily sessions may be helpful. If intensity is kept low to moderate, sedentary but otherwise healthy adults may be able to start with sessions of 20 minutes, and experienced exercisers or high fitness athletes may begin with 30–40 minutes.

The exercise session itself may be modified during the initial stage of training by expanding the warm-up period, using it to inventory possible signs of failure to adapt ("Let's stretch out our quadriceps now; is anyone sore here?"), providing information, and answering questions. The initial stage of training generally lasts 3–6 weeks but may be expanded for those requiring additional time to adapt. The ability to conduct an exercise session independently and as prescribed at the upper levels of frequency (5–6 sessions per week) and duration (30–40 minutes) for 2 weeks without signs of excessive fatigue or musculoskeletal overuse indicates that an individual is ready to progress.

Improvement Stage

In the improvement stage, expanding physiological capacities are further challenged. This stage is typified by the phrase *progressive overload*. Small increments in the FITTE factors, particularly intensity and duration, may occur nearly every week. In fact, the challenge of the improvement stage is to increase training at a rate that continues to stimulate further advancement without causing overtraining and retrogression.

Several benchmarks of progression are discussed later in the chapter, but self-observation of subjective and objective responses to training may be the most important. Failure to complete an exercise session, lack of normal interest in training, increased levels of heart rate or RPE at the same rate of external work, and an increase in minor aches and pains are all signs that progression may be too rapid (23). In an appropriately incremented improvement stage, interest and appetite for exercise normally increase in tandem with the subjective and objective impressions that progress is being made. In general, frequency, intensity, and duration should not be increased together in any single week, nor should total weekly training volume be advanced by more than 10% (20). Increasing duration by 5–10 minutes per session on a weekly basis is usually well tolerated, as is building intensity gradually through the range of 60–85% of aerobic capacity over months. Progression of both intensity and duration in a single session is not recommended.

In this stage, adjusting the training program is commonly accomplished by increasing one FITTE factor over another in a saltatory approach toward individual goals. Competitive athletes who train intensively and those encountering musculoskeletal or other physical obstacles impeding progress may benefit from the early incorporation of techniques such as cross-training, which are more typical of the maintenance stage.

The adaptive potential of physiological function is finite, and large increments in fitness, typical in the improvement stage, always taper at some point. Aerobic capacity can be expected to expand by approximately 10–30% in the course of a program following ACSM guidelines, while improvements of more than 30% rarely occur unless accompanied by a large reduction in body weight and fat (4). If training is discontinued, gains in fitness regress by approximately 50% within 4–12 weeks (7). After approximately 6 months of training, almost everyone makes the transition from improvement to maintenance.

The Maintenance Stage

The maintenance stage is typified by diversification of the training program and purposeful attempts to rotate and reduce the stresses of continued training. Diversification may take the form of using several modes of exercise to maintain enjoyment and explore new capabilities. This may be particularly important to lifelong programs with goals such as weight management and general health. For those with a goal of general health, frequency and duration may be reduced (up to a 50% combined reduction) without loss of functional gains if intensity is maintained (7). However, if other physical activity is not substituted, many of the health benefits of exercise, which depend upon regular repetition, may be lost (2). Therefore, reduced training frequency should be complemented by the addition of other physical activities.

For those using the maintenance phase as a sustained period of performance or competition, diversification may be used as a means of reducing the potential for overuse injuries, particularly in programs with high training volumes or for participants with musculoskeletal limitations. **Cross-training**, as this approach is often called, refers to using a variety of modes of CR endurance exercise (such as swimming, running, and biking) to main-

tain a high level of training stimulus for central aerobic adaptations such as enhanced stroke volume and expanded blood volume. This approach allows rotation of local fatigue and musculoskeletal stresses across a range of muscle groups.

Cognitively, the maintenance stage is a time for enjoyment, surveillance, and reappraisal. It is a time for enjoying the fruits of labor by competing, engaging in new activities, or reducing the demands of weekly training. Surveillance for overuse injury must continue during the maintenance phase. Equipment and footwear should be re-evaluated. Finally, the goals of the program may be re-examined, physiological or performance testing repeated, and new goals established. To advance performance and CR endurance further often requires special techniques such as periodization and isolation of performance demands.

Modifications for Sport- and Activity-Specific Conditioning

Devising specific exercise programs for athletes to reach peak personal performance comprises the profession of coaching and exceeds the scope of this chapter. However, this chapter does discuss some principles, with emphasis on modifying the components of a single training session to the demands of a particular sport or activity.

The three components of a CR conditioning session are the warm-up, the aerobic stimulus, and the cool-down. In exercise programs specifically tailored to the goals and limitations of the individual, each component of the exercise session can be modified depending on the activity.

The warm-up should provide a transition from resting state to the exercise stimulus. Specifically, it is an opportunity to identify signs or symptoms of overuse, prepare specific muscle groups, and allow the CR system to adjust and prepare for higher-intensity work. The most basic way in which the warm-up can be modified for specific activities is to use the specific muscle groups that are involved in the activity. The musculoskeletal segments should be moved through a similar range of motion as is used in the stimulus activity, both to prepare the muscles and joints for exercise and to detect any residual soreness or other signs of injury or overuse. The intensity of the warm-up should gradually be increased over 5–15 minutes to about 50% of the intensity of the aerobic activity to follow. Before simple, repetitive activities such as running or cycling, the warm-up uses the same activity as the training stimulus at a lower rate. In this type of training session, stretching may be deferred until cool-down. Before competitive events, warm-up should be expanded to include static stretching of muscle groups about to be used (after some light activity), followed by performance of the activity (at moderate intensity) prior to the start of the event.

Most sporting activities require additional warm-up to prepare for sudden changes in intensity and rapid, powerful movements of multiple muscle groups and limbs over a wide range of motion. In most cases, after some light activity, muscles that are used in such performance should be gently stretched before progressing to more intense simulations of the sport.

For racquet sports such as tennis, squash, and racquetball, an adequate precompetition warm-up takes about 15–30 minutes and includes range of motion and transitional metabolic activity for both the arms and the legs. Warm-up generally starts with gentle jogging around the court for at least 2 minutes, followed by several minutes of gentle, progressive static stretching of the major muscles of the arm and back (triceps, deltoid, pectorals, and latissimus dorsi) as well as each of the major muscles of the leg (with special attention to the gluteals and adductors, which can easily be strained during stretching for a pass or volley). After stretching, shadow tennis, performed by moving through ground and overhead strokes without a ball, is followed by noncompetitive rallying. Hitting generally progresses from soft ground strokes at the service line back to the base line and then to overheads, lobs, and volleys.

Warming up for soccer may take a similar period, but it is more focused on preparing legs for ball handling and repetitive sprints. A typical pregame warm-up starts with several minutes of light jogging around the field. Once the player is warm and loose, gentle static stretching of all the major muscle groups of the legs with special attention to the quadriceps, hamstrings, and adductors of the thigh is appropriate. Next, light work such as ball juggling, gentle dribbling in the center circle, or passing with a teammate may be followed by several wind sprints (with or without the ball) of 20–40 yards, increasing in speed and intensity.

It is the aerobic stimulus component of the exercise session that is most dramatically altered to match the patterns demanded by the sport or the limitations of the participant. Even in an individual sport such as running, the aerobic stimulus phase may range from a 3-hour continuous run at 55–60% $\dot{V}O_{2R}$ for long-distance runners to a series of six 800-m intervals at more than 95% of $\dot{V}O_{2R}$ completed in less than 25 minutes for a 3-km runner.

In general, the three basic patterns of aerobic stimulus activities are continuous, interval, and circuit (27). Continuous exercise is probably the most common form of aerobic stimulus. It is best suited for those who perform sustained, nearly single-load work during the course of a sporting activity. Walking, hiking, distance running, and cycling are all activities in which most sessions are devoted to a continuous training stimulus. Some sustained sporting activities, such as cross-country running, feature changes in work rate due to terrain or competitive tactics. Continuous training for these sports is sometimes modified to include such fluxes in intensity. Fartlek (from Swedish for *speed play*), in which segments of a continuous run are completed at varying speeds, is one example.

In interval training, intense bouts of short duration are alternated with relief periods. Interval training is classically used by intermediate and middle-distance runners as a means of providing a training stimulus to both the aerobic and anaerobic energy systems. Longer-distance athletes wishing to improve a sustainable pace can also use it less formally. For example, a recreational half-marathon runner who desires to increase pace from 9 minutes per mile to 8:45 minutes per mile, may do a workout consisting of running half-mile intervals in 4:20, with a half-mile of jogging for recovery, repeated for 3–4 total miles twice a week. After several weeks of this interval training, an 8:45 pace may be sustainable for a continuous run.

Circuit training is a similar pattern of intensive work bouts alternated with relief periods; however, the work bout features a variety of tasks. Circuit training is particularly appropriate for surge-and-recover sports that feature an array of physical qualities, such as soccer or basketball. An example of a circuit program is a six-station circuit with each station performed for 2 minutes and a 45-second recovery phase to move to the next station. This is a sample six-station circuit session for basketball:

1. A set of short (<15 yard) line drills
2. As many jump shots as 2 minutes allows from a 16-foot perimeter
3. A series of plyometric rebounding tasks
4. A recovery station of free throws
5. A series of full-court runs
6. Repetitive leaping to touch the backboard or rim

Circuit training is particularly appropriate for those in physically active occupations, such as fire fighting, for which the job is often a linked series of specific intensive tasks (28). The degree of improvement in aerobic capacity using circuit training alone is modest (about 8%), although work capacity in the specific activities may be increased to a greater degree. Therefore, in highly aerobic pursuits or programs intended to raise $\dot{V}O_{2max}$, circuit training is not recommended as the sole stimulus (7).

The cool-down need not be so specific as the warm-up or stimulus activity. The more intensive and exhausting the event or conditioning session, the greater the requirement for gradual tapering of activity to avoid signs or symptoms upon transition to rest. After routine training, deep sustained stretching may be easier and more effective during the cool-down. However, after injury or a maximal competitive event, rest, rehydration, and injury treatment usually take precedence over deep stretching. Delayed-onset muscle soreness appears to be related to muscle and connective tissue damage associated with eccentric contractions and does not seem to be prevented by stretching after the event (29).

Beyond modification of the components of a single exercise session, there are two important concepts in exer-

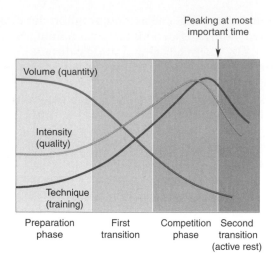

Figure 52.3. Interrelationships of volume, intensity, and technique for periodicity training.

cise programming for sports and activity. These are the concepts of isolation of specific physiological demands and periodization. Both techniques, like cross-training, may be used to advance training beyond the maintenance phase into continued progression. Each, however, has its own primary focus and range of application.

Many experienced coaches automatically do isolation of specific physiological stress. It is most appropriate in complex activities, such as sports that demand multiple physiological functions. It entails dissecting the primary functional elements of the sport and providing more intensive and focused training on each element in separate practice sessions. This isolation of distinct physiological stresses allows greater levels of overload for each element and also allows a rotation of specific stresses, which may forestall overtraining and overuse injuries.

Periodization is an advanced training technique that divides the season or annual calendar into cycles or phases (30). These phases focus adaptive development so the athlete approaches peak performance at the most advantageous time in the competitive schedule while varying exercise mode, intensity, and volume to diminish the possibility of overtraining (Fig. 52.3).

Exercise programming for sport and specific activities is clearly based on the concept of fitting the details of training to the specific performance demands of the sport or activity. As such, it serves as a fitting closing example of a primary theme in this chapter: People become fit through programs that fit them. Designing CR training programs tailored to the goals, needs, and limitations of each exerciser is a central skill of the exercise professional.

References

1. Casperson CJ, Powell KE, Christenson GM. Physical activity, exercise and physical fitness: Definitions and distinctions for health-related research. Public Health Rep 100:126, 1985.

2. Pate RR, Pratt M, Blair SN, et al. Physical activity and public health: A recommendation from the Centers for Disease Control and Prevention and the American College of Sports Medicine. JAMA 273:402, 1995.

3. Magel JR, Foglia GF, McArdle WD, et al. Specificity of swim training on maximum oxygen uptake. J Appl Physiol 38:151, 1975.

4. American College of Sports Medicine. ACSM Guidelines for Exercise Testing and Prescription. Philadelphia: Lippincott Williams & Wilkins, 2000.

5. Thomas S, Reading J, Shepard RJ. Revision of the Physical Activity Readiness Questionnaire (PAR-Q). Can J Sport Sci 17:338, 1992.

6. Fletcher GF, Balady G, Blair SN, et al. Statement on exercise: Benefits and recommendations for physical activity programs for all Americans. Circulation 94:857, 1996.

7. American College of Sports Medicine. The recommended quantity and quality of exercise for developing and maintaining CR, muscular fitness and flexibility in healthy adults. Med Sci Sports Exerc 30:975, 1998.

8. Harris SS, Caspersen CJ, DeFriese GH, et al. Physical activity counseling for healthy adults as a primary preventive intervention in the clinical setting: Report for the US Preventive Services Task Force. JAMA 261:3590, 1989.

9. NIH Consensus Development Panel. Physical activity and cardiovascular health. JAMA 276:241, 1996.

10. U.S. Surgeon General. Physical activity and health: A report of the Surgeon General. Washington: U.S. Government Printing Office, 1996.

11. McArdle WD, Katch FI, Katch VL. Exercise Physiology. Baltimore: Williams & Wilkins, 1996.

12. MacAlpin RH, Kattus AA. Adaptation to exercise in angina pectoris: The electrocardiogram during treadmill walking and coronary angiographic findings. Circulation 33:183, 1966.

13. Bouchard C, Shepard RJ, Stephens T, eds. Physical Activity, Fitness, and Health. Champaign, IL: Human Kinetics, 1994.

14. Powell KE, Thompson PD, Caspersen CJ, et al. Physical activity and the incidence of coronary heart disease. Ann Rev Public Health 8:253, 1987.

15. Blair SN, Kohl HW, Paffenbarger RS, et al. Physical fitness and all-cause mortality: A prospective study of healthy men and women. JAMA 262:2395, 1989.

16. Blair SN, Kohl HW, Barlow CE, et al. Changes in physical fitness and all-cause mortality: A prospective study of healthy and unhealthy men. JAMA 273:1093, 1995.

17. Lee IM, Hsieh CC, Paffenbarger, RS Jr. Exercise intensity and longevity in men: The Harvard alumni study. JAMA 273:1179, 1995.

18. Haskell WH. Dose-response issues from a biological perspective. In: Bouchard C, Shepard RJ, Stephens T, eds. Physical Activity, Fitness, and Health. Champaign, IL: Human Kinetics, 1994.

19. Swain DP, Leutholtz BC, King ME, et al. Relationship between % heart rate reserve and % $\dot{V}O_2$ reserve in treadmill exercise. Med Sci Sports Exerc 30:318, 1998.

20. Skinner JS. General principles of exercise prescription. In: Skinner JS, ed. Exercise Testing and Exercise Prescription. Philadelphia: Lea & Febiger, 1993.

21. Shaffrath JD, Adams WC. Effects of airflow and work load on cardiovascular drift and skin blood flow. J Appl Physiol 56:1411, 1984.

22. Nadel ER, Cafarelli E, Roberts MF. Circulatory regulation during exercise in different ambient temperatures. J Appl Physiol 46:430, 1979.

23. Lehmann M, Foster C, Keul J. Overtraining in endurance athletes: A brief review. Med Sci Sports Exerc 25:854, 1993.

24. Rowell LB. Human Circulation Regulation During Physical Stress. New York: Oxford University Press, 1986.

25. Ainsworth BE, Haskell WL, Leon AS, et al. Compendium of physical activities. Med Sci Sports Exerc 25:71, 1993.

26. Borg GA. Psychophysical bases of perceived exertion. Med Sci Sports Exerc 14:377, 1982.

27. Foss ML, Keteyian SJ. Fox's Physiological Basis for Exercise and Sport. Boston: WCB McGraw-Hill, 1998.

28. Davis PO, Dotson CO, Santa Maria DL. Relationship between simulated fire fighting tasks and physical performance measures. Med Sci Sport Exerc 14:65, 1982.

29. High DM, Howley ET. The effects of static stretching and warm-up on prevention of delayed-onset muscle soreness. Res Q 60:357, 1989.

30. Roundtable. Periodization. NSCA J 9:18, 1987.

Suggested Reading

American College of Sports Medicine. The recommended quantity and quality of exercise for developing and maintaining CR, muscular fitness and flexibility in healthy adults. Med Sci Sports Exerc 30:975, 1998.

U.S. Surgeon General. Physical activity and health: A report of the Surgeon General. Washington: U.S. Government Printing Office, 1996.

1.2.0, 1.2.5, 1.3.1, 1.8.2,   2.8.0.2, 2.8.0.9, 2.8.0.14,   4.8.6.1, 4.8.6.2,
1.8.3, 1.8.6, 1.8.15   2.8.0.19   4.8.6.3

CHAPTER **53**

MUSCULAR STRENGTH AND ENDURANCE

Cedric X. Bryant, James A. Peterson, and James E. Graves

Strength (resistance) training has become more popular over the past 15 years. Until recently, resistance training was primarily performed by selected groups of athletes and by individuals desiring to enhance physique. Resistance training has become an integral component of the exercise program for an array of individuals including those interested in fitness, competitive athletes, children, older adults, and cardiac rehabilitation patients (1–11).

Much of the increased popularity of resistance training can be attributed to successful education efforts regarding the number of positive benefits associated with it. Commonly cited reasons to engage in resistance training:

- Prevent and/or rehabilitate injury
- Control body weight
- Prevent or treat osteoporosis
- Enhance athletic performance
- Manage stress

Given the increasing body of knowledge concerning the benefits of resistance training, it is not surprising that several professional organizations and numerous members of both the exercise science and medical communities recommend that individuals of all ages and both genders participate in medically sound resistance training programs. This chapter addresses the principles and guidelines needed to develop safe and effective resistance training programs for healthy adults and certain special populations.

RESISTANCE TRAINING PROGRAM CONSIDERATIONS

Resistance training is an important component of a comprehensive fitness program. A proper resistance training program should be based on several factors, including health and fitness status, goals of the participant, proper application of the principles of training, and the training environment.

Health and Fitness Status

Before initiating resistance training, participants should take certain precautions. Minimally, a health and medical questionnaire should be completed. One of the most widely used is the Physical Activity Readiness Questionnaire (PAR-Q) (10). The PAR-Q is a relatively simple yet valid query form used for screening individuals prior to beginning an exercise program.

A muscular fitness evaluation should be considered for anyone who is to begin resistance training. Such information may serve several purposes. For example, initial level of muscular fitness can affect the magnitude and rate of improvement (12). Generally, muscularly fit individuals do not improve as much or as quickly as untrained individuals, which can be important when establishing goals or in evaluating the effectiveness of training. However, some persons may not be able to tolerate muscular fitness testing.

Goals

Once pre-exercise screening and assessment are complete, it is important to develop realistic goals and objectives. Unrealistic expectations can lead to adverse outcomes, including discouragement, poor adherence, and injury. An understanding of the physiological adaptations is important, because it enhances the likelihood that training is based on appropriate expectations. Table 53.1 summarizes the effects of resistance training on morphological, biochemical, neural, anthropometric, and performance factors (13). In addition, Chapter 19 contains an extensive discussion of the chronic adaptations to resistance training.

Principles of Training

Overload and specificity are precepts of resistance training. Both relate to the ability to adapt to stress. Adherence to these principles elicits both structural and functional adaptations, and resistance training that does not incorporate them cannot provide consistent improvement in muscular fitness.

Table 53.1. The Effects of Resistance Training on Morphology, Biochemistry, Neural Function, Body Composition, and Performance

	EFFECT		
	INCREASE	DECREASE	NO CHANGE
Morphological factors			
Size of type II (fast-twitch) muscle fibers	X		
Number of muscle fibers			X
Relative amount of muscle fibers			X
Number and size of myofibrils			X
Amount of contractile proteins	X		
Size and strength of connective tissue (e.g., tendons, ligaments, fascia)	X		
Bone mass and bone density	X		
Biochemical factors			
CP and ATP concentration	X		
Mitochondrial density		X	
Myokinase activity	X		
Neural factors			
Discharge frequency of motor neurons	X		
Motor unit recruitment	X		
Synchrony of recruitment	X		
Neural inhibitions		X	
Motor skill performance	X		
Body compositional factors			
Total body weight			X
Lean body weight	X		
Fat weight		X	
Percent body fat		X	
Performance factors			
Speed, power, balance, agility, and flexibility	X		

Overload occurs when a greater than normal physical demand is placed on muscles or muscle groups. The amount of overload required depends on the level of muscular fitness. For example, a football player requires a different level of overload from that of a sedentary person. To produce strength and endurance gains, the muscular system must be progressively overloaded. In the context of resistance training, overload can be achieved thus:

- By increasing the resistance or weight
- By increasing the repetitions
- By increasing the sets
- By decreasing the rest period between sets or exercises

By definition, overloading is dynamic (changing). In other words, as a muscle or muscle group adapts, a progressive overload is required to continue improvement. A training intensity of approximately 40–60% of one repetition maximum (1 RM) appears to be sufficient for the development of muscular strength in most normally active individuals. Intensities of 80–100%, however, have been shown to produce the most rapid gains in muscular strength (14). However, due to the possibility of overtraining or injury, caution must be used when overloading a muscle or muscle group.

Specificity relates to the nature of changes (structural and functional, systemic and local) that occur in an individual as a result of training. These adaptations are specific and occur only in the overloaded muscle groups or muscles.

The concept of specificity has other applications when applied to resistance training. Sports require specific movement patterns, which a properly designed program should consider. Although a sound resistance training program should include exercises for all of the major muscle groups, it can be modified to address the unique demands of a particular sport or activity (9, 15). The program for a pitcher, for example, should emphasize the rotator cuff, the shoulder girdle, and the upper extremities more than a soccer player's program, which focuses on the lower extremities and includes exercises to develop strength and endurance for the gluteals, quadriceps, hamstrings, abductors, adductors, and gastrocnemius.

One of the most controversial issues of specificity is the debate over how to develop muscular strength versus muscular endurance. The available literature indicates that different programs should be employed for development of muscular strength versus muscular endurance (9, 13, 14). Muscular strength is the ability to generate force at a given speed (velocity) of movement, while muscular endurance is the ability to persist in physical activity or resist muscular fatigue (4, 9). Generally, strength is developed with more resistance and fewer repetitions, while endurance requires low to moderate resistance and more repetitions (9, 13, 14). Adaptations occur at both the cellular level (metabolic adaptation) and at the fiber level (selective hypertrophy and motor unit recruitment patterns). Both strength and endurance are developed to some extent regardless of the program, because the two components exist on a continuum. However, one component may be emphasized, depending on the specific program.

Strength gains also depend on the mode of resistance training (static, dynamic, isokinetic), the type of contraction (concentric, eccentric), the speed of contraction, and the joint position (9, 14). The extent to which and how these factors should be incorporated into the design of a resistance training program remains an ongoing topic of discussion.

The Training Environment

There is a wide variety of training methods and equipment for improving muscular fitness. Methods of resistance training are typically classified according to the type of muscular contraction (static, dynamic, or isokinetic).

Types of Muscular Contractions

During static (isometric) contractions, the muscle or muscle group maintains a constant length as resistance is applied and no change in joint position occurs. Research has demonstrated that static training produces improvements in muscular strength. The strength gains, however, are limited to the specific joint angles at which the static contractions are performed (9, 16–18). As a result, static training may have limited value in enhancing functional strength. Static training has also been associated with acute elevations in blood pressure, perhaps due to increased intrathoracic pressure during static contractions. Despite the limitations, static training appears to play a positive role in physical rehabilitation. For example, it is effective for maintaining muscular strength and for preventing atrophy associated with the immobilization of a limb (e.g., application of a cast, splint, or brace) (9, 14, 17).

Dynamic (isotonic) resistance training is another common method. If movement of the joint occurs during contraction, it is dynamic. If force is sufficient to overcome resistance and the muscle shortens (e.g., the lifting phase of a biceps curl), the contraction is concentric. When resistance is greater than force and the muscle lengthens during contraction, it is eccentric (e.g., the lowering phase of the biceps curl).

Most dynamic resistance training includes both concentric and eccentric action. Significantly heavier loads can be moved eccentrically; in fact, in unfatigued muscle, the ratio of eccentric to concentric strength can be as high as 1.4:1 (9, 14). Furthermore, at the onset of fatigue, the relative level of eccentric strength and eccentric–concentric ratio increases even more. Individuals who are eccentrically trained are subject to delayed-onset muscular soreness (19, 20). Eccentric training can, however, play an important role in preventing or rehabilitating certain musculoskeletal injuries. For example, eccentric training, because it can affect deceleration capacity, has been demonstrated to be efficacious for treating hamstring strains, tennis elbow, and patellofemoral pain syndrome (21, 22).

Dynamic exercise can be further categorized into constant resistance and variable resistance. During constant resistance exercise, resistance applied does not change throughout the range of motion. Since force production can vary significantly at different points in the range of motion, gains are limited by inherent weak points on the strength curve of working muscle. On the other hand, during variable-resistance exercise, leverage advantages and disadvantages are changed over the range of motion, resulting in gains that are theoretically not restricted by variations in the strength curve of a muscle.

The other major type of resistance training, isokinetic exercise, entails constant-speed muscular contraction against accommodating resistance. The speed of movement is controlled, and the amount of resistance is proportional to the amount of force produced throughout the full range of motion. The theoretical advantage of isokinetic exercise is the development of maximal muscle tension throughout the range of motion. Research documents the effectiveness of isokinetic training (9, 17). Strength gains achieved during high-speed training (i.e., contraction velocities of 180 degrees per second or faster) appear to carry over to all speeds less than that specific speed (23, 24). Improvement in strength at slow speeds of movement, however, has not been shown to carry over to faster speeds.

Types of Resistance Training Equipment

A variety of equipment can accommodate various types of training and various training goals. Almost any type of resistance equipment enables individuals to meet training goals provided that it allows an overload and that appropriate guidelines are followed. Individuals should select equipment that is accessible and consistent with personal needs and interests. Table 53.2 compares three common types of equipment on selected criteria. More detailed discussions of resistance equipment can be found in Chapter 77 and elsewhere (2, 15).

GUIDELINES FOR DEVELOPING MUSCULAR FITNESS

Specific guidelines for achieving muscular fitness are not as widely accepted as those for aerobic fitness. Controversy regarding the most appropriate prescription for developing muscular fitness is considerable. However, there is growing awareness that moderate intensity resistance training should be an integral part of a comprehensive fitness program.

As with any exercise prescription, instructions regarding intensity, duration, and frequency; guidelines for rate of progression; and precautions are important. This information should be based on health and fitness status and personal goals and interests.

Table 53.2. Comparative Overview of Various Types of Resistance Training Equipment

	FREE WEIGHTS (BARBELLS, DUMBBELLS)	MULTISTATION MACHINES	SELECTORIZED MACHINES
Cost	Low	Somewhat high	High
Functionality	Excellent	Limited	Limited
Learning curve	Limited	Excellent	Excellent
Muscle isolation	Variable	Excellent	Excellent
Rehabilitation	Excellent	Excellent	Excellent
Safety	Relatively safe	Very safe	Very safe
Space efficiency	Variable	Excellent	Variable
Time efficiency	Variable	Excellent	Excellent
Variety	Excellent	Limited	Limited
Versatility	Excellent	Limited	Limited

Muscular fitness can be developed through either static (isometric) or dynamic (isotonic and isokinetic) exercises. Dynamic resistance is recommended for most adults who want basic resistance training. Furthermore, because the primary objective of resistance training should be to develop total body muscular fitness in a safe and time-efficient manner, individuals should be encouraged to perform 8–10 different exercises to condition major muscle groups.

Appropriate resistance training for healthy adults should be based on the following guidelines and principles:

- Use a brief warm-up prior to performing resistance exercise.
- Adhere to proper techniques for performing each exercise.
- Perform at least one set of 8–12 repetitions of each exercise to the point of volitional fatigue. There is no magic formula regarding the number of sets and repetitions that provide optimal gains in muscular fitness for all individuals.
- Increase the resistance when a predetermined number of repetitions (typically 8–12) can be completed using proper form. Increases in resistance should be made gradually (e.g., increments of approximately 5%).
- Exercise at least twice a week. Recovery time (rest) is an important component of muscular growth and strength development, and most individuals require approximately 48 hours to recover from a typical resistance training session. When training at very low loads (i.e., in certain therapeutic settings), more frequent training sessions may be tolerated.
- Perform both the lifting (concentric phase) and lowering (eccentric phase) portions in a controlled manner. Performing ballistic movements during resistance training can compromise safety and effectiveness.
- Perform each exercise through a functional range of motion. This helps ensure that joint mobility is maintained and, in some instances, enhanced.
- Maintain a normal breathing pattern; breath holding may induce excessive elevations in blood pressure through a Valsalva maneuver.
- When possible, exercise with a training partner who provides feedback, assistance, and encouragement.

An understanding of resistance training equipment and the most commonly used methods for developing strength (as well as advantages and limitations) is basic to effective modification of the prescription for resistance training for specific conditioning needs and interests. Such modification is necessary to maximize the benefits of resistance training and to avoid injury. Many standard resistance training programs are described and well illustrated in other publications (2, 15).

RESISTANCE TRAINING FOR SPECIAL POPULATIONS

Resistance training is useful for many special populations. For example, though modification is necessary, children can safely train and benefit from the positive effects (3). Resistance training has also been demonstrated to be beneficial for various age-related medical conditions and in certain types of cardiovascular disease (4, 14). Not surprisingly, there are no age or gender restrictions for resistance training. Research documents that women reap similar benefits as men and under normal circumstances do not develop large muscles (15). Furthermore, resistance training can be safely incorporated into an exercise regimen for pregnant women. In fact, the improved level of muscular fitness attendant on sound resistance training may decrease the severity and/or incidence of orthopaedic discomfort (4, 15).

Children

Until recently, the prevailing attitude among much of the medical community was that preadolescent children should not engage in resistance training because of concerns related to a lack of physical maturity. Collectively, these concerns appear to have focused on three issues:

- Whether resistance training places excess stress on the musculoskeletal systems of preadolescents
- Whether resistance training provides demonstrable benefits for children
- How resistance training programs for children should be designed to maximize benefits and minimize risks

At least three major organizations have developed position papers making formal recommendations regarding children and resistance training (1, 2, 25). Research has demonstrated that resistance training for children, when properly performed, can be productive and beneficial (i.e., benefits outweigh risks) (1–3, 25). Unfortunately, despite the benefits, resistance training for children carries some risk. One concern is the potential that inappropriate training may damage a developing skeletal system and the supportive tissues (2, 3). Lifting excessively heavy weights may significantly increase risk of growth cartilage injury. However, growth cartilage injuries associated with properly designed and supervised resistance training are rare. The risk of injury in resistance training in children is quite low if a proper lifting technique is used and only appropriate demands are placed on the child.

There are no minimum age standards for resistance training in children. Several factors should be considered before beginning resistance training in children:

- Ability to accept and follow instructions
- Desire to participate
- Basic motor skills and ability to perform exercises safely

Resistance training may be more appropriate for some children than others, depending on the aforementioned factors. Once the decision has been made, however, all programs for children must adhere to certain guidelines and principles:

- All children have developing musculoskeletal systems.
- Proper training technique for all exercises is required.
- All exercises should be performed in a controlled manner, and fast, jerky ballistic movement must be avoided.
- Resistance must be matched to the child's needs and structural limitations. Excessive resistance can damage developing skeletal and joint structures. Each set of an exercise should consist of 8–12 repetitions. Adolescents should not exercise to the point of volitional muscular fatigue.
- Overload initially by increasing the number of repetitions, subsequently by increasing the resistance.
- The array of exercises should include at least one for each major muscle group (e.g., gluteals, quadriceps, hamstrings, pectorals, latissimus dorsi, deltoids, erector spinae, and abdominals). Perform one or two sets of 8–10 different exercises.
- Perform two resistance training sessions per week with at least one rest day between sessions. Lower training volume reduces stress and allows for other forms of physical activity.
- Perform full-range multijoint exercises (e.g., leg press, lat pull-down), as opposed to single-joint exercises (e.g., leg extension, biceps curl), because such exercises facilitate development of functional strength.
- Achieve muscular balance in each session by alternating pairs of muscle groups (i.e., perform a pull exercise for each push exercise) (Table 53.3).

Appropriately trained personnel capable of providing proper strength training instruction must closely supervise all resistance training.

Seniors

Impaired muscular function has been linked to impaired functional ability in older adults. Difficulty in rising from a seated position, poor walking, and poor balance are common functional disabilities in older adults. The long-range implication of lack of strength is limited

independence. Appropriate resistance training may enhance overall function and well-being in older adults.

Resistance training may assist in effective management of osteoarthritis (26). Functional ability can be improved if surrounding muscles and unaffected joints share stress with affected joints. Stronger muscles absorb more of the attendant stress on a joint, thereby reducing stress on affected joint surfaces.

Evidence indicates that resistance training slows bone loss and can increase bone density (12, 10). Osteoporosis is characterized by decreased bone mineral content (decreased density) and may be improved by resistance training. Furthermore, training-induced improvements in muscular strength and balance may prevent falls that cause many fractures among elderly women with osteoporosis.

Resistance preserves muscle tissue during aging and may contribute to weight control by maintaining an increased metabolic rate. In addition, most daily activities require some muscular fitness. With appropriate resistance training, older adults improve the likelihood that they can maintain appropriate levels of muscular fitness and improved daily function.

Regardless of which specific resistance training protocol is adopted, several commonsense guidelines for resistance training in older adults should be followed:

- Design the program to develop sufficient muscular fitness to enhance ability to live independently.
- Closely supervise and monitor initial sessions with trained personnel who are sensitive to the special needs and capabilities of older adults.
- Use minimum levels of resistance during the first 8 weeks to allow for adaptation of connective tissue elements.
- Instruct and use proper technique for performing all exercises.
- Instruct all older participants to maintain normal breathing patterns while exercising. Teach them to avoid Valsalva maneuvers.
- Overload by increasing number of repetitions at first and only subsequently by increasing resistance.
- Use a resistance that can be comfortably lifted for at least six repetitions per set. Heavy resistance is dangerous and may damage skeletal and joint structure.
- Weights should be lifted and lowered in a slow, controlled manner. No ballistic movements should be allowed (to prevent orthopaedic trauma to joint structures).
- Perform all exercises in a pain-free range of motion, that is, the maximum range of motion that does not elicit pain or discomfort. As positive adaptations occur, individuals may gradually increase range of motion and improve flexibility.
- Perform multijoint exercises (as opposed to single-joint exercises) that tend to assist in the development of functional muscular fitness.

Table 53.3. Example of Suggested Exercise Order

	PUSH	PULL
Legs	Leg press	Leg curl
Chest, back	Bench press	Seated row
Shoulder, back	Military press	Lat pull-down
Arms	Triceps extension	Biceps curl
Trunk	Back extension	Abdominal curl

- The use of machines offers several advantages:
  - They require less skill to use.
  - They generally provide more support for the back by stabilizing body position.
  - They enable participants to start with lower levels of resistance (depending on the specific type of equipment).
  - They typically enable increased resistance level through smaller increments (not true for all resistance training machines).
  - They allow greater control of the exercise range of motion.
  - They generally provide a more time-efficient workout.
- Do not overtrain. Two resistance training sessions per week is the minimum number required to produce positive physiological adaptation. While more frequent training may elicit larger strength gains, additional improvement is relatively small.
- Resistance training must be avoided during periods of active pain or inflammation in older adults with arthritis; exercise during these periods may exacerbate the inflammation.

The resistance training program should be performed on a regular basis throughout the year. Research demonstrates that cessation of resistance training results in rapid, significant loss of strength (9). When resuming after a layoff, begin with resistance levels equivalent to or less than 50% of the intensity prior to discontinuing. As adaptation occurs, slowly and progressively increase resistance.

Cardiac Patients

Historically, cardiac rehabilitation programs have focused almost exclusively on improving cardiorespiratory fitness, despite muscular fitness requirements for all activities of daily living, especially occupational tasks. The reluctance to include resistance training has been due in part to a belief that heavy resistance exercise strains rather than stimulates the cardiovascular system. However, appropriately prescribed and supervised, regular progressive resistance exercise training may favorably affect muscle strength, cardiorespiratory endurance, hypertension, hyperlipidemia, glucose tolerance, insulin sensitivity, and psychosocial well-being (4, 6–8). Both the American College of Sports Medicine (ACSM) and the American Association of Cardiovascular and Pulmonary Rehabilitation (AACVPR) recommend resistance training as an integral part of a comprehensive exercise program for cardiac patients, particularly the following:

- Those whose occupation requires extensive arm work (e.g., laborers, construction workers, auto mechanics). Improving strength and endurance of specific muscle groups required for occupational activities allows such patients to be more capable of safely performing work-related duties while diminishing the likelihood that other bodily systems will be overtaxed.
- Those with a desire to participate in leisure or recreational activities that involve extensive use of the upper extremities (e.g., racquet sports, gardening).
- Those with a desire to engage in resistance training, either to offset the atrophy that results from a sedentary lifestyle or to enhance physical appearance by favorably altering body composition. Such changes can improve self-esteem and psychological well-being.

The decision to implement a strength-training program for a cardiac patient should be based on needs, interests, and medical and health status. After specific needs and interests have been clearly identified, the patient's physician should carefully review the medical and health history. The ACSM and AACVPR have guidelines to assist in identification of coronary-prone individuals for whom resistance training is safe and appropriate (10, 11). The ACSM and AACVPR recommend the following inclusion criteria:

- 4–6 weeks post myocardial infarction or coronary artery bypass grafting (CABG)
- 1–2 weeks following percutaneous transluminal coronary angiography or other revascularization procedure, except CABG, without myocardial infarction
- Following 4–6 weeks in a supervised cardiovascular endurance program or completion of phase II
- Resting diastolic blood pressure below 105 mm Hg
- Peak exercise capacity more than 5 METs
- Not compromised by coronary heart failure, unstable symptoms, or arrhythmias

Safety is the most important issue attendant to resistance training for cardiac patients. Specific guidelines for the safe and effective application of resistance training in cardiac patients have been developed by the AACVPR (7, 11):

- Limit resistance training to patients who are asymptomatic or only mildly symptomatic.
- Initiate resistance training after a minimum of 12 weeks of aerobic training.
- To prevent soreness and injury, select an initial resistance allowing 10–12 comfortable repetitions of an exercise. This level of resistance generally corresponds to approximately 60% of 1 RM. Training at this intensity can produce significant improvements in functional muscle strength.
- Use single-limb exercises (instead of double-limb) in patients who have an exaggerated rise in blood pressure (BP) and/or rate pressure product (systolic BP × heart rate) during resistance training.
- Two to three sets of each exercise is recommended.

- Ratings of perceived exertion (6–20 RPE scale) should not exceed fairly light (14) to somewhat hard (15) during resistance training. Patients should not strain.
- Avoid breath holding. Breathe normally at all times.
- Increase resistance by 2.5–5 lb when 10–12 repetitions can be comfortably accomplished; for high-risk adults and cardiac patients, the resistance should be increased only after at least 12–15 repetitions can be easily managed.
- Exercise muscles generally in a large-muscle to small-muscle order, 2–3 times per week. Include exercises for both the upper and lower extremities.
- Avoid excessive static contraction, hand gripping (e.g., free weight bars, dumbbells, machine handles) if possible; high-level static contraction may evoke excessive blood pressure response.
- Discontinue exercise in the event of any contraindicative warning signs or symptoms, especially dizziness, abnormal heart rhythm, unusual shortness of breath, and/or chest pain.
- Rest periods should be relatively short (about 1 minute), between both individual exercises and sets of exercises, to maximize muscular endurance and aerobic training benefits.
- Require patients to monitor and record heart rate response, RPE, and symptoms following each exercise or set of exercises.

Pregnant Women

Many women hesitate to continue resistance training during pregnancy because of the seemingly inconsistent and diverse opinions on the subject. Recently, however, specific advice for pregnant women interested in resistance training has been published (4, 15). Limited data indicate that appropriate resistance training poses little risk to either the mother or the fetus and may be beneficial. For example, proper resistance training provides a pregnant woman with an enhanced level of muscular fitness, which may help compensate for the postural adjustments typical of pregnancy that are often associated with low back pain. The activities of daily living may be performed with greater relative ease with an enhanced level of muscular fitness.

However, experts are relatively quick to note that resistance training is not advisable for all pregnant women. The following recommendations regarding resistance training and pregnancy are appropriate:

- Women with any of the American College of Obstetrics and Gynecology (ACOG) contraindications for aerobic exercise during pregnancy should not participate in resistance training (Table 53.4) (4, 10).
- Women who have never participated in resistance training should not begin during pregnancy.

Table 53.4. Contraindications for Exercising During Pregnancy

1. Pregnancy-induced hypertension
2. Preterm rupture of membrane
3. Preterm labor during previous or current pregnancy
4. Incompetent cervix
5. Persistent second- or third-trimester bleeding
6. Intrauterine growth retardation

- Ballistic exercises should be strictly avoided, since pregnancy is associated with joint and connective tissue laxity, which may increase susceptibility to injury.
- Women should be encouraged to breathe normally during resistance training, because oxygen delivery to the placenta may be reduced during breath holding (i.e., a Valsalva maneuver).
- Heavy resistance should be avoided, since it may expose the joints, connective tissue, and skeletal structures of an expectant woman to excessive forces. An exercise set consisting of at least 12–15 repetitions without undue fatigue generally ensures that the resistance is appropriate.
- As training advances, overload initially by increasing number of repetitions and only subsequently by increasing resistance.
- Resistance training on machines is usually preferred over free weights because machines require less skill and can be more easily controlled.
- If a specific exercise causes pain or discomfort, it should be discontinued and an alternative exercise used. The following warning signs or complications require consultation with a physician:
  - Vaginal bleeding
  - Abdominal pain or cramping
  - Ruptured membranes
  - Elevated blood pressure or heart rate
  - Lack of fetal movement

Limited research demonstrates that resistance training can be an integral part of a balanced exercise prescription during pregnancy. It appears that resistance training may assist in management of many of the rigors of pregnancy. Research also suggests that resistance training may not be appropriate for all pregnant women. Until more data are available, medical advice and a physician's recommendation should be obtained prior to resistance training during pregnancy. In addition, exercise prescription for resistance training during pregnancy should be individualized. As a rule, exercise professionals designing resistance training programs for pregnant women should be conservative in the approach to manipulating variables.

► SUMMARY

Resistance training programs should be an integral part of a comprehensive fitness program. Health and fitness status, individual goals, and principles of training should be considered when designing programs. Resistance training is generally safe for many special populations, including children, older adults, and cardiac patients as long as appropriate precautions are observed. Exercise professionals should be aware of both the health status and the contraindications to exercise in all clients for whom resistance training is recommended.

References

1. Cahill B, ed. Proceedings of the Conference on Strength Training and the Prepubescent. Chicago: American Orthopaedic Society for Sports Medicine, 1988.
2. Kraemer WJ, Fleck SJ. Strength Training for Young Athletes. Champaign, IL: Human Kinetics, 1993.
3. Tanner SM. Weighing the risks: Strength training for children and adolescents. Phys Sportsmed 21:105, 1993.
4. Peterson JA, Bryant CX. The StairMaster Fitness Handbook. Champaign, IL: Sagamore, 1995.
5. Munnings F. Strength training: Not only for the young. Phys Sportsmed 21:133, 1993.
6. Bryant CX, Peterson JA. Strength training for the heart? Fitness Manag 2:32, 1994.
7. Franklin BA, Bonzheim K, Gordon S, et al. Resistance training in cardiac rehabilitation. J Cardiopulm Rehab 11:99, 1991.
8. McKelvie RS, McCartney N. Weightlifting training in cardiac patients: considerations. Sports Med 10:355, 1990.
9. Fleck SJ, Kraemer WJ. Designing Resistance Training Programs. 2nd ed. Champaign, IL: Human Kinetics, 1997.
10. American College of Sports Medicine. ACSM's Guidelines for Exercise Testing and Prescription. 6th ed. Philadelphia: Lippincott Williams & Wilkins, 2000.
11. American Association of Cardiovascular and Pulmonary Rehabilitation. Guidelines for Cardiac Rehabilitation Programs. 3rd ed. Champaign, IL: Human Kinetics, 1999.
12. Hakkinen K. Factors influencing trainability of muscular strength during short term and prolonged training. Natl Strength Cond Assoc J 7:32, 1985.
13. Kraemer WJ, Deschenes MR, Fleck SJ. Physiological adaptations to resistance exercise: Implications for athletic conditioning. Sports Med 6:246, 1988.
14. DiNubile NA. Strength training. Clin Sports Med 10:33, 1991.
15. Peterson JA, Bryant CX, Peterson SL. Strength Training for Women. Champaign, IL: Human Kinetics, 1995.
16. Graves JE, Pollock ML, Jones AE, et al. Specificity of limited range of motion of variable resistance training. Med Sci Sports Exerc 21:84, 1989.
17. Knapik JJ, Mawdsley RH, Ramos NU. Angular specificity and test mode specificity of isometric and isokinetic strength training. J Orthop Sports Phys Ther 5:58, 1983.
18. Gardner G. Specificity of strength changes of the exercised and nonexercised limb following isometric training. Res Q 34:98, 1963.
19. Byrnes W. Muscle soreness following resistance exercise with and without eccentric contractions. Res Q 56:283, 1985.
20. Talag TS. Residual muscular soreness influenced by concentric, eccentric, and static contractions. Res Q 44:458, 1973.
21. Stanish WD, Rubinovich RM, Curwin S. Eccentric exercise in chronic tendinitis. Clin Orthop 208:65, 1986.
22. Fleck SJ, Falkel JE. Value of resistance training for the reduction of sports injuries. Sports Med 3:61, 1986.
23. Coyle E et al. Specificity of power improvements through slow and fast isokinetic training. J Appl Physiol 51:1437, 1981.
24. Lesme G, Costill D, Coyle E, et al. Muscle strength and power changes during maximal isokinetic training. Med Sci Sports Exerc 10:266, 1978.
25. National Strength and Conditioning Association. Position statement on prepubescent strength training. Natl Strength Condit Assoc J 7:27, 1985.
26. Ettinger WH, Burns R, Messier SP, et al. A randomized trial comparing aerobic exercise and resistance exercise with a health education program in older adults with knee osteoarthritis: The Fitness Arthritis and Seniors Trial (FAST). JAMA 277:25–31, 1997.

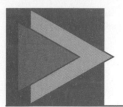

CHAPTER **54**

EXERCISE RECOMMENDATIONS FOR FLEXIBILITY AND RANGE OF MOTION

Denise M. Fredette

Flexibility is characterized by a ready capability to adapt to new and different or changing requirements and is applied more specifically to the range of motion (ROM), which occurs at a single joint or series of joints (1, 2). Increased flexibility improves fluidity, ease, coordination, and responsiveness of movement (Table 54.1).

PHYSIOLOGY OF FLEXIBILITY

Neuromuscular Factors

Four proprioceptive sensory organ systems respond to a stretch stimulus (3, 4):

- The Golgi tendon organ (GTO)
- The intrafusal muscle fibers of the muscle spindle
- The pacinian corpuscle
- The Ruffini end organs in deep connective tissue and joint capsules

These receptors are active during strong contraction or stretch. They inhibit or facilitate contraction with a coordinated effect to protect muscle from overcontraction or overstretch (4). The GTOs are located in muscle tendon, and when activated, they reflexively inhibit contraction and signal a stretched muscle to relax. Muscle spindles are sensory organs scattered throughout muscle tissue that reflexively activate muscle and concurrently inhibit the opposing, or antagonist, muscle. This response is known as the stretch reflex (4). If the stretch impulse is too great, muscle spindle input causes a protective contraction. The pacinian corpuscles and Ruffini end organs are stimulated by pressure from surrounding structures when joints are moved. Extreme pressure results in pain perception and withdrawal from a noxious stretch stimulus (3, 4).

Mechanical Factors

Mechanical properties of connective tissue, the superstructure of muscles, tendons, and joint capsules, are also important. Within connective tissue are fibroblasts that have an important role in connective tissue repair. Fi-

broblasts respond to injury by stimulating proliferation and fibrogenesis. They participate in healing of defects in connective tissue, cartilage, tendon, and adjacent connective tissue–like muscle (5). Gradual deformation of connective tissue is the goal of stretching a muscle. Microtrauma occurs in connective tissue in response to stretching, followed by recovery and repair. Repair leads to new fiber organization, thus greater extensibility (4, 6).

Connective tissue in muscle is composed of 80% plastin fibers and 20% elastin fibers, giving myofascial tissue a great potential for extensibility (5, 7, 8). Hooke's law states that the amount of stretch (deformation) is proportional to the applied force (9). Current research on the response of connective tissue to an applied stressor indicates that a slow, sustained stretch of 30–90 seconds is necessary to get beyond elastic recoil properties of skeletal muscle and produce mild deformation that stimulates fiber reorganization (7, 8). The stress–strain relationship of tissues under stretch is demonstrated in Fig. 54.1.

WHO SHOULD AND SHOULD NOT STRETCH?

Everyone can learn to stretch, regardless of age or initial flexibility. Emphasizing methods that are easy and gentle and adapting the program to individual needs is important for all ages. Children benefit from stretching as much as adults, and high levels of fitness are not required to begin a stretching program.

Some individuals have naturally loose ligaments and connective tissue, and their joint capsules, ligaments, and surface relationships may allow for excessive ROM. These hypermobile individuals should not be allowed to stretch into the extremes of ROM because joint stability should be maintained as much as possible.

During pregnancy a hormone called relaxant softens the ligaments and connective tissue, especially of the pelvis. Excessive stretching during pregnancy is not recommended. It can lead to hypermobility of the low back, sacroiliac region, and other areas during and after pregnancy. The benefits of flexibility training are listed in

Table 54.1. The Benefits of Increased Flexibility

Reduced muscle tension and increased relaxation
Ease of movement
Improved coordination through greater ease of movement
Increased range of motion
Injury prevention
Improvement and development of body awareness
Improved circulation and air exchange
Decreased muscle viscosity, causing contractions to be easier and smoother
Decreased soreness associated with other exercise

Table 54.2. Contraindications For Flexibility Training

Motion limited by bony block at a joint interface
Recent unhealed fracture
Infection and acute inflammation affecting the joint or surrounding tissues
Sharp pain associated with stretch or uncontrolled muscle cramping when attempting to stretch
Local hematoma as a result of an overstretch injury
Contracture (desired functional shortening) requiring stability to a joint capsule or ligament contracture that is intentional to improve function, particularly in clients with paralysis or severe muscle weakness (e.g., tenodesis of finger flexors to allow grasp in an individual with quadriplegia)

Table 54.3. Precautions for Flexibility Training

Stretch a joint through limits of normal ROM only.
Do not stretch at healed fracture sites for about 8–12 weeks post fracture, after which gentle stretching may be initiated.
In individuals with known or suspected osteoporosis, stretch with particular caution (e.g., men older than 80 years and women older than 65 years, older persons with spinal cord injury).
Avoid aggressive stretching of tissues that have been immobilized (e.g., cast or splinted). Tissues become dehydrated and lose tensile strength during immobilization.
Mild soreness should take no longer than 24 hours to resolve after stretching. If more recovery time is necessary, the stretching force was excessive.
Use active comfortable ROM to stretch edematous joints or soft tissue.
Do not overstretch weak muscles. Shortening in these muscles may contribute to joint support that muscles can no longer actively provide. Combine strength and stretching exercise so that gains in mobility coincide with gains in strength and stability.
Be aware that physical performance may vary from day to day.
Set individual goals.

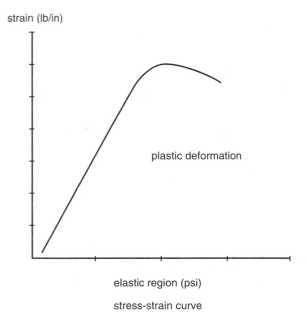

Figure 54.1. The stress-strain curve with the upward slope representing the elastic recoil zone. The curve with the downward slope portrays the plastic deformation zone.

Table 54.1. The contraindications and precautions for stretching and flexibility training are shown in Tables 54.2 and 54.3, respectively (10–12).

WHEN TO STRETCH

Individual preference determines appropriate time of day for flexibility exercise. Spontaneous stretching, done properly anywhere, is effective and desirable. Stretching before and after physical activity should be part of warm-up and cool-down. Warm-up with light activity, such as walking, before stretching is recommended. Warm muscle tissue accepts stretch easier than cold. Stretching is indicated after sitting or standing for long periods, especially during or after a long drive. Stretching can help prevent discomfort from periods of immobility.

FREQUENCY AND DURATION OF TRAINING

There is wide variation of opinion about the most effective frequency and duration for flexibility training. Beaulieu (13) states that a stretch may be held for 10–15 seconds initially and gradually increased to 45–60 seconds over 4–5 weeks. Anderson (10) suggests beginning with an easy stretch for 10–30 seconds followed by a "developmental" stretch for an additional 10–30 seconds. Moffatt (14) recommends maintaining stretching posture for about 8–12 seconds. In contrast, Feldenkrais suggests taking 3 or 4 exercises and repeating those exercises slowly 3 or 4 times for a total of 30 minutes of exercise (15). Yoga practitioners dedicate 30–45 minutes each day to stretching (16, 17). The American College of Sports Medicine proposes that a stretch should last for 10–30 seconds (18).

Connective tissue deformation and neuroinhibitory effects require 30–90 seconds to effect tissue change and

---

Table 54.4. Guidelines for Proper Stretching

Determine posture or position to be used. Ensure proper position and alignment prior to the stretch.

Emphasize proper breathing. Inhale through the nose and exhale through pursed lips during the stretch. One may stretch with the eyes closed to increase concentration and awareness.

Hold end points progressively for 30–90 seconds and take another deep breath.

Exhale and feel the muscle being stretched, relaxed, and softened so that further ROM is achieved.

Discomfort may increase slightly, but continue to focus on breathing.

Repeat the inhale–exhale–stretch cycle until the end of the available range for the day.

Do not bounce or spring while stretching.

Do not force a stretch while holding the breath.

Increased stretching range during exhalation encourages full body relaxation.

Slowly reposition from the stretch posture and allow muscles to recover at natural resting length.

---

a relaxation response (4, 7, 8). Beaulieu (13) states that stretching should be done for 10–20 minutes, 2 or 3 times per week. deVries found that stretching for 30 minutes twice a week improves flexibility within 5 weeks (19, 20). Feldenkrais and yoga practitioners recommend daily stretching because of the relaxation benefits (15, 16).

HOW TO STRETCH

The guidelines in Table 54.4 are synthesized recommendations from Anderson (10, 21), Krusen et al. (22), Kuland (23), Morris (2), Hittleman (17), and Bersin et al. (15). It is helpful to have an exercise professional observe patients during the initiation of a stretch to ensure proper alignment. Incorrect stretching can be ineffective and may be damaging. Proper alignment is defined as good biomechanical relation of each joint to the adjacent joints.

TECHNIQUES USED TO GAIN FLEXIBILITY
Static Stretching

A static stretch is slow and sustained to increase motion at a particular joint when one segment is manipulated relative to another (2, 22). The advantages of static stretching include the following (19, 23–26):

- Decreased possibility of exceeding normal range of motion
- Lower energy requirements
- Less muscle soreness
- The types of static stretching include passive, active assistive, active, and proprioceptive neuromuscular facilitation (PNF).

Passive Stretching

Passive stretch requires assistance from another person or a device. Optimal passive stretch requires relaxation of all voluntary and reflex muscular resistance, which is often hard to achieve. Trust that the partner will not go too far or too fast is essential (18). Types of passive stretching (27):

- Manual
- Prolonged mechanical
- Cyclic mechanical
- Self

Active Assistive Stretching

In active assistive stretching the muscle or joint being stretched may require assistance moving through the ROM because of weakness. The stretch requires the assistance of a partner and has the same limitations as passive stretching (18).

Active Stretching

During active stretching a muscle or joint is actively moved through the ROM. This technique requires greater energy than passive or static stretching. It may elicit a stretch reflex and thereby cause the stretch to be improperly performed (18).

Proprioceptive Neuromuscular Facilitation

Types of PNF techniques for stretching include the contract–relax (hold–relax) stretch and the contract–relax–contract (hold–relax–contract) stretch (28). For contract–relax PNF, a muscle is contracted, relaxed, then further stretched into the available ROM during this brief relaxation phase. The same procedure is used for contract–relax–contract, but subsequent contraction of the antagonist gains additional ROM. The disadvantages are the difficulty in teaching proper technique to patients, and that it is best accomplished with a partner. The end result is similar to that of passive and active assistive stretching (18). Hutton (29) compared static, contract–relax and contract–relax–contract in increasing hamstring length and demonstrated contract–relax–contract to be most effective but difficult to teach and more uncomfortable to perform. Etnyre (30) compared static stretch to contract–relax PNF and contract–relax–antagonist contract PNF stretching and found the two PNF techniques to be more effective in both men and women for increasing hip and shoulder extension ROM.

Dynamic, Phasic, or Ballistic Stretching

Dynamic, phasic, or ballistic activities refer to rapid movements requiring jerking and often bouncing movements (2). The disadvantages of this type of stretching outweigh the advantages. Ballistic movements predispose to muscle strain injury. A rapidly stretched muscle stimulates intrafusal muscle contraction (14). Ballistic movements are used to simulate sport-specific, preactivity warm-up. Static stretching and plyometrics are recommended as safer options for warm-up flexibility. Studies conclude that static stretching is safer, requires less energy, and may reduce muscle soreness associated with other exercise (19, 20, 29, 31, 32).

FLEXIBILITY EXERCISES

Specific examples of positions and postures for flexibility exercises are shown in Figures 54.2 to 54.7. These specific exercises address positions for almost every joint. Stretching techniques using props and partners are included for variety in relation to individual needs. Refer to

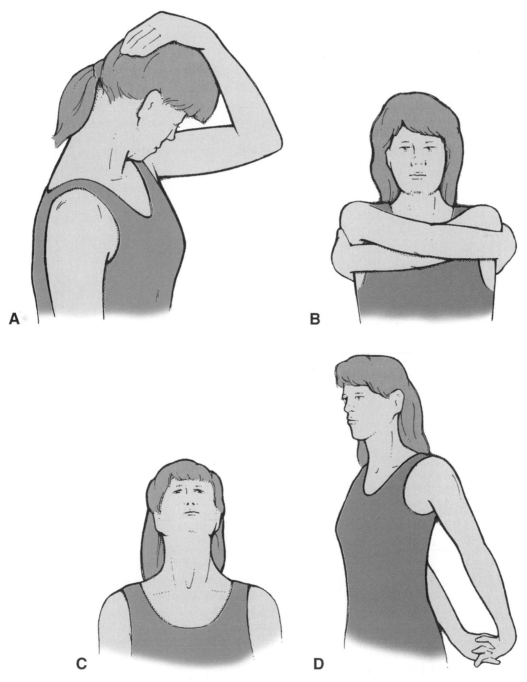

Figure 54.2. A. Neck flexion with gentle pressure. This technique can be used with side bending and a combination of side bending, flexion, and rotation. Use caution with complaints of dizziness, and avoid extension and rotation postures of the neck. **B.** Hugging and shoulder protraction stretch. Reach across the body with both arms and grasp the shoulders. Inhale deeply, focusing the sensation of stretch between the scapulae. **C.** Neck extension stretch. Neck extension with jaw thrust to increase stretch on the anterior neck and jaw musculature. Precaution: avoid complaints of dizziness. **D.** Anterior chest stretch. Shoulder extension, internal rotation, and scapular retraction with full elbow extension and hands interlocked.

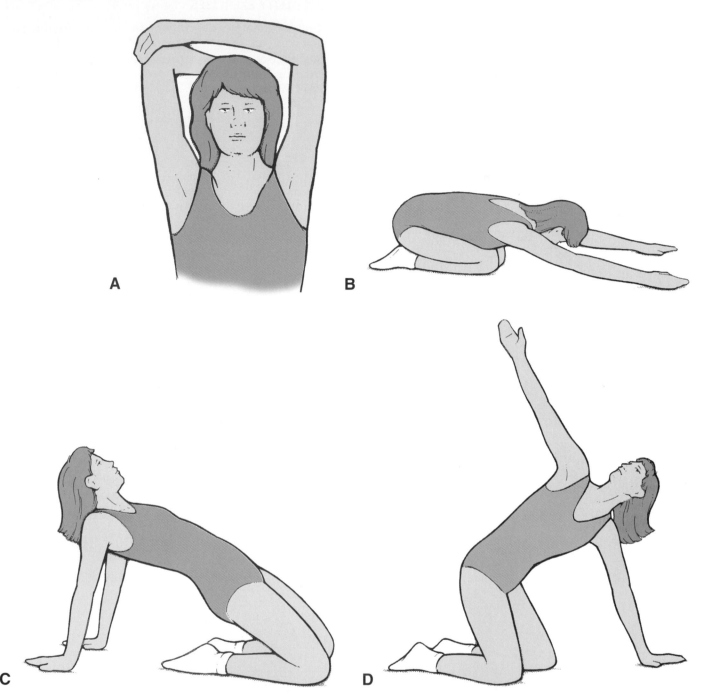

Figure 54.3. **A.** Triceps and inferior capsule stretch. Full shoulder abduction. Elbow is fully flexed and gentle overpressure is applied pulling toward the midline. Precaution: Avoid overstressing the neck anteriorly in this posture. **B.** Latissimus dorsi stretch. Begin on hands and knees. The hands stay firmly planted and the person rocks backward on hips, resting buttocks on calves. Proper position localizes stretch to low back and shoulder girdle. **C.** Thigh, abdomen, and chest stretch. Begin kneeling and reach posteriorly, extending both arms and spine, bearing weight fully on hands. Press abdomen and hips anteriorly to localize stretch to chest, abdomen, and thighs. **D.** Anterior chest and torso, mild rotation stretch. Begin on hands and knees. Reach up with one arm in extension and abduction. Allow the torso and head to rotate up, looking at the outstretched hand.

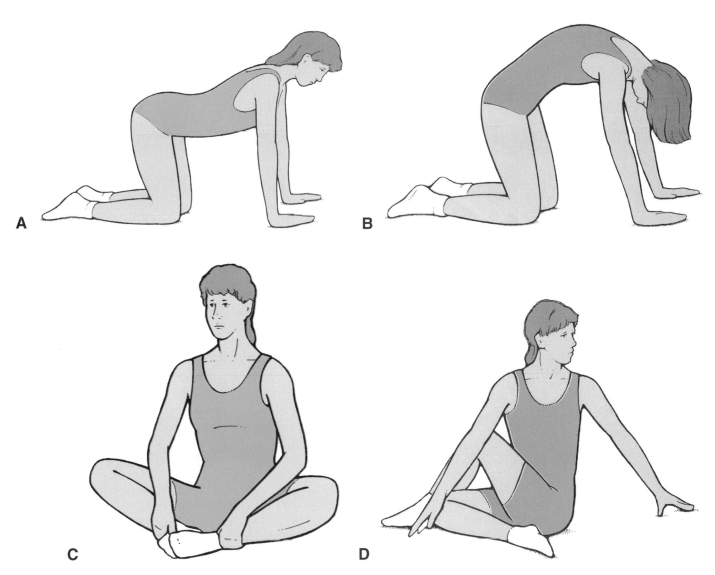

Figure 54.4. **A.** Full spinal segmental extension stretch. Begin on the hands and knees. Initiate extension of the sacrum, arching the back (extend) segment by segment, completing full extension from the lumbar to the cervical spine. **B.** Full spinal segmental flexion stretch. Begin on hands and knees. Initiate flexion of the sacrum, then lumbar, thoracic, and cervical spine. Protracting both scapulae increases flexion of the thoracic spine. **C.** Seated adductor stretch. Start in seated posture with an erect spine. Touch soles of feet together and bend knees, sliding the feet toward the midline. Allow knees to drop for increased hip abduction. With a straight back, lean forward to increase stretch in adductors. **D.** Combined spinal rotation, hip extension, and rotator stretch. Begin seated with an erect spine, both knees flexed. Cross left leg over right leg. Right arm reaches for left knee and uses the knee to assist the torso into left rotation. Inhale; on an exhalation, attempt further spinal rotation. Reverse the stretch for right rotation.

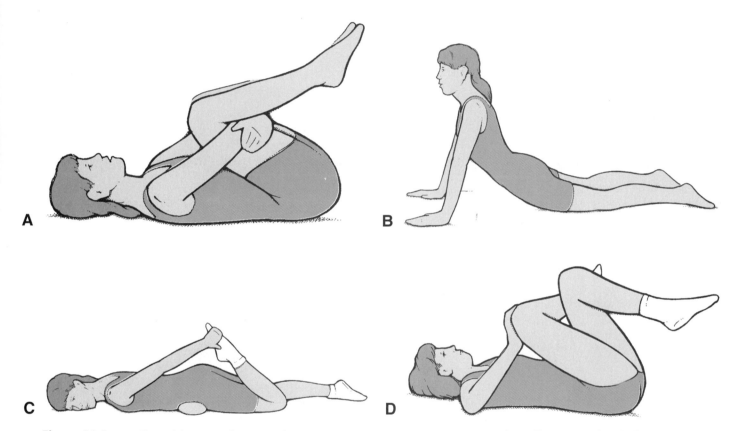

Figure 54.5. **A.** Bilateral knee to chest stretch. Begin supine. Pull both thighs to chest, supporting the back of the thigh with the hands. **B.** Full spinal extension press-up stretch. Begin prone. Place hands on the mat just below shoulder level and press up slowly. Maintain contact with the mat with front of thighs and pelvis. Evenly distribute extension throughout the entire spine. Precaution: Tightness in the thoracic spine restricts thoracic extension. This is a vulnerable area in the presence of osteoporosis. Propped on elbows is preferable for those with osteoporosis. **C.** Quadriceps stretch. Begin prone. To relieve stress on the low back, use a towel roll under the hips. Bend one knee toward the buttocks and hold the foot with one hand. A towel or rope can be used to assist reaching the lower leg. **D.** Hip rotator stretch. Begin supine. Cross one leg over, forming a figure 4, and flex both hips to or past 90°. The stretch is felt in the buttocks of the figure 4 leg.

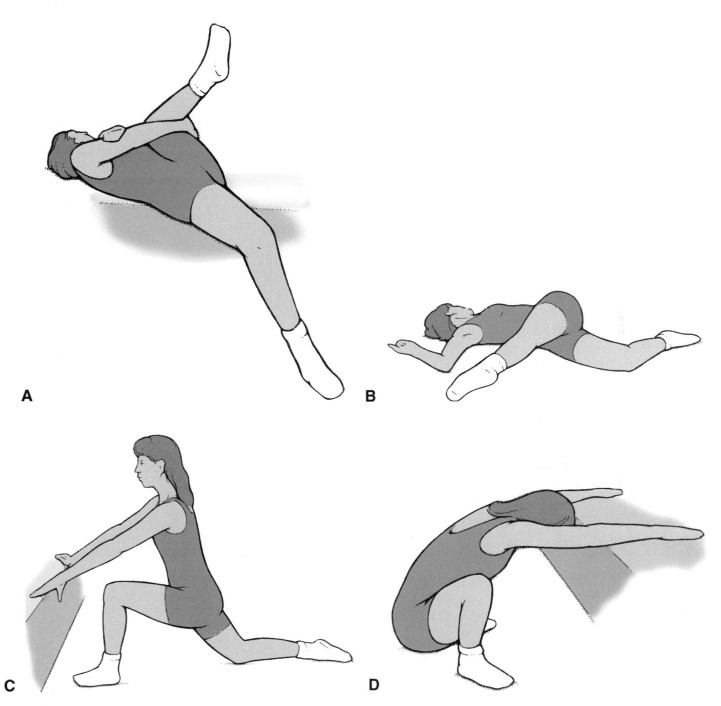

A

B

C

D

Figure 54.6. **A.** Hip flexion stretch. Begin supine. With one leg over the side of the exercise bench, flex the opposite leg as close to the chest as possible. The stretch is felt anteriorly in the hip and thigh of the hanging leg. **B.** Hip internal rotation, adduction and knee extension stretch. Begin supine. The stretch is horizontal adduction and internal rotation of the hip with fully extended knees. Rotate head in the opposite direction to aid in keeping the shoulders flat against the mat. Allowing knee flexion is a simpler technique. **C.** Forward lunge stretch. Begin standing. Step forward with one leg, leaving the trailing leg in contact with the floor. The trailing leg stretches the anterior hip and thigh. The forward leg is flexed at 90° at the knee and the hip, causing a proximal hamstring stretch. **D.** Full squat stretch. Begin standing while holding a chair or table. Allow full adduction, external rotation, and flexion at the hips. Careful attention to hip, knee, and ankle alignment is important. Try to maintain both heels in contact with the floor.

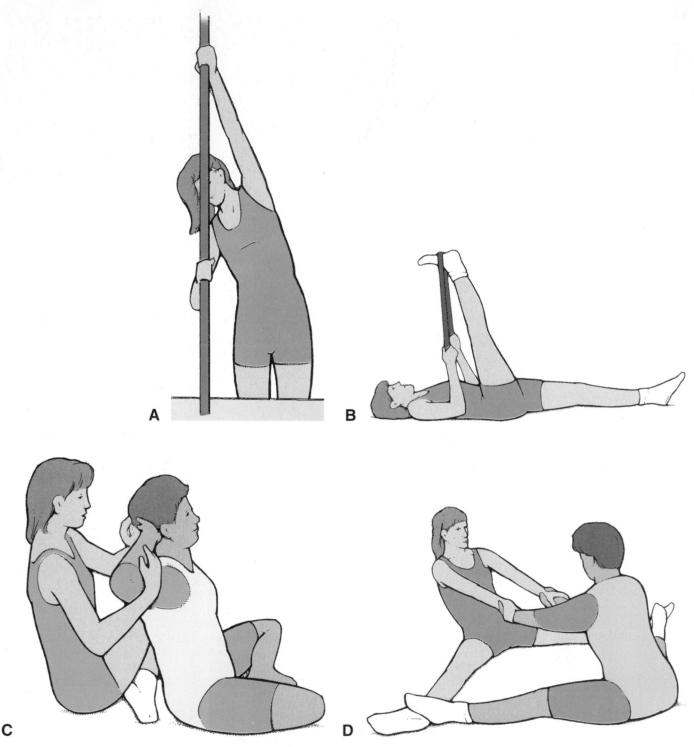

Figure 54.7. **A.** Long dowel rod prop stretch, arm and torso stretch: Begin standing. Place the pole on an exercise bench and slide the arm up the pole, lengthening the shoulder girdle, spine, torso, and ribs. Use deep breathing to increase stretch between the ribs. **B.** Assisted hamstring stretch (using a long piece of rope). Begin supine. Do a straight-leg raise with the rope hooked around the sole of the foot and pull the leg to increase hip flexion. Simpler technique requires the rope to be placed on the back of the calf. **C.** Partner-assisted pectoralis major stretch. Begin with one partner sitting behind the other. The partner re- ceiving the stretch interlocks hands behind head. The assisting partner places the knees against the stretcher's back and pulls gently on the arms, creating an extension stretch for chest and upper back. Precaution: This may be contraindicated in patients with osteoporosis. **D.** Partner-assisted stretch of the hip adduc- tors. Begin seated facing a partner in full knee extension, full hip abduction, bracing the feet against feet. One partner gently and slowly pulls forward to increase the inner thigh stretch. Alter- nate stretching between partners, asking for and giving feedback to ensure safety.

Table 54.4 and Figure 54.7 and follow illustrated and written directions for safe execution of these exercises. Also, individual exercises or some combination of these exercises may be contraindicated in a variety of populations.

PLYOMETRICS

For optimal physical performance, an athlete trains for speed, strength, power, coordination, endurance, and flexibility. Plyometrics conditions through dynamic resistance exercise. Plyometrics was first applied to lower extremities through jumping exercises. Plyometrics has now been adapted for upper extremity and torso exercise using a weighted object, such as a medicine ball. Use of a medicine ball for resistance allows the individual to move throughout the sport-specific ROM. Chu (12) describes plyometric exercises as beginning with rapid stretching (eccentric contraction) followed by shortening of the same muscle (concentric contraction). This is known as the stretch–shortening cycle. The success of plyometrics is based on the use of serial elastic properties and stretch properties of muscle. These loading conditions increase ROM and produce greater force with maximum metabolic efficiency.

► SUMMARY

Physiological changes in connective and muscle tissue accompany flexibility training. Close attention to the proper technique, precautions, and contraindications to stretching is important in prescribing and teaching a safe, effective flexibility program.

Acknowledgments

A special thanks to Dr. Elizabeth Protas, Assistant Dean, School of Physical Therapy, Texas Woman's University, Houston. She was instrumental in advising and editing this chapter. A special thanks to Elizabeth Boswell Jones, MEd., for her help as a model and exercise consultant. Ms. Jones owns and directs the Physical Conditioning Center, a Pilates-based exercise studio in Houston.

References
1. Webster's Ninth New Collegiate Dictionary. Merriam-Webster, 1991.
2. Morris HF. Sports Medicine Handbook. 1st ed. Dubuque, IA: William C. Brown 1984:45–51.
3. McNaught M, Callender L. Illustrated Physiology. 3rd ed. New York: Churchill Livingstone, 1975:241–245.
4. Per-Olof A, Rodahl K. Textbook of Work Physiology. 2nd ed. St Louis: McGraw Hill, 1977:72–79.
5. Bloom W, Fawcett DW. A Textbook of Histology. 10th ed. Philadelphia: Saunders, 1975.
6. Chamberlain G. Cyriax's friction massage: A review. J Orthop Sports Phys Ther 1982 14:16–22.
7. Garfin SR, Tipton CM, MuBarak SJ, et al. Role of fascia in maintenance of muscle tension and pressure. J Appl Physiol 51:317–319, 1981.
8. Mozam K, Lawrence J, Keagy R. Muscle relationships in functional fascia. Clin Orthop 150:403–409, 1978.
9. Bueche F. Principles of Physics. 2nd ed. St Louis: McGraw Hill, 1972:194–195.
10. Anderson B. Stretching: 20th Anniversary, Bolinas, CA: Shelter Publications, 2000.
11. Altrig Z, Hoffman J, Martin J. Clinical Exercise Testing Prescription and Rehabilitation. 5th ed. Philadelphia: Lea & Febiger, 1992:123–126.
12. Chu D. Plyometrics. Livermore, CA: Bittersweet, 1989: 8–15, 78–79.
13. Beaulieu JE. Stretching for All Sports. Pasadena, CA: Athletic, 1980:5–50.
14. Moffatt RJ. Strength and flexibility considerations for exercise prescription. In: Blair SN, Painter P, Pate R, et al., eds. Resource Manual for ACSM Guidelines for Exercise Testing and Prescription. Philadelphia: Lea & Febiger, 1988.
15. Bersin D, Bersin K, Reese M. Relaxercise Based on Feldenkrais Theory. New York: Harper & Row, 1990:3–97.
16. Satchidananda YS. Integral Yoga-Hatha. Holt, Rinehart & Winston, 1970 11–65.
17. Hittleman A. Hittleman's Yoga 28 Day Exercise Plan. New York: Workman, 1969.
18. American College of Sports Medicine. ACSM's Guidelines for Exercise Testing and Prescription. Philadelphia: Lippincott Williams & Wilkins, 2000.
19. deVries H. Evaluation of static stretching procedures for flexibility. Res Q Exerc Sport 33:222–229, 1962.
20. deVries H. Physiology of Exercise: Flexibility 1981. J Phys Ed Recreat Dance 52:41, 1980.
21. Anderson B. 8 Minute Stretch. Women Sports Fitness Nov–Dec:46–52, 1989.
22. Krusen's Handbook of Physical Medicine and Rehabilitation. 4th ed. By Frederic J. Kottke, MD, Professor Emeritus, Department of Physical Medicine and Rehabilitation, University of Minnesota Medical School, Minneapolis, MN; and Justus F. Lehmann, MD, Professor, Department of Rehabilitation Medicine, University of Washington School of Medicine, Seattle, WA.
23. Kuland D. The Injured Athlete. Philadelphia: Lippincott, 1982:165–176.
24. Karpovich PV, Hale C. Effects of warming up upon physical performance. JAMA 162:1117–1119, 1956.
25. Jensen C. Pertinent facts about warm up. Athlet J 56:72–75, 1975.
26. Martin BJ. Effects of warm up on metabolic responses to strenuous exercise. Med Sci Sports Exerc 7:146–149, 1975.
27. Kisner C, Colby LA. Therapeutic Exercise Foundations and Techniques. 2nd ed. Philadelphia: Davis, 1990.
28. Knott M, Voss D. Proprioceptive Neuromuscular Facilitation. 2nd ed. New York: Harper & Row, 1968.
29. Hutton A. Three Techniques Comparing Stretching of the Hamstrings. University of California, 1979. (Abstract reported).
30. Etnyre BR, Lee EJ. Chronic and acute flexibility of men and women using three different stretching techniques. Res Q Exerc Sport 59:222–228, 1988.
31. Agre JC. Static Stretching for Athletes. Arch Phys Med 59:561, 1978.
32. Logan H, Egstrom GH. The effects of slow and fast stretching on sacrofemoral angle. J Assoc Phys Mental Rehabil 15:85, 1988.

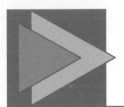

CHAPTER **55**

NUTRITION AND WEIGHT MANAGEMENT

Rosemary Riley

Approximately one-third of American adults are overweight (1). Obesity is associated with several chronic diseases, such as diabetes mellitus, hypertension, hypercholesterolemia, hyperinsulinemia, and hypertriglyceridemia, all of which increase the risk of cardiovascular disease (2). Severe obesity may limit the ability to exercise because of a low tolerance for activity or perhaps musculoskeletal problems. For individuals with severe obesity, exercise complements caloric restriction and promotes a more rapid weight loss. It can also facilitate an improvement in blood lipid profiles (3). However, complications of severe obesity may require a more aggressive clinical approach before a significant amount of physical activity can be initiated.

Exercise professionals who work in nutrition and weight management programs should understand the concepts of healthy nutrition and provide support for the behavioral changes necessary for successful weight management. A vital role for the exercise professional is to assist in the evaluation of programs to determine which are most likely to help the individual meet the weight management goals. The exercise professional should consult the state dietetic association to determine regulations regarding nutrition counseling and the practice of dietetics.

SETTING A WEIGHT GOAL

Setting a weight loss goal is a complicated task that requires negotiation and cooperation between the patient and the professional. Patients are often less concerned or motivated by health than by personal appearance. Goals should be realistic and achievable or the individual may be set up for failure.

There is little scientific consensus on the best method of setting a healthy weight goal. Body mass index (BMI) is often used to evaluate body weight. It is calculated from weight and height but is not a measure of body composition. However, BMI correlates well with body fat in many populations. Since it is relatively easy to measure, it can provide a quick assessment of body composition. The Na-

tional Institutes for Health suggested that a BMI above 27 indicates obesity and a BMI above 30 indicates morbid obesity. The BMI is not as useful in defining underweight as it is in defining obesity. Nomograms are available for converting height and weight to BMI (see Chapter 70).

Epidemiological research indicates that a BMI of 21–22 is associated with the lowest risk of cardiovascular disease (3). Individuals with diabetes mellitus, hypertension, osteoarthritis, breast cancer, or endometrial cancer or are at risk for any of these conditions may benefit from maintaining a BMI of less than 27 (4–7). Research also indicates that significant health benefits can be achieved by losing only 10–20% of body weight, even if the ideal body weight is not reached (8, 9).

The Expert Panel on Healthy Weight recommends that adults maintain a BMI of less than 25 (10). Persons with a BMI above 25 should develop a healthier weight goal, equivalent to a loss of approximately 2 BMI units (approximately 10 pounds) and maintain that weight loss 6 months before further weight loss. Obese individuals with chronic disease or who are at risk for chronic disease should consult a health care professional for weight reduction recommendations. These recommendations are suggested as an initial point for achieving goal weight. Intermediate goals for those with more ambitious objectives may prevent discouragement and failure in reaching the goal weight.

ENERGY BALANCE

Weight loss generally occurs when energy expenditure exceeds energy intake, that is, when a negative energy balance is achieved. It is generally accepted that weight loss of 1 pound per week requires a negative energy balance of about 3500 calories per week, or 500 calories per day. This can be accomplished by the following:

- Reducing daily intake by 500 calories
- Reducing daily intake by 250 calories and increasing daily energy expenditure by 250 calories, or some other

combination of decreased intake and increased expenditure equal to a loss of 500 calories a day

- Increasing caloric expenditure (physical activity) by 500 calories per day

The last option may be the most difficult for most obese individuals, who may not be able to tolerate the frequency, duration, or intensity of exercise needed to achieve this level of energy expenditure. A combination of moderate caloric restriction and moderate exercise is perhaps most likely to achieve the best result.

To improve compliance, the caloric restriction should be moderate, avoiding hunger and deprivation of favorite foods. The exercise component helps reduce stress, anxiety, and depression, which may trigger overeating. Exercise and activity can literally get you out of the kitchen or any location that contributes to unstructured eating. Individuals who exercise and conform to moderate caloric restriction achieve greater loss of fat mass and preserve lean body mass (11).

Exercise also establishes the types of behaviors required for weight maintenance. Research has shown that the best predictor of weight maintenance is continued regular exercise (12). Individuals can lose weight successfully without exercise, but successful weight maintenance without regular exercise is difficult.

DETERMINING CALORIC NEEDS

Current energy intake requirements can be determined in a number of ways, including dietary intake records and formulas that estimate daily caloric expenditure requirements for activity level and gender. Table 55.1 contains a list of factors that can be helpful in determining a person's daily energy requirements (13). Daily energy balance for weight loss can be determined using the estimated daily energy requirement, then increasing caloric expenditure (i.e., increasing physical activity) and/or reducing caloric intake proportionally.

The arbitrary assignment of caloric restriction is a third technique for meeting caloric requirements during weight reduction (14). Caloric ranges of 1200–1500 for women and 1800–2000 for men are common recommendations. Adjustments are generally made after some weeks, depending on compliance and results.

Caloric restriction plans of 1200 calories or above are considered **moderate calorie restriction programs**, or balanced calorie deficit diets. A 1200-calorie diet is believed to be the minimum level at which the recommended amounts of essential vitamins and minerals can be obtained without supplementation. Greater caloric restriction requires vitamin and mineral supplementation. Diet plans that provide 800–1200 calories are considered low-calorie diets; plans that provide less than 800 calories

Table 55.1. Estimation of Daily Energy Allowances at Various Levels of Physical Activity for Men and Women Aged 19–50

LEVEL OF ACTIVITY	ENERGY EXPENDITURE (KCAL/KG PER DAY)
Very light	
Men	31
Women	30
Light	
Men	38
Women	33
Moderate	
Men	40
Women	47
Heavy	
Men	50
Women	44

Very light activity is defined as mostly seated and standing activities such as driving, typing, ironing, cooking, and playing cards.
Light activity is defined as walking on a level surface at 2.5–3 mph, such as house cleaning, child care, golf, restaurant trades.
Moderate activity is defined as walking 3.5–4 mph, weeding and hoeing, cycling, skiing, and dancing.
Heavy activity is defined as walking with a load or uphill, heavy manual labor, basketball, climbing, football, and soccer.
Reprinted with permission from Food and Nutrition Board. Recommended Dietary Allowances, 10th ed. Washington: National Academy Press, 1989.

are considered **very low calorie diets** and should not be undertaken without medical supervision (15).

A 1200-calorie diet, though considered moderate for many individuals, is a very low calorie diet for the morbidly obese. For someone consuming 3500 calories per day, the 1200-calorie plan provides a 2300-calorie deficit. This individual can be expected to demonstrate metabolic responses (i.e., decreased thyroid hormone activity, increased diuresis, and decreased blood pressure) similar to those of a normal or thin individual on a very low calorie diet. The resulting rate of weight loss is rapid and requires medical supervision. A weight loss of 1–2 pounds per week after the first 2 weeks is considered safe. A faster rate of weight loss should be monitored by a health care professional, even when the calorie intake is considered safe.

FOOD PLANS

The foundation of any meal plan should be the *Dietary Guidelines for Americans*, fourth edition (1996), which includes the Food Guide Pyramid. The Dietary Guidelines encourage variety in intake and moderation in fat, sugar, and alcohol consumption. The Food Guide Pyramid recommends a variety of foods with particular emphasis on grains, fruits, and vegetables. To incorporate these guidelines into a weight loss program, special attention must be paid to serving size and choosing mainly from food groups appearing in the lower half of the Food Pyramid (see Chapter 3).

American Heart Association Recommendations

The American Heart Association (AHA) and the National Cholesterol Education Program (NCEP) have made more specific recommendations for a heart-healthy diet, including limiting total fat intake to less than 30% of total calories; limiting saturated fat to less than 10% of total calories, with polyunsaturated fat providing no more than 10% of total calories and the remainder of the fat intake provided by monounsaturated fat (16, 17). The AHA also recommends limiting cholesterol to less than 300 mg per day.

These recommendations for healthy individuals over age 4 do not limit total caloric intake. However, they are easily incorporated into a weight loss plan by specifying a number of grams of fat for dietary intake. Decreased fat is usually compensated for by increased intake of carbohydrates. Tables 55.2 and 55.3 illustrate details of the NCEP recommendations (17). The categories of naturally low-fat foods, such as grain products, fruits, and vegetables, allow more latitude with serving sizes, depending on caloric needs.

Table 55.2. National Cholesterol Education Program Diet Therapy Recommendations

NUTRIENT	RECOMMENDED INTAKE (% TOTAL CALORIES)	
	STEP I DIET	STEP II DIET
Total fat	30% of total calories	
Saturated FA	8–10%	7%
Polyunsaturated FA	Up to 10% of total calories	
Monounsaturated FA	Up to 15% of total calories	
Carbohydrates	≥ 55% of total calories	
Protein	Approximately 15% of total calories	
Cholesterol	< 300 mg/day	< 200 mg/day
Total calories	To achieve and maintain desirable weight	

FA, fatty acids.

Table 55.3. NCEP General Recommendations for Food Choices

Six or more servings per day of breads, cereals, pasta, potatoes, rice, dried peas, and beans
Two or three servings per day of low-fat dairy products
Up to 5–6 oz per day of lean meats, poultry, and fish
No more than 6–8 teaspoons per day of fats and oils, including fats and oils used in food preparation
Five or more servings per day of fruits and vegetables
No more than 4 egg yolks per week on Step I and no more than 2 per week on Step II

American Diabetes Association Recommendations

The American Diabetes Association (ADA) has also made dietary recommendations that can be used for weight loss (18). Although they were designed for individuals with diabetes mellitus, they present a healthy eating plan for all individuals. This eating plan, commonly known as the **exchange system**, is also the basis of many commercial weight loss plans. Food is divided into six groups (starches, milk, meat, fat, fruits, and vegetables) based on carbohydrate, protein, and fat content. Within each group, a serving size for each food that yields similar calories and macronutrients is determined. These exchanges can be switched with foods in another group. As a result, these foods can be used interchangeably in creating a meal plan. The number of servings from each group is based on caloric requirements for weight loss. The exchange system encourages a wide selection of food from different food groups and offers the advantage of providing an easy way to substitute one food for another while remaining within a caloric limit.

Counting Fat Grams

Counting fat grams has become an accepted method for weight loss. The basis is restriction of fat intake, which also helps limit total caloric intake. Fruits and vegetables are not limited, but foods high in fats (e.g., meats, cheeses, snack foods) are limited by a daily fat allowance. Although the literature supports reduced fat intake without additional caloric restriction, epidemiological data demonstrate that Americans continue to get fatter even as the percentage of total calories provided by fat decreases (19). Total caloric intake remains the most important aspect of a weight loss plan.

Counting Calories

Calorie counting may again emerge as an acceptable method of weight loss, since individuals continue to gain weight as fat intake is reduced. A detailed calorie book and attention to the new food labels may allow individuals to count total calories. This may result in lower fat intake as it becomes clear to the individual that foods high in fat are also high in calories. This method allows the individual to consume favorite foods as long as the intake of other calories is reduced proportionally. The disadvantage of calorie counting is that the nutritional quality of the diet may be inadequate if the individual fails to select from a variety of food groups.

High-Protein Diets

High-protein diets with reduced fats and carbohydrates are usually associated with a low-calorie or very low calorie diet. They are based on the premise that high protein intake preserves lean body mass during rapid weight loss. Examples of commercial variations of the high-protein diet are Medifast, Optifast, New Direction, and Health Management Resources (HMR).

The nutrient profiles of high-protein diets differ by the amount of carbohydrate and fat they contain. Some are very low in carbohydrates; the high protein–low carbohydrate profile results in mild ketosis. This type of diet, referred to as **ketogenic**, should contain 1–1.5 g of protein per kilogram of ideal body weight to preserve lean body mass and should be supervised by a physician (20).

High-protein diets provide safe, rapid weight loss with dramatic improvements in many cardiovascular risk factors. However, for the weight loss to be maintained, the programs must provide intensive behavioral counseling, exercise guidelines, and nutrition education. High-protein diet plans that limit carbohydrates until the evening meal are controversial and should be used with great caution.

General Recommendations

Health professionals should assist patients in choosing a safe and realistic weight loss plan that fits into the lifestyle of the individual. Healthy nutrition management is more than an eating plan; it requires changes in other behaviors as well. Most successful weight management programs include behavioral management in addition to a healthy eating plan. A program without record keeping, exercise, and social support should not be considered.

WEIGHT LOSS PROGRAM GUIDELINES

Selecting an appropriate weight loss program is difficult for the average consumer, given the myriad of diet and lifestyle books that promise great recipes, easy instructions, and fast results. Furthermore, there are no regulations regarding weight loss programs, although the Food and Nutrition Board recently issued guidelines to help health professionals and consumers evaluate them (20). A primary goal of the document is to shift the concern from simply weight loss to weight management and improved health. The suggested means of accomplishing this attitudinal change is by emphasizing significant improvements in health and the reduction of risk factors that result from modest weight loss, especially if the loss is maintained. Three categories of weight management programs were presented:

- Do-it-yourself programs
- Nonclinical programs
- Clinical programs

Do-It-Yourself Programs

This category includes individual or group efforts to lose weight. They include Overeaters Anonymous, Take Off Pounds Sensibly (TOPS), and the use of Richard Simmons' Deal-A-Meal Plan, among others. Books, tapes, and work site programs are included in this category. The distinguishing feature of these programs is a lack of individualization by a professional.

Nonclinical Programs

This category includes many commercial programs. The program, calorie levels, and educational materials are established by a parent company and are consistent at all company locations. Examples of nonclinical programs include Weight Watchers, Jenny Craig, Diet Centers, and Nutri-System. Educational materials and program guidelines are commonly written by health care professionals, but the personnel delivering the program are usually lay leaders trained by the program. Often successful program participants are used as group leaders or counselors.

Clinical Programs

Clinical programs and services are provided by a licensed professional who may or may not have special training in the treatment of obesity. They may be offered by a single health care professional or by a multidisciplinary team who coordinate the care. This team may include a physician, an exercise physiologist, a registered or licensed dietitian, a nurse, and a behavioral counselor. They may use a moderately reduced calorie diet, a very low calorie diet, exercise, psychological counseling, drugs, surgery, or combinations of these modalities to achieve weight loss and maintenance.

EVALUATION OF PROGRAMS

A framework for evaluating weight management programs, based both on the program and the consumer, has been developed (20).

Criterion I: Choosing the Appropriate Program

The purpose of the first criterion is to ensure that consumers choose weight management programs appropriate for their needs and that the program provides resources to meet those needs. For example, a work site program is generally not prepared to provide the medical supervision that someone with a chronic disease requires. Individuals with special needs require a program with health professionals to provide medical supervision. Work site programs can, however, provide social support, which is a critical factor in weight management.

Criterion II: Safety and Foundation of the Program

The safety and foundation of the program are considered in this criterion. Do-it-yourself and nonclinical programs should provide the following:

- Assessment of physical health and psychological status
- Nutrition information
- Physical activity
- Program safety

The minimum recommendation is that a self-administered health assessment be encouraged; optimally, the prospective participant should consult a health care professional prior to initiating a program. All programs should address both diet and physical activity. Weight loss programs without such changes cannot be successful in the long term.

Self-administered and nonclinical programs should be accompanied by minimal risk, since there is little or no monitoring of health status during the program. Clinical programs should be especially safe, considering the population served. The monitoring of participants by health care professionals makes aggressive diet and exercise strategies more reasonable. Programs should provide information about staff qualifications and training. Credentials, qualifications, and experiences in nutritional management should be clearly indicated.

Criterion III: Long-term Results

The third criterion addresses outcomes. The four components of a successful weight management program:

- Long-term weight loss
- Improvement in obesity-related comorbidities
- Improved health practices
- Monitoring for any adverse effects

It is recommended that weight loss programs be judged on these components and that consumers expect to receive information about each component when inquiring about the program. While it is unlikely that do-it-yourself programs will evaluate outcomes, they can alert the consumer to the four issues delineated in criterion III. The staff in nonclinical and clinical programs have personal contact with each participant and should monitor weight loss and changes in participant health behaviors. Weight loss programs should also teach patients with comorbidities about the possible need to adjust medications during weight loss. Furthermore, all programs should inform patients regarding the risks of weight loss as well as the benefits.

Since long-term maintenance of a large amount of weight loss remains elusive for many people, additional criteria for evaluation of weight control programs have been established. These programs should be designed to ensure the following:

- Small weight losses are maintained.
- Participants are successfully motivated to develop healthful eating habits.
- Physical activity for participants is increased.
- Obesity-related comorbidities are reduced.
- Quality of life improves.
- Positive health-related knowledge and attitudes are developed.

Evaluation of the success of a program should not be based solely on weight loss, but on a variety of health-related outcomes.

▶ SUMMARY

A variety of methods are available to help obese individuals establish realistic and achievable weight goals, to provide food plans, and to evaluate weight loss programs. The fitness professional has an important role in guiding the patient to the program most appropriate for his or her needs, providing support through exercise recommendations, and reinforcing the behavioral strategies necessary for weight loss and weight maintenance.

References

1. Kuczmarski R, Flegal K, Campbell S, et al. Increasing prevalence of overweight among US adults. JAMA 272:205, 1994.
2. Pi-Sunyer FX. Health implications of obesity. Am J Clin Nutr 53:1595S, 1991.
3. Katzel L, Bleecker E, Colman E, et al. Effects of weight loss vs aerobic exercise training on risk factors for coronary heart disease in healthy, obese, middle-aged and older men. JAMA 274:1915, 1995.
4. Pi-Sunyer FX. Weight and non-insulin-dependent diabetes mellitus. Am J Clin Nutr 63:426S, 1996.
5. McCarron D, Reusser R. Body weight and blood pressure regulation. Am J Clin Nutr 63:423S, 1996.
6. Felson D. Weight and osteoarthritis. Am J Clin Nutr 63: 430S, 1996.
7. Ballard-Barbush R, Swanson C. Body weight: Estimation of risk for breast and endometrial cancers. Am J Clin Nutr 63:437S, 1996.
8. Kannel W, D'Agostino R, Cobb J. Effect of weight on cardiovascular disease. Am J Clin Nutr 63S:419S, 1996.
9. Kanders B et al. Long-term health effects associated with significant weight loss: A study of dose-response effect. In: Blackburn G, Kanders B, eds. Obesity: Pathophysiology, Psychology and Treatment. New York: Chapman & Hall, 1994.
10. Meisler J, St. Jeor S. Summary and recommendations from the American Health Foundation's Expert Panel on Healthy Weight. Am J Clin Nutr 63:474S, 1996.
11. Svendson O et al. Effect of an energy restrictive diet, with and without exercise, on lean tissue mass, resting metabolic rate, cardiovascular risk factors, and bone in overweight postmenopausal women. Am J Med 95:131, 1993.
12. Kayman S, Bruvold W, Stern J. Maintenance and relapse after weight loss in women: Behavioral aspects. Am J Clin Nutr 52:800, 1990.
13. Food and Nutrition Board. Recommended Dietary Allowances. 10th ed. Washington: National Academy Press, 1989.
14. Lichtman S, Pisarka K, Berman E, et al. Discrepancy between self-reported and actual caloric intake and exercise in obese subjects. N Engl J Med 327:1893, 1993.
15. National Task Force on the Prevention and Treatment of Obesity. Very low calorie diets. JAMA 270:967, 1993.
16. Chait A et al. Rationale for the Diet-Heart Statement of the American Heart Association. Report of the nutrition committee. Circulation 88:3008, 1993.
17. National Cholesterol Education Program. Second report of

the Expert Panel on Detection, Evaluation, and Treatment of High Blood Cholesterol in Adults. (Adult Treatment Panel II). Circulation 89:1329, 1994.

18. Maximizing the Role of Nutrition in Diabetes Management. Arlington, VA: American Diabetes Association, 1994.

19. Allred J. Too much of a good thing? An overemphasis on eating low fat foods may be contributing to the alarming increase in overweight among US adults. J Am Diet Assoc 95:417, 1995.

20. Weighing the options: Criteria for evaluating weight management programs. Washington: National Academy Press, 1994. (Summary available in J Am Diet Assoc 95:96, 1996.)

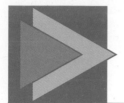

CHAPTER **56**

SPECIFICITY OF EXERCISE TRAINING AND TESTING

J. Larry Durstine and Paul G. Davis

Most athletes use training techniques that mimic movements used in competition in an attempt to train the same muscle groups required for the competitive event. For example, a soccer player spends most of the time in lower body training, while a kayak competitor requires mainly upper body training. In addition, athletes work to enhance specific energy systems used in competition.

Although the concept of specificity remains a premise of exercise training, cross-training has become particularly popular. Cross-training is the use of more than one mode of exercise (e.g., swimming and running) and/or training for more than one aspect of fitness (e.g., endurance, flexibility, and/or strength). Cross-training is often used to prevent injury, to maintain fitness while recovering from injury, or to supplement specific training. As described in this chapter, this type of training has both benefits and limitations.

Specificity also applies to exercise testing. Testing protocols that assess muscular strength do not accurately assess cardiorespiratory fitness. To test specific aspects of fitness, an activity-specific testing mode yields the most accurate results. Specificity is therefore an important consideration in testing or training for athletic competition, physical fitness, or rehabilitation after disease or injury. This chapter discusses specificity in terms of energy systems and movement and the applicability of combining different modes of exercise.

ENERGY SYSTEMS AND FIBER TYPE

Adenosine triphosphate (ATP) must be generated for movement to occur. The speed and duration of movement determine how ATP is supplied for muscle contraction: Activities requiring sudden, high-intensity work, such as throwing, primarily use stored ATP (i.e., ATP that is already in muscle cells). In short, high-speed events, such as the 100-meter run, most of the ATP is derived from the phosphocreatine system. In sustained sprint events, such as the 400-meter run, energy is derived mainly through anaerobic glycolysis. Finally, endurance

activities (e.g., cross-country skiing or a marathon) rely primarily on oxidative (aerobic) metabolism for energy. Specific training is required to enhance the energy system that is predominant in energy production for a given event or sport. Likewise, an accurate assessment of the physiological characteristics required for an event requires an exercise test protocol that is specific for that event.

Endurance Training

In his early work, Holloszy (1) examined the effects of a 3-month treadmill program on the skeletal muscle characteristics of rats and postulated the concept of specificity of training. Rats exercising 120 minutes per day 5 days per week were able to run at submaximal speeds 6 times longer than rats exercising only 10 minutes per day 5 days per week. Endurance training was accompanied by a twofold increase in Krebs cycle and electron transport activity. Gollnick and King (2) subsequently demonstrated an increase in both number and size of mitochondria in endurance-trained skeletal muscle. An increase in mitochondrial activity promotes the use of fat as an energy substrate, thus delaying glycogen depletion and enhancing performance.

Endurance training is also accompanied by enhanced oxygen and substrate transport, and increased capillary density. An increase in capillary density decreases the diffusion distance for oxygen and metabolic substrates (e.g., glucose and fatty acids) from blood to muscle. The concentration of myoglobin, which transports and stores oxygen within muscle, also increases during endurance training.

Substrate availability and use also increase by other means during endurance training. Glycogen stores may increase, and type II (fast-twitch) muscle fibers may develop characteristics of type I (slow-twitch) fibers. Specifically, an increased number of mitochondria and type IIB (fast glycolytic) fibers may convert completely to type IIA (fast oxidative) fibers (3). However, during endurance training little biochemical change occurs to improve muscle strength or anaerobic power. Increased hexokinase activity, which facilitates glucose use, may be the most significant biochemical change accompanying endurance training that may affect anaerobic power. Small increases in glycogen phosphorylase and phosphofructokinase (PFK) activity, and ATP and phosphocreatine levels have also been reported following endurance training. Creatine kinase activity does not increase.

Strength Training

The primary change in skeletal muscle structure resulting from prolonged resistance training is increased muscle size (hypertrophy) due to an increased number of myofibrils (actin and myosin) and increased amounts of connective tissue. These changes occur in all major fiber types. During the first few weeks of training, however, these changes are disproportionate to the gain in strength (4). Improved motor unit recruitment and efficiency rather than an increased amount of tissue seems to be responsible for initial gains in muscle strength (4).

As with endurance training, strength training produces evidence of muscle fiber plasticity. The percentage of type IIB fibers (fast-twitch glycolytic fibers) usually decreases during strength training, perhaps because type IIB fibers either are not recruited or are the last to be recruited (e.g., during a maximal contraction). As fiber recruitment increases, the histochemical properties of type IIB fibers may change so that they resemble the properties of type IIA (fast-twitch oxidative) fibers (4). The percentage of type I fibers usually does not change.

Because oxidative enzyme activity increases markedly during endurance training, strength training may also be expected to be accompanied by increased anaerobic enzyme activity. In contrast, resistance training is associated with little change in glycolytic (PFK or lactate dehydrogenase) or nonglycolytic (creatine kinase or myokinase) enzyme activity. Furthermore, muscle ATP and phosphocreatine levels do not increase.

Oxidative enzyme activity does not increase during strength training; in fact, the amount of mitochondria per unit of muscle weight decreases with muscle hypertrophy (5). Myoglobin concentration may also decrease with muscle hypertrophy. On the other hand, some resistance training programs have been accompanied by an increase in capillary density (4).

Endurance and Strength Training

Endurance athletes often supplement training with resistance exercise. Athletes participating in events requiring strength often add endurance exercise to their training regimen.

Effects of Endurance Training on Strength

Endurance athletes have a lower than normal vertical jump. In fact, vertical jump decreases with endurance training and increases with cessation of endurance train-

ing (6). Conversely, previously inactive subjects undergoing simultaneous endurance and resistance training of the legs demonstrate improvement in leg strength and maximal oxygen consumption ($\dot{V}O_{2max}$) (7, 8). However, these training protocols have failed to elicit strength improvements similar to improvements identified when identical resistance training programs were administered without endurance training.

These investigations used intensive interval training (3–5 repetitions of 5 minutes each near $\dot{V}O_{2max}$) to improve $\dot{V}O_{2max}$. In research conditions, less intensive interval and continuous endurance training protocols have demonstrated that combined endurance and resistance training elicits improvement in strength comparable with that seen with strength training alone (9, 10). In addition, continuous endurance training was accompanied by an increase in $\dot{V}O_{2max}$ of approximately 18%, similar to that seen with intensive interval training (8).

Effects of Strength Training on Endurance

Some studies have demonstrated that $\dot{V}O_{2max}$ increases during leg strength training, even in the absence of endurance-specific training (10, 11). However, this finding is inconsistent (Table 56.1) (12, 13). Strength training alone and the addition of strength training in endurance-trained subjects were accompanied by increased cycling and running times to exhaustion at work rates representing 100% $\dot{V}O_{2max}$ without a concomitant increase in $\dot{V}O_{2max}$ (11, 14). In addition, movement-specific resistance training increased double-poling economy in cross-country skiers (15). Sale et al. (9) demonstrated increased citrate synthase (a Krebs cycle enzyme) activity and an increased percentage of slow-twitch fibers in strength-trained vastus lateralis muscle. However, Bishop et al. (12) found no change in glycolytic or Krebs cycle enzymes in the same muscle. Increased capillary density in skeletal muscle may contribute to the enhanced endurance demonstrated in some of these studies (4).

Some endurance athletes therefore may benefit from the addition of resistance training; middle-distance athletes may benefit most, considering the increase in $\dot{V}O_{2max}$ and short-term endurance. Although power athletes do not gain strength from endurance training, low to moderate endurance training may provide benefits, such as delayed fatigue, without compromising strength. Endurance training also helps maintain a desirable body composition. Individuals exercising for health and fitness should not be discouraged from including moderate levels of both endurance and strength training in an exercise program.

SPECIFICITY OF MUSCLE GROUP

Endurance Training

Athletes often use a variety of activities to improve performance. Performance may improve through cardiovas-

Table 56.1. Effect of Strength Training on Endurance Variables

Study	Subjects, Training Duration		Cycle Ergometer $\dot{V}O_{2MAX}$ (L/MIN)	Treadmill $\dot{V}O_{2MAX}$ (mL/KG/MIN)	[a]Cycle Endurance (SEC)	[a]Treadmill Endurance (SEC)	[b]Lower Body One-Repetition Maximum (% change)	Fat-Free Mass (KG)
Bishop et al., 1999 (12)	Female cyclists, 12 weeks	Pretraining	2.97 ± 0.32				36^d	
		Posttraining	2.90 ± 0.30					
		Change	-2%					
Hickson et al., 1980 (11)	Untrained males, 10 weeks	Pretraining	3.40 ± 0.22	47.8 ± 1.5	278 ± 27	291 ± 14		[c]66.0
		Posttraining	3.54 ± 0.22^d	48.8 ± 2.0	407 ± 32^d	325 ± 12^d	$40\%^d$	68.6
		Change	4%	2%	47%	12%		4%
Hurley et al., 1984 (13)	Untrained males, 16 weeks	Pretraining		36.1 ± 1.4				66.9 ± 2.6
		Posttraining		37.8 ± 1.3			33^d	68.8 ± 2.7^d
		Change		5%				3%
McCarthy et al., 1995 (10)	Untrained males, 10 weeks	Pretraining	3.16 ± 0.12					65.9 ± 2.1
		Posttraining	3.49 ± 0.14^d				23	68.1 ± 2.6^d
		Change	10%					3%

All values are listed as mean plus or minus standard error.

[a] Endurance was measured as time to exhaustion at 100% Pretraining $\dot{V}O_{2max}$.

[b] One-repetition maximum was analyzed as the squat (10,12), the average of the squat and leg extension (11), and the average of the leg press, leg extension, and leg curl (13).

[c] Fat-free mass was not listed in (11), but was calculated from the listed body mass and percent body fat values.

[d] $P < .05$

cular, muscular, and neural changes. This section discusses how training these systems may cross over to different activities.

In addition to the metabolic changes that accompany endurance training, cardiovascular or central changes occur. Central adaptation is reflected by increased maximum cardiac output (Q_{max}), and peripheral adaptation is reflected by changed maximum arterial–venous oxygen difference (a-v D_{O2max}). An increased Q_{max} results primarily from increased stroke volume (SV); an increased a-v D_{O2max} results from increased metabolic activity and, thus, increased intracellular use of oxygen.

Cross-training benefits are probably derived through central adaptations. This is suggested by comparisons between arm and leg performances in which transfer of biochemical and neural factors is unlikely. Using arm ergometry as a training modality, Magel et al. (16) demonstrated a 16% increase in $\dot{V}O_{2max}$ measured on an arm ergometer compared to a 1% increase in $\dot{V}O_{2max}$ measured on a treadmill. The increased $\dot{V}O_{2max}$ was attributed to an increased a-v D_{O2max}, since Q_{max} and SV did not change. In another study, arm ergometer training following cessation of leg ergometer training failed to preserve a leg training–associated increase in $\dot{V}O_{2max}$ (17). In yet another study, 5 weeks of arm ergometer training in women was accompanied by an increase in a-v D_{O2max}, Q_{max}, stroke volume (SV), and arm and leg $\dot{V}O_{2max}$, though $\dot{V}O_{2max}$ assessed with arm exercises increased more than with leg exercises (18). Two 10-week swim-training studies demonstrate increased swimming $\dot{V}O_{2max}$ but failed to demonstrate a change in running $\dot{V}O_{2max}$ (19, 20). The different findings may be due to differences

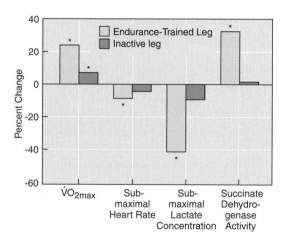

Figure 56.1. Effects of single-leg endurance training on $\dot{V}O_{2max}$, heart rate, and blood lactate concentration at a given submaximal work rate (100 watts) and succinate dehydrogenase activity in vastus lateralis biopsies. In all cases the endurance-trained leg demonstrated significantly greater change ($P < .05$) than did the untrained leg. An asterisk (*) indicates that endurance training produced significant change. (Adapted with permission from Saltin B, Nazar K, Costill DL, et al. The nature of the training response: Peripheral and central adaptations to one-legged exercise. Act Physiol Scand 96:289–305, 1976.)

in the pretraining $\dot{V}O_{2max}$ and/or differences in the training protocols (21).

Single-limb training has been used to investigate the transfer of training (Fig. 56.1). Saltin et al. (22) endurance-trained one leg for 4 weeks. The $\dot{V}O_{2max}$ increased in both the endurance-trained and inactive legs, but the increase in the trained leg was significantly greater (23% versus 7%). In addition, heart rate and blood lactate at a given submaximal workload decreased significantly when measured in the trained leg only. On the other hand, succinate dehydrogenase (a Krebs cycle enzyme) increased in the trained leg only. Results of both combined arm and leg training and single-limb training studies suggest that transfer of training does result, but not to the same extent as in a more specific training mode.

In endurance training studies using the same limbs but comparing different modes of exercise (e.g., cycling versus running), improvements in endurance were measured across modalities. Improvement may be detected more effectively by testing subjects with the same exercise mode used in training. For example, 8 weeks of treadmill training increased both treadmill and cycle ergometer $\dot{V}O_{2max}$, but cycle ergometer training increased cycle ergometer $\dot{V}O_{2max}$ more than treadmill $\dot{V}O_{2max}$ (23). Increased function appears to be more accurately assessed using a testing modality similar to the training modality.

Pierce et al. (24) trained groups with running or cycling at equal intensities (90% $\dot{V}O_{2max}$) and demonstrated similar increases in running and cycling $\dot{V}O_{2max}$. Figure 56.2 illustrates that both modes of training result in higher $\dot{V}O_2$ at lactate threshold ($\dot{V}O_{2LT}$) during cycle ergometry (cycle > running), but only run training resulted in a higher $\dot{V}O_{2LT}$ during the treadmill exercise. This change is significantly greater than the change in $\dot{V}O_{2LT}$ demonstrated when cycle ergometer testing is used after run training. While some transfer of improved performance seems apparent, this study suggests that peripheral

adaptation is more specific. Although the same muscles are used, cycling recruits fewer motor units than running. Therefore, associated biochemical changes may not carry over to an activity using more muscle mass.

These studies support both specificity and transfer of training. Although several studies indicate that central benefits gained from one mode of exercise training transfer to another mode, the extent of improvement in the training mode is usually greater. Improved $\dot{V}O_{2max}$ may be more likely to transfer from a large-muscle exercise (e.g., running) to a small-muscle exercise (e.g., cycling) than vice versa. Many studies do not investigate changes in muscle metabolism; those that do show little transfer of training (22, 24).

Although cardiovascular changes are primarily responsible for increasing $\dot{V}O_{2max}$, endurance may be enhanced more through changes in oxidative enzymes and glycogen storage. Finally, while transfer of training between different activities has been demonstrated, most studies of training transfer were conducted on previously inactive subjects. Therefore, whether cross-training (i.e., the supplementation of training with an alternative activity) enhances performance is unresolved.

Strength Training

Since resistance training does not produce cardiovascular improvement, it is logical to expect strength training to be specific, with little or no transfer among motor units. However, neural adaptations occurring early during strength training are not entirely specific.

Single-limb resistance training is accompanied by strength gains in contralateral inactive muscle groups. Moritani and deVries (25) found increased strength (35%) in trained and untrained (24%) elbow flexors. Ploutz et al. (26) demonstrated increased strength in trained (14%) and untrained (7%) knee extensors, along with limited hypertrophy in trained muscle groups and no hypertrophy in untrained muscle groups. Integrated electromyography and magnetic resonance imaging indicate that fewer motor units are recruited per unit of force applied in both trained and untrained muscle groups (25, 26). These results suggest that the transfer of strength to contralateral untrained muscle groups is due to neural adaptation. No evidence suggests that strength gain transfers to additional untrained muscle groups (e.g., legs to arms or quadriceps to gastrocnemius).

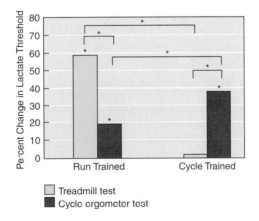

Figure 56.2. Change in oxygen consumption at lactate threshold following run training or cycle training tested on either a treadmill or cycle ergometer. An asterisk (*) above a bar indicates that oxygen consumption at lactate threshold changed significantly ($P < .05$) as a result of training. Asterisks between bars indicate different effects of training modes and testing modes. (Adapted with permission from Pierce EF, Weltman A, Seip RL, et al. Effects of training specificity on the lactate threshold and $\dot{V}O_{2peak}$. Int J Sports Med 11:267–272, 1990.)

SPECIFICITY OF MOVEMENT PATTERN

Specificity applies not only to energy systems and muscle groups but also to movement patterns. Motor units used during training demonstrate the most physiological alterations; therefore, movement patterns are also specifically trained. The following factors affect motor unit recruitment:

- Body position and movement pattern
- Static or dynamic contraction
- Concentric or eccentric contraction
- Intensity, frequency, and duration of contraction

Body Position and Movement Pattern

Strength gain is specific to the angle of the joint at which training occurs. Thorstensson et al. (27) trained subjects for 8 weeks, with free weights (squat training) and with the vertical jump and standing long jump (Fig. 56.3). Following training, a significant increase in squat strength was demonstrated, while leg press strength improved only about half as much. Leg extension strength (measured statically) did not improve.

Body position may also affect the response to endurance exercise. In the supine position, stroke volume (SV) is near maximum. Therefore, at a given submaximal work rate in this position, the passive increase in SV results in a lower heart rate and lower myocardial oxygen demand. These changes may permit some cardiac patients to exercise safely in a recumbent position at higher workloads, perhaps facilitating enhanced improvement of functional capacity.

Static Versus Dynamic Contractions

A static (isometric) contraction is applied against an immovable object, and no joint movement occurs, whereas movement accompanies a dynamic contraction because the force overcomes the resistance or vice versa. Overload training using either type of contraction in-creases strength. However, the manner in which strength increases may be different. Static training increases strength at joint angles similar to those used in training. Therefore, static training has little use for activities requiring dynamic movement. Duchateau and Hainaut (28) demonstrated greater increase in static strength of the adductor pollicis following static training than following dynamic resistance training. However, a greater increase in the speed of contraction was seen following dynamic training than following static training.

In addition, static exercise accompanied by a Valsalva maneuver is contraindicated for most high-risk populations because it can produce a marked increased in blood pressure. The prolonged contraction increases total peripheral resistance and inhibits blood flow through muscle, and the Valsalva maneuver increases intrathoracic pressure, which can reduce venous return and SV. These changes increase myocardial oxygen demand when cardiac output is reduced.

Concentric Versus Eccentric Contractions

There are two types of dynamic contraction, concentric (force is greater than the resistance, and the muscle shortens) and eccentric (force is less than the resistance, and the muscle lengthens). Lowering of a weight during a biceps curl is one example of eccentric contraction.

Although neither concentric nor eccentric contractions appear better suited for improving strength, eccentric contractions may enhance other types of adaptation. For example, both bodybuilders and ultramarathoners have large amounts of connective tissue within skeletal muscle, which may be a protective adaptation to cope with the high levels of force that must be exerted in these events (29). One disadvantage of having excess connective tissue may be that it inhibits motion in the antagonistic muscle. Excessive eccentric exercise also predisposes the athlete to overuse syndromes and muscle soreness (29).

Intensity, Frequency, and Duration of Contractions

In strength training, resistance moved and the number of repetitions and sets performed affect physiological adaptation. Competitive body builders, who typically use less resistance and more repetitions and sets than competitive weight lifters, often have greater gains in muscle girth. This may in part be due to an increased amount of connective tissue (29). Furthermore, although elite weight lifters may not have continuous hypertrophy, strength may increase substantially, perhaps because of an ability to recruit more motor units (4).

Fox et al. (30) studied 8-week interval training programs of high power (19 repetitions of 30 seconds each) and low power (7 repetitions of 120 seconds each). Figure 56.4 illustrates that both groups had similar increases in $\dot{V}O_{2max}$, and although both groups had lower blood

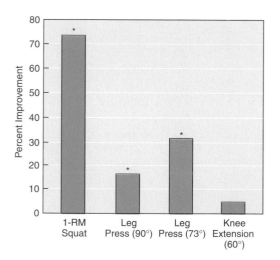

Figure 56.3. Effects of dynamic squat training on one-repetition maximum (1-RM) in squat and static strength in the leg press with the knee at 90°, the leg press with the knee at 73°, and the knee extension with the knee at 60°. An asterisk (*) indicates a significant improvement versus pretraining value ($P < .05$). (Adapted with permission from Thorstensson A, Karlsson J, Viitasalo JH, et al. Effect of strength training on EMG of human skeletal muscle. Acta Physiol Scand 98:232–236, 1976.)

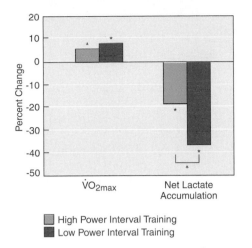

Figure 56.4. Effects of high-power (19 repetitions of 30 seconds each) and low-power (7 repetitions of 120 seconds each) treadmill interval training on $\dot{V}O_{2max}$ and net blood lactate accumulation (increased lactate concentration following a single exercise session). Similar increases occurred in $\dot{V}O_{2max}$, but net lactate accumulation decreased more as a result of low-power training than as a result of high-power training ($P < .05$). (Adapted with permission from Fox EL, Bartels RL, Klinzing J, et al. Metabolic responses to interval training programs of high and low power output. Med Sci Sports 9:191–196, 1977.)

lactate concentrations after a 2-minute posttraining run near $\dot{V}O_{2max}$, the lactate concentration in the low-power group was significantly lower than in the high-power group. Subsequently, long-duration training at a low intensity was accompanied by decreased anaerobic enzyme activity in both slow-twitch and fast-twitch muscle fibers, and increased aerobic enzyme activity in type I and type IIA muscle fibers (31). Training at a higher intensity for a shorter duration increases anaerobic capacity in type IIA muscle and type IIB muscle, and aerobic metabolism in type IIB muscle. These data indicate that intensive interval training is more beneficial for middle-distance events that rely on a blend of aerobic and anaerobic metabolism than for endurance performers, who benefit more from longer, less intensive training intervals and long-distance training. In fact, serious competitors generally apply both types of training, but the ratio depends on the event.

SPECIFICITY AND OTHER COMPONENTS OF FITNESS

There are five major categories of health-related physical fitness:

1. Cardiorespiratory endurance
2. Muscular strength
3. Muscular endurance
4. Flexibility
5. Body composition

This section discusses application of specificity to each component *in terms of both exercise testing and training.*

Cardiorespiratory Endurance

Specificity and endurance training were discussed previously in this chapter. Cross-over of training effects between one mode of endurance activity and another is limited. The most effective way to train for a particular activity is to practice that activity regularly. In addition, strength training of the same muscle group may increase endurance, but no evidence suggests that endurance training increases strength.

Specific testing protocols for assessing endurance were also discussed. A protocol inducing fatigue within 8–12 minutes assesses $\dot{V}O_{2max}$ most accurately. Uphill running on a treadmill can be used to assess $\dot{V}O_{2max}$ accurately, whereas a walking protocol is usually most appropriate for middle-aged and elderly subjects if balance is not a problem. Because of differing cardiovascular responses between upright and supine positions, posture during training should be replicated during testing whenever possible.

Muscular Endurance

Muscular endurance is the ability of a muscle or muscle group to repeat dynamic movements or to sustain static force over time. There is no clear distinction between cardiorespiratory and muscular endurance activities; both require contraction of skeletal muscle over extended time. However, cardiovascular endurance activities (e.g., distance running) are affected by cardiorespiratory limitations, and muscular endurance activities may be less affected. Muscular endurance activities (e.g., push-ups) generally require the athlete to overcome greater resistance and usually cannot be maintained as long as cardiorespiratory endurance activities. Muscular endurance activities also generally require greater anaerobic metabolic activity (anaerobic glycolysis) than aerobic metabolic activity for energy.

Training for muscular endurance can improve the efficiency of movement and acid–base buffering capacity. Trained athletes therefore often tolerate higher blood lactate concentrations than untrained persons.

Literature concerning the specificity of muscular endurance is scarce. Although some transfer from strength training is likely, optimal improvement in muscular endurance probably requires specific training. Therefore, training and testing should be activity specific. Position, movement pattern, type of contraction (i.e., static versus dynamic, concentric versus eccentric), and rate and resistance of contractions should be replicated during training.

Muscular Strength

Muscular strength is the amount of static or dynamic force that can be produced. Specificity of muscular strength was discussed earlier in this chapter. Strong evidence supports the importance of specific strength testing with respect to body position, movement pattern (including number of repetitions), and type of contraction. Single-repetition maximum testing is an excellent way of measuring strength; however, a 10-repetition maximum test may be a better indicator of muscular endurance.

Flexibility

Flexibility is the range of motion about a given joint or group of joints. Range of motion is limited primarily by the amount of soft tissue (including muscle and the joint capsule) surrounding the joint (32). Therefore, strength training resulting in hypertrophy and increased connective tissue mass may reduce the flexibility of joints involved in training. Flexibility can be increased or maintained through a regular stretching program and strength training exercises that move a *specific* joint through its full range of motion.

Body Composition

The two basic components of the body (fat and lean mass) respond differently to exercise training. Following several weeks of exercise training, the body composition may change slightly. The change is secondary to fat loss during endurance training and possibly also to increased lean mass due to muscle hypertrophy in resistance training. Methods of assessing body composition (e.g., skinfold measurements), may be sensitive to certain components of body composition and hence may produce inaccurate estimates of exercise-related changes in body composition. *Furthermore, most body density equations are biased to a specific age range, ethnicity, and gender. See Heyward and Stolarczyk (33) and Chapter 45 for more information concerning appropriate choice of a body density equation.*

For a significant amount of fat loss to occur, more energy must be expended than consumed. This is best achieved by reducing caloric intake and increasing physical activity. Endurance activity can be performed longer than resistance activity and is generally more useful for increasing caloric expenditure and fat loss. However, resistance training is more likely to preserve fat-free mass during weight loss and may help reduce fat (34). Addition of resistance training to an endurance training program enhanced the decrease in body fat percentage in hyperinsulinemic males. Improvements in systolic blood pressure and plasma insulin, glucose, and lipid concentrations were also greater (35). Therefore, weight loss programs should include both endurance and resistance training as part of the exercise program. Exercise should be prescribed to maximize total energy expenditure without undue fatigue. The optimal exercise prescription for weight control using resistance exercise remains unclear. More detailed information concerning weight control can be found elsewhere in this book.

▶ SUMMARY

A certain amount of training may be transferred between exercise training regimens. However, the need for specificity during training and performance testing is clear. In particular, the energy systems, the specific muscle groups, and the movements applied are important considerations.

Strength training may increase endurance, especially short-term endurance at high workloads. Endurance training does not increase strength, however, and may be detrimental to improvement in strength, although moderate endurance training may not impede the development of strength and should be included in exercise programs designed to improve physical fitness.

A certain amount of training adaptation can be transferred from one training mode to another. This is primarily due to cardiovascular adaptation in endurance training and neural adaptation in strength training.

Position, movement pattern, type of contraction (static versus dynamic, concentric versus eccentric), and intensity, frequency, and duration of muscle contraction are all important factors in the specificity of muscular performance. Altering these factors during exercise training may significantly alter results.

As specific as these points regarding the effects of training and training transfer may appear to be, most investigations supporting these conclusions were conducted with previously inactive subjects. The benefits of adding alternative modes of exercise to an established training regimen remain unclear.

The concept of specificity emphasizes a well-rounded program of exercise training. However, specificity also applies to testing. Task-specific testing is recommended for the assessment of both performance and performance improvement.

References

1. Holloszy JO. Biochemical adaptations in muscle. Effects of exercise on mitochondrial oxygen uptake and respiratory enzyme activity in skeletal muscle. J Biol Chem 242:2278–2282, 1967.
2. Gollnick PD, King DW. Effect of exercise and training on mitochondria of rat skeletal muscle. Am J Physiol 216:1502–1509, 1969.
3. Jansson E, Kaijser L. Muscle adaptation to extreme endurance training in man. Acta Physiol Scand 100:315–324, 1977.
4. Kraemer WJ, Fleck SJ, Evans WJ. Strength and power training: Physiological mechanisms of adaptation. Exerc Sport Sci Rev 24:363–397, 1996.
5. MacDougall JD, Sale DG, Moroz JR, et al. Mitochondrial volume density in human skeletal muscle following heavy resistance training. Med Sci Sports 11:164–166, 1979.
6. Dudley GA, Fleck SJ. Strength and endurance training: Are they mutually exclusive? Sports Med 4:79–85, 1987.

7. Hickson RC. Interface of strength development by simultaneously training for strength and endurance. Eur J Appl Physiol 45:255–263, 1980.

8. Dudley GA, Djamil R. Incompatibility of endurance- and strength-training mode of exercise. J Appl Physiol 59:1446–1451, 1985.

9. Sale DG, MacDougall JD, Jacobs I, Garner S. Interaction between concurrent strength and endurance training. J Appl Physiol 68:260–270, 1990.

10. McCarthy JP, Agre JC, Graf BK, et al. Compatibility of adaptive responses with combining strength and endurance training. Med Sci Sports Exerc 27:429–436, 1995.

11. Hickson RC, Rosenkoetter MA, Brown MM. Strength training effects on aerobic power and short-term endurance. Med Sci Sports Exerc 12:336–339, 1980.

12. Bishop D, Jenkins DG, Mackinnon LT, et al. The effects of strength training on endurance performance and muscle characteristics. Med Sci Sports Exerc 31:886–891, 1999.

13. Hurley BF, Seals DR, Ehsani AA, et al. Effects of high-intensity strength training on cardiovascular function. Med Sci Sports Exerc 16:483–488, 1984.

14. Hickson RC, Dvorak BA, Gorostiaga EM, et al. Potential for strength and endurance training to amplify endurance performance. J Appl Physiol 65:2285–2290, 1988.

15. Hoff J, Helgerud J, Wisloff U. Maximal strength training improves work economy in trained female cross-country skiers. Med Sci Sports Exerc 31:870–877, 1999.

16. Magel JR, McArdle WD, Toner M, et al. Metabolic and cardiovascular adjustment to arm training. J Appl Physiol 45:75–79, 1978.

17. Pate RR, Hughes RD, Chandler JF, et al. Effects of arm training on retention of training effects derived from leg training. Med Sci Sports Exerc 10:71–77, 1978.

18. Loftin M, Boileau RA, Massey BH, et al. Effect of arm training on central and peripheral circulatory function. Med Sci Sports Exerc 20:136–141, 1988.

19. Gergley TJ, McArdle WD, DeJesus P, et al. Specificity of arm training on aerobic power during swimming and running. Med Sci Sports Exerc 16:349–354, 1984.

20. Magel JR, Foglia GF, McArdle WD, et al. Specificity of swim training on maximum oxygen uptake. J Appl Physiol 38:151–155, 1975.

21. Franklin BA. Aerobic exercise training programs for the upper body. Med Sci Sports Exerc 21:S141–S48, 1989.

22. Saltin B, Nazar K, Costill DL, et al. The nature of the training response: Peripheral and central adaptations to bone-legged exercise. Acta Physiol Scand 96:289–305, 1976.

23. Pechar GS, McArdle WD, Katch FI, et al. Specificity of cardiorespiratory adaptation to bicycle and treadmill training. J Appl Physiol 36:753–756, 1974.

24. Pierce EF, Weltman A, Seip RL, et al. Effects of training specificity on the lactate threshold and VO_2peak. Int J Sports Med 11:267–272, 1990.

25. Moritani T, DeVries HA. Neural factors versus hypertrophy in the time course of muscle strength gain. Am J Phys Med 58:115–130, 1979.

26. Ploutz LL, Tesch PA, Biro RL, et al. Effect of resistance training on muscle use during exercise. J Appl Physiol 6:1675–1681, 1994.

27. Thorstensson A, Karlsson J, Viitasalo JH, et al. Effect of strength training on EMG of human skeletal muscle. Acta Physiol Scand 98:232–236, 1976.

28. Duchateau J, Hainaut K. Isometric or dynamic training: Differential effects on mechanical properties of a human muscle. J Appl Physiol 56:296–301, 1984.

29. Stauber WT. Eccentric action of muscles: Physiology, injury, and adaptation. Exerc Sport Sci Rev 17:157–185, 1989.

30. Fox EL, Bartels RL, Klinzing J, et al. Metabolic responses to interval training programs of high and low power output. Med Sci Sports Exerc 9:191–196, 1977.

31. Gillespie AC, Fox EL, Merola AJ. Enzyme adaptations in rat skeletal muscle after two intensities of treadmill training. Med Sci Sports Exerc 14:461–466, 1982.

32. Johns RJ, Wright V. Relative importance of various tissues in joint stiffness. J Appl Physiol 17:824–828, 1962.

33. Heyward VH, Stolarczyk LM. Applied Body Composition Assessment. Champaign, IL: Human Kinetics, 1996.

34. Walberg JL. Aerobic exercise and resistance weight-training during weight reduction: Implications for obese persons and athletes. Sports Med 47:343–346, 1989.

35. Wallace MB, Mills BD, Browning CL. Effects of cross-training on markers of insulin resistance/hyperinsulinemia. Med Sci Sports Exerc 29:1170–1175, 1997.

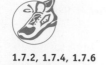
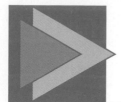

1.7.2, 1.7.4, 1.7.6

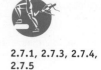

2.7.1, 2.7.3, 2.7.4, 2.7.5

CHAPTER **57**

MUSCULOSKELETAL INJURIES: RISKS, PREVENTION, AND CARE

John E. Kovaleski, Larry R. Gurchiek, and Albert W. Pearsall IV

Most types of physical activities are beneficial, because moderate exercise is an important element for general well-being. The risk of musculoskeletal injury increases for all levels of participation with increasing physical activity, intensity, and duration of training. The incidence and severity of exercise-related musculoskeletal injuries can be reduced by understanding the associated risks, preventive measures, and care of the injury. This chapter identifies and describes the incidence and severity of some exercise injuries. It also discusses several risk factors and mechanisms of recurring injury along with recommendations concerning prevention and treatment of injuries.

INCIDENCE AND RISKS OF INJURIES

With increased participation in resistance and aerobic training, there has been an increase in the frequency and severity of musculoskeletal injuries, both from acute and overuse trauma. Despite the knowledge that sprains, strains, stress fractures, and soft tissue inflammation occur frequently during training, little is known about risk factors for such injuries.

Musculoskeletal injuries are among the most common adverse effects of regular exercise and physical activity for individuals of all ages (1, 2). Running is associated with a high rate of musculoskeletal injury; 35–60% of runners report injuries that result in reduced weekly running or require medical intervention (2, 3). The patellofemoral articulation and the foot are the most common sites of injury in runners. High-impact aerobics and dance also are associated with a high incidence of injury (4). The incidence of injury in aerobic dance is reported to be approximately 45% of students and 75% of instructors (5). Four-fifths of these injuries affect the lower leg and are related to high frequency of exercise (>3 times per week), improper footwear, and/or exercise on a hard, nonresilient surface (6).

Musculoskeletal injuries can be attributed to the complex interaction of **intrinsic risk factors** (Table 57.1) and **extrinsic risk factors** (Table 57.2) that predispose physically active individuals to specific types of injuries (7–9). Poor biomechanics is a common cause of microtrauma and is associated with overuse and fatigue injuries. Past physical activity, poor baseline physical fitness, and present level of training also affect the incidence of injury.

Knowledge of risk factors is essential for reducing most injury rates. Both the sports medicine professional and the participant must have a good understanding of the short- and long-term risks of exercise. Improved understanding and identification of modifiable risk factors may lead to strategies and intervention to alter risk factors, which may help prevent injury. The following discussion focuses on several fitness activities and associated risk factors that can be encountered within the exercise setting.

Fitness Activity Risk Factors

Repetitive bouts of **microtrauma** leading to overt tissue injury cause **overuse injuries**. The overuse injury of running is one of the most common (10, 11). The causation of musculoskeletal running injuries is related to the runner, the running, and the environment (3). Most investigations of running-related injuries examined cross-sections of runners at various levels of training (11, 12). Musculoskeletal injury increases exponentially with increased frequency and total volume of training (3, 6, 13). Pollock et al. (14) reported that with beginning joggers and runners who trained 30 minutes a day for 1, 3, or 5 days per week, 1 day of rest between exercise days helps prevent injury. As functional capacity improves, frequency can be increased or jogging alternated with lower-impact modes of exercise. Another common risk factor for overuse is training errors. Training errors, which are reported in 60–80% of injuries to runners, are commonly caused by exceeding limits of duration or intensity, high rates of progression, and excessive hill running (15).

Decreased flexibility is an intrinsic risk factor for musculoskeletal injury (7). People with decreased flexibility are at particular risk for muscle strain and musculoskeletal injury (16). Jones et al. (17) examined injuries associ-

Table 57.1. Intrinsic Risk Factors Associated with Musculoskeletal Injury

Bony alignment abnormalities
Leg length discrepancy
Muscle weakness and imbalance
Restricted range of motion, inflexibility
Joint laxity
Predisposing musculoskeletal disease
Previous injury
Body composition
Gender
Previous physical activity
Performing warming-up exercises
Performing stretching exercises

Table 57.2. Extrinsic Risk Factors Associated with Musculoskeletal Injury

Excessive load on the body
  Type of movement
  Speed of movement
  Number of repetitions
  Footwear
  Surface
Training errors
  Excessive distances
  Fast progression
  High intensity
  Running on hills
  Poor technique
  Monotonous or asymmetrical training
  Fatigue
Adverse environmental conditions
  Darkness
  Heat or cold
  High humidity
  Altitude
  Wind
Faulty equipment

Modified with permission from Strauss RH, ed. Sports Medicine. Philadelphia: Saunders, 1992.

ated with physical training among young men and observed that the most flexible and least flexible individuals are at higher risk for lower body injury than moderately flexible individuals. Increased flexibility decreases the incidence of musculoskeletal injury, minimizes or alleviates muscle soreness, and contributes to improved performance (18). Stretching is important because it lengthens the musculotendinous unit, increasing flexibility and range of motion.

Muscle that is not properly warmed is susceptible to injury (19). Warmth improves elasticity of intramuscular connective tissue, speeds metabolism, and increases potential magnitude and speed of contraction. Warmth and the concomitant increase in connective tissue elasticity

may explain why warmed-up muscles can stretch more and resist injury at greater force. Warm-up, therefore, reduces the risk of muscle injury. Despite the theoretical support for warm-up, studies of warm-up do not demonstrate a clear advantage (7, 20, 21). For example, Walter et al. (20) reported that runners who never warm up have significantly less risk of running injuries than those who always, usually, or sometimes warm up. There are some indications that training programs using stretching and warm-up can decrease the incidence of injury. However, these programs incorporated several confounding variables, and the effect of single factors has not been determined. At present, it appears that warm-up may be more important in performance than injury prevention.

Other Risk Factors

Age is not associated with risk of exercise-related injury. Although several studies have concluded that there are no differences in the rate of injury between men and women, women appear to be at greater risk for exercise injury during endurance training (2, 3, 22, 23). For both genders, contact sports cause more injuries than noncontact sports, with sprains and strains cited as the most common (24). Whether injury rates are sport or exercise specific rather than gender specific is not clear. Nevertheless, gender differences in musculoskeletal anatomy (e.g., lower leg alignment, patellofemoral disorders), characteristics of training, and baseline fitness levels may play a role in injury incidence and type (10, 25).

Physiological variables, such as low body fat and certain body stature characteristics, may be risk factors for exercise and running-related injuries (e.g., stress fractures in females). No relationship between anthropometric data, physical fitness characteristics, and sports injuries have been reported (13, 22, 26). Therefore, definitive conclusions about the relationship between anthropometry and injury remain unclear.

Orthopaedic Risk Factors

Disorders of the musculoskeletal system may directly increase the risk of acute or chronic injury by interrupting normal structure and function of bone, joint, and soft tissue. The most common musculoskeletal risk factors include osteoarthritis, osteoporosis, chondromalacia, age-related musculotendinous degeneration, and malalignments of the lower extremity (7).

Past exercise injury and low physical activity are associated with a risk of musculoskeletal injury. Excessive weight has been found to predispose individuals to acute and overuse injuries as well as **osteoarthritic changes** of the hip and knee with weight-bearing recreational activities (27, 28). Weight loss reduces the risk of developing knee osteoarthritis, but its effect on the progression of the disease is unknown (29). In addition, vigorous physical activity may predispose to osteoarthritis by means of mechanical trauma to the joint (27). For example, an increased risk of osteoarthritis has been shown for competitive sports and running but not recreational running (30).

Obesity, a poor sitting posture that duplicates the fully flexed standing posture, frequent back flexion, loss of back extension, and low physical activity are among proposed risk factors of **low back pain** (31, 32). Episodes of low back pain are usually related to acute trauma or overuse. However, individual age, specific sport, and activity level are also covariables. Movements such as a poor lifting position and fatigue have also been reported in incidence and recurrence of low back pain (31).

Recommendations for Exercise Testing and Programming

A complex interaction of risk factors exists between musculoskeletal injury and exercise. To reduce the incidence and severity of injury, it is important to alter predisposing risk factors through education and clinical intervention. Behavior modifications with regard to early detection of symptoms of overuse injuries and full rehabilitation after injury are important for prevention. Participants should be encouraged to report injuries and symptoms, since untreated musculoskeletal injuries are likely to worsen the problem or predispose to future exercise-related injuries (25). Strenuous exercise is contraindicated in the presence of acute joint injury, chronic joint inflammation (osteoarthritis), or uncontrolled joint systemic disease (rheumatoid arthritis). Under medical management, submaximal and subjective symptom-limited fitness testing along with participation in regular conditioning exercise to improve health and physical fitness should be possible. The goal of exercise programs for individuals with orthopaedic disease and disability should be to prevent debilitation due to inactivity and to improve endurance, exercise tolerance, strength, and flexibility (33). The progression and level of physical activity must be individualized and determined largely by the pain and medical limitations of the condition.

PREVENTION OF INJURIES

Attempts to maintain or improve fitness require awareness of injury prevention. The expanded participation of a larger population in exercise potentiates the incidence of injury as the number of participants and volume of training increase. Increased injuries have prompted the development and promotion of several methods to prevent injuries.

Preparticipation Screening

Exercise professionals should be encouraged to use health and fitness screening before patients begin an exercise program. Most pre-exercise screening is used to de-

tect cardiopulmonary and metabolic contraindications to exercise. The American Academy of Family Physicians guidelines and objectives for **preparticipation evaluation** were developed for athletes in high school and college sports programs (34). It may be appropriate to consider similar tools to document any history of musculoskeletal injury prior to implementation of an exercise program (35).

Prevention of musculoskeletal injury can begin with preparticipation evaluation (Table 57.3). Identification of conditions, symptoms, and risk factors for injury along with a complete evaluation and musculoskeletal testing by a sports medicine professional should be part of preparticipation screening.

Basic Physical Fitness and Training

A well-rounded exercise program includes warm-up, cool-down, flexibility training, muscular strengthening, and aerobic conditioning. Proper training techniques require attention to the principles of specificity of exercise, overload, progressive resistance, and progression. Each program must be tailored for the mode of activity, intensity, duration, and frequency. In addition, proper equipment (clothing and shoes) plays an important role in safe participation and injury prevention.

Warming up and Cooling Down

The cardiovascular, respiratory, and neuromuscular systems can be put in a state of readiness for vigorous activity through warm-up exercises. Warm-up exercises gradually increase in intensity until myocardial blood flow and deep muscle temperature are suitable for exercise. Each exercise session should be preceded by a warm-up and followed by a cool-down. These periods generally require 5–10 minutes each. Prior to undertaking any exercise regimen, **general** and **specific warm-ups** are essential. **General warm-up** increases internal temperature through active movement. General warm-up includes light activity, such as jogging, stationary cycling, or calisthenics, and is followed by static stretching to enhance flexibility. **Specific warm-up** increases body and muscle temperature with movements similar to those used in the

Table 57.3. Objectives of the Musculoskeletal Pre-participation Evaluation

PRIMARY OBJECTIVES	SECONDARY OBJECTIVES
Detect conditions that limit or contraindicate participation	Determine general health
Detect conditions that predispose to injury	Counsel on health-related issues
Meet legal and insurance requirements	Assess physical maturity
Recommend preventive measures to optimize health	Assess fitness level and performance

activity. Cool-down includes light general exercise, such as walking or calisthenics, followed by stretching to maintain joint range of motion in muscle groups used in the activity.

Flexibility Training

Flexibility is the ability of soft-tissue structures, such as muscle, tendon, and connective tissue, to elongate through the available range of motion. The muscle sheath and connective tissue framework provide most of the resistance to the stretching of normal muscle, although if there is a previous injury, scarring, adhesions, and fibrotic contractures may also diminish flexibility. Stretching is an important aspect of the exercise-specific program, and it should be performed before and after the exercise session.

Flexibility training is a planned, regular exercise routine used to increase range of motion of a joint or system of joints. Flexibility warm-up is a deliberate and regular exercise performed immediately before activity to improve performance or reduce risk of injury. Although it is difficult to determine the ideal level of flexibility, a level that permits efficient movement and reduces the likelihood of musculoskeletal injury is recommended.

Resistance Training

Resistance training supplements health and fitness programs to enhance muscle conditioning and strength (7, 36). Muscles and other soft tissues subjected to resistance training exhibit an increased ability to absorb mechanical loads during activity. A pre-exercise evaluation is important to quantify and identify muscular strength, muscle imbalances, and flexibility deficits that predispose to injury. The first step when prescribing resistance exercise is to understand the components of the resistance exercise prescription. Along with a needs analysis, exercise resistance sequence, number of sets, repetitions, and length of rest between sets should be considered. Proper technique should be reinforced to avoid injury and improve program effectiveness. Periodic review of the resistance training routine can prevent overtraining and enhance effectiveness by ensuring appropriate progression. In addition, periodic alterations in the exercise program (e.g., sequence of exercises, volume, muscle groups worked) can enhance the program's effectiveness.

RECOGNITION AND CARE OF INJURIES

The exercise professional is often asked for advice regarding an injury or the need for referral for more specific care. It is important to understand the role of unlicensed individuals in the evaluation of an injury. Because of the unique nature of each situation, this chapter provides only general guidelines for the injury recognition process (37). Tables 57.4 and 57.5 contain a summary of common injuries, their signs and symptoms, and associated causes and mechanisms.

Table 57.4. General Injury Classifications and Conditions

MUSCLE INJURIES	MAJOR SIGNS AND SYMPTOMS
Acute	
Contusions	Soft tissue hemorrhage, hematoma, ecchymosis, movement restriction
Strains	Movement pain, local tenderness, loss of strength, range of motion
Tendon injuries	Pain; strength & range of motion loss; palpable defect
Muscle cramps, spasms	Involuntary muscle contraction; muscle pain
Acute-onset muscle soreness	Muscle pain, fatigue; resolve when exercise has ceased
Delayed-onset muscle soreness	Muscle stiffness 24–48 hours after exercise; tenderness and pain
Chronic	
Myositis, fasciitis	Local swelling and tenderness; stiffness
Tendinitis	Gradual onset, diffuse or local tenderness, swelling, pain
Tenosynovitis	Crepitus, diffuse swelling, pain
Bursitis	Swelling, pain, some loss of function
JOINT INJURIES	
Acute	
Sprains	Swelling, pain, joint instability, loss of function
Acute joint synovitis	Pain during motion, swelling, pain
Subluxation, dislocation	Loss of limb function, deformity, swelling, point tenderness
Chronic	
Capsulitis, synovitis	Joint edema, reduced range of motion, joint crepitus
Osteochondrosis	Joint locking, swelling, pain, disability
Osteoarthritis	Joint pain, articular crepitus, stiffness, reduced range of motion; cartilage destruction
Rheumatoid arthritis	Morning stiffness > 30 min; chronic pain; loss of joint integrity
Gouty arthritis	Joint inflammation, pain, low-grade fever
BONE INJURIES	
Periostitis	Pain over bone, especially under pressure
Acute fracture	Deformity, bone point tenderness, swelling, ecchymosis
Stress fracture	Vague pain that persists when attempting activity; local tenderness
Osteoporosis	Silent; becomes apparent on progression to stage at which a bone fractures

Table 57.5. Common Acute and Chronic Exercise and Sport Injuries and Causes

SITE	CONDITION	MECHANISM
Upper extremity		
Shoulder region	Rotator cuff strain	Throwing; swimming freestyle
	Rotator cuff tendinitis	Use of arm above horizontal; repetitive overhead activities
	Acromioclavicular joint sprain	Direct blow to tip of shoulder
	Anterior glenohumeral dislocation	Forced abduction, external rotation
Upper arm	Bicipital tenosynovitis	Repeated forceful external rotation of arm
Elbow	Lateral epicondylitis	Repeated forceful extension of the elbow (tennis elbow)
	Medial epicondylitis	Repeated forceful flexion of the elbow
Wrist and hand	Carpal tunnel syndrome	Activities that require repeated wrist flexion
	Strains and sprains	Falling on the wrist
	Fractures	Falling on the outstretched hand
Lower extremity		
Foot	Heel bruise	Contusion; sudden stop-and-go movements in running
	Plantar fasciitis	Unequal leg length; inflexible longitudinal arch; tight gastrocnemius–soleus muscle
	Retrocalcaneal bursitis	Pressure, rubbing by upper edge of shoe
	Metatarsalgia	Excessive pressure under the forefoot; fallen metatarsal arch
	Metatarsal stress fracture	Abusive training or overload; unequal leg length; hyperpronation of foot
Ankle, lower leg	Inversion ankle sprain	Foot forced into inversion-plantar flexion
	Achilles tendon strain	Sudden excessive dorsiflexion of foot
	Achilles tendinitis	Training errors; tight gastrocnemius–soleus muscle
	Anterior, posterior tibial tendinitis	Faulty posture alignment; falling arches; overuse stress
	Stress fracture of the tibia, fibula	Overuse stress; biomechanical foot problems
	Shin splints	Overtraining; running on hard surface; malaligned lower leg
Knee	Patellar femoral pain syndrome	Overuse, e.g., long training sessions, hill running; patellar compression
	Joint sprain	Direct straight-line or rotary forces
	Meniscal lesion	Excessive pressure (squatting); shear forces
	Patellar subluxation, dislocation	Alignment abnormalities; quadriceps weakness
	Chondromalacia patella	Abnormal patellar tracking; anatomical variation
	Degenerative arthritis	Overuse stress; obesity
	Patellar or quadriceps tendinitis	Sudden or repetitive forceful extension of knee
	Iliotibial band friction syndrome	Overuse stress associated with running, cycling
Upper leg	Quadriceps muscle strain	Weak muscles; sudden contraction, as during jumping
	Hamstring muscle strain	Strength imbalance; tightness; explosive movements
Hip	Trochanteric bursitis	Increased Q-angle; unequal leg length
Trunk		
Abdomen	Muscle strain	Sudden twisting of the trunk; reaching overhead
Spine	Lumbar strain and sprain	Poor posture; lumbar lordosis; sudden abrupt extension contraction, sometimes with trunk rotation
	Low back pain	Acute traumatic event; overuse; poor sitting posture; static or repeated flexion activities

Management of musculoskeletal injuries follows a logical sequence outlined in Table 57.6. The use of **HOPS** (history, observation, palpation, special tests) is especially important in obtaining information about the injury. A pertinent history along with systematic observation and palpation of the injured area frequently provide invaluable information. Highly specific examinations are beyond the clinical skill base of exercise professionals and should be performed by a physician or health care professional specifically trained in injury examination (38).

Injury management requires planning. Each acute or chronic injury should be evaluated and managed on an individual basis. This may entail immediate first aid and referral to a physician or simply advice about training and modifications in the exercise program. If a musculoskeletal complaint is beyond the expertise of the exercise professional, the individual should be referred to another health care professional for further examination. Prompt referral is imperative when medical safety may be in question. For example, a report of knee and calf pain with accompanying edema, localized tenderness, and venous distension justifies immediate referral to a physician for vascular evaluation. However, the exercise professional may elect to help an individual with minor musculoskeletal complaints. However, the athlete should be referred for further evaluation if the complaints do not resolve within a reasonable period or if they increase in severity.

Table 57.6. The Injury Recognition Process

1. Check vital signs and perform immediate first aid, if necessary
2. Stabilize the individual and/or injury
3. Identify injury
   History: Subjective statements by the injured person that include major complaints and injury history; for example, description of mechanism, functional impairments, pain, previous injury, training level and changes, equipment used, and prior rehabilitation
   Observation: Inspect or look at the individual and the injured part. Note variation in size, swelling, skin discoloration, posture, gait, limping, joint range of motion, instability or deformity, and atrophy. Compare the injured part with the uninjured part and so on.
   Palpation: Using the fingers, carefully and gently feel the affected part, including soft and bony structures. Examine for edema, skin temperature variations, deformity, point tenderness, and so on.
   Special tests: Detect specific conditions, such as joint stability, muscle strength, neurological status, and circulation
4. Decide your course of action
   RICES
   Referral to physician
   Return to activity
5. Administrative procedures
   Record injury or incident in file
   Inform immediate supervisor

Physiology of Injured Tissue

To optimize treatment, the exercise professional must know the basics of tissue healing and restraints related to the exercise program. Most activity-related injuries result from macrotrauma (tension, shear, or compression) and/or microtrauma (**overuse** or **cyclic loading**). When forces exceed the limits of tissues, injury results, and the response is a physiologically systematic process to resolve the injury. This process is similar for all types of soft tissue injuries.

At the time of injury, mechanical trauma damages cells. Because damaged cells cannot transport or process oxygen, nutrients, waste, and metabolites, cellular necrosis occurs. Blood vessels are commonly damaged, causing hemorrhage. The immediate response to hemorrhage is to activate coagulation and decrease blood flow to the area. Damage to tissues and cells from direct trauma is the **primary injury**. With the exception of controlling hemorrhage, treatment procedures have little effect on the extent or severity of primary injury. Additional swelling and tissue damage, known as **secondary hypoxic injury**, may continue even after bleeding is controlled. Secondary hypoxic injury is likely to occur without proper treatment and care.

Secondary hypoxic injury results from the reduction of the oxygen supply to undamaged cells and tissues adjacent to the site of injury. Metabolic changes in undamaged cells may result in further necrosis of tissue not directly affected by the primary injury. This causes cell fluid loss and blood plasma escape, which produce tissue edema and swelling, sometimes hours after the injury. Proper treatment to control the extent and amount of tissue damage and edema includes rest, ice, compression, elevation, and stabilization (**RICES**).

The Healing Process

The three phases of soft tissue healing are inflammation, repair, and remodeling (37, 39). Each phase consists of a systematic sequence of events. Optimal resolution of the injury allows a return to the preinjury level of activity. However, the outcome and the time necessary to achieve this stage depend not only on the severity of the injury but also on the type of treatment during each phase of the healing process.

Inflammatory Phase of Healing

The physiological reaction to tissue injury is **inflammation**. Signs and symptoms of inflammation include redness, local heat, swelling, pain, and loss of function. The purpose of inflammation is to localize injury, protect tissues from further damage, rid tissue of injurious agents and dead cells, and prepare for the repair phase. White blood cells are attracted by chemotactic factors. Other cells that migrate to the area form new capillaries and connective tissue. Though inflammation is a necessary part of healing, it should not last long, and chronic inflammation may result when the cause of an injury is not eliminated (39, 40).

Repair Phase of Healing

The repair process begins within the initial hours after injury, and it depends on resolution of the inflammatory phase. During the repair phase, proliferative and regenerative activity lead to scar formation and repair of injured tissue. Most soft tissues (muscle, tendon, and joint tissue) cannot regenerate the specific tissue that was damaged. Healing occurs by the formation of scar tissue. Initially, fragile and highly vascularized collagen fibers forming scar tissue are randomly laid down. Eventually, the fibrous connective tissue aligns along the lines of stress and grows significantly stronger. However, despite the strength of scar tissue, it generally remains an inadequate substitute for original tissue. In most cases, scar tissue is not as structurally sound or elastic as original tissue. Signs and symptoms associated with inflammation often disappear at the end of this phase of scar formation.

Remodeling Phase of Healing

The remodeling phase overlaps the repair phase. While certain areas of the injury form scar, others are remodeling scar. Remodeling entails the realignment of collagen fibers so that scar tissue becomes stronger according to the tensile forces to which it is subjected. Strengthening of scar tissue often continues for several months following injury. It is fairly common for ligaments to take a year or longer to become completely remodeled. If excessive strain is placed on scar tissue during remodeling, the duration of the healing may be extended. If, however, an optimal level of stress is placed on remodeling fibers, stronger and more viable scar tissue is the result. As healing progresses, controlled activities, including strengthening exercise, should be combined with protective support or bracing. Recommendations from a sports medicine professional regarding the appropriate time to begin activity and the type and intensity of exercise following injury may be helpful for full resolution.

Treatment for Exercise-Related Injuries

Standard treatment is divided into initial (first aid) and follow-up treatment. Initial treatment for acute musculoskeletal injuries is designated by the acronym **RICES** (39, 40). Initial treatment should be administered for the first 24–72 hours, depending on the severity of the injury. The purpose of RICES is to limit the amount of secondary hypoxic injury, control edema, and aid physiology of the inflammatory response.

Rest

Rest allows time to control the effects of trauma and to avoid additional tissue damage. Rest is a continuum ranging from complete rest to restricted activity (relative rest). The approximate rest time is relative to the severity of the injury. Rest can be accomplished by immobilization or with assistive devices such as a cane or crutches. Premature movement may increase hemorrhage and the extent of injury, thus prolonging recovery time. Generally, pain and swelling should guide treatment, and excessively painful movements should be avoided.

Ice

The application of ice is the first step in treatment. Ice or some form of cold application lowers the temperature of tissue, slowing cell metabolism. Subsequent metabolic demands are reduced, which enables healthy surrounding tissue to survive diminished blood flow and hypoxia. This in turn decreases secondary hypoxic injury and edema formation (40). Cold applications also are beneficial for reducing pain and muscle spasm that accompany musculoskeletal injury.

Ice is usually applied in a plastic bag, but commercial ice bags, chemical cold packs, and reusable ice packs are appropriate. An ice bag should be applied for 20–30 minutes approximately every 2 hours during the day. This procedure should be followed for the first 24 hours (40).

Compression

Compression controls edema and prevents fluid from accumulating in the injured area by creating a pressure gradient that facilitates the resorption of fluid. In addition, the support offered by a compression wrap decreases unwanted movement and may help relieve pain. Compression is accomplished with an elastic wrap or bandage.

Elevation

Elevation of the injured area above the level of the heart (when possible) limits swelling and increases venous return by lowering capillary hydrostatic pressure and decreasing capillary filtration pressure. Controlling edema associated with injury also decreases tissue damage, resulting in a smaller area of damaged tissue to be repaired.

Stabilization

Muscular spasm (termed muscle guarding) and pain, both undesirable responses to injury, often result from an attempt to protect the injured area. Muscle spasm increases pressure on nerve endings, which increases pain, which in turn can lead to more spasm. This vicious circle is commonly called the **pain–spasm cycle**. Stabilization supports the injured area so surrounding muscles can relax. Early stabilization through the use of braces and splints allows the muscle to relax, thus decreasing the pain–spasm cycle.

Follow-up Treatment

Therapeutic modalities and exercise procedures that follow the initial treatment are designed to allow return to functional activity. Application of heat is often prescribed after initial treatment is complete. Heat should not be applied during the acute inflammatory phase or when additional hemorrhage or swelling is likely. The purpose of heat is to increase circulation and reduce pain. Diminished pain allows movement of the injured part to begin more quickly with a greater pain-free range of motion (39, 40).

While both heat and cold application are beneficial, exercise is the most important follow-up treatment (40). Exercise is the most effective method to increase blood flow to an injured area; therefore, ice and heat should always be combined with exercise. The physician or sports medicine professional should direct follow-up treatment.

Medications

Several medications are available for treatment of joint and muscle inflammation and pain caused by direct trauma, overuse injury, and orthopaedic disease (36). Medications prescribed by the physician include aspirin, nonsteroidal anti-inflammatory drugs (NSAIDs), disease-modifying drugs (DMARDs), and newer immunosuppressive agents for the treatment of inflammatory rheumatic disease. In osteoarthritis and minor joint inflammations, NSAIDs and acetaminophen are often prescribed to manage stiffness and pain. Pharmacological management to control the discomfort associated with low back injuries includes the use of acetaminophen to manage pain, muscle relaxants, and NSAIDs.

The three nonprescription drugs most often used are aspirin, ibuprofen, and acetaminophen. Aspirin and ibuprofen are NSAIDs with analgesic, antipyretic, and anti-inflammatory properties. Aspirin, a salicylate drug, and ibuprofen, reduce pain, fever, and inflammation. Aspirin and various other NSAIDs have been associated with a variety of adverse reactions, including nausea, gastric discomfort, and decreased platelet aggregation. Although most individuals tolerate ibuprofen, gastric discomfort and stomach pains indicate poor tolerance. Acetaminophen has both analgesic and antipyretic effects but does not have significant anti-inflammatory properties. Aspirin-sensitive individuals should consult a physician before taking these pain relievers because they may encounter cross-reactivity with other medications.

Medications fulfill legitimate needs to relieve minor pain and discomfort. However, if dosage instructions are not followed, these products can be harmful. Use of nonprescription and prescription medications should be discussed with a physician or pharmacist. Individuals with persistent pain or injuries that do not resolve despite pharmacological intervention should consult a physician.

▶ SUMMARY

Musculoskeletal injury often results from a complex interaction of several identifiable intrinsic and extrinsic risk factors. Individuals must be educated about preventive measures to minimize the incidence and severity of exercise injuries. When injury does occur, the exercise professional contributes by participating in education, physical conditioning, and referral of the individual. Only through educational efforts and clinical interaction between exercise professionals and sports injury specialists can prevention and reduction of exercise-related injuries occur.

References

1. Bijur PE, Tumble A, Harel Y, et al. Sports and recreation injuries in U.S. children and adolescents. Arch Pediatr Adolesc Med 149:1009–1116, 1995.
2. Koplan JP, Powell KE, Sikes RK, et al. An epidemiologic study of the benefits and risks of running. JAMA 248:3118–3121, 1982.
3. Powell KE, Kohl HW, Caspersen CJ, et al. An epidemiologic perspective on the causes of running injuries. Phys Sports Med 14:100–114, 1986.
4. Garrick JG, Gillien DM, Whiteside P. The epidemic of aerobic dance injuries. Am J Sports Med 14:67–72, 1986.
5. Mutoh Y, Sawai S, Takanashi Y, et al. Aerobic dance injuries among instructors and students. Phys Sports Med 16:81–88, 1988.
6. Richie DH, Kelso SF, Bellucci PA. Aerobic dance injuries: A retrospective study of instructors and participants. Phys Sports Med 13:130–140, 1985.
7. Renstrom P, ed. The Encyclopedia of Sports Medicine: Sports Injuries. Oxford: Blackwell Scientific, 1993.
8. Renstrom P, Kannus P. Prevention of Sports Injuries. In: Strauss RH, ed. Sports Medicine. Philadelphia: Saunders, 1992.
9. Shephard RJ, Astrand PO, eds. The Encyclopedia of Sports Medicine: Endurance in Sport. Oxford: Blackwell Scientific, 1992.
10. Arendt EA. Common musculoskeletal injuries in women. Phys Sports Med 7:39–48, 1996.
11. Andrews JR. Overuse syndromes of the lower extremity. Clin Sports Med 2:137–148, 1983.
12. Nieman DC. Fitness and Sports Medicine: An Introduction. Palo Alto, CA: Bull, 1990.
13. Blair SN, Kohl HW, Goodyear NN. Rates and risks for running and exercise injuries: Studies in three populations. Res Q Sport Exerc 58:221–228, 1987.
14. Pollock ML, Gettman LR, Milesis CA, et al. Effects of frequency and duration of training on attrition and incidence of injury. Med Sci Sports Exerc 9:31–36, 1977.
15. James SL, Bates BT, Osternig LR. Injuries to runners. Am J Sports Med 6:40–50, 1978.
16. Liemohn W. Factors related to hamstring strains. J Sports Med 18:71–76, 1978.
17. Jones BH, Cowan DN, Tomlinson JP, et al. Epidemiology of injuries associated with physical training among young men in the army. Med Sci Sports Exerc 2:197–203, 1993.
18. Worrell TW, Perrin DH, Gansneder B, et al. Comparison of isokinetic strength and flexibility measures between hamstring injured and non-injured. J Orthop Sports Phys Ther 13:118–125, 1991.
19. Zarins B, Ciullo J. Acute muscle and tendon injuries in athletes. Clin Sports Med 2:167–182, 1983.
20. Walter SD, Hart LE, McIntosh JM. The Ontario Cohort Study of running-related injuries. Arch Intern Med 149:2561–2564, 1989.
21. van Mechelen W, Hlobil H, Kemper H, et al. Prevention of running injuries by warm-up, cool-down, and stretching exercises. Am J Sports Med 21:711–719, 1993.
22. Macera CA, Jackson KL, Hagenmaier GW, et al. Age, physical activity, physical fitness, body composition, and incidence of orthopedic problems. Res Q Sport Exerc 60:225–233, 1989.
23. Kowal DM. Nature and causes of injuries in women resulting from an endurance training program. Am J Sports Med 8:265–269, 1980.
24. DeHaven KE, Lintner DM. Athletic injuries: Comparison by age, sport, and gender. Am J Sport Med 14:218–224, 1986.
25. Almeida SA, Trone DW, Leone DM, et al. Gender differences in musculoskeletal injury rates: A function of symptom reporting? Med Sci Sports Exerc 31:1807–1812, 1999.
26. Jones BH, Bovee MW, Harris JM, et al. Intrinsic risk factors for exercise-related injuries among male and female army trainees. Am J Sports Med 21:705–710, 1993.
27. Felson DT, Zhang Y, Hannan MT, et al. Risk factors for incident radiographic knee osteoarthritis in the elderly: The Framingham Study. Arthritis Rheum 40:728–733, 1997.
28. Ettinger WH, Burns R, Messier SP, et al. A randomized trial comparing aerobic exercise and resistance exercise with a health education program in older adults with knee osteoarthritis: The Fitness Arthritis and Seniors Trial (FAST). JAMA 277:25–31, 1997.
29. Felson DT, Zhang Y, Anthony JM, et al. Weight loss reduces the risk for symptomatic knee osteoarthritis in women. Ann Intern Med 116:535–539, 1992.
30. Lane NE. Physical activity at leisure and risk of osteoarthritis. Ann Rheum Dis 55:682–684, 1996.

31. Heistaro SE, Vartiainen E, Heliovaara M, et al. Trends in back pain in eastern Finland, 1972–1992, in relation to socioeconomic status and behavioral risk factors. Am J Epidemiol 148:671–682, 1998.

32. Carpenter DM, Nelson BW. Low back strengthening for the prevention and treatment of low back pain. Med Sci Sports Exerc 31:18–24, 1999.

33. Durstine JL, ed. ACSM's Exercise Management for Persons with Chronic Diseases and Disabilities. Champaign IL: Human Kinetics,1997.

34. American Academy of Family Physicians. Preparticipation Physical Evaluation. Chicago: American Academy of Family Physicians, 1996.

35. Peltz JE, Haskell WL, Matheson GO. A comprehensive and cost-effective preparticipation exam implemented on the World Wide Web. Med Sci Sports Exerc 31: 1727–1740, 1999.

36. Soukup JT, Maynard TS, Kovaleski JE. Resistance training guidelines for individuals with diabetes mellitus. Diabetes Educ 20:129–137, 1994.

37. Arnheim DD, Prentice WE. Principles of Athletic Training. 10th ed. Boston: McGraw-Hill, 2000.

38. American Academy of Orthopaedic Surgeons. Athletic Training and Sports Medicine. 3rd ed. Park Ridge, IL: American Academy of Orthopaedic Surgeons, 1999.

39. Prentice WE. Therapeutic Modalities in Sports Medicine. 4th ed. Boston: WCB/McGraw-Hill, 1999.

40. Knight KL. Cryotherapy in Sport Injury Management. Champaign, IL: Human Kinetics, 1995.

Suggested Reading

American Academy of Orthopaedic Surgeons. Athletic Training and Sports Medicine. 3rd ed. Park Ridge, IL: American Academy of Orthopaedic Surgeons, 1999.

ACSM's Exercise Management for Persons with Chronic Diseases and Disabilities. Champaign IL: Human Kinetics, 1997.

Whiting WC. Biomechanics of Musculoskeletal Injury. Champaign, IL: Human Kinetics, 1998.

1.3.0, 1.7.5

2.7.4, 2.7.5

4.8.8, 4.8.9

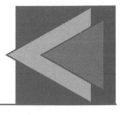

CHAPTER **58**

MEDICAL COMPLICATIONS OF EXERCISE

Ben Levine, Julie Hanson-Zuckerman, and Chris Cole

The possible medical complications of exercise are numerous (Table 58.1) (1). Fortunately, serious complications are rare, and common complications are minor. Musculoskeletal and traumatic injuries, the most frequent hazards of exercise, are usually self-limited, with only 10–20% requiring medical attention (2, 3). However, serious and even fatal events do occur during increased levels of activity, particularly in individuals who are not habitually active. This chapter focuses on these complications.

CARDIOVASCULAR COMPLICATIONS OF EXERCISE

Cardiovascular complications are cause for the most concern. Almost all such complications occur in individuals with underlying acquired heart disease or congenital abnormalities; individuals without heart disease have a low risk of a cardiac event during exercise. These complications can be divided into two general groups based on age. Cardiac problems in those older than 35 tend to be due to coronary heart disease (CHD), while those that occur in persons younger than 35 are usually secondary to cardiovascular structural abnormalities (4–6) (Fig. 58.1 and Table 58.2).

Complications in Those With Coronary Heart Disease

Coronary heart disease (CHD) is the leading cause of serious morbidity and mortality during high activity levels in those over 35 years of age. In a healthy population, a cardiac event during exercise is uncommon, but in those with underlying CHD, exercise may trigger an acute myocardial infarction (MI) and/or sudden cardiac death (4, 7–9). Albert has recently evaluated the risk of sudden death during exercise in a large cohort of 21,481 men enrolled in the Physicians Health Study (4). The participants were asked about their frequency of vigorous exercise at enrollment in the study and then prospectively followed. After 12 years of follow-up there were 122 deaths of which 23 had occured either during or in the 30 minutes following vigorous activity. The risk of dying during or immediately following exercise was increased by a factor of 16.9 compared to sedentary periods. However, the absolute risk during any given episode of vigorous exercise was very low with only 1 sudden death occuring for every 1.51 million episodes of exercise. Additionally, those who participated in regular exercise had a lower risk of death during vigorous activity although it was still higher than at rest. The group at higher risk was those men who only sporadically participated in vigorous exercise. This group had a 74-fold increase in risk of death during vigorous exertion (4).

In the presence of CHD, competitive activity places the older athlete at a particularly high risk for sudden death (4, 5, 10). Competition is defined as any event in which external pressures, such as motivation to win and/or team participation, inhibit the athlete from appropriately ceasing exercise in spite of warning symptoms (e.g., chest pain or light-headedness) (11). This problem was demonstrated in a review of sudden deaths among older athletes, among whom more than three-quarters of the fatalities occurred during competition (7). Competitive activity was also a factor in one-third of the jogging-related deaths in the Rhode Island study. Furthermore, in a series by Noakes, 20 of 28 marathon runners who died suddenly had reported symptoms of nausea, abdominal discomfort, dizziness, severe fatigue, and even angina, but they continued running (4, 12). It is therefore essential that all exercising adults be informed of the symptoms of cardiac ischemia and instructed to stop exertion in the face of pain.

Recommendations for participation in competitive activities for athletes with CHD are found in the 26th Bethesda Conference report (11). This report suggests that athletes with CHD can be stratified into groups with mildly and substantially increased risk based on the following:

- Left ventricular systolic function
- Exercise tolerance
- Exercise-induced ischemia or complex ventricular arrhythmias
- Hemodynamically significant coronary artery stenosis

Table 58.1. Possible Medical Complications of Exercise

Cardiovascular Complications
Cardiac arrest
Ischemia
  Angina
  Myocardial infarction
Arrhythmias
  Supraventricular tachycardia
  Atrial fibrillation
  Ventricular tachycardia
  Ventricular fibrillation
  Bradyarrhythmias
  Bundle branch blocks
  Atrioventricular nodal blocks
Congestive heart failure
Hypertension
Hypotension
Aneurysm rupture
Underlying medical conditions
  predisposing to increased
  complications
  Hypertrophic cardiomyopathy
  Coronary artery anomalies
  Idiopathic left ventricular
    hypertrophy
  Marfan syndrome
  Aortic stenosis
  Right ventricular dysplasia
  Congenital heart defects
  Myocarditis
  Pericarditis
  Amyloidosis
  Sarcoidosis
  Long QT syndrome
  Sickle-cell trait
Metabolic Complications
Volume depletion
Dehydration
Rhabdomyolysis
  Renal failure
Electrolyte disturbances
Thermal Complications
Hyperthermia
  Heat rash
  Heat cramps
  Heat syncope
  Heat exhaustion
  Heat stroke
Hypothermia
Frostbite
Pulmonary Complications
Exercise-induced asthma
Bronchospasm
Pulmonary embolism
Pulmonary edema

Pneumothorax
Exercise-induced anaphylaxis
Exacerbation of underlying
  pulmonary disease
Gastrointestinal Complications
Vomiting
Cramps
Diarrhea
Endocrine Complications
Amenorrhea
Complications in diabetics
  Hypoglycemia
  Hyperglycemia
  Retinal hemorrhage
Osteoporosis
Neurological Complications
Dizziness
Syncope (fainting)
Cerebral vascular accident
  (stroke)
Insomnia
Musculoskeletal Complications
Mechanical injuries
Back injuries
Stress fractures
Carpal tunnel syndrome
Joint pain/injury
Muscle cramps/spasms
Tendonitis
Exacerbation of musculoskeletal
  diseases
Overuse Complications
Overuse syndromes
Over-training
Over-exercising
Shin splints
Plantar fasciitis
Traumatic Injuries
Bruises
Strains and sprains
Muscle and tendon tears and
  ruptures
Fractures
Contusions and lacerations
Bleeding
Crush injuries
Blunt trauma
Internal organ injury
  Splenic rupture
  Myocardial contusion
Drowning
Head injuries
Eye injuries
Death

Table 58.2. Cardiovascular Abnormalities in 134 Young Competitive Athletes Who Died Suddenly

Primary Cardiovascular Lesion	No. (%) of Athletes	Median Age (range)
Hypertrophic cardiomyopathy	48 (36.0)	17.0 (13–28)
Unexplained increase in cardiac mass[a]	14 (10.0)	17.0 (14–24)
Aberrant coronary arteries[b]	17 (13.5)	15.0 (12–23)
Other coronary anomalies	8 (6.0)	17.5 (14–40)
Ruptured aortic aneurysms[c]	6 (5.0)	17.0 (16–31)
Tunneled left anterior descending coronary artery	6 (5.0)	17.5 (14–20)
Aortic valve stenosis	5 (4.0)	14.0 (14–17)
Lesion consistent with myocarditis	4 (3.0)	15.5 (13–16)
Idiopathic dilated cardiomyopathy	4 (3.0)	18.0 (18–21)
Arrhythmogenic right ventricular dysplasia	4 (3.0)	16.0 (15–17)
Idiopathic myocardial scarring	4 (3.0)	20.0 (14–27)
Mitral valve prolapse[c]	3 (2.0)	16.0 (15–23)
Atherosclerotic coronary artery disease	3 (2.0)	19.0 (14–28)
Other congenital heart disease[d]	2 (1.5)	13.5 (12–15)
Long QT syndrome[e]	1 (0.5)	
Sarcoidosis	1 (0.5)	
Sickle cell trait[f]	1 (0.5)	
"Normal" heart[g]	3 (2.0)	18 (16–21)

[a] Includes 1 athlete with grossly normal heart but distinctly abnormal histological architecture with marked disorganization of cardiac muscle cells and bundles. Also, 2 of the 13 athletes with mildly increased mass had associated tunneled left anterior descending artery.
[b] Anomalous origin of the left main coronary artery from the right sinus of Valsalva in 13 (1 of these also showed acute-angle takeoff of the right coronary artery, and 1 had a tunneled segment of left anterior descending artery). Anomalous origin of the right coronary artery from the left sinus of Valsalva in 2. Anomalous origin of the left margin coronary artery from between the left and posterior cusps with acute-angle takeoff in 1. Origin of the left anterior descending coronary artery from the pulmonary trunk in 1.
[c] Marfan syndrome was also present in 3 athletes with ruptured aortic aneurysm and in 1 with mitral valve prolapse.
[d] One athlete with secundum atrial septal defect and 1 with coarctation of the aorta.
[e] Also had anomalous origin of the right coronary artery from the left sinus of Valsalva.
[f] Judged to be the probable cause of death in the absence of any identifiable structural cardiovascular abnormality.
[g] Absence of structural heart disease on standard autopsy examination.
Reprinted with permission from Maron BJ et al. Sudden death in young competitive athletes. JAMA 276:199–204, 1996.

competition. Those in the substantially increased risk group should restrict activities to low-intensity competitive sports. The Bethesda report offers a complete discussion of this topic, including criteria for risk stratification (11).

Although more frequently seen in those over 35 years, coronary artery disease is occasionally identified as the cause of death in young athletes. For example, Maron (6) identified three individuals aged 14, 19, and 28 years who died of atherosclerotic coronary artery disease. Eliciting a family history of premature atherosclerotic disease or unexplained death at an early age is crucial in screening. In addition, cholesterol screening can help identify those at risk.

Having documented CHD does not imply that all ex-

Athletes in the mildly increased risk group may participate in low dynamic and low or moderate static competitive activity, but generally should not participate in intensely competitive activities. However, it was acknowledged that specific individuals with preserved left ventricular function, high exercise capacity, and no evidence of inducible ischemia could be cleared for higher-intensity

Causes of Sudden Death in Athletes

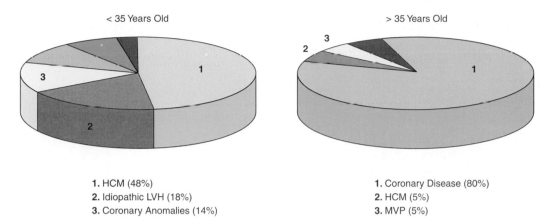

< 35 Years Old

1. HCM (48%)
2. Idiopathic LVH (18%)
3. Coronary Anomalies (14%)

> 35 Years Old

1. Coronary Disease (80%)
2. HCM (5%)
3. MVP (5%)

Figure 58.1. HCM-hypertrophic cardiomyopathy, LVH-left ventricular hypertrophy, MVP-mitral valve prolapse. Causes of sudden death in athletes divided by age. (Reprinted with permission from Maron BJ et al. Causes of sudden death in competitive athletes. *J Am Coll Cardiol* 7:204–214, 1996.)

ercise must be curtailed. In fact, the risk of an adverse cardiovascular event is reduced by regular physical activity (8, 13, 14). This was demonstrated by Siscovick et al. (13), who retrospectively examined 133 deaths due to cardiac arrest and classified them according to activity level at time of cardiac arrest and by the amount of habitual vigorous activity. He documented that the overall risk of sudden cardiac death in habitually vigorous men was 40% less than in sedentary men. A similar reduction has been identified for the risk of acute MI. Mittleman et al. (8) interviewed 1228 patients following MI and classified them according to frequency of heavy physical exertion per week. Those who were the most active had a risk of onset of MI during heavy physical exertion that was only about 1% that of the sedentary group, demonstrating the benefits of exercise in persons with CHD (8). Finally, regular exercise has been clearly shown to be an important factor in reducing the risk of CHD mortality and is to be encouraged in virtually all able individuals (14).

Complications in Those With Cardiac Structural Defects

While CHD is the leading cause of death during exercise in the elderly, anatomical defects are the foremost cause of sudden death in young athletes. All of these congenital abnormalities are rare; the most common are hypertrophic cardiomyopathy, coronary artery anomalies, and Marfan syndrome. These three defects account for almost three-quarters of 158 deaths in young competitive athletes examined by Maron et al. (6) between 1985 and 1995 (Fig. 58.1).

Hypertrophic Cardiomyopathy

Hypertrophic cardiomyopathy (HCM), along with the closely related idiopathic concentric left ventricular hypertrophy, is the single most common abnormality found on autopsy in young athletes who die suddenly (5, 6).

HCM is a genetic condition resulting in asymmetrical thickening of the left ventricle, particularly the septum; it occurs in about 0.1% of the general population (15). Diastolic filling is impaired and in about 25% of cases is accompanied by left ventricular outflow tract obstruction. Symptoms, which may or may not be present, include dyspnea, angina, light-headedness, and syncope during exertion. Even when symptoms are absent, HCM may be detected by physical examination. Physical findings include right-sided fourth heart sound, systolic ejection murmur along the left sternal border, and systolic murmur at the apex, increasing with amyl nitrate inhalation, assuming upright posture, or Valsalva maneuver.

HCM has a variable clinical course because of its wide spectrum of severity. Many individuals with HCM are asymptomatic and unaware of it. There is, however, a definite increase in the risk of death with HCM; annual mortality reaches 1% (15). Heavy physical exertion increases this risk. The mechanism whereby activity leads to sudden death is complex; arrhythmias (ventricular tachycardia, ventricular fibrillation) resulting from myofibrillar disarray and hypotension precipitated by exercise-related tachycardia both play a role. Arrhythmias occur at the same rate in those with and without left ventricular outflow tract obstruction and with and without symptoms, even after surgical correction. Because of the high risk of a cardiac event during strenuous exercise, patients with HCM should not participate in most competitive sports except those of low intensity. For additional information, review the Bethesda guidelines for high-risk subsets (11).

Anomalous Coronary Artery

The second-largest group of structural defects in young athletes who die suddenly are anomalous coronary arteries (Fig. 58.2). These arteries arise from and/or course through atypical locations, and occasionally, because of their anatomical position, an interruption of blood flow

Causes of Sudden Death in High School/College Athletes
(1983-93)

Cardiovascular Conditions

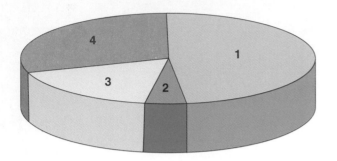

Coronary Artery Anomalies

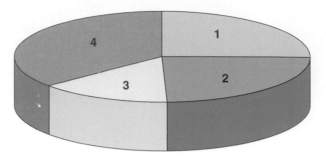

1. Hypertrophic Cardiomyopathy (48%)
2. Probable Hypertrophic Cardiomyopathy (5%)
3. Coronary Artery anomaly (14%)
4. Other (33%)

1. Intramural LAD (25%)
2. Anomalous Origin of LCA from R Sinus of Valsalva (24%)
3. Anomalous Origin of LCA from PA (13%)
4. Other (38%)

*22% of all deaths due to noncardiovascular causes

Figure 58.2. LAD, left anterior descending; LCA, left coronary artery; PA, pulmonary artery. Causes of sudden death in high school/college athletes (1983–93). (Reprinted with permission from Van Camp SP et al. Nontraumatic sports deaths in high school and college athletes. *Med Sci Sports Exerc* 27:641–647, 1995.)

results in sudden death. The risk of occlusion (blockage) is particularly high during and immediately after exercise. All coronary artery anomalies are rare, but most common are the following:

1. Left coronary artery arising from the anterior sinus of Valsalva (right cusp of the aortic valve) and coursing between the aorta and pulmonary trunk (Fig. 58.3) (16).
2. Mural left anterior descending artery (artery tunneled into the ventricular wall) (17).

Less common coronary artery anomalies resulting in sudden death include the following:

1. Single artery
2. Hypoplasia (small size or short course)
3. Intussusception (inward convulsion)
4. Aneurysm
5. Acute-angled takeoff of the left main coronary artery (18, 19)

Marfan Syndrome

Marfan syndrome is an inherited connective tissue disease that predisposes affected individuals to develop aortic aneurysm. It is suspected in tall, thin individuals, such as basketball and volleyball players, with physical characteristics consistent with Marfan's and a family history of

sudden death. Possible physical findings include an outflow murmur and the presence of a pulsatile mass in the abdomen. If suspected, aneurysms can be screened with ultrasound. If undetected, these aneurysms may rupture during vigorous activity and cause death (20).

Diagnosis

Most underlying congenital conditions are difficult to detect. Of 134 athletes who died suddenly, only 4 (3%) were suspected of having cardiovascular disease on routine prescreening physical examination, and the cardiovascular abnormality responsible for death was correctly identified in only 1 (0.9%) prior to death (6). Hypertrophic cardiomyopathy may be suspected on finding an outflow murmur during physical examination or from a family history of sudden death at a young age and can be confirmed with echocardiography. However, routine screening of athletes with echocardiography is not cost-effective (21).

Coronary artery anomalies are difficult to identify prospectively. However, there may be prior episodes of syncope, exertional angina, or resting electrocardiographic (ECG) abnormalities (16). Some types of anomalous arteries may be excluded by echocardiography but may be clearly visualized with magnetic resonance imaging. Those who are identified, particularly with the left coronary artery arising from the right cusp of the aorta, should not participate in competitive sports unless they have undergone surgical correction (11).

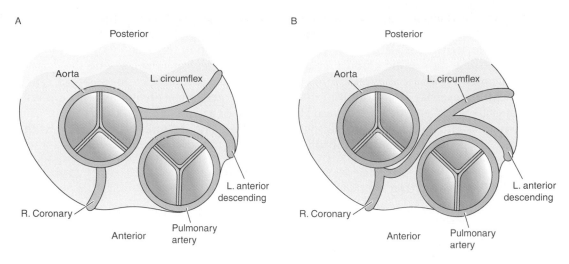

Figure 58.3. **A** and **B.** Anomalous coronary arteries.

COMPLICATIONS OF EXERCISE TESTING

An exercise test is heavy physical exertion by an individual in a controlled setting. As such, the same complications seen in the general population during increased activity may occur. Most of these complications are, as in the general population, rare, and range from minor to serious. To measure the level of risk, Atterhog et al. (22) prospectively studied 50,000 exercise tests in an unselected clinical population. Documented complications were as follows: 2 deaths (0.4/10,000 tests); 2 cardiac arrests (0.4/10,000 tests), one of which was fatal; 7 MIs (1.4/10,000), including one death; 2 cases of pulmonary edema (0.4/10,000 tests); and 2 cerebrovascular events (0.4/10,000 tests) (22). These rates were higher than those of a large retrospective study of more than 1.7 million exercise tests done in the general population, which reported 0.11 MIs and 0.02 fatal MIs per 10,000 tests (23). Almost 90% of patients with complications had suspected or proven heart disease, reinforcing that those with CHD are at increased risk for cardiac events during exercise (22, 23).

In those without known heart disease, exercise testing is a very low risk procedure. For example, no complications occurred in 380,000 exercise tests done in young individuals presumed to be free of heart disease (23). In addition, in 71,914 exercise tests performed at a single institution as part of a preventive medicine program, only one cardiac complication occurred among persons without known CHD (24).

Arrhythmic Complications

Arrhythmias can be precipitated by exercise and so may be encountered during exercise testing and cardiac rehabilitation. Two of the most serious arrhythmias are ventricular fibrillation and ventricular tachycardia. Most cases of ventricular fibrillation during exercise in the gen-

eral population are fatal because they are not identified and treated. During exercise testing and cardiac rehabilitation, however, participants are closely monitored, and ventricular fibrillation may be identified and its prevalence determined.

Ventricular tachycardia is a rapid arrhythmia of the ventricles that can degenerate to ventricular fibrillation which usually suggests myocardial scar rather than myocardial ischemia. It is slightly more common than ventricular fibrillation and was found to arise 29 times in 50,000 exercise tests (5.8/10,000 tests) (22). Both ventricular tachycardia and ventricular fibrillation require immediate treatment with direct current cardioversion with a defibrillator.

Other arrhythmias that may occur during exercise testing are atrial tachycardia (2/10,000 tests), sinus bradycardia (0.8/10,000 tests), atrial fibrillation (0.8/10,000 tests), atrioventricular nodal tachycardia (0.4/10,000 tests), atrial flutter, second-degree atrioventricular block, and left bundle branch block (0.2/10,000 tests) (22). Arrhythmias are most likely to occur in those with a history of arrhythmia. Of 263 patients with a prior arrhythmia, 24 (9.1%) had an arrhythmia during maximal exercise testing. In 3444 patients with no history of conduction disturbance, only 4 (0.1%) had sustained tachyarrhythmia or bradycardia during testing (25). Therefore, for maximum safety, persons trained in recognition and treatment of arrhythmias should be present during exercise testing and rehabilitation of high-risk individuals.

Hemodynamic Complications

Blood pressure should also be monitored during exercise testing. During dynamic upright exercise on a treadmill, systolic blood pressure normally rises, and diastolic blood pressure remains the same or decreases slightly. Monitoring may reveal either a hypertensive (high blood pressure) or hypotensive (low blood pressure) response. A hypertensive response to exercise may occur in individuals with underlying hypertension. Relative indications to terminate exercise testing are systolic blood pressure above 260 or diastolic blood pressure above 115mm Hg (26). Hypotension during exercise is a more ominous finding. A drop in systolic blood pressure of ≥ 10mm Hg or a drop below resting standing blood pressure strongly suggests extensive myocardial ischemia and is an absolute indication to stop the test (27).

Contraindications to Exercise Testing

Because exercise testing can be dangerous, it is crucial to identify those who are at increased risk for complications and exclude them when necessary. All personnel involved in performing exercise testing should be familiar with contraindications and precautions. There are published guidelines for contraindications to exercise testing (26, 27).

In general, contraindications are conditions that may be aggravated by exercise or that may affect exercise performance. For example, exercise testing in an individual with unstable angina may precipitate MI or fatal arrhythmia. Severe aortic stenosis, dissecting aneurysm, and myocarditis increase the risk of a fatal complication. These contraindications are empirical rather than based on clinical studies.

The experience level of the personnel conducting the test, access to emergency medical equipment and services, and the benefit of testing should be considered in the decision as to whether a safe exercise test can be performed on persons whose health indicates precautions. In some cases, a decision to defer testing until the individual is treated and more stable is appropriate. Changes in the mode and protocol for exercise and/or end points for stopping the test can contribute to the safety of the test in some cases. The ability to monitor changes in the ECG and blood pressure is critical, and the presence of a health care professional with extensive experience in exercise testing and a low threshold for stopping the test is crucial for testing.

Absolute and Relative Indications to Stop an Exercise Test

Indications to stop an exercise test are categorized as relative and absolute (26, 28, 29). Terminating a test depends on the expertise and judgment of those supervising it. As with contraindications, the setting and indications for the test may influence termination. Increasing angina, hypotension, signs and symptoms of myocardial ischemia, and serious arrhythmias are grave problems that may precipitate test termination. Other reasons, such as the technical inability to monitor the ECG and request by the patient, are self-evident.

Relative indications for termination of an exercise test are findings that increase the level of concern and vigilance in those administering the test. Relative indications for termination rely heavily on the judgment of the personnel supervising the test, and the decision to continue with the test should be made by an experienced health care professional, preferably with a physician in attendance or accessible during the test. In general, high-risk patients should be treated cautiously, with a tendency to stop the test soon rather than late. In contrast, for low-risk patients, interpretation of the relative indications may be more liberal.

Follow-Up After Terminating an Exercise Test

If an exercise test is terminated, the health care personnel supervising the test must carry out the appropriate course of action. Appropriate follow-up may include any or all of the following:

1. Notification of and attendance by a physician if one was not present during the exercise test
2. Careful observation of ECG, blood pressure, and other signs and symptoms until the condition subsides or stabilizes
3. Treatment (i.e., of arrhythmias or angina) when qualified medical personnel are in attendance
4. Phone contact with primary and/or referring physicians
5. Transport to an emergency department or physician's office
6. Access to the emergency medical system

Regardless of the course of action, documentation, including ECG tracings, blood pressure recordings, and all test results, should be provided to the physician.

COMPLICATIONS OF CARDIAC REHABILITATION

As previously discussed, habitual exercise decreases the risk of a cardiac event in those with CHD (8, 9). This important principle forms the basis for cardiac rehabilitation. Cardiac rehabilitation is an important aspect of postischemic care (patients who have unstable angina, have had MI, or have undergone coronary artery bypass grafting), because it not only restores lost functional capacity, but also improves life expectancy. Because all of these individuals have CHD, the risk of complications is higher than in the general population but is still generally low (30).

At one cardiac rehabilitation program, there were 5 episodes of exercise-induced ventricular fibrillation during 75,000 person-hours of supervised exercise (31). This would translate to one episode of ventricular fibrillation a year for a program with 100 participants that met three times a week for an hour. All of these individuals had un-

Table 58.3. Risk of Sudden Cardiac Arrest During Exercise Training

STUDY	STATUS	ACTIVITY	MONITORING	SUPERVISION	SUDDEN CARDIAC ARRESTS EVENTS PER HOUR
In the general population					
Vuori et al. (32)	normal	cross-country skiing	none	none	1/600,000
Gibbons et al. (33)	normal	jogging, swimming, tennis	none	none	1/375,000
Thompson et al. (34)	normal	jogging	none	none	1/396,000
Vander (35)	normal	court games, jogging	none	none	1/888,000
Average for general population					1/565,000
Individuals with known heart disease					
Fletcher and Cantwell (25)	cardiac	jogging	intermittent	present	1/6000
Leach et al. (36)	cardiac	jogging	intermittent		1/12,000
Mead et al. (37)	cardiac	jogging	intermittent	present	1/6000
Hartley (38)	cardiac	jogging	intermittent	present	1/6000
Hossack and Hartwig (39)	cardiac	jogging	none	present	1/65,185
Haskell (31)	cardiac	mixed	intermittent	present	1/22,028
Van Camp and Peterson (40)	cardiac	mixed	continuous	present	1/117,333
Hartley*	cardiac	bicycling, walking	intermittent	none	1/70,000
Fletcher*	cardiac	mixed	intermittent	present	0/70,200
Average all cardiac					1/59,142

*unpublished data
Reprinted with permission from Fletcher GF et al. Exercise Standards: A statement for healthcare professionals from the American Heart Association. Circulation 91(2):580-615, 1995.

derlying CHD; in healthy participants, ventricular fibrillation would be much less common.

Table 58.3 lists studies that have examined the risks of exercise in apparently healthy individuals and in participants in cardiac rehabilitation programs (28). Two of the larger studies rely on data collected from surveys of cardiac rehabilitation centers. One 1978 survey found 1 nonfatal cardiac event per 34,673 person-hours of cardiac rehabilitation activity and one death per 116,402 hours of activity (29). The risk has since decreased. In a recent survey, the rates of nonfatal and fatal cardiac complications were 1 event per 90,458 hours of activity and 1 event per 783,972 hours of activity, respectively—a further indication of the low risk of rehabilitation-induced complications (43). These events generally occurred when heart rate guidelines were exceeded, giving support to the importance of supervised, monitored exercise in high-risk patients.

NONCARDIOVASCULAR COMPLICATIONS OF EXERCISE
Heat Complications

Overheating is a leading cause of noncardiovascular deaths in young athletes (5). Heat injury is a function of environment, degree of exposure, intensity of exercise, prior conditioning, and pre-existing physical illness. Athletes are most prone to develop heat illness when they are not acclimated to hot weather, are wearing heavy clothing (such as full football gear), are dehydrated, have sickle cell trait, and/or are in a hot and humid climate (41).

Under these conditions complications range from mi-

nor to fatal. The illnesses that may be precipitated by exercise in warm climates are heat rash, heat cramps, heat syncope, heat exhaustion, and exertional heat stroke. Most of these problems are benign and self-limited, but heat exhaustion and exertional heat stroke may be fatal if not properly treated.

Heat exhaustion is characterized by intense thirst, gooseflesh, dizziness, fatigue, rapid pulse, muscle cramps, nausea, vomiting, syncope, and, in advanced stages, circulatory failure. Heavy sweating usually persists throughout the course of illness. Core temperature remains below 40°C (104°F) and there is no tissue injury. Heat exhaustion may progress to heat stroke.

Heat stroke is different from heat exhaustion in that core temperature rises above 41°C (105.8°F), resulting in significant tissue injury. The skin may feel cool and the athlete often shivers, making it important to measure core temperature for the diagnosis. Sweating may cease in heat stroke, in contrast to heat exhaustion. When this occurs, body temperature regulation is lost and a true medical emergency arises. There may be mental status changes; victims sometime progress to convulsions and/or coma. Rhabdomyolysis, acute renal failure, hemolysis, myocardial infarction, hyperkalemia, and hepatic necrosis can also develop, and, if untreated, death often follows (42).

To treat heat exhaustion and exertional heat stroke, the victim should be moved to a cooler environment and the body cooled with fans, ice, and wet cloths. Excessive clothing must be removed and the feet elevated. Intake of oral fluids should be encouraged. Heat stroke requires additional more intensive treatment (chilled intravenous saline and possibly hospitalization), but these actions may be performed until trained medical personnel are present.

Heat illness may be prevented by avoiding the extremes of weather or by gradual adaptation to activity in hot climates. It is recommended that athletes curtail activities when the wet bulb–globe temperature, an index of temperature, humidity, and radiation, is greater than 28°C (82°F) (43). In addition, maintaining adequate hydration is an important aspect of prevention.

Hydration-Related Complications

To maintain body temperature in a physiological range during exercise, sweating is necessary to promote heat loss. Water and electrolytes, mainly sodium and chloride, are lost in sweat. During prolonged exercise, this loss leads to dehydration (a loss of more water than sodium with a resulting rise in serum sodium), which impairs exercise performance. The amount lost is determined by the rate of sweating (which depends on the intensity of exertion), ambient temperature, humidity, amount of clothing, and acclimation level of the athlete, as well as individual variation. Depending on these factors, sweat rates can range from 0.5 to 3.7 L/hour. Children have lower sweat rates than adults.

Fluid ingestion during prolonged exercise is recommended to prevent significant dehydration (43). The ideal fluid is an isotonic carbohydrate–electrolyte solution that fulfills dual purposes of replacing sweat loss and providing carbohydrate fuel, such as glucose, to supplement tissue stores. Fluid replacement is generally not necessary for exercise lasting less than 30 minutes, but it becomes more important with prolonged activity (44).

The exact amount of fluid that should be ingested during exercise is not established. The American College of Sports Medicine "Position Paper on the Prevention of Thermal Injuries During Distance Running" (43) recommends that participants in foot races be encouraged to drink 100–200 mL of water every 2–3 km of the race. This is only a guideline; it may be too much or too little, depending on the environment and the pace and sweat rate of the athlete. Overconsumption of water can lead to hyponatremia (low serum sodium), a rare condition that may cause medical problems (45). Thus, correct fluid intake, neither too much nor too little, is key to optimal performance and avoidance of medical complications. Guidelines to help achieve this balance are presented in Table 58.4.

COMPLICATIONS IN SPECIAL POPULATIONS

Exercise considerations in special populations, such as those with chronic disease and pulmonary complications (asthma, exercise-induced bronchospasm), are addressed elsewhere in this book. Complications in special populations, diabetes for example (see Chapter 31), are specific to the population and the disease state. First aid for these and other common complications is listed in Table 58.5.

Besides knowledge of first aid, it is imperative that all persons working in exercise testing and rehabilitation be trained in cardiopulmonary resuscitation. Certification may be obtained through the American Heart Association or the American Red Cross. Classes are available in most cities.

Some members of these special populations require medical evaluation before beginning a physical activity program. All persons at high risk for complications during exercise should be screened before making significant changes in activity level. The *ACSM Guidelines* gives further criteria for risk stratification and pretest evaluation (27).

Table 58.4. Suggested Guidelines for Fluid Replacement During Prolonged Exercise

1. Immediately prior to exercise or during warm-up, ingest up to 300 mL of cool (about 10°C) flavored water.
2. For the initial 60–75 min of exercise, ingest 100–150 mL of a cool, dilute (5 g/100 mL) glucose polymer solution at regular (10–15 minute) intervals. It seems unwarranted to consume CHO in amounts much greater than 30 g during this period, since only 20 g of ingested CHO are oxidized in the first hour of moderate-intensity exercise, irrespective of the type of CHO consumed or the drinking regimen.
3. After 75–90 min of exercise, increase concentration of ingested glucose polymer solution to 10–12 g/100 mL plus 20 mEq/L sodium. Higher sodium concentrations, although possibly may promote rapid intestinal fluid absorption, are not palatable to most athletes. Small amounts of potassium (2–4 mEq/L), which may facilitate rehydration of the intracellular fluid compartment, may be included. For the remainder of the exercise, consume 100–150 mL of this solution at 10–15-min intervals. Such a regimen ensures optimal rates of fluid and energy delivery, limiting any dehydration-induced decreases in plasma volume and maintaining the rate on ingested CHO oxidation at about 1 g/min late in exercise.

CHO, carbohydrate.
Reprinted with permission from Nokes TD et al. Fluid and energy replacement during prolonged exercise. Curr Ther Sport Med 517–520, 1995.

► SUMMARY

Despite the many potential complications of exercise, the risk for most individuals is low. Those who are at increased risk for complications should be carefully screened and appropriately treated. For the remainder of the population, the benefits that may be gained from increased activity, such as improved cardiovascular, respiratory, and musculoskeletal fitness; weight loss; reduced blood pressure; and increased sense of well-being, far outweigh the risks.

Table 58.5. Possible Medical Emergencies and Suggested First Aid

PROBLEM	FIRST AID PROCEDURE
Heat cramps	Replace fluids, sodium, and potassium lost through excessive sweating.
Heat exhaustion and heat stroke	Move victim to shade; have victim lie down with feet elevated above the level of the heart.
	Remove excess clothing.
	Cool victim with sips of cool fluid; sprinkle water on face and body; rub ice pack over major vessels in armpits, groin, and neck.
	Victim should seek immediate medical attention and be given intravenous fluids as soon as possible.
Fainting (syncope)	Leave the victim lying down. Turn on the side if vomiting occurs.
	Maintain an open airway.
	Loosen any tight clothing.
	Take blood pressure and pulse if possible.
	Seek medical attention; syncope may be life threatening, and the cause must be determined.
Hypoglycemia (symptoms include diaphoresis, pallor, tremor, tachycardia, palpitations, visual disturbances, mental confusion, weakness, light-headedness, fatigue, headache, memory loss, seizure, coma)	May become life threatening. Seek medical attention to treat cause.
	Give oral glucose solution such as Kool-Aid with sugar, nondiet soft drinks, juice, milk.
	If patient is able to ingest solids, gelatin sweetened with sugar, mild chocolate, or fruit may be given.
Hyperglycemia (symptoms include dehydration, hypotension, and reflex tachycardia, osmotic diuresis, impaired consciousness, nausea, vomiting, abdominal pain, hyperventilation, odor of acetone on breath)	May be life threatening if it leads to diabetic ketoacidosis.
	Seek immediate medical attention.
	Rehydrate with intravenous normal saline.
	Correct electrolyte loss (K^+).
	Victim should receive insulin.
Sprains, strains	No weight bearing on affected extremity.
	Loosen shoes; apply a pillow or blanket splint around extremity.
	Elevate the extremity.
	Apply bag of crushed ice to the affected area.
	Seek medical attention if pain or swelling persists.
Simple or compound fracture	Immobilize the extremity.
	Splint the extremity to prevent further injury to the bone or soft tissue.
	Use anything at hand as a splint.
	Do not attempt to reduce any dislocation in the field unless there is danger of losing life or limb.
	Seek immediate medical attention.
	Protect the victim from further injury.
Bronchospasm	Maintain open airway.
	Give bronchodilator via nebulizer if prescribed for patient.
	Give oxygen by nasal cannula if available.
Hypotension, shock	Lay the victim down with feet elevated.
	Maintain open airway.
	Monitor vital signs (pulse, blood pressure).
	Call for immediate advanced life support measures; this is a life-threatening emergency that requires intensive monitoring of vital signs, administration of intravenous fluids and drugs to maintain adequate tissue perfusion during diagnosis (e.g., hypovolemia, cardiogenesis, sepsis).
Bleeding	Apply direct pressure over the site to stop the bleeding.
Lacerations	Protect the wound from contamination and infection.
Incisions	Possibly seek medical attention; victim may need stitches, tetanus toxoid.
Puncture wounds	If bleeding is severe, in addition to direct pressure, elevate the injured part of the body, and if an artery is
Abrasions	severed, apply direct pressure over the main artery to the affected limb and seek immediate medical
Contusions	attention.

Reprinted with permission from Strauss WE et al. Emergency plans and procedures for an exercise facility. ACSM Resource Manual for Guidelines for Exercise Testing and Prescription. 2nd ed. Philadelphia: Lea & Febiger, 1993:373.

References

1. Levine BD, Stray Gundersen J. The medical care of competitive athletes: The role of the individual and the individual assumption of risk. Med Sci Sports Exerc 26:1190–1192, 1994.
2. Kraus JF, Conroy C. Mortality and morbidity from injuries in sports and recreation. Ann Rev Pub Health 5:163–192, 1984.
3. Koplan JP, Siscovick DS, Goldbaum GM. The risks of exercise: A public health view of injuries and hazards. Pub Health Rep 100:189–195, 1985.
4. Albert CM, Mittleman MA, Chae CU, Lee IM, Hennekens CH, Manson JE. Triggering of sudden death from cardiac causes by vigorous exertion. N Engl J Med 343:1355–1361, 2000.

5. Van Camp SP, Bloor CM, Mueller FU, et al. Nontraumatic sports deaths in high school and college athletes. Med Sci Sports Exerc 27:641–647, 1995.

6. Maron BJ, Shirani J, Poliac LC, et al. Sudden death in young competitive athletes. JAMA 276:199–204, 1996.

7. Opie LH. Sudden death and sport. Lancet 1:263–266, 1975.

8. Mittleman MA, MaClure M, Tofler GH, et al. Triggering of acute myocardial infarction by heavy physical exertion. N Engl J Med 329:1677–1683, 1993.

9. Willich SN, Lewis M, Lowel H, et al. Physical exertion as a trigger of acute myocardial infarction. N Engl J Med 329:1684–1690, 1993.

10. Thompson PD, Klocke FJ, Levine BD, et al. 26th Bethesda Conference. Recommendations for determining eligibility for competition in athletes with cardiovascular abnormalities. Task Force 5: Coronary artery disease. J Am Coll Cardiol 4:845–899, 1994.

11. Maron BJ, Mitchell JH. 26th Bethesda Conference. Recommendations for determining eligibility for competition in athletes with cardiovascular abnormalities. Revised recommendations for competitive athletes with cardiovascular abnormalities. J Am Coll Cardiol 24:845–899, 1994.

12. Noakes TD. Heart disease in marathon runners: A review. Med Sci Sports Exerc 19:187–194, 1987.

13. Siscovick DS, Weiss NS, Fletcher RH, et al. The incidence of primary cardiac arrest during vigorous exercise. N Engl J Med 311:874–877, 1984.

14. Blair SN, Kampert JB, Kuhl HW, et al. Influences of cardiorespiratory fitness and other precursors on cardiovascular disease and all-cause mortality in men and women. JAMA 276:205–210, 1996.

15. Wigle ED, Rakowski H, Kimball BP, et al. Hypertrophic cardiomyopathy, clinical spectrum and treatment. Circulation 92:1680–1692, 1995.

16. Barth CW, Roberts WC. Left main coronary artery originating from the right sinus of Valsalva and coursing between the aorta and pulmonary trunk. J Am Coll Cardiol 7:366–373, 1986.

17. Morales AR, Romanelli R, Bovcek RJ. The mural left anterior descending coronary artery, strenuous exercise and sudden death. Circulation 62:230–237, 1980.

18. Roberts WC, Glick BN. Congenital hypoplasia of both right and left circumflex coronary arteries. Am J Cardiol 70:121–123, 1992.

19. Roberts WC, Silver MA, Sapala JC. Intussusception of a coronary artery associated with sudden death in a college football player. Am J Cardiol 57:179–180, 1986.

20. Tahernia AC. Cardiovascular anomalies in Marfan's syndrome: The role of echocardiography and beta-blockers. South Med J 86:305–310, 1993.

21. Maron BJ, Bodison SA, Wesley YE, et al. Results of screening a large group of intercollegiate competitive athletes for cardiovascular disease. J Am Coll Cardiol 10:1214–1221, 1987.

22. Atterhog JH, Bjorn J, Samuelsson R. Exercise testing: A prospective study of complication rates. Am Heart J 98:572–579, 1979.

23. Wendt TH, Scherer D, Kaltenbach M. Life-threatening complications in 1,741,106 ergometries. Dtsch Med Wochenschr 109:123–127, 1984.

24. Gibbons L, Blair SN, Kohl HW, et al. The safety of maximal exercise testing. Circulation 80:846–852, 1989.

25. Fletcher GF, Cantwell JD. Ventricular fibrillation in a medically supervised cardiac exercise program. JAMA 238:2627–2629, 1977.

26. Young DZ, Lampert S, Graboys TB, et al. Safety of maximal exercise testing in patients at high risk for ventricular arrhythmias. Circulation 70:184–191, 1984.

27. American College of Sports Medicine. ACSM's Guidelines for Exercise Testing and Prescription. 6th ed. Philadelphia: Lippincott Williams & Wilkins, 2000.

28. Dubach P, Froelicher VF, Klein J, et al. Exercise-induced hypotension in a male population. Circulation 78: 1380–1387, 1988.

29. Fletcher GF, Balady G, Froelicher VF, et al. Exercise standards: A statement for healthcare professionals from the American Heart Association. Circulation 91:580–615, 1995.

30. Haskell WL. The efficacy and safety of exercise programs in cardiac rehabilitation. Med Sci Sports Exerc 26:815–823, 1994.

31. Haskell WL. Cardiovascular complications during exercise training of cardiac patients. Circulation 57:920–924, 1978.

32. Vuori I, Jaaskelainen A. Sudden death and physical activity. Cardiology. 63:287–304, 1978.

33. Gibbons LW, Cooper KH, Meyer BM, Ellison RC. The acute cardiac risk of strenuous exercise. JAMA 244:1799–1801, 1980.

34. Thompson PD, Funk EJ, Carleton RA, Sturner WO. Incidence of death during jogging in Rhode Island from 1975 through 1980. JAMA 247:2535–2538, 1982.

35. Vander L. Cardiovascular complications of recreational physical activity. Physic Sports Med. 10:89–98, 1982.

36. Leach CN Jr, Sands MJ Jr, Lachman AS, Skinner W. Cardiac arrest during exercise training after myocardial infarction. Conn Med. 46:239–243, 1982.

37. Mead WF, Pyfer HR, Thrombold JC, Frederick RC. Successful resuscitation of two near simultaneous cases of cardiac arrest with a review of fifteen cases occuring during supervised exercise. Circulation 53:187–189, 1976.

38. Hartley LH. Exercise and cardiac rehabilitation. Proc N Engl Cardiovasc Soc. 28:37–40, 1976.

39. Hossack KF, Hartwig R. Cardiac arrest associated with supervised cardiac rehabilitation. J Cardiac Rehabil 2:402–408, 1982.

40. VanCamp SP, Peterson RA. Cardiovascular complications of outpatient cardiac rehabilitation programs. JAMA 256:1160–1163, 1986.

41. Kark JA, Posey DM, Schumacher HR, et al. Sickle-cell trait as a risk factor for sudden death in physical training. N Engl J Med 317:781–787, 1987.

42. Knochel JP. Pathophysiology of heat stroke. In: Hopkins, Ellis, eds. Hyperthermia and Hypermetabolic Disorders. Cambridge, UK: Cambridge University Press, 1996:42–62.

43. American College of Sports Medicine. Position statement on the prevention of thermal injuries during distance running. Med Sci Sports Exerc 19:529–533, 1987.

44. Noakes TD. Dehydration during exercise, what are the real dangers. J Clin Sport Med 5:123–128, 1995.

45. Frizell RT, Lang GH, Lowance DC, et al. Hyponatremia and ultramarathon running. JAMA 255:772–774, 1986.

SECTION ELEVEN
HUMAN DEVELOPMENT

SECTION EDITOR: Matt Herridge, PhD

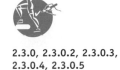

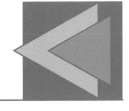

CHAPTER **59**

HUMAN DEVELOPMENT AND AGING

Mark A. Williams

Changes in human physiology over a life span are often categorized into periods based on calendar age to assist physicians, exercise professionals, and other health and fitness practitioners in the evaluation of growth, changes in physiological function with aging, and interventions that may affect function. Although these distinctions can provide guidance, variations in growth and development, environment, aging, and disease often lead to wide discrepancies between calendar and biological age (1).

THE IMPACT OF AGING

The aging categories in Table 59.1 facilitate the following review of physiological changes associated with aging. This chapter provides an overview of the effect of aging on selected physiological parameters important to exercise testing and prescription.

The Heart

The major limitation in attempting to describe structural changes in the heart associated with aging is that most investigations have included individuals with cardiovascular disease. Thus, it is possible that changes associated with aging may be related in part to cardiovascular disease. Nevertheless, in studies of normal men and women, aging-related increased left ventricular hypertrophy has been demonstrated between the second and seventh decades (2, 3). With aging, elasticity of major blood vessels, including those within the peripheral vasculature, declines. These age-related changes in the blood vessels may limit cardiac performance. Substantial evidence suggests that resistance to ventricular emptying increases with age. Increased afterload (the pressure that must be overcome by the left ventricle to allow for ejection of blood into the periphery) resulting from increased peripheral resistance appears to be the primary mechanism for ventricular hypertrophy (4). However, the degree of left ventricular hypertrophy seen with advancing age is mild compared with that of disease (3). Hemodynamic changes in the heart due to age-related increased aortic

stiffness also require greater left ventricular stroke volume, resulting in increased wall tension and myocardial oxygen consumption during systole. This often leads to increased blood pressure at rest and during exercise. In addition, pulse wave velocity is consistently found to increase with age, indicating decreased arterial compliance (5).

Several studies over the past 25 years show that resting cardiac output and stroke volume decrease with age. Results suggest that cardiac output decreases about 1% per year, from a mean of 6.5 L per minute in the third decade to a mean of 3.9 L per minute in the ninth decade (6). From 25 to 85 years, resting stroke volume decreases 30%, from 85 mL to 60 mL (6, 7). However, in subjects who have been carefully screened for coronary artery disease, investigators have demonstrated that overall left ventricular function, using resting ejection fraction as an index, does not decline between 25 and 80 years (8). Estimates of volume made by echocardiography and gaited radionuclide scintigraphy demonstrate that resting stroke volume also does not decline with age. Since resting heart rate is also not age related, these data suggest that resting cardiac output does not decline with age in healthy individuals. Other work assessing intrinsic cardiac muscle function also indicates that resting myocardial performance is not affected by aging (2). In general, variability in activity level, training status, and methods of screening for any underlying disease have led to confounding results regarding the effect of chronological aging (9).

Although cardiac output increases with growth in children, at any given level of work, cardiac output is somewhat lower in children than in adults primarily because of lower stroke volume (10, 11). It is not clear whether these findings are the result of smaller heart size, limitations in cardiac function, or both. Lower sympathetic stimulation in children than in adults has been suggested as a cause of lower stroke volume. However, during modest submaximal exercise, increases in stroke volume do not seem to be related to aging, although in boys, stroke volume is higher and heart rate lower than in girls at given absolute sub-

Table 59.1. Stages of Aging

Neonatal	Birth to 3 weeks
Infancy	3 weeks to 1 year
Childhood	
Early	1–6 years
Middle	7–10 years
Later	Prepubertal
	Girls 9–15 years
	Boys 12–16 years
Adolescence	6 years following puberty
Adulthood	
Early	20–29 years
Middle	30–44 years
Later	45–64 years
Senescence	
Elderly	65–74 years
Older elderly	75–84 years
Very old	85 years and above

maximal work rates (12). With aging, however, smaller increases in stroke volume and ejection fraction and greater left ventricular end-diastolic pressure are observed with increasing workloads. This phenomenon is a result of greater reliance on the Frank-Starling mechanism to compensate for a reduced number of pacemaker cells and impaired beta-adrenergic chronotropic function (7, 13). Maximal cardiac output in a 65-year-old person is 10–30% less than in a young adult (9, 14, 15). Decreases in both maximal heart rate and maximal stroke volume contribute to decreased maximal cardiac output. By contrast, in the period immediately after high-intensity exercise, heart rate recovery, return of oxygen uptake to baseline, and muscle power recovery occur faster in children than in young adults and adults (16–18).

Early left ventricular diastolic function is significantly lower with increased age than is systolic function (2, 19, 20). This impairment of left ventricular filling may be related to age-related left ventricular hypertrophy that diminishes ventricular diastolic compliance.

Heart Rate

In children, heart rate is often high at rest (80–100 beats per minute, or bpm), apparently as a result of reduced stroke volume relative to body size (1). This reduced stroke volume generally disappears with growth and increased levels of physical activity. In combination with an increase in the capacity of blood to carry oxygen (hemoglobin increases through the late teens), resting heart rate decreases to approximately 65–75 bpm.

A decline in maximal exercise heart rate with aging has been suggested (predicted maximum heart rate = 220 − age [±10 beats]), although there is considerable variation. A decrease in myocardial sensitivity to catecholamines and the effect of prolonged diastolic filling

with aging appear to be responsible for this decline in heart rate. Decreased maximal heart rate with aging results in a 30–50% reduction in maximal exercise cardiac output from 25 to 85 years (21). Children, endurance-trained athletes, and active older adults are among those who frequently evidence variations from predicted maximum heart rate response. Maximum heart rates of 210–215 bpm have been observed in children, even though motivating children for a sustained effort to determine maximal heart rate is difficult. In endurance athletes, values 5–10 bpm lower than predicted have been observed (22). Finally, many healthy older persons who maintain a lifelong commitment to physical activity can achieve heart rates higher than those predicted (23).

Maximal Oxygen Uptake

Aerobic capacity, assessed by maximal oxygen uptake ($\dot{V}O_{2max}$) appears to remain constant through childhood. There is, however, controversy concerning an apparent loss of $\dot{V}O_{2max}$ beginning about age 12, perhaps related to decreased levels of physical activity (24). At adulthood, a steady age-related decline in $\dot{V}O_{2max}$, averaging about 1% per year between 25 and 75 years (about 5 mL O_2/kg/minute with each decade of aging), has been observed (25, 26). However, the degree to which this decline occurs is significantly affected by amount and intensity of physical activity. The decline parallels reduced maximal work capacity and is attributed to decreased maximal cardiac output and reduced maximal arterial–venous oxygen difference (a-vDO$_2$), as well as a loss of skeletal muscle mass (27, 28). Microstructural changes, including myofilament disorganization and changes in mitochondrial structure and distribution resulting in reduced oxidative capacity, may explain a reduced maximal a-vDO$_2$ (29). Additionally, physical limitations resulting from a sedentary lifestyle, loss of coordination, lack of familiarity with required skills, and disabling diseases such as arthritis and obesity may also play a role in limiting $\dot{V}O_{2max}$ (30, 31). Conversely, individuals who are habitually active throughout life do not seem to demonstrate the level of reduction of $\dot{V}O_{2max}$ observed in sedentary individuals.

Pulmonary System

Lung compliance increases with age, while the ability to expand the chest cavity becomes limited (32). This is particularly evident by age 65. There is progressive decrease in both maximal expiratory flow and lung volume reserve with aging. Residual volume increases by 30–50% and vital capacity decreases by 40–50% by age 70 (33). With exertion, increased ventilation depends more on frequency than depth. The overall net effect is a 20% increase in the work of respiratory muscles (34). Despite these changes, respiratory function does not limit exercise capacity or the ability to benefit from exercise training unless lung function is severely impaired. However, because of the increase in work of respiratory muscles, the elderly may complain of breathing discomfort during exertion and increased ventilatory demand, even in those with normal cardiopulmonary function (35).

Skeletal Muscle and Strength

The relative proportion of fast- and slow-twitch fibers is largely determined at birth (1). The total number of muscle fibers is fixed at an early age, although considerable enlargement of muscle remains possible by fiber splitting and hypertrophy of existing fibers. Both boys and girls are capable of increasing the ability to generate muscular force, although children exhibit disproportionately less ability to generate upper body muscular force than adults. At adolescence, boys exhibit rapid hypertrophy of muscle that is disproportionately greater than observed in girls at puberty. Thus, although ability to generate muscular force in active boys is similar to that of girls, men are approximately 40% stronger than women. Both genders reach maximum levels of strength in the early 20s, followed by a plateau maintained into the mid-40s. Subsequently, accelerated loss of lean tissue is associated with decrements in static and dynamic force generation as well as contractile speed. Thus, by 65 years, most people have changes in the musculoskeletal system, in terms of both skeletal muscle mass and decreased levels of physical activity (30, 36).

Muscle function decreases approximately 25% by age 65 and by as much as 40% over a life span (37–39). Loss of muscle function appears to be due to decreased total fibers, decreased muscle fiber size, impaired excitation–contraction coupling mechanism, and decreased high-threshold motor units. There may also be selective loss or atrophy (particularly after 70 years) of fast-twitch (type II) fibers, although this is controversial and the cause unclear (40). At all ages, females appear to be more vulnerable to loss of lean tissue than males. As a result, the elderly must use a high proportion of available muscle mass for exercise, which may result in overuse and strain, expressed as decreased strength and early onset of fatigue.

It remains uncertain how much age-related loss of muscle function is an inevitable consequence of aging and how much it reflects decline in physical activity (40). Some data suggest that lean tissue mass can be sustained well into the seventh decade with an active lifestyle; others note than lean tissue can be maintained and function restored even into the ninth (41, 42). Evidence also suggests significant improvement in strength and to a lesser degree in muscle mass as the elderly participate in programs for strength improvement (42–44). Nonetheless, muscle function decline is the direct result of progressive decrease in the number of muscle fibers and cross-sectional area and decline in neuromuscular function resulting from disuse or loss of motoneurons (40, 45).

Anaerobic power develops in parallel with changes in muscle mass through childhood into young adulthood, deteriorating in middle age corresponding to loss of muscle mass (1). Decreases of 45–60% from 25 to 65 years are observed in both genders, although such losses may be from physical inactivity, decreased neuromuscular coordination, decreased efficiency of movement, and decreased motivation.

Anaerobic capacity as described by peak blood lactate levels also develops through young adulthood. Blood lactate concentrations during submaximal exercise at standardized work intensities are typically lower in children than adults owing to a number of factors related to muscle metabolism (46). After exhaustive exercise, lactate concentrations in blood and muscle are greater in adults than in children, the latter having reduced levels of glycolytic enzymes and a smaller ratio of muscle mass to blood volume (47). Decreased motivation and neuromuscular coordination probably also contribute to reduced anaerobic capacity in children. Both sexes maintain a plateau of anaerobic capacity through about age 35, at which time there is increased loss of function. By age 65, anaerobic capacity declines to essentially the level of childhood even when subjects are highly motivated for testing.

Bone

The exact timing of peak bone mass attainment is unclear. Although genetic predisposition appears to be the principle determinant of bone mass in adults, several other factors, including physical activity, body composition, hormonal status, nutritional status, and any chronic disease play roles in this process, particularly with aging (48). Bone growth during childhood presents two primary problems because the epiphysis is not united with the bone shaft. First, overuse can result in epiphysitis during this growth period. Second, fracture may pass through the epiphyseal plate, sometimes leading to disruption of normal growth (1). Beginning at age 30 in women and age 40 in men, calcium content progressively decreases, leading to progressive bone loss with aging, although less rapidly in men. In women, loss occurs at a rate of approximately 1% per year after age 35 and is particularly rapid during the 5 years after menopause. In addition, low levels of estrogen with amenorrhea such as are observed in women athletes is also associated with bone loss (49). Men lose 10–15% by age 70 and 20% by age 80 (50, 51). In women the loss amounts to about 20% by age 65 and 30% by age 80. In both genders, by age 65 bone loss has generally progressed to the point of predisposition to fractures. Bone fracture is a significant cause of morbidity and mortality in the elderly. Decreasing dietary calcium intake, diabetes mellitus, renal impairment, and physical inactivity may accelerate bone loss. It appears that adequate mineral intake and progressive weight-bearing activity can stabilize calcium loss in various age groups (52–54). In addition, hormone replacement therapy in women appears effective in limiting bone mass loss.

Degeneration or damage to articular cartilage results in a significant increase in incidence of osteoarthritis with aging (1). By age 60, as much as 80% of the population shows such evidence, although only about 15% have symptoms. The contributions of overuse or trauma to this problem remain unclear.

Joints and Flexibility

A progressive loss of flexibility, resulting from a number of factors including disuse, deterioration of joint structures, and progressive degeneration of collagen fibers, begins during young adulthood (1). Increased incidence of knee and back problems from osteoarthritis has been observed beginning with middle age and progressing through old age. Degeneration of joints, especially the spine, is often found in elderly persons (31). Weight-bearing activity may accelerate this onset. Healthy lifestyle, including appropriate nutrition and body composition coupled with exercise training to promote strength, may decelerate it (30, 31). Along with loss of strength, loss of flexibility plays a significant role in increased risk of falls and other injuries. The rate of deterioration accelerates beyond age 65, but few specific findings are available for this age group.

Aging is also associated with changes in connective tissue (55). Connective tissue, including fascia, ligaments, and tendons, becomes less extensible. Range of motion, both active and passive, declines with age. It is not clear whether this decreased flexibility is a consequence of biological aging, degenerative disease, inactivity, or some combination of these factors.

Body Composition and Metabolism

In young children, the proportion of body fat ranges from 10–15%, with girls carrying slightly more body fat than boys of similar age (1). In addition, the ratio of body surface area to mass is greater in children than adults (10). In adolescence and into young adulthood, body fat percentage generally increases to 15–20% in males and 20–25% in females. In the moderately obese person, body fat that accumulates beyond normal is generally a result of imbalance of calorie intake and energy expenditure, the latter often decreasing with aging. Contributing to the decline of energy expenditure are several metabolic changes. The basal metabolic rate gradually decreases with aging as lean body mass decreases, while relative body fat increases (29, 56). In addition, glucose tolerance diminishes with age and is accompanied by increasing likelihood of developing non–insulin dependent diabetes mellitus (36). Thus, by middle age, body fat percentage may continue to increase beyond 20–25% in men

and 25–30% in women. These values may continue to increase with age.

Renal Function, Fluid Regulation, and Thermoregulation

Renal function declines approximately 30–50% between ages 30 and 70 years (1). Along with this decline, acid-base control, glucose tolerance, and drug clearance decrease. A general reduction in total cellular water occurs with aging, with a decline of 10–50% in total body water.

The primary maturational characteristics related to exercise in heat occur in late puberty or early adulthood. Prior to that time, children have a consistently lower sweat rate characterized by lower absolute and relative amounts along with increased core temperature required to start sweating. Composition of sweat, particularly increased chloride in children, also differs (57, 58). Additionally, children tend to rely more on radiation and convection for heat dissipation than adults (10). Aging is also associated with attenuated skin and blood flow, which may contribute to a reduced ability to thermoregulate (59). Furthermore, the effects of aging predispose older individuals to rapid dehydration that may become particularly important during exercise through evaporative water loss and perspiration (60). In addition, many older adults take a variety of medications that may further confound limitations of thermoregulation.

Children have a greater ratio of surface area to mass than adults, which enhances convective and radiative heat transfer between skin and the environment, making adaptation to cold more difficult (61). However, it has been suggested that other factors that mature with aging, such as thermogenic and vasoconstrictive responses, may also limit thermoregulation to cold in children. Beyond childhood, it has been demonstrated that core temperature regulation is detrimentally affected by aging (62–64).

Nervous System

Infants and very young children undergo intensive learning to develop motor skills for function and performance. It has been recognized that the central nervous system is the predominant center for determining the outcomes of this learning. The process includes the integration of movement patterns that minimize physiological cost, asymmetry, and variability of body segment coordination (65). The improvement in economy of movement may actually decrease oxygen consumption at given absolute workloads (66). Changes in the central and peripheral nervous systems over time include slowed conduction velocities and reaction times, which drop 15% by age 70 (67). Both incidence of sensory deficits, particularly hearing and vision, and threshold of perception for many stimuli increase. Changes such as these may be related to a 35–40% increase in falls by persons over age 60 (14, 29).

Immune System Function

Aging significantly impairs immune system function (68–69). From peak immune system activity around puberty, an overall decline of 5–30% over a normal life span is expected, with some functional indices dropping to 5–10% of young adult function. However, it remains unclear how much the age-related impairment is a function of aging, environmental factors, or more likely both (70). The end result is reduced resistance to pathogens and increased incidence of both tumors and autoimmune disorders.

Exercise Prescription and Exercise Training Response

The interplay of frequency, intensity, and duration of exercise training is responsible for the effectiveness of exercise training, but it is apparent that the age of the subject also affects the relationship of these variables (1). Young children have difficulty sustaining duration of effort, so frequency and intensity of training should be emphasized. There is no clear evidence that prepubescent children do not respond to aerobic training, nor is there any apparent physiological basis for suggesting that children are less suitable than adults to prolonged bouts of exercise, apart from some possible limitations described in Table 59.2 (71). The limitations related to sustained activity are probably related to preference for short-term intermittent activity, which are more fun than those that tend to be prolonged and monotonous.

As one ages, higher intensities of effort are required to maintain or increase conditioning level. Such increasing intensity is not realistic for most of the population, primarily because of decreased motivation and increased risk of injury associated with high-intensity exercise in an aging, often sedentary population, especially in those with a history of injury. Additional factors that may also affect the ability to maintain or increase one's conditioning level include increased body mass index, perceived time limitations to exercise, and degree of various negative psychosocial behavior traits, such as "type A" behavior, anxiety, and depression (72). Thus, increased duration and frequency of exercise training take precedence, emphasizing caloric expenditure, particularly when

Table 59.2. Potential Limitations to Prolonged Exercise in Children

Mechanical inefficiencies in movement
General limitations in the cardiovascular response to exercise
Low capacity to sweat
General limitations in ability to acclimate
Limitations on exercising in climatic extremes:
    Heat intolerance as a result of high metabolic rate leading to excessive body heat
    Intolerance to cold

health as opposed to fitness is the primary consideration (73, 74).

► SUMMARY

Human growth and development have a clear effect upon the ability to take exercise. An understanding of expected changes in physiology as a result of these processes allows evaluation of both normal and abnormal responses to physical activity throughout life. The changes associated with aging may be a direct result of aging itself or may be a consequence of other aspects that are superimposed on the aging process. With aging, there is often a decline in habitual physical activity, poor nutrition, cumulative effects of long-term smoking, and increased chronic disease and depression, all of which adversely affect quantity and quality of life (68, 75). The contribution of appropriate health practices to offsetting the rapidity and degree of aging remains unclear.

References

1. Shephard RJ. Physiologic changes over the years. In: ACSM's Resource Manual for Guidelines for Exercise Testing and Prescription. 2nd ed. Philadelphia: Lea & Febiger, 1993.
2. Gerstenblith G, Frederiksen J, Yin FCP. Echocardiography assessment of a normal adult aging population. Circulation 56:273–278, 1977.
3. Sjogren AL. Left ventricular wall thickness in patients with circulatory overload of the left ventricle. Clin Res 4:310–318, 1972.
4. Fleg JL, Gerstenblith G, Lakatta EG. Pathophysiology of the aging heart and circulation. In: Messeril FH, ed. Cardiovascular Disease in the Elderly. Boston: Martinus Nijhoff, 1988.
5. Avolio AP, Deng FQ, Li WQ, et al. Effects of aging on arterial distensibility in populations with high and low prevalence of hypertension, comparison between urban and rural communities. Circulation 71:202–210, 1985.
6. Schulman SP, Lakatta EG, Fleg JL, et al. Age related decline in left ventricular filling at rest and exercise. Am J Physiol 263:H1932–H1938, 1992.
7. Lakatta EG. Cardiovascular regulatory mechanisms in advanced age. Physiol Rev 73:413–467, 1993.
8. Rodeheffer RJ, Gerstenblith G, Becker LC, et al. Exercise cardiac output is maintained with advancing age in healthy human subjects: Cardiac dilatation and increased stroke volume compensate for a diminished heart rate. Circulation 69:203–213, 1984.
9. Minson CT, Kenney WL. Age and cardiac output during cycle exercise in thermoneutral and warm environments. Med Sci Sports Exerc 29:75–81, 1997.
10. Falk B, Bar-Or O, MacDougall JD. Thermoregulatory responses of pre-, mid-, and late-pubertal boys to exercise in dry heat. Med Sci Sport Exerc 24:688–694, 1992.
11. Rowland T, Popowski B Ferrone L. Cardiac responses to maximal upright exercise in healthy boys and men. Med Sci Sports Exerc 29:1146–1151, 1997.
12. Turley KR, Wilmore JH. Cardiovascular responses to sub-

maximal exercise in 7- to 9-yr-old boys and girls. Med Sci Sports Exerc 29:824–832, 1997.

13. Tate CA, Hyek MF, Taffett GE. Mechanisms for the responses of cardiac muscle to physical activity. Med Sci Sports Exerc 26:561–567, 1994.

14. Ogawa T, Spina RJ, Martin WH, et al. Effects of aging, sex, and physical training on cardiovascular response to exercise. Circulation 86:494–503, 1992.

15. Fleg JL, Schulman SP, O'Connor FC. Cardiovascular responses to exhausting upright cycle exercise in healthy highly trained older men. J Appl Physiol 77:1500–1506, 1994.

16. Hebestreet H, Mimura KI, Bar-Or O. Recovery of muscle power after high-intensity short-term exercise: Comparing boys and men. J Appl Physiol 74:2875–2880, 1993.

17. Baraldi E, Cooper DM, Zanconato S, et al. Heart rate recovery from 1 minute of exercise in children and adults. Pediatr Res 29:575–579, 1991.

18. Zamconato S, Cooper DM, Armon Y. Oxygen cost and oxygen uptake dynamics and recovery with 1 minutes of exercise in children and adults. J Appl Physiol 71:993–998, 1991.

19. Gardin JM, Henry WL, Savage DD, et al. Echocardiographic measurements in normal subjects: Evaluation of an adult population without clinically apparent heart disease. J Clin Ultrasound 7:349–447, 1979.

20. Gledhill N, Cox D, Jamnik V. Endurance athletes' stroke volume does not plateau: Major advantage in diastolic function. Med Sci Sports Exerc 26:1116–1121, 1994.

21. Wiebe CG, Gledhill N, Jamnik VK, Ferguson S. Exercise cardiac function in young through elderly endurance trained women. Med Sci Sports Exerc 31:684–691, 1999.

22. Dal Monte A, Faina M, Menchinelli C. Sport-specific equipment. In: Shephard RJ, Astrand PO, eds. Sports and Human Endurance. Oxford: Blackwell Scientific, 1992.

23. Sidney KH, Shephard RJ. Maximum and submaximum exercise tests in men and women in seventh, eighth, and ninth decades of life. J Appl Physiol 43:280–287, 1977.

24. Shephard RJ. Maximal oxygen intake. In: Shephard RJ, Astrand PO, eds. Sports and Human Endurance. Oxford: Blackwell Scientific, 1992.

25. Jackson AS, Wier LT, Ayers GW, et al. Changes in aerobic power of women ages 20, 64 yr. Med Sci Sports Exerc 28:884–891, 1996.

26. Shvartz E, Reibold RC. Aerobic fitness norms for males and females aged 6, 75 years: A review. Aviat Space Environ Med 61:3–11, 1990.

27. Granath A, Jonsson B, Strandell T. Circulation in healthy old men studied by right heart catheterization at rest and during exercise in a supine and sitting position. Acta Med Scand 176:425–446, 1964.

28. Julius S, Amery A, Whitlock LS, et al. Influence of age on a hemodynamic response to exercise. Circulation 36:222–230, 1967.

29. Shock NW. Physiological aspects of aging in man. Ann Rev Physiol 23:97–122, 1961.

30. Fitzgerald PL. Exercise for the elderly. Med Clin North Am 69:189–196, 1985.

31. Ike RW, Lampman RM, Castor CW. Arthritis and aerobic exercise. Phys Sportsmed 17:128–139, 1989.

32. Babb TG. Mechanical ventilatory constraints in aging, lung disease, and obesity: Perspectives and brief review. Med Sci Sports Exerc 31(Suppl 1):S12–S22, 1999.

33. Smith EL, Serfass RC. Exercise and Aging: The Scientific Basis. Hillside, NJ: Enslow, 1981.

34. deVries HA, Adams GM. Comparison of exercise responses in old and young men. J Gerontol 27:344–348, 1972.

35. Babb TG. Ventilatory response to exercise in subjects breathing CO_2 or HcO_2. J Appl Physiol 82:746–754, 1997.

36. Rosenthal M, Doberne L, Greenfield M, et al. Effect of age on glucose tolerance, insulin secretion, and in vivo insulin action. J Am Geriatr Soc 30:562–567, 1982.

37. Shephard RJ. Body Composition in Biological Anthropology. London: Cambridge University, 1991.

38. Aoyagi Y, Shephard RJ. Aging and muscle function. Sports Med 14:376–396, 1992.

39. Shephard RJ, Montelpare W, Plyley M, et al. Handgrip dynamometry, Cybex measurements and lean mass as markers of the ageing of muscle. Br J Sports Med 25:204–208, 1991.

40. Rogers MA, Evans WJ. Changes in skeletal muscle with aging: Effects of exercise training. In: Holloszy J, ed. Exercise and Sport Science Reviews. Baltimore: Williams & Wilkins, 1993:65–102.

41. Kavanagh T, Shephard RJ. Can regular sports participation slow the aging process? Data on masters athletes. Phys Sportsmed 18(6):94–104, 1990.

42. Fiatarone MA, Marks EC, Ryan ND, et al. High-intensity strength training in nonagenarians: Effects on skeletal muscle. JAMA 263:3029–3034, 1990.

43. Ghilarducci LE, Holly RG, Amsterdam EA. Effects of high resistance training in coronary artery disease. Am J Cardiol 64:866–870, 1989.

44. Kauffman TL. Strength training effect in young and aged women. Arch Phys Med Rehabil 65:223–226, 1985.

45. Bemben MG, Massey BH, Bemben DA, et al. Isometric intermittent endurance of four muscle groups in men aged 20–74. Med Sci Sports Exerc 28:145–154, 1996.

46. Mahon AD, Duncan GE, Howe CA, Del Corral P. Blood lactate and perceived exertion relative to ventilatory threshold: Boys versus men. Med Sci Sports Exerc 29:1332–1337, 1997.

47. Falk B, Bar-Or O, MacDougall JD, et al. Sweat lactate in exercising children and adolescents of varying physical maturity. J Appl Physiol 71:1735–1740, 1991.

48. Madsen KL, Adams WC, Van Loan MD. Effects of physical activity, body weight and composition, and muscular strength on bone density in young women. Med Sci Sports Exerc 30:114–120, 1998.

49. Petit MA, Prior JC, Barr SI. Running and ovulation positively change cancellous bone in premenopausal women. Med Sci Sports Exerc 31:780–787, 1999.

50. Aloia JF, Cohn SH, Ostuni JD, et al. Prevention of involutional bone loss by exercise. Ann Intern Med 89:356–358, 1978.

51. Smith DM, Khairi MR, Norton J. Age and activity effects on rate of bone mineral loss. J Clin Invest 58:716–721, 1976.

52. Nickols-Richardson SM, Modlesky CM, O'Connor PJ, Lewis RD. Premenarcheal gymnasts possess higher bone mineral density than controls. Med Sci Sports Exerc 32:63–69, 2000.

53. Bass S, Pearce G, Bradney M. Exercise before puberty may confer residual benefits in bone density: studies in active prepubertal and retired female gymnasts. J Bone Miner Res 13:500–507, 1998.

54. Taafe DR, Duret C, Cooper CS, Marcus R. Comparison of calcaneal ultrasound and DXA in young women. Med Sci Sports Exerc 31:1484–1489, 1999.

55. Ippolito E, Natali PG, Postacchini F, et al. Morphological, immunochemical, and biochemical study of rabbit Achilles tendon at various ages. J Bone Joint Surg 62A:583–598, 1980.

56. Novak LP. Aging, total body potassium, fat free mass, and cell mass in males and females between ages 18 and 85 years. J Gerontol 27:438–443, 1972.

57. Meyer F, Bar-Or O, MacDougall D, et al. Drink composition and the electrolyte balance of children exercising in the heat. Med Sci Sport Exerc 27:882–887, 1995.

58. Falk B, Bar-Or O, MacDougall JD. Aldosterone and prolactin response to exercise in the heat in circumpubertal boys. J Appl Physiol 71:1741–1745, 1991.

59. Kenney WL. Control of heat-induced vasodilation in relation to age. Eur J Appl Physiol 57:120–125, 1988.

60. Kenney WL, Tankersley CG, Newswanger DL, et al. Age and hypohydration independently influence the peripheral vascular response to hear stress. J Appl Physiol 68:1902–1908, 1990.

61. Smolander J, Bar-Or O, Korhonen O, et al. Thermoregulation during rest and exercise in the cold in pre- and early pubescent boys and in young men. J Appl Physiol 72:1589–1594, 1992.

62. Falk B, Bar-Or O, Smolander J, et al. Response to rest and exercise in the cold: Effects of age and aerobic fitness. J Appl Physiol 76:72–78, 1994.

63. Tankersley CG, Smolander J, Kenney WL, et al. Sweating and skin blood flow during exercise: Effects of age and maximal oxygen uptake. J Appl Physiol 71:236–242, 1991.

64. Young A. Effects of aging on human cold tolerance. Exp Aging Res 17:205–213, 1991.

65. Jeng SF, Liao HF, Lai JS, Hou JW. Optimization of walking in children. Med Sci Sports Exerc 29:370–376, 1997.

66. Unnithan VB, Dowling JJ, Frost G, Bar-Or O. Role of mechanical power estimates in the O_2 cost of walking in children with cerebral palsy. Med Sci Sports Exerc 31:1703–1708, 1999.

67. Elia EA. Exercise and the elderly. Clin Sports Med 10:141–155, 1991.

68. Shephard RJ, Shek PN. Exercise, aging and immune function. Int J Sports Med 16:1–6, 1995.

69. Rall LC, Roubenoff R, Cannon JG, et al. Effects of progressive resistance training on immune response in aging and chronic inflammation. Med Sci Sports Exerc 28:1356–1365, 1996.

70. Nieman DC, Henson DA. Role of endurance exercise in immune senescence. Med Sci Sports Exerc 26:172–181, 1994.

71. Shephard RJ. Effectiveness of training programmes for prepubescent children. Sports Med 13:194–213, 1992.

72. Van Mechelen W, Twisk J, Molenduk A, et al. Subject-related risk factors for sports injuries: A one year prospective study in young adults. Med Sci Sports Exerc 28:1171–1179, 1996.

73. Fletcher GF, Balady G, Froelicher VF, et al. Exercise standards: A statement for health care professionals from the American Heart Association. Circulation 91:580–615, 1995.

74. US Centers for Disease Control and Prevention, American College of Sports Medicine. Physical activity and public health. Sports Med Bull 28:7, 1993.

75. Hallfrisch J, Muller D, Drinkwater D, et al. Continuing diet trends in men: The Baltimore Longitudinal Study of Aging (1961–1987). J Gerontol 45:M186–M191, 1990.

1.3.0, 1.3.2   **2.3.0, 2.3.0.1, 2.3.0.2, 2.3.0.4, 2.3.0.5**   **4.3.0, 4.3.0.1**   **5.3.1**

CHAPTER **60**

Exercise Testing and Prescription Considerations Throughout Childhood

Linda D. Zwiren

This chapter generally refers to childhood as the period that ends with adulthood and that includes preadolescence and adolescence. In accordance with the recent International Consensus Conference on Physical Activity Guidelines for Adolescence, adolescence is defined as age 11–21 years (1). Data on preadolescents are limited by the fact that many experimental procedures are not appropriate for use with children. The advent of noninvasive methods to study subcellular responses, such as phosphorus magnetic resonance imaging and the use of stable isotopes to study muscle metabolism may lead to significant increases in what is known about these responses in preadolescents (2, 3). There is substantial variation in growth status and maturity level for any given chronological age, making the distinction between preadolescence and adolescence imprecise. The first portion of this chapter focuses on activity guidelines for children and adolescents of all ranges of physical ability, while the latter part covers various aspects of pediatric exercise testing.

While the terms *physical activity*, *physical fitness*, and *sports* are sometimes used interchangeably, each term has a unique meaning and refers to a different concept (4). *Physical activity* is a process or lifestyle behavior. Physical activity involves any bodily movement that causes moderate increases in energy expenditure. Increases in physical activity can be a result of walking, gardening, chopping wood, swimming, vacuuming, climbing stairs, riding a bicycle to school, and so on. Physical activity can be performed at various intensity levels. Reductions in the time children are lying down or sitting and increases in the time they are moving raise physical activity levels.

Physical fitness refers to a person's set of physical attributes, which can be improved by engaging in the appropriate exercise programs. Health-related fitness includes cardiovascular endurance, muscular strength, endurance, flexibility, and the ability to attain and maintain a healthy body weight (4).

Sports are activities that require specific skilled movements performed during organized games. To participate in sports, children need a certain level of motor or skill-related physical fitness and the ability to perform the specific skilled movements. Motor fitness includes such factors as agility, balance, coordination, power, speed, and reaction time (4).

PHYSIOLOGICAL ASPECTS

Preadolescents and adults differ significantly in physiological responses to exercise (5). These differences and the implications for exercise are presented in Table 60.1. Apart from low movement economy and limitations of exercising in climatic extremes, no apparent underlying physiological factors that make preadolescents less suitable than adults for prolonged, continuous activities have been identified (6).

Although preadolescents can perform exercise over a wide variety of intensities and durations, they spontaneously prefer short-term intermittent activities with a high recreational component and variety rather than monotonous, prolonged activities. Physiologically, preadolescents may use oxygen more efficiently than adults do, but they are less able to facilitate anaerobic pathways. Therefore, preadolescent children have greater oxygen-dependent adenosine triphosphate (ATP) generation and higher pH during exercise. In accordance with their physiological profile and from a psychological viewpoint, children seem best suited to repeated activities of varying intensities that last a few seconds, interspersed with short rest periods. In addition, this pattern of activity characterized by short bursts may optimize the anabolic effect of exercise in the growing child (2). The physiologically least suitable forms of exercise for preadolescent children are intensive activities lasting 10–90 seconds (7).

Since adolescent children can be pubescent, pubertal, or postpubertal, it is hard to identify specific physiological responses of the adolescent. The pubescent has a physiological profile similar to that of a preadolescent. The postpubertal child is physiologically similar to an adult.

Table 60.1. **Physiological Characteristics of the Exercising Child**

FUNCTION	COMPARISON TO ADULTS	IMPLICATIONS FOR EXERCISE PRESCRIPTION
Metabolic		
Aerobic		
$\dot{V}O_{2peak}$ ($L \cdot min^{-1}$)	Lower related to smaller body mass	
$\dot{V}O_{2peak}$ ($mL \cdot kg^{-1} \cdot min^{-1}$)	Similar	Can perform endurance tasks reasonably well
Submaximal oxygen demand (economy)	Cycling: similar (18–30% mechanical efficiency); walking and running: higher metabolic cost	Greater fatigability in prolonged high-intensity tasks (running and walking); greater heat production in children at a given speed of walking or running
$\dot{V}CO_2$	Time required to increase $\dot{V}CO_2$ at onset of activity and to return to baseline is markedly faster in preadolescents.	
Anaerobic		
Glycogen stores	Lower concentration and rate of utilization of muscle glycogen. Increase with age, similar to adult levels by about age 16.	
Phosphofructokinase (PFK) concentration	Glycolysis limited because of low level of PFK. For children aged 11–14 years a variety of glycolytic enzymes are the same as for adults at maximal exercise.	Ability of preadolescent children to perform *intensive* anaerobic tasks that last 10–90 sec is distinctly lower than for adults. Same ability to deal metabolically with very brief intensive exercise.
Phosphagen stores	Stores and breakdown of ATP and CP are the same.	Same ability to deal metabolically with very brief intensive exercise.
Oxygen transient	Faster reaching of steady state than adults. Shorter half-time of oxygen increase in children.	Preadolescent children reach metabolic steady state faster. Children contract a lower oxygen deficit. Children therefore are well suited to intermittent activities. Faster recovery.
LA_{peak}	Lower blood lactate levels at $\dot{V}O_{2peak}$	Individual variation is wide.
LA_{submax}	Lower at a given percent of $\dot{V}O_{2peak}$	May be reason children perceive a given workload as easier.
HR at lactate threshold	Higher	Children can exercise closer to peak exercise levels than adults before LT is reached.
Cardiovascular		
Q_{max}	Lower due to size difference	Immature cardiovascular system means child is limited in bringing internal heat to surface for dissipation when exercising intensively in the heat
Q at a given $\dot{V}O_2$	Somewhate lower	
SV_{max}	Lower because of size and heart volume difference	
SV at given $\dot{V}O_2$	Lower	
HR_{max}	Higher	Up to maturity HR_{max} is between 195 and 215 beats/min
HR at submaximal work	At given power output and at relative metabolic load, child has higher HR	Higher HR compensates for lower SV
Oxygen-carrying capacity	Blood volume, hemoglobin concentration, and total hemoglobin are lower in children.	
C_aO_2–C_vO_2	Somewhat higher	Potential deficiency of peripheral blood supply during maximal exertion in hot climates
Blood flow to active muscle	Higher	
Systolic and diastolic pressures	Lower maximal and submaximal	No known beneficial or detrimental effects on working capacity of child
Pulmonary Response		
V_{Emax} ($L \cdot min^{-1}$)	Lower	Early fatigability in tasks that require large respiratory minute volumes
V_{Emax} ($mL \cdot kg^{-1} \cdot min^{-1}$)	Smaller	Less efficient ventilation, therefore greater oxygen cost of ventilation. May explain relatively high metabolic cost of submaximal exercise.
$V_{Esubmax}$	V_E at any given $\dot{V}O_2$ is higher in children	Same as in adolescents and young adults

Table 60.1. *Continued*

FUNCTION	COMPARISON TO ADULTS	IMPLICATIONS FOR EXERCISE PRESCRIPTION
Respiratory frequency and tidal volume	Marked by higher rate—tachypnea—and shallow breathing	Physiological dead space is smaller than adults; therefore, alveolar ventilation is adequate for gas exchange.
VT	VT occurs at a higher percentage of $\dot{V}O_{2max}$ in children	Additional indicators that children may rely more on aerobic metabolism to meet enery demands
R_{max} ($\dot{V}CO_2/\dot{V}O_2$)	Lower in children	
Perception		
RPE	Exercising at a given physiological strain is perceived by children to be easier.	Implications for initial phase of heat acclimation
Thermoregulatory		
SA	Per unit mass is approx. 36% greater in children (percentage depends on size of child, i.e., SA per mass may be higher in younger children and lower in older)	Greater rate of heat exchange between skin and environment. In climatic extremes, children are at increased risk for stress.
Sweating rate	Lower absolute amount per unit of SA. Greater increase in core temperature required to start sweating.	Greater risk of heat-related illness on hot, humid days because of reduced capacity to evaporate sweat. Lower tolerance time in extreme heat.
Acclimation to heat	Slower physiologically; faster subjectively	Children require longer and more gradual program of acclimation; special attention during early stages of acclimation.
Body cooling in water	Faster cooling due to higher SA per heat-producing unit mass, lower thickness of subcutaneous fat	Potential for hypothermia
Body core heating during dehydration	Greater	Prolonged activity; hydrate well before and force fluid intake during activity

Qmax, maximal cardiac output; SV_{max}, maximal stroke volume; HR_{max}, maximal heart rate; C_aO_2–C_vO_2, oxygen content in arterial and venous blood; V_{Emax}, maximal minute ventilation; VT, ventilatory threshold; RPE, rating of perceived exertion; SA, surface area.
Reprinted with permission from Zwiren LD. Exercise prescription for children. In: ACSM Resource Manual for Guidelines for Testing and Prescription. 3rd ed. Baltimore: Williams & Wilkins, 1998.

The precise physiological response during puberty, therefore, depends on the status of somatic **growth** and biological maturation.

SOMATIC GROWTH AND BIOLOGICAL MATURATION

It is important to keep children naturally active. If activity level falls below a biological threshold, somatic growth is impaired (2). There is little evidence that raising levels of physical activity above this biological threshold increases age at peak height velocity, skeletal maturation, or sexual maturation (7, 8). However, some evidence indicates that excessive training, especially in gymnastics, may have *adverse* effects resulting in a reduction of growth potential (8). In addition, if food lacking in nutritional value is used to increase caloric consumption, or if calories are restricted to control body weight, nutrition may be inadequate to support normal growth.

Bone Mass

While there is little research regarding physical activity and increasing bone mass to genetic potential, adolescence is a crucial time in terms of bone density maximization. Therefore, the International Consensus on Physical Activity Guidelines for Adolescents (9) declares that physical activity and exercise, especially weight-bearing exercise, are necessary, in combination with adequate nutrition and appropriate hormonal status, for attainment of maximal bone density.

It is important to monitor menstrual status in postmenarchal females, since amenorrhea can have severe consequences, especially with respect to bone density. The American Academy of Pediatrics recommends intervention after onset of amenorrhea in physically active females to preserve normal bone development and to prevent skeletal demineralization (10).

The current recommendation is that females be encouraged to engage in a variety of activities at a range of intensities. However, since disordered eating (inadequate caloric intake compared to energy expended) coupled with intensive exercise can lead to amenorrhea, it is imperative that adequate caloric intake of nutrient-dense foods is promoted in active adolescents (11). Table 60.2 lists signs associated with eating disorders.

PRECAUTIONS FOR EXERCISING IN CLIMATIC EXTREMES

Preadolescent children have a high energy expenditure ($\dot{V}O_2$) at any given submaximal walking or running speed and therefore produce disproportionate metabolic heat during exercise. This higher metabolic load, combined

Table 60.2. Danger Signals

ANOREXIA NERVOSA	BULIMIA NERVOSA
Has lost a great deal of weight in a relatively short period	Develops eating rituals and eats small amounts of food (e.g., cuts food into tiny pieces or measures everything before eating extremely small amounts)
Continues to diet although already thin	Prefers to eat alone
Reaches weight goal and immediately sets another goal for further weight loss	Becomes obsessive about exercising
Remains dissatisfied with appearance, claims to feel fat	Appears unhappy much of the time
Loses menstrual periods	Exercises often but retains or regains weight
Appears depressed much of the time	Disappears into the bathroom for long periods
	Binges regularly (eats large amounts of food, empties refrigerator; food disappears)
	Purges regularly (uses diet pills, caffeine, water pills, diuretics)

Reprinted with permission from Casper RC. Fear of fatness and anorexia nervosa in children. In: Cheung LWY, Richmond JB, eds. Child Health, Nutrition, and Physical Activity. Champaign, IL: Human Kinetics, 1995.

with decreased ability to regulate temperature in extreme heat, large surface-to-mass ratio, and immature cardiovascular system (Table 60.1), decreases tolerance for exercise in the heat (7). The American Academy of Pediatrics (AAP) recommends lightweight clothing limited to one layer of absorbent material to expose skin and facilitate evaporation of sweat. Wet clothing should be replaced by dry, and rubberized sweat suits should not be used (12).

Children have low tolerance to extreme heat or cold. However, when exercising in neutral or moderately warm climates, they can regulate temperature as effectively as adults, and depending on the degree of maturation of sweat glands and cardiorespiratory organs, mechanical efficiency, physical fitness, and body composition, they may exhibit exercise heat tolerance similar to that of adults (13, 14). The AAP emphasizes that "heat related disorders are particularly pronounced in races that exceed 30 minutes" (6). Activities lasting 30 minutes or longer should be reduced when relative humidity and air temperature are above critical levels (Table 60.3).

While preadolescent children do have characteristics that increase risk of heat illness, it is not dangerous for children to exercise in hot and humid environments. Preadolescent children are more likely to have heat exhaustion than other heat illness. Adolescents are most likely to have heat stroke at stressful temperatures (14).

Acclimation

Preadolescent children may lag behind adults in the *rate* of physiological acclimation and therefore should have a longer, more gradual period of acclimation. The AAP recommends that intensity and duration should begin low and gradually increase over 10–14 days (12). Children can acclimate to some extent when they exercise in neutral environments and when they rest in hot climates; however, *subjectively* they acclimate faster than adults. Therefore, especially during early stages of acclimation, children may feel capable of performing exercise

Table 60.3. Weather Guide for Prevention of Heat Illness

AIR TEMPERATURE (°F)	DANGER ZONE (% RELATIVE HUMIDITY)	CRITICAL ZONE (% RELATIVE HUMIDITY)
70	80	100
75	70	100
80	50	80
85	40	68
90	30	55
95	20	40
100	10	30

Reprinted with permission from Haymes EM, Wells CL. Environment and Human Performance. Champaign, IL: Human Kinetics, 1986.

in the heat despite significant heat stress.

Fluid Replacement

During continuous activity lasting longer than 30 minutes, fluid should be replaced at a rate of 100–150 mL every 15–30 minutes even if thirst is not apparent (12, 13). Bar-Or (13) recommends that replacement fluids for children not exceed 5 mEq/L Na^+ (0.3 g/L NaCl), 4 mEq/L K^+ (0.28 g/L KCl), and 25 g/L sugar. Haymes and Wells (15) suggest that a 40-kg child should ingest 150 mL of cold water every 30 minutes during activity. Carbohydrate drinks (i.e., sport drinks) appear to offer no inherent benefit over water in preadolescent children who are well hydrated (16), although sport drinks may enhance voluntary drinking because of their taste or ability to induce thirst (17).

OVERUSE INJURY

Increasing numbers of children have overuse injuries (18). Overuse injuries are caused by repetitive microtrauma to the musculoskeletal system (19). Risk factors for overuse injury:

- Significant changes in the intensity, duration, frequency, or type of training (including attending youth summer camps)
- Musculotendinous tautness in early adolescence
- Imbalance in strength and flexibility
- Anatomical malalignment of lower extremities
- Incorrect biomechanics
- Improper footwear
- Training on a hard surface
- Excessive loading of the back during growth spurts (18–20)

It is estimated that 50% of overuse injuries in children are preventable (20). Prevention entails the following:

- Improvement in musculoskeletal fitness and sport-specific skills
- Monitoring of growth rate to identify periods of accelerated growth, when vulnerability may be greatest and therefore training regimens should be modified
- Gradual progression in training, with no more than a 10% increase in the amount of training time, distance covered, or number of repetitions performed at any progression (20).

The American Academy of Pediatrics recommends that pediatricians consider the risks of distance running when advising parents and children. At present, however, evidence does not indicate that children should refrain from distance running (6). For a complete description of sports injuries that children and adolescents may incur, consult Micheli and d'Hemecourt (21).

ACTIVITY GUIDELINES: LARGE-MUSCLE ACTIVITY

The National Association for Sport and Physical Education has developed activity guidelines for children. The following is a summary of those guidelines (22):

1. Elementary school–aged children should accumulate at least *30 to 60 minutes* of age-appropriate physical activity from a variety of physical activities on most or all days of the week.
2. An accumulation of *more than 60 minutes and up to several hours a day* of age- and developmentally appropriate activity is encouraged for elementary school–aged children.
3. Some physical activity each day should be in periods lasting 10–15 minutes or more and include moderate to vigorous physical activity. This activity typically is intermittent, alternating periods of moderate to vigorous activity with *brief periods* of rest and recovery.
4. *Extended periods of inactivity are inappropriate* for children.

5. A variety of physical activities are recommended for elementary school children.

The recommendation of 30 minutes to an hour of *accumulated* activity per day (6–8 Kcal/kg/day) is to ensure that children meet the adult standard when they mature (11). Because children have different preferences for exercise and activity, an "adult" exercise prescription for sustained large-muscle activity for a minimum of 20 minutes may be discouraging and interfere with the enjoyment of movement and activity (22). Increased energy expenditure and reduction in sedentary time, coupled with appropriate eating habits, are major components of multidisciplinary programs for obese children and for the prevention of obesity (23).

The primary goal for preadolescent children is to keep them active, so that they enjoy moving and develop lifelong activity habits. To accomplish these goals, preadolescent children should be:

- Allowed to control the intensity and duration of their activity (22)
- Allowed to be naturally active
- Enjoying activity: children should have a voice in the choice of physical activity and sports
- Encouraged to play outside and away from the television and computer (22) to decrease sedentary time
- Involved in programs that emphasize gaining basic motor and sport skills so they may participate in these activities throughout life

Parents, guardians, and family members must support and encourage activity and should provide active role models for children. Multidisciplinary intervention programs should be implemented for children who are sedentary, obese, or disabled. Girls may require more support to be physically active (23). Sedentary children with disability may have the most to gain from increased activity through increased functional level and decreased risk of secondary infection.

For adolescent children, acquiring motor and sport skills should also be emphasized. Specific recommendations for activity and exercise to improve health-related fitness comes from the International Consensus Conference on Physical Activity Guidelines for Adolescents (24) as follows:

1. *All adolescents should be physically active daily nearly every day, as part of play, games, sports, work, transportation, recreation, physical education, or planned exercise, in the context of family, school, and community activities. Adolescents should do a variety of enjoyable physical activities, including some weight-bearing activities, as part of their daily lives. The intensity and duration of the activity are probably less important than the fact*

that energy is expended and a habit of daily activity is established. Such activities as walking up stairs, walking or riding a bicycle for errands, having conversation while walking with friends, parking at the far end of parking lots, and doing household chores are examples of ways to increase activity level.

2. *Adolescents should engage in three or more sessions per week of activities that last 20 minutes or more at one time and that require moderate to vigorous levels of exertion.* Moderate to vigorous activities are those that require at least as much effort as brisk or fast walking. A diversity of activities that use large muscle groups are recommended as part of sports, recreation, chores, transportation, work, school, physical education, or planned exercise. Examples include brisk walking, jogging, stair climbing, basketball, racquet sports, soccer, dance, swimming laps, skating, strength (resistance) training, lawn mowing, strenuous housework, cross-country skiing, and cycling.

The promotion of active lifestyles and lowering of obesity rates also depend on community support and availability of safe and accessible facilities, media exposure and advertising, socioeconomic and political factors. Therefore, it is imperative to promote activity for minorities, individuals with disabilities, and those in low socioeconomic levels, where safety of facilities and other cost-related factors may prohibit children from engaging in activity. Children with illness or disability may require a specific or modified exercise prescription (5, 13, 25–28). Specific prescriptions may also be provided for hypokinetic children and those who have two or more risk factors for coronary artery disease.

RESISTANCE TRAINING

Muscular strength is the maximal force or torque developed by a muscle or muscle group during a single maximal voluntary action. Muscular endurance is the ability to exert force continuously without producing movement or repeatedly while producing or resisting movement. Power is the rate at which work is performed. Resistance training is the use of equipment to increase muscular strength and/or endurance (11, 29). Isokinetic resistance can be used; however, resistance training usually entails a series of repetitions against some resistance (30). High-repetition, low-resistance training improves endurance, whereas high-resistance, low-repetition training increases strength (31).

Consideration of the benefits of training (e.g., strength gains, injury protection, improved sports performance, psychological benefits) should be weighed against the risks (e.g., low back injury, growth plate injury in adolescents, and other acute and chronic musculoskeletal injuries) (32). Available evidence suggests that resistance training programs can be performed safely and appropriately by both children and adolescents. Recommendations for resistance training in youth are as follows:

- Resistance testing and training equipment should be adapted to children.
- Close, continuous, trained supervision is required.
- Adequate warm-up is necessary.
- High-repetition training is the most appropriate choice (>6–8 repetitions per set).
- Adequate recovery (2 or 3 days) between training sessions is important.
- Multijoint exercises should be used.
- Exercises must be performed in a controlled manner throughout a full range of movement.
- Proper form and correct technique must be emphasized.
- Flexibility exercises should be included in the program (5, 32–35).

In the early stages of a program, the following recommendations are useful:

- Using body weight as resistance can be effective.
- New exercises using little or no load should be introduced.
- Intensity progression should be gradual.
- Proper technique is more important initially than application of resistance.
- Overload should initially be achieved by increasing repetitions, then by increasing resistance.

Children should avoid competitive weight lifting, power lifting, and bodybuilding until Tanner stage 5 level of developmental maturity (34). Resistance training should be one component of the exercise program for increasing fitness or performance in children but should not be the sole component. Field and laboratory tests for muscular strength and endurance are described in the literature (29).

Resistance training can be accomplished with minimal risk of injury in pubescent and pubertal children and in fact can be used to minimize sports injuries when appropriate adult supervision is available (33). Preadolescents make similar relative improvement but smaller absolute strength gains than adolescents and young adults. As with adults, improvement depends on overload (32). Training-induced gains in muscular strength and endurance are lost during detraining (32). Resistance training may have value beyond physiological and neurological muscular adaptation, since improved self-esteem and enhanced body image have been reported after resistance training in obese children (36).

GRADED EXERCISE TESTS

Rationale for Exercise Testing

Reasons for using exercise testing in children are listed in Table 60.4 and in the *ACSM Guidelines* (5). Application of graded exercise testing to specific diseases or problems is beyond the scope of this chapter, but other reviews are available (37, 38). In many cases, the graded exercise test is used most successfully as an affirmation that exercise can be performed safely at high intensity. For research purposes, the legality and ethics of testing children should be considered and informed consent of both the parent and child should be obtained (39).

Mode of Testing

Similar modes of testing can be used with children and adults, though children, especially those younger than 7 years, should be tested on a treadmill. Local muscle fatigue and inability to maintain required pedaling cadence prevent many children from reaching maximal values on a cycle ergometer. Children should be instructed about using ergometers. Cardiorespiratory measurements must be directly assessed, since estimation of maximal values from submaximal tests is not reliable (13). Handrails on the treadmill and the support system for gas analysis equipment must be modified to fit children (40, 41).

Table 60.4. Rationale for Exercise Testing in Pediatric Diagnosis

---

Measure physical working capacity
1. Assess daily function: establish whether daily activities are within physiological functioning level.
2. Identify deficiency in specific fitness component: muscular endurance and strength may limit daily performance rather than aerobic capacity (e.g., muscular dystrophy).
3. Establish a baseline before onset of an intervention program.
4. Assess effectiveness of an exercise prescription.
5. Chart the course of any progressive disease (e.g., cystic fibrosis, Duchenne muscular dystrophy)

Exercise as a provocation test
1. Amplify pathophysiological changes.
2. Trigger changes otherwise not seen in the resting child.

Exercise as an adjunct diagnostic test
1. Noninvasive exercise test can be used for screening to determine the need for an invasive test.
2. Assess the severity of dysrhythmias.
3. Assess functional success of surgical correction.
4. Assess adequacy of drug regimens at varying exercise intensities.

Assessment and differentiation of symptoms
1. Chest pains (asthma from myocardial infarction)
2. Breathlessness (bronchoconstriction from low physical capacity)
3. Coughing
4. Easy fatigability

Instill confidence in child and parent.

Assess motivation or compliance in intervention program

Adapted from Bar-Or O. Exercise in pediatric assessment and diagnosis. Scand J Sport Sci; 7:35–39, 1985.

Electronically braked cycle ergometers are preferred because power output does not depend on pedaling rate. Pedaling rates of 50–60 rpm are recommended for mechanically braked ergometers (13). Special models for children should be used, or existing cycle ergometers can be modified for children under 9 years or under 125 cm (50 inches). The handlebars, seat height, and pedal crank length should be individualized (13, 38). In addition, smaller resistance increments may be required; therefore, resistance indicators should be in 5-watt gradations. Some special populations may require an arm ergometer for testing. Some test procedures (e.g., radionuclide imaging and echocardiography) are more conveniently determined on a cycle ergometer (38).

Protocol

A variety of protocols are appropriate for children (5, 13, 37–39, 42). Some are similar to those used in adults, but in some instances, modification of initial power output and subsequent incremental increases are necessary. Recently, Rowland (42) made a compelling case for the use of the modified Balke Treadmill Protocol in clinical testing of children. The specific protocol selected depends on the following:

- The goals and objectives of the test
- The measurements to be obtained
- Whether submaximal and/or maximal data are required
- The abilities and limitations of the subject

A graded exercise test is not required prior to initiating an exercise program for asymptomatic children. Guidelines for screening young athletes for risk of cardiovascular disease are available (43).

Supervisory Personnel

A physician trained in exercise testing in general and in clinical exercise testing in children should assume responsibility for diagnostic testing, although the actual conduct of the test may be delegated to other qualified personnel (38). A physician should be directly involved in testing children with the following clinical conditions (13, 38):

- Serious rhythm disorders
- Aortic stenosis with gradients above 50 mm Hg
- Myocardial disease
- Cyanotic heart disease
- Advanced pulmonary vascular disease
- Ventricular dysrhythmia with heart disease
- Coronary artery disease

ACSM-certified professional can perform or supervise maximal exercise testing in normal children for research purposes (38).

Contraindications to Exercise Testing

In addition to the contraindications listed in the *ACSM Guidelines*, the following are contraindications to exercise testing of children (5, 13, 38):

1. Dyspnea at rest; 1-second forced expiratory volume (FEV_1) or peak expiratory flow less than 60% of predicted value
2. Acute renal disease or hepatitis
3. Insulin-dependent diabetes in someone who did not take insulin as prescribed or who is ketoacidotic
4. Acute rheumatic fever with myocarditis or pericarditis
5. Severe pulmonary vascular disease
6. Poorly compensated heart failure
7. Severe aortic or mitral stenosis
8. Hypotrophic cardiomyopathy with syncope

Criteria For Termination Of Test

Criteria for stopping an exercise test are similar to those for adults included in the *ACSM's Guidelines for Exercise Testing and Prescription* (5). Attainment of peak oxygen consumption ($\dot{V}O_{2peak}$) and/or maximal heart rate is one criterion for terminating a child's exercise test.

Maximal Oxygen Uptake

Evidence for a plateau in maximal oxygen uptake ($\dot{V}O_{2max}$) in children is less common than in adults, so $\dot{V}O_{2peak}$ values are acceptable (41). Data on intraindividual variation in $\dot{V}O_{2max}$ indicate, however, that acceptable data can be obtained even if criteria for identifying a plateau in $\dot{V}O_{2max}$ are not always satisfied (13, 41). Determination of the respiratory exchange ratio and ventilatory threshold may be helpful for test interpretation if maximal effort was not attained (5).

Maximal Heart Rate

Children with weak or atrophied peripheral musculature (e.g., muscular dystrophy or cerebral palsy), congenital heart block and a number of other congenital heart defects, anorexia, and those receiving beta-blocker therapy may have low maximal heart rate (5, 13). Young children attain a higher maximal heart rate than adults (Table 60.1). Maximal heart rates usually do not change in children until after puberty, when there is a decrease of 0.7 or 0.8 beats per minute per year of age. Treadmill exercise results in a slightly higher maximal heart rate than does cycle ergometry (38).

References

1. Sallis JF, Patrick K, Long BJ. Overview of the International Consensus Conference on Physical Activity Guidelines for Adolescents. Pediatr Exerc Sci 6:299–301, 1994.
2. Cooper DM. New horizons in pediatric exercise research. In: Cameron CJR, Bar-Or O, eds. New Horizons in Pediatr Exerc Sci. Champaign, IL: Human Kinetics, 1995:1–24.
3. Bar-Or O. Pediatric Exercise Sciences: Why and where to? Sportsmedicine Bulletin, 35(2):8, 2000.
4. Corbin CB, Pangrazi RP, Franks BD. Definitions: Health, fitness, and physical activity. President's Council on Physical Fitness and Sports Research Digest, Series 3, No. 9:1–8, March 2000.
5. American College of Sports Medicine. ACSM's Guidelines for Exercise Testing and Prescription. 6th ed. Baltimore: Lippincott Williams & Wilkins, 2000.
6. American Academy of Pediatrics Committee on Sports Medicine. Risks in running for children. Pediatrics 86:656–657, 1990 (reaffirmed 1994).
7. Bar-Or O. Exercise in childhood. In: Walsh RP, Shephard RJ, eds. Current Therapy in Sport Medicine, 1985–1986. Toronto: Mosby, 1985.
8. Malina RM. Growth and maturation of young athletes: Is training for sport a factor? In: Chan KM, Micheli LJ, eds. Sport and Children. Hong Kong: Williams & Wilkins, 1998:133–161.
9. Bailey DA, Martin AD. Physical activity and skeletal health in adolescents. Pediatr Exerc Sci 6:424–433, 1994.
10. American Academy of Pediatrics. AAP Committee on Sports Medicine. Amenorrhea in adolescent athletes. Pediatrics 84:394–395, 1989.
11. Rowland TW. Exercise and Children's Health. Champaign, IL: Human Kinetics, 1990.
12. American Academy of Pediatrics. Climatic heat stress and the exercising child. Phys Sport Med 11:155, 159, 1983.
13. Bar-Or O. Pediatric Sports Medicine for the Practitioner: From Physiologic Principles to Clinical Applications. New York: Springer, 1983.
14. Armstrong LE, Maresh CM. Exercise-heat tolerance of children and adolescents. Pediatr Exerc Sci 7:239–252, 1995.
15. Haymes EM, Wells CL. Environment and Human Performance. Champaign, IL: Human Kinetics, 1986.
16. Meyer F, Bar-Or O, MacDougall D, Heighenhauser GJF. Drink composition and the electrolyte balance of children exercising in the heat. Med Sci Sports Exerc 27:882–887, 1995.
17. Rivera-Brown AM, Guttierrez R, Guttierrez JC. Drink composition, voluntary drinking and fluid balance in exercising, trained, heat-acclimated boys. J Appl Physiol 86:78–84, 1999.
18. Macera CA, Wooten W. Epidemiology of sports and recreation injuries among adolescents. Pediatr Exerc Sci 6:424–433, 1994.
19. American Academy of Pediatrics, Committee on Sports Medicine and Fitness. Sports Medicine: Health Care for Young Athletes. Elk Grove Village, IL: AAP, 1991.
20. American College of Sports Medicine. The prevention of sport injuries of children and adolescents. Med Sci Sports Exerc 25(8):1, 1993 (supplement).
21. Micheli LJ, d'Hemecourt PA. Sports injuries in the child and adolescent. In: Chan KM, Micheli LJ, eds. Sports and Children. Hong Kong: Williams & Wilkins, 1998:178–209.
22. Pate RR. Physical activity for young children. President's Council on Physical Fitness and Sport Research Digest, Series 3, No. 3:1–8, 1998.
23. Bar-Or O, Foreyt J, Bouchard C, et al. Physical activity, genetic, and nutritional considerations in childhood weight management. Med Sci Exerc Sports 30(1): 2–10, 1998.

24. Sallis JF, Patrick K. Physical activity guidelines for adolescents: Consensus statement. Pediatr Exerc Sci 6:302–314, 1994.

25. Ganley T, Sherman C. Exercise and children's health. Phys Sportsmed 28(2):85–92, 2000.

26. Goldberg B, ed. Sports and Exercise for Children With Chronic Health Conditions. Champaign, IL: Human Kinetics, 1995.

27. Small E, Bar-Or O. The young athlete with chronic disease. Clin Sports Med 14:709–726, 1995.

28. American Diabetes Association. Position statement on diabetes mellitus and exercise. Diabetes Care 18(1); 30–37, 1997.

29. Gaul CA. Muscular strength and endurance. In: Docherty D, ed. Measurement in Pediatric Exercise Science. Champaign, IL: Human Kinetics, 1996:225–258.

30. Baltzopoulos V, Kellis E. Isokinetic strength during childhood and adolescence. In: Van Praagh E, ed. Pediatric Anaerobic Performance. Champaign, IL: Human Kinetics, 1998:225–240.

31. Wathen D. Load assignment. In: Baechle TR, ed. Essentials of Strength Training and Conditioning. Champaign, IL: Human Kinetics, 1994.

32. Blimkie CJR. Resistance training during preadolescence: Issues and controversies. Sports Med 15:389–407, 1993.

33. FIMS. Resistance training for children and adolescents: Position statement by the International Federation of Sports medicine. In: Chan KM, Micheli LJ, eds. Sports and Children. Hong Kong: Williams & Wilkins, 1998:265–270.

34. American Academy of Pediatrics Committee on Sports Medicine. Strength, training, weight and power lifting, and body building by children and adolescents. Pediatrics 86:801, 1990.

35. Freedson PS, Ward A, Rippe JM. Resistance training for youth. In: Grana, WA, Lombardo JA, Sharkey BJ, Stone JA, eds. Advances in Sports Medicine and Fitness, vol 3. Chicago: Year Book Medical, 1990:57–65.

36. Isaacs LD. Status of research in prepubescent strength training. American Alliance for Health, Physical Education, Recreation, and Dance Research Consortium News 19(1):1–2, 1997.

37. Rowland TW. Aerobic exercise testing protocols. In: Roland TW, ed. Pediatric Laboratory Exercise Testing: Clinical Guidelines. Champaign, IL: Human Kinetics, 1993:19–41.

38. Gibbons RJ, Balady GJ, Beasley JW, et al. ACC/AHA guidelines for exercise testing. A report of the American College of Cardiology/American Heart Association Task Force. J Am Coll Cardiol 30:260–315, 1997.

39. Armstrong N, Welsman JR. Assessment and interpretation of aerobic fitness in children and adolescents. Exerc Sport Sci Rev 22:435–476, 1994.

40. Docherty D, ed. Introduction. In: Docherty D, ed. Measurement in Pediatric Exercise Science. Windsor, Ontario: Human Kinetics, 1996:1–13.

41. Léger L. Aerobic performance. In: Docherty D, ed. Measurement in Pediatric Exercise Science. Windsor, Ontario: Human Kinetics, 1996:183–224.

42. Rowland TW. Crusading for the Balke Protocol: Editor's notes. Pediatr Exerc Sci 11(3):189–192, 1999.

43. Rowland TW. Screening for risk of cardiac death in young athletes. Gatorade Sports Science Institute, Sports Science Exchange 12(3):1–5, 1999.

1.3.1, 1.3.2

2.3.0, 2.3.0.2, 2.3.0.4, 2.3.0.5

4.3.0, 4.3.0.1

5.3.0, 5.3.1

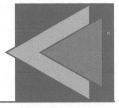

CHAPTER 61

EXERCISE PROGRAMMING FOR OLDER ADULTS

David E. Corbin

DEMOGRAPHICS

The United States, along with most of the developed countries of the world, is undergoing an age wave. In 1998 there were more than 34 million people 65 years of age and over in the United States. That constitutes 12.7% of the U.S. population, or about one in every eight Americans. The number of older Americans has increased 10% since 1990, compared to an increase of 8% for the under-65 population (1).

In 1998, there were more than 20 million older women and more than 14 million older men, or a gender ratio of about 10 women per 7 men. The older people get, the greater the ratio of women to men. For those over age 85 there are 10 women for every 5.5 men (1). In 1997, 65-year-olds had an average life expectancy of an additional 17.6 years (19.0 years for women and 15.8 years for men). A child born in 1997 can expect to live 76.5 years, about 29 years longer than a child born in 1900 (1).

Almost 1.9 million persons (5190 per day) celebrated their 65th birthday in 1998. In the same year, about 1.75 million people 65 or older died, so that the population of those over 65 increased by about 396 per day (1). This dramatic growth in older adults, which is projected to continue well into this century, combined with an increased knowledge of the benefits of exercise for older adults, has set the scene for more exercise and fitness programs for older adults.

BENEFITS OF EXERCISE FOR OLDER ADULTS

Unfortunately, while the population of older adults has increased, the growth of qualified exercise professionals has not. Indeed, exercise leaders in aerobics classes for younger people are more likely to be certified to teach than exercise leaders for older adults. Certification for most aerobics teachers does not include specialization for working with older adults, and many gerontologists are not trained to plan, implement, or evaluate exercise programs for older adults. Certainly the lack of exercise pro-

fessionals is not because the benefits of exercise for older adults are not proved. The research is conclusive with respect to the importance of exercise for older adults (2–8). Table 61.1 summarizes the benefits of exercise from the U.S. Surgeon General's report.

Research since the Surgeon General's report suggests that regular exercise can decrease the risks of gallstone disease in women (9). There is even evidence that exercise can decrease the risks of certain hearing problems and can help people with Alzheimer's disease to maintain physical health and reduce agitation (10–12). In addition, exercise is vital for rehabilitation from certain surgeries, such as mastectomy and hip replacement. Table 61.2 summarizes some of the national organizations that publish materials related to their special interests and the benefits of exercise.

It is beyond the scope of this chapter to document all of the benefits of exercise for older adults, but many reports and books summarize the research and practice in this field. Some of the most significant are ACSM's position stand entitled *Exercise and Physical Activity for Older Adults* (5), The President's Council on Physical Fitness and Sport Research Digest's *Physical Activity and Aging: Implications for Health and Quality of Life in Older Persons* (13), and Spirduso's Physical Dimensions of Aging (14).

The U.S. Department of Health and Human Services' *Promoting Physical Activity: A Guide for Community Action* (15) and the World Health Organization's *Heidelberg Guidelines for Promoting Physical Activity Among Older Adults* (16) offer additional information about the benefits of exercise and tips on how to engage older adults in exercise (15, 16). For example, The Heidelberg Guidelines encourage " . . . the development of strategic policies and both population and community-based interventions aimed at maintaining and/or increasing the level of physical activity for all older adults (16)." These guidelines provide a list of the physiological, psychological, and social benefits of exercise for older adults. The emergence of the *Journal of Aging and Physical Activity* is evidence of increased interest in research in exercise and aging.

Table 61.1. How Physical Activity Affects Health

Regular physical activity that is performed on most days of the week reduces the risk of developing or dying from some of the leading causes of illness and death in the United States. Regular physical activity improves health in the following ways:

- Reduces the risk of dying prematurely
- Reduces the risk of dying prematurely of heart disease
- Reduces the risk of developing diabetes.
- Reduces the risk of developing high blood pressure
- Helps reduce blood pressure in people who already have high blood pressure
- Reduces the risk of developing colon cancer
- Reduces feelings of depression and anxiety
- Helps control weight
- Helps build and maintain healthy bones, muscles, and joints
- Helps older adults become stronger and better able to move about without falling
- Helps people with chronic, disabling conditions improve their stamina and muscle strength
- Helps control joint swelling and pain associated with arthritis

Reprinted from Physical Activity and Health: A Report of the Surgeon General. Atlanta: National Center for Chronic Disease Prevention and Health Promotion, 1996.

Despite the overwhelming evidence that exercise is beneficial to older adults: "Inactivity increases with age. By age 75, about one in three men and one in two women engage in no physical activity (17)."

LEADERSHIP TIPS

The challenge for exercise professionals and program design is to motivate increased numbers of older adults to exercise and to provide programs that meet their needs over a long time. The need for individualized exercise programs increases with age. For example, most older adults have at least one chronic disease, and many have several. In 1996, 36.3% of older adults reported limitations because of chronic conditions. Among all older adults, 10.5% were unable to carry on a major activity. In comparison, only 10.3% of the population under 65 years was limited in their activities, and 3.5% were unable to accomplish a major activity (1). Exercise programs must make accommodations for these conditions. There is evidence that carefully planned exercise programs can prevent or diminish the severity of many common chronic health problems that affect older people.

Table 61.2. Organizations That Publish Materials on the Benefits of Exercise

LIFE-THREATENING AND DEBILITATING DISEASES	EXERCISE BENEFITS PREVENTION AND/OR CONTROL	ORGANIZATIONS	MATERIALS	CONTACTS
Cardiovascular and cerebrovascular diseases	Helps prevent and control CV disease and stroke, lowers risk of atherosclerosis, lowers BP	American Heart Association	*Just Move, Walking for a Healthy Heart, Exercise and Your Heart, How Can Physical Activity Become a Way of Life?*	800-AHA-USA1 (800-242-8721)
Cancer	Exercise can help prevent colon cancer and rehabilitate after certain cancer surgeries	National Cancer Institute, American Cancer Society	Pertain to rehabilitation rather than prevention, e.g., exercise after surgery	800-4-CANCER (800-422-6237) 800-ACS-2345 (800-227-2345)
NIDDM	Decreases risk of developing NIDDM, helps control weight, increases cells' sensitivity to insulin	American Diabetes Association	*The Fitness Book for People With Diabetes*	800-DIABETES (800-342-2383)
Arthritis	Can increase mobility and decrease need for medication	Arthritis Foundation	*Exercise and Your Arthritis*, PEP video, *PACE* classes and video, *Joint Efforts*	800-283-7800
Depression and mental health	Clinically depressed people are helped by exercise, perhaps because of endorphins	American Psychological Association	*Exercise Therapy for Patients With Psychiatric Disorders: Research and Clinical Implications*	http://www.apa. org/journals/ pro/pro303275. html
Osteoporosis	Weight-bearing exercise helps prevent bone loss	National Osteoporosis Foundation	*Be BoneWise: NOF's Official Exercise Video*	http://store. yahoo.com/ nof/ bebonexnofof. html
Parkinson's disease	Helps control tremors, stiffness, and rigidity of the muscles	National Parkinson Foundation	*Fitness Counts*	http://www. parkinson.org/ fc3.htm

Contrary to popular belief, older adults are a heterogeneous group. Therefore, exercise options should be broad. The FITT principle (frequency, intensity, time, and type) varies according to the exercise history, medical history (including the types of drugs being taken), exercise environment (e.g., temperature, lighting, floor surface), community resources (e.g., public trails, community fitness centers, malls that allow walking programs), and personal likes and dislikes.

There are some excellent resources for planning and implementing exercise programs for older adults. Three books that address issues of safety, guidelines, and exercise theories are *Promoting Physical Activity: A Guide for Community Action* (15), *Exercise and Fitness for the Older Adult* (18), and *Exercise for Older Adults* (19).

SAFETY AND GUIDELINES

Older adults must have medical clearance to begin what may eventually become a vigorous exercise program. Men older than 40 and women older than 50 are advised to obtain a medical evaluation before engaging in vigorous physical activity (20). The Physical Activity Readiness Questionnaire (PAR-Q) is a simple screening tool to identify those who should not participate in physical activity without a physician's evaluation (21). The Council on Aging and Adult Development of the American Alliance for Health, Physical Education, Recreation and Dance has developed *Medical/Exercise Assessment for Older Adults*, also a useful tool (21). In the booklet *Exercise: A Guide from the National Institute on Aging and NASA* (22), it is recommended that if an older adult has any of the following, a physician should be consulted prior to participating:

- Any new, undiagnosed symptom
- Chest pain
- Irregular, rapid, or fluttery heart beat
- Severe shortness of breath
- Significant ongoing weight loss that has not been diagnosed
- Infections, such as pneumonia, accompanied by fever
- Fever itself, which can cause dehydration and a rapid heartbeat
- Acute deep-vein thrombosis (blood clot)
- A hernia that is causing symptoms
- Foot or ankle sores that do not heal
- Joint swelling
- Persistent pain or a disturbance in walking after falling
- Certain eye conditions, such as bleeding in the retina or detached retina
- After a cataract or lens implant or after laser treatment or other eye surgery

There is considerable debate among professionals about what type of medical clearance is needed before an older adult can engage in a moderate exercise program. Part of the qualifications of the exercise professional should be to be able to make informed and intelligent decisions about requirements for participation in activity. A professional with background in both gerontology and exercise is most likely to be able to determine the needs of participants. Certainly, every exercise program should have a well-defined emergency plan for professionals to follow in the event of a medical emergency.

Exercise professionals should be trained in cardiopulmonary resuscitation (CPR). They should familiarize participants with how to calculate target heart rate zones, teach them to rate perceived exertion, and about the talk test as measures of intensity and ways to avoid overexertion. Leaders should always be vigilant for fatigue, pallor, breathlessness, discomfort, and pain (23). When these occur, the participant should stop. "No pain, no gain" is never an appropriate guideline in an exercise program for older adults.

The types of formations and equipment used for exercise also affect safety. For example, a circle formation for group exercise allows the leader to observe participants at all times. Adaptations should be readily offered, such as a sturdy chair or a wall to aid in balance, the option to stand or sit during the exercise, and the option to exercise at half tempo, regular tempo, or double tempo. Participants should be taught to monitor symptoms and report adverse symptoms to the leader immediately. Participants should be encouraged to breathe deeply and rhythmically during the exercise and not to hold their breath. They should wear well-fitting nonslip shoes and loose clothing. A 5- to 10-minute warm-up period should be conducted prior to the main exercise program and a 5- to 10-minute cool down should follow. Stretching exercises should not include ballistic stretches (bouncing); stretches should be held. If shakiness or tremors occur during the stretch, the participant should ease back to hold the stretch at a more comfortable position. If the participant cannot chat (talk test), sing a song, or whistle while performing the exercise, it is too strenuous. Target heart rate formulas are based on younger people, so the older the participant, the less likely the formula is appropriate; hence the importance of perceived exertion and close monitoring by the leader. Age and prescription drugs may undermine the premise of the target heart zone in these participants.

Safety should not be confused with overprotection. Many older adults, even those who have been active for a lifetime, are sometimes encouraged to limit activity drastically as they get older. They may be told to take it easy or not to do too much for fear of hurting themselves. Consequently, some older adults become overcautious and afraid to exert themselves. The result is a further loss of function stemming from a sedentary lifestyle. Fiatarone et. al. (4) put an end to some of these myths by demonstrating that people 90 and older in institutions could significantly improve strength with resistance training. The temptation is to do things for older people rather than providing programs to help them be and remain independent. A key to any exercise program for older adults is to accentuate the movements they can do rather than to dwell on the activities they cannot do. For example, physical functioning of older adults can fall into the following categories that determine the type of exercise program that is best suited to them:

- Physically elite
- Physically fit
- Physically independent
- Physically frail
- Physically dependent (14)

These categories, along with medical and exercise histories, help the exercise professional design a program with activities best suited the to the participants.

FUNCTIONAL FITNESS ASSESSMENTS

There are two batteries of functional fitness tests for older adults. These assessments can serve several purposes:

1. Assess the fitness levels of older adults and determine which types of fitness should be emphasized in individualized exercise programs
2. Evaluate the progress of participants by comparing results over time. Help motivate participants, particularly if progress is evident. Contribute to a database to establish age group norms

The Council on Aging and Adult Development Functional Fitness Assessments for Adults Over 60 Years includes measures of body composition, trunk and leg flexibility, agility and dynamic balance, hand–eye coordination, arm strength and endurance, and aerobic endurance (23). The Functional Fitness Test for Older Adults developed by Rikli and Jones (24, 25) includes assessments of lower body strength, upper body strength, two options for aerobic endurance, lower body flexibility, upper shoulder flexibility, agility, and dynamic balance. Of course, other fitness assessments are more appropriate for older adults who are already elite or fit.

THEORIES OF EXERCISE AND BEHAVIORAL CHANGE

There are several theories of behavioral change upon which exercise programs can be based. The most common:

- Health belief model
- Transtheoretical model

- Relapse prevention theory
- Social cognitive theory
- Theory of planned behavior
- Social support theory
- Ecological perspective theory

These are summarized in *Physical Activity and Health: A Report of the Surgeon General* (17). A theoretical basis can add to the success of the program in many ways, including the following:

1. Establishing the importance of exercise
2. Motivating the participants to get started
3. Meeting the physical, psychological, and social needs of the exercisers
4. Providing the resources and environment needed to start and maintain exercise practices
5. Retaining people in exercise programs once they have started
6. Helping people to plan and implement their own exercise programs
7. Providing both internal and external incentives for exercising

A minimal level of knowledge about behavior change is required to decide which theory may work best for particular individuals or groups of older adults. Considerable additional research is needed to determine the best ways to match theory to practice.

SPECIFIC EXERCISES

The history of the exerciser and the desired fitness outcomes are used to determine the most appropriate types of exercise. Several publications describe and illustrate specific types of exercises for older adults, including resistance, flexibility, balance, and cardiovascular exercises. Several of these resources are related to specific medical conditions (Table 61.2). More general exercises ranging from warm-up to cool-down are summarized in several books and booklets, such as *Exercise for Older Adults: ACE's Guide for Fitness Professionals* (19), *Reach for It: A Handbook of Health, Exercise and Dance Activities for Older Adults* (21), and *Exercise: A Guide from the National Institute on Aging and NASA* (22).

INCENTIVES AND MOTIVATORS

The attractiveness of exercise programs is not determined solely by the exercises and the leader. The ambiance should welcome older adults, and social opportunities are important. The music selection is also important. Leaders can poll participants to determine the type of music that they prefer. A cool-down session with partner massage is a powerful and pleasant motivator for many participants. Intergenerational exercise programs, pairing children, high school, and/or college students with older adults, can motivate both generations and help to bridge communication gaps between the generations. Awards can sometimes keep people motivated to continue an exercise program. The President's Council on Physical Fitness and Sports sponsors the Sports Fitness Awards for participation in more than 70 different categories (telephone 800-780-4048). Fitness assessments can also serve as motivators if fitness levels are improved or maintained.

► SUMMARY

As the rate of population growth of older adults continues to exceed that of younger people, as surveys indicate the relative lack of exercise participation by older adults, and as research continues to verify the value of exercise to the health of older adults, it is paramount that qualified exercise professionals keep up with the need for sound exercise programs. Fortunately, numerous resources are available to assist this endeavor. The volume of research on exercise and older adults is growing. Governmental and volunteer health agencies are on board in the movement to increase exercise among older adults, and numerous professional organizations, such as ACSM, are focusing resources toward building a healthier, fitter population of older adults.

References

1. A profile of older Americans—1999. Washington: American Association of Retired Persons and Administration on Aging, 1999.
2. Bennett J, Carmach MA, Gardner VJ. The effect of a program of physical exercise on depression in older adults. Phys Educ 39:21–24, 1982.
3. Exercise Therapy for Patients With Psychiatric Disorders: Research and Clinical Implications. American Psychological Association. Online: http://www.apa.org/journals/pro/pro303275.html
4. Fiatarone M, Marks E, Ryan ND, et al. High-intensity strength training in nonagenarians. JAMA 263:3030–3034, 1990.
5. Mazzeo RS, Cavanagh P, Evans WJ, et al. Exercise and physical activity for older adults. Med Sci Sports Exerc 30:992–1008, 1998. Online: http://www.ms-se.com/
6. Paffenbarger RS, Hyde RT, Hsieh C, Wing AL. Physical activity, other life-style patterns, cardiovascular disease and longevity. Acta Med Scand (Suppl) 711:85–91, 1986.
7. Paffenbarger RS, Hyde RT, Wing AL, Hsieh C. Physical activity, all-cause mortality, and longevity of college alumni. N Engl J Med 314:605–613,1986.
8. Salles JF, Haskell WL, Wood PD, et al. Physical activity assessment methodology in the five-city project. Am J Epidemiol 121:91–106, 1985.
9. Leitzmann MF, Rimm EB, Willett WC, et al. Recreational physical activity and the risk of cholecystectomy in women. N Engl J Med 341:777–784, 1999.
10. Cristell M, Hutchinson KM, Allessio HM. Effects of exercise training on hearing ability. Scand Audiol 27:219–224, 1998.
11. Manson J, Alessio HM, Cristell M, Hutchinson KM. Does cardiovascular health mediate hearing ability? Med Sci Sports Exerc 26: 866–871, 1994.
12. Schnelle JF, MacRae PG, Giacobassi K, et al. Exercise with physically restrained nursing home residents maximizing benefits of restraint reduction. J Am Geriatr Soc 44:507–512, 1996.
13. Chodzko-Zajko WJ, ed. Physical Activity and Aging: Implications for Health and Quality of Life in Older Persons. President's Council on Physical Fitness and Sports Research Digest, Series 3, No. 4, Dec. 1998.
14. Spirduso WW. Physical dimensions of aging. Champaign, IL: Human Kinetics, 1995.
15. National Center for Chronic Disease Prevention and Health Promotion. Promoting Physical Activity: A Guide for Community Action. Champaign, IL: Human Kinetics, 1999.
16. World Health Organization. The Heidelberg Guidelines for Promoting Physical activity Among Older Adults 1:1–8, 1997. not a journal
17. Physical Activity and Health: A Report of the Surgeon General. Atlanta: National Center for Chronic Disease Prevention and Health Promotion, 1996.
18. Osness WH, ed. Exercise and Fitness for the Older Adult. Dubuque, IA: Kendall/Hunt, 1998.
19. Cotton RT, Ekerorth CJ, Yancy H, eds. Exercise for Older Adults: ACE's Guide for Fitness Professionals. San Diego: American Council on Exercise, 1998.
20. AHA/ACSM Joint statement: Recommendations for cardiovascular screening, staffing, and emergency policies at health/fitness facilities. 30:1009–1018, 1998. Online: http://www.ms-se.com/
21. Corbin DE, Metal-Corbin J. Reach for It: A Handbook of Health, Exercise and Dance Activities for Older Adults. Dubuque, IA: Eddie Bowers, 1997.
22. Exercise: A Guide from the National Institute on Aging and the National Aeronautics and Space Administration. Online: http://stellar.arc.nasa.gov/exerciseandaging/cover.html
23. Osness WH, Clark B, Hoeger W, et al., eds. Functional Fitness Assessment for Adults over 60 Years: A Field Based Assessment. Dubuque, IA: Kendall/Hunt, 1996.
24. Rikli RE, Jones CJ. Development and validation of a functional fitness test for community-residing older adults. J Aging Phys Act 7:129–161, 1999.
25. Rikli RE, Jones CJ. Functional Fitness Normative Scores for community-residing older adults, ages 60–94. J Aging Phys Act 7:162–181, 1999.

SECTION TWELVE
MODIFICATIONS OF HEALTH BEHAVIOR

SECTION EDITOR: Matt Herridge, PhD

1.5.0, 1.5.1, 1.5.4   2.5.1   4.5.2   5.50

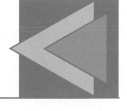

CHAPTER **62**

HEALTH COUNSELING SKILLS

Douglas R. Southard and Barbara H. Southard

Chapters in this section on psychology and behavior modification provide resource material useful to counselors in health and fitness settings. This initial chapter presents an overview and addresses interpersonal communication issues common to all health counseling environments. Chapter 63 examines the concept of adaptive versus maladaptive mechanisms of coping with life stressors. Chapter 64 describes common forms of psychopathology often associated with an inability to cope in an adaptive manner. Principles of modifying behavior, along with elements of stress management and social support, critical components in all lifestyle interventions, are presented in Chapters 65–67. The remaining chapters cover counseling issues specific to exercise promotion, dietary intervention, and smoking cessation.

HEALTH COUNSELING SKILLS

Counselors in health promotion settings serve four significant functions. The first is to **develop rapport and convey a sense of empathy** for the challenges participants confront in making and maintaining lifestyle changes. The second function is to **assess health-related behaviors** with respect to the effect on optimal functioning and risk of disease, which includes understanding the perspective of the participant on how these behaviors contribute to health and quality of life. This second function also includes **assessing the state of readiness for change**. The third function is to **facilitate change** through discussion of potential benefits and problems associated with implementing a lifestyle change. This function allows participants to make informed decisions consistent with personal values. Finally, the counselor is in a key position to assist the participant in **managing transient life crises**, which may include allowing the participant to ventilate feelings while skillfully expressing empathy. The counselor must also know enough about psychopathology to identify participants needing referral for further evaluation and possible treatment.

Function 1: Developing Rapport and Conveying Empathy

Acceptance

The counselor should set a tone of openness and acceptance during initial conversations with the participant. It is particularly important to refrain from appearing to make judgments about lifestyle or health history. Such a perception on the part of the participant may affect the type of information the participant is willing to disclose and/or the accuracy of the information. To behave neutrally is not easy, particularly if values conflict, as is often the case in the area of health behaviors. Therefore, it is important for the counselor to separate personal values and beliefs from those of the participant. Only then can the counselor respond in an objective and empathic manner, both verbally and nonverbally.

Expressing Empathy Through Active Listening

Empathy has been defined as the ability to understand people from their frame of reference rather than your own (1). Cold, unempathic counselors tend to skip over events that are distressing the patient (e.g., recent death of an old friend, marital discord) to focus on the "important" clinical issues (e.g., what was your heart rate when you exercised yesterday?). Failure to acknowledge the importance of personal events in the life of a participant can diminish understanding of the emotional state and its effect on health-related behaviors.

There are a number of barriers to discussing such sensitive issues for both participants and counselors (2). These may include cultural expectations that the interview focus on medical issues only, logistical concerns about wasting time, and personal preferences not to address emotional issues. To be an effective counselor, however, the practitioner must make an effort to understand what the person feels and convey to the participant that desire to comprehend.

Empathy can be conveyed through the use of active listening responses. This entails having participants describe experiences, after which the counselor responds by rephrasing what has been said. Such paraphrasing ensures that the counselor has made an accurate interpretation and also conveys that the counselor is attempting to listen and understand what is being said. For example, a counselor might respond to complaints by saying, "You seem frustrated with not being able to jog as fast as you would like." This response is particularly effective, as it identifies and reflects the emotional component of the experience. Such statements facilitate the development of rapport and self-disclosure.

In contrast, expressing sympathy conveys an attempt to share another's feelings (e.g., "I've had the same thing happen to me") or to imply pity for the experience (e.g., "I'm sorry you are having a problem"). Although such responses are useful in some limited situations, in general counselors should be careful not to convey that their personal experiences are exactly the same as the participant's or that an expression of sympathy is only given because it is socially appropriate. However, an empathic response is almost always helpful.

Active listening can also be conveyed through the use of questions designed to clarify a statement or probe for additional information. For example, a participant may say, "I've tried to stop smoking, but every time I do I gain a ton of weight and go right back to smoking again anyway. The only thing I change is my weight, and that's not a good change."

A clarifying response would be, "When you say a ton of weight, just how much do you mean?" A more probing response would be, "Can you tell me how you tried to stop smoking? Did you take a class, use a transdermal patch, or go cold turkey?"

At times, the counselor may wish to summarize the interview with the intention of identifying a general theme or succinctly rephrasing a story. Using the smoking example, a summarizing response might be, "So you've tried unsuccessfully to stop smoking, and as a result you weigh more than before you tried to quit." Alternatively, an interpretative response may be used. An interpretative response offers insight regarding the problem that goes beyond what has been stated. For example, an interpretative response to the same example would be, "You've tried to quit smoking, ended up gaining weight, and now maybe you're a little afraid that if you try again, you'll end up gaining even more weight." Interpretations are a little riskier than summarizing statements and generally are used once good rapport and a comfortable counseling relationship has been established.

Nonverbal Communication

Communication between counselor and participant includes both verbal and nonverbal components. Although the verbal portion of a message is often easiest to describe, the nonverbal component is also extremely important (1). Nonverbal communication, such as maintaining good eye contact, is essential to the development of rapport and expression of empathy. Humans respond to nonverbal communication, even if they are not specifically aware of what they are sensing and responding to. Experienced counselors, however, are particularly alert to seeing and hearing nonverbal communication. For example, when asked about his diet, a participant may report, "I kept up with it fairly well." The verbal report may suggest that the participant is doing well. However, poor eye contact, inflections in the tone of voice, and hesitant, low-energy speech may suggest that compliance with the prescribed diet was less than fairly good. Such incongruence between verbal and nonverbal components should prompt the counselor to consider a gentle, inquisitive confrontation regarding the issue (e.g., "You say you are keeping up with your diet, but you seem hesitant when talking about it. I'm wondering if you could share with me any problems you might be having.").

Nonverbal communication can be divided into three main categories. **Kinesics** refers to body movements that convey information, such as eye contact, hand gestures, winking, body position, and facial expressions. Poor eye contact, extremely low levels of body movement, or a flat or sad facial expression are particularly important cues. Characteristics of speech, such as voice inflections and changes in volume, are collectively referred to as **paralinguistics.** These characteristics often modify the meaning of the verbal content. The example at the beginning of this section, in which the voice inflection conflicts with verbal statements regarding dietary compliance, provides an example of how important it is to be aware of paralinguistics to understand the complete message.

Finally, characteristics of interpersonal space, such as seating arrangements and interpersonal distance, are included in the nonverbal component of **proxemics.** Awareness of proxemics is vital to achieving an atmosphere conducive to successful counseling. For example, a participant is more likely to feel comfortable during individual counseling when the counselor uses a small private room where there are minimal barriers (e.g., having only the corner of a desk rather than a large desk between counselor and participant) and where the chairs, temperature, noise level, and so on are comfortable and appropriate. In a group counseling session, the room should be larger to accommodate more people. In addition, a room that is noisy or lacking in privacy may hinder open sharing and communication. The counselor should arrange chairs in a circle so that all participants can make eye contact with each other to facilitate open discussion.

Function 2: Assessing Health-Related Behaviors
Behavioral Assessment

The importance of obtaining a comprehensive history of health-related behaviors cannot be overemphasized. In addition to self-report, a particularly useful strategy for gathering data during the assessment phase is to have the participant track or self-monitor health behaviors, preferably in a graphic format over a prescribed period. It may also be helpful to involve family members and significant others in the interview process. Frequently, people close to the participant have valuable insight into health behaviors and can provide information that the participant may not be aware of or is not able, willing, or ready to disclose. Thus, these supplementary sources often fill in holes in what a counselor has been able to glean. Such input can also provide the counselor with a better understanding of the social environment in which the participant will attempt to make lifestyle changes.

Motivational Assessment

Health-related behaviors must be understood in the context of the values and overall lifestyle of the participant. Whereas one cannot motivate individuals directly, one can appeal to what motivates them. Motivations for health-related behavior change may not be the same for the participant and the health professional. The challenge is to find common ground where health-enhancing recommendations also meet a participant's goal. For instance, the counselor may suggest a regimen of regular aerobic exercise to increase cardiopulmonary endurance. The initial response may be a lack of perception of a significant need to engage in such activity, since the participant can perform most daily activities. Careful questioning, however, may reveal that the participant discontinued hunting several years ago because of lack of strength and endurance. In this case, the task would be to connect the need for cardiopulmonary endurance with the desire to participate once again in a valued recreational activity. Once this match is realized and appreciated, the task is to help the participant develop clear goals and a well-designed program to achieve them within a specific time.

Function 3: Facilitating Change
Counselor's Role

The task of the counselor is to facilitate change rather than simply to prescribe it. Thus, the counselor and participant should work together to discuss, develop, and agree on a plan for change. In doing so, the counselor should be wary of the tendency to overwhelm the participant with a barrage of verbal instructions and written materials designed to promote compliance. Simplicity is often a key to success.

During this partnership the counselor should always keep in mind that the ultimate goal for the participant is to accept and maintain responsibility for personal behavior. Dependency on the counselor is a real threat to long-term maintenance, one that is not readily apparent to those new to the counselor role. Therefore, it is critical that the counselor encourage independence. For example, the counselor may facilitate social support and link rewards for success to family and friends rather than solely to the counselor. In addition, the participant must be encouraged to accept personal responsibility for making the change and solving related problems that arise on a day-to-day basis.

In preparing for behavior change, it is often helpful to assist the participant in identifying all of the benefits as well as the costs of the behavior change. Consider having the participant list the benefits on one side and costs on the other side of a piece of paper. Then ask the individual to compare and to determine whether the benefits truly outweigh the costs. The role of the counselor during this process is to help the participant explore all of the possibilities in terms of costs and benefits, including those that have not been considered. Once they are identified, discussion can be focused on methods to decrease the costs and improve the benefits. Unfortunately, although this exercise puts the behavior change into perspective and provides a frame of reference that can be used to advantage during difficult times in the process, it is often bypassed in the haste to get on with the behavior change. For instance, the written list can be saved for use during relapse, when the participant may have lost perspective, to bring back the original frame of reference in terms of the cost–benefit ratio.

Participants often have mixed feelings regarding the adoption of a new behavior (e.g., exercise) or cessation of a valued behavior (e.g., smoking, high-fat diet). It is therefore fairly common to hear a participant say, "I want to lose weight," only later to admit that he or she doesn't want to change eating habits. When the counselor suspects a conflict, gentle confrontation may be a very useful technique. This entails restating the two conflicting points and probing for clarification. For example, "Mary, I need you to help me. You've said that you really want to exercise more often and that 5:30 P.M. is the best time for you. Still, you rarely are able to make it. What are you saying to yourself when you are making the decision not to exercise?" Although an extremely useful technique, confrontation, if not carefully worded, can be uncomfortable for both participant and counselor. Hence, gentle confrontation is generally employed once rapport has been established. Chapter 64 provides an overview of additional techniques relevant to modifying health-related behaviors.

Working in Groups

Group counseling is an alternative or supplement to individual counseling. Groups can be designed specifically for the efficient conveyance of information or for a combination of information and social support. Some groups address a variety of related issues (e.g., ongoing cardiac rehabilitation support group); others are more time limited and focused on a specific topic (e.g., weight loss, anger control). Small-group formats offer several advantages over individual counseling. First and foremost is social support. Participants sometimes receive information and advice better from other participants than from professional counselors. They may also see themselves in other participants and begin to understand their own problems. Participants can also offer important feedback to other group members in a way that counselors cannot. Additionally, a small group allows participants to give support, encouragement, feedback, and so on, in an altruistic manner, a gesture that has significant psychological benefit (3).

Powerful as these small groups can be, it is important that the counselor be prepared to deal with problems that may arise. This requires informing the group from the beginning of the rules of confidentiality, instructing them to speak about their own challenges using "I" statements, and cautioning them against giving extensive advice to others on how to solve their problems.

Function 4: Managing Transient Life Crises
Types of Crises

Counselors in health and fitness settings routinely encounter participants in one or more life crises. Some of the more common types include interpersonal stress involving spouse, family, and significant others; financial stress involving changes in job status or outstanding medical bills; crises due to loss of health or function; and crises involving legal problems (see Chapters 63 and 64). Crisis management can be conceptualized as a series of five basic steps.

1. Listen actively and express empathy. Do not take responsibility for or try to solve problems quickly unless related to a safety issue under your control.
2. Assess for imminent danger (harm to self or others). Notify appropriate authorities or refer to other health care providers as necessary.
3. Assist the client in clarifying problems and identifying options.
4. Facilitate the development of a plan of action using individual, family, community, and/or professional resources.
5. Follow up with the participant in person or by phone to determine the effectiveness of your counseling and/or referral.

Managing Crises in Small Groups

While groups offer an excellent environment for facilitating behavior change, they may be uncomfortable for both counselor and participants if significant emotional distress is present. Episodes of crying, anger outbursts, and interpersonal conflict are particularly uncomfortable. Knee-jerk reactions either to ignore the event or to take immediate action to restore a peaceful environment may

not be the most effective. Rather, it may be more appropriate to use active listening skills that focus on the process (e.g., "John, this seems to make you angry" or "Helen, you seem upset when talking about this issue") and to acknowledge that such feelings are reasonable and/or acceptable (e.g., "it's OK to cry; these are difficult issues"). Tissues should be available in case they are needed. Interpersonal conflict within the group can also be openly acknowledged; however, it is essential to minimize escalation through the use of facilitator input (e.g., "Bob, can you describe what it is about Henry's behavior that bothers you without verbally attacking him?").

▶ SUMMARY

Health counselors can enhance the development of rapport and facilitate behavior change through the use of active listening responses and by paying careful attention to nonverbal and verbal forms of communication. Assessment of health-related behaviors should include self-monitoring data and reports from significant others when possible. It is also important to identify and appeal to aspects of the behavior change that the participant finds inherently motivating. Counselors can facilitate change by gently confronting participants when they express conflicting thoughts or feelings regarding behavior. Long-term success is increased when counselors promote self-reliance and emphasize the development of problem solving skills. Counselors also have an important role in assisting individuals as they attempt to make behavior changes while coping with common life crises. Therapeutic success can be enhanced through the use of small-group work as a supplement or alternative to individual counseling.

References
1. Cormier WH, Cormier LS. Interviewing Strategies for Helpers: Fundamental Skills and Cognitive Behavioral Interventions. Pacific Grove, CA: Brooks/Cole, 1993.
2. Egener B. Empathy. In: Feldman MD, Christensen JF, eds. Behavioral Medicine in Primary Care: A Practical Guide. Stamford, CT: Appleton & Lange, 1997:8–14.
3. Yalom ID. The Theory and Practice of Group Psychotherapy. 3rd ed. New York: Basic Books, 1985.

Suggested Reading
Coulehan JL, Block MR. The Medical Interview: Mastering Skills for Clinical Practice. 3rd ed. Philadelphia: FA Davis, 1997.
Lewis JA, Sperry L, Carlson J. Health Counseling. Pacific Grove, CA: Brooks/Cole, 1993.
Sotile WM. Psychosocial Interventions for Cardiopulmonary Patients: A Guide for Health Professionals. Champaign, IL: Human Kinetics, 1996.

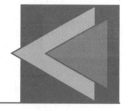

CHAPTER **63**

STRESS AND COPING

Wesley E. Sime and Kathryn Hellweg

From the moment of birth, humans experience a wide range of personal challenges that result in substantial physical and emotional stress. Physical stress (i.e., exertional and environmental stress) can be the stimulus for strength, endurance, and acclimatization when presented at an appropriate duration, frequency, and intensity. An overload of physical stress in any one or more of these dimensions, however, can cause illness or injury (e.g., arthritis, carpal tunnel syndrome, and back pain). In the same way, emotional stress can have positive or negative outcomes. In both forms of stress, it is the physical and emotional constitution of the individual, together with training and conditioning, that determine how well the individual adapts to a new stressor. In fact, total absence of physical or emotional challenge is neither optimal nor healthy.

Healthy, vibrant working adults who become ill suddenly and unexpectedly (e.g., cardiac patients) are likely to be highly stressed. The change in lifestyle (e.g., diet, exercise), temporary limitations in work capability and threat to the identity (e.g., loss of a sense of physical prowess) induced by the sudden change in health status are substantive stressors. For men in particular, the ego-threatening compromise in physical ability can be devastating and depressing. Many patients become self-conscious about the medical attention required and resist acknowledging the disease state. Family members who sincerely express concern and put forth reminders to help the patient follow medical orders or maintain limits or restrictions on eating and working may become the target of angry, defensive reactions.

Family members are likely to have a variety of emotional responses, ranging from fear of losing a close relative to irritability over failure to follow prescribed behavioral changes. Special efforts are recommended to provide emotional support for spouses and to elicit their cooperation in both understanding the patient and in reinforcing positive behavioral changes as needed. Social support

from family and friends has a buffering effect on cardiovascular response (e.g., reduced blood pressure and heart rate) to stressful challenges (1, 2).

This chapter describes many healthy and appropriate stress coping principles, including the accurate appraisal of an undesirable event (e.g., a heart attack) as a means of developing physical and emotional hardiness and participation in a well-designed rehabilitation program. Some of these principles are based on pioneering work on the psychophysiological effects of stress and the stress-reducing effects of exercise (36).

STRESS AS A CHALLENGE FOR POSITIVE OR NEGATIVE OUTCOMES

Considerable empirical experience shows that a program of progressively increasing emotional or cognitive challenge is both healthy and invigorating. Individuals who are confronted with reasonable task demands and who meet such demands usually feel personally satisfied as well as better able to cope with new challenges. The ability to adapt to new circumstances and to cope with apparent threats is most important for emotional as well as physical health, especially cardiovascular health. "The coping process has been described as one of constant change in cognitive and behavioral reactions to manage external or internal demands that the individual appraises as taxing to existing resources" (8).

Coping with stress can be either positive or negative (Figure 63.1). Using a work stress model, this figure shows how a healthy, capable employee who is beset by overwhelming burdens, challenges, or demands can emerge from the travail successfully with increased confidence, higher self-esteem, and a sense of hardiness gained from having faced a difficult challenge and being committed to having a positive outcome. The figure also shows how the person who views the task as burdensome, who gains little satisfaction from the work, who worries

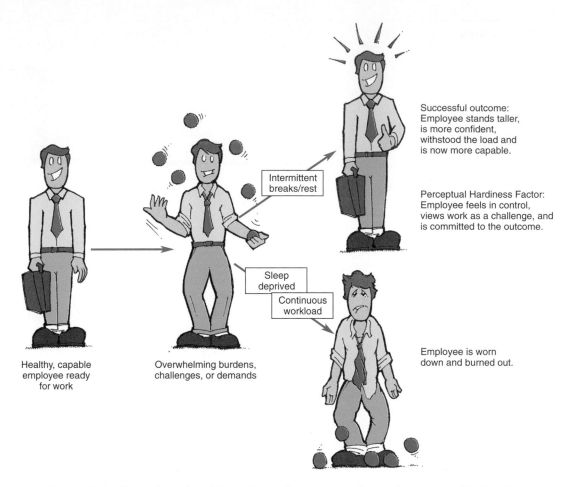

Figure 63.1. Illustration of positive and negative outcomes in reaction to stressful situations.

and frets and gets little substantive relaxation (i.e., recreation), and who may also be sleep-deprived is more likely to burn out. While the model presented in this illustration is oversimplified, it provides patients with a clear picture of the effects of overwork coupled with little personal satisfaction.

The concept of emotional stress or distress is controversial, partly because the stimulus load of the stressful event or circumstance is difficult to describe objectively. In exertional and environmental stress, the units of load are clear and generally universal (e.g., foot-pounds, kilocalories, and atmospheric pressure); in humans, however, emotional load is determined in part by personal interpretation, which is influenced greatly by personality and experience. Personality variables can be assessed objectively and are discussed in detail throughout this chapter. However, experiences are more difficult to assess objectively and vary widely with the degree of traumatization and accumulation over time. For example, some individuals exhibit remarkable tolerance for prior traumas, while others are extremely sensitive to even a single distressing event (e.g., events causing embarrassment, terror, anger, or hopelessness), allowing it to cause substantial distress.

Individual variation in coping styles may account for variations in sensitivity to stressful events. The response to stress may be unique. Ordinarily, a stressful circumstance may be thought of as an immediate threat or acute challenge. For a cardiac patient, the stress is initially acute because of the fear of death. The initial period is followed by the long-term uncertainty of other possible compromises (e.g., inability to work) and complications. A heart attack is perhaps most worrisome to patients because a quick and fatal incident is always a serious possibility. The irony is that when patients worry about future ills and when they are prone to emotional outbursts, their risk of coronary disease increases (9). As a result, it is extremely important to make patients aware of the risks associated with acute and chronic stress exposure and help them develop coping skills.

COPING WITH STRESS

A number of situational and personality factors influence the appraisal of stress. A description of factors associated with job stress is provided in Tables 63.1 and 63.2. These items are presented as a concept (e. g., novelty) fol-

Table 63.1. Situational Factors That Influence Appraisal of Stress Using Job Stress Examples

SITUATIONAL FACTORS	DESCRIPTION	EXAMPLE
Novelty (with negative history)	Facing a new situation with a history of harm, danger, or loss in similar experiences	New job assignment while having been embarrassed or failed in previous assignments
Predictability (consequence, no control)	Recognizing warning signals of impending threat without option to prevent it	Seeing indications that a bad outcome may result from a new job assignment
Imminent threat with time to worry	Knowing that harm, danger, or loss will likely occur, but not knowing when it will occur	Receive notice that job layoffs are expected in the near future
Incubation period and length of exposure	Time prior to stressful event and duration of exposure	Job layoffs will occur in 30 days and may last 3–6 months or longer
Anticipation of a time limited event	Not knowing when an event is going to occur, but knowing that it won't last very long	Rumors that a layoff is inevitable in the near future, but layoffs never last more than a week or two
Acute versus chronic exposure	Immediate short-term exposure contrasted with regular intermittent threats of extended losses	Taking a cut in pay to obtain a stable, secure job versus keeping a lucrative job risking frequent layoffs
Situational ambiguity	Lack of clarity or insufficient information to make an appraisal of degree of threat	Rumors threaten job security, but no one knows which areas will be affected

Adapted with permission from Lazarus R, Folkman S. Stress, Appraisal and Coping. New York: Spring, 1984:55–115.

Table 63.2. Personality Factors that Influence Appraisal of Stress Using Job Stress Examples

PERSONALITY FACTORS	DESCRIPTION	EXAMPLE
Personal uncertainty	Confusion in one's mind about the meaning of the warning signals or the degree of threat	Received notice of promotion or transfer, but not able to evaluate the risks versus the benefits
Commitment and risk-taking	Level of drive, determination, motivation, investment, persistence, planning, e.g., will to live	Making the choice to continue battling against adversity despite being vulnerable to embarrassment or disappointment
Belief system	Perceptual lens through which the events or circumstances are viewed and interpreted	Interpreting new opportunities in light of past experiences, personal values, etc.
Cognitive appraisal	The evaluation process of taking inventory; assessing loss or gain and options for future risk	Lost my job, but what advantages, disadvantages, result, e.g., more time to look for better job or to start a new business or profession
Stress coping	Individuals differ widely in sensitivity and vulnerability to various exposures to stressful circumstances	Anger, depression, anxiety, denial, guilt, challenge, vengefulness, persistence, helplessness

Adapted with permission from Lazarus R, Folkman S. Stress, Appraisal and Coping. New York: Spring, 1984:55–115.

lowed by a description (e.g., a new situation complicated by negative experiences in similar situations) and an example of how each factor influences the ability to cope with stress in a job setting. The situational factors include novelty, predictability, imminent threat (with time available to worry), incubation, exposures, anticipation of time-limited events, acute versus chronic exposure, and ambiguity.

The personality factors that influence the degree of stress reaction include the following:

- Personal uncertainty (confusion)
- Commitment and risk taking
- Personal belief system (perception)
- Cognitive appraisal (taking inventory of advantages, disadvantages, and options when facing a crisis)

- Inherent stress coping strategies (denial versus feeling guilty; challenged versus feeling helpless).

People can have situational ambiguity, but know exactly what decision to make when the stressor occurs; that is, an individual can have situational ambiguity without personal uncertainty. The greater the situational ambiguity, the more strongly personality factors influence the effect of stressful situations. Careful examination of the job examples (Table 63.1) reveals a wide variety of unique individual outcomes that emanate from the peculiar threat of each situational and personality variable as it relates to job security. Many cardiac patients have a history of high job stress preceding the onset of disease and can expect some difficulty returning to the same level of job performance after treatment (10).

The relationship of stress to illness includes a critical role for cognitive appraisal. As described by Lazarus et al., it is the foundation of the specificity of illness model, which suggests that any personal environmental stressor is first mediated by individual appraisal, which then determines the extent to which physiological disturbance and possibly illness occur (11). Emotions vary with the way an individual constructs and evaluates events or relationships in light of personal goals and expectations. Conflicts and adverse events affect the individual to the degree that cognitive interpretation of the event allows. This theory serves as the basis for several stress management techniques presented in Chapter 66 (2).

INHERENT STRESS COPING REACTIONS

Several additional inherent stress coping reactions distinguish stress coping from coping techniques specifically used to change attitudes or behaviors to manage stress. The limited discussion in this chapter focuses on denial, emotion-focused coping, problem-focused coping, and social-focused coping.

Denial

Interestingly, denial is sometimes a healthy response to stress. While denial appears to be negative and unproductive (i.e., a closed-minded effort to minimize the problem), it has a few benefits. For example, if no constructive solution to an immediate problem is possible, denial can temporarily alleviate distress. In the instance of an anticipated job layoff, for example, worry becomes needless if no immediate action can be taken. Denial can also be viewed as a strange mode of positive thinking (it will never happen to me), as long as it does not interfere with the ability to perform necessary job functions. On the other hand, denial is risky for cardiac patients when it precludes an early diagnosis and proper treatment. Regardless, denial can be beneficial as long as necessary therapy and medications are not neglected.

Emotion-Focused Coping

Emotion-focused coping is one of several natural reactions to an overwhelmingly stressful experience. Classic examples of emotion-focused coping include anger (toward self or others), avoidance, rationalization, rejection, and distancing. These are nonphysical, passive responses to stress; however, it is possible that an active response, such as exercise, may facilitate emotional coping. For example, exercise allows patients to distance themselves from stressful issues and allows them to work through their thoughts while working off physical tension. If anger is the predominant emotion, then some form of ballistic, vigorous exercise (e.g., punching a bag or stomping on a stair climber) can help dissipate the tension associated with emotion. Ironically, some individuals seem to need

to embellish an angry response before the stressor can be overcome and recovery ensues. Relief comes only after a period of self-blame or self-punishment that allows the individual to fully experience the distress.

Problem-Focused Coping

Problem-focused coping is a far more appropriate means of responding to a crisis or any seriously distressing situation when a solution is available. The process includes both external and internal analysis. The **external analysis** includes the following steps:

1. Defining the problem
2. Generating alternative solutions
3. Weighing the alternatives
4. Choosing the best alternative

The internal analysis, which is designed for introspection of inherent self-defeating attitudes and behaviors, involves the following steps:

1. Changing goals to eliminate the problem
2. Reducing ego involvement in the outcome
3. Learning new skills to overcome the problem
4. Developing new behaviors and new reinforcers to maintain those behaviors

These essential steps in crisis management should be offered as a part of the rehabilitation process.

Social-Focused Coping

Social-focused coping includes other people in the coping process. It also requires a minimum level of social skills. Individuals must be able to express their needs effectively and behave somewhat appropriately to elicit the cooperation and support that is required. This method of coping also tends to generate problem-solving options and facilitates the use of group activity to negotiate potential solutions. One critical issue is to determine whether a personality problem tends to bring on unnecessary challenges. If so, a referral to a psychologist or family counselor may be appropriate.

Interpretation, personality, and experience cloud the ability to measure emotional workloads or the demands of a particular task or experience. Therefore, the combination of physical, behavioral, cognitive, and emotional responses to a realistic stressor becomes the only measurable factor in the stress–illness equation, with physical and behavioral responses being the most objective and reliable factors.

OBJECTIVE INDICATORS OF FAILURE TO COPE

Physical responses indicating failure to cope include measures common in cardiac rehabilitation (e.g., increased heart rate, blood pressure, rate–pressure product) and other less familiar parameters of heart health (e.g., peripheral resistance, peripheral blood flow, electrodermal response, and electromyography). Other common physical signs and symptoms of stress are listed in Chapter 5 (12).

The most common and observable behavioral indicators of inadequate stress coping skills include irritability, fear, anger, anxiety, and depression. To some extent, these phenomena are observable and as such can be recorded and documented in event-provoked circumstances, such as a structured interview for type A behavior patterns. Similarly, depression can be measured objectively through observation during an interview or by using a psychological screening instrument, such as the Beck Depression Inventory (13). Staff who suspect depression should refer the patient to a psychologist for testing and possible counseling, since depression is an important predictor of survival (14). For a comprehensive assessment, the entire array of behavioral and cognitive–emotional elements of stress can be determined through self assessment using a battery of questionnaires, such as the state–trait measures of anxiety, anger, hostility, self-deception, type A personality, and hardiness (Table 63.3).

Self-reports of stress coping are often influenced by situational factors and are subject to personal openness, honesty, and perceptual awareness. More specifically, some individuals fail to report behaviors that appear to be socially undesirable or reflect badly upon their character. Others are candidly honest, but inaccurate in their reporting, failing to report certain moods (e.g., depression) and behaviors (e.g., hostility) that are obvious to others, but not to themselves. Thus, it is important to interview the spouse and perhaps other family members to obtain more detailed information about the true coping ability of the individual in stress to determine the role of personality in the disease process.

STRESS HARDINESS AND COPING

Hardiness is an internal resource facilitating resistance to stress. This personality construct applies to individuals who have a sense of commitment and a feeling of control, which allows them to view problems as mere challenges. Recent evidence suggests that hardiness is a valid indicator of long-term psychosocial adjustment in patients with coronary heart disease (15).

Several discrete personality subtypes (hardy, distressed, inhibited, repressed) have also been useful in predicting future risk of coronary heart disease (16). Hardy individuals tend to use active coping techniques; they are self-assured and resilient, which helps them to adjust easily to stressful difficulties. A higher risk of heart disease is found in individuals who are distressed (dissatisfied with self and others), inhibited (insecure and low in self-expression), or repressed (avoid confrontation and deny emotions). Overall, the difference between hardy individuals and others seems to lie in their appraisal of adverse events. In hardy individuals, events appraised as less threatening and more controllable elicit less stress reactivity (9). Likewise, hardy individuals tend to have a strong sense of coherence, such that life circumstances are relatively comprehensible, manageable, and meaningful for them (17).

Table 63.3. Measures of Stress and Coping Appropriate for Cardiac Rehabilitation Patients

State–trait anxiety (23)	State anxiety is the acute experience of distress at the moment, while trait anxiety is the tendency to feel anxious in general for no apparent reason.
Depression (13)	Feeling dejected, with loss of interest and possible change in weight, appetite, increased fatigue, agitation, fatigue guilt, shame, low self-esteem, and self-destructive tendencies.
State–trait anger (23)	The short-term immediate reaction to a provocation eliciting an emotional response is state anger. By contrast, the tendency to hold back the outward expression of severe disgruntlement and to turn the expression of anger inward is the trait anger measure.
Hostility measures (25)	The experience of severe annoyance and anger compounded by profound verbal display or cynicism portrayed with resentment, unpleasantness, and discourteousness.
Shapiro Control Inventory (17)	Patients who feel in control or having the ability to gain control as needed versus those who fear losing control, have no control, emotions, ability, power, etc.
Jenkins Activity Survey-Questionnaire (26)	Assessment of type A behavior pattern featuring three essential components: 1. Speed and impatience 2. Hard driving and aggressiveness 3. High job involvement
The Stress Profile (21)	The Stress Profile is a comprehensive measurement instrument that features elements of personal vulnerability to stress as well as strengths in coping by emotion-focused and problem-focused methods. It includes an appraisal of the patients' work stress situation.
Kobasa's Hardiness Scale (27)	The concept of hardiness is defined as an internal resource facilitating stress resistance. This personality construct describes individuals who have three important personality qualities: (1) a sense of commitment, (2) a feeling of control, and (3) the ability to view problems as mere challenges.

FACILITATING RESILIENCE AND STRESS COPING CONTROL

The amount of stress induced by a heart attack or a recent diagnosis of cardiac disease may vary with several personality factors. For some individuals, the fear of dying may compound the reaction to ordinary treatment and therapy; for others, a heart attack or surgery may be an acceptable reason to avoid a noxious job or strong justification for needing help with a marginally unbearable workload. As such, the convalescence period may produce some unintentionally rewarding experiences, known commonly as secondary gain. Initially, a patient may be in emotional shock due to a crisis that occurs without warning. Form a psychological standpoint, the patient may feel helpless, panicky, and confused, then tend to go through withdrawal and denial. Hopefully, during the recovery phase, there will be an opportunity for reality testing, wherein the best and the worst of the situation are recognized so that a healthy recovery can be pursued.

In general, coping is described as the continuous process of adjusting thoughts and behaviors to avoid, manage, or ignore some form of threat or challenge (Fig. 63.1). Unfortunately, numerous inherent constraints can compromise effectiveness of coping, including fear of public embarrassment; fear of failure; fear of success; feeling helpless, guilty, or distrustful; and not wanting to appear needy. In the worst cases, some individuals are so personally conscientious that they never seek assistance because they would feel obliged to return the assistance, and the sense of personal indebtedness is simply intolerable.

Issues of control or lack thereof also tend to compromise the effectiveness of various coping instincts. Some individuals have a greater need for control than others, especially when coping with stress. Some interesting manifestations of control must be considered in light of coping among patients.

1. Primary control is an attempt to change the environment.
2. Secondary control is an effort to fit in better.
3. Predictive control involves guessing about future risks to avoid distress.
4. Illusory control involves aligning with the most likely outcome to share in the success for stress relief.
5. Interpretive control involves developing a logical rationale, so that understanding why bad things happen provides some stress relief.
6. Vicarious control involves becoming associated with other powerful influences to share in their success.

Efforts to assess several dimensions of control related to cardiovascular risk have been made (18). Some individuals have a sense of either being in control or having the ability to gain control as needed. At the other extreme are individuals who have either a fear of losing control or a sense of having no control over such things as emotions, ability, and power. The Shapiro Control Inventory describes four specific dimensions of controlling behavior:

- Positive assertive (decisive leader)
- Negative assertive (manipulative or overcontrolling)
- Negative yielding (timid, indecisive)
- Positive yielding (trusting, accepting)

Unfortunately, no single homogeneous control profile in cardiovascular disease has been clarified; rather, several combinations of these profiles are associated with increased risk (18).

Patients often feel out of control following a heart attack or bypass surgery. However, those who view a problem as a challenge and who feel commitment to family and a sense of control over their destiny are most likely to survive and thrive (19). Fortunately, it is possible to assess these and other psychosocial coping behaviors using a comprehensive stress profile in rehabilitation (20).

The Stress Profile is a comprehensive instrument that can elicit candid patient responses to personal and professional areas of concern for stress and coping (Fig. 63.2) (21). It is designed to screen both elements of personality that are vulnerable to stress and coping strengths while assessing work stress concerns. Results of the assessment are provided in graphic illustrations by category (psychosocial, work environment, family relationships, major life events, hassles versus satisfactions, self-perception, coherence, coping skills, stress reactions, and burnout). Each patient is encouraged to review the results with a staff member to confirm the accuracy of the assessment and to make a plan of action that reduces the causes of stress and enhances coping skills.

Several other complicating factors must be dealt with to strengthen coping behaviors. Many patients are emotionally challenged by exercise tolerance testing used for diagnosis and for exercise prescription. Even an exercise training program can be viewed as a stage for performance and evaluation. By comparison, these experiences are similar to having test anxiety. Fortunately, it has been possible to reduce test anxiety and improve performance (22).

Getting patients to communicate well and socialize among themselves may be one of the most important ways of reducing situational anxiety in the clinical testing and training environment. Finally, many patients have a legitimate fear of dying. While death is inevitable, it is often hard to recognize and accept the fact that cardiovascular function is compromised and that risk of death, in a number of months or years, is high.

STRESS PROFILE
Sample output

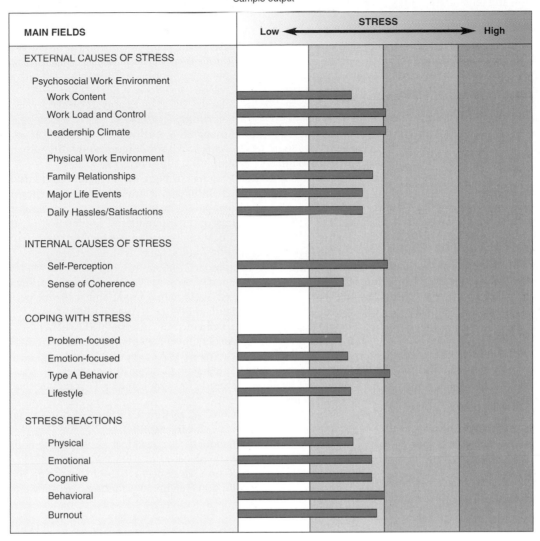

Figure 63.2. Main field output from the Stress Profile.

► SUMMARY

This chapter is an attempt to provide a realistic and meaningful discourse on the most relevant issues related to coping with stress. That stress is a challenge which can be met in widely diverging ways is clearly evident from the illustration in Figure 63.1. A variety of situational and personality variables (Tables 63.1 and 63.2) influence perception and appraisal of the degree to which a stressful event provokes a distressful outcome. Several inherent coping reactions (denial, emotion, social, and problem-focused coping) interact within persons, making them more or less vulnerable (or hardy) in the face of difficult circumstances. Recognizing the need for control (with positive and negative implications for assertiveness or manipulative behavior) among cardiac patients is critical to long-term survival. Last, the use of an interactive interview and a plan of action for coping with real-world stressors is strongly recommended.

References
1. Gerin W, Pickering T. Social support as moderator of cardiovascular reactivity: A test of the direct effects and buffering hypothesis. Proceedings of the Society of Behavioral Medicine Meeting. Boston, MA, April 1994.
2. Sotile W. Stress management. Resource manual for guidelines for exercise testing and prescription. In: Roitman J, ed. Resource Manual for Guidelines for Exercise Testing and Prescription. 3rd ed. Philadelphia: Lea & Febiger, 1998.

3. Sime W, McKinney M. Stress management applications in the prevention and rehabiliation of coronary heart disease. In: Blair S, Painter P, Pate R, et al., eds. Resource Manual for Guidelines for Exercise Testing and Prescription. Philadelphia: Lea & Febiger, 1988.

4. Sime W, McGahan M, Eliot R. Stress management and coronary heart disease: Risk assessment and intervention. In: Durstine JL, King A, Painter P, et al., eds. Resource Manual for Guidelines for Exercise Testing and Prescription. 2nd ed. Philadelphia: Lea & Febiger, 1993.

5. Sime W. Psychophysiologlcal (emotional) stress testing for assessing coronary risk. J Cardiovasc Pulm Tech 8:27, 1980.

6. Sime W. Psychological benefits of exercise. Adv Inst Health 1(4):15–29, 1984.

7. Reference deleted.

8. Lazarus R. Progress on a cognitive-motivational-relational theory of emotion. Am J Psychol 46:819–834, 1991.

9. Eliot RS. From Stress to Strength: How to Lighten Your Load and Save Your Life. New York: Bantam, 1994: 24–42.

10. Maschewsky W. Psychosocial working conditions in industry and coronary heart disease. Proceedings of the First International Symposium on Work Environment and Cardiovascular Disease. Copenhagen, Denmark, June 1995.

11. Lazarus R, Folkman S. Stress, Appraisal and Coping. New York: Springer, 1984:55–115.

12. Sime W, Eliot RS, Solberg EE. Stress and coronary heart disease: Epidemiology and risk assessment. In: Roitman JL et al, eds. Resource Manual for Guidelines for Exercise Testing and Prescription. 3rd ed. Baltimore: Williams & Wilkins, 1998.

13. Beck AT. Depression. Causes and Treatment. Philadelphia: University of Pennsylvania, 1972.

14. Frazure-Smith N, Lesperance F, Talajic M. Depression following myocardial infarction. JAMA 270:1819–1825, 1993.

15. Drory Y, Florian Y. Long-term psychosocial adjustment to coronary artery disease. Arch Phys Med Rehab 72:326–331, 1991.

16. Denollet J. Biobehavioral research on coronary heart disease: where is the person? J Behav Med 16:115–141, 1993.

17. Antonovsky A. Personality and health: Testing the sense of coherence model. In: Friedman HS, ed. Personality and Disease. New York: Wiley, 1990:155–177.

18. Shapiro DH. The Shapiro Control Inventory. New York: Behaviordyne, 1994.

19. Rosengren A, Orth-Gomor K, Wedel H, et al. Stressful life events social support and mortality in men born in 1933. BMJ 307:1102–1110, 1993.

20. Lisspers J, Hallgren D, Hallgren I, Setterlund S. Changes in rehabilitation factors after a comprehensive program for rehabilitation and secondary prevention of CHD. Proceedings of the International Conference on Stress and Health. Stockholm, Sweden, September 1996.

21. Setterlund S, Larsson G. The stress profile: A psychological approach to measuring stress. Stress Med 2:85–92, 1995.

22. Sime W, Ansorge C, Olson J, et al. Coping with math anxiety: Stress management and academic performance. J Coll Student Pers 28:421–437, 1987.

23. Spielberger CD, Gorsuch RL, Lushene R. The State–Trait Anxiety Inventory Manual. Palo Alto, CA: Consulting Psychologist, 1970.

24. Spielberger C, Grier K, Greenfield G. Major dimension of stress in law enforcement. Fl Frat Order Pol J 10–12, spring 1982.

25. Cook W, Medley D. Proposed hostility and phasic-virtue scales for the MMPI. J Appl Psych 38:414–418, 1954.

26. Jenkins C, Zyzanski S, Rosenman R. Jenkins Activity Survey Manual. New York: Psychological, 1979.

27. Kahn S. Fact Sheet for Third Generation Hardiness Test. Arlington Heights, IL: Hardiness Institute, 1986.

1.9.0

2.5.1

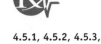
4.5.1, 4.5.2, 4.5.3,
4.5.4, 4.5.5

5.5.0, 5.5.1, 5.5.2

CHAPTER **64**

PSYCHOPATHOLOGY

C. Barr Taylor and Nancy Houston Miller

Exercise professionals encounter a variety of psychological issues and problems in leading and conducting exercise programs. Many of these problems affect not only participation, but also other aspects of the participant's life. This chapter provides an overview of some of the important issues and problems and discusses how to deal with them. Exercise professionals should be able to identify major psychopathological problems and provide referral as needed.

CRISIS

Perhaps the most general psychological event affecting participants in exercise programs is a personal crisis. A crisis can be defined as a usually brief period when demands of an event exceed the ability and resources to cope, leading to distress (1). People in crisis may feel hopeless, anxious, and tense. Other common feelings are fear, anger, guilt, embarrassment, and shame. The high level of anxiety often impedes thinking and impairs coping. A crisis is necessarily a very stressful period in life, and stress coping techniques, as described in Chapter 63, may be useful to help the patient cope.

The most common crises are situations such as physical illness, status and role change, rape, physical abuse, divorce, and loss of a loved one. People in crises should not be considered mentally ill, yet their distress should be taken seriously. Frasure-Smith and Prince (2) telephoned myocardial infarction patients on a regular basis following the event. Patients were assessed at each phone call with a brief psychological screen to determine level of distress. Those exhibiting extreme distress were visited at home and helped to deal with what was most commonly a crisis. This relatively simple intervention had significantly improved survival.

Determining whether a person is in crisis is usually not difficult, since most people show their distress. People may cope with a crisis by avoiding customary habits, such as attending an exercise program. Thus, unplanned absence may be caused by or indicate a crisis.

Crisis Management

There are four general steps in crisis management. The exercise professional should become familiar with these steps to assist patients with coping in crisis. The steps in crisis management:

- Psychosocial assessment
- Development of a plan
- Implementation of the plan
- Follow-up

Psychosocial Assessment

The purpose of assessment is to determine the origin of the problem and get a sense of the cause and how effectively the patient is coping. It is important to determine whether the individual has adequate resources (e.g., financial, social) to get through the crisis. Attempts should be made to determine whether an individual is suicidal or might harm someone else. The key risk factors for suicide are found in Table 64.1 (3).

Prediction of suicide is difficult, but the possibility should be entertained when any of the features listed in Table 64.1 are exhibited. If the exercise professional suspects depression or suicidal tendencies, the participant should be asked directly whether he or she is contemplating suicide. One might say, "You seem pretty down. Have you had any recent thoughts of hurting yourself or even killing yourself?" Participants with physical illness who feel helpless and hopeless are at particularly high risk for suicide. Any suggestion that suicide is a possibility should be followed up to determine the seriousness of the intent. A common belief is that asking about suicide may plant the idea; this is not true. An open discussion about suicidal feelings is helpful in and of itself and can set the stage for referral. Participants who are suicidal or dangerous and unable to take care of themselves should be referred for immediate professional treatment. Suicide crisis centers and community mental health centers can provide advice and recommendations about referral. Participants may also be taken to hospital emergency departments.

Table 64.1. Risk Factors For Suicide

1. Previous suicide attempt
2. Overt or indirect suicide talk or threats
3. Current plan for how to commit suicide
4. Has a means to commit suicide
5. Depressed mood
6. Significant recent loss, e.g., spouse, job
7. Unexpected change in behavior or attitude
8. Being elderly, male, isolated, with chronic illness
9. Sense of hopelessness, helplessness, loneliness, exhaustion, "unbearable" psychological pain
10. Alcohol or drug abuse or intoxication
11. Failing health, particularly if previously independent

One should ensure that there is an immediate safe place and transportation. Suicidal individuals should not transport themselves for treatment but rather should be accompanied.

Occasionally the exercise professional encounters a potentially violent patient or client. Some groups, such as young males, violent urban cultural subgroups, and alcohol or drug users or abusers, are at high risk for becoming violent. Individual predictors include history of violence, active use of alcohol, physical abuse as a child, and history of brain injury. All threats of violence should be taken seriously. The exercise professional must be willing to seek assistance from police as necessary for reasons of security and safety. Most crises, however, are not accompanied by emergencies. Further assessment includes answering questions such as these:

- To what extent has the crisis disrupted normal life patterns?
- Is the person able to hold a job?
- Can the person handle the responsibility of daily living?
- Has the crisis disrupted the lives of others?
- Has the crisis distorted perception of reality?
- Is the usual support system present, absent, or exhausted?
- What are the available resources?

Development of a Plan

Crisis management entails the development and assistance in management of a plan. For exercise professionals the focus is usually on referral and follow-up and on helping the person continue with an exercise program.

Implementation of the Plan

The third step in crisis management is drawing on personal, social, and material resources to help overcome the crisis. This role is usually left to the mental health professional; the role of the exercise professional is assistance with referral.

Follow-up

Continued support and reinforcement of the plan and support of positive actions are the final, critical stage of the plan. Support in the environment of the patient is important to maintaining the plan and to resolution of the crisis.

DEATH AND DYING

Most exercise programs have participants who lose or have lost a loved one. Grieving individuals are at increased risk for relapse to old habits, dropping out of exercise programs, illness, injury, and even death. Support from an exercise professional can help prevent or minimize these outcomes. The exercise professional should be aware of the basic processes affecting a grieving individual.

While the nature and course of grief are complex, individual, and strongly affected by background, psychology, culture, beliefs, and experience, many aspects of grieving are universal (4). Immediately upon loss of a loved one, grieving individuals appear emotionally numb, seeming to disbelieve the loss. This period is followed by pangs of grief—periods of crying and yearning—interspersed with longer periods of anxiety, despair, and a sense of unreality. The grieving person may feel anger, self-reproach, bewilderment, and many other emotions in the struggle to make sense of the loss. In addition, appetite falls off. Sometimes anxiety escalates to full-blown panic attacks or hyperventilation and despair to serious depression. The grieving person may have transitory hallucinations of the lost one being near at hand or even speaking to them. As time passes, the intensity and frequency of the grief diminish and there are longer periods of apathy and despair. The grieving person avoids thinking about the future and may remain disengaged. The death of a loved one forces most people to re-evaluate many of their assumptions and habits, and new roles have to be adopted. The transition to this new role is often resisted. Eventually, reorganization, recovery, and perhaps new insight and meaning take place.

The exercise professional should be aware of the course of changing moods during bereavement. Some studies suggest that those who repress grief are more likely to remain depressed and disabled than those who express it. The exercise professional should be supportive and communicative, allowing the expression of grief, but still respecting privacy. While there is no single normal grieving process, these symptoms or behaviors may indicate problems:

- Not exhibiting a sense of loss (at least in the first month or so after loss of the loved one)
- Symptoms of illness like those of the deceased
- Increase of psychosomatic illnesses
- Excessive withdrawal

- Excessive hostility or fury
- Deep depression

In fact, grieving individuals are at high risk for depression; grief is a significant risk factor for suicide. Exercise professionals may want to monitor how well the grieving participant is doing, particularly with respect to the final two domains. Participants who are having extreme trouble with grieving or exhibit depression or suicidal tendencies should be referred to mental health counselors.

Exercise programs may also have participants who are dying of a terminal illness or who die during the course of participation in the program. This is true especially when programs deal with medically ill populations. When deaths occur, the exercise professional should inform the group and perhaps acknowledge the contributions the participant brought. Support for those close to the participant is particularly important. Sending a sympathy card or a brief note to grieving family members may help bring closure.

PSYCHOSOCIAL ASSESSMENT

A general psychosocial assessment may be helpful in routine evaluation of participants. Some simple screening tools can help identify major problems. These tools can be followed up with more sophisticated instruments or assessments as required. Although the variety of important problems is wide, the general domains for assessment include the following:

- Depression
- Anxiety
- Drug and alcohol abuse
- Eating disorders
- Stress, coping, type A behavior
- Family and social support

One approach is the use of a simple screening tool that may help identify individuals requiring assistance. Table 64.2 provides an overview of a psychosocial screening tool used in the Stanford Cardiac Rehabilitation Program (5). A score of 5 or greater on the first four items indicates a possible problem requiring follow-up. Questions 7–10 are the CAGE questionnaire, an instrument widely used to screen for alcohol abuse (6). Two or more positive answers suggest alcohol abuse or dependence and indicate the need for follow-up. Follow-up clinical questions should be guided by criteria described hereafter. Questions 14 and 15 are used to determine degree of social isolation; however, there is no simple instrument that adequately assesses social isolation. Social isolation is often defined as the absence of social support. Social support includes emotional, physical, monetary, and instrumental (e.g., availability of transportation) support. Each of these domains should be assessed in anyone who may be isolated. The American As-

sociation of Cardiovascular and Pulmonary Rehabilitation (AACVPR) has published outcome measures for cardiac and pulmonary rehabilitation programs (7). Many of those described can be used to provide more information about depression, anxiety, and other psychological factors.

DEPRESSION

Depression affects 5–10% of adults during their lifetime (8, 9). In addition to feeling down, depression is often accompanied by somatic symptoms (Table 64.3). Depression following a myocardial infarction (MI) has been associated with poor prognosis, including increased mortality and morbidity (10–12). Depressed patients may exhibit psychomotor retardation, tearfulness, and a sad face. They often feel helpless and hopeless and express self-reproach. Especially relevant to assessment is that depression is frequently accompanied by suicidal feelings. Depressed patients should be asked if they have been feeling like hurting themselves or if they have been having suicidal thoughts, and if so, they should be referred for care, following the aforementioned guidelines for crises.

Hospitalization for psychiatric care is sometimes necessary, but more often depressed patients recover with outpatient professional help, medication, and the passage of time. The symptoms of depression make exercising difficult, but exercise appears to be beneficial (13).

Patients hospitalized with MI often feel depressed. This feeling usually resolves after return home. Moderate or worsening depression, persisting 2–3 weeks after returning home and resuming usual activities, requires further evaluation. Such patients should be considered for referral to a mental health professional or their primary care physician.

ANXIETY DISORDERS

Anxiety affects everyone at some time (14). Severe anxiety can lead to avoidance and restriction of activities and may be associated with severe depression and panic attacks. Acute anxiety can often be resolved with reassurance or brief periods of psychotherapy. Chronic anxiety is sometimes secondary to depression, but it may be a primary anxiety disorder. The three most common clinical anxiety disorders:

- Generalized anxiety disorder
- Panic disorder (with or without agoraphobia)
- Social phobia

Generalized anxiety disorder is characterized by excessive worry and signs of motor tension (e.g., trembling, muscle tension, restlessness), autonomic hyperactivity (e.g., sweating, dry mouth, and frequent urination), vigilance, and scanning (e.g., feeling keyed up or on edge all the time). Panic disorder is characterized by recurrent

Table 64.2. Psychosocial Questionnaire

Name _____ Date _____

For the first four questions, please circle a number on the scale following each item to show how much you are troubled now by each emotion.

1. Feeling miserable or depressed

1	2	3	4	5	6	7	8	9
Hardly		Slightly		Moderately		Markedly		Very Severely

2. Feeling irritable or angry

1	2	3	4	5	6	7	8	9
Hardly		Slightly		Moderately		Markedly		Very Severely

3. Feeling tense, anxious, or panicky

1	2	3	4	5	6	7	8	9
Hardly		Slightly		Moderately		Markedly		Very Severely

4. Feeling under stress or pressure at work or at home

1	2	3	4	5	6	7	8	9
Hardly		Slightly		Moderately		Markedly		Very Severely

5. Would you like help with any of these areas?

   Depression: No _____ Yes _____   Anxiety: No _____ Yes _____

   Anger: No _____ Yes _____   Stress: No _____ Yes _____

6. Do you ever drink alcohol?

   _____ No (go to #13) _____ Yes

	No	Yes
7. Have you ever felt you ought to cut down on your drinking?	_____	_____
8. Have people ever annoyed you by criticizing your drinking?	_____	_____
9. Have you ever felt bad or guilty about your drinking?	_____	_____
10. Have you ever had a drink first thing in the morning ("eye opener") to steady you nerves or get rid of a hangover?	_____	_____

11. About how often do you drink alcohol?

   1 Daily or almost every day   4 Once or twice per month

   2 3 or 4 times per week   5 Less often than once per month

   3 Once or twice per week   6 Never

12. How many of these alcoholic beverages do you drink during an average **WEEK**?

   _____ # of 12-oz bottles or cans of beer, ale, etc.

   _____ # of 4-oz glasses of wine, sherry, port, etc.

   _____ # of shots (one shot = 1.5 oz) of vodka, rum, scotch, whiskey, bourbon, tequila, or gin (including mixed drinks and cocktails)

   _____ # of after-dinner drinks or liqueurs

13. Do you ever use illegal drugs?

   _____ No _____ Yes

14. Do you live alone?

   _____ No _____ Yes

15. Do you have enough help at home? _____

Thank you for your responses to these questions. This information will remain confidential.

Table 64.3. Symptoms of Depression

Emotional features
  Depressed mood, feeling blue
  Irritability, anxiety
  Loss of interest
  Withdrawal from others
  Preoccupation with death
Cognitive features
  Feeling of worthlessness or guilt
  Hopelessness, despair
  Poor concentration
  Indecision
  Suicide feelings
Vegetative features
  Fatigue, lack of energy
  Trouble sleeping
  Loss of appetite
  Weight loss or gain
  Lack of interest in sex
  Depressed look

panic attacks, which are discrete periods of apprehension or fear accompanied by symptoms such as dyspnea, palpitations, choking, chest pain or discomfort, sweating, dizziness, fear of going crazy, and/or fear of doing something uncontrolled. The initial panic attack usually occurs in the early 20s and may be spontaneous. Many patients with panic disorder develop avoidance of public places and spaces. Such patients are not likely to be able to participate in an exercise program, but participation can be very beneficial to them.

Social phobia is characterized by fear of social situations. Participants who appear shy or unnecessarily embarrassed in public may need special encouragement to participate in exercise programs.

Chronic anxiety can be secondary to psychiatric problems other than depression, such as alcoholism, drug abuse, or schizophrenia. It can also be caused by medical problems such as hyperthyroidism, hypoglycemia, and temporal lobe epilepsy.

Some patients with anxiety report unpleasant symptoms with exercise. Use of a diagnostic treadmill test can reassure anxious patients that exercise is safe and can help the exercise professional identify any contraindications to exercise (15). Furthermore, exercise may reduce symptoms in patients with severe anxiety disorders (13).

ALCOHOL AND DRUG ABUSE

Alcohol or drug abuse is indicated by a maladaptive pattern of use leading to clinically significant impairment or distress manifested by the following:

- Tolerance (a need to increase amounts of the substance to achieve intoxication or desired effect or markedly di-

minished effect with continued use of the same amount of the substance)
- Withdrawal
- Use of larger amounts or over a longer period than intended
- Persistent desire or unsuccessful efforts to cut down or control use
- Extensive time and effort spent to obtain the substance
- Impairment of social, occupational, or recreation activities because of substance use
- Continued use despite knowledge of having a persistent or recurrent problem related to use

Confrontation may be necessary if the exercise professional suspects abuse (e.g., the patient smells of alcohol, reports blackout periods, or seems preoccupied with alcohol). This entails directing attention to something that the client may not be aware of or is reluctant to admit. Confrontation should only address observable facts and not infer motives or emotional state. For example, a post-MI participant who is intoxicated at the time of an exercise session and is disruptive requires confrontation. An example of an overaggressive confrontation follows:

Exercise professional: You have been drinking. You had better not drink before you come here.

A more appropriate confrontation might be:

Exercise professional: You seem to be acting funny today. Have you been drinking?
Participant: Nah.
Exercise professional: I can smell alcohol on your breath. When did you last have something to drink?
Participant: Oh, a couple of beers about an hour ago.
Exercise professional: I can't allow people to exercise here if they have been drinking. Will you make sure you have not been drinking before you come next time?

Most of us are uncomfortable with direct confrontation, but sometimes it is necessary. Choosing the appropriate time and circumstance are important, particularly if a participant may become violent; generally the time to confront is not when a participant is intoxicated.

Participants who appear to be or admit to abusing alcohol may benefit from referral. The Yellow Pages under Alcoholism Information or Drug Abuse and Addiction Information is an excellent place to look for treatment resources. Alcoholics Anonymous and Narcotics Anonymous are good resources available in most communities. The National Clearinghouse for Alcohol and Drug Information (telephone 800-729-6686) can also provide local or state alcohol treatment resources.

DISORDERED EATING
Bulimia Nervosa

Bulimia nervosa is characterized by the following (16):

- Recurrent episodes of binge eating (rapid consumption of a large amount of food over a short period)
- Feeling a lack of control over eating during the binges
- Self-induced vomiting; use of laxatives or diuretics
- Strict dieting or fasting or vigorous exercise to prevent weight gain
- Persistent overconcern with body shape and weight

Food consumed during a binge is usually high in calories, sweet, and easy to swallow. Binges generally take place in secret, and the food is eaten quite rapidly, with little chewing. A binge ends with abdominal discomfort, sleep, social interruption, extreme guilt, or induced vomiting. Bulimia is more common among exercisers than nonexercisers. Bulimic patients often feel guilty about vomiting, laxative, and/or diuretic abuse and are likely to have some depression. Frequent vomiting can lead to dental erosion and other health problems. Electrolyte imbalance and dehydration may occur and can lead to serious physical complications (17).

Cognitive–behavioral psychological interventions are effective in assisting bulimic patients reduce symptoms, and treatment should be encouraged. The National Association of Anorexia Nervosa and Associated Disorders (telephone 708-831-3438) is a good resource.

Anorexia Nervosa

Anorexia nervosa is a rare, life-threatening eating disorder. Table 64.4 provides a clinical description of anorexia nervosa (16, 18). Most patients exercise to excess. If anorexia is suspected, weight and dietary history should be obtained, and if possible the percentage of body fat should be measured. Weight should be monitored weekly.

Professionals specializing in eating disorders can best help these patients, but the exercise professional can play an important role through confrontation about the seriousness of the disorder and by insisting that the person seek help. Once therapy has begun, the exercise profes-

sional can assist in designing a program for normal eating and activity that emphasizes health and proper nutrition, not weight, and by providing psychological support.

ORGANIC BRAIN DISEASE

Organic brain disease is rarely encountered in most exercise programs, but the exercise professional should be aware of the signs of organic brain disease:

- Sudden, unexplained change in personality or behavior, including a significant change in personal appearance
- Difficulty remembering information, particularly newly presented information
- Confusion
- Difficulty finding words
- Impairment in planning and organizing

Sudden onset of such symptoms may indicate an acute, serious medical condition.

HOW TO MAKE A REFERRAL

Referrals from the exercise professional to a mental health professional may be most effective if:

- The participant believes the exercise professional cares about and understands the problem
- The participant accepts the need for the referral and the referral is likely to lead to improvement
- The exercise professional is familiar with the mental health professional to whom the referral is being made
- Follow-up is obtained

Empathically listening to concerns and being supportive are important parts of the referral process. Most depressed and anxious patients suffer, and many desire to seek treatment. The alcoholic or drug abuser who denies or minimizes the problem is more difficult to refer. Such patients may require confrontation in a clear, directive fashion. Finally, follow-up to determine whether the referral occurred and treatment has ensued is important.

► **SUMMARY**

The role of the exercise professional in psychopathology is both evaluative and supportive. Evaluation and assessment require fundamental knowledge of basic situations and problems that may arise and the ability to propose and guide participants to referral. Support requires empathy, reinforcement of positive behavior, and ongoing rapport to gain trust and confidence of all participants.

Table 64.4. Clinical Picture of Anorexia Nervosa

Loss of more than 25% premorbid body weight
Distorted body image
Fears of weight gain or of loss of control over eating
Adolescent and young adult women primarily affected
Perfectionist behavior
Refusal to maintain normal body weight
No known physical illness to account for weight loss

References

1. Hoff LA. People in Crisis. 2nd ed. Menlo Park, CA: Addison-Wesley, 1984.
2. Frasure-Smith N, Prince R. Long-term follow-up of the ischemic heart disease life stress monitoring program. Psychol Med 51:485, 1989.
3. Ghosh TB, Victor BS. Suicide. In: Hales RE, Yudofsky SC, eds. Synopsis of Psychiatry. Washington: American Psychiatric Press, 1994.
4. Parke CM. Bereavement. In Doyle D, Hanks GWC, MacDonald N, eds. The Oxford Textbook of Palliative Medicine. Oxford, UK: Oxford University, 1994.
5. Miller NH, Taylor CB. Lifestyle Management in Patients with Coronary Heart Disease. Champaign, IL: Human Kinetics, 1995.
6. Ewing JA. Detecting alcoholism: The CAGE Questionnaire. JAMA 252:1905, 1984.
7. AACVPR Outcomes Committee. Outcome measurement in cardiac and pulmonary rehabilitation. J Cardiopulm Rehabil 15:394–405, 1995.
8. American Psychiatric Association. Diagnostic and Statistical Manual of Mental Disorders. 4th ed, revised. Washington: APA, 1994.
9. AHCPR. Depression in Primary Care, Vol 1 and 2. Rockville, MD: Agency for Health Care Policy and Research Pub. 93-0551, 1993.
10. Carney RM, Rich MW, Freedland KE, et al. Major depressive disorder predicts cardiac events in patients with coronary artery disease. Psychosom Med 50:627, 1988.
11. Levine JB, Covino NA, Slack WV, et al. Psychological predictors of subsequent medical care among patients hospitalized with cardiac disease. J Cardiopulm Rehabil 16:109, 1996.
12. Allison TG, Williams DE, Miller TD, et al. Medical and economic costs of psychologic distress in patients with coronary artery disease. Mayo Clin Proc 70:734–742, 1995.
13. Benight CC, Taylor CB. The effects of exercise on improving anxiety, depression, emotional well-being and elements of type A behavior. In: Elliot DL, Goldberg L, eds. Exercise as Medical Therapy. Philadelphia: FA Davis, 1994:319–332.
14. Taylor CB, Arnow B. The Nature and Treatment of Anxiety Disorders. New York: Free Press, 1988.
15. Taylor CB, King R, Ehlers A, et al. Treadmill exercise testing and ambulatory heart rate measures in patients with panic attacks. Am J Cardiol 60:48J, 1987.
16. Agras WS. Eating Disorders: Management of Obesity, Bulimia, and Anorexia Nervosa. New York: Pergamon, 1987.
17. Harris RT. Bulimarexia and related serious eating disorders with medical complications. Ann Intern Med 99:800, 1983.
18. Garfinkel PE, Garner DM. Anorexia Nervosa: A Multidimensional Perspective. New York: Brunner/Mazel, 1982.

Suggested Reading

Gonda TA, Ruark JE. Dying Dignified. Menlo Park, CA: Addison-Wesley, 1984.

Rando TA. How to Go on Living When Someone You Love Dies. Bantam Books, Random House, NY, NY 1991.

1.5.0, 1.5.3   2.5.0   3.5.0, 3.5.1   4.5.0

CHAPTER **65**

PRINCIPLES OF HEALTH BEHAVIOR CHANGE

C. Barr Taylor and Nancy Houston Miller

Assisting people to begin and maintain health behavior change is a challenge for the most experienced counselor. Nevertheless, behavioral scientists have identified strategies that if systematically applied, are useful in helping an individual begin and sustain health behavior change (1). The transtheoretical model, developed by Prochaska and DiClimente, has had the greatest influence in recent years on designing exercise interventions and has been applied to a number of health behavior change areas (2–4). This model predicts a progression of behavior change through a series of stages: precontemplation (no intent and no exercise), contemplation (intent, but no exercise), preparation (intent and occasional exercise), action (regular exercise), and maintenance (exercising for 6 months or more). Progression through these stages is related to use of various behavior change strategies, the expected outcomes of exercise (both pros and cons), and self-confidence, or self-efficacy. Marcus et al. (5) showed that a work site exercise program designed to account for a level of motivation had a significantly stronger effect than one that did not.

The transtheoretical model is partly derived from social learning theory, a comprehensive analysis of human functioning in which human behavior is assumed to be developed and maintained on the basis of three interacting systems: behavioral, cognitive, and environmental (6). Social learning theory emphasizes the human capacity for self-directed behavior change. Willingness to change is related to self-confidence, which is influenced by four main factors: persuasion from an authority, observation of others, successful performance of the behavior, and physiological feedback. Social learning theory is a useful model to help in the understanding of why people change; behavioral therapy provides the methods and strategies for effecting and maintaining behavior change. Many excellent and detailed discussions of behavior change programs are available (7–10).

Other theoretical models have added useful ideas for conceptualizing behavior change. The theory of reasoned action and the theory of planned behavior describe the re-

lations among health beliefs, attitudes, intentions, behavior, and perceived behavioral control as applied to exercise and other behaviors (11–13). The health belief model also emphasizes the role of beliefs in determining health care behavior (14). In this model, the important variables influencing behavior include the readiness to make a change, the perceived benefit of the change, cues to action, and modifying factors, such as knowledge and socioeconomic background. Also, the cognitive and behavioral processes used in changing health behaviors have been examined, particularly in relation to exercise (4). Finally, comprehensive models of behavior change, including systems and even community factors, may provide helpful ideas for designing more effective programs (15, 16).

HEALTH BEHAVIOR CHANGE MODEL

Health behavior change can be conceptualized as occurring in stages, arbitrarily divided into the antecedent, adoption, and maintenance phases (Fig. 65.1). The antecedent stage includes the precontemplation, contemplation, and preparation components of the transtheoretical model (3). Antecedents refer to all conditions that can assist, initiate, hinder, or support change. For example, observing the benefits a friend receives from exercising may serve as an antecedent or stimulus for motivation to begin an exercise program. Adoption (or the action phase in the transtheoretical model) comprises the early phases of a behavior change program. Maintenance applies to later phases, when the participant is undergoing behavior change.

Antecedents

People sometimes decide to change for reasons that they do not understand or that are beyond their control. A chance encounter with a friend who has made important changes and looks better, an illness, a caustic remark from a coworker, and loose clothes that become tight are all events that may initiate a health behavior change. Nev-

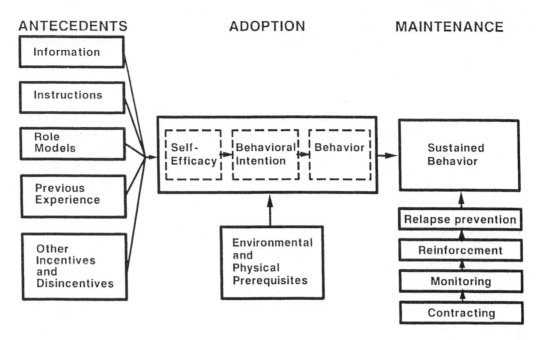

Figure 65.1. Health behavior change can be conceptualized as occurring in stages, arbitrarily divided into antecedent, adoption, and maintenance phases.

ertheless, social learning theory and the transtheoretical model predict that certain antecedents to behavior change are useful in increasing intention to change. If you ask a person to rate intention on a scale from 0 to 10 in which 0 indicates no intention to change and 10 indicates certainty, people with little intention are not likely to change, whereas those persons with higher scores of intention are more likely to change (17). Intentions frequently change and can be influenced by the factors listed in Figure 65.1. For motivated individuals, environmental cues such as posters or notes on bulletin boards may stimulate a behavior change.

Information

Intention to change often begins with information, which should be presented in simple and clear ways using language that is understandable. About 30–40% of the public read at a seventh-grade level or lower. Information is most effective when combined with instructions about how to make the changes. Information about benefits to change rather than risks from no change may be emphasized for more impact. Although pamphlets, self-help books, and handouts are often used to communicate health information, most people read no more than 10–15% of such material unless they are extremely interested or are held accountable. Some audiences who would seem to benefit most from information may ignore it. For instance, smokers ignore messages about the risks of smoking, nonexercisers know less about the benefits of physical activity than exercisers, and poorly educated groups may not read long or complicated materials. Knowledge critical to behavior change should be tested

prior to the program so myths and misperceptions can be corrected.

Instructions

Instructions to change a particular behavior (persuasion) from a person of authority are a powerful antecedent to behavior change. The public considers health care professionals the most credible source of information. Persuasion from an authoritative figure should occur in a kind, but firm manner. People reluctant to make health behavior change listen for ambivalence in the message. They are not, for example, likely to follow this message: "Smoking is bad for your health; you should think about stopping." They are more likely to be affected by this: "You must stop smoking." Instructions should be clear, achievable, and accompanied by necessary information about how to bring about change. In addition, reminders and feedback should reinforce instructions. Participants should be asked to repeat the critical information.

Models

Role models, whether family, friends, or other credible sources (e.g., health professionals), can facilitate change by allowing the participant to see how other individuals make change, react to change, generalize change to different types of situations (e.g., how people practice food changes at home, in restaurants, and in grocery stores), and cope with difficult situations to maintain healthy habits. People undergoing health behavior change can benefit from being asked to think of persons they know or admire who have made changes. Videotapes or films demonstrating how individuals have made changes and the effect of change can be effective in increasing intention to change.

Experience

Experience is a major factor in determining initiation of a new health behavior. People are more likely to repeat a behavior if it was helpful in the past. Experience may also lead to superstitious health traps. A cold that seemed to resolve more rapidly than usual may, for example, be associated with taking a vitamin whether or not the vitamin is helpful. The level of confidence to try a new behavior is largely determined by experience. Review of previous success or failure may assist with the change process. Examination of a previously unsuccessful attempt at exercise, for example, may reveal ways to encourage adoption of the behavior in a future attempt. People often need to develop new skills to be more effective before change can occur. Developing new skills leads to increased confidence and intention to change.

Other Incentives and Disincentives

Other incentives and disincentives are important antecedents for health behavior change. Incentives should be built into a program and should outweigh the disincentives. Clients should be encouraged to answer the question, "How can I make sure that I benefit from this program?" Some of the benefits may be obvious, such as exercising to feel and look better, while other benefits may not be as obvious, such as exercising to prevent disease. Reducing disincentives when beginning a health program is equally important. Participants may begin exercise at an inconvenient time, in a place that does not appeal to them, or with an activity that is not enjoyable. Such disincentives almost ensure that a program will be short lived.

Careful attention to antecedents can influence intention to adopt behavior change. With sufficient information, compelling instructions, appropriate models to change, positive physiological feedback, increased confidence to change, and maximized incentives and minimized disincentives, a health behavior change is likely to be adopted. An examination of the antecedents for change answers these questions:

- What does the participant need to know about the reasons for and methods of bringing about the desired change?
- What instructions (persuasion) have been given from significant people about the importance of making changes?
- What are existing and potential models for change?
- What has been the past success with making this or comparable changes?
- How confident is the participant that change can be accomplished this time?

- What can be done to increase confidence?
- What are the incentives and disincentives?

Adoption

When to intervene or encourage adoption of a new behavior should be guided by clinical experience and science and facilitated by carefully listening to the participant's needs and interests. Continued gentle reminders may be useful, even for a chronic smoker who has refused to quit many times in the past. Simply asking a person to try a new behavior (e.g., increase activity or alter diet) may be sufficient to instigate change. Medical or personal crises may present an incentive and often an opportunity for change. However, at times it is important not to push the participant beyond willingness to change. Questions such as, "Are you ready to try to stop smoking?" or "Do you want to consider a healthier diet?" may tell the exercise professional whether to encourage further change.

Goal setting is an important part of the adoption phase. Asking participants to list goals and to identify areas where assistance is needed may be effective. A number of studies have demonstrated that flexible, individually tailored, achievable goals increase adherence to change. Goals should be specific, not global, and short term, but linked to longer-term goals. A useful way to determine whether a goal is likely to be achieved is to determine level of confidence (using a scale from 0-100%, no confidence to entirely certain) for attaining the goal in a given time frame. Participants reporting 70% or more are likely to be able to do so. In setting goals it is important to ensure that needs, goals, and preferences are included in the goal-setting process.

Once a person intends to make a behavior change and is confident of success, the adoption of change is often precipitated by cues to action. For instance, many people begin a health care program on the basis of symptoms or general state of being. Such physiological and emotional feedback cues people to change and is critical in influencing maintenance. Smoking relapse often occurs in the first few days after quitting because withdrawal symptoms overwhelm intentions. Poorly conditioned people may stop exercising at the beginning of an exercise program because of unpleasant feelings, such as shortness of breath.

Certain environmental and physical prerequisites are often necessary for health behavior change and should be discussed with participants. Such prerequisites for exercising:

- Clothing and equipment
- Access to facilities
- Necessary written materials
- A release from a physician if appropriate

The early stages of change are often the most difficult. Replacing one activity, even a self-destructive one, with another involves many subtle and important shifts in life. Cigarette smokers who quit often say they feel as if they have lost a good friend. Support is particularly important at such times.

MAINTENANCE

Once a behavior is adopted, other factors determine maintenance. Behavior that satisfies (reinforcing) or reduces discomfort is likely to be maintained. Four strategies may prove useful in enhancing maintenance:

1. Monitoring and feedback of change (monitoring)
2. Making the activity as satisfying as possible (reinforcement)
3. Anticipating relapse or interruptions (relapse prevention)
4. Making a formal commitment (a contract)

Monitoring

Self-report, diary, physiological, or other types of monitoring are useful for maintaining behavior change and assisting exercise professionals in determining progress. Monitoring forms may be used by exercise professionals for review and problem solving. In addition, monitoring through use of self-reports and diaries provides participants with important feedback that may increase the likelihood of maintenance. Goals vary, but cognitive-behavioral and physiological goals should be developed as appropriate. Monitoring forms should be simple and convenient.

Reinforcement

Positive reinforcement is a powerful factor for sustaining change. Many environmental stimuli, such as food, water, sexual activity, and warmth, are natural reinforcers. Social and/or symbolic reinforcers include attention, praise, money, and awards. Recognition from peers or games and competition can help maintain a behavior. However, it is important to realize that reinforcers are idiosyncratic, that is, reinforcement to one participant may not be reinforcement to another person. Several excellent discussions of reinforcement are available (18–20).

Relapse Prevention

Various techniques assist participants with relapse or prepare for interruptions or other events that may cause discontinuation of a program. The relapse prevention model is derived from studies of alcoholics and smokers attempting to change. Marlatt and Gordon observed that even one cigarette might lead to total relapse and that preparation for the situations in which the cigarette urge is strongest (e.g., while drinking or under stress) could help to prevent this relapse (20). The model can be applied to other behaviors. For instance, the Stanford Cardiac Rehabilitation Program staff encourages people to

monitor exercise to improve maintenance and identify clear signals for relapse, such as an actual or anticipated reduction in exercise frequency, and to develop strategies to deal with possible relapse (4).

Upon initiation of an exercise program, participants are encouraged to write what they will do when illness, injury, or changes in schedule interrupt exercise. Some examples:

- Asking a jogging partner for a reminder after return from vacation
- Leaving a money deposit with a friend that is refundable when restarting exercise after an illness
- Asking an exercise professional to call periodically to inquire about exercise

Participants who stop exercising for an extended time may require additional effort to overcome the lapse, but the principles are similar. Note that relapse prevention focuses on decreasing rather than increasing behavior.

Contracts

Written contracts are also extremely useful to maintain change and to help with maintenance. Exercise professionals should not make contracts that are unrealistic or unlikely to be achieved. Behavior change is dynamic, and goals should be assessed, updated, and revised as necessary. Problem solving may be important for goals that are not achieved. In problem solving, a participant identifies a list of possible solutions, develops a plan for implementing these solutions, tries them, evaluates results, and repeats the process if the initial solutions are not successful.

DEVELOPING A PROGRAM

A program consists of the antecedent, adoption, and maintenance phases of behavioral change, how the interventions associated with this phase are sequenced and integrated, and the interaction between the exercise professional and the client. An example of the components integrated into the Stanford exercise studies of moderate exercise is detailed in Table 65.1 (8).

Organization

Implementing behavior change takes time. Programs should ensure that such time is available for both the exercise professional and the participant. A session immediately prior to exercise class devoted to education and behavior change may be helpful. This session can be used to present new information, review progress toward goals, share solutions for problems, and so on. It is also important to allow exercise professionals time with peers and administrators for formal review of behavioral aspects of the program. Such sessions can be spent evaluating educational material, reviewing progress of clients, solving problems, and designing new aspects of intervention.

Table 65.1. Elements of Exercise Program Design

Antecedents and adoption
  Written description of benefits of exercise
  Assessment of expectations
  Review of expectations to make them realistic
  Assessment of confidence
  Skills training to enhance confidence
  Videotape instruction on warming up and keeping heart rate within guidelines
  Physical examination, treadmill, weight, and skinfold assessment
  Experimentation to identify most enjoyable locations
Maintenance
  Monitoring
    Weekly diaries of exercise duration and intensity
    Heart rate monitor with auditory feedback
  Reinforcement
    Social
      Biweekly phone calls from staff
      Group meetings
    Monetary: None built into program
    Physical: 3- and 6-month treadmill test and weight assessment
    Symbolic: T-shirts
    Accomplishment: Monitoring confidence, psychological variables
    Contracts: None built into program
  Relapse prevention
    Participant develops own plans for coping with interruptions of exercise

The components listed in Table 65.1 can be easily organized into a step-by-step approach to a behavior change program. The initial step is asking a participant to consider change. Often people intend to adopt one behavior, but recommending additional health behavior changes may be important, such as recommending that an exerciser also stop smoking. Suggesting such changes can be difficult, but few people resent a thoughtful attempt to assist in improving health.

The second and perhaps most important step is to provide information, instructions, and models for change. This includes reviewing the past, building confidence for change, reducing disincentives, and increasing incentives to change.

The third step is to request a commitment that is specific in time and place for when the new behavior will occur. The final step is to develop, with the participant, a way to monitor progress of the new behavior and to determine when and how progress will be reviewed. Early in the adoption phase, the participant should be trained in relapse prevention. Problem solving should be used as necessary to help overcome difficulties. Such problem solving can occur in the whole group, at the beginning or the end of a session, via telephone, or in a face-to-face counseling session.

Exercise Professional Qualities

Different exercise professionals achieve different outcomes, even within the same program. Exercise professionals seem to be most effective when participants feel that the exercise professional is competent, likes them, understands them, and is interested. This relationship translates into a bond between exercise professional and participant that helps to make the program effective. Role playing of typical participant situations with peers and receiving feedback is a particularly good way for exercise professionals to develop interpersonal skills.

Overpersistence with an unwilling participant is a problem for some exercise professionals. Exercise professionals who assume too much responsibility for the actions of another person are particularly likely to be overpersistent. Unfortunately, overpersistent exercise professionals often begin to resent inaction, feel chronic frustration, or devote too much time to that participant. To avoid these problems, exercise professionals should have guidelines about when a program or request for change may be discontinued. In one YMCA program, participants meet with the coordinator to review reasons for noncompliance, to solve problems, and to set measurable compliance goals. A second meeting is scheduled if the participant continues to be noncompliant. If the participant fails to comply after a second meeting, a termination meeting is scheduled to discontinue the program. During the termination meeting, the coordinator explains that this program is not appropriate for the participant and that in light of the hazard of noncompliance both to the participant and to persons who might be influenced by noncompliance (e.g., overexerting), the participant should not continue in the program.

▶ SUMMARY

Social learning theory is the basis for a model for understanding behavior change. Behavior therapy helps to develop many effective change procedures. Information, instructions, models, increasing confidence in performing exercise, and maximizing incentives and minimizing disincentives can increase intention to change and may lead to actual adoption of the behavior. Once adopted, monitoring and feedback, reinforcement, relapse prevention, and the use of contracts can improve maintenance.

References

1. Elder JP, Ayala GX, Harris S. Theories and intervention approaches to health-behavior change in primary care. Am J Prev Med 17:275–284, 1999.
2. Prochaska JO, DiClimente CC. Stage process of self-change of smoking: Toward an integrative model of change. J Consul Clin Psych 51:390, 1983.
3. Prochaska JO, Velicer WF, Rossi JS, et al. Stages of change and decisional balance for 12 problem behaviors. Health Psychol 13:39, 1994.
4. Marcus BH, Simkin LR. The transtheoretical model: Applications to exercise behavior. Med Sci Sports Exerc 26:1400, 1994.

5. Marcus BH, Emmons KM, Simkin-Silverman LR, et al. Evaluation of motivationally tailored vs. standard self-help physical activity interventions at the workplace. Am J Health Promot 12:246, 1998.

6. Bandura A. Self-Efficacy: The Exercise of Control. San Francisco: WH Freeman, 1997.

7. Agras WS, Kazdin AE, Wilson CT. Behavior Therapy: Toward an Applied Clinical Science. San Francisco: WH Freeman, 1979.

8. Miller NH, Taylor CB. Lifestyle Management in Patients with Coronary Heart Disease. Champaign, IL: Human Kinetics, 1995.

9. Watson DL, Tharp RC. Self-Directed Behavior Change. Monterey, CA: Brooks/Cole, 1981.

10. Blumenthal JA, McKee DC. Applications in Behavioral Medicine and Health Psychology: A Clinician's Source Book. Sarasota, FL: Professional Resource Exchange, 1987.

11. Fishbein M, Ajzen I. Belief, Attitudes, Intention and Behavior. Reading, MA: Addison-Wesley, 1975.

12. Ajzen I. From intentions to actions: A theory of planned behavior (pp. 11–40). In: Kuhl J, Beckmann J, eds. Actional Control: From Cognition to Behavior. New York: Springer-Verlag, 1985.

13. Courneya KS. Understanding readiness for regular physical activity in older adults: An application of the theory of planned behavior. Health Psychol 14:80, 1995.

14. Becker MH, Maiman LA. Sociobehavioral determinants of compliance with health and medical care recommendations. Med Care 13:10, 1975.

15. Winett RA, King AC, Altman D. Psychology and Public Health: An Integrative Approach. New York: Pergamon, 1989.

16. Green LW, Kreuter MW. Health Promotion and Planning: An Education and Environmental Approach. Mountain View, CA: Mayfield, 1991.

17. Taylor CB, Houston-Miller N, Killen JD, DeBusk RF. Smoking cessation after acute myocardial infarction: Effects of a nurse-managed intervention. Ann Intern Med 113:118, 1990.

18. Goldfried M, Davison CC. Clinical Behavior Therapy. New York: Holt, Rinehart & Winston, 1976.

19. Cautela JR, Kastenbaum RA. Reinforcement survey schedule for use in therapy, training, and research. Psychol Rep 29:115, 1967.

20. Marlatt GA, Gordon JR, eds. Relapse Prevention. Maintenance Strategies in the Treatment of Addiction. New York: Guilford, 1985.

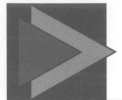

CHAPTER **66**

STRESS MANAGEMENT

Wayne M. Sotile

The rubric and techniques of stress management training can be effectively used to address many goals and problems of rehabilitation and health promotion. A plethora of interventions have been described in stress management literature, and no single model is universally accepted. The effective emotional management (EEM) model depicted in Figure 66.1 is an effort to organize this disparate body of information into a set of practical guidelines for providing brief counseling in medical settings (1). This model integrates key components for promoting stress hardiness in both healthy and rehabilitating populations. This is only one of many ways of structuring stress management efforts.

THE EFFECTIVE EMOTIONAL MANAGEMENT MODEL

As illustrated in Figure 66.1, a comprehensive stress management program should address five areas:

1. The physiological and psychological aspects of stress
2. Relaxation methods
3. Ways to manage personality-based coping patterns
4. Relationship skills
5. Cognitive control

The EEM model proposes that stress management should focus on helping the patient in two broad ways. First, teach patients to disrupt problematic coping progressions by making more-adaptive cognitive, behavioral, physiological, or interpersonal choices. Second, assist patients in creating supportive environments and social networks. Stress hardiness is enhanced when the territory in which an individual lives provides a reasonable fit between daily demands and inner needs, wants, and values. Living territory can be defined by three factors:

- *Where* the patient spends time, including the community, neighborhood, job setting, church, clubs, and health care facilities

- *What* the patient does by way of self-care; physically, psychologically, emotionally, and spiritually
- *Whom* the patient affiliates with and how he or she manages these relationships with intimate others, friends, health care providers, colleagues, and acquaintances

Through supportive interaction, psychoeducation, and coaching, stress management training should help patients create situations (the where factor), processes (the what factor), and relationships (the who factor) that enhance functioning. In this way, health care providers become part of the nurturing influence in patients' lives.

PRACTICAL APPLICATIONS

Stress management training is implemented in various treatment venues, ranging from brief, informal consultation delivered during administration of typical medical care to formal presentation of a systematically delivered program. Depending on the treatment format, interventions may focus on some or all of the factors discussed hereafter.

Clarification of Emotional and Psychological Symptoms

Being stressed is typically equated with being anxious. However, the stress response actually yields a variety of physical and emotional manifestations. Table 66.1 illustrates various emotional concomitants that may accompany different stages of the stress response. Explaining this fact can highlight the need for stress management training.

Identify the Causes of Stress

Most patients perceive that major causes of stress lie outside of their realm of control. Effective emotional management hinges on learning to identify and manage the aspects of the coping process that are controllable, even when faced with uncontrollable external circum-

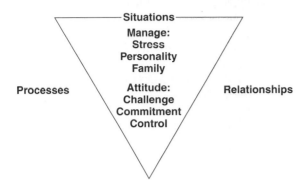

**Keys to Effective Emotional Management
Nurturing & Affirming**

Situations
Manage:
Stress
Personality
Family
Attitude:
Challenge
Commitment
Control

Processes   Relationships

Figure 66.1. Effective emotional management. (Reprinted with permission from Sotile W. *Psychosocial Interventions for Cardiopulmonary Patients: Guidelines for Health Professionals.* Champaign, IL: Human Kinetics, 1992.)

Table 66.1. Physical and Emotional Aspects of Stress

PHYSIOLOGICAL ASPECTS	EMOTIONAL CORRELATES
Fight or flight	Anxiety
	Alarm
	Anger
Conservation withdrawal	Numbness
	Vulnerability
General adaptation syndrome	Depression and problems in each of the following areas:
	Physical
	Emotional
	Cognitive
Neurochemical depletion, or "jamming"	Clinical depression or anxiety disorders

Reprinted with permission from Sotile W. Psychosocial Interventions for Cardiopulmonary Patients: A Guide for Health Professionals. Champaign, IL: Human Kinetics, 1996.

stances. Various standardized or clinician-developed inventories and exercises facilitate this aspect of stress management training.

For example, the numbers and types of transitions faced by the patient may be assessed with the Holmes-Rahe Social Readjustment Scale, or a thought diary can be used to track cognitive coping patterns (1, 2). A values inventory can assess behavioral choices made in daily life that are (or are not) harmonious with inner needs and wants (3). Finally, patients can be reassured that even if they face many stressors, overall well-being and stress management will be enhanced if they commit to increasing the frequency of uplifting experiences in their daily life. Examples of uplifts include engaging in healthy pleasures, receiving or giving interpersonal support, and praying (3).

Assist with Pinpointing Reactions to Stressors

Comprehensive stress management training includes teaching about the ways that cognitions and personality mediate stress responses.

Thinking Patterns

In addition to teaching ways to monitor and disrupt maladaptive thinking habits, stress management counseling should help patients and significant others clarify attitudinal paradigms that shape world views and influence the approaches to fitness or rehabilitation. The importance of maintaining or developing an optimistic outlook and its accompanying cognitive habits should be emphasized (4).

In addition, patients should be instructed in the importance of embracing the **three C's of stress hardiness** suggested by Kobasa et al. (5). Stress management capability is enhanced if a given stressor is viewed as a **challenge**, if the individual is **committed** to facing that challenge, and if the individual learns what is necessary to gain a reasonable sense of **control** over the coping process. Patients should be asked to define stressors. For example, is the situation being faced a punishment, a relief, an opportunity, a beginning, an ending, a warning, or a tragedy?

Personality-Based Coping Patterns

Comprehensive stress management requires disrupting stress-generating personality-based coping patterns. Discussion of this important topic need not be esoteric or extensive. Table 66.2 outlines a concise commonsense model for conceptualizing personality-based coping patterns and the underlying hopes and pitfalls that come with corresponding modes of coping. Medical input should be delivered in language matching the personality-based coping style and its corresponding underlying

Table 66.2. What Drives You? Coping Patterns and Pitfalls

DRIVER	UNDERLYING HOPE	COPING PITFALLS
Being strong	To be nurtured	Numbness, loneliness, anger
Being perfect	To feel good enough	Guilt, anxiety, obsessive preoccupation, aloofness
Trying hard	To feel deserving of rest and enjoyment	Exhaustion, stress, depression, joylessness
Pleasing others	To feel understood and appreciated	Exhaustion, withdrawal, guilt
Hurrying	To feel finished	Frazzled and chaotic feelings
Being careful	To feel safe	Free floating, fear, obsessive worrying

Reprinted with permission from Sotile W. Heart Illness and Intimacy: How Caring Relationships Aid Recovery. Baltimore: Johns Hopkins University Press, 1992.

hope. Extensive guidelines for incorporating this information into the delivery of medical care are available (1, 6).

Type A Behavior Pattern

Type A behavior patterns amplify any coping tendency. This is not a one-dimensional coping pattern, and no one evidences all of the characteristics of this syndrome; however, it is estimated that upward of 70% of individuals evidence at least one pronounced type A coping habit. It is prudent to integrate information regarding this syndrome into a stress management program. Comprehensive treatment programs for type A behavior have been described (7, 8). Minimally, intervention should focus on teaching the importance of managing hostility and coaching hostility management behavior, a topic to be discussed hereafter.

Relaxation Techniques and Use of the Relaxation Response

The term *relaxation training* is used in the health literature to refer to various processes, including yoga, training in self-hypnosis, progressive muscular relaxation, breathing exercises, and biofeedback. There is no convincing evidence that one form of relaxation therapy is more effective than others (1). Relaxation can be quickly learned through instruction in identification of naturally occurring or previously learned relaxation strategies. For example, recalling sensations and/or techniques employed during Lamaze methods for childbirth, past classes in yoga or meditation, or prayer can help a person relax. Instructing the patient to concentrate on a multisensory memory of such a time—elaborating the sights, smells, sounds, and bodily sensations of the experience—can produce a deepened state of hypnotic-type relaxation (1).

Biofeedback is another method for learning control of voluntary and involuntary physiological functions using visual or auditory cues. Digital displays, auditory feedback, and/or graphic representations of the effects of emotional arousal on various physiological functions, such as heart rate, blood pressure, skin temperature, and palmar sweating, are commonly used (9, 10). Through trial and error, patients learn cognitive strategies for controlling these functions. Biofeedback is typically offered in 2 to 5 sessions as an adjunct to stress management training.

In clinical practice, combinations of relaxation strategies are most often taught. For example, diaphragmatic breathing may be paired with progressive muscular relaxation and guided imagery. In guided imagery, a relaxed patient is encouraged to replace distressing images with images that enhance a sense of well-being. This may include visualizing the healing or strengthening of certain body parts or systems. Comprehensive guidelines for such healing imagery are available (11).

The relaxation state is a fertile time for use of cognitive rehearsal that can bolster confidence in stress management skills. This method pairs the state of relaxation with imagery of upcoming events during which a relaxation response would enhance adaptive coping (1). Similarly, through imagery, the state of relaxation can be deepened with specific verbal, kinesthetic, or visual cues, which can then be used repeatedly (e.g., throughout the day) to trigger brief periods of relaxation. This is an effective method of pattern disruption in stress management training.

Use of Exercise as a Tool for Stress Management

Although whether regular exercise in and of itself leads to lasting psychosocial benefits is controversial, clinical experience strongly suggests that exercise is an effective way for stressed individuals to enhance sense of self-control and coping efficacy (1, 12). Thus, regular exercise should be incorporated into stress management efforts. Aerobic exercise of moderate intensity and duration decreases muscle tension acutely and should therefore be recommended as a prelude to relaxation training (9).

Interpersonal Skill Training

No program of stress management is complete without psychoeducation and skill building of interpersonal factors. Sensitizing individuals to their effects on others, teaching appropriate assertive behavior, and teaching anger management strategies should also be considered. Individuals locked into type A coping habits may create especially taxing interpersonal environments (6, 13). Highly hostile patients are likely be motivated to learn new interpersonal skills if they are presented with facts that implicate hostility and anger as dangerous to health (1). Excellent summaries of this information are available (14–16). In addition, the construct of high hostility actually contains three distinct components (15):

- Anger: an unpleasant emotion ranging from irritation to rage
- Aggression: overt behavior such as attacking or destructive or hurtful actions
- Hostility: anger that perpetuates a tendency to distrust others and to wish to inflict harm on them

The cognitive mediators of hostility can be treated with various cognitive retraining strategies. Aggressive behavior is best treated by training in the use of alternative adaptive behaviors, such as methods of assertion and conflict resolution. Extensive guidelines for assertion training are available (17). In addition, through role playing or with the aid of audiovisual or videotaped interactions, patients can learn to attend to various aspects of communication style, such as what is said (words and nonverbal sounds) and how it is said (voice quality, tone, and volume), body movements, facial expressions, and gestures. Extensive models for structuring anger management interventions are available (1, 14, 16).

OUTCOMES

The positive effects of various forms of stress management training have been documented in broad-based research literature (1). Relaxation techniques have been shown to reduce anxiety, heart rate, respiratory rate, and muscle tension in normal populations and to be useful in treating medical disorders such as headache, insomnia, and hypertension. The benefits of providing brief relaxation training to patients anticipating surgery have also been documented. Sime et al. (9) discussed the fact that training in relaxation can enhance response to exercise. Benson et al. (18) found that oxygen consumption at a fixed workload is significantly lower (4%) when subjects use relaxation during exercise on a bicycle ergometer.

Stress management interventions of various types have been shown to be effective in reducing systolic blood pressure and anxiety (19). Cognitive therapy is effective for reducing anger (16). Biofeedback, especially in conjunction with relaxation training, is effective in treating hypertension and for individuals who show exaggerated type A behavior (20, 21).

In nonmedical populations, regular aerobic exercise has been found to reduce the cardiovascular effect of emotional stressors; to diminish anxiety, muscular tension, and depression; and to increase stress management ability and general feelings of well-being and self-esteem (1).

The importance of supportive family relationships, especially spouse support, has been demonstrated in research on smoking cessation, dietary modification, and adherence to exercise programs (22). In addition, spouse support has been shown to be a crucial component in effective management of various psychosocial issues for recovering medical patients (23, 24).

Combination approaches to stress management have been found to be especially effective for both healthy populations and those with cardiopulmonary disease (1). Stress management intervention emphasizing exercise has been shown to reduce exaggerated cardiovascular reactivity and to enhance control of arrhythmias and psychosocial functioning (25). Van Dixhoorn et al. (26) demonstrated the benefits of incorporating relaxation therapy, consisting of systematic breathing therapy, into formal cardiac rehabilitation through decreased failure rates (up to 50%). Finally, marked positive changes in type A behavior have been documented from extensive treatment programs combining group support and stress management in both healthy and cardiac populations (7, 8).

STRESS MANAGEMENT TRAINING AND THE FORMAL REHABILITATION PROGRAM

Following is a curriculum for a model stress management training program that can be incorporated into the educational portion of a rehabilitation program. It is based on clinical experiences and relevant literature (9, 27). This program entails four weekly lecture–discussion group sessions of an hour each and a 20–30-minute relaxation training session conducted immediately after exercise once a week. The relaxation training is tape-recorded, and patients should be encouraged to use the tape during a daily relaxation practice session of 10–20 minutes. Patients should also be encouraged to invite a significant other to attend all sessions, especially session 3. Videotaped and audiotaped material can be used to stimulate discussion.

Week 1

Topics
> Overview of the program
> Physiology and psychology of stress
> Self-directed exercises for pinpointing stressors

Audiovisuals
> Video about emotional reactions to illness

Sample discussion questions
> What are your major stressors at this time?
> What changes have you faced in the past 2 years?
> What are your physical and emotional signs of stress?
> What do you typically do next when these stress symptoms occur?

Homework
> Listen to selected audiotape regarding stress management.
> Practice relaxation exercise daily for 20–30 minutes.
> Keep a thinking journal.

Week 2

Topics
> Brief overview of personality-based coping patterns
> Brief discussion of type A behavior pattern
> Outline of anger and assertion training skills

Audiovisuals
> Video about coping strategies and type A behavior

Sample discussion questions
> What did you learn from your thinking log?
> How does your personality compel you to cope when stressed?
> How are you type A? Your loved ones?
> What small changes can you make to disrupt your typical stress-generating coping patterns?

Homework
> Listen to audiotape about relationship issues.
> Practice relaxation and monitor type A coping styles.

Week 3

Topics
> The importance of social support
> Description of families as teams
> The importance of daily uplifts to counter the stress effects of daily hassles

What support means

Audiovisuals

Videos about relationship issues and the importance of social support after illness.

Sample discussion questions

In facing illness, what problems do patients and their spouses or other significant partners share?

What problems are unique to each group?

How are children or grandchildren affected?

Which family reactions are helpful to the patient?

Which are not helpful?

Where do you get your support?

Homework

Discuss with loved ones exactly *how* they can be supportive.

Listen to audiotape about guidelines for managing intimate relationships.

Week 4

Topics

Review of progress

Ways to use relaxation and cognitive strategies to cope

Pinpointing desired areas of change in relationships

Goal setting regarding overall emotional management

Sample discussion questions

How would your life have to be 6 months from now for you to feel satisfied that you have learned to manage stress better?

List two specific stress management goals that you will address in the upcoming weeks.

What challenges face you, individually and in your family, in the immediate future?

What resources for facing these challenges do you have?

References

1. Sotile WM. Psychosocial Interventions for Cardiopulmonary Patients: A Guide for Health Professionals. Champaign, IL: Human Kinetics, 1996.
2. Holmes TH, Rahe RH. The social readjustment scale. J Psychosomatic Res 11:213, 1967.
3. Kanner AD, Coyne JC, Shaefer C, Lazarus RS. Comparison of two modes of stress measurement: Daily hassles and uplifts versus major life events. J Behav Med 4:1–39, 1981.
4. Seligman ME. Learned Optimism. New York: Knopf, 1991.
5. Kobasa SC, Maddi SR, Puccetti MC, et al. Effectiveness of hardiness, exercise and social support as resources against illness. J Psychosomatic Res 29:525, 1985.
6. Sotile WM, Sotile MO. Beat Stress Together: The BEST Way to a Passionate Marriage, a Healthy Family, and a Productive Life. New York: Wiley, 1999.
7. Friedman M, Ulmer D. Treating Type A Behavior and Your Heart. New York: Knopf, 1984.
8. Roskies E. Stress Management for the Healthy Type A: Theory and Practice. New York: Guilford, 1987.
9. Sime WE, McGahan M, Eliot RS. Stress management and coronary heart disease: Risk assessment and intervention. In: ACSM's Resource Manual for Guidelines for Exercise Testing and Prescription. Philadelphia: Lea & Febiger, 1993:489–506.
10. Schwartz MS. Biofeedback: A Practitioner's Guide. New York: Guilford, 1987.
11. Naparstek B. Staying Well With Guided Imagery. New York: Warner, 1994.
12. Emery CF, Pinder SL, Blumenthal JA. Psychological effects of exercise among elderly cardiac patients. J Cardiopulm Rehab 9:1989.
13. Smith TW, Anderson NB. Models of personality and disease: An interactional approach to type A behavior and cardiovascular risk. J Person Soc Psych 50:1166, 1986.
14. McKay M, Rogers P, McKay J. When Anger Hurts. San Francisco: New Harbinger, 1989.
15. Smith TW. Hostility and health: Current status of a psychosomatic hypothesis. Health Psych 11:139, 1992.
16. Williams R, Williams V. Anger Kills. New York: Harper, 1993.
17. Alberti R, Emmons M. A Guide to Assertive Living: Your Perfect Right. San Luis Obispo, CA: Impact, 1982.
18. Benson H, Dryer T, Hartley H. Decreased VO_2 consumption during exercise with elicitation of the relaxation response. J Hum Stress 4:38, 1978.
19. Bosley F, Allen TW. Stress management training for hypertensives: Cognitive and physiological effects. J Behav Med 12:77, 1989.
20. Kaufman PG, Jacob RG, Ewart CK. Hypertension intervention pooling project. Health Psych 7:209, 1988.
21. Stoney CM, Langer AW, Stutterer JR, et al. A comparison of biofeedback assisted cardiodeceleration in type A and B men: Modification of stress-associated cardiopulmonary and hemodynamic adjustments. J Psychosomat Med 49:79, 1987.
22. Sotile WM, Sotile MO, Ewen GS, et al. Marriage and family factors relevant to effective cardiac rehabilitation: A review of the risk factor literature. Sport Med Train Rehab 4:115, 1993.
23. Sotile WM, Sotile MO, Sotile LJ, et al. Marriage and family factors relevant to cardiac rehabilitation: An integrative review of the psychosocial literature. Sport Med Train Rehab 4:217, 1993.
24. Sotile WM. The intimacy factor in cardiopulmonary illness: A practical model for structuring interventions. J Cardiopulm Rehab 13:237, 1993.
25. Blumenthal JA, Emery CF, Walsh MA, et al. Exercise training in healthy type A middle-aged men: Effects on behavioral and cardiovascular responses. Psychosomatic Med 50:418, 1988.
26. Van Dixhoorn J, Duivenvoorden HJ, Staal HA, et al. Physical training and relaxation therapy in cardiac rehabilitation assessed through a composite criterion for training. Am Heart J 118:545, 1989.
27. Dracup K, Meleis A, Baker K, et al. Family focused cardiac rehabilitation: A role supplementation program for cardiac patients and spouses. Nurs Clin North Am 19:113, 1984.

Suggested Reading

American Heart Association. Healthy Heart. American Heart Association, 7320 Greenville Ave., Dallas, TX (video series) 1996.

Levin R. Portrait of a Heartmate. Minneapolis: Heartmates (video series).

Naparstek B. Health Journeys. Audiotape series. Los Angeles: Time Warner AudioBooks (audiotape series).

Sotile WM. Controlling Yourself During Uncontrollable Times. Winston-Salem, NC: (audiotape).

Sotile WM. Coping With Heart Illness. Human Kinetics, Champaign, IL (video series).

Sotile WM. High-Powered Lives Need High-Powered Relationships. Winston-Salem, NC: (audiotape).

Sotile WM. Thriving, Not Just Surviving. Winston-Salem, NC: (audiotape).

For an extensive list of audiovisual aids for rehabilitation settings, contact the American Association of Cardiovascular and Pulmonary Rehabilitation, 7611 Elmwood Avenue, Suite 201, Middleton, WI 53562.

1.5.0, 1.5.2, 1.5.3   2.5.0   4.5.0

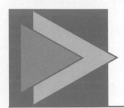

CHAPTER **67**

ENHANCING SOCIAL SUPPORT AND GROUP DYNAMICS

Paul M. Ribisl and Sally A. Shumaker

Measurement of social support and understanding its role in influencing physical activity outcomes in preventive and rehabilitative programs has not received the attention that it perhaps deserves. Yet oddly enough, social support has the potential to be one of the most influential factors affecting the success of intervention in preventive and rehabilitative programs because it has a direct effect on adherence. Well-designed programs with state-of-the-art facilities and equipment conducted by well-trained staff may be compromised or even fail if social support of participants or patients is inadequate.

DEFINITION

Social support has been defined as "the comfort, assistance, and/or information one receives through formal or informal contacts with individuals or groups" (1). It can also describe both the **structure** of the social environment and the **resources** or functions such environments provide. Structural support refers to the size, density, complexity, symmetry, and stability of family, friends, coworkers, health professionals, and community resources (i.e., the social network). Resources refer to the perception of the availability of support and of the resources provided (i.e., social support). The two dimensions are often combined in measures of social support.

IMPORTANCE OF SOCIAL SUPPORT

Social support has a significant role in both the causation of and the recovery from illness and disease. Considerable literature links social support to health outcomes (2–4). Two major theories have been proposed regarding the role of social support in disease causation:

- The **direct hypothesis**
- The **buffering hypothesis**

The direct hypothesis infers creation of a positive effect, improved self-esteem, and a sense of stability and control. These lead to the development of healthful behaviors, such as smoking cessation, improved diet, and increased physical activity. In the buffering hypothesis, people are protected from the pathogenic effects of stress by instilling coping behaviors and reducing reactivity to perceived stress (5).

In preventive and rehabilitative programming, the focus should be on understanding how social support interacts with the intervention strategies used in these programs to promote positive outcomes. Specific interventions typically include smoking cessation, dietary intervention and weight control, psychosocial stress management, physical activity, education, and adherence to prescribed medications. Unfortunately, the prevailing literature provides us with an incomplete understanding of how social support may influence outcomes associated with these intervention programs.

SOCIAL MILIEU IN HEALTH BEHAVIORS: AN OVERVIEW

Efforts to use social support in intervention programs must capitalize on the different forms that social support takes at different ages. Research on parental influence on physical activity patterns of children is inconsistent; however, several studies demonstrate that parental social influence is effective (6–8).

For **preschool children**, parents appear to be most influential in the development of positive health behaviors, while siblings and playmates play a minor role. Parental prompting to play outdoors instead of playing video games or watching television increases level of activity (9). Programs developed in preschool may influence these behaviors as well. Taylor et al. (6) give examples of how social support can be used to increase physical activity in children:

- Providing information on physical activity
- Viewing a child at play or practice
- Discussing physical activity with the child

568

- Offering to exercise with the child
- Assisting the child in physical activity interests by providing transportation to practice and games

For **elementary school children** parents continue to be the most influential source of support, but classmates and school programs begin to play a greater role. The widespread loss of scheduled physical education classes in American public schools, along with increased attraction of passive activity, such as television and computer games, has significantly diminished the opportunity for daily physical activity in this age group. While young children are fairly active, the level of physical activity actually declines about 50% during the school years (10).

These same forces continue to operate in **secondary school**; however, influence from classmates and friends assumes a greater role than that of parents during adolescence. Nevertheless, Anderson and Wold have demonstrated that parental encouragement is closely correlated with physical activity level in adolescents (11). However, Sallis points out that if adolescents identify with a peer group that values and participates in activity, the group creates a supportive environment; in contrast, the group becomes a deterrent if it devalues physical activity (12). For most adolescents, organized sports and school programs are the major opportunities for regular physical activity, and both coaches and team members provide a significant source of social support for continued participation.

In the young adult of **college age**, peers or classmates exert the primary influence and provide the major source of support for healthful behaviors. While alcohol, tobacco, and other drug use may be initiated in middle school or high school, early adulthood is a critical time for maintenance of good health habits, because peers can exert a powerful influence on these behaviors during a vulnerable time. This may also be the first time that individuals live away from home and make personal food choices without parental influence or control. While some colleges offer courses on healthful lifestyles, the exposure is brief and peer influence has a greater potential to affect behavior.

For most **middle-aged adults**, a spouse, friends, or coworkers are the major sources of support in the form of encouragement, participation in physical activities, and assistance, such as child care (12). Challenges to individuals in the workforce are different from those of persons who are at home raising families. Finding the time and setting to exercise during the workday is difficult for most, especially the blue-collar worker, while for mothers with children at home, there is the challenge of finding time to exercise in addition to the expense of child care. These barriers are sufficient to cause a large proportion of the middle-aged to remain physically inactive. Social support in the form of coworkers to exercise with at work, or in the case of the mother at home, having friends or family to assist with child care, may make the difference between being active and inactive. Also, Danielson and Wanzel indicate that women have better attendance in fitness classes when with a companion, while Wankel found that a buddy system positively influences adherence in exercise settings (13, 14).

The major sources of social support for the **older adult** are the spouse, friends, and community social systems. Physical activity benefits to older individuals are substantial, and this group may need physical activity more than any other age group. Disability due to chronic disease is most prevalent in this group, and maintaining independence for activities of daily living is closely linked with an active lifestyle. Yet Cousins points out that this group may encounter a number of factors that increase the difficulty of becoming active, such as disapproval from a spouse, lack of peer involvement, discouragement from the immediate family, and inadequate encouragement from physicians (15). Older adults face other barriers to being physically active. Shephard cites the following that must be recognized and overcome (16):

- Absence of a suitable companion
- Lack of transportation to the exercise site
- Limited sight or hearing
- Cognitive, emotional, or behavioral problems

GROUP DYNAMICS IN EXERCISE PROGRAMS: ENHANCING THE SUPPORTIVE ATMOSPHERE

Formal exercise programs have various sources of social support, including exercise professionals and participants. Both have the potential to exert positive or negative influences. Exercise professionals are crucial to a supportive atmosphere and perhaps offer the dominant influence on compliance of participants. Individuals often, but not always prefer to be among participants who are similar in age, gender, fitness level, and physique. Older adults do not want to feel out of place, and as Shephard and Sidney and Shephard point out, it is often better for the sake of role modeling to use an older person to lead an exercise class, since research suggests that a very fit class leader may further weaken self-reliance and motivation among the frail elderly (16, 17).

Sometimes certain participants have a negative social influence on the conduct of group exercise classes. The following discussion addresses some of the more common types of negative influence that may be encountered.

Chronic Complainers

Chronic complainers should be interviewed carefully to determine whether the cause of the complaint is physical. It is possible that there are legitimate physical ailments (e.g., arthritis, joint problems, back problems) that make exercise uncomfortable, and medical attention may be warranted. If the complaints are due to dissatisfaction with the program or leadership, address them directly. Some individuals are general malcontents and are often tolerated; however, if the person is disruptive to the program, ask him or her either to modify the behavior or to find another program.

Disrupters and Comedians

Disrupters and comedians must be dealt with at the first sign of disruption to minimize the effects on other participants. Usually, the need for attention can be channeled into productive activity by having them take a leadership role in the class. Allowing them to lead warm-up exercises or help in another way may satisfy attention-getting needs that otherwise lead to disruptive behavior. Depending on the class makeup, a comedian participant may enhance the mood of the class. However, if the behavior poses a danger to other participants or detracts from the program, the comedian should be dealt with directly about modifying the behavior.

Noncompliers

Noncompliers may either underexert or overexert during the activity portion of a program. Those who fail to comply by exercising under the prescribed threshold should be taught the benefits of overload and encouraged to exercise at appropriate levels. However, since program dropout rates are higher from vigorous activity than from moderate activity, there is a downside to pushing individuals beyond a certain point (18). In addition, the sedentary person who has rarely exercised requires a gradual period of adjustment to learn to tolerate levels of discomfort that are commonly accepted by a veteran exerciser. A discussion with a sympathetic exercise professional, along with matching the person with another participant who can share experiences may help such participants.

In contrast, those who overexert pose a significant safety hazard to themselves (19). The value of pacing should be emphasized. They may also be paired with another patient, preferably a former overexerter who has modified exercise style. As Sotile has pointed out, the overexerter's orientation to hurry up and try harder than the next person is counterproductive to a safe, individualized exercise threshold (20).

RESEARCH ON SOCIAL SUPPORT IN CARDIOPULMONARY REHABILITATION

Evidence that social support protects cardiovascular health is convincing. Orth-Gomer cites both cross-sectional and longitudinal studies demonstrating that lack of social support and weak social integration are associated with elevated risk of myocardial infarction (21). In one study, the influence of stressful life events on all-cause mortality in middle-aged men was examined (22). Only men with adequate emotional support seemed to be protected. Further work substantiates that when standard risk factors for coronary artery disease are controlled, two factors emerge as the strongest independent risk contributors to myocardial infarction in middle-aged men: smoking and lack of social support (23).

The literature on social support in cardiac rehabilitation has been directed primarily at influences on adherence to physical activity. Much of this research focuses exclusively on spouse support rather than on a full network or the support available within a formal program (i.e., other participants and professional staff) (24–26). Most studies are retrospective, examining multiple factors, including social support, that influence compliance in the form of attendance or adherence to a healthful behavior. Most findings support the notion that social support is positively related to adherence to healthful behaviors. However, experimental research in which social support is manipulated to determine whether it is an independent variable and has significant influence on improving outcomes (adoption or maintenance of healthful behaviors) is lacking.

According to Dracup (27), the evidence suggests that enhanced social support is a relatively powerful, but relatively untested component of cardiac rehabilitation and that a major problem with the research is that it is difficult to differentiate the effects of social support from the other interventions in a cardiopulmonary rehabilitation program. Patients receiving social support from family and friends are more likely to comply with modification of behaviors associated with risk factors, and spousal support is a known predictor of program adherence in cardiac rehabilitation (28, 29). A recent pilot study demonstrated that even a brief session with family members teaching them how to support exercise behavior can get patients to be more physically active outside the formal program (30). Other supportive evidence from the Heart Smart Family Health Promotion focuses on the entire family system rather than individuals (31). The format minimizes lecture and maximizes awareness, skills development, problem solving, and real-life application over a 12–16 week agenda. This program has demonstrated positive changes in cardiovascular risk factors, and it can be applied to both clinical and health promotion settings.

OUTCOMES AND MEASUREMENT OF SOCIAL SUPPORT

To provide evidence that a specific intervention is effective, outcomes that reflect change in important parameters of social support should be defined and measured. Kaplan discusses the complex issues associated with the measurement of health outcomes in social support research and concludes that while social support is associated with a lower rate of mortality from cardiovascular disease, studies linking social support to health are problematic (4). This is partly due to problems associated with conceptualization and measurement and to lack of a consensual definition of social support. While efforts to develop valid and acceptably reliable measures of social support in the cardiopulmonary rehabilitation literature continue, the consensus is that the phenomenon of social support is sufficiently robust to warrant inclusion as an important psychosocial parameter in cardiopulmonary rehabilitation.

Despite continuing debate regarding specific instruments, it makes sense to use the best of what is available until further research yields more definitive measures of social support and its influence on the course of patient treatment in cardiopulmonary rehabilitation. Several measures of social support are considered appropriate.

The MOS Social Support Survey

The MOS Social Support Survey is a brief, multidimensional self-administered social support survey that has been used in both healthy populations and in patients with chronic disease (32). It identifies four functional support scales, including **tangible**, **affectionate**, **positive social interaction**, and **emotional–informational** support. The instrument has excellent psychometric properties and has been used extensively in clinical research. Brief descriptions of the four types of support:

- Tangible support: Someone to help you if you are confined to bed, take you to a doctor if needed, prepare meals, help with daily chores
- Affection support: Someone who shows you love and affection, hugs you, and makes you feel wanted
- Positive social interaction: Someone to have a good time with, get together with for relaxation, and do something enjoyable with
- Emotional support: Someone to listen when you need to talk, give advice in a crisis, confide in and share private worries and fears, and who understands your problems

This survey provides a total score and separate ratings of each of the four types of support that can identify those who lack sufficient social support.

The Health Support Index

Evidence suggests that success rates of programs designed to change health-related behaviors (diet, exercise, and smoking habits) may be influenced by the availability of social support for these targeted changes (33, 34). In an effort to focus on how social network members provide support related to desired behavioral changes, the Health Support Index (HSI) is used to assess existing social support for planned changes in health-related behaviors. It measures two theoretically distinct aspects of social and environmental support for health-related behavior change: supportiveness and modeling. A subscale of the HSI assesses each component. The validity and reliability of the HSI indicate that it may be a promising tool for evaluating social support for the modification of health-related behaviors (34).

The Social Provisions Scale

The Social Provisions Scale measures six provisions related to social support received from friends, family members, and coworkers (35):

- Attachment
- Social integration
- Reassurance of worth
- Guidance
- Opportunity for nurturance
- Reliable alliance

This scale can also be modified to indicate support for specific health-related behaviors such as smoking, dietary intake, stress management, and physical activity.

RECOMMENDATIONS FOR PRACTICE

How measures of social support should be used to improve outcomes in cardiopulmonary rehabilitation requires speculation, because there is little published research for guidance. It is prudent to assess level of social support at entry using instruments such as the **MOS Scale** or the **Social Provisions Scale** to determine whether levels of social support present a threat to compliance. While it may not be possible to alter the social support and network involving family, friends, and coworkers, it may be feasible to look for ways to provide supplemental social support for those who have the greatest need. This may be in the form of increased attention during program participation, written materials for home use, periodic phone calls and/or mailings to encourage compliance, and establishing support groups that meet outside of regular program hours.

▶ **SUMMARY**

While the research on social support continues to provide more scientific evidence of its effectiveness, clinical experiences over the past two decades provide empirical evidence that social support in many forms is a powerful factor for promoting and sustaining health behavior change. Assessing social support at entry and providing mechanisms within the preventive or rehabilitative program may help improve compliance and adherence.

References
1. Wallston BS, Alagna SW, DeVellis BM, et al. Social support and physical health. Health Psych 2:367–391, 1983.
2. Cohen S, Syme SL, eds. Social Support and Health. New York: Academic, 1985.
3. Shumaker SA, Czajkowski SM, eds. Social Support and Cardiovascular Disease. New York: Plenum, 1994.

4. Kaplan RM. Measures of health outcome in social support research. In: Shumaker SA, Czajkowski SM, eds. Social Support and Cardiovascular Disease. New York: Plenum, 1994.

5. Cohen S, Kaplan JR, Manuck SB. Social support and coronary heart disease: Underlying psychological and biological mechanisms. In: Shumaker SA, Czajkowski SM, eds. Social Support and Cardiovascular Disease. New York: Plenum Press, 1994.

6. Taylor WC, Baranowski T, Sallis JF. Family determinants of childhood physical activity: A social-cognitive model. In: Dishman RK, ed. Advances in Exercise Adherence. Champaign, IL: Human Kinetics, 1994.

7. McKenzie TL, Sallis JF, Nader PR, et al. Beaches: An observational system for assessing children's eating and physical activity behaviors and associated events. J Appl Behav Anal 24:141–151, 1991.

8. Dennison BA, Straus JH, Mellits E, et al. Childhood physical fitness tests: Predictor of adult physical activity levels? Pediatrics 82:324–330, 1988.

9. Epstein LH, Smith JA, Vara LS, et al. Behavioral economic analysis of activity choice in obese children. Health Psych 10:311–316, 1991.

10. Sallis JF, Nader PR, Broyles SL, et al. Correlates of physical activity at home in Mexican-American and Anglo-American preschool children. Health Psych 12:390–398, 1983.

11. Anderssen N, Wold B. Parental and peer influences on leisure-time physical activity in young adolescents. Res Q Exerc Sport 63:341–348, 1992.

12. Sallis JF. Influences on physical activity of children, adolescents, and adults or determinants of active living. Phys Activity Fitness Res Dig 1(7):3, 1994.

13. Danielson R, Wanzel R. Exercise objectives of fitness program dropouts. In: Landers D, Christina R, eds. Psychology of Motor Behavior and Sport. Champaign, IL: Human Kinetics, 1977:310–320.

14. Wankel LM. Decision-making and social-support strategies for increasing exercise involvement. J Cardiac Rehab 4:124–135, 1984.

15. Cousins SO. The role of social support in later life physical activity. In: Quinney HA, Gauvin L, Wall AE, eds. Toward Active Living. Champaign, IL: Human Kinetics, 1994.

16. Shephard RJ. Determinants of exercise in people aged 65 years and older. In: Dishman RK, ed. Advances in Exercise Adherence. Champaign, IL: Human Kinetics, 1994.

17. Sidney KH, Shephard RJ. Attitudes towards health and physical activity in the elderly: Effects of a physical training programme. Med Sci Sport 8:246–252, 1977.

18. Dishman RK, Sallis JF. Determinants and interventions for physical activity and exercise. In: Bouchard C, Shephard RJ, Stephens T, eds. Physical Activity, Fitness, and Health: International Proceedings and Consensus Statement. Champaign, IL: Human Kinetics, 1984:214–238.

19. American College of Sports Medicine. ACSM's Guidelines for Exercise Testing and Prescription. 5th ed. Baltimore: Williams & Wilkins, 1995.

20. Sotile WM. Psychosocial Interventions for Cardiopulmonary Patients. Champaign, IL: Human Kinetics, 1996.

21. Orth-Gomer K. International epidemiological evidence for a relationship between social support and cardiovascular disease. In: Shumaker SA, Czajkowski SM, eds. Social Support and Cardiovascular Disease. New York: Plenum, 1994.

22. Rosengren A, Orth-Gomer K, Wedel H, et al. Stressful life events, social support, and mortality in men born in 1933. Br Med J 307:1102–1105, 1983.

23. Orth-Gomer K, Rosengren A, Wilhelmsen L. Lack of social support and incidence of coronary heart disease in middle-aged Swedish men. Psychosomatic Med 55:37–43, 1993.

24. Knapp D, Gutmann M, Foster C, et al. Exercise adherence among coronary artery bypass surgery (CABS) patients. Med Sci Sport Exerc 15:120, 1983.

25. Burkett PA. Practical issues for increasing exercise adherence. J Cardiopulm Rehab 12:18–19, 1992.

26. Oldridge N, Ragowski B, Gottlieb M. Use of outpatient cardiac rehabilitation services: Factors associated with attendance. J Cardiopulm Rehab 12:25–31, 1992.

27. Dracup K. Cardiac rehabilitation: The role of social support in recovery and compliance. In: Shumaker SA, Czajkowski SM, eds. Social Support and Cardiovascular Disease. New York: Plenum, 1994.

28. Gianetti VJ, Reynolds J, Rign T. Factors which differentiate smokers from ex-smokers among cardiovascular patients: A discriminant analysis. Soc Sci Med 20:241–245, 1985.

29. Andrew GM, Oldridge NB, Parker JO, et al. Reasons for dropout from exercise programs in post-coronary patients. Med Sci Sport Exerc 11:376–378, 1979.

30. Dominick KL, Ribisl PM, Rejeski WJ, et al. Social support strategies improve physical activity outcomes in cardiac rehabilitation. J Cardiopulm Rehab 14:335, 1994.

31. Johnson CC, Nicklas TA. Health ahead: The Heart Smart Family approach to prevention of cardiovascular disease. Am J Med Sci 310(Suppl 1):S127–S132, 1995.

32. Sherbourne CD, Stewart AL. The MOS social support survey. Soc Sci Med 32:705–714, 1991.

33. Robbins SR, Slavin LA. A measure of social support for health-related behavior change. Health Education 19(3):36–39, 1988.

34. Colletti G, Brownell KD. The physical and emotional benefits of social support: Applications to obesity, smoking, and alcoholism. In: Hersen M, Eisler RM, Miller PM, eds. Progress in Behavior Modification. New York: Academic, 1982:110–179.

35. Russell D, Cutrona CE. The provisions of social relationships and adaptation to stress. In: Jones WH, Perleman D, eds. Advances in Personal Relationships. Greenwich, CT: JAI, 1987.

CHAPTER **68**

PHYSICAL ACTIVITY PROMOTION: ANTECEDENTS

Abby C. King and Michaela Kiernan

An explosion of interest by both the public and health professionals in physical activity as a means for achieving goals related to health, functioning, and quality of life has occurred. Despite this increased interest and beliefs of personal benefit, available evidence indicates that one-third or more of Americans do not exercise regularly (i.e., on three or more days per week) and one-fourth or more do not exercise at all. Over the past decade there has been an increase in leisure time physical activity in many industrialized nations, including the United States; however, a number of subgroups remain underactive (1). Population segments notably underrepresented among those engaging in regular physical activity include individuals who are older (particularly women), less educated, smokers, and the overweight. Of the 10% (or fewer) of sedentary adults who begin regular physical activity in a year (and those already participating), approximately one-half drop out within 3 to 6 months. Half of individuals enrolled in secondary prevention programs drop out within 12 months.

Such statistics indicate that assisting individuals to stay regularly involved in physical activity is a challenge requiring creativity and patience. In addition, finding ways to encourage the extremely sedentary to adopt a more active lifestyle is an increasingly important public health goal. Exercise professionals can take advantage of the current public enthusiasm for becoming more active and the growing literature suggesting strategies than can be effective for enhancing participation in physical activity.

THE ADHERENCE PROBLEM

In some ways, physical activity may be a unique health behavior, governed by factors that differ somewhat from other health behaviors (2–4). Certainly the demand for regularity in performing physical activity to benefit throughout life calls for innovative methods of studying the process that makes regular exercise habitual. Additionally, factors influencing initial adoption and early participation in exercise may differ from those affecting maintenance. Stages of change models may better identify strategies that will work for individuals in different stages and levels of exercise participation, such as persons contemplating joining an exercise program, those in the early stage of exercise adoption, or those committed to maintaining a program across the long term. Such models draw extensively from social cognitive theory and other theories of behavior change (5, 6). Although the understanding of this process is generally not extensive, a number of potentially important variables have been identified (6).

Social Cognitive Theory

Though no single theory fully explains why individuals become or stay active, efforts to understand such health behaviors by placing them in the context of a social learning–social cognitive model of health behavior change has helped. The social cognitive approach, broadly defined, views such behavior as being initiated and maintained through a complex interaction of personal, behavioral, and environmental factors and conditions. Past experiences with physical activity; views of physical activity in general and different forms of activity in particular; the extent of activity-related knowledge, skills, and beliefs; and how the surrounding environment either helps or hinders efforts to increase physical activity all play a role in influencing how active the individual is and will remain.

The social learning–social cognitive theoretical approach emphasizes ability to regulate behavior through setting goals, monitoring progress toward these goals, and modifying the physical and social environment to support the goals. Observational learning and modeling by others is an important influence on behavior. Self efficacy (i.e., belief in one's ability to perform a specific behavior or activity) and outcome expectancies (i.e., belief that the behavior leads to a desired outcome) are identified as the critical factors influencing which behaviors are attempted and with what level of effort before a person gives up.

In addition to social cognitive theory, other conceptual models or approaches include the health belief model, the locus of control model, relapse prevention models, the theory of reasoned action, and expectancy–value decision theories (7). To date few have been as heuristic as the social cognitive perspective in helping to shape effective intervention.

Social cognitive and related approaches to understanding physical activity behavior have been supplemented in recent years with increased appreciation for the place of psychological readiness in changing physical activity patterns. Such psychological readiness interacts with and can be influenced by the types of personal, behavioral, program-related, and environmental factors described next.

Personal Factors

Among the demographic factors found to be associated with physical activity participation are the following:

- Gender. Women participate less in vigorous activity, especially at younger ages.
- Age. Increasing age is associated with lower levels of physical activity.
- Educational attainment. Educational level is positively associated with leisure time physical activity.

Meanwhile, demographic factors, such as occupation and race or ethnicity, have less consistent relationships with leisure time physical activity. Though few studies have specifically examined differences by race, some have demonstrated that African American women are consistently less active than white women (7). There is some evidence that physical activity levels may to some extent run in families; however, reasons (i.e., genetic, behavioral, environmental, or some combination of these factors) are unclear.

Health factors have been shown to have consistent relationships with physical activity level. People with medical problems or disabilities are likely to be inactive. Smoking status is related to low levels of physical activity in some, although not all, populations and is associated with high dropout rates from vigorous leisure time exercise programs.

Overweight and obese individuals have been consistently found to be less active in a range of activities, including both leisure time and routine activity, such as walking and taking stairs. It is, however, unknown why overweight and obese individuals are less active. It is possible that engaging in physical activity is more aerobically challenging and physically difficult due to weight. However, it may also be that attending exercise classes or engaging in physical activity is stressful for some subgroups of overweight individuals who are dissatisfied with physical appearance. People may be more dissatisfied about appearance when in situations eliciting thoughts about appearance and may actively avoid situations that exacer-

bate feelings of dissatisfaction (8). Exercise, especially in a group with a focus on appearance and social comparison, may be one such situation. Cognitive strategies including correcting size and weight estimates of self relative to peers, norms, and objective standards, and behavioral strategies such as incremental exposure to a target situation, have been demonstrated to improve body image for normal weight individuals (9, 10). Such approaches may also be helpful for overweight individuals who have extreme body dissatisfaction and indicate the desire to engage in increased physical activity.

In addition to demographic and health factors, variables influencing initial participation in regular physical activity include the following:

- Past experiences with physical activity
- Perceptions of health status, exercise ability, and skills
- Self-efficacy beliefs, defined as the level of confidence in the ability to perform a specific physical activity regimen
- Outcome efficacy beliefs (i.e., belief that physical activity has value for health, fitness, or related outcomes)
- Perceived enjoyment and satisfaction
- Perceptions related to access to exercise facilities, lack of time, and exercise intensity
- Understanding of how increased physical activity relates to personal benefits, in both the short and the long term

In addition, rating of self-motivation may be related to continued participation in exercise. Self-motivation may be learned when defined as an ability to find rewards for behavior independent of external rewards available for that behavior. This concept is preferable to definitions of motivation that place responsibility for nonadherence on internal processes related to personality or similar constructs. These latter definitions, aside from being unfair because they ignore extrapersonal influences on behavior (e.g., the environment), do not provide the exercise professional with a firm direction for intervention.

Though many of the aforementioned factors are associated with initial participation in physical activity, relatively few appear to substantially influence length of maintenance of an exercise regimen. Influential factors may be smoking status, weight, self-efficacy, and perceived lack of time. Other factors likely to have an effect on continued participation are ongoing enjoyment of the physical activity and the perception of barriers such as scheduling, illness, travel, and other factors that can impede physical activity.

Behavioral Factors

Behavioral factors include the skills to carry out physical activity to facilitate exercise-related benefits while minimizing injury and boredom. Such skills include knowledge and use of behavioral and psychological strategies that assist negotiation of barriers and pitfalls, which inevitably interfere with regular activity.

A useful behavioral skill may be as simple as knowing how to plan by identifying and preparing for periods when disruption to exercise is likely (e.g., during holidays). This type of strategy is known as relapse prevention (11). Studies applying relapse prevention strategies, either alone or in combination with other behavioral strategies, suggest their utility in promotion, adoption, and maintenance of physical activity (11–13). Another potentially effective strategy is implementation of a decision balance sheet, whereby careful evaluation of expected or experienced benefits and costs of participating are compared. Other self-regulatory skills that appear to promote physical activity participation, if used regularly, are self-monitoring of progress, realistic short- and longer-term goal setting coupled with ongoing feedback related to success, and the use of self-rewards (7).

Environmental and Program Factors

A number of environmental and program-based factors can influence initial participation as well as longer term adherence. These include the following:

- Family influences and support (spouses of individuals reported to be neutral or unsupportive of physical activity are likely to drop out)
- Proximity and access to facilities (for persons preferring facility-based activities)
- Weather
- Regimen flexibility
- Convenience of activity (real or perceived)
- Immediate cues and prompts in the environment promoting physical activity (e.g., reminders to exercise)
- Immediate consequences of activity

The social environment can have major impact on both adoption and maintenance of physical activity. Family participation and support and parental level of physical activity are associated with increased physical activity in some population groups. Social support from friends or coworkers may also have a positive effect. In addition, physicians and other health professionals can positively influence physical activity behavior. Although surveys suggest that physician advice is considered to be potentially important with respect to health behaviors, relatively few physicians discuss physical activity practices with patients. Barriers to physician counseling on physical activity include lack of confidence in ability to effectively advise patients (often stemming from lack of knowledge and/or training), lack of time, lack of knowledge related to the most appropriate referral sources in the community, and limited reimbursement for these services. As part of Project PACE, funded by the Centers for Disease Control and Prevention, a physician-based brief physical activity assessment and counseling protocol is available for use in the clinical setting (14).

The type of physical activity (e.g., swimming, brisk walking, aerobic dance), as well as intensity, duration, and frequency, can influence participation levels. The format in which the activity is offered (e.g., class, home-based, with or without partners) may also have an important effect on both initial participation and longer-term adherence. Although most exercise programs are offered in a class or group format, evidence indicates that the public generally prefers programs offered outside a formal group. There are important benefits to long-term adherence with adequately structured home-based regimens (13). The mode, intensity, frequency, duration, and location of physical activity must meet the needs of differing groups of individuals. For example, women report stronger preference for videotaped exercise and aerobic dance than men. Similarly, the workplace has been shown to be preferred for physical activity in some groups (7).

Immediate consequences, including observance of physical activity–related benefits and enjoyability of activity, are other program-related factors likely to have a strong impact on adherence. Conversely, sedentary people persist principally because it is immediately reinforcing, and attempts to become physically active are likely to result in immediate aversive consequences. Thus, the task of the health professional is to ensure that initial attempts to exercise are painless, enjoyable, and reinforcing. Although time constraints are typically noted as major reasons for inactivity, regular exercisers complain as much as persons who are not regularly active. Thus, perceived available time may reflect in large part the priority on being active rather than actual time limitations.

In light of the substantial prevalence of inactivity, there is growing interest in physical and psychological health benefits of moderate-intensity physical activity. Traditionally, research examining health benefits of exercise focuses on the relationship between exercise training and physical fitness. It was assumed that health improved as a result of exercise only if requisite increases in physical fitness (i.e., mainly cardiorespiratory fitness) occurred. To achieve increased cardiorespiratory fitness, it is necessary to participate in exercise that is relatively vigorous, continuous, and aerobic. Recommendations for exercise involved the rhythmical and aerobic use of large muscle groups, 3–5 days/week, at 60–90% of maximum heart rate, for 20–60 minutes. These recommendations have been considered a **threshold** exercise prescription for health benefits.

However, a new conceptual paradigm based on epidemiological data broadens the focus to include health benefits from activity (15). It is now assumed that health benefits can be gained from diverse types of physical activity, such as walking, stair climbing, gardening, and household tasks rather than only from aerobic exercise.

Additionally, the dose of physical activity includes moderate-intensity (not just vigorous) activities and the utility of activity accumulated intermittently rather than continuously. The current recommendations also acknowledge that increased health benefits are likely to accrue with increased amounts and/or intensity of physical activity. However, a growing body of research demonstrates that moderate-intensity physical activity, such as walking, is more appealing to many than more vigorous programs (7).

The results from a recent 2-year study of 269 healthy, initially sedentary middle-aged men and women who had been randomly assigned to one of three physical activity programs suggested six clinically meaningful subgroups of people who were at low, moderate, or high risk of poor adherence by the second year of their physical activity program (16). For instance, persons who had been assigned initially to a community-based exercise class offered three times per week throughout the study period and who had a body mass index (i.e., body weight in kilogram per height in square meters) of 27 or greater were at particularly high risk for poor adherence throughout the 2-year study period (i.e., only 7.7% of this subgroup achieved exercise adherence rates of at least 66% or greater by the second year). In contrast, individuals who had been initially assigned to a supervised home-based physical activity program and who reported low initial stress levels were at relatively low risk for poor exercise adherence throughout the 2-year study period (i.e., more than half of this subgroup achieved exercise adherence rates of at least 66% across the 2-year period). Continued research in this area using applications of such clinical decision-making approaches will help to refine our understanding of those subgroups of people, defined through a combination of biological, psychosocial, behavioral, and exercise program–specific factors, for whom tailored interventions are particularly indicated.

SIGNAL DETECTION

Signal detection methods were originally used by engineers to detect physical stimuli (e.g., auditory signals). They have been applied in medicine to develop diagnostic methods and tests. Signal detection can be used to define, through application of algorithms consisting of a series of simple and/or decision rules, distinct groups that are mutually exclusive and maximally discriminated from each other. More recently, applications of signal detection methods that define a signal as a behavioral outcome (e.g., presence or absence of smoking or regular exercise participation) have been discussed (17). A strength of signal detection in behavioral research is that it allows for full use of all data available for each variable being evaluated, thereby eliminating problems related to missing data that accompany the use of multiple regression approaches (17).

► SUMMARY

The factors that most strongly influence initial adoption are probably different from those that affect maintenance (18). Currently noted variables clearly constitute part of the factors relevant in affecting activity levels, many of which have yet to be identified. Because of the complex interrelationships among these variables, many individuals may have difficulty explaining problems with starting or maintaining exercise without monitoring activity. Some factors identified as predictive of inactivity (e.g., smoking status or being overweight) are present in those who may reap the most benefit from regular physical activity, those who are least likely to adopt or maintain an activity program. Finally, the variety of factors implicated indicates the importance of developing programs and strategies that fit the needs and preferences of various population groups. This tailoring can be contrasted with more typical methods of fitting individuals into existing programs. By tailoring physical activity to the population or individual, exercise professionals may positively influence initial dropout rate (during the critical period, i.e., the first 3–6 months) and during later periods. Systematic research evaluating specific methods of tailoring programs is increasingly indicated. In addition, applications knowledge of endurance exercise should be systematically applied to other dimensions of physical activity, including strength and flexibility training.

The use of linear regression method to define factors associated with physical activity participation offers limited understanding of the manner in which various personal, behavioral, program-specific, and environmental factors combine to identify subgroups at particular risk for poor physical activity adherence. Recent applications of clinical decision-making approaches, such as signal detection analysis, show promise in helping to define in a meaningful way subgroups of people at risk for poor exercise adherence, thus for whom tailored programs may be able especially effective (17).

ACKNOWLEDGMENTS

This work was supported in part by PHS grant AG-12358 from the National Institute on Aging awarded to Dr. King.

References
1. Stephens T, Caspersen CJ. The demography of physical activity. In: Bouchard C, Shephard RJ, Stephens T, eds. Physical Activity, Fitness, and Health: International Proceedings and Consensus Statement. Champaign, IL: Human Kinetics, 1994:239–256.
2. Dishman RK. Compliance/adherence in health-related exercise. Health Psychol 1:237–267, 1982.
3. Oldridge NB. Compliance with exercise rehabilitation. In: Dishman RK, ed. Exercise and Public Health. Champaign, IL: Human Kinetics, 1988:283–304.

4. Martin JE, Dubbert PM. Exercise adherence. Exerc Sport Sci Rev 13:137–167, 1985.
5. Bandura A. Social Foundations of Thought and Action: A Social Cognitive Theory. Englewood Cliffs, NJ: Prentice Hall, 1986.
6. Marcus BH, Takowski W, Rossi JS. Assessing motivational readiness and decision making for exercise. Health Psych 11:257–261, 1992.
7. King AC, Blair SN, Bild DE, et al. Determination of physical activity and intervention in adults. Med Sci Sports Exerc 24: S221–S236, 1992.
8. Haimovitz D, Lansky LM, O'Reilly P. Fluctuations in body satisfaction across situations. Int J Eating Dis 13:77–84, 1993.
9. Rosen JC, Saltzberg E, Srebnik D. Cognitive behavior therapy for negative body image. Behav Ther 20:393–404, 1989.
10. Butters JW, Cash TF. Cognitive-behavioral treatment of women's body image dissatisfaction. J Consult Clin Psych 55:889–897, 1987.
11. King AC, Frederiksen LW. Low-cost strategies for increasing exercise behavior: The effects of relapse preparation training and social support. Behav Modif 4:3–21, 1984.
12. Belisle M, Roskies E, Levesque JM. Improving adherence to physical activity. Health Psychol 6:159–172, 1987.
13. King AC, Haskell WL, Taylor CB, et al. Group vs home-based exercise training in healthy older men and women: A community-based clinical trial. JAMA 266:1535–1542, 1991.
14. Calfas KJ, Long BJ, Sallis JF, et al. A controlled trial of physician counseling to promote the adoption of physical activity. Prevent Med 25(3):225–233, 1996.
15. Pate RR, Pratt M, Blair S, et al. Physical activity and public health: A recommendation from the Centers for Disease Control and Prevention and the American College of Sports Medicine. JAMA 273:402–407, 1995.
16. King AC. Using signal detection methods to predict exercise adherence in adults (abstract). Ann Behav Med 17(Suppl): S041, 1995.
17. Kraemer HC. Assessment of 2×2 association: Generalization of signal detection methods. Am Stat 42:37–49, 1988.
18. Saltis JF, Haskell WL, Fortmann SP, et al. Predictors of adoption and maintenance of physical activity in a community sample. Prev Med 15:331–341, 1986.

1.5.0, 1.5.2, 1.5.3   2.5.0   3.5.0, 3.5.1   4.5.0

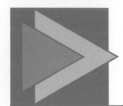

CHAPTER **69**

PHYSICAL ACTIVITY PROMOTION: ADOPTION AND MAINTENANCE

Abby C. King and John E. Martin

A growing number of theories and models of ways to change health behavior have been applied to physical activity behavior with varying results (1). Among the most heuristic of these approaches is the application of social learning–social cognitive theories (2). These theories (see Chapter 68) focus on the dynamic relationships among personal attributes and resources, the behavior targeted for change, and influences of the physical and social environment in shaping adoption and maintenance of the targeted behavior. Along with similar conceptual approaches, they provide a framework for development of physical activity interventions.

In recent years, such theories have been augmented with both stage-based and readiness approaches, such as the motivational interviewing approach and the transtheoretical model, in which phases and processes that may be employed in the acquisition and maintenance of health behaviors are described (3, 4). In combination with social learning–social cognitive theories and similar approaches, such stage-sensitive models may help identify groups of people at varying levels of psychological readiness for change, allowing targeted intervention. However, social cognitive theory and similar approaches, as well as stage-based approaches to intervention, have not often been applied in a comprehensive fashion in physical activity intervention research. In addition, most physical activity intervention studies focus on endurance exercise, often ignoring other forms of activity, such as strength and flexibility training, that are important components of fitness. While more systematic work is needed in this area, some promising strategies—drawn primarily from social learning–social cognitive approaches—for facilitating participation in early and later stages of physical activity have been clarified.

INCREASING ADOPTION AND EARLY ADHERENCE

Adoption of increased physical activity patterns can be enhanced through paying particular attention to factors in personal, behavioral, environmental, and program-related spheres.

Personal and Behavioral Factors

Previous experience with physical activity should be explored along with unreasonable beliefs and misconceptions about exercise (e.g., "no pain, no gain" and the notion that older individuals should not be active because they need to conserve their energy). For example, many potential exercisers believe that exercise is inherently painful and therefore aversive; these individuals must be told and shown that this statement is untrue. Sedentary individuals are often unaware of the utility of moderate activities (e.g., brisk walking) that may be more appealing than more structured, vigorous regimens. Many sedentary individuals benefit from specific instruction (accompanied by actual rehearsal and feedback) on appropriate ways of performing specific activities (e.g., jogging, striding, cycling, and warm-up exercises) to obtain health-related benefits while avoiding injury.

In addition to physical activity–related attitudes, knowledge, and skills, a physical activity program should be personally relevant, in terms of both type of activities and goals. For example, if stress reduction is a motivating factor, activities that can be helpful in reducing stress (i.e., not too competitive, noisy, or demanding) should be selected. Examples of such activities include brisk walking, jogging, or bicycling conducted outdoors in pleasant surroundings that allow time to get away from it all.

Additional useful measures include structuring appropriate expectations concerning physical activity (what can and cannot be accomplished) as early as possible, stressing the many benefits of making change, as well as exploring perceived barriers to increasing physical activity (e.g., unreasonable expectations, fear of embarrassment, failure, boredom). A simple questionnaire regarding expectations can provide an exercise professional with early clues to such expectations.

Environmental and Program-Related Factors

Numerous environmental and program-related variables enhance initial adoption and early adherence to physical activity. These include the factors discussed in the following sections.

Convenience

Three factors related to convenience are important to successful initiation and maintenance of an exercise program.

- The greater the effort required to prepare for physical activity (i.e., a long drive to an exercise facility), the greater the potential for dropping out (up to twice the dropout and half the initial participation rates for inconvenient facilities). Facilities should be easily accessible. Alternatively, encouraging methods of being physically active in or around the home (the place where many people prefer to exercise) can make convenience less of a deterrent to adherence. Participation in an exercise program (i.e., joining a spa or health club) close to home or work or conveniently between these settings should be encouraged.
- Time is often the primary factor. If a program has a class structure, several time options may be helpful. For some with extreme time constraints (e.g., working mothers), alternatives to a class format are often necessary if child care is not available at home or at the fitness site.
- Modes of exercise requiring special, costly, or time-consuming preparation (e.g., skiing and even swimming) may adversely affect adherence.

Thus, location or facility, time, and mode can be critical during early stages of behavior change. Before initiating an exercise program, both the participant and the exercise professional should carefully evaluate the choices.

Behavioral Shaping

For sedentary persons, the major objective is to establish a physical activity habit while decreasing opportunities for failure. The initial activity prescription may be less vigorous than some guidelines recommend, and it should be easy to do, given preferences, motivation, skills, and life circumstances. For some individuals, shaping may translate to a simple initial increase in activities of daily living, such as walking or taking stairs more at work and at home. For others, the initial prescription may involve some less frequent, but structured endurance activity with a concomitant increase in routine activity until more vigorous activity is indicated.

The key consideration in all exercise prescriptions and programs should be gradual shaping of successive steps toward the ultimate goal. When behavior shaping is violated, adherence is almost always impaired. The rates of injury and dropout significantly increase when beginning exercisers are exposed to high intensity (85% or more of aerobic capacity), frequency (5 or more days per week), and/or duration (45 or more minutes per session). This may affect as many as 50% of participants. In contrast, once an individual is beyond initial stages and has an increased level of fitness, higher intensity, frequency, and duration may become tolerable.

Thus, the exercise regimen should be easy and gradually incremented, ensuring success at each stage. Most important, exercise professionals and beginning exercisers should focus primarily on shaping and maintaining the exercise habit for approximately 6–12 weeks, rather than on rapid establishment of the optimal regimen for desired benefits. Remember, benefits of even the most successful exercise program are lost unless a habit is solidly established. This approach of first establishing behavioral control of the habit implies that exercise professionals should encourage early participants to show up ("No matter how little you may feel like doing or can do, remember that we are reinforcing the habit of exercise; the benefits will come if you can form the habit").

Several methods may be considered in properly shaping to avoid excessive exercise during the early stages of a program. Maintaining an intensity during which talking is possible is one method. The participant and the exercise professional can easily monitor this level. However, simply telling participants to take it easy when the instructor and most of the class are working at a higher level of intensity is often ineffective. A more effective strategy is to provide an additional role model demonstrating a lower-intensity alternative. Individuals can also be taught distraction techniques, when relevant, to help refocus attention from aversive aspects of activity (e.g., increased exertion and sweating).

Heart rate is a good index of physiological intensity. Pulse rates can be monitored manually or with portable heart rate monitors. Rating of perceived exertion (RPE) tracks perception of intensity, which may be as important as physical work (5). In practice, these measures can be used together. For example, an initial RPE of 12 or less and a heart rate of 70% or less of maximum is recommended in sedentary participants for optimal enjoyment and establishment of a lifetime habit. In fact, it has recently been demonstrated that even relatively low levels of exercise intensity (e.g., less than 60% of maximal heart rate) are associated with significant health improvements and disease risk reduction. This is true particularly in special populations, such as older individuals and those with hypertension (6).

Enjoyability

It is critically important to adherence that the activity be enjoyable and immediately beneficial. The physical discomfort that often accompanies early stages of increased activity should be minimized, or at least moderated by positive factors, if habit is to be maintained.

Methods for enhancing enjoyability include tailoring of the types of activity, the actual exercise regimen, and the format of the regimen (group versus individual, facility- versus home-based). One method of assessing enjoyability is to ask participants to note level of enjoyment on a range of values from very unenjoyable to very enjoyable (e.g., 1–5 scale). If two or more sessions are unenjoyable, the regimen should be modified or varied, perhaps with additional reinforcement.

External Rewards and Incentives

The initial steps involved in becoming more physically active are found by many persons to be anything but rewarding. Often it is not until several months into a regular physical activity program that participants begin to report experiencing positive benefits from physical activity on a regular basis. In fact, the longer the period of inactivity and the more unfit the individual, the longer it may take before any physical activity feels good. Therefore, beginners may need external rewards early in the program for encouragement and motivation.

This is consistent with the theory of behavioral shaping, in which early approximations of end goal or target behavior require ample reinforcement or rewards for optimal adoption. For highly unfit overweight smokers, beginner status may extend to 6 months or a year, and special external incentives may have to be programmed throughout that time. For fitter persons, the beginner phase may last perhaps as little as 2–3 weeks.

One valuable and reinforcing form of reward is social support, a powerful motivator for many people. Social support can be delivered through an instructor, exercise partners, and family members who encourage increased activity and through telephone contacts and letter prompts from a health professional. Praise is a critical component of social support, especially for beginning exercisers and completely relapsed former exercisers. To be most effective, this vocal encouragement should be both immediate (during or very shortly after the exercise) and specific. For example: "Your effort level is great. You'll be able to keep that pace for some time." or "Great going. Your attendance has been perfect over the past month." Praise from exercise professionals, family members, and fellow participants should be consistent and frequent during the early stages. Families of neophyte exercisers should also be encouraged to exercise with them, or at least to accompany them whenever possible, to enhance support. When support from significant others is active and ongoing, exercisers are two to three times as likely to persist as those with little or no family support. Counselors, family members, and helpers should all be cautioned, however, against even well-intentioned nagging or use of other aversive procedures (e.g., using guilt) designed to induce a reluctant person to exercise. These counterproductive actions almost inevitably increase the punishing characteristics of exercise and may even impair the partnership between the individual and the supportive agent, further upsetting the delicate balance between motivation to exercise and remaining inactive.

The use of social support can also be extended and formalized using written contracts between the individual and a significant person. Contracts are written, signed agreements that specify the activity-related goals in a public format and for which there is value exchange much as with a legal contract. They typically specify short-term, concrete goals and the types of rewards that ensue upon reaching the goals. The contract should be flexible, so that rigid daily goals are avoided (see following section). In the earlier stages of a program, an appropriate goal might be for attendance rather than performance. These contracts often work best if developed in tandem with an interested person or helper. Such contracts can help to increase personal responsibility and commitment. Those managing physical activity behavior should also consider using contingency management, in which more highly rewarding or preferred activities are made contingent on achieving a particular goal, such as watching a favorite television program only after an exercise session.

An alternative to the value exchange contract is a written agreement in which the participant agrees to perform or complete certain behaviors. Although less effective than a formal contract, an agreement can be useful for those who refuse or are reluctant to sign a behavioral contract.

The use of appropriate and consistent physical activity models in the environment (i.e., other individuals who may be observed exercising) can also motivate people to begin and continue exercise. These models should be as similar as possible to the targeted individuals (some programs use successful graduates as future participant assistants for maximal effectiveness) (7, 8). Furthermore, when possible, the exercise professional or therapist should set an appropriate example by exercising with participants.

Another important type of incentive is feedback regarding progress in relevant or important dimensions of activity. Feedback stimulates a positive reactive effect on a wide variety of behaviors. For example, monitoring of caloric intake usually results in a short-term reduction. Similarly, the physical activity habit is frequently enhanced when attendance, general exercise adherence or performance, and results of exercise are systematically monitored. One simple way to bring this reactive effect of feedback to bear, especially in those who cannot engage in a systematic program, is to provide an inexpensive pedometer or movement sensor (e.g., Caltrac) to track walking and physical activity levels.

Feedback can also be delivered by another person or generated through use of self-recorded monitoring sheets, an activity diary, and/or a graph showing progress in one or more variables, such as plotted heart rates, attendance, and adherence across time. Computer-generated letters of feedback are promising as an efficient, systematic method of providing personalized feedback on a regular basis. When used in conjunction with goals that are reasonable, personally relevant, and short term, feedback can be a powerfully motivating factor.

BEHAVIORAL SUCCESS

Continued adherence usually results from success rather than education. Engaging in an activity on a regular basis shapes beliefs and attitudes about continuing the activity rather than vice versa. This may help explain why many individuals, despite being knowledgeable about exercise, are not active. Exercise professionals can help by pointing out the changes and gains, no matter how modest. Participants should be shaped such that they engage in exercise regardless of subjective feelings (barring illness or injury) or attitude. Eventually, this regular, successful participation produces appropriate feelings of mastery, perhaps enjoyment, and positive attitudes toward exercise, a process that enhances the probability of maintaining exercise.

Self-Management

Success in behavior change correlates with early training in self-management strategies and an understanding of the importance of taking personal responsibility for physical activity. Individuals must recognize the importance of taking charge of physical activity as a lifelong goal rather than as something that ends when a 12-week class or program is over. Such programs are a vehicle for establishing a lifelong habit and are not the means by which physical activity should be defined. Early in all programs, methods to prompt and successfully engage participants in activity in a variety of settings and under a variety of circumstances should be outlined (Table 69.1).

Table 69.1. Methods of Engaging Participants in Exercise

Suggestions for planning exercise
    Carry exercise clothes in the car.
    Leave exercise clothes by the bed.
    Spend time with other exercisers.
    Park the car and walk.
    Make decisions concerning whether or not to exercise or how much to exercise only after arriving at the exercise site or locale.
Suggestions for a missed session (relapse prevention)
    Admit responsibility for the slip.
    Develop a restart plan, including appropriate goals.
    Call exercise buddy.
    Arrange reinforcement.
    Simplify or change regimen.
    Begin by simply visiting the usual exercise place or locale.

ENHANCING MAINTENANCE: RECOMMENDED STRATEGIES

In addition to sedentary individuals, who may have difficulty initiating physical activity, some individuals spend significant time restarting exercise programs that have terminated for various reasons. Often individuals stop exercising completely after an inevitable break because of illness or injury, travel, holidays, inclement weather, or increased demands at work. One useful step is to prepare in advance (both psychologically and behaviorally) for breaks or slips in activity that may lead to full-blown relapse and a return to previous sedentary lifestyle (9). It should be emphasized that such breaks are inevitable and do not indicate laziness or failure. Early identification of high-risk situations that may lead to inactivity, along with devising strategies to prepare for slips, can be effective.

Useful plans include identification of alternative activities (e.g., brisk walking), planning to exercise as soon as possible after a break, arranging to exercise with someone else, and resetting goals to an easier level to avoid discouragement. Other methods that may be used for enhancing maintenance include those discussed in the next sections.

Reminders of Benefits

Provide continued evidence of relevant personal physical, social, and psychological benefits from regular exercise. Exercise professionals may regularly ask about benefits and positive outcomes of a physical activity program. For persons at particular risk for dropping out, these questions should be posed frequently (e.g., once a month or more). If an individual cannot define the positive aspects of exercise or provides a number of negatives, there is serious risk of dropout. These participants are targets for increased attention.

Generalization Training

Generalization training entails expanding behavior from one setting or set of circumstances to a different setting to link the behavior with cues or stimuli in the second setting that may help to facilitate adherence. To ensure adherence, the exercise habit must be generalized or re-established in new (e.g., home) environments prior to discontinuing programmed sessions. Generalization may be accomplished in several ways:

- Requiring home exercise sessions from the beginning or at an early stage of the program (stimulus generalization)
- Including family or significant others in exercise sessions
- Before graduation, adding exercises that are easily maintained at home (response generalization)

Avoid discontinuing exercise programs suddenly, especially if no generalization training has been provided. Ideally, responsibility for session supervision, reinforcement, and feedback should be gradually transferred from the instructor to the participants and to home environment or helpers as the change date approaches. This more closely approximates the conditions likely to prevail in the maintenance setting.

Reassessment of Goals

Reassessment of goals provides opportunity to verify that they are relevant, realistic, and motivating. Goals that are too long term or vague do not provide sufficient motivation to maintain behavior through difficult periods. During the early stages of an exercise program (1–6 months), goals should be adjusted as frequently as necessary (e.g., every 2 weeks) to maintain exercise behavior.

Social Support

Continued use of a variety of social supports is valuable. If the format is a class or group, the leader should call participants who miss two classes in a row (one class in high-risk participants). The purpose of such calls is to let individuals know they are missed and others notice and care. Other individuals in the class can assume this type of responsibility as well (a buddy system). If exercise is conducted outside of a formal class or group, the exercise professional may continue support in the form of periodic telephone calls, letters, and/or newsletters. Family members, coworkers, and friends should continue to encourage and support exercise. In addition, it may be helpful to schedule special sessions to train helpers in supporting (prompting, modeling, and reinforcing) physical activity.

Relevant Rewards

Rewards should change periodically to maintain motivating influence if used in conjunction with physical activity goals. Reward systems may include such things as points accumulated as exercise continues to be maintained. Material rewards (e.g., a new exercise outfit, dinner out, a small trip) or small rewards such as time off (to read or engage in other enjoyable activities) may ensue from the accumulation of points. Other examples are requiring a monetary deposit that is returned upon achievement of goals (especially behavioral goals, such as attendance and participation) or reducing program fees on good adherence to the program.

Feedback

Self-monitoring and other forms of feedback are useful for noting progress and enhancing motivation. For some, feedback may take the additional form of self-administered (e.g., field) or professional fitness assessments. Such fitness assessments compare current to past levels of fitness.

Contracts

Contracts should be updated and changed frequently, if necessary, and should include specific goals, rewards, and helpers. Contracts that are too easy do not provide the challenge needed to motivate many individuals. In contrast, contracts that are too difficult lead to frustration, discouragement, and perhaps injury.

Boredom

Individuals should be encouraged to monitor enjoyment and to be responsible for making activity more enjoyable, especially if it is not meeting needs or expectations. The exercise professional should collaborate to achieve this goal, such as through implementation of new activities, environments, goals, and/or partners. With a wide variety of aerobic activities and a diversity of settings in which to conduct activities, "I'm bored" should not be allowed to persist and extinguish behavior. Some individuals can resolve boredom through a regimen involving a variety of activities. For others, one activity conducted in varied settings and formats may be more appropriate. Enjoyable competition (e.g., fun runs or walkathons) may stimulate maintenance.

Importance of Routine Activities

An increase in activities of daily living can help maintain individual fitness, especially when more vigorous activity is not performed. Health benefits obtained from activity can be more effectively realized by becoming more active in a variety of ways, both within and outside of formal programs.

General Motivational Counseling to Enhance Probability of Exercising

Attention has recently been paid to the application of brief motivational counseling approaches for health behaviors such as exercise (3). Motivational interviewing was developed initially as a brief and effective method of helping those with addictive behaviors (primarily alcohol and subsequently smoking) to increase readiness to change. Some promising work with such techniques has recently begun to occur in the exercise area as well. Key components of this approach include acknowledging, normalizing, and gently working through ambivalence concerning physical activity; stressing the freedom to choose not to exercise while encouraging acceptance of responsibility for change and the consequences of not changing; developing internal discrepancy for remaining inactive through strategic reflections, feedback, and questions from the counselor; and encouraging the client to evaluate the pros and cons (decision balance) of remaining inactive versus becoming more active (3).

▶ SUMMARY

Assisting individuals to initiate and maintain increased levels of physical activity can be a challenge to even the most enterprising exercise professional. Such a task requires continued creativity and flexibility in developing and modifying programs to meet the changing needs of participants. Exercise professionals may become more effective in these efforts by applying the following guidelines for changing and maintaining behavior:

- Behavior, including physical activity, is strongly influenced by its immediate consequences.
- Increasing the immediately rewarding aspects of behavior and decreasing the negative or punishing aspects increases the likelihood that a behavior will occur.
- Individual choice of reward is personally motivating.
- Set appropriate activity-related goals and modify goals as necessary.
- Encourage individual tailoring of, and flexibility in, exercise goal setting; emphasize adherence and attendance initially rather than performance.
- Provide relevant feedback whenever possible. Encourage and teach exercisers to plot and display progress for visual motivation.
- Gradually shape initially difficult behavior; have individuals start with less demanding activity goals to ease into the habit of being physically active.
- Structure appropriate expectations during the early stages of a program.
- Prepare participants for inevitable lapses or breaks in exercise by encouraging planning; unexpected breaks in programs should be put into perspective.
- When possible, offer choices as a means of tailoring exercise programs to fit individual needs and preferences.
- Encourage public expression of commitment to exercise through the use of written contracts, decision balance sheets, and other strategies.
- Teach participants how to use environmental or social prompts and reminders to set the stage for regular adherence.
- Foster self-management of exercise, including ongoing use of decision balance, public declarations, and other strategies.
- Use as many types of social support as feasible; when relevant, prepare individuals for changes in leadership to minimize disruptions to the class or group.
- Use the exercise program as an opportunity to model and promote a healthy lifestyle.
- When appropriate, consider the application of motivational interviewing strategies and other client-centered approaches to counsel and interact with inactive individuals struggling with ambivalence.

The use of a public health perspective for exercise adoption and adherence problems provides a valuable perspective that emphasizes the importance of inspiring a large number of individuals in a community to engage in some physical activity. The use of a traditional exercise prescription of three times per week for 30–40 minutes at a prescribed intensity is a useful general goal for some, but for many individuals it is unreachable. Striving to motivate the sedentary to increase general activity through more moderate, convenient activities of daily living can be a worthwhile and in fact is the focus of the most recent recommendations supported by the Centers for Disease Control and Prevention, the American College of Sports Medicine, and the Surgeon General's report (10). Health professionals must remain open to various options for enhancing physical activity, particularly on a community-wide, cost-efficient basis.

ACKNOWLEDGMENT

This work was supported in part by PHS grants #AG-12358 and #AG16587 from the National Institute on Aging awarded to Dr. King.

References

1. King AC, Blair SN, Bild DE, et al. Determinants of physical activity and interventions in adults. Med Sci Sports Exerc 24:S221–226, 1992.
2. Bandura A. Social Foundations of Thought and Action: A Social Cognitive Theory. Englewood Cliffs, NJ: Prentice Hall, 1986.
3. Rollnick S, Mason P, Butler C. Health Behavior Change: A Guide for Practitioners. London: Churchill Livingstone, 1999.
4. Marcus BH, Rossi JS, Selby VC, et al. The stages and process of exercise adoption and maintenance in a worksite sample. Health Psych 11:386–395, 1992.
5. Borg GV. Perceived exertion as an indicator of somatic stress. Scand J Rehabil Med 2:92–98, 1970.
6. Patten CA, Martin JE. Exercise interventions for older adults with high blood pressure: From efficacy to adherence. J Prevent Intervent Commun 13:111–142, 1996.
7. Chance P. Learning and Behavior. 3rd ed. Pacific Grove, CA: Brooks-Cole, 1994.
8. Martin JE, Dubbert PM, Katell AD, et al. Behavioral control of exercise in sedentary adults: Studies 1 through 6. J Consult Clin Psych 52:795–811, 1984.
9. Sallis JF, Haskell WL, Fortmann SP, et al. Predictors of adoption and maintenance of physical activity in a community sample. Prev Med 15:331–341, 1986.
10. Pate RR, Pratt M, Blair S, Haskell WL, et al. Physical activity and public health: A recommendation from the Centers for Disease Control and Prevention and the American College of Sports Medicine. JAMA 273:402–407, 1995.

1.9.0, 1.9.1, 1.9.2, 1.9.3   2.9.0, 2.9.0.1, 2.9.0.2

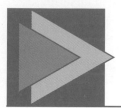

CHAPTER **70**

INTERVENTIONS FOR WEIGHT MANAGEMENT

Carlos M. Grilo and Kelly D. Brownell

Obesity is a serious, prevalent, and growing public health problem (1, 2). Excessive weight is associated with increased risk of mortality and morbidity, including coronary heart disease, non–insulin dependent (type II) diabetes, hypertension, and other illnesses (3, 4). Despite the known seriousness of obesity, increased public concern, and record rates of dieting, obesity remains a common problem. Some 97 million Americans are believed to be overweight or obese, and this figure is increasing (1, 5).

DEFINITION

Obesity is a surplus of adipose tissue–containing fat stored in triglyceride form, resulting from excessive energy intake relative to energy expenditure. The point at which excessive fat constitutes obesity is arbitrary. Overweight is defined as deviation in body weight from some standard or "ideal" weight related to height. In 1959 the Metropolitan Life Insurance Company published what used to be the most frequently used standard. Although the precise point at which increasing weight exceeds the threshold for good health is unclear, a figure of 20% above the standard was adopted at the 1985 NIH Consensus Conference on the Health Risks of Obesity.

Overweight does not always reflect obesity; for example, athletes can weigh more than the "ideal" weight yet be quite lean. The various weight-for height-measures (e.g., percent overweight, weight for height, and body mass index) have correlation coefficients of approximately 0.7 with body fat measured directly.

Increasingly, body mass index (BMI) has been adopted as the standard for expressing body weight. BMI is expressed as weight in kilograms divided by height squared in meters. Figure 70.1*A* is a nomogram for calculation of body mass index and recommendations for assessment and intervention (6). In 1998 the National Institutes of Health adopted a lower threshold for overweight (BMI > 25) and retained BMI > 30 for obesity (5).

Fat distributed in the abdomen, called upper body or android-type obesity because it occurs most often in men,

is associated with greater morbidity and mortality than is body fat distributed below the waist, called lower body or gynoid obesity. The ratio of waist to hip (WHR) circumference is a stronger predictor of cardiovascular risk than is body weight, body fat, or body mass index. Figure 70.1*B* shows a nomogram for assessment of WHR and associated risk (7). The waist measurement is considered a proxy for intra-abdominal obesity, which carries greater risk than peripheral fat distribution. Sophisticated measurement is necessary to assess intra-abdominal fat; therefore, circumference measurements are more practical for developing an index of body fat distribution.

PSYCHOLOGY AND PHYSIOLOGY OF WEIGHT REGULATION

Many health professionals (and the public) incorrectly believe that excessive weight reflects lack of willpower, poor self-concept, and deep-seated psychological problems. Excessive weight results from a complex interaction of cultural, social, genetic, physiological, behavioral, and psychological factors. Although it is likely that overeating accounts in part for overweight, eating behaviors should be considered with biological (e.g., genetics, metabolism) and behavioral (e.g., physical activity) factors (8, 9). Most research on the psychological aspects of obesity reveals few significant differences between overweight and average-weight persons (10). Even when psychological distress occurs in overweight persons, the distress may be either cause or consequence. Recent research has, however, identified two psychological factors that may be especially salient among overweight persons: body image dissatisfaction and binge eating (10, 11).

Overweight persons tend to suffer more from negative body image and are more likely to have problems with binge eating than average-weight peers. Binge eating is associated with increased risk of psychological problems and may merit consideration with specialized treatments (11–14).

NOMOGRAM FOR BODY MASS INDEX

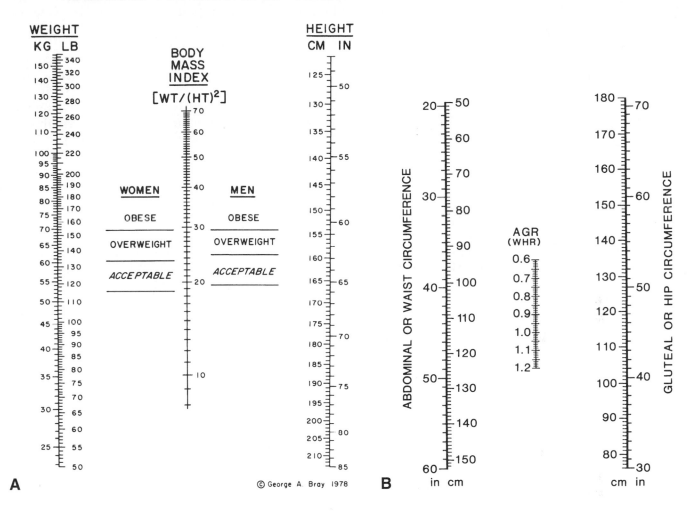

© George A. Bray 1978

A

B

Adult Intervention Guidelines		
BMI kg/m^2		
19–34 years	>35 years	
< 25	< 27	Normal; refer to waist-to-hip ratio
25–27	—	Intervention indicated if there is a family history or presence of heart disease, type II diabetes, hypercholesterolemia, or hypertension.
> 27	> 27	Intervention indicated even in the absence of another risk factor

C

Figure 70.1. Nomograms. **A.** Body mass index (BMI). **B.** Waist-to-hip ratio (WHR). **C.** Recommendations for adult interventions based on BMI and classification of health risk based on WHR. (A reprinted with permission from Bray GA. Definitions, measurements, and classification of the syndrome of obesity. Int J Obes 2:99, 1978. B reprinted with permission from Bray GA, Gray DS. Obesity: Part I. Pathogenesis. West J Med 149:429, 1988.)

Interest in physiological factors dates to the concept of a body weight **set point**. The set point theory proposes a natural weight for each individual, that is, the weight the body seeks to protect against pressures to be too heavy or too thin. A set point above the ideal predicts a battle against physiology in an attempt to lose weight. The concept of set point is appealing because it leads a search for factors that regulate body weight, but whether a set point exists remains controversial (15). Working with overweight individuals requires walking a fine line between acknowledging the importance of biology and painting a pessimistic physiological picture of weight change (16).

Body weight is in part controlled genetically (17, 18). It is estimated that approximately 25–40% of the variance in body weight is explained by genetics. Moreover, the pattern of body fat distribution (e.g., upper or lower body) also appears to be genetically influenced. Studies also indicate that resting metabolic rate (RMR), which accounts for roughly 70% of daily expenditure, but varies considerably is also influenced by genetics.

Genetic investigations of obesity, bolstered by recent technological advances, represent a particularly promising avenue that may soon contribute to a better understanding of obesity (17). A specific gene believed to contribute to obesity has recently been identified and cloned (19). In mice, this gene mutates and appears to produce extreme obesity and type II diabetes. Evidence also suggests that a specific secreted protein, leptin, may function as part of a signaling system that regulates the size of body fat deposits. Such research may someday lead to the development of pharmacological interventions for weight and fat regulation.

The findings that weight and fat distribution seem to be strongly influenced by biological and genetic factors, do not, however, suggest that environmental influences are unimportant or that dieting is ineffective (16, 20). They do suggest that individuals should adopt more **reasonable** goals and should avoid wholesale pursuit of aesthetic or even health "ideals." Overweight individuals **inherit only the tendency for obesity, and diet and exercise can influence the extent of its expression**.

EXERCISE AND WEIGHT CONTROL

Evidence demonstrates the importance of exercise in weight control (21). First, most overweight persons are not physically active; however, inactivity may be either the cause or consequence of overweight. People in weight loss programs who maintain the loss are most likely to exercise. Many, but not all, experimental controlled studies demonstrate that exercise in combination with diet produces greater weight loss than diet alone. The available controlled studies of exercise and diet that include posttreatment follow-up assessments are consistent—exercise facilitates long-term weight loss (22). Since successful weight loss maintenance, rather than short-lived weight loss, is viewed as the biggest challenge faced by obese persons, available data suggest that exercise should be included in weight control programs.

Exercise has been used as a component of weight control programs for years, but it is generally treated as a formality. The prospect of exercise to someone with the physical burden of excessive weight may be daunting. There are compelling reasons, however, to **emphasize physical activity**. Exercise professionals should be aware of the benefits of exercise and enthusiastic about the role of exercise in weight control. Describing the benefits to those attempting to lose weight can provide an added incentive to become more physically active.

Exercise Expends Energy

Exercise uses calories. It is a mistake to believe that caloric expenditure from low-level activity is adequate to permit increased food intake. However, the cumulative effects of exercise over long periods are substantial, so even modest levels of activity can be beneficial.

Exercise May Suppress Appetite

There is more animal than human evidence of this, but exercise may help to suppress appetite in some persons, while others increase caloric intake to offset increased expenditure. The effects of exercise on appetite, therefore, may be either neutral or positive. It may be helpful to schedule exercise at times of day when overeating is common.

Exercise Counteracts the Ill Effects of Obesity

Exercise reduces morbidity and mortality via a number of possible mechanisms (21). Exercise has positive effects on blood pressure, serum cholesterol, body composition, and cardiorespiratory function, and obese persons are at increased risk for abnormalities in these areas (23). Some of the benefits of exercise are independent of weight loss. Some research indicates that exercise may be necessary to achieve desired health outcomes of dietary interventions.

Exercise Improves Psychological Functioning

Changes in anxiety, depression, general mood, and self-concept are noted in those who maintain an exercise program, perhaps through increased sense of personal control. These psychological changes may enhance dietary compliance in someone attempting to lose weight.

Exercise Can Minimize Loss of Lean Body Mass

Up to 25% of weight lost through dieting alone is lean body mass (LBM). Overweight people typically have increased LBM as well as fat, but loss of LBM during dieting can be dangerous if protein reserves in essential areas of the body are depleted. LBM loss decreases when diet is combined with exercise (24). Aerobic exercise and resistance training have both been found to minimize the loss of LBM. The potential for decelerating loss of LBM via resistance weight training is an important area for further research.

Exercise May Counteract the Metabolic Decline Produced by Dieting

Caloric restriction produces a rapid reduction of resting metabolic rate (RMR). The decline may be up to 20%, and because RMR accounts for 60–70% of total energy expenditure, this phenomenon may be important. This reduction in RMR may partly account for the plateau at which weight loss slows or stops even if caloric intake is stable. Exercise increases RMR, but the magnitude and duration of increase are unknown. How the type, frequency, intensity, and duration of exercise can be altered to offset the metabolic decline produced by dieting is not clear.

EXERCISE ADHERENCE

As is the case with dieting, compliance with exercise is a major challenge. In addition to teaching clients the importance of exercise for weight control, the professional can enhance compliance in several ways.

Emphasize Psychological Benefits

The psychological benefits of exercise can be substantial. In addition to expending energy and improving health, exercise can enhance self-esteem, provide motivation, decrease anxiety, and buffer individuals against stress. The exercise professional can do much to enhance adherence by stressing that every time some form of physical activity is performed, it is a positive step. Motivationally, it is important to keep track of such success (e.g., parking on the outer edge of the lot and walking to the mall), which may contribute to a feeling of greater **personal control**.

Be Sensitive to the Excessive Weight

When sedentary people say what prevents them from exercising, it commonly includes being too busy. This barrier to exercise can often be overcome by creative scheduling and by alerting people to the benefits of exercise. This reason, however, often masks other more important barriers. One such barrier is excessive weight itself. Becoming active can be difficult, tiring, and painful under the added workload of obesity. People should be assisted with setting reasonable exercise goals and expecting reasonable amounts of time to elapse before high levels of activity can be accomplished.

Negative self-image is another obstacle to exercise. It involves associations that plague many people, particularly those who have been overweight since childhood and/or are characterized by negative body image. They are likely to be self-conscious and embarrassed about their body, and the mere prospect of exercise evokes negative feelings.

Prescription of levels of activity consistent with abilities and fitness, assisting individuals to select enjoyable activities, and sensitivity to body image concerns are essential.

Emphasize Consistency and Lifestyle Activity

A common question is, "How much exercise should I do?" Public health guidelines developed by the Centers for Disease Control and the American College of Sports Medicine recommend that adults accumulate 30 minutes or more of moderate physical activity on most days of the week, and experts suggest that overweight patients should aim for 60 or more minutes per day (25). These new guidelines followed research findings that modest physical activity and modest weight loss both have significant health benefits. Relatively low levels of activity are associated with improved health and decreased mortality (26, 27). Modest lifestyle exercise also predicts weight loss (28).

Exercise professionals should make a specific point about exercise and activity: **any exercise or activity is better than none**. Moreover, such an effort represents a positive commitment. **Consistency and regular lifestyle physical activity may be more important than the type or amount of exercise.** Research continues to investigate the benefits of various exercise prescriptions (29, 30).

Select the Right Exercise

The selection of a realistic and appropriate exercise program is a key predictor of adherence. People are most likely to continue activities that are enjoyable. Two questions can be asked as a starting point: **"Is it fun?"** and **"Will you do it regularly?"** The exercise professional can assist in choosing activities that match lifestyle and schedule. For obese individuals, the choice of low-impact activities is particularly important. For many, obese or lean, regular walking is a potentially rewarding option (26).

Prevent Injury

Physical discomfort and injury are frequent reasons for attrition from exercise. Exercise professionals should assist patients in establishing gradually progressive exercise programs that minimize discomfort and potential for injury, including attention to appropriate clothing and footwear. Care should be taken to prevent overheating and dehydration.

A COMPREHENSIVE APPROACH TO WEIGHT CONTROL

Overweight is not easily remedied by simple advice to eat less and exercise more. Important elements of programs should have a broad base addressing three factors: nutrition, exercise, and behavior change (31).

There is a wide range of options for weight control programs. Self-directed approaches, self-help groups, commercial programs, behavioral approaches, hospital-based programs (including very low calorie diets), professional counseling, pharmacological treatments, and surgery are among the approaches that can be successful. Although some treatments produce significant short-term weight loss, average weight losses are far from optimal and are difficult to maintain over time. Obesity is increasingly viewed as a chronic, ongoing problem that for many people requires lifestyle change, not simply short-term efforts.

Therefore, well-selected referrals are an important aspect of working with overweight persons. Unfortunately, clinical judgment must be relied upon for making such referrals, because research does not provide clear guidelines about matching patients to effective treatment. A **stepped-care** approach prescribes the least intensive interventions first (e.g., self-directed programs), especially for persons who are not significantly overweight, followed by more intensive treatment for those who have been unable to succeed in other programs. Matching individuals to specific treatments is based on personal needs and program characteristics. For example, psychological counseling combined with methods that address weight might be indicated in someone with significant distress or for binge eaters (11).

COMPONENTS OF EFFECTIVE TREATMENT

Behavior change, exercise, and nutrition are three key elements of weight control programs (31). The integration of behavioral components into comprehensive weight control programs seems to produce improvements in general well-being and result in fewer negative psychological effects than dieting alone.

Behavior Change

Lifestyle and behavior change are cornerstones of effective treatment. Behavioral interventions are critical to ensure such changes and should focus on more than eating and exercise habits. They involve teaching individuals the relation between **antecedents** (i.e., events, thoughts, and feelings leading up to eating), **behaviors** (i.e., eating, binging), and **consequences** (i.e., events, thoughts, and feelings that follow eating and can determine subsequent problematic eating). In addition, individuals can be taught specific **coping skills** to change eating and exercise patterns and to overcome problems that interfere with change. Teaching coping skills to overcome difficult situations and prevent negative reactions is perhaps the most important treatment intervention.

Exercise

Consistency, adherence, and enjoyment, rather than intensity or mode of exercise, are the goals of exercise for weight control. Exercise professionals should work with patients to set reasonable short-term physical activity goals that contribute to achieving intermediate-term goals of consistent lifestyle activity coupled with regular bouts of moderate exercise.

Nutrition

Adequate nutrition and decreased calorie intake relative to expenditure (negative energy balance) are general goals of dietary intervention (28). There are three primary methods for monitoring caloric intake. First, count calories. The person is instructed about specific servings and portion sizes from basic food groups with a defined total calorie intake. A second method is the American Dietetic Association (and the American Diabetic Association) food exchange plan. Individuals are taught about exchanges within food groups; each exchange is a specific amount of food within group. Exchanges are equivalent in nutrition and calories. Finally, the Food Guide Pyramid, recently developed by the U.S. Department of Agriculture, encourages specific servings from various food groups. Each approach may be acceptable in appropriate circumstances. Personal preference of patient and professional can be used to select one method. Reducing both overall caloric intake and fat intake appears to be more effective than fat reduction alone. Research continues to address relative merits of specific diets (32).

Negative Energy Balance

Although there are numerous ways to arrive at a recommendation for caloric intake, the following approach is recommended. Generally, 1500 kcal/day for men and 1200 kcal/day for women is used as a starting point. Modify caloric consumption depending on the individual and activity and a weekly goal of 1–2 pounds of weight loss. Calorie intakes below 1000 kcal/day should be medically monitored.

Determination of caloric intake necessary to produce 1–2 pounds of weight loss per week can be difficult because various, complex factors can influence metabolic requirements. For example, reducing calorie intake by 500 per day (3500/week) is associated with a 1-pound (per week) weight loss only over large population groups, but there is considerable variability among individuals. Thus, a dietary record may aid in adjusting intake to help establish specific calorie goals.

Adequate Nutrition

Nutrition requirements should be carefully considered when selecting the approach to weight reduction. Inadequate nutrition during weight reduction can have serious medical consequences. Hypocaloric diets must be nutritionally adequate, especially with respect to protein, vitamin, and mineral intake. Moreover, diet composition may influence various mechanisms relevant to weight control, such as diuresis, appetite, and satiety.

Very Low Calorie Diets

A particularly aggressive approach to weight loss is the very low calorie diet (33). These diets entail fasting with either a powdered supplement or small amounts of lean meat, fish, or fowl. Intake ranges from 400–800 kcal/day, and programs vary considerably in the quality of behavioral and nutritional intervention. Research has indicated that there is little advantage to diets with less than 800 calories/day.

These diets are typically used in individuals 40% or more over ideal weight and should be medically supervised. They are appealing because weight loss is rapid (2–3 pounds per week for women, 3–5 pounds per week for men) and because food choice is not an issue. Long-term maintenance, however, can be a problem. The initial studies with 1-year follow-up demonstrated good maintenance of weight loss when a very low calorie diet is combined with a high-quality behavioral program. Results from 3- and 5-year follow-up, however, indicate nearly total recidivism. While it may be premature to abandon these diets, persons contemplating them should be cautioned about the probability of relapse. In the meantime, research examining methods for sustaining impressive losses produced by these diets is needed.

Cognitive Change

Thoughts and attitudes about self, nutrition, and exercise play key roles in weight maintenance. It is important to assist people to become **actively** aware of thoughts. Often **automatic** thoughts, or overlearned responses to particular situations, influence feelings and have a profound influence on dietary compliance. Examples are self-deprecating thoughts following dietary violations, adoption of unreasonable goals, and all-or-none thinking (e.g., foods are legal or illegal, or being on or off a diet). Teaching awareness of these thoughts and ways to substitute more objective thoughts can be effective. The exercise professional can also help individuals **focus on progress** (not shortcomings) and look for **problems in behaviors and situations** (not character defects).

Social Support

The social environment influences health behavior. Social support can be a positive resource for dietary change; however, some individuals benefit from social support and others do not. Some prefer privacy in weight loss programs, whereas others benefit from social support. It is helpful to examine this issue with individuals and to teach those who would profit from such reinforcement methods for eliciting and sustaining the support.

Relapse Prevention

Maintaining weight loss is the greatest challenge facing those attempting to lose weight. Many individuals lose weight numerous times, only to regain it. This problem of relapse and repeated fluctuations in weight may have negative psychological and medical consequences. Research demonstrates that individuals whose body weight fluctuates repeatedly over time (cycles of weight loss and gain) may be at higher risk for coronary heart disease than those with stable weight.

We view relapse as a process, not an outcome. Those attempting to lose weight, regardless of motivation, commitment, or level of success, inevitably are tempted and almost universally have episodes of overeating. How a dieter **copes** with such situations may determine whether that isolated event (temptation or lapse) escalates into repeated overeating (relapse), leads to abandonment of the diet (collapse), or ideally, leads to increased confidence and continued maintenance. Relapse prevention techniques have been developed to identify **high-risk** situations and develop **coping skills** to overcome those situations. When lapses do occur, individuals must be taught to avoid negative reactions and to react instead with an attempt to learn from the lapse, solve problems for future events, and renew commitment to the program.

PHARMACOLOGICAL TREATMENTS

Recent advances in biology and genetics, coupled with a shift toward viewing obesity as a chronic biobehavioral disorder of energy regulation and metabolism, have led to an explosion of interest in pharmacological approaches to treatment. There are 12 U.S. Food and Drug Administration (FDA) approved medications for weight control. Of them, 10 are centrally active adrenergic drugs (amphetaminelike compounds), one (sibutramine) is a centrally active combined adrenergic and serotonergic drug, and one (orlistat) is the first approved locally active medication that works by altering fat absorption.

Two previously FDA-approved drugs, dexfenfluramine and fenfluramine, which influence the serotonergic system, were removed from the market and are no longer approved for treatment of obesity. One of these drugs (fenfluramine) was part of the popular fen-phen combination with phentermine, a centrally acting adrenergic drug with low abuse potential that remains on the market. A series of studies identified two major health risks associated with those two medications: primary pulmonary hypertension and heart valve abnormalities (34, 35).

The adrenergic drugs are generally associated with about 1 kg/week weight loss that is regained soon after discontinuation. Such drugs are generally not recommended because of the potential for abuse. Sibutramine has demonstrated efficacy for acute weight loss in several randomized placebo-controlled trials (36, 37), with doses of 10 and 15 mg daily similar in efficacy and tolerability and superior to placebo (roughly 5 kg versus 1.5 kg weight loss over 12-week trials). Orlistat has demonstrated efficacy for acute and longer-term (over 2 years) weight control (38, 39). In these two multicenter controlled trials, obese patients treated with orlistat 120 mg three times a day plus diet lost significantly more weight (an average of 5.8 kg more) than patients receiving placebo plus diet during acute treatment. Moreover, during the second year of weight maintenance diets, patients randomly and blindly assigned orlistat regained significantly less weight than patients assigned placebo.

Medications are only one part of a comprehensive weight control program. Indeed, the recent pharmacological treatment studies with sibutramine and orlistat have examined the possible benefits of the medications above and beyond behavioral dietary interventions. The advantages of drug treatments must be balanced against side effects and risks (40). However, the risks of obesity also should be considered and balanced against the risk of drug treatments. Severe obesity with resultant medical complications may warrant consideration of the risks and benefits. The recent fen-phen problem also demonstrated that obesity drugs should not be prescribed for persons who are not obese. The FDA and the federal guidelines recommend that approved obesity medications be used only in persons with BMI above 30, or above 27 if at least two obesity-related medical comorbidities are present (5). Moreover, the federal guidelines recommend attempting a comprehensive lifestyle behavioral approach for at least 6 months before initiating an obesity medication trial.

▶ SUMMARY

Obesity is a significant health problem. Complex physiological, genetic, cultural, and psychological factors contribute to the problem and it cannot be attributed solely to weak willpower or personal deficit. Exercise is an important predictor of success for weight reduction, therefore increased physical activity is a key goal for those who wish to lose weight. Compliance may be jeopardized, however, if special physical and psychological burdens of being overweight are not considered. Regardless of the level of intervention, a comprehensive program involving nutrition, behavior, cognitions, and social support, in addition to exercise, appears to hold the greatest promise for long-term results. The high frequency of relapse and potential psychological and medical consequences emphasize the need for aggressive work in relapse prevention.

Continued research to better understand the complex biological and psychological aspects of weight regulation is important and may lead to the identification of pharmacological approaches to enhance the effectiveness of treatment components. Recent studies have suggested the potential efficacy of two new medications for enhancing the outcomes of behavioral and dietary treatments for obese patients. Consistency and lifestyle change are key goals in all weight reduction programs.

References

1. Flegal KM, Carroll MD, Kuczmarski R, Johnson CL. Overweight and obesity in the United States: Prevalence and trends, 1960–1994. Int J Obes Relat Metab Disord 22: 39–47, 1998.
2. Wolf AM, Colditz GA. Current estimates of the economic costs of obesity in the United States. Obes Res 6: 97–106, 1998.
3. Eckel RH. Obesity in heart disease: A statement for healthcare professionals from the Nutrition Committee, American Heart Association. JAMA 96:3248–3250, 1997.
4. Manson JE, Willett WC, Stampher MJ, et al. Body weight and mortality among women. N Engl J Med 333:677–685, 1995.
5. National Institutes of Health and the National Heart, Lung and Blood Institute. Clinical Guidelines on the Identification, Evaluation and Treatment of Overweight and Obesity in Adults: The Evidence Reports, 1998.
6. Bray GA. Definitions, measurements, and classification of the syndrome of obesity. Int J Obes 2: 99, 1978.
7. Bray GA, Gray DS. Obesity: Part I. Pathogenesis. West J Med 149:429, 1988.
8. Brownell KD, Wadden TA. Etiology and treatment of obesity: Towards understanding a serious, prevalent, and refractory disorder. J Consult Clin Psychol 60:505, 1992.
9. Wilson GT. Behavioral treatment of obesity: Thirty years and counting. Adv Behav Res Ther 16:31, 1994.
10. Friedman MA, Brownell KD. Psychological correlates of obesity: Moving to the next research generation. Psychol Bull 117:3, 1995.
11. Grilo CM. The assessment and treatment of binge eating disorder. J Pract Psychiatry Behav Health 4: 191–201, 1998.
12. Grilo CM. Self-help and guided self-help treatments for bulimia nervosa and binge eating disorder. J Pract Psychiatry 6: 18–26, 2000.
13. Yanovski SZ. Binge eating disorder: Current knowledge and future directions. Obesity Res 1:306, 1993.
14. Agras WS, Telch CF, Arnow B, et al. Weight loss, cognitive-behavioral, and desipramine treatments in binge eating disorder: An additive design. Behav Ther 25:225, 1994.
15. Brownell KD, Fairburn CG, eds. Eating Disorders and Obesity: A Comprehensive Handbook. New York: Guilford, 1995.
16. Brownell KD, Rodin J. The dieting maelstrom: Is it possible and advisable to lose weight? Am Psychol 49:781, 1994.
17. Comuzzie AG, Allison DB. The search for human obesity genes. Science 280:1374–1377, 1998.
18. Vogler GP, Sorensen TIA, Stunkard AJ, et al. Influences of genes and shared family environment on adult body mass index assessed in an adoption study by a comprehensive path model. Int J Obes 19:40, 1995.
19. Zhang Y, Proenca R, Maffei M, et al. Positional cloning of the mouse obese gene and its human homologue. Nature 372:425, 1994.
20. Grilo CM, Pogue-Geile M. The nature of environmental influences on obesity: A behavior genetic analysis. Psychol Bull 110:520, 1991.
21. Grilo CM. The role of physical activity in weight loss and weight loss management. Med Exerc Nutr Health 4:60, 1995.
22. Pavlou KN, Krey S, Steffee WP. Exercise as an adjunct to weight loss and maintenance in moderately obese subjects. Am J Clin Nutr 49:1115–1123, 1989.
23. Wood PD, Stefanick ML, Williams PT, et al. The effects on plasma lipoproteins of a prudent weight-reducing diet, with

or without exercise, in overweight men and women. N Engl J Med 325:461–466, 1991.

24. Ballor DL, Katch VI, Becque MD, et al. Resistance weight training during caloric restriction enhances lean body weight maintenance. Am J Clin Nutr 47:19–25, 1988.

25. Pate RR, Pratt M, Blair SN, et al. Physical activity and public health: A recommendation from the Centers for Disease Control and Prevention and the American College of Sports Medicine. JAMA 273:402–407, 1995.

26. Rippe JM, Ward A, Porcari JP, et al. Walking for health and fitness. JAMA 259:2720–2724, 1988.

27. Dunn AL, Marcus SH, Kampert JB, et al. Comparison of lifestyle and structured interventions to increase physical activity and cardiorespiratory fitness: A randomized trial. JAMA 281:327–334, 1999.

28. Andersen RE, Wadden TA, Bartlett SJ, et al. Lifestyle activity versus structured aerobic exercise to change body composition and cardiovascular risk factors in obese women: A randomized trial. JAMA 281:335–340, 1999.

29. Jakicic JM, Wing RR, Butler BA, Robertson RJ. Prescribing exercise in multiple short bouts versus one continuous bout. Int J Obes 19:893–901, 1995.

30. Jakicic JM, Winters C, Lang W, Wing RR. Effects of intermittent exercise and use of home exercise equipment on adherence, weight loss, and fitness in overweight women. JAMA 282:1554–1560, 1999.

31. Brownell KD. The LEARN Program for Weight Management 2000. Dallas: American Health, 2000.

32. Schlundt DG, Hill JO, Pope-Cordle J, et al. Randomized evaluation of a lowfat and libitum carbohydrate diet for weight reduction. Int J Obes 17:623, 1993.

33. Wadden TA, Van Itallie TB, Blackburn GL. Responsible and irresponsible use of very-low-calorie diets in the treatment of obesity. JAMA 263:83, 1990.

34. Abenhaim L, Moride Y, Brenot F, et al. Appetite-suppressant drugs and the risk of primary pulmonary hypertension. N Engl J Med 335:606–616, 1996.

35. Kurz X, Van Ermen A. Valvular heart disease associated with fenfluramine-phentermine. N Engl J Med 337:1772–1773, 1997.

36. Drouin P, Hanotin C, Courcier S, Leutenegger E. A dose ranging study: Efficacy and tolerability of sibutramine in weight loss. Int J Obes 18:60, 1994.

37. Hanotin C, Thomas F, Jones SP, et al. Efficacy and tolerability of sibutramine in obese patients: A dose-ranging study. Int J Obes 22:32–38, 1998.

38. Davidson MH, Hauptman J, DiGirolamo M, et al. Weight control and risk factor reduction in obese subjects treated for two years with orlistat: a randomized controlled trial. JAMA 281:235–242, 1999.

39. Sjostrom L, Rissanen A, Anderson T, et al. Randomized placebo-controlled trial of orlistat for weight loss and prevention of weight regain in obese patients. Lancet 352:167–172, 1998.

40. Manson JE, Faich GA. Pharmacotherapy for obesity: Do the benefits outweigh the risks? N Engl J Med 335:659–660, 1996.

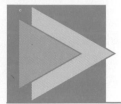

CHAPTER **71**

SMOKING CESSATION

Andrew M. Gottlieb

HEALTH RISKS OF SMOKING

Cigarette smoking is the leading preventable cause of premature death from heart disease, lung disease, and cancer. Of the 46 million Americans who smoke regularly, approximately 420,000 die of premature illness each year. Worldwide, the damage cigarette smoking does to health is staggering. According to a recent survey conducted by the World Health Organization (WHO), 3 million people die each year of smoking-related illnesses (1). By 2020, the death toll will rise to 10 million per year. Of the people alive today, roughly half a billion will die of tobacco-related causes. U.S. women are disproportionately affected. Though only 5% of women live in the United States, 50% of women worldwide who die of smoking-related causes live in the United States.

Although most people are aware of the link between smoking and cancer, far fewer individuals understand the causal relationship between smoking and heart disease. The risk of heart disease is directly related to the number of cigarettes smoked. Smoking one pack per day doubles the risk compared to nonsmoking; smoking more than one pack per day triples the risk. The main mechanisms that affect the development of heart disease are the effects of carbon monoxide. Nicotine in tobacco smoke causes increases in heart rate and blood pressure, which increases the work of the heart. It also may increase platelet adhesiveness, changing blood viscosity. Carbon monoxide interferes with the ability of red blood cells to carry oxygen, thereby reducing oxygen delivered to the heart muscle.

HEALTH BENEFITS OF QUITTING SMOKING

The health benefits of quitting smoking are immediate and substantial. They extend to young and old and to those with and without smoking-related disease. Smoking cessation is the single most important step that smokers can take to enhance length and quality of life (2).

Although risk from smoking is cumulative, risks of cancer and heart disease drop rapidly after stopping smoking, even if the person has smoked for many years (3, 4). After 2.5 years of not smoking, risk of lung cancer is reduced by 50%. Within 3–5 years of not smoking, risk of a heart attack is similar to that of a nonsmoker, and within 5–10 years, risk of major health problems decreases to levels only slightly greater than for those who have never smoked. Other benefits include increased energy, improved sense of smell, the ability to exercise more easily, and higher self-esteem.

WHY PEOPLE SMOKE

To counsel smokers effectively, it is useful to understand that both physical and psychological components drive smoking (5, 6). Physical dependence on nicotine is one major factor. Each cigarette puff delivers a hit of nicotine to the brain within 7 seconds, making smoking one of the most effective drug delivery systems known. The average smoker may self-administer 50,000–70,000 nicotine doses a year. Nicotine appears to have both stimulating and tranquilizing effects, depending on dosage. Some evidence suggests that nicotine may increase the production of brain hormones, such as beta-endorphins. This effect may explain why nicotine can reduce the perception of pain and increase feelings of well-being. Smokers can fine-tune emotional responses by varying puff rate and depth to control the amount of nicotine delivered to the brain. Thus, a smoker literally has fingertip control of emotional and physical responses, reducing the need for other coping techniques. Once a person becomes dependent on these effects to function normally, quitting becomes extremely difficult.

The other major component is conditioned psychological dependence. The thousands of nicotine doses received each year are linked to situations and emotional states. Each of these situations and emotional states becomes a cue to the smoker that it is time for a puff. Situational cues include such things as drinking coffee or an alcoholic beverage, talking on the phone, watching TV, finishing a meal, and driving. Other cues are negative emotions, such as anger, frustration, stress, or boredom. Furthermore, diminishing blood levels of nicotine trigger withdrawal symptoms that also encourage smoking.

CESSATION

The Quitting Process

The experience of quitting varies considerably among smokers. Some smokers quit easily and report surprise at how much easier than expected it was; some report that quitting was the most difficult thing that they ever attempted; others report some degree of difficulty between these two extremes. Some report the physical factors being the primary difficulty; some, the psychological factors; and others, both.

Withdrawal from nicotine can produce a variety of effects, including craving for tobacco, anxiety, irritability, restlessness, difficulty concentrating, headache, drowsiness, and gastrointestinal disturbances. These symptoms are generally most intense for the first 2–3 days after cessation, then decrease, but they increase again around day 10 and finally decrease gradually thereafter. The acute phase of nicotine withdrawal is generally over within 2–4 weeks, although some withdrawal symptoms, such as the urge to smoke, can continue for months or even years (7). The number of reported withdrawal symptoms varies from none to many and severity, from mild to severe. (Nearly 90% of smokers have at least one withdrawal symptom.)

Most smokers quit a number of times before achieving long-term abstinence. Most smokers who relapse do so within 6 months of quitting; some relapse years after cessation, but this is the exception. As the duration of abstinence increases, relapse becomes less likely (2). Many smokers are able to quit for short periods, but maintaining cessation is a major challenge.

Approaches to Smoking Cessation

Most people who have quit smoking report doing so without the help of a health professional. Formal smoking cessation programs can be helpful to smokers who cannot quit on their own, often including those who smoke heavily and are strongly addicted (8, 9).

To guide a smoker to appropriate assistance for smoking cessation, it is important to know the options available, their effectiveness, and any barriers to participation (cost, location, time, cultural biases) (8). The appropriateness of a group program versus individual sessions with a health professional should be considered. When examining effectiveness, one must look at the long-term quit rate of a strategy or program, since relapse is common. Some programs boast high initial quit rates but fail to report long-term relapse rates. There is no magic bullet at any cost that can guarantee long-term quitting. However, there is help in a variety of forms to assist any

smoker who would like to quit. Smoking cessation techniques include the following:

- Pharmacological interventions
- Behavioral interventions
- Other strategies, such as acupuncture and hypnosis

Stop smoking programs are available in a variety of formats:

- Self-help materials, with or without minimal contact
- Group meetings
- Individual sessions with a health professional

Many studies evaluating various behavioral and pharmacological approaches to cessation have been conducted, allowing some confidence in identifying approaches that are most effective.

Pharmacological Interventions
Overview of Nicotine Replacement Medications

An apparently effective pharmacological intervention in widespread use is nicotine replacement via nicotine polacrilex (Nicorette), transdermal patch (Habitrol, Nicoderm, Nicotrol, and ProStep), or nasal spray (Nicotrol NS). The gum and patches are available over the counter. They are designed to provide a partial substitute for the nicotine obtained from cigarettes to make the initial phase of tobacco withdrawal less unpleasant, allowing the person to learn new ways of coping with the behavioral aspects of smoking cessation (unlinking smoking-related cues from actual cigarette smoking). Nicotine nasal spray is available by prescription only. Nicotine replacement treatment should be used for at least 10–12 weeks following quitting; many smokers require 6 months' treatment, and some need treatment for 1–2 years before successfully tapering off nicotine medication.

NICOTINE GUM. Nicotine polacrilex 2 mg and 4 mg, available since 1984 by prescription and over the counter since 1996, contains nicotine bound to a resin base, that is, nicotine gum. When the gum is chewed, nicotine is released and absorbed through the oral mucosa. For maximum benefit, the patient has to chew 12 or more pieces of gum a day. The suggested dosing is as follows:

- Weeks 1–6: one piece every hour
- Weeks 7–10: tapering
- Week 12: discontinuing use

Patients should be instructed carefully in how to chew the gum, since optimal use is quite different from that of regular chewing gum. Over-the-counter costs are about $50 ($0.46 per piece) for the 2-mg starter kit, which includes information on quitting and 108 pieces of gum. The 4-mg starter kit is about $60 ($0.56 per piece). Refills cost about $30 ($0.62 per piece) for 48 pieces of 2-mg gum and $35 ($0.72 per piece) for 4-mg gum. Thus, with use of 12 pieces a day, the cost of 12 weeks of treatment is about $465. (One suggestion to patients is to buy the starter kits rather than the refill kits, as the gum is up to 43% cheaper that way.)

Researchers have reported impressive improvements in quit rates, but primarily when combined with some behavioral counseling or follow-up. The 4-mg gum is more effective than 2-mg gum for highly nicotine dependent smokers (those who smoke more than 25 cigarettes a day), yielding 2-year quit rates of 34% (4 mg) versus 6% (2 mg) (10).

Researchers continue to examine ways to increase the effectiveness of nicotine polacrilex. Clear chewing instructions and a behavioral change component should accompany a prescription (11, 12). When advising a smoker, one must steer the individual to either a behavioral program in which nicotine polacrilex use is an integral part or to a physician who will provide good follow-up care along with this medication.

Studies show that the effectiveness of nicotine polacrilex 2 mg is influenced by the behavioral intervention that accompanies it (5, 6). If there is no behavioral component and if a physician simply phones in a prescription to a pharmacy, nicotine polacrilex is no more effective than placebo at the 1-year follow-up; however, even with minimal behavioral intervention, a significant effect can be expected. Studies indicate that including a physician's advice with nicotine polacrilex increases the 1-year quit rate from approximately 5% to 9%; adding a physician's advice and follow-up increases quit rates from 15% to 27%; and adding comprehensive group counseling increases quit rates from 16% to 38%. Studies in which behavior modification is combined with nicotine polacrilex are associated with 1-year quit rates above 40%. Now that nicotine polacrilex is available without prescription, it is even more important that some type of behavioral support or follow-up be encouraged.

NICOTINE PATCH. The nicotine patch was approved in the United States in late 1991 and is available over the counter. Patches are a much easier route for nicotine delivery than gum, making both smokers and health professionals happy they are available. Nicotine patches are no magic bullet, however.

Patches come in three sizes, 30 cm^2, 20 cm^2, and 10 cm^2, delivering nicotine 24 hours a day (Habitrol, Nicoderm, ProStep) or 16 hours a day (Nicotrol). The 24-hour patches deliver 21, 14, and 7 mg nicotine a day (30 cm^2, 20 cm^2, and 10 cm^2 respectively), while the 16-hour patches deliver 15, 10, and 5 mg nicotine a day. Nicotine patches are applied once a day. Most smokers who use the 24-hour patches begin with the 21-mg patch and taper to 14- and 7-mg patches. Most smokers who use the 16-hour patches start with the 15-mg patch and taper to the 10- and 5-mg patches. Cost is about $4 per day of treatment. Recommended duration of treatment is 8 weeks for light smokers and 10 weeks for heavy smokers, for a total cost of about $225–$280. Smokers reduce nicotine intake by using a 21-mg patch for 6 weeks, then tapering to 14 and 7 mg over the next 4 weeks.

Whether to use a 24-hour or 16-hour patch probably depends on the strength of the craving for cigarettes in the morning. Those with intense morning craving may do better on a 24-hour patch, but a 16-hour patch produces less sleep disruption and fewer nightmares. In a study of 935 participants, 6-month sustained abstinence rates for those receiving the nicotine patch were significantly higher than for those receiving placebo (26% versus 12%, respectively). Good results have been found with nicotine patch therapy as long as there is regular contact with the patient. Nine group counseling sessions over 12 weeks of patch therapy resulted in 26% nonsmoking rates at 6 months (13). Seven regular physician visits over 18 weeks of patch therapy produced 34% cessation rates at 6 months (14). Even brief weekly telephone follow-ups during 6 weeks of patch therapy yielded a 21% quit rate at 6 months (15).

Combining gum with patch provides better relief of nicotine withdrawal symptoms than either drug alone (16–18), and may increase the odds of 12-month cessation by a factor of 1.8 (19). Used this way, the nicotine patch provides baseline levels of nicotine, while the gum adds nicotine in high-risk situations and may provide a higher level of nicotine replacement. But the overall dose of nicotine would still be less than that attained by smoking.

NICOTINE NASAL SPRAY. Nicotine nasal spray (Nicotrol NS) is simply aqueous nicotine delivered into the nasal pathways using a device similar to that used to deliver intranasal steroids. Nasal spray may be helpful for heavy smokers who do not get adequate relief using gum or patches. Available by prescription, nasal spray delivers nicotine in a quickly absorbed form, resulting in blood levels that peak within 4–15 minutes at a level of 2–12 ng/mL. Some 20% of users achieve a blood level similar to that derived from smoking one cigarette. Dosing is 1 mg nicotine per two sprays (one in each nostril). Maximum daily dose is 5 per hour, or 40 per day, with a treatment time of 3 months. However, according to the package insert, 32% of spray users reported feeling dependent, so the potential for addiction may be higher than with patch or gum (20).

Cost is approximately $46 per 10 mg, about 100 doses. At the recommended rate of one to two doses per hour, cost for 10 weeks of treatment is $515–$1030. One study found that combining nasal spray with patch more than doubled abstinence rates at 6 months (31% versus 16%), 1 year (27% versus 11%), and 6 years (16% versus 9%) compared to the patch alone (19).

All of these medications seem to be safe. The most common side effects are local, such as skin irritation from patches, heartburn from gum, and nasal irritation from spray. Contrary to press reports from July 1992, the nicotine patch does not cause heart attacks (21).

Cigarettes deliver nicotine more rapidly than any of the medications. Next is nicotine nasal spray, followed by nicotine policrex, and slowest (but steadiest), a nicotine patch. Thus it may be that nicotine nasal spray best simulates the nicotine bolus effect of smoking cigarettes, but whether this makes it difficult to give up the spray remains to be seen (21).

Other Pharmacological Approaches: Buspirone and Bupropion

Buspirone (BuSpar) is a nonbenzodiazepine antianxiety medication. One randomized, double blind, placebo-controlled trial demonstrated that participants using buspirone had 4-week abstinence rates of 47% compared to 16% for placebo (22). Buspirone may be useful either alone or in combination with nicotine gum or patches, especially with smokers who use cigarettes to cope with anxiety.

A series of interesting findings relate cigarette smoking and depression. The lifetime prevalence of major depression is 3.7–6.7%. However, it is 27% in the smoking population and 46–61% in smokers who present for treatment. Of those with major depression, 74% smoke, in contrast to only 26% of the general population. Furthermore, the quit rate of those with major depression is about half that for smokers with no psychiatric diagnosis (23, 24).

Thus it appears that some smokers may use smoking to control depression. For those smokers, concomitant treatment with an antidepressant may be helpful. The best published studies on antidepressants and smoking are on sustained-release bupropion (Wellbutrin or Zyban). One found 55% of patients treated with bupropion abstinent at 6 months as compared to none treated with placebo (25). Another study of 190 people showed 40% of bupropion-treated patients abstinent at 4 weeks compared with 24% of placebo-treated subjects (26). A large-scale study using 244 subjects compared four treatment conditions: bupropion, nicotine patch, bupropion combined with patch, and placebo. Cessation rates at 12 months were respectively 30.3%, 16.4%, 35.5%, and 15.6%, which suggests that the combination of bupropion and nicotine patch is an effective treatment (27). Evaluating smokers for depression using the Beck Depression Inventory (Center for Cognitive Therapy, Philadelphia) or other similar instruments and concomitant treatment for depression may significantly improve smoking cessation results.

No single pharmacological intervention used alone seems to be significantly more effective than the rest. One randomized study of nicotine gum, patch, nasal spray, and nasal inhaler found 12 week quit rates of 20%, 21%, 24%, and 24%, respectively, with high compliance with use of patch, lower compliance for gum, and very low compliance for nicotine spray or inhaler (28).

Behavioral Interventions

Behavioral interventions, including components such as self-monitoring, contracts, and assertiveness skills training, are often included in stop smoking programs. As previously stated, these components may increase long-term effectiveness. One of the most effective techniques is rapid smoking; when properly administered, this approach has had long-term abstinence rates of 64–70%. Rapid smoking entails several elements, including relapse prevention training (see subsequent discussion) and rapid smoking, in which patients inhale smoke from a cigarette every 6 seconds until they no longer want another puff. The procedure creates an aversion to smoking that leads to good cessation outcomes when combined with skills training. This technique must not be attempted without support and guidance from a health professional. It is used rarely now, because it requires close medical support and because nonaversive methods have become more widely available.

Relapse prevention is a useful behavioral approach to maintaining cessation. Relapse prevention teaches anticipation of situations in which temptation to smoke may be present and development of new coping methods for avoiding relapse in these situations (29, 30). Simple questionnaires can be used to measure confidence in ability to resist smoking in high-risk situations (31). These questionnaires may be helpful in determining the types of coping skills on which to focus attention. The relapse prevention approach is particularly valuable in smoking cessation. As Mark Twain said, "Quitting smoking is easy; I have done it many times." Staying quit is difficult.

Other Techniques

Smokers are often attracted to acupuncture or hypnosis as the magic bullet or as an easy way to achieve long-term smoking cessation. Controlled studies fail to show any positive correlation between acupuncture and smoking cessation (32). Hypnosis can be provided individually or in groups for one or multiple sessions and is often combined with other behavioral techniques. However, no controlled studies of hypnosis for smoking cessation demonstrate a significant long-term treatment effect.

Stop Smoking Programs

Programs are available in a variety of formats. In a self-help or minimal-intervention format, a smoker works to quit smoking without the continued assistance of health professionals, trained leaders, or organizations; reliance on self is the primary method with a self-help book or guide to assist in devising ways to quit and stay off cigarettes. A study using the American Lung Association's Freedom From Smoking in 20 Days (one of the many manuals available), reports a 1-year quit rate of 5% versus 2% for controls. Generally, self-help programs report substantially lower quit rates than more formal programs, but are inexpensive and generally widely available. Efforts to maximize effectiveness of self-help programs are under way (33).

Programs in a group format provide a support group, which some smokers find helpful. The content, cost, and providers of these programs vary, but generally health organizations and commercial groups offer them. Few well-designed studies have evaluated this type of program. When specific programs advertise high success rates, it is important to inquire about long-term (ideally a year, but minimally 6 months) rates and the method for determining those rates.

Some smokers prefer working with a health professional on an individual basis. In this case it is important to inquire about approaches used and qualifications of the health professional. Typically the health professional is a physician, nurse, or counselor of some type. Research projects at medical schools, universities, and other medical facilities can provide another resource for smokers.

HOW TO HELP SOMEONE STOP SMOKING

Exercise professionals are often asked to help with smoking cessation in individual cases. The following guidelines may be useful as aids to promote successful quitting.

Advise The Smoker To Quit

Advice to quit from a health professional with good rapport may have substantial influence. For example, studies show that 60 seconds of definitive advice from a physician has substantial impact on long-term (1 year) quit rate, increasing it 17-fold in one study (34). Advice should clearly, succinctly, and unequivocally state the dangers of smoking and the benefits of quitting. Timing the discussion to occur when a patient is having symptoms caused by, attributed to, or exacerbated by smoking, such as coughing, shortness of breath, or angina, may be especially effective. Avoidance of moralism or punitive action is important. Emphasize the benefits of quitting and advise the patient to eliminate tobacco products. There are **no** healthful tobacco products, and virtually no one can smoke in a limited way.

Help Develop a Specific Plan for Cessation

Help the smoker choose a specific quit date. A specific quit date helps prepare for not smoking. Review prior quit attempts to evaluate what was helpful and identify problems. Reframe past relapses in a positive light by emphasizing that past attempts can teach something useful. Say that most successful long-term quitters have made more than one attempt to quit.

Inform the smoker about resources in the community, such as self-help or minimal contact programs, group programs, and individual health professionals who work in smoking cessation. A list of the programs, with names and phone numbers for additional information, is help-

ful, as is information about the components, format, cost, and effectiveness of the intervention. Good sources of information concerning local programs:

- Local universities
- Medical groups, hospitals
- Agencies such as American Cancer Society, American Lung Association and the American Heart Association
- Commercially available over-the-counter nicotine replacement options, such as nicotine gum or patches

Encourage Quitting Efforts and Provide Support During Difficult Times

Help motivate by asking about positive health benefits and other positive occurrences resulting from quitting, such as increased stamina, better breathing, less coughing, and improved sense of smell. Point out that withdrawal symptoms are temporary and are signs that dependence on nicotine is diminishing. Since relapse is common after quitting, ask about difficult times and help identify ways to cope.

Some smokers are not ready to quit immediately but express readiness later. Those not ready to quit are sometimes concerned about the disadvantages of quitting or their ability to succeed; these factors should be addressed if they are clearly expressed. Gentle, firm reminders about the importance of quitting can influence motivation to make the attempt.

Respond To Concerns About Weight Gain

Smokers may express concern about weight gain, either as a reason not to quit or after cessation. Approximately 80% of those who quit gain weight after cessation. The average weight gain is approximately 5 pounds. Increased food intake and/or decreased energy expenditure may be partially responsible for this weight gain. The health benefits of smoking cessation far exceed any risks from the average weight gain (2). It is useful to tell the patient that 100 pounds would have to be gained before the health effect of the weight equaled that of continued smoking. Suggestions such as increasing physical activity, eating low-fat sweets in response to an increased desire for sweet foods, and having low-calorie snacks available may be helpful. The best way to avoid excessive weight gain is to increase levels of physical activity and exercise. Also, using bupropion (Zyban) during cessation can reduce weight gain (27).

▶ SUMMARY

Cigarette smoking is the leading preventable cause of death. Smoking cessation has major and immediate health benefits. Advice to quit smoking from a health professional with good rapport may have substantial effect. Millions of smokers have quit successfully; however, for some, quitting is difficult. Both physical and psychological factors contribute to cigarette smoking. There is no magic bullet, but help is available. Most smokers quit without assistance, and most successful long-term quitters have made many short-term quit attempts before achieving long-term abstinence.

A variety of techniques provided in a variety of formats are available to help smokers who want to quit, but are unable to do without assistance. Programs that include nicotine replacement in combination with behavioral interventions seem to provide the best results. There are a number of options for nicotine replacement, and both nicotine gum and nicotine patches are available without a prescription. Bupropion (Zyban) is a useful adjunct treatment, especially when combined with nicotine replacement.

It is important to encourage smokers to quit and to provide clear information and support to help increase chances of success. The good news is that even small interventions seem to have large effects, especially compared with no intervention. Thus, with a little knowledge and persistence, a professional can have a powerful positive effect on the health of patients.

References

1. University of California at Berkeley Wellness Letter 12(5) Feb. 1996.
2. U.S. Department of Health and Human Services. The Health Benefits of Smoking Cessation. DHHS Pub (CDC) 90-8416, 1990.
3. Sachs DPL. Cigarette smoking: Health effects and cessation strategies. Clin Geriatr Med 2:337–362, 1986.
4. Schuman LM. The benefits of cessation of smoking. Chest 59:421–427, 1971.
5. Sachs DPL, Leischow SJ. Pharmacologic approaches to smoking cessation. Clin Chest Med 12:769–791, 1991.
6. Sachs DPL. Advances in smoking cessation treatment. Curr Pulmonol 12:139–198, 1991.
7. Gottlieb A, Killen J, Marlatt GA, Taylor CB. Psychological and pharmacological influences in cigarette smoking withdrawal: Effects of nicotine gum and expectancies on smoking withdrawal symptoms and relapse. J Consult Clinic Psychol 55:606–608, 1987.
8. Fiore MC, Novotny TE, Pierce JP, et al. Methods used to quit smoking in the United States: Do cessation programs help? JAMA 263:2760–2765, 1990.
9. Glynn TJ. Methods of smoking cessation: Finally some answers. JAMA 263:2795–2796, 1990 (editorial).
10. Tonnesen P, Fryd V, Hansen M, et al. Effect of nicotine chewing gum in combination with group counseling on the cessation of smoking. N Engl J Med 318:15–18, 1988.
11. Pomerleau OF, Pomerleau CS, eds. Nicotine Replacement: A Critical Evaluation. Progress in Clinical and Biological Research, vol 261. New York: Alan R. Liss, 1988.
12. Sachs DPL. Nicotine polacrilex: Practical use requirements. Curr Pulmonol 10:141–158, 1989.
13. Transdermal Nicotine Study Group. Transdermal nicotine for smoking cessation: 6-month results from two multicenter controlled clinical trials. JAMA 266:3133–3138, 1991.
14. Sachs DPL, Sawe U, Leischow SL. Effectiveness of a 16 hour transdermal nicotine patch in a medical practice setting, without intensive group counseling. Arch Intern Med 153:1881–1890, 1993.
15. Westman E, Levin E, Rose J. The nicotine patch in smoking cessation: A randomized trial with telephone counseling. Arch Intern Med 153:1917–1923, 1993.
16. Fagerstom KO, Schneider N, Lunelle E. Effectiveness of nicotine patch and nicotine gum as individual versus combined treatments for tobacco withdrawal symptoms. Psychopharmacology 111:271–277, 1993.
17. Stapleton J. Commentary: Progress on nicotine replacement therapy for smokers. BMJ 318:289–290, 1999.
18. Kornitzer M, Boutsen M, Dramaix M, et al. Combined use of nicotine patch and gum in smoking cessation: A placebo-controlled clinical trial. Prev Med 24:41–47, 1995.
19. Blondal T, Gudmundsson LJ, Olafsdottir I, et al. Nicotine nasal spray with nicotine patch for smoking cessation: Randomised trial with six year follow up. BMJ 318:285–288, 1999.
20. Package insert, Nicotrol NS. Pharmacia AB, Sweden.
21. Sachs PL, Fagerstom KO. Medical management of tobacco dependence: Practical office considerations. Curr Pulmonol 16:239–249, 1995.
22. West R, Hajek P, McNeill A. Effect of buspirone on cigarette withdrawal symptoms and short term abstinence rates in a smokers clinic. Psychopharmacology (Berl) 104:91–96, 1991.
23. Hall SM, Munoz, RF, Reus VI, et al. Nicotine, negative affect, and depression. J Consult Clin Psychol 61:761–767, 1993.
24. Glassman AH, Helzer JE, Covey LS, et al. Smoking, smoking cessation and major depression. JAMA 264:1546–1549, 1990.
25. Ferry LH, Robbins AS, Scariati PD, et al. Enhancement of smoking cessation using the antidepressant bupropion hydrochochloride. Circulation 86:I-167, 1992.
26. Ferry LH, Burchette RJ. Evaluation of bupropion versus placebo for treatment of nicotine dependence. Oral paper presented at the 147th meeting of the American Psychiatric Association, Philadelphia, May 26, 1994.
27. Jorenby DE, Leischow SJ, Nides MA, et al. A controlled trial of sustained-release bupropion, a nicotine patch, or both for smoking cessation. N Engl J Med 340:685–691, 1999.
28. Hajek P, West R, Foulds J, et al. Randomized comparative trial of nicotine polacrilex, a transdermal patch, nasal spray, and an inhaler. Arch Intern Med 159:2033–2038, 1999.
29. Marlatt GA, Gordon J. Relapse Prevention: Maintenance Strategies in the Treatment of Addictive Behaviors. New York: Guilford, 1985.
30. Brownell KD, Glynn TJ, Glasgow R, et al. Interventions to Prevent Relapse. Health Psychol 5(suppl.):53–68, 1986.
31. Condiotte MM, Lichtenstein E. Self-efficacy and relapse in smoking cessation programs. J Consult Clin Psychol 49:648–658, 1981.
32. Ter Riet G, Kleijnen J, Knipschild P. A meta-analysis of studies into the effect of acupuncture on addiction. Br J Gen Pract 40:379–382, 1990.
33. Glynn TJ, Boyd GM, Gruman JC. Essential elements of self-help/minimal intervention strategies for smoking cessation. Health Educ Q 17:329–345, 1990.
34. Russell MAH, Wilson C, Taylor C, et al. Effect of general practitioners' advice against smoking. BMJ 2:231–235,1979.

SECTION THIRTEEN

PROGRAM MANAGEMENT

SECTION EDITOR: *Tracy York, MS*

2.10.0, 2.10.0.1,
2.10.0.7

3.10.0.2 3.10.6.2,
3.10.6.3

5.10.0

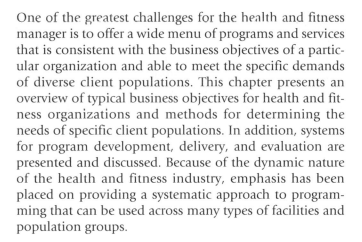

CHAPTER **72**

HEALTH AND FITNESS PROGRAM DEVELOPMENT

Sandra L. Minor

One of the greatest challenges for the health and fitness manager is to offer a wide menu of programs and services that is consistent with the business objectives of a particular organization and able to meet the specific demands of diverse client populations. This chapter presents an overview of typical business objectives for health and fitness organizations and methods for determining the needs of specific client populations. In addition, systems for program development, delivery, and evaluation are presented and discussed. Because of the dynamic nature of the health and fitness industry, emphasis has been placed on providing a systematic approach to programming that can be used across many types of facilities and population groups.

PROGRAMMING BASED ON ORGANIZATIONAL OBJECTIVES

As the health and fitness industry has matured over the past decade, facilities have become more similar with respect to general design characteristics and types of equipment. It is likely, for example, that a prospective participant will find a similar range of cardiovascular equipment (treadmills, stair machines, bicycles, and rowers) available at both community and commercial fitness facilities. As a result of this lack of differentiation with regard to facilities and equipment, health and fitness programming has become the primary product that differentiates organizations in the marketplace. Therefore, it is important that the menu of programs offered by a health and fitness facility be carefully designed to match specific facility and program goals and objectives.

The following section outlines four general categories of organizational settings in the health and fitness industry. A description of typical business objectives in each of these categories has been presented to provide the health and fitness manager with a point of reference. In reality, regardless of the category, there is likely to be a combination of objectives within the business plan of a given organization. It is the responsibility of the health and fitness

manager to identify clearly the specific objectives of the facility. The four general categories of organizational settings in the health and fitness industry are commercial, community, work site, and clinical.

Commercial Settings

Commercial health and fitness organizations are usually operated with the intention of generating a profit. Private health and fitness clubs, country clubs, and spas are examples of commercial organizations. Health and fitness programming contributes to the profitability of commercial organizations in several ways. Programs can generate revenue directly through assessment of fees for specific services (fee-for-service programs). These fees are often charged in addition to the fees that are collected monthly or annually for use of the facility. Personal fitness training is an example of a highly profitable revenue-generating program that is popular in many commercial organizations. In addition to fee-for-service programs, complimentary programs also contribute to the profit-generating objectives of a commercial organization.

Complimentary programs are often packaged into the general membership fees that participants are charged for use of the facility. In many cases, participants make decisions to join facilities based on the types of complimentary programs and services offered. In addition, the decision to continue paying dues is based largely on individual assessment of the value received for the money expended. A client who uses the facility and participates regularly in the programs and services offered is likely to meet individual goals and perceive membership as having value. Programs that encourage regular participation and effective facility use can improve member retention and therefore profitability.

Community Settings

The objective of most community health and fitness organizations is to provide services to the members of a specific community group. YMCAs, Jewish Community Centers, community recreation centers, and university recreation centers are examples. Health and fitness programs in these organizations typically target a specific market and attempt to provide services to as many members of that market as resources will allow. Most community organizations receive some level of outside funding and are classified as not-for-profit organizations. These favorable financial circumstances can allow community organizations to offer programs at low cost, increasing access for many segments of a given community. It is fairly common for some programs in a community organization to be offered on a for-profit basis as a way of generating revenue to deliver other programs at little or no cost to participants. In many YMCAs, for example, fitness memberships are sold to the public as a way to generating revenue to offset the cost of non–profit generating programs such as children's summer camps, senior exercise classes, and programs for individuals with special needs.

Work Site Settings

Work site health and fitness organizations typically are intended to reduce health care costs and/or increase productivity, morale, and recruitment. Work site settings may include traditional fitness facilities or may simply be health and fitness programs in existing space at the work site. Health and fitness programs in these settings can be funded entirely by the company, but in various models individual employees share at least a portion of the program costs. The programs provided in work sites are quite broad. Wellness-oriented programs (e.g. health education classes, smoking cessation, nutrition, stress management) are often given emphasis equal to that of fitness programs. Outdoor activities, such as walking, running, and cycling, are also popular programs that can be offered at the work site without the benefit of additional facilities. Programs offered in the work site are often directly tied to the objective of creating a healthier employee population.

Clinical Setting

Clinical health and fitness organizations are a broad category of businesses that operate with many objectives. Examples of clinical organizations include health and fitness facilities at hospitals, satellite clinics, physical therapy offices, and chiropractic offices. If a clinical health and fitness organization operates as a for-profit business, programs are conducted with similar objectives to those in a commercial setting. If the business model is not-for-profit, objectives are more similar to those of a community or work site setting. As an example, a hospital may operate a work site business for its employees in an attempt to control health care costs and to improve productivity and morale. The facility may also operate as a community business for health insurance subscribers with the objective of helping clients maintain healthy lifestyles and reduce use of medical services. Finally, the hospital may operate commercially, offering health and fitness programs as a way to position itself as a wellness-oriented health care provider, thus improving health insurance sales to subscribers and increasing profitability.

As can be seen from these examples, it has become increasingly difficult to define an appropriate menu of health and fitness programs for an organization based solely upon business setting (e.g., commercial, community, work site, or clinical). The business objectives of an organization provide important guidance, but for programming to be successful, the specific needs of individual participants must also be considered.

PROGRAMMING BASED ON PARTICIPANT GOALS

Regardless of the business setting, each individual participant has specific needs (goals) related to health and fitness. Understanding and identifying the range of goals within the target population for a particular organization is an essential step in programming. The following section describes three categories of goals for individuals who are considering participation in a health and fitness program. Participant goals are rarely limited to a single category, however, and often change over time. It is important to identify the range of participant goals in a particular setting and offer a variety of programs and services to address as many of these goals as possible without compromising quality for quantity. In this manner, as the goals of individuals change over time, the organization will adjust programs and services so as to continue to address participants' goals. Individual goals related to health and fitness programs can be categorized as wellness goals, physical health and fitness goals, and performance goals.

Wellness Goals

People often consider participation in a health and fitness program as a way of improving the overall feeling of wellness. Wellness is an expanded idea of health that goes beyond physical fitness or absence of disease. Wellness is a feeling of optimal health and vitality that encompasses physical, emotional, intellectual, social, mental, and spiritual dimensions (1). Health and fitness settings offer numerous opportunities for wellness programming. Classes directed at lifetime learning, social interaction, travel adventures, relaxation, and meditation are several examples of programs that can help participants meet wellness goals. In addition, educational programs can be offered to assist individuals with achieving positive health behavior changes such as quitting smoking, changing nutritional habits, or beginning an exercise program.

In the case of a participant who is new to exercise, initial assessments, such as health risk appraisals, provide important information about health status and risk of chronic disease. Fitness assessments can also provide valuable information regarding baseline fitness levels. Exercise prescription for this population should emphasize the adoption of regular physical activity at a level consistent with recommendations in the 1996 U.S. Surgeon General's report that all people accumulate 30 minutes of moderate activity on most, if not all days of the week (2).

As with any exercise program design, recommendations with the beginning exerciser should be provided in three distinct phases: the initial phase, improvement phase, and maintenance phase. The initial phase is a gentle introduction to activity emphasizing regular participation and proper technique. The improvement phase is a progressive increase in frequency, intensity, and duration of the activity. The maintenance phase includes variations in program design in a manner that maintains the level of fitness and assists in long-term adherence. Beginning exercisers may need to spend considerable time in the initial phase before proceeding to the improvement phase. Incentive programs may also prove helpful for beginning exercisers, particularly when they have reached the maintenance phase of a program.

Physical Fitness Goals

Many people participate in health and fitness programs to accomplish specific physical fitness goals such as losing weight or getting in shape. Programming opportunities for physical fitness goals are numerous, and new ideas are continually emerging. Group exercise classes, personal fitness training, cardiovascular equipment, weight training machines, free weights, stretching programs, yoga, and martial arts are just a few examples of popular programs that can help individuals meet physical fitness goals.

Regardless of initial fitness levels, all participants with physical fitness goals should have a complete health screening prior to initiating a program. Fitness assessments can also provide baseline information for each component of fitness. Exercise prescription for this population should focus on the ACSM guidelines "Quantity and Quality of Exercise for Developing and Maintaining Cardiorespiratory and Muscular Fitness in Healthy Adults" (3). Programming for this population should involve individualized exercise prescriptions based on the participant's specific goals. Emphasis is placed on the improvement phase of exercise programming.

Performance Goals

In addition to wellness and physical fitness, people participate in health and fitness programs to achieve specific performance goals. Participants may desire to improve ability in a specific sport or type of activity. The range of abilities and skill levels among individuals with performance goals is broad. Some individuals may wish to learn techniques that allow them to take part in a new sport, such as tennis or golf. Others may wish to achieve a high level of performance in a particular competition. Still others may be looking to rehabilitate from an injury and reach a performance goal of getting back to a particular baseline of physical ability. Programming opportuni-

ties are very broad in this category. Examples of programs that can be offered at health and fitness facilities include sport technique training, such as tennis, fly-fishing, or golf; specialty conditioning classes, such as ski conditioning, rowing, or swimming; and educational classes on topics such as nutrition and advanced exercise program design. Specific exercise prescription with frequent re-evaluation is necessary when working with individuals who have performance goals. Measuring outcomes is essential to assess the effectiveness of the programs being offered.

EFFECTIVE PROGRAM PLANNING MODELS

Developing a menu of programs to meet the specific goals of a particular client population is a four-step process that involves needs assessment, program planning, program implementation, and program evaluation (Fig. 72.1).

The Needs Assessment

The purpose of the needs assessment is to determine the specific goals and interests of the client population. This information, combined with industry trends and organizational objectives, can help define an appropriate menu of programs and services. Options for conducting the needs assessment include the following.

Target Market Surveys

The purpose of a target market survey is to determine levels of interest among prospective participants. The target market survey should be conducted early in the planning process. Surveys can be administered though personal distribution of questionnaires, mailing surveys to homes, or interviewing individuals by telephone. Questions must be carefully constructed, and sample groups must be selected at random to obtain accurate and relevant information. In the case of a start-up operation, with which initial programming decisions may have a significant financial influence on facility design, facilities should consider hiring a professional consultant for a

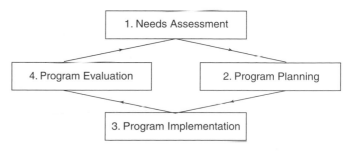

Figure 72.1. Outline for development of effective programs. (Reprinted with permission from Patton B et al. Developing and Managing Health/Fitness Facilities. Champaign IL: Human Kinetics, 1989.)

thorough market analysis. Consultation fees may seem high initially, but the relative cost of renovating a facility to accommodate programming needs that were not initially discovered usually justifies the investment.

Focus Groups

Focus groups are informal discussions conducted with small groups of participants. The group is usually selected according to common characteristics, such as age, sex, or previous participation. A skilled facilitator who tries to obtain information on participants' reactions or attitudes to specific topics typically leads focus group discussions. Before designing a health and fitness facility, focus groups can be an effective way to obtain detailed information regarding prospective participants' interests. Focus groups can also be used to obtain information regarding appropriate pricing, scheduling, and other details related to specific program plans. In an existing facility, focus groups can be used to learn about current programs and clients' interests for expansion. The involvement of a third party in the interview can make participants more comfortable and less reluctant to express their views.

Participant Surveys

If new programming is being considered in an existing facility, a survey of current participants can provide valuable insight. These surveys can be distributed through billing statements, at specific programs, or as part of registration for other activities in the facility. Regardless of the method used, participation is likely to increase if an incentive is offered for completion of the survey. It is important to recognize that any programming changes in a facility affects all other programming. If scheduling changes are involved, some participants will be displaced. If a new program is added, some participants will switch activities and may leave another program undersubscribed.

Evaluation of Current Programs

As part of complete program delivery, evaluations of all programs offered within a facility should be conducted from time to time (see next section for further details). These program evaluations provide valuable information regarding adaptations of existing programs and can detect opportunities for new program development. This process should be ongoing and should include budgetary analysis of revenue and expenses, attendance records, participants' satisfaction, and attainment of program goals and objectives.

Surveys of Staff, Management, and Advisory Committees

Input from staff, management, and other experts can provide important insight for program development. In addition, these individuals can provide an important base of support for marketing during the implementation phase of the program. Individuals who are involved in the planning phase of a program are likely to feel a sense of ownership and high level of support and excitement. Staff members who have direct contact with participants can often provide the most insightful feedback regarding participant needs. These staff members are regularly exposed to informal suggestions and complaints, many of which never are written down or placed on survey questionnaires. Managers often have important input as well regarding operational issues and financial considerations related to overall business objectives. Finally, expert advisers from the community provide an unbiased outside perspective.

Health Screening and Fitness Assessment

Establishing specific program goals and objectives is an essential step in programming. Health appraisal questionnaires and fitness assessment tests can provide specific and detailed information on the baseline status of a given population group. As an example, a specific work site may implement an employee exercise program as a way to lower the incidence of hypertension and obesity in the population. Initial testing for resting blood pressure, body mass index, and body composition could provide important baseline data by which this program could be monitored and evaluated in the future. Initial health risk appraisals can also be used as a way to identify program priorities for the population.

Health Care Usage Reports

Reports on health care usage can also assist an organization in identifying priorities for health and fitness programming. For example, a health insurance company may identify a particular work site that has a large number of claims related to back pain and injury. In this particular facility, educational programs, stretching classes, and ergonomic workstation adjustments may be identified as priority areas of health and fitness programming.

Community Agency Data

Organizations and agencies such as the American Heart Association, American Lung Association, American Red Cross, Centers for Disease Control, and local public health departments provide a wealth of information regarding prevalence of specific diseases and risk factors in the population. In addition, these agencies can provide a wealth of resources, such as written materials, web sites, programs, and consultants.

Program Planning

Once the needs assessment phase has been completed and program needs have been clearly defined, the second phase of program development begins. Program planning is the phase of development in which program details are clearly defined and put into operation. All program planning should include a long-term vision so that short-term planning becomes a means by which the long-term vision is achieved. The following steps should be included in the planning process:

Defining the Target Market

The first step in the program planning phase is to define the target market for the specific program under consideration. Needs assessment data should be used to identify the specific characteristics of people who are likely to participate. In addition, this information can help to determine whether the market size is adequate to meet the specific program objectives.

Identifying Program Goals and Objectives

The next step is to define the specific goals and objectives for the program. Clearly defined goals and objectives provide the foundation for all future planning decisions. In addition, program objectives provide a basis for program evaluation. Examples of program goals for a health and fitness facility include the following:

- Generating net revenue
- Acquiring new participants
- Improving participant retention
- Providing community service

Program objectives are more specific than program goals. Examples of program objectives:

- Decreasing the average body fat level of program participants from 32% to 28% as measured by skinfold caliper tests
- Increasing program participants' knowledge of general nutritional guidelines as measured by change in scores on a nutritional knowledge test
- Reducing cardiovascular risk factors among exercise program participants at a work site as measured by scores on a health risk appraisal instrument

Organizing Programming Staff

An essential step in program planning is the selection of members for the programming team. Programs are most successful when different types of staff members are involved in the planning process. The planning team should include management personnel and staff from other departments in the facility. Special care should be taken with the selection of personnel to handle the actual program delivery. It is important to define the knowledge, skills, and experience required in order for these individuals to meet the program goals and objectives. During the initial planning meeting a project leader should be selected and specific responsibilities should be designated to individual team members. A project plan is a helpful document for establishing specific target dates for each task and tracking progress. This document should include a master list of all tasks to be completed, the name of the staff member who is responsible, a target date for completion, and an indication of when a given task has been successfully accomplished.

Developing Program Content

Once program goals and objectives are established, specific program content can be developed. Program content decisions include the identification of specific materials, equipment, documents, and reference materials to be used and the specific knowledge and skills to be presented. In addition, program content should clearly identify any procedures that are required before participation, such as health screenings, informed consent, and signatures on waivers. The amount of time available, participants' initial knowledge and skill, facility resources, budgetary guidelines, and staff qualifications are among the many issues that must be considered when planning program content.

Establishing a Delivery Model

The delivery model for a program includes decisions related to the location, time of day, duration of sessions, length of the program, number of participants, and instructional techniques to be used. These decisions depend on the specific goals and objectives for the program, characteristics of the target market, projected number of participants, availability of qualified staff, and program budget.

- **Location:** The location must be accessible and convenient for the target market. In addition, the facility must be appropriate for the program content.
- **Scheduling:** The program must be scheduled at a time that is convenient for participants and consistent with the overall business objectives for the facility. Consider scheduling of other programs that serve this target market, including programs and events outside of the facility, such as school vacations and public holidays.
- **Staff-to-participant ratio:** Establishing these ratios in advance allows for establishing enrollment limits, accurate budgeting, and identification of facility requirements. These limits ensure that the program content can be effectively delivered.

Developing Marketing and Sales Plans

The marketing plan defines the message that will be communicated to potential participants about the program. The marketing plan also identifies the specific methods that will be used to inform potential participants about the program. The sales plan outlines the direct action that will be taken to get participants to sign up for the program. Since marketing and sales activities have serious financial implications for the success or failure of a program, it is especially important that the target market be clearly identified and understood in advance. Typical marketing activities include newsletter articles, e-mail messages, voice mail messages, brochures, fliers, bulletin board displays, posters, information sessions, program demonstrations, and direct staff interaction with potential participants. Sales activities involve instructing staff on effective communication techniques. This can be accomplished through role playing and the use of scripts. These activities can help staff gain confidence and be more effective communicating program benefits and registering participants.

Developing a Budget and Establishing Pricing

Once program planning is complete, specific pricing and budgets can be established. Typical program expenses include salaries, payroll taxes and benefits, marketing expenses, sales commissions, program materials, equipment, and facility use charges. Pricing is typically established through consideration of a number of factors. It is essential to consider the general program objectives (e.g., profit, overall retention, improved health status of participants) and the projected number of participants. If the program has been designed with the objective of generating a profit, it is important that minimum and maximum participant numbers be projected and program fees established at a level that adequately covers program costs. Sometimes it is appropriate to offer a program at a loss initially as a way of building a base of support, refining program content and delivery issues, and marketing the program for the future. In such cases, however, it is important to have established timelines and target dates for programs to reach profitable levels. To conduct programs within established budgetary guidelines, revenues and expenses should be reviewed throughout all phases of program delivery, not just at the completion of the program.

Program Implementation

Program implementation entails hiring staff, implementing marketing and sales plans, registering participants, and finally, delivering the program components as planned. The implementation phase is a dynamic process that continually rolls back into small planning phases as new needs of participants are identified. The most effective programs are created with enough flexibility to make immediate changes in the delivery model as new needs are identified.

Program Evaluation

Program evaluation should be conducted throughout the implementation phase (process evaluation) and immediately upon conclusion of the program (impact evaluation). In some cases, long-term follow-up is also appropriate (outcome evaluation). Process evaluations provide insight into delivery. Process evaluations can demonstrate whether procedures were followed and whether they are appropriate and effective. Impact and outcome evaluations assess effectiveness by measuring whether goals and objectives have been met.

Process Evaluation

Process evaluation is the assessment of the ability to carry out specific components of the program. Process evaluation should be conducted throughout the implementation phase. Techniques for process evaluation include direct supervision, soliciting participants' suggestions (Fig. 72.2), surveys of staff members, and tracking of daily participation levels. Once needs are identified, changes in delivery should be made immediately. Waiting until the next session to implement changes may drive away current participants and preclude recruitment of new ones.

Impact and Outcome Evaluation

The first step in evaluating the outcome of a program is to refer to the original program goals and objectives. Goals and objectives provide the standard for measuring success. Table 72.1 illustrates examples of goals and objectives and appropriate methods of evaluation. A cost–benefit analysis can also be conducted as a method of evaluation. This process requires identification of all expenses and assignment of a dollar value to all benefits. The overall cost, savings, or profit that a program produced can then be calculated.

Computers

The use of computers and various software packages is essential for effective management of health and fitness programs. Desktop publishing allows for cost-effective marketing, and participant management software allows for data collection, tracking, and reporting. A number of software programs designed specifically for the health and fitness industry are available through many vendors. A fully integrated package allows for input of participant data such as health history, fitness assessment, goals, interests, and participation records. This can provide important needs assessment information for program planning and development. Many participant management packages produce summary reports on topics such as primary goals and interests of the clients in a given facility. Reports can also be generated on participation levels for specific programs, health risk factors among specific groups, and improvements in specific fitness measures. Finally, group reports can be generated and used for communication with corporations and health maintenance organizations regarding outcomes for particular client groups. These reports can provide important information on program effectiveness while protecting the confidentiality of individual clients.

SPECIFIC PROGRAM PLANNING

The following section provides an overview of some common programs that are found in health and fitness settings. This list is by no means exhaustive. Program offerings in health and fitness facilities are continually in

Please help us evaluate the effectiveness of this program by completing the following questions:

Name of program: _____   **Date:** _____

Instructor: _____

How did you hear about this program? _____

Circle the appropriate number:
1   Strongly disagree
2   Disagree
3   No opinion
4   Agree
5   Strongly agree

1)	This program met my expectations	1	2	3	4	5
2)	The facility location was appropriate and convenient	1	2	3	4	5
3)	The time allowed for this program was appropriate	1	2	3	4	5
4)	The program was scheduled at a convenient time	1	2	3	4	5
5)	The instructor was an effective communicator	1	2	3	4	5
6)	The instructor allowed time for participant questions	1	2	3	4	5
7)	I would recommend this program to other potential participants	1	2	3	4	5

Comments: _____
_____
_____
_____

Optional:

Name: _____   Phone #: _____

Figure 72.2. Sample participant questionnaire.

Table 72.1. Program Evaluation

Evaluation of program goals	
Generate net revenue	Financial analysis of revenues and expenses
Improve client retention	Analysis of length membership in the facility for program participants vs. nonparticipants
Acquisition of new clients	Questionnaire that gathers information on reasons given by clients for joining the facility
Provide community service	Track the number of participants served by the program and their satisfaction levels
Evaluation of program objectives	
Improving performance	Pre/post measurements of performance on specific tasks
Improving fitness level	Pre/post fitness measures
Increasing knowledge	Pre/post knowledge assessments
Decreasing risk factors	Pre/post health risk appraisals and screenings

transition. As new information is made available, programs must be adjusted. As clients become complacent, creative strategies must be developed. The purpose of this section is to highlight some of the programs that have been successful at meeting specific program objectives.

Health Screening and Fitness Assessment

Individualized health screenings and fitness assessments should be made available to participants in all health and fitness facilities. There are a variety of options for screening and assessment programs. Protocol selection should be based on the target population and the specific objectives for the program. The most basic screening tool is the PAR-Q (Physical Activity Readiness Questionnaire), a self administered questionnaire designed to detect medical contraindications to exercise. Customized questionnaires and health risk appraisal instruments can provide more detailed information regarding risk factors, personal medical history, family history, lifestyle factors, and exercise history. Fitness assessment can provide more detailed information regarding the specific components of fitness: aerobic capacity, muscular strength and endurance, body composition, and flexibility. This information can provide an important foundation for other individual and group exercise programs offered in the facility.

Health screenings and fitness assessments can be offered free or for a fee. This decision should be based on the specific objectives of the program. Objectives for screenings and assessments include revenue production, client safety, and client retention. In addition, assessments can identify contraindications to exercise, establish baseline fitness levels, and assist in evaluating program effectiveness. Only experienced health and fitness professionals should conduct screenings and assessments. These professionals must be able to obtain accurate results, recognize abnormal responses, adapt tests for specific participants' needs, properly interpret data, and communicate effectively with clients. It is important for a program manager to interview and screen these professionals, validate the accuracy of data collection techniques, and ensure consistency with other staff members. It is also important to establish policies and procedures that ensure confidentiality.

A variety of computer software programs allow for easy interpretation of data and the production of user-friendly reports. These software programs also allow for risk factor screenings to be conducted with large population groups. These large-scale risk factor screenings are often used as marketing tools to promote health and fitness programming at community and corporate health fairs.

Personal Fitness Training

Offering fitness professional services on a fee-for-service basis has grown into a significant revenue-generating business for many health and fitness facilities. Most facilities have a staff of fitness professionals who are available to participants on a complimentary basis for introductory appointments and basic fitness information. A second group of staff members are usually designated as personal fitness trainers. These staff members are for hire on a fee-for-service basis.

There are several models for personal training programs in health and fitness facilities. Some facilities pay trainers a percentage of the revenue generated by the services they deliver. Other facilities hire personal trainers as full-time salaried employees with designated work shifts and pay the trainers an additional commission for services rendered. Individual salaries or commission rates for trainers are often determined by specific evaluation criteria, such as education, certification, experience, seniority, job performance, and volume of revenue produced. Regardless of the type of employee compensation model, it is important that all program costs be considered during planning. Additional costs for marketing, ad-

ministrative support, meetings, uniforms, payroll taxes, liability insurance, and continuing education can dramatically affect the profitability of the personal training program.

Skills required for the position of personal trainer are similar to those required for other health and fitness professionals. Emphasis should be placed on communication and leadership skills. A strong knowledge base in health screening, fitness assessment, and exercise program design for all population groups is essential. Successful trainers typically have strong business skills in sales, marketing, administration, and time management. Facilities should require all trainers to be certified by a nationally recognized organization. The American College of Sports Medicine's Health/Fitness Instructor certification is appropriate for the personal training position. Other national organizations offer more specialized certification programs that may be appropriate for specific population groups. It is the responsibility of the health and fitness manager to know about various certifications and decide which are appropriate for their particular facility.

Wellness Education Programs

Most fitness facilities offer a variety of programs to enhance knowledge on a range of health topics. The range of wellness programs offered in health and fitness facilities is broad. Programs may address any of the various dimensions of health, namely, physical, emotional, intellectual, spiritual, and social. Examples of wellness education programs include cardiopulmonary resuscitation and first aid, stress management and relaxation, smoking cessation, nutrition, back care, injury prevention, relationships, and a variety of other social, family-oriented, and personal development programs. Depending on the topic, programs can be offered in a variety of formats, such as single-session lectures, ongoing workshops, and off-site retreats. Programs offered with the objective of improving participant retention and adherence are usually presented free or at a minimal cost to cover expenses. Programs offered with the objective of revenue production are usually presented on a fee-for-service basis with pricing based on projected expenses and desired profit margins.

An advisory board of wellness professionals from the community can assist in identifying appropriate topics, approving content, and recommending instructors. Many community agencies and private businesses are willing to trade services for the opportunity to market products and services to the members.

Nutrition and Weight Management

Scientifically based nutrition and weight management programs are important programs for most health and fitness facilities, since many participants have specific weight loss goals. Weight management programs should be consistent with the ACSM position statement "Proper and Improper Weight Loss Programs" (4). Emphasis should be placed on education, the development of lifetime habits, and the benefits of exercise.

Nutrition programs vary in size and scope depending on facility and staff resources. A number of programming models are available for nutrition programs in health and fitness facilities. Many facilities have a registered dietitian as an independent contractor. The facility provides office space and other administrative resources and in exchange is able to offer nutritional services to participants without making a large financial investment. The registered dietitian typically charges fees for services rendered and is paid a commission on the revenue that is generated. If a registered dietitian is contracted, it is important to interview and screen this individual carefully to ensure that his or her philosophy is consistent with the philosophy of the facility and other professional staff.

There are also a number of models for weight management programs in health and fitness facilities. One popular model provides options for participants to purchase a number of related programs and services, including nutrition consultations, dietary analysis, fitness assessments, exercise prescriptions, educational lectures, grocery shopping trips, healthy cooking demonstrations, and personal fitness training sessions. Services can be offered à la carte or in structured packages. A typical package may include a 12-week program with before-and-after fitness assessments, access to the related services, and weekly group exercise training sessions. Such programs require detailed planning and coordination. Planning this kind of specialized program requires an advisory board of wellness professionals.

Other models for nutrition and weight management programs include the sale of food and nutritional supplements. These programs are popular in many fitness facilities because they have the potential to produce large amounts of revenue. It is important that a health and fitness manager fully investigate these products prior to the implementation of such a strategy. It is imperative that all product claims be accurate and that all products be safe and effective.

Group Exercise Classes

Group exercise classes can add an important dimension to health and fitness programming in a facility. Group exercise classes allow facilities to provide instruction, motivation, and guidance to participants at a relatively low cost. Most health and fitness facilities have an extensive menu of group exercise classes that include traditional aerobics classes and aerobics classes that use equipment such as steps and bikes. Other popular program offerings include resistance training, body sculpting, flexibility, sport-specific conditioning, prenatal and postnatal programs, programs for children and older adults, martial arts, yoga, and various types of dance.

Program schedules vary with the facility's resources and the number of participants. For example, small facilities may offer a limited number of the most popular group exercise classes during prime hours. A larger facility with several studios may offer a wider variety of programs concurrently. The health and fitness manager must stay current on programming trends by attending conferences, reading journals, and attending continuing education programs. Successful group exercise programs regularly survey participants to assess satisfaction levels, interest areas, and appropriateness of scheduling.

Skills required for the position of group exercise instructor are similar to those for other exercise professionals. Emphasis is placed on strong group leadership qualities. Instructors should know about health risk factors, be able to conduct appropriate screenings, and design programs that meet the needs of members. The ability to modify programs for special populations is also essential. Facilities should require group exercise instructors to hold appropriate certifications from nationally recognized organizations, such as the American College of Sports Medicine's Group Exercise Leader certification. As with the personal training staff, the health and fitness manager is responsible for being informed about various certifications and deciding which will be required or accepted by the organization.

▶ SUMMARY

The development of programs for health and fitness facilities is a complex process that demands the consideration of many factors. Program development requires needs assessment, program planning, program implementation, and program evaluation. Programming should be designed in a manner that is consistent with the specific goals and objectives of the facility and the participants. Following a systematic approach to programming is the most effective way to ensure that these goals and objectives are met.

References

1. Greenberg, J. Health and wellness: A conceptual differentiation. Health Educ 16:4–6, 1985.
2. U.S. Department of Health and Human Services. Physical activity and health: A report of the surgeon general executive summary. Washington: U.S. Government Printing Office, 1996.
3. American College of Sports Medicine. The recommended quantity and quality of exercise for developing and maintaining cardiorespiratory and muscular fitness, and flexibility in healthy adults. Med Sci Sports Exerc 30:975–991, 1998.
4. American College of Sports Medicine. Proper and Improper Weight Loss Programs. Med Sci Sports Exerc 15:ix–xiii, 1983.

Suggested Reading

American College of Sports Medicine. ACSM's Guidelines for Exercise Testing and Prescription. 6th ed. Baltimore: Lippincott Williams & Wilkins, 2000.

Gilmore GD, Campbell MD. Needs assessment strategies for health education and health promotion. 2nd ed. Madison, WI: Brown & Benchmark, 1996.

Green LW, Kreuter MW. Health promotion planning: An educational and environmental approach. Palo Alto, CA: Mayfield, 1991.

Kern D. Everyday wellness for women. Moulton, AL: Slaton, 1999.

Patton B et al. Developing and Managing Health/Fitness Facilities. Champaign, IL: Human Kinetics, 1989.

CHAPTER **73**

PERSONNEL ISSUES

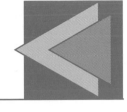

Brent Darden

The greatest asset of a successful company is its people. The collective talents of a diverse group of individuals constitute the defining characteristics of any organization. Employees who know and understand their job responsibilities and relation to the overall mission of the business can provide better performance and better services than if these matters are unclear (1). Although facilities and programs may initially draw participants, the staff dramatically influences customer satisfaction and retention. Creating a culture that maximizes human potential through effective leadership, empowerment, and accountability is of paramount importance.

HIRING

Effective hiring is critical to success, particularly in a service-oriented business. A systematic, well-organized, and positive approach to selection increases the chances of a mutually beneficial relationship between employer and employee. Time and preparation invested prior to hiring result in more satisfied employees and better-functioning organizations. In addition, the substantial direct and indirect costs associated with employee turnover can be minimized.

Developing Job Descriptions

Creating a useful job description begins with defining the responsibilities and expectations that accompany the position. A properly constructed job description helps to ensure that the best person is hired and serves as a valuable reference throughout the term of employment. Key points for developing a job description:

- Fit the job title to the job.
- Identify reporting relationships.
- Include a summary statement of the job.
- Describe essential duties and responsibilities.
- State the qualifications required.
- State the physical requirements if appropriate.
- Specify hours, shifts, and work schedule.

- Specify the role of the position within the organization.
- Assign responsibility for upholding mission statement and core values.

Recruitment

Once the job description is complete, soliciting applicants is the next step in the hiring process. It can be a challenge to find health and fitness professionals who are technically qualified and who possess excellent people skills. Although traditional methods of advertising positions (e.g., local newspapers) may provide viable candidates, networking through fitness industry contacts and seeking referrals through current employees usually produce better results. Posting the position with local colleges, professional associations, placement services, and professional trade journals may also prove useful.

Selection

A systematic comparison of applicants' qualifications and the job's requirements helps to narrow the pool of candidates for interview. A thorough evaluation of educational background, certification, experience, references, and personality is important.

Educational Background

A minimum of a bachelor's degree should be required for most positions. There are many health and fitness degrees, and although the degree title is typically based on a specialization, the differences between them are often negligible and rarely should be a determining factor when processing applications. Health and fitness professionals usually have expertise in either health promotion or exercise physiology. Health promotion specialists are generally competent in needs assessment, program planning, implementation, and evaluation in a variety of health-related areas. Exercise physiologists may be more proficient in exercise testing and prescription, fitness training, and exercise class leadership (2). Proficient exercise professionals may possess skills and/or experience in both areas.

Certification

Some type of certification has become standard for most positions. The benefits of certification obtained through a credible provider can be of great value. Acknowledgment of nationally recognized and widely accepted certification programs is prudent. Recommended standards for various positions can be found in *ACSM's Health and Fitness Facility Standards and Guidelines* (1) (Table 73.1).

Experience

Beyond the obvious advantages of previous employment in the health and fitness industry, look for related skills that may be beneficial. Customer service, sales, teaching, management, supervisory experience, and many other such skills are transferable.

Table 73.1. Organizations Offering Health and Fitness Professional Certifications

ORGANIZATION	CERTIFICATIONS
American College of Sports Medicine Box 1440 Indianapolis, IN 46206-1440 317-637-9200	Program director Exercise specialist Group exercise leader Health fitness instructor Health fitness director
American Council on Exercise P.O. Box 910449 San Diego, CA 92191-0449 800-825-3636	Aerobics instructor Personal trainer
Aerobics and Fitness Association of America 15250 Ventura Blvd. #200 Sherman Oaks, CA 91403 818-905-0040	Personal training workshops Weight training Basic aerobics instructor Advanced step aerobics instructor
Cooper Institute for Aerobics Research 12330 Preston Road Dallas, TX 75230 800-635-7050	Health promotion director Physical fitness specialist Specialty Certifications Providing dietary guidance Older adults Aquatics Special populations martial arts Indoor cycling Biomechanics of resistance training Total well being-physicians Group exercise leadership
National Strength and Conditioning Association P.O. Box 38909 Colorado Springs, CO 80937-8909 719-632-6722	Strength conditioning Personal training
YMCA of USA 101 North Wacker Drive Chicago, IL 60606 312-977-0031	Resistance exercise programming Physical fitness specialist

References

Most applicants carefully select only positive references. Nevertheless, it is important to check all references. The nature of the adjectives used to describe the candidate may provide useful insight. For example, describing someone as dependable with a strong work ethic and attention to detail is quite different from describing someone as creative, outgoing, and resourceful.

Interviewing

The interview is perhaps the most important part of the hiring process. The paramount skill for effective interviewing is listening. The 85/15 principle is a good rule of thumb: the candidate should do 85% of the talking, the interviewer 15%. Ideally, at least three or four top candidates should be interviewed in a consistent manner. Prepare in advance, set aside uninterrupted time, develop a set of questions relating to the position, and avoid rushed hiring decisions.

Multiple interview sessions should be scheduled, and the interviews should include a panel consisting of several staff members. A standard interview report facilitates objectivity. Structure the interview by asking all applicants the same questions in the same manner. Table 73.2 provides a sample of interview questions. Avoid the tendency to jump to conclusions based on first impressions. Ensure that the questions are legally permissible. Equal Employment Opportunity Commission, affirmative action, and the Americans with Disabilities Act strictly prohibit discrimination (3). Each interview session should include the following:

- Introduction: Establish rapport, tour the facility, and sell the organization.
- Explain the interview process: Include the time, length, and format.
- Interviewer questions: Ask open-ended questions.
- Candidate questions
- Closing remarks: Thank applicants for applying and let them know the next step.

Once the selection has been made, draft an offer letter that includes the following:

- Job title
- Start date
- Rate of pay (expressed in dollars per hour or amount per pay period for salaried employees)
- Acceptance deadline

Retain a signed offer letter to keep in the employee's file. Do not overstate the responsibilities or opportunities associated with the position. After a position has been

---

Table 73.2. Interview Questions

What part of your work has given you the greatest feeling of achievement and satisfaction?

What part of your work have you found the most frustrating or unsatisfying?

How do you determine which activities and responsibilities should have top priority?

Under what kinds of conditions do you do your best work?

Describe the best or worst person for whom you have worked. Why did you have this reaction?

How do you keep informed about what's happening in your profession?

What is the greatest thing that distinguishes a superior employee from someone who gives typical good performance?

Why did you choose this career?

What do you consider to be your greatest strengths and weaknesses?

What motivates you to put forth your greatest effort?

What two or three accomplishments have given you the most satisfaction? Why?

Why did you decide to seek a position with this company?

How does this job fit into your career path?

What did you like and dislike most about your previous job?

How do you think your present (past) superior would describe you?

What traits or qualities do you most admire in someone who is your immediate superior?

What is most important to you in a job?

Why did you leave your prior job or jobs? (Get full explanation)

How would you define customer service?

What qualities and characteristics do you believe are most important for this position?

What are some general tactics you might use when dealing with an upset customer?

What are your short- and long-term career goals? Why are you the best choice for this job?

---

filled, candidates who were not selected should be notified and thanked for their time and interest.

Compensation

Payroll costs are typically the highest expense associated with operating a business. A sensible and fair salary should be commensurate with the job and required skills. A comparison of salaries for similar positions outside the organization can help govern compensation decisions. Consider the following factors when making comparisons:

- Type of business (corporate, commercial, hospital, nonprofit, university)
- Type of facility (multipurpose, fitness, medical)
- Size of facility
- Location of facility (region of country, city, suburb, or rural)
- Financial status (yearly revenue generated)

Incentive-based compensation management is viable in many settings. This method is based on the philosophy that employees are motivated to perform and financially rewarded for achieving specific or measurable goals. Some form of commission structure may be applicable in many departments and at virtually all levels of staffing. Careful review of the incentive structure, with assistance from a financial expert if possible, should occur before implementation of such a system. Important points include the following:

- Incentives should be based on factors over which the individual has control.
- Use a relatively short interval for reward (e.g., monthly, quarterly).
- Use simple methods for calculating earned commissions and bonuses.
- Level of incentive should mirror level of performance.
- Reward system should encourage teamwork.

Sources of information regarding personnel issues include state employment commissions, local human resource associations, and health and fitness professional organizations.

EMPLOYEE BENEFITS

The significance of the benefits program cannot be overstated. Although most benefits are not required by law, they are generally essential to attract good employees. The extent of benefits offered by an organization is one indicator of care and concern for individuals. While fair compensation is certainly the primary concern, vacation and sick days, paid holidays, insurance, 401K plans, continuing education, and some form of recognition program are standard items in a benefits package. Some form of employee wellness program should be a prerequisite for organizations in the health and fitness industry. A quality benefits program detailed in writing will help attract and retain quality employees.

STAFF DEVELOPMENT

Investing in the development of employees is good business. It is imperative to the health and success of both the individual and the organization that staff development include training, supervision, recognition, and the potential for growth (2). The attention and energy dedicated to these objectives should be conscientious and consistent.

Staff Training

A well-thought-out training program for all employees is critical, and training should be viewed as an ongoing process, regardless of position or tenure. The groundwork for peak performance begins with the new employees' orientation. Introducing the mission statement, core values, philosophy of service, organizational structure, coworkers, responsibilities, and customers is requisite. Orientation should welcome employees and familiarize them with daily operations, responsibilities, expectations, and their role in the team environment. Introduction to various departments, services, equipment, facilities, and personnel helps establish a broad base of understanding and knowledge that facilitates delivery of service to the customer. A checklist can provide direction to the orientation process and ensure that all areas are covered (Table 73.3).

Table 73.3. New Employee Checklist

HR REPRESENTATIVE:

	Welcome gift basket		Membership information
	Offer letter (signed)		Certification courses
	Policy manual		Employee directory form
	Policy manual receipt form signed		Name tag
	D.L. & S.S. Card Copied		Notification form
	Payroll		W-4 form
	Direct deposit		I-9
	Parking policy (sticker)		Emergency contact
	Employee wellness program		Mission statement
	Informed of scheduled meetings		Core values
	Phone list		Insurance
	Employee recognition		401K
	Tour		

SUPERVISOR

	Review job description		Attended traditions training
	On the job training		CPR certification
	Review departmental policies		Business cards (if applicable)
	Phone system operations		Computer training (if applicable)
	Voice mail extension		Certifications recorded (if applicable)
	Uniform		Dept. policies & procedures
	Offer letter		Keys made (if applicable)

Date completed: _____

Supervisor's signature: _____

Employee's signature: _____

Employees should be encouraged to learn through industry periodicals, training videos, seminars, workshops, conferences, and any other avenue possible. The health and fitness industry is constantly changing with new research findings, improved training techniques, and state-of-the-art equipment, requiring that exercise professionals remain informed and up-to-date.

Supervision

Personnel leadership can be one of the most rewarding and challenging aspects of supervision. Open, effective communication is paramount during the initial phases of training and throughout the employee's tenure. Providing opportunities for exchange of information through staff meetings, group discussions, one-on-one meetings, and an open-door philosophy fosters a sense of cooperation.

LEADERSHIP

Providing guidance to employees is challenging and complex. It has been said that things can be managed, but people must be led. A wide variety of management philosophies, each having advantages and disadvantages, have been successfully demonstrated. No single theory is best in every situation. Optimally, managers should understand and incorporate sound management principles into strategies that fit their own leadership styles. People generally respond well to leaders who have a positive attitude, high expectations, and genuine confidence in them. An effective leader provides direction, channels employee efforts toward a common desired outcome, and empowers staff. A basic five-step plan for coaching people is as follows (4):

- Tell employees what you want them to do.
- Show what good performance looks like.
- Let the employees do it.
- Observe employees' performance.
- Praise progress and/or redirect efforts.

A common tenet of good management is to catch people doing something right and recognize their contribution. Companies that offer money as the sole motivation for work are destined to lose good people. Praising accomplishments provides psychological rewards critical to satisfaction in any professional setting. The manager should strive to develop win–win agreements that are mutually beneficial. Creating an environment that is result oriented and based on a standard of excellence requires attention to detail and constant awareness of opportunities for improvement. Treating staff with respect, valuing opinions, and following the golden rule will help ensure a content and well-motivated staff. It is also interesting to note that admirable characteristics most often cited in a leader are based on attitude rather than aptitude. Traits such as a positive attitude, enthusiasm, determination, and confidence are seen as most desirable (5).

GROWTH

Almost all employees are interested in the opportunity for personal and professional growth. Promotion, increased pay, expanded responsibilities, continuing education, professional affiliation, attendance at industry conferences, public speaking, and committee service are all viable options. Growth typically mirrors experience and is a result of learning and change (2). Continual growth requires a conscious and cooperative effort by the employee and supervisor or employer.

TIME MANAGEMENT

Personal time management significantly affects performance. Success often can be attributed to the ability to distinguish what is urgent from what is important. The ongoing challenge to use time wisely requires the ability to focus on goals, objectives, and priorities, both personal and organizational. There are many systems and philosophies for time management. Choose an approach that matches personal management style and evaluate merits regularly. Make a conscious choice to handle telephone calls, meetings, paperwork, unannounced visitors, and other potential time wasters efficiently. By objectively analyzing how time is spent and recognizing that time-related problems can typically be controlled, steps can be taken to improve time management skills. An excellent source on time management is *First Things First* by Stephen R. Covey (6).

PERFORMANCE REVIEWS

A performance appraisal allows the supervisor and the employee each to discuss expectations and how well those expectations are being met. Performance appraisals should not be viewed as adversarial proceedings or opportunities for socialization but rather as a forum for communication between people with a common purpose (3). Employees need to know their level of performance and cannot be expected to improve if coaching is not provided. Preparation for the performance review should focus on desired outcomes of the appraisal session. Feedback should be based on what has been seen, heard, and measured about performance. The overall objective of a productive performance review is to bridge the gap between present and ideal performance (Table 73.4).

A meaningful performance review allows the supervisor to reinforce positive behavior and correct unsatisfactory performance. Appraisals should address the future within the organization and lay the groundwork for upcoming reviews. In an appraisal discussion, four fundamental areas should be covered (7):

Table 73.4. Performance Review Tips

If a review will focus on areas needing improvement, schedule it when the employee can start taking action immediately.
Schedule meetings when both parties can give their undivided attention.
Create a formal, but unthreatening environment.
Focus the discussion on the job, not the person.
Ensure that the employee contributes to meaningful discussion.
Use open-ended questions whenever possible.
Practice active listening.
Emphasize the importance of employee's contributions.
Clearly communicate expectations.
Balance positive and negative feedback.
Encourage the employee to give feedback and express expectations.
Provide a copy of the review to employee.

- Measurement of performance against goals, expectations, and standards
- Recognition of contributions and achievements
- Identification of specific areas needing improvement
- Establishment of goals and/or expectations for the next appraisal period

MANAGING CONFLICT

Most people prefer to avoid conflict whenever possible. However, since conflicts are often inevitable, steps should be taken to learn to deal with them in the most productive manner possible. Developing a management style based on mutual achievement and win–win agreements fosters an atmosphere of cooperation. Covey's philosophy of conflict resolution begins with a win–win performance agreement that clarifies expectations by making the following five elements explicit (6):

- Desired results
- Guidelines
- Resources
- Accountability
- Consequences

By approaching conflicts with an open mind and exploring options, both parties can formulate a mutually desirable outcome. Taking a thoughtful stance with employees or customers by using questions rather than accusations helps avoid defensiveness and redirects anger into communication and understanding. Investing time and effort toward enhancing conflict resolution skills is extremely worthwhile.

TERMINATION

If repeated attempts to correct unfavorable behavior are not successful, termination may be the best option. The discharge of an employee should not come as a surprise to either party if performance evaluations have been handled conscientiously and a progressive system of discipline has been followed. A sequence of warnings and disciplinary actions designed to allow the employee to correct areas needing improvement should be documented. Graduated steps include an oral warning, written warning, probation, and ultimately termination. Termination is rarely a pleasant experience. Every effort should be made to treat the employee fairly and with respect. In a confidential and formal atmosphere, the employee should be told directly that he or she is being discharged with a concise explanation of the reasons. Although it is appropriate to listen to the employee's response and carefully answer questions, avoid arguing and leave no doubt that the decision is final. Before concluding the meeting, explain any severance considerations, including extended medical benefits. A human resource representative if available or a second member of the management team should be included in termination proceedings to assist with communicating details of the severance package and for support throughout the process. Careful review of the reasons for termination may help avoid legal action for wrongful termination by an employee. Exit interviews should be conducted with all employees to gain insight that may aid in reducing future employee turnover.

ORGANIZATIONAL STRUCTURE

The organizational structure, such as the one depicted in Figure 73.1, identifies responsibilities, reporting relationships, and the framework for accomplishing organizational objectives. Depending on the size and scope of the program, a wide variety of department director positions may be needed. Departments may include administration, marketing, programming, fitness, youth, mature market, recreation, operations, spa, group exercise, and so on.

Medical support may be provided directly by a staff medical director (rarely found outside hospital-based programs) or indirectly by a medical adviser. This physician can offer guidance, evaluate policies and procedures, and assist with special cases as required. The director of the program should work closely with the medical liaison or referring physician to ensure that appropriate protocols are followed, restrictions are adhered to, and follow-up, including documentation, is thorough. An advisory committee adds credibility and contributes expertise to a comprehensive program.

Commercial, nonprofit, corporate, hospital, clinical, church, and university-based programs, though similar in many regards, require different mixes of professional staff.

EXTERNAL SERVICES

It is often appropriate to seek outside services for assistance in delivering comprehensive programs. Consultants, subcontractors, interns, and volunteers often help

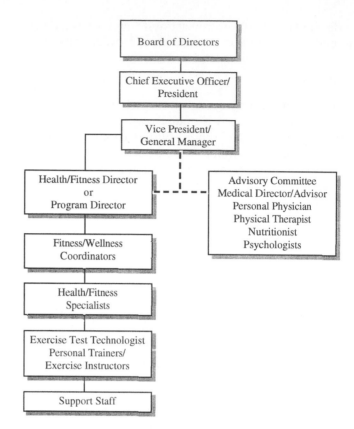

Figure 73.1. Sample organizational structure.

provide these services in a cost-effective manner. In addition to avoiding the overhead cost of having permanent staff on the payroll, external sources offer special expertise and can supply trained personnel quickly. Outside services that are frequently used:

- Medical and fitness testing
- Group exercise class instruction
- Educational seminars
- Needs assessments
- Equipment maintenance
- Housekeeping
- Computer support
- Health intervention programs

Prior to engaging an outside service, define the scope of assistance required, and afterward, monitor the quality of service provided. Volunteers frequently supply assistance with special events, fitness programs, walks or runs, tournaments, and promotions. Actively recruiting volunteers often provides a needed support network.

EMPLOYEE ASSISTANCE PROGRAMS

One mission of health promotion and wellness programs is to increase awareness of health issues. A desire to educate and motivate the public to take personal responsibility for their health lies at the core of wellness strategy. Prevention and early detection of health-related problems is a common goal of health promotion services and employee assistance programs (EAPs). While wellness initiatives invariably emphasize care for physical health, a holistic approach must include emotional and psychological health (the fundamental concern of EAPs). Speakers, counseling, and other services focusing on such topics as stress, parenting, relationships, managing change, dependency, and spirituality are frequently addressed in EAPs. Cross-promotion between these organizations is mutually beneficial, especially since many companies actively encourage employees to use EAP self-referral services on a confidential basis.

► SUMMARY

Taking steps to ensure the highest-quality staff requires a strategic approach and an ongoing commitment to develop human potential. Hiring the best person for the job is paramount and should be given great consideration. A positive, nurturing work environment is the foundation of a successful organization. Remember that as employees are treated, so employees treat the customer.

References

1. Sol N, Foster C. Organizational Structure and Professional Staffing. American College of Sports Medicine Health/Fitness Facility Standards and Guidelines. Champaign, IL: Human Kinetics, 1992.
2. Patton RW, Grantham WC, Gerson RF, et al. Staff selection and development. In: Wilmoth S, Mount C, Gilly H, eds. Developing and Managing Health/Fitness Facilities. Champaign, IL: Human Kinetics, 1989.
3. Maddux RB. Are you ready for better appraisals? In: Crisp MG, ed. Effective Performance Appraisals. 3rd ed. Menlo Park, CA: Crisp, 1993.
4. Shula D, Blanchard K. Overlearning. In: Cryderman L, ed. Everyone's A Coach. New York: Zondervan, 1995.
5. O'Dooley P. Medical Certificates. Flight Plan for Living: The Art of Self-Encouragement. New York: Master Media, 1992.
6. Covey SR, Merrill AR, Merrill RR. Empowerment from the inside out. In: Covey SR, ed. First Things First. New York: Simon & Schuster, 1994.
7. Maddux RB. How to prepare for more effective appraisals. In: Crisp MG, ed. Effective Performance Appraisals. 3rd ed. Menlo Park, CA: Crisp, 1993.

Suggested Reading

Blanchard K, Bowles S. Gung Ho!: Turn on the People in Any Organization. New York: William Morrow & Co., 1997.

Blanchard K, Shula D. Everyone's a Coach. Grand Rapids, MI: Zondervan Publishing House, 1996.

Freiberg K, Freiberg J, Peters T. Nuts!: Southwest Airlines' Crazy Recipe for Business and Personal Success. New York: Bantam, 1988.

2.10.0.1

3.10.2, 3.10.2.1, 3.10.2.2,
3.10.2.3, 3.10.2.4,
3.10.2.5, 3.10.2.6,
3.10.2.7, 3.10.2.8

5.10.0, 5.10.10

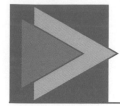

CHAPTER **74**

FINANCIAL CONSIDERATIONS

Frank Ancharski

The financial considerations of any organization, whether for-profit or not-for-profit, in a university or community setting, corporation or private health club, is often the driving force behind major decisions. Fitness professionals too often view the bottom line as a necessary evil for which someone else is responsible. The exercise professional is often preoccupied with the work of fitness and may have little understanding and appreciation for the contribution of dues or programming fees to revenue. A corporate fitness director may favor public relations and staff morale rather than annual capital improvements. Certainly, the public perception of an organization and the satisfaction of employees in the work environment are vital to the success of an organization. However, the importance of sound financial decision making by the fitness professional cannot be underestimated. This chapter concerns the need to embrace and understand basic fiduciary issues rather than allowing accountants, business managers, and corporate higher-ups to be solely responsible.

BASIC TERMS AND PRINCIPLES

Financial management in the health and fitness field is essentially no different from that of any major corporation. The most notable difference is the responsibility a publicly held corporation may have to stockholders. Few companies in the health and fitness industry have such an obligation. Recently, however, firms such as Bally's Total Fitness and Sports Club Company of Los Angeles have made initial public offerings (IPO) with limited success (1). The industry is relatively young and other firms are likely to follow.

Typically, an ACSM-certified health and fitness director or program director is employed by a private or public entity with no publicly held stock. If the parent company trades on the market, the health facility only remotely affects the performance of the company in the stockholders' eyes. Some include corporate fitness facilities (e.g., Johnson & Johnson, Ford Motor Company). University recreation centers, not-for-profit hospital programs, and com-

mercial health clubs are not usually concerned with stockholder obligations. In either case, the following basic terms of finance apply (2).

Real Assets

Tangible assets are such things as furniture, fixtures, equipment (FF&E), and buildings. Intangible assets such as technical expertise, trademarks, and patents are considered real assets.

Financial Assets

Sometimes referred to as securities, financial assets are likely to be shares of stock, cash, accounts receivable, bonds, bank loans, and lease obligations.

Value

Whether an organization is deciding to build a facility, finance capital improvements, or provide working capital, it should begin by valuing the investment, that is, determining the return on investment (ROI). Unless the ROI is very near or better than what an investor can get in the market, obtaining private or bank financing is difficult. An investor generally decides on a balance between risk and reward. A high ROI with limited risk and/or investment is generally preferred. ROI is determined by dividing the average annual cash flow over the life of the project by the initial investment outlay. ROI is sometimes referred to as ROA (return on assets) (3).

For example, if the average annual cash flow is $80,000 (over 5 years, $50,000, $60,000, $70,000, $100,000, $120,000) and the initial investment is $400,000, the ROI is $80,000 ÷ $400,000 = 20%. An average ROI of 15–20% is considered excellent.

Net Profit or Loss

Net profit or loss is calculated using information for costs (variable and fixed) and revenue as illustrated thus:

- Operating profit equals revenue minus variable costs (costs that may change).
- Net profit equals operating profit minus fixed costs

(costs that remain the same) when revenues exceed variable costs and fixed costs.

- Net loss occurs when variable costs and fixed costs exceed revenues.

Capital

Capital is money available for new equipment and facility improvements. When capital is invested in a lump sum, it is considered a fixed cost and is debt to an investor, who may use an ROI valuation to determine whether the return is worth the investment. A facility may consider borrowing or leasing equipment if available capital is insufficient to buy it. In either case, both a lease payment and a bank loan debt are usually reflected in fixed costs.

Working Capital

Working capital is defined as current assets minus current liabilities. Equity, or owner's equity, is not included when determining working capital. On a balance sheet, total assets must equal total liabilities (4). Current assets, including cash in the bank and accounts receivable, make up a portion of total assets (Table 74.1). Accounts receivable are assets that have been earned for a performed service or delivered product, but have not been received. Current liabilities, such as accounts payable, taxes, salaries, and wages are considered a part of total liabilities. Accounts payable are liabilities payable to a party who has performed a service or has delivered a product to a recipient of those services or products.

Working capital is a primary concern early in a project because of the possibility of a net loss (variable costs and fixed costs exceeding revenue). Working capital must be obtained through investors, donations, personal savings, or bank loans to finance a net loss until revenues exceed variable and fixed expenses. Unlike capital, which is used for real assets such as FF&E, working capital can take the form of cash or accounts receivable and can be used to finance operating costs.

Break-Even

In many settings such as a not-for-profit, hospital, corporate, or university, a break-even point analysis is reserved for evaluating wellness (e.g., weight loss or smoking cessation) or usage incentive programs (e.g., "rowing the Colorado River" using a rowing machine or "climbing Mount Everest" using a stair climber). When valuing a facility, break-even point occurs when revenue is equal to expenses. As illustrated in Figure 74.1, the break-even point for a program or facility occurs when revenue and expenses are equal or when revenue exceeds expenses. In Figure 74.1, break-even occurs in year 2. This also coincides with the point at which working capital is no longer necessary and a net profit results. A net surplus is a synonym for net profit in not-for-profit facilities.

Time and Opportunity

The principle of time and opportunity is analogous to spending more than income allows in the short term. An opportunity with obvious long-term benefit may arise when short-term financing is unavailable. Sometimes when such an opportunity arises, it pays over the long term to undertake the expenses even in the absence of sufficient revenue to cover them. A director must face the inevitable fact that windows of opportunity can be small, and moving forward on a program or a project is important to the overall mission and goals of an institution.

People

The principles of finance include people, because real assets and financial assets alone do not constitute a suc-

Table 74.1. **Sample Balance Sheet**

Assets	Liabilities
Short-term	Short-term
Cash	Accounts payable
Marketable securities	Short-term debt (notes payable)
Accounts receivable	Accruals (taxes due, salaries, wages)
Inventory	
Long-term	Long-term
FF&E, plant	Debt
Less: Depreciation	Preferred stock
Net, FF&E, plant	Equity (owner's equity)
	Stock
	Retained earnings
Total Assets	**Total Liabilities**

FF&E furniture, fixtures, and equipment.

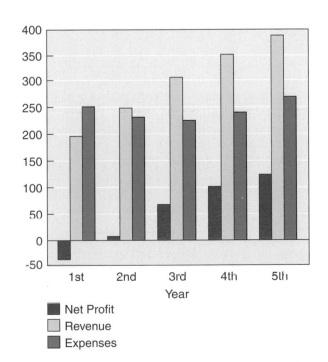

Figure 74.1. Sample break-even profitability graph.

cessful facility. Assets, though tangible, are not brought to life without cooperation, teamwork, and support of people who must carry out the business. While there is a fiduciary responsibility to understand and manage the financial aspects of a business, the director must not lose sight of the people-driven dynamics of business.

Business Organization

There are various types of business organizations. The influence of taxes and personal risk weigh heavily in the process of deciding which type should be used. The main types are listed in the following sections.

Sole Proprietorship

The name defines the sole proprietorship: a single person owns the business. This is the simplest, least expensive form of business to start. Often, only a license or registration is required to begin operation. Few government regulations apply, and earnings are subject to personal income tax. A major disadvantage is the difficulty in obtaining significant capital to start or expand such a business. Also, the personal liability for debt is extensive.

Partnership

A partnership can be either an informal agreement or a formal written document filed with the state government. Partnerships have limited governmental constraints, and the partners are personally taxed in proportion to their share of ownership. This form of business can consolidate the skills and resources of each partner, but transfer of ownership or the death of a partner can cause problems. Partnership does carry financial liability, including exposure to risk of loss of personal assets if other partners cannot meet obligations.

Corporation

The corporation is a formal establishment and is heavily influenced by laws, regulations, and stockholders, who are free from debt liabilities. The charter and bylaws govern the operations of a corporation. The risk to owners is limited, and a wide variety of investors may be attracted to the business. Transfer of ownership is easier than with either a partnership or a sole proprietorship. The corporation is a legal entity that is completely separate from managers and owners. Changes in management and ownership do not affect the charter or bylaws.

Subchapter S Corporation

The subchapter S corporation, or S corporation, is a hybrid of a partnership and corporation. At times, a small business with grand growth plans begins as an S corporation. This entity combines the advantages of the sole proprietorship, the partnership, and the corporation without the accompanying disadvantages. There is limited risk and exposure of personal assets, and partners cannot be taxed twice on salary and business income. A partner is free to distribute dividends, avoiding the complexities of a partnership.

BUDGET DEVELOPMENT AND FORECASTING

Budgets are necessary to forecast financial expectations and goals, provide accountability, track progress of actual versus projected results, and allow for justification and scrutiny. Completing an accurate, reliable budget without a computer is virtually impossible.

Capital Budget

The difference between a capital budget and an operational budget is in the purpose. A capital budget is developed to plan for FF&E and cosmetic improvements generally for 1 year, but multiyear projections may be made. Exercise equipment, renovations, and expansion plans are addressed in this type of budget. Major changes planned for a facility are detailed in the capital budget and should be carefully monitored and implemented. Costs should be tracked, time lines adhered to, and final audits and evaluation made. Competitive bids should be procured to obtain favorable prices.

Depreciation

The costs of capital expenditures are depreciated or amortized over the useful life of the equipment or by the amount permitted using generally accepted accounting principles, a formal set of rules established by the accounting profession. The depreciation cost is often found on the financial statements under fixed expenses. The director should encourage owners and investors to regularly reinvest a portion of profits (often 1–5% of gross revenues) to maintain the facility.

Operating Budget

An operating budget is a plan detailing goals for expected revenues and expenses to operate a facility. Operating costs are the costs of doing business. Ideally, in most if not all settings, revenues for participant use (e.g., membership fees and ancillary income, wellness programs, pro shops, personal training) should exceed projected expenses. Start-up facilities and not-for-profit facilities may be the exception. Expenses are usually broken into two categories, operating and fixed. See Table 74.2 for a sample budget. A reliable litmus test against industry norms would be to compare the budget against key ratios (Table 74.3).

Assumptions for the Budget

A critical portion of the budget is development of assumptions, and one major assumption is that expenses increase continually. In this attachment to the budget, an item-by-item (e.g., enrollment fees, payroll increases, cost of uniforms) explanation with supporting calculations is critical. Table 74.4 shows an example of assumptions that correspond to line items on the budget.

Table 74.2. Sample Budget

ACSM FITNESS CENTER							
	EXISTING CLIENTS	MONTHLY	NEW	AVG FEE	CANCELS	TOTAL CLIENTS	TOTAL REVENUE
ENROLLMENT PROJECTIONS							
Jan	700	$ 45	50	$ 150	0	750	$ 39,000
Feb	750	$ 45	75	$ 150	22	803	$ 44,010
Mar	803	$ 45	75	$ 150	25	853	$ 46,260
Apr	853	$ 45	65	$ 150	25	893	$ 47,010
May	893	$ 45	55	$ 150	27	921	$ 47,220
June	921	$ 45	50	$ 150	28	943	$ 47,685
July	943	$ 45	50	$ 150	28	965	$ 48,675
Aug	965	$ 45	50	$ 150	29	986	$ 49,620
Sept	986	$ 45	60	$ 150	29	1017	$ 52,065
Oct	1017	$ 45	65	$ 150	31	1051	$ 54,120
Nov	1051	$ 45	70	$ 150	31	1090	$ 56,400
Dec	1090	$ 45	50	$ 150	33	1107	$ 55,065
TOTAL MEMBERSHIP REVENUE:							**$ 587,130**

OTHER REVENUE

Smoking cessation	$ 1,200
Massage	$ 16,200
Guest Fees	$ 35,000
1–1 Training	$ 32,400
Weight management	$ 12,000
Pro-shop	$ 1,200
Rest	$ 3,000
Welness programs	$ 1,200
Misc.	$ 10,000
TOTAL OTHER REVENUE	**$ 112,200**
MEMBERSHIP REVENUE	$ 587,130
TOTAL REVENUE	**$ 699,330**

PAYROLL PROJECTIONS

General Manager	$ 35,000
Sales 1	$ 35,000
Administrator	$ 20,000
Fitness Director	$ 26,000
FT Fitness 1	$ 22,000
FT Fitness 2	$ 20,000
PT Fitness	$ 21,840
Receptionist	$ 25,000
Aerobics	$ 18,000
Nutrition	$ 9,500
Cleaning	$ 24,000
Bonus	$ 8,000
TOTAL PAYROLL	**$ 264,340**
TAXES	$ 34,364
BENEFITS	$ 18,240
TOTAL SALARIES	**$ 316,944**

TOTAL OPERATING EXPENSES

Salary, Tax & Benefits		$ 316,944
Marketing		$ 48,000
Maintenance/Repair		
HVAC	$ 1,500	
Equipment	$ 2,400	
Exterminate	$ 1,200	
Other	$ 500	
TOTAL MAINTENANCE		$ 5,600
Operating Supplies		
Cleaning	$ 1,200	
Locker Rm	$ 3,000	
Other	$ 1,500	
Towels	$ 2,000	
TOTAL SUPPLIES		$ 7,700
Utilities		
Electric	$ 36,000	
Gas	$ 4,800	
Water	$ 2,000	
TOTAL UTILITIES		$ 42,800
Rent		$ 70,705
Other Expenses		
Printing	$ 3,600	
Postage	$ 3,000	
Travel	$ 2,000	
Uniforms	$ 6,000	
Programs	$ 500	
Office Supp.	$ 600	
Telephone	$ 7,200	
Misc	$ 1,000	
TOTAL OTHER EXPENSES		$ 23,900
Corporate Expenses		
Amort/Dep	$ 24,000	
Debt		
Insurance		
Leasing		
Mgmt Fees		
TOTAL CORPORATE		$ 108,400
TOTAL EXPENSES		**$ 624,049**
NET PROFIT/(LOSS)		**$ 75,281**

Table 74.3. Key Ratios, 1997–1998

Revenue growth (annual)	9.6%
Payroll (% of gross revenue)	42.0%
Retention (annual)	69.0%
Net membership growth (annual)	8.4%
Revenue/member ($)	$871.00
Sq. ft./member	23
Revenue/sq. ft. ($)	$45.00
Revenue not from dues	27.0%

Adapted with permission from Profiles of Success: Industry Data Survey. Boston, 2000.

Though perhaps initially tedious, the process is worth the effort. (During budgetary approval, all parties privileged to the justification of the numbers make better decisions.) This process is useful for preparing the budget, explanation of variances throughout the year, and planning for the next year.

Development, evaluation, revision, and approval of a budget are usually lengthy processes, and adequate time must be allotted. If the fiscal year matches the calendar year, September through November is an acceptable timetable for the budget process, allowing for all levels of approval. Prior to each budget meeting, the director should gather general ledgers (line item explanation of paid invoices), current financial statements, and assumption pages for current year and projected year (5).

Including department supervisors, administrators, and key personnel in the budget development process helps employees buy into the expectations, and well-informed employees contribute to success. Each supervisor who participated in the process should be given a final copy of the operating budget. Monthly financial statements should be distributed to supervisors to compare actual numbers to budget. A monthly action plan is established to remain on budget, make adjustments for the coming month, and adjust for any revenue shortfall or extra expense.

FINANCIAL INDUSTRY TRENDS

The fitness industry has many organizations that monitor and support financial performance. The International Health Racquet Sports Association (IHRSA) is well recognized by commercial for-profit facilities. They perform and provide analysis of industry trends to clubs. Some of the more significant trends noted in 1998 (6):

- Some 12% of the population exercises in facilities.
- There are 15,372 clubs.
- California, Texas, New York, Florida, and Pennsylvania have the most participants.
- California, Colorado, Minnesota, Nevada. and Virginia have the highest rates of participation.
- The most popular class forms of exercise are aerobics, dance, cardiopulmonary and kickboxing classes, yoga,

Table 74.4. Assumptions for Budget Preparation

LINE ITEM	ASSUMPTIONS
Revenue	
New enrollment fees	Each new member pays 50% of current months dues plus one full month and an average enrollment fee of $75 each.
Guest fees	Project 10 members/day paying $10/visit 7 days/week for 52 weeks.
Expenses	
Payroll: reception	4 part-time employees, each working 20 hours for $6.00/hr for 52 wk. Each will receive a 5% raise in June.
Uniforms	10 new full uniforms at $50/uniform (jacket, pants, shorts, shirt) three times/year. Staff pays via payroll deduction for seconds.
Insurance	Increased $100/month compared to last year at $1,500/month.

and studio or group cycling. Other popular activities are the pump, t'ai chi, and Pilates (posture, isolation, lengthen, alignment, torso stabilization, energize, and strengthen).

- The most popular special needs programs are physical therapy, cardiac rehabilitation, arthritis, and diabetes programs.
- The most popular "other services" are massage, social programs, day spa, and full-service restaurant.
- The largest age group, 53% of those exercising in facilities in 1987, was 35–54. By 1998 that figure was reduced to 36%, nearly equal to the over-55 group.
- Some 35% of the industry comes from the senior market (55+) as compared to 30% in 1987.
- Some 27% of revenue comes from programming not covered by dues.
- The most profitable clubs have low attrition rates and high-revenue-generating participants.
- Average attrition rate is 31%.
- Payroll is 42% of gross revenue.
- Net growth in membership from 1996–1998 was 23%.
- Revenue per member per year is $871.
- Revenue per square foot is $45, a 7% 3-year growth trend.

Expense Model

In the 9-year period 1980–1989, the industry expense model changed. The following model (Table 74.5) is determined by using line item expense as a percentage of total gross revenue (e.g., gross revenues = $100,000; payroll = $40,000. Payroll is 40% of gross revenues).

The former model, a 60/40 ratio of operations to fixed expense, has slowly evolved. The model noted in 1998 according to IHRSA's 1999 Industry Data Survey, Profiles of Success, is a 66/34 model. Profits have risen to account for 11.6% of the total fixed amount. This model clearly represents the challenge to maintain conservative profit

Table 74.5. Expense Model

	1980			1989	
	RANGE (%)	AVG. (%)		RANGE (%)	AVG. (%)
Operating expenses					
Payroll	24–26	25.0		33–37	35.0
Utilities	7–9	8.0		7–9	8.0
Repairs & maint.	6–8	7.0		5–7	6.0
Marketing	4–6	5.0		4–8	6.0
Admin. equip. & supplies	2–4	3.0		2–3	2.5
Club equip. supply	2–4	3.0		2–3	2.5
Legal, accounting	2–4	3.0		1–3	2.0
Cost of goods[a]	5–7	6.0	Insurance[a]	2–4	3.0
Total operating expense	51–69	60.0		56–74	65.0
Fixed expenses					
Debt service[b]	14–16	15.0		14–16	15.0
Depreciation[c]	8–10	9.0	Reserve, replace[c]	4–6	5.0
Real estate taxes[b]	2–4	3.0		2–3	2.5
Insurance[b]	2–4	3.0		2–3	2.5
Profit (Loss)	8–12	10.0		8–12	10.0
Total fixed expense	34–46	40.0		30–40	35.0

1998 industry benchmarks & key ratios: Total operated department expense + Total undistributed operating expense = 66%. Earnings before interest taxes depreciation amortization + earnings before income taxes = 34%.
[a] Referred to pro shop, restaurant and massage, personal trainers, seminar, lessons performed by independent contractors. These items deleted in 1989 to compare equally.
[b] Occupancy cost is used in place of debt service, real estate taxes, and insurance for leasehold facilities.
[c] Reserve for replacement replaces depreciation as genuine fixed cash expense. (7)
Reprinted with permission from McCarthy J. Fund allocation has become critical. Club Business International 1990.

margins (10–11.6%). Profit is considered a fixed expense because the model is a zero sum model. However, it is clear from Figure 74.1 (break-even chart) that net profit is not always fixed. The primary factor in the change to the expense model is usually payroll (wages and benefits). Because of the litigious society in the United States, the cost of insurance also contributes to the challenge of producing a profit.

Taxes

A noteworthy trend is the attention the Internal Revenue Service (IRS) is paying to tax-exempt organizations. Fitness facilities may be organized as either taxable or tax-exempt (7). The primary advantage a tax-exempt entity enjoys is simply in tax savings, which are often significant and carry a competitive advantage over commercial facilities. However, certain restrictions are placed on tax-exempt organizations, including continuing proof of benefit to the community. In addition, they should provide services that cannot be found in for-profit settings within the community. Furthermore, organizations labeled as 501C(3) must restrict activity for ancillary income (8).

FINANCIAL STATEMENTS AND EXPENSE MANAGEMENT

Analysis of financial statements should be conducted monthly, with written variance reports and action for the coming month. Assumption pages and general ledgers can be used to explain variances and to generate action points. Information should be shared with supervisors who help prepare budgets and are accountable for line items within specific departments. The financial statement should include a comparison of actual revenues and expenses versus budgeted amounts for both current year to date and previous year.

Comparisons of actual financial results to budget should be used as a guide for evaluating performance. Most directors do not carry forward excess profit or earmark net profit. Such discipline ensures that profits are not used for future expenses. Each month should be evaluated separately and profit reserved for times when profit may be minimal (e.g., summer or year's end) or when year-to-date profit may be depleted.

Financial statements reflect both revenue- and expense-related problems. Over time, reducing expenses to offset revenue shortfalls becomes a serious problem of diminishing returns. Continual expense cutting affects service, customer satisfaction, retention, and ultimately, revenue.

When faced with such a challenge, the sense of urgency to generate revenue cannot be overstated. Often, enrollment or membership revenue accounts for 80% or more of total income (9). This is an area where much of the manager's time and effort should be concentrated. If marketing efforts are not planned properly or the results tracked diligently, effectiveness cannot be determined. The critical precursor to membership revenue is marketing (outflow). Planning for marketing programs (e.g., direct mail, newspaper ads, health fairs) and enhancing sales skills through training are paramount to correcting a revenue shortfall. Other revenue sources can be enhanced by creating profit centers, such as Pilates or t'ai chi classes, ballroom or line dancing, spa services, scuba lessons, or group trips, such as sporting or theater events, to fill revenue gaps (10).

Allocation of operating costs may be dictated by industry norms, historical information, and management style. These variable costs usually rise each year. Control of such costs can be ensured by methods such as using a budget bank. Similar to home budgeting and checkbook balancing techniques, this is an example of a budget bank:

Income − recurring or fixed expenses = operating or variable expense

where income is projected revenue from budget; recurring expenses include mortgage, utilities, depreciation, payroll, and so on; operating expenses include marketing, uniforms, seminars, training, printing, telephone, office, pool and laundry supplies, and so on.

The amount left for operating or variable expenses should be treated as the remaining expenses for a given period. Each check is deducted from the previous balance. When the budget bank balance reaches zero, all ordering ceases until the next budget month. This process repeats monthly. The key benefit of using this type of process is to manage expenses when incurred (at the point of ordering), not when invoices arrive or after financial statements are produced. This is a prospective tool to manage expenses, whereas financial statements are a retrospective tool. If used correctly and carefully, the budget bank should never bounce.

There are many other ways to manage expenses, all of which require a director to understand the details of financial statements. A thorough understanding of general ledgers, assumption pages, and operational cost issues improves fiscal fitness. The following are some techniques used by industry professionals to diagnose problems and confront expense management are listed (9–12).

Services

- Review heating, ventilation, air conditioning, accountant, pool, attorney, and equipment contracts semiannually.
- Tabulate class attendance weekly. Cut low-attendance classes.
- Track use of day care and courts.
- Keep track of exercise equipment, laundry, and other equipment parts in an on-site inventory.
- Employee money savers: use staff to recruit interns from colleges; offer incentives to staff to recommend employees and recruit at job fairs.

Supplies

- Restrict use of copier and mail meter or use coded keypad access.
- Lock storage areas for office supplies, pro shop goods, and uniforms, and limit key distribution.
- Bid 1–3 vendors for major purchases or supplies.
- Stick to a budget bank and record when order is placed, not when invoice is received.
- Use a purchase order system with organized procedures and approval processes.
- Check unit costs regularly. Watch for abrupt increases with regular vendors. Ask for price lists semiannually.

Fixed Costs

- Confirm property taxes with local assessment board. Be willing to ask tax authorities for a reassessment.
- Ask utility suppliers to audit use and recommend changes and improvements.
- Shop insurance costs yearly.

Advertising and Marketing

- Purchase graphic software and hire and train staff for in-house newsletter production and promotion.
- Comarket with restaurants, schools, and community or national events (e.g., smoking cessation class that coincides with the Great American Smokeout).
- Use independent market feasibility analysis to determine site of facility. Superior services, equipment, facilities, and staff cannot overcome a poor location (12).
- Purchase demographic report on target market.
- Investigate vendors whose service can be accessed through the Internet.

Hidden Expenses

- Block access to directory information and shop all long distance *and* local carriers.
- Look for carriers who bill on the lowest incremental time, and audit number of phone lines in use.
- Check postal rates for options on presort, zip code +4, and bar codes.
- Shop credit card fees.
- Negotiate bank charges.
- Use brokers to shop for disability insurance.
- Contest unemployment claims. Not doing so shows precedent to existing staff, and rate increases with each successful claim.
- Change job classification categories (laundry attendant to housekeeping personnel) and add as many as possible to lower worker compensation insurance.

FACTORS AFFECTING DECISIONS

Not every decision can or should be made in a purely financial fashion, using only budgetary or financial data. Haste in decision making leads to some of the biggest mistakes. The day-to-day process of dealing with multiple situations, being consumed by multiple priorities, and having days filled with endless interruptions lends credence to the axiom that haste makes waste.

Lack of planning contributes to poor decisions. Little time dedicated to thinking about planning precipitates disregard for planning. With the tasks required of a director including budgeting, financial statement review, program evaluation, staff allocation, market analysis, and community development (to name a few), planning cannot be successfully performed without quiet planning time.

There follow two examples of how this quiet time might be used to make important decisions concerning operations that contain financial consideration but for which finances may not be the determining factor.

- **Decision 1:** Staff positions can be examined for level of contribution and whether hiring or layoff is necessary. Examine performance reviews and scheduling grids to ensure maximum staffing levels. Hire fewer people and expect more from them. Higher pay may be possible to help retain key personnel. Brainstorming such as this can generate ideas that may lead to solutions.
- **Decision 2:** The marketing department may project from competitive market analysis that bicycle spinning classes would create a competitive advantage and attract new members. If the number of new enrollments due to spinning classes exceeds the cost of the bikes, instructors, and other equipment within a short time, the decision is clear. The major variable is the confidence in enrollment projections. However, the capital budget may be reduced by 10%, forcing close scrutiny of spinning over, for example, replacing a chlorinating system for the pool. Space may be at a premium, so a program, though financially beneficial, may not be possible. Formal planned evaluations of programs are necessary to justify the time and money being used. Attendance, cost of materials, and revenue generated should be considered during evaluation of a program.

Another kink in this spin scenario is that current members may prefer another use for the space. If staff is not in tune with existing and prospective members' needs, the addition of such classes may be a mistake. Also, if retention improves because existing members' needs are met or exceeded by adding space for stretching weight bars, resistance balls, or spinning classes, this additional revenue may be made available for other capital items.

The constant barrage of decisions for a facility is no small job. It can be an adventure to seek feedback of superiors, subordinates, and members. Once all such input is digested, a director sometimes uses instinct to make the right decision.

Consider obligations to the community. Hospitals,

universities, and health clubs are giving back to the community and educating the public. If the fitness industry is to be a torchbearer for exercise and health, proactive involvement with local charities or business chambers must occur.

▶ SUMMARY

The competition among and between profit and not-for-profit organizations and hospitals, recreation, and university fitness centers is increasing. Each entity is under scrutiny from constituents. Shareholders, taxpayers (in some cases), and investors in commercial facilities all demand justification for dollars spent. The pressure to justify costs and enhance financial performance is shared by all directors, despite location.

It is no longer sufficient to be the best fitness person on the floor, to influence morale and productivity of an organization, or to decrease absenteeism and health care costs of participants. The bottom line knows no bias when it comes to facilities and organizations. Success may depend on open mind, basic financial knowledge, and fear that a poor bottom line may be exorcised. Financial considerations have become as important as influencing behavior to increase exercise habit. The more this is accepted, the better all facets of the organization can be coordinated and directed toward success.

References

1. Caro R, King D, Davis N. Developing an Exit Strategy. San Diego, CA: International Health Racquet Sports Association National Convention, 1996.
2. Healy RA, Myers SC. Principles of Corporate Finance. New York: McGraw-Hill, 1988.
3. Weston JF, Copeland TE. Managerial Finance. New York: CBS College, 1986.
4. Lowery AJ. How To Become Financially Successful By Owning Your Own Business: A Step-by-Step Guide To Independence and Profits. New York: Simon & Schuster, 1981.
5. Krieger G. The Budget Process: "The Right Stuff." San Diego, CA: International Health Racquet Sports Association National Convention, 1996.
6. Profiles of Success: Industry Data Survey: IRHSA. Boston, 2000.
7. McCarthy J. Fund allocation has become critical. Club Bus Int 1990.
8. Coopers & Lybrand. Tax Implications of Hospital Owned Fitness Facilities: IRHSA. Boston, 1996.
9. Handley A. Setting up new profit centers. Club Indus January 1995.
10. Sattler TP, Doniek CA. Trim the extra fat from your facility. Fitness Manage April 1996.
11. Morris BA. Cost Control Tactics For The 90's. Club Indus April 1995.
12. Caro R. Attacking hidden expenses. Parts I–IV. Club Insider June 1994, July 1994, October 1995. (Cioletti J. Stay on target. Club Industry Feb 2:27–32, 1999.)

2.6.0.4, 2.7.3   3.7.3, 3.10.4.6   5.7.1

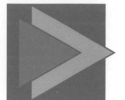

CHAPTER **75**

LEGAL CONSIDERATIONS

David L. Herbert and William G. Herbert

Legal considerations constitute an important dimension of service for those administering fitness evaluations and exercise tests, engaging in physical activity counseling and exercise prescription, or providing fitness programs for apparently healthy adults or individuals with stable chronic diseases. One area of paramount concern to exercise leaders, fitness instructors, rehabilitation specialists, and program administrators is the professional–client relationship and activities performed within the confines of that relationship. Other considerations with special significance in law include the physical setting and areas in which program activities are conducted, the specific purpose for which exercise services are performed, the equipment used, and the techniques employed with the exerciser.

The law influences exercise professionals in each of these domains and in others. Furthermore, expectations are substantially affected by the exercise environment—recreational, commercial, or clinical—and by the type of clientele being served. Regardless of the situation, sensitivity to issues of law and rigorous application of risk management principles may enhance the quality of service and client satisfaction. Moreover, practicing with a risk management perspective may reduce service-related injuries, the likelihood of personal injury litigation, and the extent of damage to the provider in the event of claim and lawsuit.

Laws affecting these matters vary considerably from state to state. Nonetheless, certain legal principles have broad application to pre-exercise screening, exercise testing, prescription, and activity supervision. All exercise program personnel should know these principles, endeavor to develop practices aimed at reducing risks of negligence litigation, and maintain safe care of clients.

In carefully screened and supervised adult populations, the risks of serious cardiovascular accidents in exercise programs are very low. Even for those with some signs of disease who undergo clinical tests, the cardiovascular complication rate is about 2/10,000, and for selected cardiac patients following moderate-intensity exer-

cise the rate is less than 1/35,000 (1, 2). Recent survey findings indicate that facility readiness and staff practice for serious adverse events in the health and fitness industry is abysmal, despite the fact that more and more such facilities accept older clients and those with controlled chronic diseases (3). More than 75% of these facilities reported that they had summoned emergency medical services at least once in 5 years. This suggests a high potential for personal injury lawsuit (3). Until the 1990s, only a fraction of personal injury cases resulted in claims against exercise professionals. In recent years, however, there has been a definite increase in exercise-related claims processed through the legal system, especially claims against health and fitness facilities (4, 5). Although tort reform proposals may help stem this trend, the future portends an ever-increasing risk of claim and suit for health care professionals generally; exercise professionals are not likely to escape the problem.

TERMINOLOGY AND CONCEPTS

Generally, claims against exercise professionals center on alleged violations of either contract or tort law. These two broad concepts, along with written and statutory laws, define and govern most legal relationships between individuals, including activities of exercise professionals with clients.

Contract Law

The law of contracts defines undertakings that may be specified among individuals. A contract is simply a promise or performance bargained for and given in exchange for another promise or performance, all of which is supported by adequate consideration (i.e., something of value).

In examining exercise testing and prescription activities, the law of contracts affects the relationship between exercise professionals and clients. The client may receive physical fitness information and recommendations on exercise training. Likewise, the professional may perform exercise testing in exchange for payment, or some other consideration of value. This contract relationship also encompasses any related activities that occur before and after exercise testing, such as health screening prior to testing, exercise prescription, and first aid and basic emergency care that arises from exercises temporally associated with on-site provider services. If expectations during this relationship are not fulfilled, lawsuit for breach of contract may be instituted. Such potential suits allege nonfulfillment of certain promises or a breach of alleged warranties that the law sometimes imposes on many contractual relationships. Apart from the professional–client relationships, contract law also has implications for interprofessional relations, such as those with equipment companies, independent service contractors, and employees.

Informed Consent

Aside from breach of contract claims arising from a lack of promise fulfillment, claims against exercise professionals can be based upon a type of breach of contract for failure to obtain adequate informed consent from exercise participants. Although claims based on lack of informed consent, founded upon contract principles, are somewhat archaic, suits based upon such failures are still put forth in some jurisdictions. More frequently today, however, such claims are brought forth in connection with negligence actions rather than breach of contract suits. Before an exercise professional subjects a client to a specific exercise procedure both properly and lawfully, the client must give informed consent to the procedure. Informed consent is intended to ensure that the client entered into the procedure with full knowledge of the material, relevant risks, any alternative procedures that might satisfy certain of the objectives, and the benefits associated with that activity. This consent can be express (written) or implied by law simply as a function of how the two parties to the procedure conducted themselves. To give valid consent to a procedure, the person must be of age, not be mentally incapacitated, know and fully understand the importance and relevance of the material risks and benefits, and give consent voluntarily and not under any mistake of fact or duress (6). Written consent is certainly preferable to any oral or implied form of consent; it expressly demonstrates the process, should questions arise later as to whether that was the case.

In many states, adequate information must be provided to ensure that the participant knows and understands the risks and circumstances associated with the procedure before informed consent can be given. In such states, a so-called subjective test is used to determine whether that person understood and comprehended the risks and procedures associated with the matter at hand. Other states have adopted a less rigid rule and provide an objective test to determine consent to a procedure or

treatment. Under this test, the determination centers on whether the participant, as a reasonable and ordinary person, understood the facts and circumstances associated with the procedure so as to give voluntary consent. Although some states do not require the use of informed consent for nonsurgical procedures or when a test is performed for health care–related purposes, adherence to the process is a desired approach. Examples of informed consent documents for exercise testing and training programs are available elsewhere (6–9).

In suits arising from the informed consent process, an injured party commonly claims that a professional was negligent in the explanation of the procedure, including the risks, and that the participant would not, but for the negligence of the professional, have undergone the procedure. These cases are often decided upon the testimony of expert witnesses who determine whether the professional engaged in substandard conduct in securing the informed consent. These cases can involve claims related to contract law, warranties, negligence, and malpractice. Suits arising from alleged deficiencies in the informed consent process related to testing, exercise prescription, or physical activity have become more commonplace. The law is moving toward a broadening requirement for disclosure of risk to participants. Some courts have even gone so far as to require the disclosure of all possible risks, as opposed to those that are simply material (10). Such a requirement imposes unusual burdens on programs and raises substantial medicolegal concern (11). These concerns require individual analysis and response.

One element of the informed consent process relates to confidentiality and disclosure of personal and sensitive information that may be gathered from the client in the course of evaluating health status or delivering services. Provision should be made in the informed consent or other documentation to secure the written authorization to disclose specific test results, exercise progress reports, and so on, to health care professionals who have a need to know, such as a primary care physician. Written authorization may also be secured from clients if there is an intent to use data in reporting group statistics for program evaluation or research purposes, even when such information is only to be presented in ways not identifiable with the client. Many states and the federal government have promulgated privacy statutes that may affect the release of personally identifiable material regarding a program participant. The application of these laws to a program and rights to release information will depend on a variety of factors that only a local counsel can properly address.

Tort Law

A tort is simply a civil wrong. Most tort claims affecting exercise professionals are based on allegations of negligence or malpractice causing personal injury or death.

Negligence

Although negligence has no precise definition in law, it is regarded as failure to conform one's conduct to a generally accepted standard or duty. A legal cause of action based on claims of negligence may be established given proof of certain facts, specifically that one person failed to provide due care to protect another to whom the former owed some duty or responsibility and that such failure proximately caused some injury to the latter person (6). Thus, the validity of negligence claims is typically established through a specific process that examines certain facts and establishes whether:

- A defendant owed a particular duty or had specific responsibilities to some person who has issued a claim of negligence
- One or more failures (breaches) occurred in the performance of that duty, as compared to a particular set of behaviors that were expected (due care, standard of care)
- The injury or damage in question was attributable to the established performance failure or failures; that is, they were the proximate cause of the injury or damage

When negligence claims arise, whether an exercise professional provided due care is critically important. Once a duty is established, the nature and scope of expected performance are usually determined by reference to published standards and guidelines from peer professional associations. Standards of care are discussed in a different section of this chapter. Ultimately, the most effective shield against claims of negligence may be the daily pattern of adhering to and documenting compliance with the most rigorous published guidelines that are relevant.

Malpractice

Malpractice is a specific type of negligence action involving claims against defined professionals. Malpractice actions generally involve claims against professionals who have public authority to practice (arising from specific state statutes) for alleged breaches of professional duties and responsibilities toward patients or other persons to whom they owed a particular standard of care or duty (6). Historically, malpractice claims have been confined to actions against physicians and lawyers. By statute or case law, however, some states have expanded this group to include nurses, physical therapists, dentists, psychologists, and other health professionals. In 1995, Louisiana became the first state to pass legislation to license and regulate exercise practitioners who work under the authority of physicians with patients in cardiopulmonary rehabilitation treatment programs (12, 13). The Louisiana State Board of Medical Examiners now provides regulatory management for this practitioner group. As yet, no published reports have addressed the effect of this relatively new public regulation on cardiac rehabilitation professionals in Louisiana. The more obvious possibilities of effect include level of autonomy in practice, changes in provisions of liability insurance, costs of such insurance, and exposure to claims of malpractice.

DEFENSES TO NEGLIGENCE OR MALPRACTICE ACTIONS

Properly given informed consent can sometimes be used as defense against claims based on either tort or contract principles. In such cases, defense counsel may seek to characterize consent as an assumption of risks by the plaintiff. Assumption of risks of the procedure, however, is often difficult to establish without an explicit written statement or clear conduct that demonstrates such an assumption. In addition, an assumption of risks never relieves the exercise professional of the duty to perform in a competent and professional manner. Even where a valid informed consent with assumption of risks obtained, a spouse, children, and/or heirs can sometimes independently file suits against the exercise professional for loss of consortium-type claims, even when the participant could not have asserted these claims because of his or her own assumption of risks (14).

In some jurisdictions, it may be advisable or even necessary to obtain consent from a participant, a spouse, and perhaps, in a limited number of states, to make it binding on any children or the executor, administrators, and heirs to an estate. Certainly such consents should be binding on estates if certain of these negligence and malpractice claims from those quarters are to be successfully avoided (15, 16).

Informed consent often is confused with so-called releases. Releases are statements sometimes written into consent-type documents that contain exculpatory language, that is, wording that professes to relieve the provider of any legal responsibility in the event of an injury or death due to any error or omission or even negligence. These releases, sometimes called prospective waivers of responsibility, in some states may be disfavored. Moreover, in a medical setting the use of such releases, with certain limited exceptions, has been declared invalid and against public policy. In nonmedical settings, however, particularly with certain ultra-hazardous activities, such as auto racing, sky diving, and certain exercise-related activities, the use of such releases may be valid in some jurisdictions and certain circumstances, if properly drafted and used. In fact, when well defined and properly written, such documents may have substantial benefit to programs. In recent years, there has been a definite trend toward increased use of waivers in health and fitness and recreational exercise settings to reduce providers' exposure to damage and loss arising from negligence actions. Improperly developed waivers can fail to protect providers. Consequently, a qualified attorney with a license in the jurisdiction of application should be consulted to determine their applicability and to prepare these documents.

Several other defenses to claims of negligence or malpractice are available. In some states, for example, proof of negligence by the participant, referred to in law as contributory negligence, can preclude any recovery of damages from a defendant. In many states, however, this rule has been modified by adoption of a so-called system of comparative negligence. Under this rule, negligence of the injured party is compared with negligence of all defendants in the case. Then, if the negligence of the injured party is found to be less than that of all defendants in the case, or in some states in any defendant in the case, the plaintiff is allowed to recover, although in an amount reduced by the contribution of negligence by the injured party (6).

Liability insurance is an effective mechanism to protect against financial loss in the event of claim and suit. Such insurance policies pay for defense of any covered claims and suits and provide indemnification from any judgment or settlement that is not excluded from the terms of coverage—up to the limits of said coverage.

STANDARDS OF PRACTICE

Standards of practice (or care) express how contemporary services should be delivered to give reasonable assurance that desired outcomes will be achieved in a safe manner. In most professions, such standards are developed and periodically revised by consensus among professionals or national associations of providers. Standards documents address what are considered to be benchmark methods, procedures, processes, and so on, that are applied in almost all settings regardless of location, resources, or training of the provider.

In reality, the national standard of practice at any time typically is influenced by a variety of sources, including published statements from professional associations, government policies, state and national government regulations, and so on. In recent years, the promulgation of standards for fitness and health care has increased dramatically. This circumstance mandates that professionals stay abreast of new pronouncements and regulations. Without knowledge of the most relevant and current standards and incorporation of those tenets into the operating protocols and records of service fulfillment, the individual practitioner becomes vulnerable to damage and loss in the event of legal challenges arising from personal injury lawsuits.

The reason for this derives from the critical role of standards of care in the legal arena. Consider that in law, proof of negligence consequent to injury of a client (plaintiff) often depends on whether it can be established that there was a clear causal connection between the injury to the client and what the professional did (commission) or failed to do (omission). To establish what should or should not have been done in a given case, the court relies heavily upon interpretations from these standards. The use of these standards in certain cases dealing with exercise testing and exercise leadership has already occurred (4).

Several organizations have published documents that influence the standard of care in the health and fitness and exercise rehabilitation fields. Some of the most important are those of the American College of Sports Medicine (ACSM), the American Heart Association (AHA), American Association of Cardiovascular and Pulmonary Rehabilitation (AACVPR), the Agency for Health Care Policy and Research, the American College of Cardiology, the American Medical Association, the International Health Racquet & Sportsclub Association, and the Aerobics and Fitness Association of America (7–9, 17–25). Documents from these organizations vary in scope and applicability. Professionals should carefully examine services, uses of technologies and procedures, and clientele before deciding which standards and guidelines are most applicable.

Published guidelines may be incomplete or not entirely uniform. In the event of injury or death of a participant, such deficits may create confusion rather than define the professional behavior expected in a specific setting. In the area of exercise testing, standards of the ACSM, AACVPR, and AHA are inconsistent with regard to the need for significant involvement of a physician during graded exercise testing (7–9, 17–19).

On the matter of exercise prescription, one AHA publication explicitly identifies the nurse as an individual who may "assess physical activity habits, prescribe exercise, and monitor responses in healthy persons and cardiac patients" (17). Another contemporary AHA source acknowledges that exercise by cardiac patients may be appropriately supervised by physicians, nurses, or exercise physiologists, as long as supervisors are trained and their duties are consistent with state statutes governing the practice of medicine and certain other allied health care professions (18). If deficiencies or disparities in the published guidelines have implications for safety and legal exposure in a particular situation, the development of low-risk protocols and procedures may be a matter of critical importance that requires advice of local counsel.

Health care professions are in the midst of a movement that will eventually see written standards and guidelines covering nearly every major dimension of care. Fitness and rehabilitation professionals are in similar circumstances and must keep up to date with consensus publications that affect services. To reduce medicolegal risks, it is prudent to adopt the most stringent standards possible. Fulfillment is equally important: practitioners should not only update program operating manuals to verify adoption of current standards but also document day-to-day client records of service delivery to show what was done and how it was done.

In fact, documentation is vital to many aspects of risk management, not just verification of adherence to standards. Documentation should include contemporaneous recording of critical response levels that arise in exercise testing or training (e.g., important symptoms, estimations of effort, and activity demand, along with signs suggesting myocardial ischemia or poor ventricular response) and annotations about how these are referred to appropriate health care providers in a timely way. It also encompasses notations on program incidents, especially care delivered in emergencies (perhaps the most important setting in which to demonstrate after the fact what and when essential steps were performed). Follow-up should always be performed and program records maintained to verify the outcome of the situation whenever emergency and nonemergency incidents occur.

Very recently, the AHA and ACSM released a joint position statement recommending certain basic policies and procedures for pre-exercise screening and emergency readiness in all health and fitness facilities, even in hotels offering only unsupervised access (20). Every health club and recreational fitness center should evaluate the key features of its organization and clientele, finding how best to structure written policies, procedures, and fulfillment relative to these important safety functions so as to adhere to this new recommendation (20). From a risk management point of view the adequacy of any policy or procedure is a function of its being committed to written form, kept up to date relative to changing professional guidelines, and linked to ongoing evidence of fulfillment. With regard to emergency readiness, fulfillment may be partially shown by keeping dated records of regular emergency drills. Another dimension of documenting fulfillment may be achieved by maintaining records that show names of staff members who practiced in emergency drills and notations on staff performance and any improvements made in the emergency drills. These formal drills prepare staff for rapid and effective response when a genuine emergency arises. If a legal challenge should ever occur, this record of fulfillment may be quite helpful in establishing that a particular standard was adopted and routinely followed.

Forms also may be developed for staff to use routinely in ensuring standardization in areas in which injury and/or legal risks are considered significant. Examples of these situations include forms for pre-exercise screening and consultation, instruction of new clients in exercise routines, specific cautions for avoidance of injury to the client, and staff inspection of equipment and facilities. Effective forms demonstrate how a facility has linked an important standard to a critical area of service. Use of such forms along with routine annotation of client records shows consistency of fulfillment.

UNAUTHORIZED PRACTICE OF MEDICINE AND ALLIED HEALTH PROFESSIONAL STATUTES

In recent years, the growing prominence of exercise testing and other health and fitness services increasingly places exercise professionals in collaborative roles with licensed health care providers. This evolution has stimulated a variety of initiatives to clarify roles and responsibilities, promote professionalism, and increase professional opportunities. Competency credentials of the ACSM (e.g., ACSM Exercise Specialist®, ACSM Program Director[SM], ACSM Group Exercise Leader[SM], ACSM Health/Fitness Instructor[SM], ACSM Health/Fitness Director®, and ACSM Registered Clinical Exercise Physiologist[SM]), the AACVPR core competency position statement for cardiac rehabilitation specialists, and efforts to establish licensure are illustrations of initiatives that affect positioning of specialists and/or greater role delineation (13, 21).

Providing exercise services with some degree of independence in collaboration with licensed providers can create legally precarious circumstances for the exercise professional. A prime example of confusion in this area is reflected in questions that often arise about the competency and legal authority needed to provide emergency cardiac care in community or clinic-based settings for exercising cardiac patients. The emergency response standard in this situation is clear and universal. It calls for a defibrillator, crash cart with artificial airways, suction pump, emergency drugs, and so on, and competency of an on-site provider who can administer advanced cardiac life support skills of the AHA when needed (7, 9, 19). The provider of emergency services, however, must understand that he or she cannot assume such duties unless the physician in charge has given written standing orders to that effect and the individual has legal authorization under state statutes to accept such standing orders. This is almost never the case for the unlicensed exercise professional, with or without current successful training in an ACLS program of the AHA. Very recent advances in technology and new state and federal statutes are changing public expectations regarding use of automated external defibrillation. This evolution may soon alter the standard of care for emergency service in the health and fitness setting, at least for larger clubs that specifically define their clientele to include members who have known cardiovascular disease, but who are classified as being at low risk for exercise-related adverse events.

The continuing evolution of health care reform further confuses the roles of health care providers. This often may be problematic for the exercise professional working in diagnostic exercise laboratories or rehabilitation centers. A significant part of this evolution has been aimed at reducing costs by using paraprofessionals in increasingly important treatment roles. In fact, various states have undertaken efforts to expand nursing practice and other medical practice laws beyond mere observation, reporting, and recording of the patient's signs and symptoms. Various physician assistant and similar paraprofessional laws allow expanded treatment authority to nonphysicians.

Until health care reform is complete, however, some nonphysicians engage in certain practices that might be characterized as the practice of medicine or some other statutorily defined and controlled allied health profession. In such situations the unlicensed provider runs the risk of engaging in unauthorized practices that could lead to both criminal and civil sanctions. Many states have defined the practice of medicine broadly so that persons engaged in exercise testing and prescription activities could under some circumstances fall within the ambits of such statutes.

As previously indicated in this chapter, published standards are not always definitive in expressing roles and responsibilities for exercise professionals, particularly with regard to services for clients with documented diseases or even those with no outward signs of disease (e.g., silent myocardial ischemia). Thus, without the presence or assistance of a licensed physician or other allied health professional for certain aspects of these exercise services, claims as to the unauthorized practice of medicine could be put forth. Under some of these state statutes, such practices are often classified as crimes, usually misdemeanors, punishable by imprisonment for less than 1 year and/or a fine.

In addition, a person found to have engaged in the unauthorized practice of medicine or some other allied health profession faces (after the fact) the legal expectation to provide an elevated standard of care in the event of injury or death of a participant. Under this rule, the actions of an exercise professional are compared to an assumed standard of care of a physician or other allied health professional acting under the same or similar circumstances. In the event that the actions do not meet this standard (which the nonphysician or allied health professional cannot meet because of inadequacies of knowledge, skill, authorization, and experience), liability may result.

► SUMMARY

As more and more participants are exposed to organized exercise programs, the actual number of untoward events, avoidable or otherwise, will inevitably rise. Increased numbers of these occurrences will result in negligence claims that will ultimately find resolution in court. The probabilities of such traumatic actions are low, particularly for individuals and organizations that operate programs in a manner commensurate with accepted professional standards. Awareness of the areas of special legal vulnerability and adoption of legally sensitive practices, however, will keep the risks of litigation low and lead to safer and more efficacious programs. Professionals are advised to keep current concerning developments in this ever-changing medicolegal field (6).

References

1. Rochmis P, Blackburn H. Exercise tests: A survey of procedures, safety and litigation experience in approximately 170,000 tests. JAMA 217:1061, 1971.
2. Haskell WL. Cardiovascular complications of outpatient cardiac rehabilitation programs. JAMA 57:920, 1978.
3. McInnis KJ, Hayakawa S, Balady GJ. Cardiovascular screening and emergency procedures at health clubs and fitness centers. Am J Cardiol 80:380, 1997.
4. *Mathis v. New York Health Club, Inc.*, 690 N.Y.S.2d 433, 1999.
5. *Mandel v. Canyon Ranch, Inc., et al.* Superior Court of the State of Arizona, Puma County, Case No.3122777, 1998.
6. Herbert DL, Herbert WG. Legal Aspects of Preventive and Rehabilitative Exercise Programs. 3rd ed. Canton, OH: Professional Reports Corporation, 1993.
7. American College of Sports Medicine. ACSM's Guidelines for Exercise Testing and Prescription. 6th ed. Philadelphia: Lippincott Williams & Wilkins, 2000.
8. American College of Sports Medicine. ACSM's Health/Fitness Facility Standards & Guidelines. 2nd ed. Champaign, IL: Human Kinetics, 1997.
9. American Association for Cardiovascular and Pulmonary Rehabilitation. Guidelines for Cardiac Rehabilitation and Secondary Prevention Programs. 3rd ed. Champaign, IL: Human Kinetics, 1998.
10. *Hedgecorth v. United States.* 618 F. Supp.627 (E.D. Mo, 1985).
11. Herbert DL. Informed Consent Documents for Stress Testing to Comport With *Hedgecorth v. United States.* Exerc Stand Malpract Rep 1:81, 1987.
12. Louisiana licenses clinical exercise physiologists! Exerc Stand Malpract Rep 9:56 (editorial) 1995. (Reproduction of the licensing act included.)
13. Herbert WG. Licensure of clinical exercise physiologists: Impressions concerning the new law in Louisiana. Exerc Stand Malpract Rep 9:65, 1995.
14. Child sues for "loss of consortium." Lawyers Alert 3:249, 1984.
15. Herbert WG, Herbert DL. Exercise testing in adults: Legal and procedural considerations for the physical educator and exercise professionals. JOHPER 46:17, 1975.
16. Koeberle BE. Legal Aspects of Personal Fitness Training. Canton, OH: Professional Reports, 1990:35–38.
17. American Heart Association. The AHA medical/scientific statement on exercise. Circulation 86:340, 1992.
18. American Heart Association. The AHA medical/scientific statement on cardiac rehabilitation programs. Circulation 90:1602, 1994.
19. American Heart Association. Guidelines for cardiopulmonary resuscitation and emergency cardiac care. JAMA 268:2171, 1992.
20. Balady GJ, Chaitman B, Driscoll D, et al. American College of Sports Medicine and American Heart Association joint position statement: Recommendations for cardiovascular screening, staffing, and emergency policies at health/fitness facilities. Circulation 97:2283, 1998.
21. American Association for Cardiovascular and Pulmonary Rehabilitation. Core competencies for cardiac rehabilitation specialists. J Cardiopulm Rehabil 14:87, 1994.

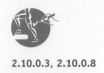

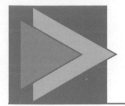

CHAPTER **76**

OPERATIONS

Victoria McGrath and Nestor Fernandez II

Managing the operations of a health and fitness facility requires a thorough understanding of the financial statements, daily operations, and customer service. A detailed operational plan that identifies key areas and potential problems is necessary in operating a well-managed facility. This chapter describes areas that require attention to manage a facility well.

FINANCIAL STATEMENTS
Market Analysis

A detailed operational plan must be built on a current market analysis. An annual market analysis can be provided by an outside marketing consultant or simply by the club, which provides the research information. Key elements for a market analysis:

- Demographic breakdown
- Analysis of competitors
- Primary market analysis: consumer survey
- Secondary market analysis: referral sources
- Demand projections
- Financial considerations
- Recommendations

A market analysis may also include member surveys, comment cards, and focus group information.

Budgets

The annual operating budget is based on the information obtained in the market analysis. This information provides the baseline data to build the budget from the ground up. It should not be assumed that prior year trends or financial statements determine the annual operating budget. Health and fitness organizations traditionally begin with determining sales goals. The sales goals are set by determining the number of members joining over the course of a year multiplied by all associated membership fees. This total is broken down into monthly, quarterly, and annual sales goals.

Income accounts for most health clubs include membership fees, locker revenues, guest fees, lesson fees, pro shop income, café income, and special program fees. Expense accounts include payroll, utilities, maintenance, supplies, outside services, marketing, and advertising. A separate budget addresses capital expenditures. Most successful club operations spend 4–7% of revenue on capital improvements. Capital improvements should include 1-year, 3-year, and 5 year plans and concentrate on the long-term goals of the organization.

DAILY OPERATIONS
Manager On Duty Procedures

The use of a manager on duty (MOD) system provides a consistently high level of service during all operating hours. The MOD system is composed of specific senior staff with proven leadership skills to support and execute service strategies and standards. This is accomplished by providing a constant level of communication, visibility, and responsibility. The MOD should be in communication with all areas of the club by means of a two-way radio or paging system. The MOD should also be trained in CPR and first aid and all areas of operations. These include the following:

- Knowledge of all departmental daily operations
- Emergency procedures
- Computer systems: point of purchase, member check-in, alarm
- Schedule of events and programs

The MOD may be required to respond to an accident or incident in the club. The appropriate procedures must be followed for the safety of the members and employees alike. A detailed report must be completed and kept on file for legal purposes.

Emergency Procedures

Most states require that employees undergo job-specific safety training. Prudent safety training includes proper operation of equipment and training in lifting and back health. Consult with local government offices and/or business insurance carriers to determine specific state and local requirements.

Detailed facility evacuation plans should be developed, communicated, and reviewed with staff quarterly. An evacuation plan covers all necessary steps to evacuate the facility, emphasizing safety of members and staff. All required information (e.g., phone numbers, contact names) should be maintained in a central location (usually the front desk) for easy, quick access. Regular review and update of the information and procedures and ongoing staff training ensure a safe environment for members and staff.

Opening and Closing Procedures

Clients' expectations require that businesses be accessible during scheduled hours of operation. The appropriate management staff, preferably a MOD, should staff the opening and closing shifts. A checklist completed by the opening MOD prepares the facility for use prior to admitting clients into the facility. It identifies basic safety issues (e.g., lighting, equipment, alarms, and all prepresentation preparation, starting computer systems, daily signage, cash register count, restocking supplies, and cleanliness). A walk-through of the entire facility before presentation is required to ensure that the building, equipment, and common areas are visually presentable and ready for use.

In the event that problems keep the facility from opening, a backup plan should be in place. The opening MOD should have access to telephone and pager numbers of staff who can open in an emergency.

Closing checklist procedures are similar to those for opening, except that special attention is placed on securing the facility (Fig. 76.1). All points of entry, including windows, elevators, and maintenance doors, should be secure. All electrical equipment, including computers, televisions, and stereos, should be turned off. The closing MOD should be the last person to leave the building. He or she has final responsibility for securing the facility, engaging alarms, and locking up.

The opening MOD should review the closing checklist from the prior evening for problems or areas of concern before opening. Once the facility is open for business and adequately staffed for operations, a supervisor or department head should review the opening and closing checklists. Problem areas should be reviewed and corrected. All corrective actions should be communicated to the reporting employees.

FACILITY MANAGEMENT
Operating Procedures

Procedures establish guidelines to address operational demands. Their main purpose is to establish guidelines for safety, cleanliness, member satisfaction, and employee support. Procedures should be thorough, clearly defined, easily performed and tracked, communicated to employees at all levels and departments, and regularly reviewed to evaluate effectiveness. Most procedures should be invisible to the customer, and rather than presenting obstacles, they should ensure delivery of outstanding customer service.

Quality Control

The highest standard of cleanliness and safety and a visually appealing environment are the responsibility of every employee. These standards are met by developing a systematic approach that will maintain the property and prevent any problems. This highly organized system includes daily, weekly, monthly, quarterly, and annual checklists developed for specific areas of operations. The head housekeeper, operations director, department manager, or general manager (depending on distribution of responsibility and size of the facility) reviews all checklists.

The facility should be inspected quarterly to evaluate every component. All areas of presentation and safety, both interior and exterior, should be reviewed. Checklists should cover a variety of components, including the following:

- Wall repairs
- Paint condition
- Cleanliness of heating, ventilation, and air conditioning (HVAC) systems
- Carpeting, rubber floors
- Light fixtures
- Condition and cleanliness of fitness equipment

Inspections may take place daily for general housekeeping and presentation and monthly for larger projects, such as patching and painting of walls, equipment replacement, lighting, and ventilation (Fig. 76.2). Regardless of frequency, the goal is to ensure that responsible staff are examining all aspects of the facility with a discriminating eye, seeing potential problems, and observing each component of the facility from a customer's point of view.

Many facilities schedule annual club shutdowns, when the facility is closed for deep cleaning. In addition, large projects that may be difficult to accomplish while members are present and facilities are in use can be completed. Projects commonly completed during these closures:

- Court resurfacing
- Area renovations
- Extensive painting
- Swimming pool resurfacing or cleaning
- HVAC and plumbing repairs

_____Announce the Club will be closing 1 hour before the Club closes and repeat every 15-minutes.

_____Clean Sports Desk area.

_____Stock supplies for the next day: In and Out Sheet, Guest Registration, office supplies, etc...

_____Log-in remaining Lost & Found items.

_____Check out all remaining members and guests.

_____Count cash register, make "X" report, "Z" report, and prepare drop bag.

_____Turn off the computer.

_____Lock main doors.

_____Close handicap entrance doors.

_____Lock women's locker room entrance. Turn off all lights in the women's locker room.

_____Check aerobics studio doors and lights.

_____Turn off basketball court, free weight, and pool hallway lights.

_____Lock pool door.

_____Lock double doors in cardio room.

_____Turn off all lights in men's locker room.

_____Turn off all lights on third and second floors, making sure that marketing office door is locked.

_____Put the safe drop bag in the safe and punch out.

_____Turn off the lights in Sports Desk area, making sure that Child Care and Pro Shop doors are locked.

_____Return Allen wrench to lock box, and lock the lock box.

_____Set the alarm.

_____Exit through main doors and push doors in securely at the bottom.

_____Drive home safely.

ALL AREAS OF THE BUILDING MUST BE CHECKED FOR CLEANLINESS AND/OR MAINTENANCE ISSUES.
PLEASE INDICATE ANYTHING THAT NEEDS IMMEDIATE ATTENTION BELOW:

Figure 76.1. Sample closing checklist.

DATE:

STATUS

CARDIO ROOM

Carpet	
Ceiling Tiles	
Air Vents	
Mirrors	
Mats	
Baseboards	
Walls - patching	
Walls - paint	
Trash Cans	
Water Fountain	
Equipment - cleanliness	
Equipment - repair	
Televisions	
Newspaper Racks	

FITNESS TESTING OFFICE

Carpet	
Ceiling Tiles	
Air Vents	
Baseboards	
Walls - patching	
Walls - paint	
Trash Cans	
Telephone	
Office Furniture	

FITNESS OFFICE

Carpet	
Ceiling Tiles	
Air Vents	
Baseboards	
Walls - patching	
Walls - paint	
Trash Cans	
Telephone	
Office Furniture	

POOL HALLWAY

Carpet	
Ceiling Tiles	
Air Vents	
Baseboards	
Walls - patching	
Walls - paint	
Handicap Ramp	
Pool Doors	
Women's Locker Room Door	
Men's Locker Room Door	

SWIMMING POOL

Perimeter Landscaping	
Flower Pots	
Pool Deck	
Pool Deck Matting	
Running Track	
Pool Furniture - repair	
Pool Furniture - cleanliness	
Aquatics Equipment	
Shower	
Walls - patching	
Walls - paint	
Rear Gates	

Figure 76.2. Club walk-through.

FREE WEIGHT ROOM

Carpet	
Ceiling Tiles	
Air Vents	
Baseboards	
Walls - patching	
Walls - paint	
Mirrors	

RACQUETBALL COURTS

Floors	
Walls	
Air Vents	
Lighting	

BASKETBALL COURTS

Floors	
Walls	
Air Vents	
Lighting	
Score board	
Basketball nets, rims and backboard	
Emergency exit door	

CHILD CARE ROOM

Carpet	
Ceiling Tiles	
Air Vents	
Vinyl floor	
Bathroom	
Baseboards	
Walls - patching	
Walls - paint	
Sink	
Equipment - cleanliness	

SPORTS DESK/LOBBY

Floors	
Ceiling Tiles	
Air Vents	
Countertops	
Baseboards	
Walls - patching	
Walls - paint	
Telephones	
Lighting	
Stairs	
Handicap hallway	
Porter Room	

WOMEN'S LOCKER ROOM

Carpet	
Ceiling Tiles	
Air Vents	
Mirrors	
Mats	
Baseboards	
Walls - patching	
Walls - paint	
Trash Cans	
Water Fountain	
Cardio equipment - cleanliness	
Cardio equipment - repair	
Television	
Restroom stalls	
Toilets	
Restroom dispensers	

Figure 76.2. *Continued.*

Lighting	
Vanity dispensers	
Telephones	
Bulletin boards	
Signage	
Tanning room - supplies	
Tanning room - equipment	
Tanning room - walls	
Tanning room - floors	
Jacuzzi	
Cold dip	
Showers - tile	
Showers - dispensers	
Showers - lighting	
Showers - air vents	
Showers - partitions	
Shower heads	

MEN'S LOCKER ROOM

Carpet	
Ceiling Tiles	
Air Vents	
Mirrors	
Mats	
Baseboards	
Walls - patching	
Walls - paint	
Trash Cans	
Water Fountain	
Cardio equipment - cleanliness	
Cardio equipment - repair	
Television	
Restroom stalls	
Toilets	
Restroom dispensers	
Lighting	
Vanity dispensers	
Telephones	
Bulletin boards	
Signage	
Tanning room - supplies	
Tanning room - equipment	
Tanning room - walls	
Tanning room - floors	
Jacuzzi	
Cold dip	
Showers - tile	
Showers - dispensers	
Showers - lighting	
Showers - air vents	
Showers - partitions	
Shower heads	

ACTION ITEMS:

Figure 76.2. *Continued.*

Because the facility is closed to normal operations, these projects can be completed without disturbing clients. In the long run this contributes to maintaining the quality of the facility.

PLANNING

Facilities should establish an annual plan to determine staffing requirements and scheduling for special programs and events. Staffing requirements address several factors:

- Seasonal requirements
- Vacation scheduling
- Dates when all staff are expected to be available
- Annual facility closing for comprehensive maintenance and cleaning

Developing an annual programming calendar prepares for extraordinary demands on facility and staff and prevents scheduling conflicts.

Seasonal Usage

The annual operational plan complements the annual budget. Forecasting demands on staff and facility resources creates a clear picture of the costs associated with each. Planning for seasonal help is important for clubs with summer programs, outdoor pools, catering operations, and other specialty departments or programs.

Seasonal help must be hired and trained in advance. Advertising and recruiting staff with specific skills that are in demand during peak seasons should be anticipated prior to the beginning of the season. Although these staff may be temporary, regular orientation (similar to that for permanent employees) is important. Performance standards should be similar to those for other employees to ensure seamless service delivery.

Facilities that have extraordinary use during peak seasons should prepare by developing a preventive maintenance checklist to address needs specific to that season. Repairs and maintenance should be completed prior to the peak period so that service is not interrupted. Commonly replaced parts and components should be stocked in anticipation of repair or maintenance necessitated by high use.

Scheduling

An annual operations plan not only accounts for additional staff, but also schedules to meet the needs of peak use. Careful tracking of traffic through the facility and anticipation of planned programs and events helps organize scheduling. Scheduling vacations and block-out times is important to efficient operation. An operations calendar outlines events and programs that may require full or additional staffing. This allows staff to request vacation time around block-out times.

CUSTOMER SERVICE

Every business must determine the level of service that customers expect—and must exceed it. A business that delivers consistently good service outperforms the competition and satisfies the customers. Facilities should evaluate customers' expectations and the facility's ability to deliver those services, then organize operations to support delivery of services up to those standards. Standards, determined from customer feedback, are the blueprint for the training, implementation, and continuous revision of a service delivery system. More detailed discussions of program planning and marketing can be found in Chapters 72 and 80.

Identify Member Expectations

Customer expectations drive the facility, programs, planning, and budget. An organization must seek and facilitate input from membership. Annual questionnaires and focus groups covering every component of the facility, including cleanliness, staff responsiveness, customer service, program offerings, and facility improvements, can produce useful information, which must be carefully reviewed to form an overall picture representing customers' expectations. Reporting results to the customers is important.

Focus groups can be organized around specific programs or areas of the facility. Focus groups can and should be composed of staff as well as customers. Once members' expectations are identified, they must be integrated into training and communication of service standards (Table 76.1).

Customer Service

Payment of monthly membership dues indicates that members are satisfied with the service they received the previous month. Because members speak with their feet, if they are happy they will stay, but if they are not satisfied, they will go elsewhere. This is why it is so important

Table 76.1. Service Standard

We provide all that enter with a sense of home. The club is a place where people feel safe, secure, comfortable, and sheltered from the stresses of the outside world.

- Remember to be an amiable host at the club and encourage the staff to do the same (e.g., smile, have eye contact, say hello, good morning).
- Stay agreeable, friendly, and helpful even when being confronted.
- Coach the staff in maintaining a friendly, calm, helpful attitude.
- Encourage and coach the staff to treat the member as their personal guest at all times.
- Coach and assist the staff in solving members' problems in a swift and friendly manner.
- Take the initiative and authority to do whatever you think is appropriate to satisfy members' needs.
- Encourage and coach the staff to empathize with the members' plight or situation at all times.

to provide world-class service from the moment the members walk through the door.

The customer service model begins and ends with the member service desk, the hub of club operations. This is the customers' first and last impression of the club. Because they are the first and last to touch the members, the member service staff must be trained to provide the highest level of customer service. The member service staff must have a complete working knowledge of club procedures and operating systems.

The service delivery system should be specific and detailed, yet flexible enough to allow employees to solve unexpected problems. Policies and procedures should guide employees' actions. However, employees should be

I. Review of last week's meeting:

II. Program/Operational Concerns:

- • • •
- • • •
- • • •

III. Current Week's "To Do List"

	TASK	COMPLETION DATE	STATUS	COMMENTS
1	_____	( )	( )	
2	_____	( )	( )	
3	_____	( )	( )	
4	_____	( )	( )	
5	_____	( )	( )	
6	_____	( )	( )	
7	_____	( )	( )	
8	_____	( )	( )	
9	_____	( )	( )	
10	_____	( )	( )	

IV. Schedule: week beginning:_____

MONDAY	_____
TUESDAY	_____
WEDNESDAY	_____
THURSDAY	_____
FRIDAY	_____
SATURDAY	_____
SUNDAY	_____

**MUST BE RECEIVED BY THE GENERAL MANAGER BY 10:00 AM
EVERY MONDAY.**

Figure 76.3. Weekly objectives.

empowered to make decisions in keeping with the spirit of the service standards. In addition, senior staff must convey a sense of leadership that not only reviews and enforces service standards but also models them through behavior and action.

World-class customer service comes from responding to the needs of the members in a timely fashion. Nothing frustrates a member more than no response from management to the suggestion card they took the time to complete. It is important to respond to all suggestion cards within 24 hours or less. All member calls should be responded to the same day. The most important point is to respond to the members in a timely fashion.

CLUB MANAGEMENT SYSTEMS

To organize the member service desk and all operating systems of the club, many companies offer comprehensive club management systems designed to satisfy all levels of club services. These services include member service desk check-in with photo verification, automated reservations (accessed by touch screen kiosks, personal PCs, or in-club Internet-powered cardiovascular equipment), guest maintenance, locker management, e-mail servers, fitness tracking systems, billing, and point of sale. These total club operating systems take advantage of a wired communication system between the members' PCs, in-club Internet-driven equipment, and club-based kiosks. These ports allow members to check in, pay fees, schedule appointments, and check fitness levels. These systems are the future of club operations, because they provide unlimited integration of service, hence convenience and communication between all club systems.

COMMUNICATION

Continued maintenance of a well-managed facility requires ongoing communication of operational demands between all departments and staff. Management must facilitate information sharing from all sources as procedures are performed, member expectations are identified, and operational plans are executed. This information can be used to develop the best action plans for continued growth and development.

Daily communication focused on issues and items in the day-to-day operation requires attention. These are typically reported from opening and closing checklists, inspection reports, and/or MOD reports. The problems should be resolved quickly. Operational concerns should also be addressed during weekly managers' meetings or regular department heads' or supervisors' meetings. Each department head should have a clear understanding of the operational condition of his or her area and its influence on customer satisfaction (Fig. 76.3). Changes and improvements in operations can be communicated through regularly scheduled clubwide staff meetings to ensure that all staff receive important information. Continual clear communication between all levels of the organization helps to maintain a high level of customer satisfaction and employee morale. Ultimately, this can contribute to a good bottom line.

▶ **SUMMARY**

Operation of a facility includes all aspects important to daily and continuous management of the facility. Procedures and checklists for operating all aspects of the facility are critical to efficient and effective management. Customer service is crucial to the success of any facility and is part of the operational plan. Planning and communication for operations and management of a facility help ensure ability to meet customers' needs and thereby satisfy customers' expectations.

Suggested Reading
Patton RW, Grantham WC, Gerson RF, et al. Staff selection and development. In: Wilmoth S, Mount C, Gilly H, eds. Developing and Managing Health/Fitness Facilities. Champaign, IL: Human Kinetics, 1989.
Peterson JA, Tharrett SJ, et al. American College of Sports Medicine Health/Fitness Facility Standards and Guidelines. Champaign, IL: Human Kinetics, 1992.
Storlie J, Baun WB, Horton WL. Guidelines for Employee Health Promotion Programs: Association for Fitness in Business, 1992. Champaign, IL: Human Kinetics, 1992.
Grantham WC, Patton RW, York TD, et al. Health Fitness Management. Champaign, IL: Human Kinetics, 1998.

2.7.2, 2.7.6   3.10.4.1, 3.10.4.3

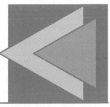

CHAPTER **77**

SELECTION, PURCHASE, AND MAINTENANCE OF EQUIPMENT

Mike Caton

Selecting, purchasing, and maintaining exercise equipment can be a challenge. The growing number of equipment options, advancements in technology, and monetary risks make purchasing equipment increasingly difficult. This chapter provides basic information about equipment selection, purchase, and maintenance, whether stocking a new facility, replacing existing equipment, or considering a new product on the market.

EQUIPMENT SELECTION

New equipment may be requested for several reasons:

- Long waiting lines at existing equipment
- High repair costs of outdated equipment
- Member requests
- An intriguing piece seen in a trade journal
- Improved ergonomic and biomechanical design

In any case, it is vital to make an informed decision without allowing emotions to lead to a costly mistake (Table 77.1).

Need

Before purchasing any equipment, the first step is to confirm the need. Ask the following questions:

- Is this equipment necessary?
- Is the product in question a legitimate option or a fad?
- Is the equipment suited for the demographics of membership?
- Is it affordable?

Space

Evaluate availability of space by examining dimensions of the equipment and the available space. For example, a treadmill may not be the best choice if the space is narrow or near a walkway. A climber, because of the small space requirements, may be more desirable. Equipment layout is another factor that must be considered, in-cluding the location of the appropriate electrical outlets. It is also important to allow for traffic flow and to avoid blocking access to an emergency exit. Refer to *ACSM's Health/Fitness Facility Standards and Guidelines* for additional information regarding spacing of equipment.

Gathering Information

Gathering product information is the next step. Review and compare as many equipment choices as possible. Trade magazines, trade shows, and equipment vendors are excellent sources of this information. Trade magazines and journals provide reader service cards and often publish an annual guide listing names and numbers for all equipment manufacturers. In addition to advertisements featuring a variety of brand names, monthly issues also have an advertising index in each issue.

Trade shows facilitate gathering information. The differences between brands are more obvious and choices become clearer and narrow quickly when direct comparison is possible.

CARDIOVASCULAR EQUIPMENT

Cardiovascular equipment is no longer limited to bikes, treadmills, and rowers. The marketplace has an array of cardiovascular machines from which to choose. Each has advantages, and there is no best choice for every environment or situation. This section reviews and discusses popular choices of cardiovascular exercise equipment and discusses advantages and disadvantages.

Treadmills

Treadmills are consistently among the favorites in fitness settings. Treadmills have distinct advantages. Most people do not require time to learn the activity because walking and running are natural activities. Walking is a weight-bearing activity, and the large muscles of the leg require significant energy production for exercise, so heart rate can be raised and maintained in the target range, leading to sustained training for an increased length of

Table 77.1. Equipment Selection Checklist

Determine needs, validity, and budget.
Evaluate facility for space, safety, and power requirements.
Gather product information from resources such as trade journals, trade shows, and distributors.
Evaluate products for safety in terms of design, ergonomics, biomechanics, and electrical circuitry.
Investigate reputation of manufacturers for quality, service history, financial stability.
Compare cost of products.
Evaluate products on basis of aesthetics.
Check references of current users. Lists can be obtained from manufacturers.
Compare warranties for length and comprehensiveness.
Determine service points provided by manufacturers in terms of availability of local service and parts.
Use product.
Compare products in terms of learning curves, familiarity of movements, and accessibility.
Determine most effective purchase plan.
Purchase equipment.

time without extensive local fatigue. Intensity of exercise can be changed easily by increasing speed or elevation. Treadmills also have some disadvantages. Weight-bearing exercise may be difficult for those with weight problems or orthopaedic injury. In these cases, non–weight-bearing exercise may be more appropriate. Also, treadmills take up considerable space. Finally, treadmills are the most expensive type of cardiovascular equipment.

Stationary Bikes

The stationary bicycle is popular and time tested. Among its advantages:

- Cycling is a motion that most people are comfortable performing.
- Little time is required for habituation.
- It is non–weight bearing and therefore nonimpact.

Therefore, a stationary bicycle can be an ideal mode of exercise in rehabilitative settings. However, because of lack of habituation, fatigue of leg muscles may cause difficulty achieving and maintaining a target heart rate for those using a bicycle ergometer.

Recumbent Bikes

Recumbent and semirecumbent bicycles are popular and have become standard in many facilities. The seat is more comfortable than traditional bicycle seats. These bicycles may be beneficial for special populations because they give back support. Safety is increased because of the wide base of support and the ease of mounting and dismounting.

The disadvantages are similar to those of other stationary bicycles. Maintaining target heart rate may be more

difficult than on upright bicycles because of the supine position. Local fatigue can also be a consistent problem on these bicycles.

Stair Climbers

Stair climbers, or stair steppers, are another popular cardiovascular exercise option. The advantages of stair climbers include the following:

- The motion of stepping or climbing is familiar, making it easy to learn.
- It is weight-bearing, which makes it relatively easy to maintain target heart rate.
- It is low impact.
- Climbers occupy less space than many other types of equipment.

Elliptical Trainers

Elliptical trainers are the newest type of cardiovascular machines in the industry, but they are already a popular piece in most health and fitness environments. As with stair climbers, they have the advantage of being weight-bearing and nonimpact. Their perceived benefit is the elliptical movement of the pedals, attempting to mimic the natural movement of the lower body. Some also have variable elevations, further enhancing the resistance options. Like treadmills, elliptical trainers are large, so they are space intensive, and they are relatively expensive.

Rowers

Though a legitimate form of cardiovascular exercise, rowing machines have never enjoyed the popularity of most other modalities and have decreased in popularity recently. Rowing uses large muscles of the legs as well as the large upper body muscles of the arms and back; raising and sustaining target heart rate is relatively easy. Rowing is a non–weight-bearing, nonimpact exercise.

On the negative side, the rowing motion is unfamiliar to most users, making it more difficult to learn. Emphasis on proper instruction is required. Also, rowers require significant floor space (especially in length) and may require specially shaped space.

Cross-Country Skiers

Cross-country ski machines have become commonplace in fitness centers. Skiers offer some advantages. Large muscle mass (upper and lower body muscle groups are used) is used during exercise, and therefore target heart rate range is easily reached and sustained. Though it is weight-bearing, cross-country skiing is nonimpact.

Most people are unaccustomed to this activity and have difficulty learning the skill. Despite the disadvantage, ski machines enjoy a great deal of positive press as well as very effective marketing. Consequently, many exercisers try skiers more than once in an attempt to learn the skill.

RESISTANCE TRAINING EQUIPMENT

In recent years, resistance training has become one of the most popular forms of exercise. This growing popularity has compelled manufacturers to extend the market and types of equipment. Where there was once a single multistation unit with one exercise option per muscle group, there are now multiple machines and free weights, offering several exercise options for each muscle group. Expanding demographics of the exercising population have caused manufacturers to change the appearance of equipment, creating broader market appeal.

Types of Equipment

Manufacturers of resistance training equipment offer three types: isotonic, variable resistance, and isokinetic. **Isotonic resistance training**, in which the *resistance remains constant throughout the range of motion*, is performed using free weights and some machines. **Variable resistance** machines, by changing the radius of a cam, *increase the resistance through part of the range of motion* coinciding with the biomechanics of contraction. **Isokinetic** machines *increase resistance at the point of maximum force while controlling the speed of contraction*. This is accomplished through the use of systems including hydraulics or motors.

Resistance training machines come in a variety of styles and shapes. Although the majority are "selectorized" (using a weight stack), some manufacturers offer plate-loaded equipment with manually placed weight plates instead of weight stacks. In many cases this plate-loaded equipment looks and feels similar to the selectorized counterparts. This type of machine can be purchased at a much lower cost than selectorized machines.

Although the increased popularity of variable resistance machines has diminished the demand for free weight training, barbells and dumbbells continue to be cost-effective resistance training equipment. Most recently, developers have added dual-axis machines, which offer resistance in multiple planes. This type of exercise is consistent with natural movement patterns.

Fitness Networking

A recent addition to exercise equipment is fitness networking. This is defined as networking some or all of the pieces of strength and cardiovascular pieces of a facility to a computer. With the use of specific computer hardware and software, information about the exerciser, staff, and equipment can be shared. The shared information enables the fitness professional to manage larger numbers of users than conventional systems. Other benefits of fitness networking are limited to the potential of the specific software, but they can include enhanced exercise adherence on the part of the exerciser.

SAFETY CONSIDERATIONS

Safety has primary importance in selection of fitness equipment. Health and fitness facilities are legally obligated to provide a safe exercise environment.

1. Ensure that all electrical plugs are secured, grounded, and covered or removed in all traffic areas.
2. Treadmills should have easily accessible emergency cutoff switches.
3. Mount safety instructions on all equipment.
4. Ensure that equipment accommodates various body sizes and types. Adjustable seats, back pads, and leg pads should be available.
5. The machines must restrict joint movements beyond normal range of motion.
6. Back pads should never force loss of the natural curve of the spine.
7. Bench width should provide support without restricting the movement of the upper arm in supine exercises.
8. Free weight racks must be wide enough to accommodate the width of an Olympic bar, decreasing the risk of pinching a hand when reracking a weight. The apparatus must be constructed properly to sustain adequate amounts of weight.

Equipment trials in the fitness center may be important to the decision-making process. Purchasing equipment based on advertisements is not recommended. Direct experience to determine workmanship, comfort, and biomechanical appropriateness is imperative. An exercise session on the equipment provides an accurate feel for the machine.

DECISION-MAKING FACTORS

Once needs are determined and product information has been gathered, evaluation begins. Factors in evaluation include cost, aesthetics, references, warranty, support and training, and maintenance.

Cost

The cost of a product is often the first question. If the product costs more than the budget allows, buying the equipment is not feasible. However, though cost is a major factor, it should not be the only one, and purchasing a piece of equipment because it is the least expensive may be a mistake. Many factors determine cost, including quality of the materials used, manner of assembly, and sales volume.

Aesthetics

Appearance of equipment is rightfully a consideration. It is important that all equipment fit with the desired look of a facility. Beyond decor, some equipment may particularly appeal to certain demographic groups. For example, large, high-profile pieces of weight lifting equipment might appeal to members interested and skilled in weight lifting but may intimidate members of a wellness facility.

References

When considering any exercise equipment, request references from current owners, including familiar companies if the product in question is unfamiliar or new to the facility. An equipment manufacturer may make quality treadmills but inferior bicycle ergometers.

Warranty

Manufacturer's warranty is another important issue. The length and terms of the warranty (exactly what is covered) are important considerations. Most manufacturer warranties on strength equipment place a different warranty period on moving parts and upholstery than on metal frames. One way to determine practical life of any piece of equipment prior to need for replacement, repair, or refurbishing is to determine the warranty period.

Support and Training

Many companies provide a representative to help set up equipment and train staff and members on proper usage. Amount, speed, and quality of support provided are also important. Some equipment may require minimal support after installation and training, while other types (e.g., computer-based or automated equipment) may require continued support. For some types of equipment, these may be critical factors in purchasing.

Maintenance

All equipment requires maintenance. Determining the level of local service is a concern. Most major companies train local technicians to service and stock parts. Review the local company and obtain references.

Demonstration Period

Some equipment manufacturers offer trial periods or demonstrations. In these situations, facilities may allow members to assist in the decision, although some managers believe this is undesirable, as some members may become attached to a piece of equipment that ultimately is not purchased.

After potential suppliers are identified, request a bid and layout. At this point, with a narrowed field, a decision may be based on cost. Bids may be formal or informal and may involve some negotiating. A minimum of three bids should be obtained for all purchases.

EQUIPMENT PURCHASING OPTIONS

Before making a final decision, some purchasing options should be considered: buying new, buying used, or leasing.

Buying New Equipment

The first option is buying new equipment outright. Although payment structures can be negotiated, most manufacturers require 50% down and the balance at installation. It is important to know whether freight and installation are included in the purchase price. Some facilities withhold 10% of the cost for 30 days to ensure satisfactory installation, training, and support.

Buying Used or Refurbished Equipment

A second option is buying used or refurbished equipment. Many equipment dealers specialize in refurbished and used equipment. They resell at prices of up to 30–50% less than new equipment. This is a good option, especially for resistance equipment, which is well made and sturdy; many used pieces are considered as good as new. The same is generally not true of cardiovascular equipment. The warranty on most cardiovascular equipment is 2 years, as opposed to 10 or more for resistance equipment. Most fitness facilities maintain resistance equipment at least that long. Older equipment is considered outdated and is likely to have excessive wear and tear.

Leasing

Leasing equipment may be a consideration if funds to buy the equipment outright are not available. Some manufacturers work through leasing companies to make this possible. Leasing requires a smaller initial cash outlay, allowing the organization to acquire more equipment. Leasing to own often provides better selection, better warranty, and sometimes buyback options. In addition, tax credits may be available for leased equipment. However, leasing is usually considered high risk, and interest rates may be high.

EQUIPMENT MAINTENANCE

A maintenance program can extend the life of equipment. Some facilities have staff that are knowledgeable and experienced in repairing equipment or dedicated to maintenance. Others use the services of an outside person or company for preventive maintenance and repair. The advantage of on-staff employees to service equipment is that response time is shorter. The disadvantage is that a staff maintenance worker, because of lack of training on intricacies of equipment, may misdiagnose a problem and delay the repair. In addition, facilities rarely stock adequate parts and must order them, resulting in more delay. Regardless of the approach, exercise equipment must undergo regular preventive maintenance to extend life and save repair costs.

Internal Maintenance

While some maintenance is suited for a trained professional, designated staff can regularly perform other tasks

Table 77.2. Cardiovascular Equipment Maintenance Checklist

Treadmills
  Check tension and alignment of walking belt monthly
  Check speed calibration monthly
  Check grade calibration monthly
  Lube drive belt monthly
  Lube elevation gears monthly
  Wax walking deck semiannually
Bicycles
  Lube chain semiannually
  Check crank bearings monthly
  Check seat monthly
  Check tension and RPM sensor monthly
  Lube pedals bimonthly
Steppers
  Lube pivots quarterly
  Grease sprockets quarterly
  Lube chains quarterly
  Check chain tension quarterly
  Tighten drive belt quarterly
Rowers
  Oil chains quarterly
  Check RPM sensors quarterly
  Inspect seat bearings quarterly

In addition, it is important that all pieces be cleaned throughout each day to remove perspiration, dust, dirt, and other elements that may come into contact with equipment and people.

that reduce cost. This is internal maintenance. Much of internal maintenance is cleaning, which is the single most effective means of preventing premature breakdown. Some claim that cleaning can double the life of a piece of cardiovascular equipment. A preventive maintenance program can cut expenses as much as 50%; therefore, an effective internal maintenance program is critical. The checklist in Table 77.2 is an example of an effective maintenance schedule.

UPHOLSTERY

Upholstery on resistance training equipment is one of the most important parts of the equipment because it is the point of contact between the user and the equipment. Regular disinfecting is essential. Some forms of herpes skin virus have been shown to survive on a warm, moist surface for up to 6 hours. Regular cleaning also prevents drying and cracking caused by oils and salts from perspiration. The most common areas for cracking are the points at which the head and elbows are supported. Another cause of upholstery damage is the buckles of weight-lifting belts. The use of belts on this equipment should be avoided. It is easy and cost-effective to replace upholstery on high-use areas. Other steps that

can prolong the life of the equipment are listed in Table 77.3.

It is important to track repairs of all equipment. Figure 77.1 is an example of a repair log for fitness equipment. These forms can be an important tool in communicating with a repair company. In addition, with good records, the upkeep cost of each piece of equipment can be determined. One commonly accepted rule of thumb can help determine when to replace equipment that requires constant and costly upkeep. If the cost of repair over 2 years is greater than the cost of a new unit or if a single repair costs 50% of the cost of a new unit, replace the unit.

After it is determined that a single piece or an entire line of equipment is too costly to maintain, there are two options: replace or refurbish. Refurbishing is a viable alternative to replacing equipment because of the cost savings, although it is not always the best decision. Refurbishing cardiovascular equipment may not be a good decision because life span is comparatively short. However, refurbishing resistance training equipment, especially free weight and plate-loaded equipment, is a good investment because of the long life span. Another consideration is the amount of structural damage sustained. If the frame has been exposed to large amounts of rust or heat (e.g., from a fire), refurbishing is not a good idea. High levels of rust or heat can weaken stress joints and make a unit unstable.

Table 77.3. Resistance Training Equipment Checklist

General
  Wax upholstery with a hard floor wax monthly.
  Remove pads at first sign of cracking.
  Stock backup pads.
Frames
  Inspect for cracks in welds monthly.
  Apply factory touch-up paint to chipped areas to prevent spreading as needed.
  Inspect for loose nuts and bolts monthly.
  Clean chrome parts with a chrome polish monthly. Household cleaners will fade the finish.
  Apply car polish to painted surfaces quarterly.
  Remove rust with fine steel wool and apply polish to surface as needed.
  Replace worn or missing warning decals.
Replace worn hand grips and seat belts.
Moving parts
  Inspect all parts and connections monthly.
  Replace any worn, stretched, or frayed cables, belts, or chains.
  Lubricate bearings and bushings with a Teflon type-lubricant when metallic dust or shavings or when squeaking or grinding sounds appear.
  Lubricate chains with chain lubricant monthly.
Weight Stack
  Clean guide rods with an aerosol cleaner that leaves no residue weekly.
  Apply a light coating of a Teflon lubricant to the guide rods weekly.
  Clean chrome weight stacks with a chrome polish weekly.

Fitness Equipment Repair Chart

Date	Equipment	Serial No.	Problem	Date Repaired	Order #	Cost

Figure 77.1. Fitness equipment repair chart.

EXERCISE TESTING AREAS

An area should be set aside for exercise testing to ensure privacy and comfort. The space should be quiet and well ventilated. Although the type of test, protocol, and equipment may vary, Table 77.4 describes equipment that should be incorporated into an exercise testing area. A crash cart, an electrocardiographic defibrillator or an automatic defibrillator (AED), and a spine board should be kept in the testing area if maximal graded tests are performed. A physician or other legally authorized individual must have authority to use the emergency equipment.

An air handling system that ensures negative air pressure should be designed and installed to ensure constant circulation in all fitness testing, health promotion, and wellness areas. Appropriate temperature, humidity, and air circulation levels should be maintained in the fitness testing area. The following levels are recommended:

- Air temperature: 68 72°F
- Humidity: 60% or less
- Air circulation: 6–8 exchanges per hour

► SUMMARY

Selection, purchase, and maintenance of equipment are all critical to the effective operation of a fitness facil-

Table 77.4. Fitness Testing Area Equipment

Bicycle ergometer or treadmill
Body composition measuring device
Sit and reach bench or goniometer
Tensiometer or other device for measuring muscular strength/endurance
Perceived exertion chart
Clock
Metronome
Sphygmomanometer (blood pressure cuff)
Stethoscope
Tape measure
Scale
First aid kit

Adapted with permission from ACSM. ACSM Fitness Facility Standards and Guidelines. Champaign IL: Human Kinetics, 1992.

ity. In addition, they contribute to member satisfaction, marketing, and attracting new members. All exercise professionals should be familiar with various types of equipment and maintenance and proper use of it.

Suggested Reading

American College of Sports Medicine. ACSM Fitness Facility Standards and Guidelines. Champaign, IL: Human Kinetics, 1989.

Patton R et al. Developing and Managing Health/Fitness Facilities. Champaign, IL: Human Kinetics, 1989.

3.10.0.3   5.10.1, 5.10.3, 5.10.4

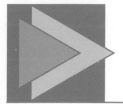

CHAPTER **78**

POLICIES AND PROCEDURES FOR CLINICAL PROGRAMS

Valerie Bishop and Linda K. Hall

Probably every health care organization in the United States today has undergone the panic-stricken year preceding a visit from the Joint Commission on Accreditation of Healthcare Organizations (JCAHO) or another accrediting organization. The JCAHO is an accrediting organization to which any health care organization (meeting the following definitions) may apply for accreditation to provide services and meet reimbursement criteria from federal agencies (1):

- Hospitals
- Non–hospital-based psychiatric and substance abuse organizations, including community mental health centers, free-standing chemical dependency providers, and organizations that serve persons with mental retardation and other developmental disabilities
- Long-term care organizations
- Home-care organizations
- Ambulatory care organizations
- Organization-based pathology and clinical laboratory services
- Health care networks

Additionally, the American Public Health Association, the Commission on Accreditation of Rehabilitation Facilities (CARF), the American Association of Cardiovascular and Pulmonary Rehabilitation, and state agencies provide some level of certification for institutions. All of these organizations have or are developing certification procedures for facilities and programs that examine quality control, licensure, appropriateness of care, policies, and procedures—in essence, everything in the conduct of business.

These review and accreditation processes require organizations delivering rehabilitation, fitness, health enhancement, and preventive programs to establish an operational design. This design must include individualized policies and procedures for activities, application of therapies, and programming. Policies and procedures should be developed using standards of care promulgated by pro-

fessional organizations and associations. Also, appropriate medical and legal personnel should review the policies and procedures so that they may serve as the immediate line of defense for a program in the event of legal claim and lawsuit (2).

DESIGN AND STRUCTURE

Several steps should be taken when developing a program, re-engineering an existing program, or designing the physical structure of a new fitness or wellness center before writing policies and procedures:

- Develop vision and mission statements that define the philosophy and purpose of the program or center.
- Find centers of excellence that have developed similar programs and centers.
- Review published standards and guidelines.
- Review policy and procedure manuals in use within the organization.

Vision and Mission Statements

The development of vision and mission statements is a group effort. Every level of employee should be involved in the process to ensure success. "Ownership" by all levels within the organization is required to carry out the statements. A vision statement is a broad, powerful, forward-looking description of the ideal state that a center may achieve. The mission statement is a broad, powerful, forward-looking description of the way the vision will be accomplished. If the program or center is a part of a large organization, such as a hospital system or a company, the vision and mission statements reflect a similar philosophical direction.

Sample Vision Statement: "Baptist Memorial Hospital will be THE leader in health care quality, value and service in this region, and one of the leading health care providers in the world" (3).

Sample Mission Statement: "Ford Motor Company is a world wide leader in automotive and automotive-related products and services as well as in newer industries such as aerospace, communications, and financial services. Our mission is to improve continually our products and services to meet our customers' needs, allowing us to prosper as a business and to provide a reasonable return for our stockholders, the owners of our business" (4).

Vision and mission statements are fluid and should be reviewed regularly and rewritten as required by changing circumstances within or outside the organization. If new programs have been added, the direction of services has changed, or other therapies are included in delivery of services, these statements may be rewritten. Furthermore, reviewing them is an important step to help remind staff of the vision and mission and may renew vigor and enthusiasm. The major thrust of the vision and mission should be to provide the best possible programs, producing positive outcomes that may be benchmarked against local, regional, and national programs.

Centers of Excellence

During design of a program, center, or facility, it is important to see what others have done. Some programs, deemed centers of excellence, should be used as models for program development. Reading journals from professional organizations such as the ACSM and the American Association of Cardiovascular and Pulmonary Rehabilitation can identify such centers. These journals contain articles written by national leaders about programs or research that may assist in structuring programs. Attending regional or national meetings also can help identify centers of excellence. Visiting these centers and talking with leaders can help with program and facility design and equipment purchase. Some centers may be willing to share actual policies and procedures.

Published Standards and Guidelines

Collect and review the most recent publications of standards and guidelines promulgated by national organizations, such as *ACSM's Guidelines for Graded Exercise Testing and Exercise Prescription*, 6th edition (American College of Sports Medicine); *Guidelines for Cardiovascular Rehabilitation and Secondary Prevention Programs, Guidelines for Pulmonary Rehabilitation Programs* 3rd edition (American Association of Cardiovascular and Pulmonary Rehabilitation), and *Health/Fitness Facility Standards and Guidelines* (American College of Sports Medicine). There are also federal, state, and local agency documents and standards to which a program or facility may be held accountable.

The policies and procedures for programs and facilities should not have standards lower than local, state, regional, or national standards. When legal liability may be in question, these gold standards have been and continue to be used as the baseline for determination of a standard of care against which the issue in question will be compared.

Organizational Policies and Procedures

Collect policy and procedural manuals within the parent organization. For example, in most hospitals, the following policy and procedural manuals are generally available:

- Infection control and hazardous waste
- Human resource management
- Emergency preparedness
- Hospital policy and procedure manual
- Standards of nursing practice

Comprehensively review these manuals before attempting to write policies and procedures for programs, facilities, or staff. If a standard or guideline in these manuals or in the state, regional, or national guideline is exactly what will be followed, there is no need for duplication; rather, cite it in the departmental policy manual. Establish a central location where all staff have access to program and facility policy and procedure manuals, as well as state, regional, and national guidelines and standards. This area contains the directional atlas for the facility, programs, and staff.

PREVENTIVE AND REHABILITATIVE EXERCISE PROGRAMS

Several key areas must be considered when identifying and writing policies for delivering preventive and rehabilitative exercise programs. These key areas contain basic standards of care and program implementation. The policies should not hold staff or facility to a level of practice less than found in any state, regional, or national guideline regarding the same practice. These policies and procedures become standard operating procedure for all staff in operating the facility, dealing with clients, and applying therapy. During orientation, new staff should read the policy and procedure manual and be trained to apply it. This manual must identify the right thing to do and define how to do it. Leadership must ensure that the staff follows these procedures (5). Once training is complete, a competency checklist should be completed and placed in the personnel file.

Leadership

Providing excellent services to clients requires effective leadership. Effective leadership is based on planning, designing, and evaluating programs, facility use, staff growth, marketing, and program development. Leadership is responsible for directing, integrating, and coordinating services. Possible types of leadership include a board of directors or a president or vice president, a medical director, and/or a board of medical advisers. The leadership is responsible for coordinating meetings, setting agendas, and carrying out decisions and recommendations from these boards. An organizational chart designating lines of authority should be placed at the beginning of the policies and procedures manual. Generally, the medical director or board is responsible for establishing guidelines and processes for clinical practice. The medical director or board approves the process of evaluating clients and prescribing exercise. The board of directors or president or vice president establishes business policies and practices. The manager or director carries out the policies and processes instituted by these governing bodies.

Effective leadership creates a clear vision for the future and defines values that underlie day-to-day operations. This type of leadership is evaluated by an accrediting organization, such as JCAHO or CARF, for being inclusive, not exclusive, and for encouraging staff participation in shaping the vision and values that are the backbone of excellent program delivery. Effective leadership is guided by the principle of leadership development at every level of the organization. This type of leadership is reflected in the development of the chain of command that in modern management practice is more horizontal than vertical.

Effective leadership accurately assesses the needs of present and future clients so as to shape and reshape programs to meet their needs. The program should foster a culture in which the staff is focused on continuous customer service and quality improvement of processes. The responsibility of the program and facility includes awareness of issues related to the community in which it resides. Furthermore, leadership ensures that all services within the scope of the program or facility are integrated and imbued with the same culture and theme of safe, high-quality provision of care.

Environmental Concerns

Policies and procedures regarding management of the environment are aimed at providing safe, functional, and effective surroundings for program delivery. The components of the policies should include the following:

- Planning use of space
- Acquisition and maintenance of equipment and dispersal of resources
- Reduction and control of environmental hazards and risks
- Prevention of accidents and injuries
- Maintenance of safe conditions
- Provision for emergency treatment, training, and practice programs
- Training staff for emergencies such as disaster, bomb threats, fire, earthquake, hazardous waste, and power failures
- Climate control
- Smoking policy

- Storage, control, and emergency management of hazardous waste and materials
- Ongoing records of safety and security management

These policies should reflect national, state, and local regulations, and all staff should be aware of them. If they are described in the parent organization policy and procedure manual, only those that apply specifically must be written.

Improving Performance

The success of any program, organization, or company is predicated on the delivery of excellent services, using new and innovative techniques, with the application of science-based information aimed at producing proven outcomes. The mechanism for achieving this success is continual analysis and evaluation of performance within the context of scientific knowledge. This is managed through designing a process for examination of efficacy, appropriateness, and availability of programs. The mechanism for continual performance improvement, which should mirror the plan within the parent organization, includes the following:

- Regular review of policy and procedure manuals to ensure comprehensiveness and accuracy
- Evaluation of performance dimensions (e.g., timeliness, effectiveness, continuity, safety, and efficiency)
- Evaluation of clients' satisfaction
- Continued scrutiny of national, regional, and local programs for benchmarking outcomes
- Demonstration of continuing evaluation of performance, outcomes, and processes, both as a whole facility and in individual departments, as required by regulating agencies and accrediting organizations

Clients' Rights and Organizational Ethics

- Introduce clients and families to advanced directives.
- Plan for maintaining confidential patient records.
- Provide written statement of patient rights.
- Plan for client orientation.
- Inform clients of the availability of pastoral counselors.
- Plan for clients' grievances and complaints.

Safety and Emergency Protocols

- Guidelines concerning the philosophy of prevention of medical emergencies within the program
- Guidelines and proper protocol for an emergency during a session
- Guidelines for the institution of emergency drills, both medical and nonmedical, in the rehabilitation continuum

Information Management

This section describes how to manage the storage, transmission, use, and tracking of information related to operation. Included are policies and procedures with regard to the following:

- Clients' records, clients' privacy and confidentiality, storage, and outcome data
- Financial records, analysis, budget allocation, and capital and operational expenses
- Insurance billing, precertification, and reimbursement
- Provision of charity and scaled remunerative services
- Client registration and procedure scheduling
- Program outcomes and ongoing progress toward program goals

Policies for information management are usually determined by the parent organization. An information services department coordinates tracking programs, billing and registration processes, and client records and is responsible for developing organizationwide policies related to client records, data collection, clinical outcomes, and reporting channels. Individual services, such as cardiac rehabilitation and preventive services, may write program-specific guidelines unique to the application of those services and consistent with policies of the parent organization.

Human Resources

The program should have a master staffing plan, including an evaluation of the complexity of client care and delivery of services, information management, fiscal management (including purchasing, billing, insurance precertification, and financial resource management), facility maintenance, and other areas involved in facility and program management. Policies and procedures should include the following:

- Job descriptions for each position with baseline educational requirements and knowledge. The job description outlines primary responsibilities and required competencies and includes a description of the physical demands and working conditions (e.g., Occupational Safety and Health Administration rules, bloodborne pathogens, lifting, carrying, job classification).
- An orientation process and formal 90-day evaluation to ensure proper training of new employees.
- The annual performance appraisal of employees and a mechanism of remuneration in each employee's file.
- Required staff certifications and licenses; current staff should have copies of credentials on file.
- Clearly delineated staff rights.
- Completed competency and skills checklist particular to specific job description. Competence must be as-

sessed, maintained, demonstrated, and continually improved.

- A written grievance policy outlining proper process and specific lines of communication.
- Regularly scheduled and documented staff meetings with attendance records.

Staff Education and In-Service Training

Continuing education for staff is critical to providing quality programs and facilities. Policies must state required continuing education, in-service training, and education. A number of national guidelines require monthly in-service training for emergency education and skill training. Surveying agencies may review documentation of department meetings, agendas, in-service training, educational programs, and certifications. The policy and procedure manual should describe what, when, how, and where these should be delivered, evaluated, and recorded. Included are policies for staff performance review and evaluation and perhaps advancement and promotion.

Clients' Rights

Preventive, rehabilitative, and exercise programs and facilities survive by the volume of clients they serve, either temporarily or through continuing membership. Maintaining client loyalty and satisfaction is an optimum requirement. The client has rights that must be posted within the facility. The client has the right to:

- Considerate care that safeguards personal dignity
- Respect for cultural, psychosocial, and spiritual values
- Knowledge of the personal responsibility in the care process

Policies and procedures should establish guidelines that ensure clients' privacy and confidentiality. The delivery of care should improve outcomes by respecting individual rights and conducting the business of the program or facility ethically. This includes promoting consideration of clients' values and preferences, recognizing the facility or program's responsibility, and comprehensive communication and record keeping. Record keeping includes informing the client of risks and processes in the provision of evaluation, exercise prescription, rehabilitation and exercise programs, and receiving informed consent to provide these services.

Client Assessment and Provision of Care

Provision of comprehensive services to the client occurs only when initial and ongoing assessments are the basis for determining and addressing specific care needs. This assessment is accomplished by collecting data specific to physical and psychosocial status and health history, analyzing the data, and making care decisions based on the data. In ongoing assessment, specific guidelines delineate the client's participation in goal setting for personal health and lifestyle achievements. The major phases for delivery of services are assessment, development and application of a care plan, monitoring, determining outcomes and end points, modification of the plan, and coordination of follow-up. Included in these policies should be these specific guidelines:

- Assessment of the client's medications and potential for interaction with application of therapy
- Consideration and assessment of the medication's efficacy, effect on function, and side effects
- Communication with referring physicians regarding the client's compliance with medication regimen
- Assessment of nutrition and dietary needs and establishment of a diet plan appropriate to the diagnosis and treatment plan

Rehabilitative Care

This area outlines tasks after completion of the assessment. It includes the following areas:

- A description of the risk stratification process and assignment of risk status
- A decision concerning monitoring and supervision in light of risk status (e.g., continuous or intermittent electrocardiography, blood pressure, heart rate, signs and symptoms, rating of perceived exertion)
- Exercise prescription methodology, including mode, time, intensity, frequency, and progression
- Risk factor evaluation, goal setting, and expected outcomes
- Vocational retraining
- Discharge planning and follow-up

The objective is to establish a protocol in which the client achieves optimal functioning, self-care and responsibility, independence, and an acceptable quality of life. It is also important to recognize that projected outcomes are based on national norms and scientific data with the objective of reducing future clinical events and minimizing development or exacerbation of chronic illness.

Client and Family Education

Because education promotes healthy behavior, educational programs are a key function of any wellness, rehabilitative, or preventive center. It is important to establish policies regarding development of and referral to educational programs dealing with risk factors that are common across the chronic and acute disease spectrum, such as smoking cessation, stress management, control of hypertension, dietary programs for diabetes, cholesterol, weight loss, pulmonary disease, sports nutrition, and relaxation, as well as exercise training and behavior man-

agement. The goals of the educational programs should be to help people:

- Change lifestyle to bring about a positive health status
- Exchange negative for positive health behaviors
- Reduce risk of chronic and acute disease
- Develop and use skills for coping with chronic disease
- Acquire physical skills
- Optimize health status
- Optimally function in vocational and avocational activities

Policies and procedures establish protocols for the client to become self-directed, participate in the decision-making process, and use experience and problem solving skills as a learning resource. The educational policies should be based on principles of adult education, evaluation of readiness to learn, and principles of lapse and relapse prevention.

The intent of educational programs is to improve health outcomes by promoting healthy behavior and involving clients in care and life decisions. The basis of this education is founded in encouraging acceptance of personal responsibility for self-teaching. The educational program should provide materials and knowledge that clients are unable to obtain for themselves.

Continuum of Care and Services

Policies describing the integration of settings for all phases of the care continuum from entry through discharge should be in place. The needs of clients should be matched with appropriate services, appraisals, and programs. Policies in this section:

- Appointment scheduling
- Parking
- Registration
- Insurance precertification and enrollment
- Informed consent
- Program evaluation
- Referral to other disciplines as needed (e.g., occupational and physical therapy)
- Intermittent progress evaluations
- Discharge planning and follow-up

This section should establish the process by which the client is able to move within the rehabilitative system and facility from parking through registration with a minimum of difficulty or excessive time and with a clear understanding of the process.

▶ SUMMARY

As with the vision and mission statements, policies and procedures are fluid. They should be reviewed regularly and updated similarly to any new application or process. The rapidly changing nature of health care delivery and reimbursement, coupled with the increasing number of preventive and rehabilitation programs, makes regular review and revision of the policies and procedures (every 6–12 months) prudent. This should ensure adherence to national standards and guidelines and satisfy accrediting organizations.

The baseline of a comprehensive policy and procedure document is the goals and objectives of the program. A written statement describing the process—to whom, when, where, why, and how delivery of services occurs—is the content. Finally, those policies must be aligned with existing national, regional, state, and local standards and guidelines.

References
1. Joint Commission on Accreditation of Healthcare Organizations, 1996. Comprehensive Accreditation Manual for Hospitals. Oakbrook Terrace, IL: JCAHO, 1995.
2. Herbert DL, Herbert WG. Medicolegal aspects of rehabilitation of the coronary patient. In: Wenger NK, Hellerstein HK, eds. Rehabilitation of the Coronary Patient. New York: Churchill, Livingstone, Inc.
3. Baptist Memorial Hospital. Vision Statement, 1996. Baptist Memorial Hospital, Memphis, TN.
4. Ford Motor Company. Mission Statement, 1988. Detroit, MI.
5. Deming WE. Quality Productivity and Competitive Position. Cambridge: Massachusetts Institute of Technology, Center for Advanced Engineering Study, 1982.

Suggested Reading
Monthly

Hospitals and Health Networks. American Hospital Publishing, Chicago.

Circulation. American Heart Association, Dallas.

Medicine and Science in Sports and Exercise. ACSM, Indianapolis, IN.

Journal of Cardiopulmonary Rehabilitation. Lippincott, Philadelphia.

Books

Froelicher VF. Manual of Exercise Testing. 2nd ed. St. Louis: Mosby–Year Book, 1994.

Heggestad J. Cardiac Health and Rehabilitation and Graded Exercise Testing Policies and Procedures Guidelines. 3rd ed. Academy Medical Systems, 1998.

Pollock ML, Schmidt DH, eds. Heart Disease and Rehabilitation. Champaign, IL: Human Kinetics, 1995.

1.7.1, 1.7.2, 1.7.3,
1.7.8

2.7.1, 2.7.2, 2.7.3,
2.7.4, 2.7.5

3.10.4.1, 3.10.4.3

4.7.1, 4.7.3

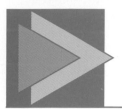

CHAPTER **79**

EMERGENCY PROCEDURES AND EXERCISE SAFETY

Sue Beckham

Although there is always risk with exercise programs, most health and fitness professionals believe the benefits outweigh the risks. However, vigorous exercise entails a variety of risks, including musculoskeletal injury and cardiovascular complications. The risk of injury and myocardial infarction associated with exercise and exercise testing can be reduced through appropriate screening and risk stratification procedures, exercise prescription techniques, and facility safety standards. Furthermore, rehearsing emergency procedures reduces the risk of serious complications in the event of an emergency. Staff training and client orientation sessions maximize safety and minimize liability. The information in this chapter is intended as a template for developing policies and procedures specific to facility, clientele, staff, and community medical resources. Numerous resources are available to assist in the development of safe and effective exercise programs for clientele and staff.

DEATH AND CARDIAC ARREST

Many researchers have investigated the incidence of sudden death and cardiac arrest during exercise. In cases of sudden cardiac death in persons under age 20, coronary artery disease is rare; congenital or other abnormalities such as hypertrophic cardiomyopathy, myocarditis, and conduction system abnormalities are often associated with these exercise-related deaths (1). Thompson et al. showed men 30–64 years of age who jog at least 2 days a week had a yearly sudden death rate of 1/7620 (2). Excluding men with known heart disease reduced the death rate to 1/15,200 joggers per year. The incidence of sudden cardiac death in women is lower at all ages (3). Studies report that the incidence of heart attack during exercise is less than 10/100,000 men/year (4). Many of these victims already had heart disease and were sedentary. The relative risk of heart attack is 5.9 times greater in men and women who are habitually inactive than in those who exercise regularly (5). As the frequency of regular, vigorous exercise increases, the risk of heart attack with exertion de-

creases significantly. These studies emphasize the need for risk factor stratification; appropriate medical screening, such as graded exercise tests; and a data-based exercise prescription to reduce the risk of complications and death.

Exercise-related risk should be examined relative to the risks associated with physical inactivity. Physical inactivity is a major risk factor for coronary artery disease. The average relative risk for coronary artery disease in inactive individuals is 1.9 times the risk for an active person (6). This is similar to the relative risk associated with smoking, hypertension, and hypercholesterolemia. Only modest amounts of regular activity are required for significant reductions in mortality rates from heart disease and cancer. Blair et al. reported that the greatest reduction (about 50%) in all-cause mortality rates occurred when an individual moves from the lowest level of fitness ($\leq$ 6 METs) to the next lowest level (7 METs) (7). No additional reduction in mortality rate was associated with aerobic capacities greater than 9–10 METs. According to the Surgeon General's report, more than 60% of American adults and 50% of youth are not physically active on a regular basis; this exceeds the percentages of adults with risk factors for hypertension, hypercholesterolemia, or smoking, suggesting that physical activity should be vigorously targeted for intervention (7, 8). In view of this epidemiological evidence, the benefits of moderate exercise outweigh the risks in most individuals, assuming that American College of Sports Medicine (ACSM) guidelines for health screening, risk stratification, and exercise prescription are followed.

MUSCULOSKELETAL INJURY

Epidemiological studies investigating the incidence of injury during vigorous activity provide valuable information for the selection of appropriate activities, based on health history and fitness evaluation. More epidemiological data are available for running than for other exercise. Studies investigating the incidence of running injuries report yearly rates of 24–77%, or 2.5–12 injuries per 1000 hours of running; generally, lower rates are reported in recreational runners and higher rates in competitive athletes (9, 10). Differences in the definition of injury among studies also contribute to variation in the incidence of injury. Injury rates for other weight-bearing activities, such as aerobic dance classes, are approximately 45% for students (1/1000 hours of aerobic dance) and 75% for instructors (11–13). Most of the classes studied were high-impact and many of the reported injuries resulted in discomfort, but little alteration in participation. During the late 1980s, low-impact and high–low-impact classes replaced many of the traditional high-impact classes. A more recent study reported an injury rate of 35% for students and 53% for instructors; injury rates for low-impact (24%) were lower than for high-impact (38%) aerobics (14). Studies investigating injury rates associated with other types of popular group exercise classes, such as kickboxing, yoga, Pilates, resistance training, and indoor cycling are lacking. The injury rates are lower in non–weight-bearing activities, such as swimming (15).

Risk Factors for Musculoskeletal Injury

Risk factors associated with injury can be classified as environmental, individual, or program factors. With regard to distance running, the most consistent predictors of injury are previous injury, high weekly mileage, lack of experience, and running to compete (9, 16–18). Pollock et al. reported that the incidence of injury in 70 men 20–35 years of age increased as the frequency and duration of training increased (19). The incidence of injury was 22%, 24%, and 54% in the 15, 30, and 45 minutes per session groups, respectively; incidence of injury was 0%, 12%, and 39% for the 1, 3, and 5 days a week groups, respectively. Training intensity was 85–90% of maximal heart rate for all groups. This study suggests that the incidence of injury in novice runners increases significantly with more than 30 minutes of exercise or more than 3 days a week. With regard to aerobic dance, factors such as a history of orthopaedic problems, type of class (high versus low impact), use of upper body weights, and frequency of participation (4 or more classes a week) were associated with increases in injury rates (11–14).

EXERCISE-RELATED INJURIES

Exercise-related injuries fall into two categories, traumatic and overuse. Traumatic injuries usually occur in a single violent event. Injuries such as strains, sprains, tears, and fractures are considered traumatic injuries. Conversely, overuse injuries are caused by chronic, repetitive submaximal forces leading to inflammation and pain (20). Common overuse injuries include tendinitis, strains, shin splints, stress fractures, and blisters. Acute

treatments for common injuries are outlined in Table 79.1. Many of the following conditions and injuries are discussed in other chapters in this book. The reader is encouraged to review each of those chapters for detailed information about specific topics of interest. Chapter 57 provides an extensive discussion of musculoskeletal injuries related to exercise.

Skin Wounds

Skin wounds, including blisters, corns, abrasions, lacerations, punctures, sunburn, and infections, are caused by mechanical trauma, environmental factors, or transmission of infectious organisms. Blisters are caused by friction between the surface of the skin and athletic wear or equipment, resulting in fluid accumulation. The blister itself provides a protective dressing and should be covered with a sterile dressing, which promotes rapid healing and reduces the risk of infection (20). Blisters often rupture because of their location in areas such as feet or require drainage for other reasons. To drain a blister, puncture it with a sterile needle, treat with antibiotic ointment, and cover with a sterile dressing. Properly fitting sport-specific socks, gloves, and shoes help prevent blisters.

Bleeding open skin wounds, such as lacerations, may require direct application of pressure and elevation to stop bleeding. It is important to prevent the transfer of blood-borne pathogens during cleaning of the wound. Medical evaluation is indicated for deep or large wounds or if signs of infection, such as swelling, redness, or pain, are present.

Contusions

Contusions are bruises with intact skin. Common in contact sports, muscle contusions incite an inflammatory response and may cause formation of a hematoma. The treatment of choice is rest, ice, compression, elevation, and stabilization (RICES) (Table 79.2). A physician should evaluate severe, painful contusions, especially when accompanied by hematoma formation.

Strains and Sprains

Strain is stretching or tearing of the musculotendinous unit, and sprain is injury to a ligament. Strains and sprains are classified as grade I, II, or III, depending on the severity of tissue tearing. Grade I strains and sprains are stretching or minor tearing of connective tissue. Grade II strains and sprains result from partial tearing; grade III strains and sprains involve extensive tearing or complete rupture of tissue and generally require surgery. The RICES protocol is appropriate for acute strains and sprains.

Following joint injury, proprioception, or the ability to perceive position in space and respond, is often affected; mechanoreceptor function and proprioceptive feedback

Table 79.1. Acute Responses for Common Injuries/Emergencies

INJURY OR EMERGENCY	SIGNS AND SYMPTOMS	ACUTE CARE
Closed skin wounds (blisters, corns)	Pain, swelling, infection	Clean with antiseptic soap; apply sterile dressing, antibiotic ointment
Open skin wounds (lacerations, abrasions)	Pain, redness, bleeding, swelling, headache, mild fever	Apply pressure to stop bleeding; clean with soap or sterile saline; apply sterile dressing; refer to physician for stitches, tetanus toxoid
Contusions (bruises)	Swelling, local pain, loss of function if severe	RICES; apply padding if necessary for protection
Strains*a*		
Grade I	Pain, local tenderness, tightness	RICES
Grade II	Loss of function, hemorrhage	RICES, refer for physician evaluation if impaired function
Grade III	Palpable defect	Immobilization, RICES, immediate referral to physician
Sprains*a*		
Grade I	Pain, point tenderness, strength loss, edema	RICES
Grade II	Hemorrhage, measurable laxity	RICES, evaluation by a physician
Grade III	Palpable or observable defect	Immobilization, RICES, evaluation by a physician
Fractures		
Stress	Pain, point tenderness	Evaluation by a physician, rest, non–weight-bearing activities
Simple	Swelling, disability, pain	Immobilize with splint; evaluation by a physician; radiography
Compound	Bleeding, swelling, pain, disability	Immobilize; control bleeding; apply sterile dressing; immediate evaluation by a physician
Dizziness, syncope	Disoriented, confused, pale skin	Determine responsiveness; place supine with legs elevated; administer fluids if conscious; begin emergency ventilation and/or compressions as needed
Hypoglycemia	Profuse sweating, tachycardia, hunger, double vision, tremors, headache, disorientation, seizure	Administer 10–30 g carbohydrate (regular soda, orange juice, or 3 glucose tablets) if conscious; follow with protein; if recovery requires more than 1–2 min, activate EMS; if unconscious, place sugar granules under tongue and activate EMS
Hyperglycemia	Lethargy; weakness; confusion; nausea; headache; sweet, fruity breath; thirst; abdominal pain and vomiting; hyperventilation	Activate EMS; administer fluids if conscious; turn head to side if vomiting
Hypothermia	Shivering, but may stop with extreme drops in core temperature; loss of coordination, muscle stiffness, lethargy	Activate EMS and transport to hospital; remove wet clothing; replace with dry, warm clothing
Hyperthermia		
Heat cramps	Involuntary isolated muscle spasms	Administer fluids with electrolytes; apply direct pressure to spasm and release; massage cramping area with ice
Heat exhaustion	Profuse sweating; pale, clammy skin; multiple muscle spasms; headache; nausea; loss of consciousness; dizziness; tachycardia; hypotension	Move to cool area; place supine with feet elevated; remove clothes; cool with fans, cold water, or ice but avoid chilling the victim; administer fluids; monitor body temperature; refer for evaluation by a physician
Heat stroke	Hot, dry skin, but can be sweating; dyspnea; confusion; unconsciousness common	Activate EMS and transport to hospital immediately; remove clothing; douse with cool water (ice water baths preferred) or wrap in cool wet sheets; administer fluids if conscious
Exertional rhabdomyolysis	Muscle pain, swelling and weakness, dark urine	Activate EMS and transport to hospital immediately; cool and administer fluids if conscious
Angina	Pain or pressure in the chest, neck, jaw, arm and/or back; sweating; denial of medical problem; nausea; shortness of breath	Stop activity; place in seated or supine position (whichever is more comfortable), activate EMS if pain is not relieved
Sudden cardiac arrest	No breathing or pulse	If AED is immediately available, defibrillate if appropriate; if not, activate EMS, begin CPR as needed
Dyspnea, labored breathing	Hyperventilation, dizziness, wheezing, coughing, loss of coordination	Maintain open airway; administer bronchodilator if prescribed; try pursed lip breathing; if no relief, activate EMS and transport

a Signs and symptoms for each grade include those for grades below the one listed: grade II includes those of grade I; Grade III includes those of grades I and II.

Table 79.2. RICES Protocol for Acute Injuries

TREATMENT	PURPOSE	APPLICATION
Rest	Pain control, prevention of reinjury	Complete rest, immobilization, or reduction in training intensity, duration, frequency; or non–weight-bearing activities, depending on severity of injury
Ice	Reduction of pain, swelling, inflammation and bleeding	Immediately post-injury, 2–4 times daily, 20–30 min: plastic bag filled with crushed ice and secured with an elastic bandage; ice massage for small areas, such as tendons and strains, for 10–20 min
Compression	Reduction of swelling	Elastic wrap or compression sleeve
Elevation	Reduction of swelling	Elevate extremity above heart level
Stabilization	Reduce muscle spasm	Use of brace, splint, wrap to stabilize area around joint injury

to the brain are decreased (20). Therefore, proprioceptive exercises should be included in the rehabilitation program to restore kinesthetic awareness, coordination, and agility in addition to flexibility and strength.

Fractures

Fractures include three types: stress, simple, and compound. Stress fractures, or microfractures in the bone surface, are caused by repetitive stress. The bone remains within the skin in simple fractures, while compound or open fractures involve external exposure of bone, increasing the risk of infection. Common in runners, stress fractures are often related to sudden increases in running distance and/or intensity (21). Point tenderness and pain with weight bearing are characteristic of stress fractures, which may not appear on radiographs. Non–weight-bearing and partial weight-bearing activities, such as swimming and bicycling, are recommended for maintenance of cardiovascular fitness until pain-free activity is possible.

Dizziness and Syncope

Dizziness or syncope (temporary loss of consciousness) during exercise may be caused by hyperventilation, cardiac arrhythmias, heat stress, cardiomyopathy, aortic stenosis (narrowing of aortic valve), anomalous coronary arteries, or coronary artery disease (20). Acute care should always include evaluation of the airway, breathing, and pulse if the individual is unresponsive. Cessation of exercise is paramount, and evaluation by a physician is essential to determine whether an underlying condition is present.

Hypotension can also cause dizziness and fainting. Postexercise hypotension occurs when blood pools in the lower extremities because of inadequate cool-down. A 5–10-minute low-intensity cool-down using large muscle groups is effective in preventing postexercise hypotension. Antihypertensive medications may exacerbate postexercise hypotension, necessitating a longer cool-down period. **Orthostatic hypotension**, a drop in blood pressure with changes in posture, may occur when mov-

ing from lying to standing. Gradual movement with momentary sitting often prevents orthostatic hypotension. Plasma volume depletion caused by dehydration or diuretic medication is also a causative factor in hypotension; adequate hydration should always be encouraged.

Hypoglycemia and Hyperglycemia

Hypoglycemia is low blood glucose. Symptoms may occur at various blood glucose levels, especially in insulin-dependent diabetics (22). Hypoglycemic reactions, which may occur during or after exercise in diabetics, are associated with strenuous exercise, inadequate caloric intake, and inadequate adjustment of insulin dosage (23). Hypoglycemia may occur in nondiabetic individuals who are not eating appropriately, especially with respect to activity level. Hypoglycemia and hyperglycemia are medical emergencies that, if not treated immediately, may lead to seizures, coma, or death. Signs and symptoms of hypoglycemia and hyperglycemia may be similar; however, symptoms of hypoglycemia develop rapidly, while signs and symptoms associated with hyperglycemia are slower to manifest. A more detailed discussion of glycemic control during exercise can be found in Chapter 31.

Hypothermia and Hyperthermia

Hypothermia, or cold injury, is a decrease in core temperature that occurs when metabolic heat production is inadequate to match the rate of heat lost through evaporation of sweat, radiation, conduction, and convection. Factors such as wind chill (wind speed) and moisture increase the risk of hypothermia. Most hypothermia can be prevented if exercise intensity is controlled, adequate clothing made of fabric designed to wick moisture is worn, and alcohol and drugs that impair thermoregulation are avoided. Elderly persons, children, and individuals with ischemic heart disease or poor aerobic capacity should limit physical activity in the cold.

Hyperthermia, or heat injury, is a category of heat-related disorders, including heat cramps, exhaustion, stroke, and exertional rhabdomyolysis (breakdown of skeletal muscle due to excessive exercise in the heat). The combination of high ambient temperatures, humidity, and metabolic heat leads to increases in core temperature, increased sweat rate, and dehydration, which may result in circulatory collapse and death. The wet bulb–globe temperature heat stress index, an index of temperature and humidity, should be used to determine the risk of heat stress. Prevention of heat-related injuries includes acclimation to heat, avoidance of exercise if the heat index is in the high-risk zone, replacement of electrolytes and fluids, monitoring of body weight, and use of light clothing that promotes cooling and evaporation. Obesity, sleep deprivation, illness, poor physical fitness, a history of heat stroke, and certain medications are risk factors for heat illness (24).

Heat cramps, though uncomfortable, are benign; however, exercise should be discontinued and rehydration initiated immediately. Heat exhaustion, characterized by profuse sweating and pale, clammy skin with nearly normal body temperatures, can rapidly deteriorate into heat stroke, which is distinguished by hot, red, dry skin, tachycardia, and disorientation or loss of consciousness. Any mechanisms available to reduce core temperature should be attempted immediately. Heat syncope, which may accompany heat injury, should be treated as described earlier. Exertional rhabdomyolysis, although less common, is characterized by dark urine and muscle pain, swelling, and weakness. This is also a life-threatening event that can lead to renal failure and death. Chapter 24 provides more detailed information about environmental considerations during exercise.

Angina

Pain or discomfort in the chest, jaw, neck, arms, or other areas during exercise that is not altered by movement of the involved areas or extremity may require immediate medical attention. Individuals with anginal type of discomfort should discontinue exercise immediately and rest sitting or recumbent until the discomfort is resolved. Individuals with medication for anginal symptoms should be encouraged to carry the medication at all times and use it as directed.

Sudden Cardiac Arrest

Sudden cardiac arrest, caused by factors such as heart disease and rhythm and congenital abnormalities, results in 250,000 deaths annually (25). During sudden cardiac arrest, the victim usually develops an abnormal heart rhythm called ventricular fibrillation, causing the heart to beat in an uncoordinated fashion. Since blood is not effectively pumped, the pulse and subsequently the breathing stop. If the heart is electrically shocked soon thereafter, normal rhythm may be restored. Cardiopulmonary resuscitation (CPR) alone can add only a few minutes to the time available for successful defibrilla-

tion. However, when defibrillation is performed during the first 3 minutes after collapse, survival rates can be as high as 70–80%; for every minute that defibrillation is delayed, there is a 7–10% reduction in the chance of survival (26). The automated external defibrillator (AED) is a portable device that identifies heart rhythms amenable to defibrillation, uses audiovisual prompts to direct the correct response, and delivers the appropriate shock. Even children can be trained to operate AEDs safely and effectively (27). Courses that incorporate AED training into traditional CPR training are available to the public. The Cardiac Arrest Survival Act extends good Samaritan protections to AED users. The limited number of trial court verdicts on AEDs suggest that organizations adopting AED programs have a lower risk of liability than those who do not.

Dyspnea

Dyspnea (abnormal shortness of breath or labored breathing) may occur in response to bronchospasm, which can be triggered by allergens, cold air, airborne irritants, and respiratory infection. Prescription bronchodilators are often used to resolve such episodes.

TREATMENT OF EXERCISE-RELATED INJURIES

The immediate treatment for acute traumatic and overuse injuries follows the RICES protocol. Anti-inflammatory drugs, such as aspirin and ibuprofen, may be useful in treatment of chronic and acute injuries. Acetaminophen may be used for pain relief, but is not considered anti-inflammatory. For a detailed discussion of RICES, see Chapter 57.

INJURY PREVENTION

Many injuries occurring in the fitness setting can be prevented with regular maintenance of equipment, training of personnel, and formal member orientations regarding equipment use, weight room etiquette, and safety policies. Outlined hereafter are precautions to ensure members' and employees' safety. *ACSM's Health/Fitness Facility Standards and Guidelines* contains a detailed list of guidelines (28). The following recommendations for maintenance and safety apply to fitness facilities of many types:

1. Free-weight exercises, such as squats and bench presses, should be performed with a properly trained spotter. Two spotters are recommended for heavily loaded free-weight exercises.
2. The buddy system is ideal for resistance training. One individual monitors form and biomechanics and provides feedback to the partner. In the event of an emergency, a rapid response is ensured.

CONTRAINDICTATED/HIGH-RISK EXERCISE		ALTERNATIVE EXERCISE
Straight leg or bent knee full sit-ups with hands behind neck 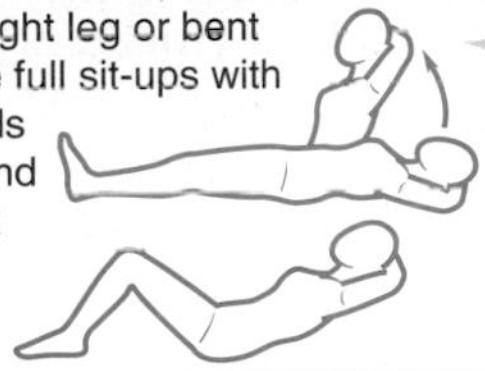	Risk: Stress on low back places high compressional forces on spinal discs, exercise primarily targets hip flexors, loaded neck flexion can sprain cervical ligaments and damage discs	Curls, Hands Under Lumbar Region, Lift Shoulder Blades but not Low Back off Floor 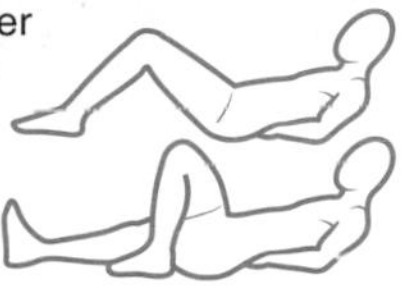
Double Leg Raises 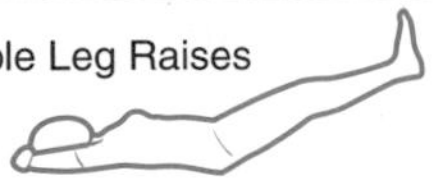	Risk: Hyperextends low back due to utilization of hip flexors with origin in the lumbar spine	Single Leg Raises-Opposite Knee Flexed 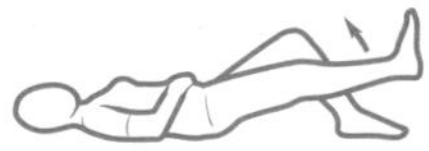
Full Squats 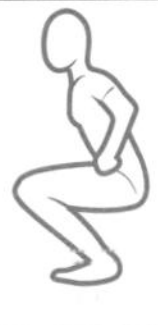	Risk: Patellar tendon forces during deep knee bending are 7.6 times body weight increasing the risk of chondromalacia and meniscal tears;	Squats to ≥90 Degrees of Knee Flexion-Knee Over Ankle 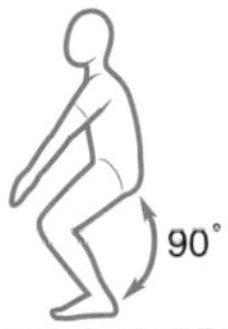
Hurdler's Stretch for quadriceps (leaning backwards) 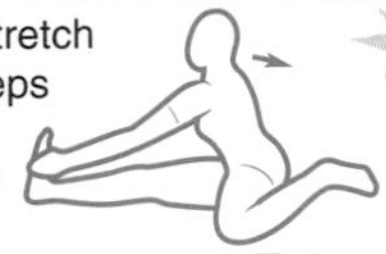	Risk: Knee flexion at end range of motion with rotational forces on hinge joint may stress the medial collateral ligament and menisci, also hyperextension of lumbar spine	Standing Quadricep Stretch, with Torso Upright; Hold Ankle, not Foot, with Opposite Hand; Avoid Hip Abduction 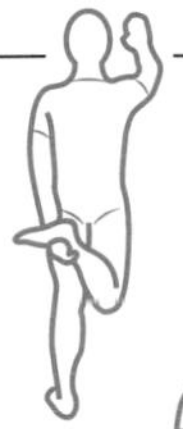
Standing quadricep stretch (same arm to ankle with hip abducted 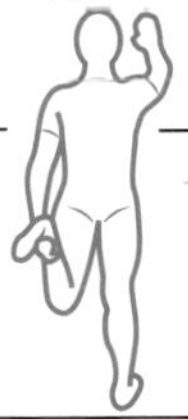	Risk: Hip abduction places rotational forces on knee and stresses the medial collateral ligament and menisci	Standing Quadricep Stretch, with Torso Upright; Hold Ankle, not Foot, with Opposite Hand; Avoid Hip Abduction 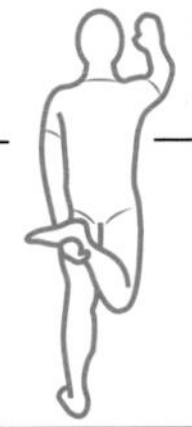
Hurdler's Stretch for hamstrings 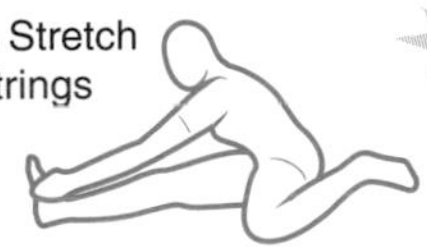	Risk: Knee flexion at end range of motion with rotational forces on hinge joint may stress the medial collateral ligament and menisci	Seated Hamstring Stretch, Back Flat with One Knee Flexed, Arms Behind Back 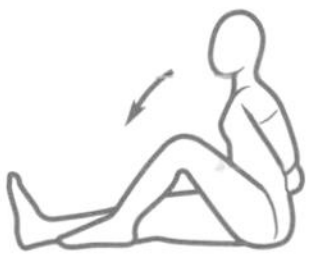
Plough 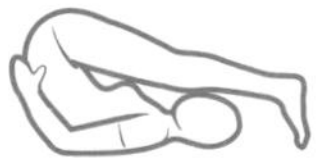	Risk: Loaded neck flexion can sprain cervical ligaments and damage discs, especially in those with spinal osteoporosis and arthritis	Double Knee to Chest 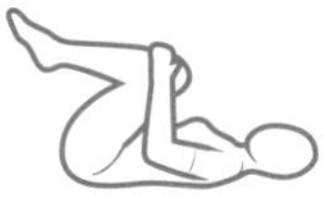
Back Hyperextension to increase strength 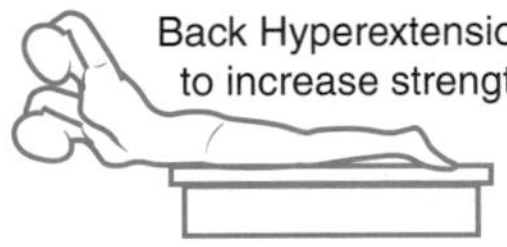	Risk: Uncontrolled, ballistic hyperextension of the lumbar spine can damage the vertebrae and spinal discs	Controlled Lumbar Extension to Normal Standing Lumbar Lordosis 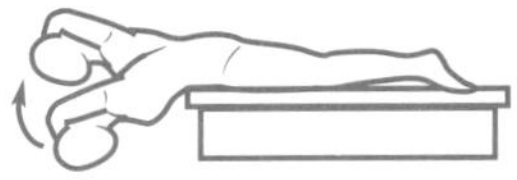
Full neck rolls 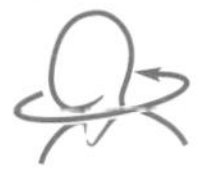	Risk: Compression of nerves and vessels which can lead to dizziness, disc damage	Slow, Controlled Lateral and Extension Neck Stretches Performed Separately 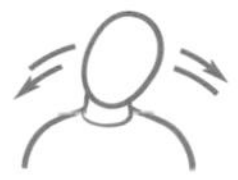
Loaded spinal flexion with rotation 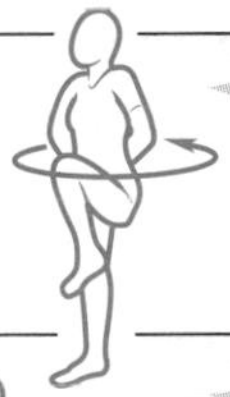	Risk: Loaded spinal flexion with rotation increases pressure and shear forces on spinal discs, common cause of low back injuries	Supine Crunches with Flexion followed by Rotation 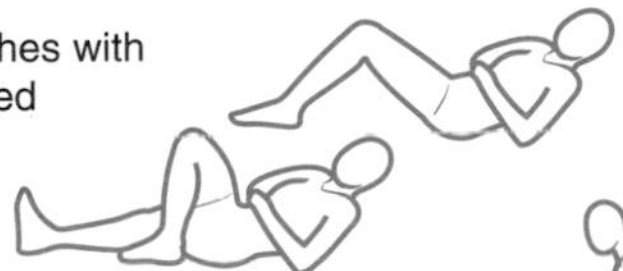
Standing toe touch 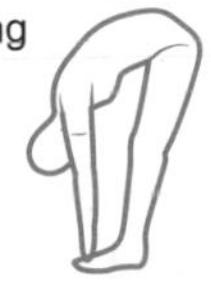	Risk: Increases pressure in lumbar disks and overstretches lumbar ligament	Standing Hamstring Stretch with Foot at a Height that Allows Maintenance of Flat Back as Hip Is Flexed, Arms Behind Back 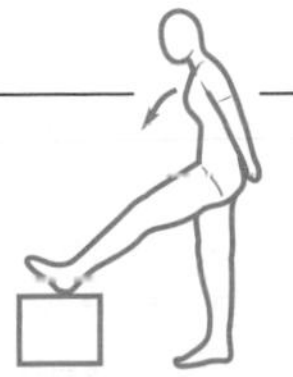

Figure 79.1. Common high-risk exercises and recommendations for alternative exercises. Adapted with permission from Frankel VH, Hang YS. Recent advances in the biomechanics of sports injuries. Acta Orthop Scand 46:484, 1975, and Wendell L, Haydu T, Phillips D. Questionable Exercises. President's Council on Physical Fitness and Sports Research Digest 3:8, 1–8, 1999.

3. Routine inspection and maintenance of resistance and cardiovascular equipment are necessary to reduce risk of injury resulting from equipment malfunction.

4. Passageways between equipment should be sufficient (approximately 3 feet) to allow safe movement at all times (28).

5. Weights and other accessories (pads, attachments, collars, and pins) must be racked or properly stored after use.

6. Members should be oriented to equipment, including proper lifting technique, controlled speed of movement, adjustments required for proper alignment, appropriate amount of weight, and number of sets and repetitions.

7. Weight room etiquette should be shared with members to facilitate courteous flow of members through the weight room. Allowing others to rotate in during the rest period, racking weights, and wiping equipment with towels to decrease the risk of transmitting viral or bacterial infections are examples of such courtesy.

8. Staff should clean all pads daily with antifungal and antibacterial agents.

9. Equipment should be arranged in a manner consistent with the appropriate order of training.

EMERGENCY PROCEDURES

All facilities should have a written emergency plan for medical complications. This plan should list specific responsibilities of each staff member, required equipment, and a predetermined contact for emergency response. Emergency plans including telephone numbers for EMS, police, and fire should be posted next to all telephones. First aid kits, first responder blood-borne pathogen kits, latex gloves, AED, CPR mouthpieces, and resuscitation bags must be readily available and transportable. The areas where first aid equipment is stored should be clearly labeled and supplies checked monthly. Regular periodic review of the emergency plan by a medical professional is recommended to ensure that all appropriate steps are outlined. The plan should be practiced with both announced and unannounced drills on a quarterly basis. Strategies for coping with potential and common injuries in the exercise and fitness testing setting should be rehearsed. Completion of a written report, including an evaluation of the drill and recommendations for any necessary changes, should follow each emergency drill.

Emergency plans specific to both minor and major medical incidents are required. Minor medical events are not life- or limb-threatening and can be initially managed within the facility, but may be referred to a medical resource. Major medical emergencies require an initial response by the staff followed by immediate transport to a medical facility. Since a medical emergency may arise at any time and any location, all employees, including secretarial, janitorial, and child care staff, should be certified in CPR and first aid. *ACSM's Guidelines for Exercise Testing and Prescription* detail emergency plans for nonemergency and life-threatening situations (29). Emergency plans may vary according to the facility size, staff, and local emergency response.

EVALUATION SKILLS

A critical responsibility of the exercise professional is evaluation of technique and body position during resistance, flexibility, and cardiovascular training. Early recognition and correction of poor technique may help reduce the risk of injury and ensure that the client receives the maximum benefit possible. Participants are usually appreciative and respectful if approached in a friendly, knowledgeable manner. The utmost concern for client safety and science-based information should be emphasized when correcting form or technique. Clients should be discouraged from selecting high-risk exercises.

CONTRAINDICATED AND HIGH-RISK EXERCISES

Much controversy surrounds the decision to label specific exercises as contraindicated or inappropriate for everyone. Factors such as age, flexibility, strength, type of exercise, pre-existing orthopaedic problems, and individual ability to perform an exercise properly make it difficult to label exercises as acceptable or unacceptable for all persons. Therefore, the term *high-risk* may be more appropriate than *contraindicated*, since an exercise may be appropriate for an athlete in sports requiring high-risk movements, such as gymnastics but inappropriate for the general fitness setting. Figure 79.1 is a list of commonly performed high-risk exercises and some alternatives.

In a group exercise setting when all individuals are performing the same exercise, caution in selecting appropriate exercises for all ages, disabilities, and skill levels is crucial. Demonstration of a modified form of an exercise is always appropriate in a group, since individuals in advanced classes may exhibit high levels of cardiovascular fitness, but poor levels of flexibility, agility, strength, and/or muscular endurance. Since many popular group exercise classes (e.g., kickboxing, boot camp) involve high-intensity ballistic movements that require above-average flexibility and agility, the fitness professional should provide a mechanism for screening participants prior to participation. Selection of the most effective and safe exercises is important, as most exercise classes attempt to provide multiple fitness components within a limited (45–60 minutes) time. When selecting exercises appropriate for the group or individuals, the following evaluation is recommended; a yes answer to all questions is required to maximize participants' safety.

- Is the exercise safe for all participants based on age and health status?
- If the exercise is safe, are the participants able to perform the exercise properly?
- Is this exercise an effective way to increase flexibility, strength, coordination, balance, or cardiovascular endurance?

If any questions are answered with a no, replace the activity with a safe exercise that is more effective in achieving the ultimate goal.

The personal trainer or fitness instructor working one-on-one has to make decisions regarding the safety and effectiveness of exercises for only one client at a time. This task is easier than evaluating a group exercise class; however, the same procedure should be used.

▶ SUMMARY

First and foremost, the exercise professional should attempt to prevent injury through careful review of the medical and injury history and fitness level. An exercise prescription based on this information can be developed to prevent exercise-related injuries, improve specific fitness components, and assist in meeting clients' goals. The exercise professional and the client should monitor warning signs of overtraining (fatigue, insomnia, loss of appetite, or a decline in performance) and injury. Early recognition and appropriate modification of the exercise program may prevent serious overuse injuries. If an injury does occur, prompt recognition and application of acute care treatments minimize the time required to return to full activity. If the injury is serious, the exercise professional should refer clients for medical evaluation and diagnosis.

References

1. Drory Y, Turetz Y, Hiss Y, et al. Sudden unexpected death in persons less than 40 years of age. Am J Cardiol 68:1388–1392, 1991.
2. Thompson PD, Funk EJ, Carleton RA, Sturner WQ. Incidence of death during jogging in Rhode Island from 1975 through 1980. JAMA 247:2535, 1982.
3. Cupples LA, Gagnon DR, Kannel WB. Long- and short-term risk of sudden coronary death. Circulation 85:I11–I18, 1992.
4. Nieman DC. Exercise Testing and Prescription. 4th ed. Mountain View, CA: Mayfield, 1999.
5. Mittleman MA, Maclure M, Tofler GH, et al. Triggering of acute myocardial infarction by heavy physical exertion: Protection against triggering by regular exertion. N Engl J Med 329:1677–1683, 1993.
6. Powell KE, Thompson PD, Caspersen CJ, Kendrick JS. Physical activity and the incidence of heart disease. Ann Rev Publ Health 8:253–287, 1987.
7. Blair SE, Kohl HW, Paffenbarger RS, et al. Physical fitness and all cause mortality: A prospective study of health and unhealthy men. JAMA 262:2395–2401, 1989.
8. U.S. Dept. of Health and Human Services. Physical Activity and Health: A Report of the Surgeon General. Atlanta: National Center for Chronic Disease Prevention and Health Promotion, 1996.
9. Caspersen CJ. Physical inactivity and coronary heart disease. Phys Sportsmed 15:11, 43–44, 1987.
10. Pate RR, Macera CA. Risk of exercising: Musculo-skeletal injuries. In: Bouchard C, Shephard RJ, eds. Exercise, Fitness, and Health: A Consensus of Current Knowledge. Champaign, IL: Human Kinetics, 1994.
11. Van Mechelen W. Running injuries: A review of epidemiological literature. Sports Med 14:320, 1992.
12. Garrick JG, Requa RK. Aerobic dance: A review. Sports Med 6:169–179, 1988.
13. Richie DH, Kelso SF, Bellucci PA. Aerobic dance injuries: A retrospective study of instructors and participants. Physician Sportsmed 13:130–140, 1991.
14. Rothenberger LA, Chang JI, Cable TA. Prevalence and types of injuries in aerobic dancers. Am J Sports Med 16:403–407, 1988.
15. Janis LR. Aerobic dance survey: A study of high-impact versus low-impact injuries. J Am Podiatr Med Assoc 80:419–423, 1990.
16. Baxter-Jones A, Maffulli N, Helms P. Low injury rates in elite athletes. Arch Dis Child 68:130–132, 1993.
17. Hoeberigs JH. Factors related to the incidence of running injuries: A review. Sports Med 13:408–422, 1992.
18. Van Mechelen W. Can running injuries be effectively prevented? Sports Med 19:161–165, 1995.
19. Pollock ML et al. Effects of frequency and duration of training on attrition and incidence of injury. Med Sci Sport Exerc 9:31, 1977.
20. Grana WA, Kalenak A, eds. Clinical Sports Medicine. Philadelphia: Saunders, 1991.
21. McKeag DB, Dolan C. Overuse syndromes of the lower extremity. Phys Sportsmed 17:108, 1989.
22. Skinner JS. Exercise Testing and Exercise Prescription for Special Cases. Philadelphia: Lea & Febiger, 1987.
23. Konick-McMahan J. Riding out a diabetic emergency. Nursing 29(9):34–39, 1999.
24. American College of Sports Medicine. Position stand on heat and cold illnesses during distance running. Med Sci Sports Exerc 27:i–x, 1996.
25. American Heart Association. 1998 Heart and Stroke statistical update. Dallas: AHA, 1997.
26. American Heart Association. Operation Heartbeat Implementation Guide. Dallas: AHA, 1998.
27. Gundry JW, Comess KA, DeRook FA, et al. Comparison of naive sixth-grade children with trained professionals in the use of an automated external defibrillator. Circulation 100:1703–1707, 1999.
28. American College of Sports Medicine. ACSM's Health/Fitness Facility Standards and Guidelines. 2nd ed. Cham-

paign, IL: Human Kinetics, 1992.

29. American College of Sports Medicine. ACSM's Guidelines for Exercise Testing and Prescription. 6th ed. Baltimore: Lippincott Williams & Wilkins, 2000.

30. Corbin B, Lindsey R. Concepts of Physical Fitness With Laboratories. 5th ed. Dubuque: Brown, 1985.

Suggested Reading

Nieman D. Exercise Testing and Prescription. Mountain View, CA: Mayfield, 1999.

American College of Sports Medicine. ACSM's Health/Fitness Facility Standards and Guidelines. 2nd ed. Champaign, IL: Human Kinetics, 1992.

2.10.0.3

3.10.0.1, 3.10.0.2,
3.10.3, 3.10.3.1,
3.10.3, 3.10.3.4,
3.10.3.5

CHAPTER **80**

SALES AND MARKETING

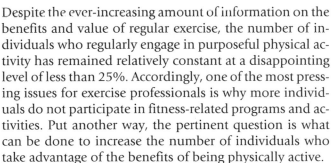

James A. Peterson, Cedric X. Bryant, and Barry A. Franklin

Despite the ever-increasing amount of information on the benefits and value of regular exercise, the number of individuals who regularly engage in purposeful physical activity has remained relatively constant at a disappointing level of less than 25%. Accordingly, one of the most pressing issues for exercise professionals is why more individuals do not participate in fitness-related programs and activities. Put another way, the pertinent question is what can be done to increase the number of individuals who take advantage of the benefits of being physically active.

One logical step is to encourage various agencies and organizations (e.g., health–fitness clubs, YMCA) that offer fitness-related programs and activities to be more marketing oriented in efforts to entice participation in their offerings. Unfortunately, some surmise that for such participation to occur, all the exercise professional must do is to compile a formidable list of fitness-related programs and activities and sit back and wait for prospective members to sign up. In reality, however, individual participation in such offerings does not occur automatically. Positive steps are required to bring the product to the attention of individuals concerned with the problem and to convince them that the product has superior qualities. These steps take planning, energy, and judgment—precisely the qualities that constitute the core of sound business practices. The framework for these efforts is a proper understanding and efficient application of fundamental marketing principles.

Almost every individual in the field of exercise and fitness is cast, by the very nature of the voluntary aspect of fitness-related programs, into the role of marketing manager. As such, not only is it necessary for an exercise professional to develop an inclusive offering of fitness-related activities and programs, it is also a professional responsibility to encourage participation through whatever managerial means are appropriate.

What is meant by the term appropriate managerial means? The literature suggests that administrative efforts are most effective when planned and carried out on an integrated basis. To achieve this goal, exercise professionals must answer an extremely difficult and sometimes complex question: **What is the product the organization offers to potential clients?** The response to this question provides the focal point of the marketing effort. Is the product merely an opportunity to participate in any of a vast listing of fitness-related activities? The point can be made that anyone who tenders this severely narrow interpretation of exercise has a seriously limited view of the health–fitness profession. Someone once asked Charles Revson, the cosmetic king, about his product, and he replied, "In the factory we make cosmetics, but in the drugstore, we sell hope."

Like Revson, exercise professionals offer more than the obvious prepackaged product. In a real and yet somewhat abstract sense, participation in fitness-related activities and programs serves as the means by which different participants achieve different ends: health, fun, excitement, diversion, weight control, mental health, friendship, self-esteem, peer acceptance, and rehabilitation, to name just a few. In one major way, whatever view of a product a potential participant has is critical only to the extent that it affects the desire to become actively involved with the product. Fortunately, for whatever reason an individual engages in a fitness-related program, the benefits of exercising on a regular basis accrue regardless of awareness or interest in those benefits.

The key point is that as more professionals understand and are sensitive to how others view the product, the better able they will be to influence the behavior of those individuals toward a particular objective (e.g., sign up for a membership, purchase a special service). Affecting behavior, however, can be difficult. Consciously arranging sales and promotional efforts through a variety of messages and a choice of specific channels to achieve a calculated effect on the attitude or behavior of a specific audience or individual is a complicated task at best. Unfortunately, this task is sometimes further complicated when exercise professionals fail to employ fundamental marketing principles.

This chapter illustrates how marketing theory can aid

exercise professionals in the discharge of their professional responsibilities. Five broad areas are examined:

1. Conceptualizing marketing management
2. Analyzing marketing opportunities
3. Organizing for marketing
4. Targeting a particular market
5. Planning a successful marketing program

CONCEPTUALIZING MARKETING MANAGEMENT

Americans are subjected to a wide variety of marketing efforts. From coast to coast, these efforts permeate almost every facet of daily life. However, recent marketing efforts have spread far beyond the traditional abode of giant corporations such as Coca Cola, General Motors, and Microsoft. In fact, the practice of product marketing has become fashionable in a variety of endeavors. Cultural concerns are turning to marketing. Increasingly, museums, symphonies, and libraries are redefining services and products in terms of what people desire and are turning to more sophisticated approaches to packaging, distributing, promoting, and communicating in reaching out to the public. A listing of examples to show the relevance of marketing efforts could be endless, but the basic implication is the same: whenever ideas and causes compete for attention or any other specified response, marketing can be useful.

Once exercise professionals accept the precept that marketing is an essential aspect of everyday duties, one of the initial steps is to develop a fundamental definition of marketing and market management. Although a variety of definitions and perspectives of marketing are possible, a core definition of marketing is as follows: **Marketing is the set of human activities directed at facilitating and consummating exchanges.** This definition suggests (intuitively) that at least three elements must be present to define a marketing situation:

- Two or more parties are or may be interested in exchange.
- Each party possesses things of value to the other.
- Each party is capable of communication and delivery.

Certainly, the setting of a commercial fitness organization can accommodate these criteria. The parties who are interested in exchange are the staff (as either a total or partial entity) and the various elements of the community that the organization is attempting to serve (young professionals, overweight individuals, women, older adults, and so on).

Note that the suggested definition of marketing deliberately avoids specifying what is being exchanged. Each participant exchanges (in varying degrees) several things, including time, energy, commitment, sociopsychological attachments, and in most cases, money.

The pertinence of the third and last element of marketing is obvious. If the segments of a market were unable to communicate and unable to exchange their goods and services, commercial fitness organizations would simply not exist.

Once the core premise of marketing is identified as centering on exchange, market management can be interpreted as an action approach based on principles for improving the effectiveness of exchange. A more explicit definition of market management is that **marketing management consists of the analysis, planning, implementation, and control of programs designed to bring about desired exchanges with target audiences for the purpose of personal or mutual gain.** In other words, for the exercise professional, sound marketing management is the collective efforts to enhance the carrying out of exchange relationships.

Within commercial fitness organizations, a variety of attitudes and philosophies are often held by various staff members regarding marketing management and its importance in the total picture of daily operations. Exercise professionals, for example, may view marketing as largely a problem of influencing others or as an issue of serving others; marketing may be perceived as a small or a large part of the job; they can see it as a commonsense task or as a skilled practice. All of these attitudes are influenced (and therefore explained) to some extent by the goals, resources, and particular circumstances attendant to each role within an organization.

ANALYZING MARKET OPPORTUNITIES

Before exercise professionals can organize and plan a marketing program, an analysis of market opportunities is required. This responsibility has at least four elements:

- Identifying and applying the marketing concept
- Examining the marketing environment of the organization
- Appraising the concept of marketing opportunity
- Analyzing the dimensions of a commercial fitness organization's market

The Marketing Concept

On a broad basis, the marketing concept is an administrative approach to achieving organizational goals by meeting customer needs and generating customer satisfaction. This concept contrasts with the traditional sales approach, which focuses on the product rather than on needs of the customer. The basic differences between the two approaches in a commercial fitness organization setting are illustrated in Figure 80.1. Obviously, the choice between the two concepts as a basis for marketing efforts has a significant effect on the methods employed to operate the organization. For example, the traditional sales approach starts with an existing program of activity offerings

FOCUS	MEANS	END
Traditional "sales" concept		
Traditional activity and program offering	Drop-in signups, flyers to organized groups, etc.	Involvement through inherent attractiveness of the activities
Marketing concept		
Customer needs	Integrated marketing	Involvement through customer satisfaction

Figure 80.1. A contrast between the traditional sales concept and the marketing concept in a commercial fitness organization.

and considers the primary task to be using promotional means to stimulate member participation. The marketing concept, on the other hand, starts with existing and potential participants and their needs, designs a coordinated set of services and programs to serve those needs, and attempts to build member involvement by creating meaningful value satisfactions within those services and programs.

Since adhering to a marketing approach may be a novel undertaking for many exercise professionals, the three pillars of the marketing concept should be examined in more detail. The first cornerstone is **customer orientation**. The marketing concept requires a basic reorientation by a commercial fitness organization from looking inward at various activity and program offerings to looking outward toward the needs of potential clients. Several steps can be undertaken by exercise professionals who truly wish to use a customer-oriented approach, including the following:

- Defining the basic needs that the commercial fitness organization intends to serve and satisfy customers within particular segments of a community.
- Identifying groups and specific needs within each group that the organization will attempt to serve while taking into consideration limitations, such as finances, facility, or personnel, that may affect the efforts of any organization to achieve stated goals. This practice (described in marketing theory as target groups definition) may be used to establish an orderly determination of organizational priorities.
- Developing a variety of services, activities, and programs to meet the needs of groups selected as targets. For example, if a commercial fitness organization wants to attract and involve individuals who have previously been almost totally sedentary, the marketing efforts should be designed and implemented in a manner conducive to this specific group.
- Measuring, evaluating, and interpreting wants, attitudes, and behaviors of the target groups. Although a

number of actions can be undertaken to help accomplish this, one of the most positive steps is to work with and seek input from outside professionals who can help interpret data collected on the target groups (e.g., aging specialists, psychologists, wellness experts, marketing theorists).

The second pillar of the marketing concept, **integrated marketing**, involves several factors. First, all staff and personnel within an organization should appreciate the fact that customer (member) satisfaction is everyone's responsibility. The key point is that **everyone** within a fitness organization has a profound effect on the efforts to attract and sustain member participation. Integrated marketing also implies that exercise professionals should rationally and logically coordinate organizational efforts to facilitate the exchange relationship. For example, all promotional efforts for an activity or program should be planned to occur at the most effective time and in the most conducive manner to maximize participation levels.

The third and last pillar of the marketing concept is the amount of **customer satisfaction** that an organization can generate. The barometer for this factor must be more than just a cursory examination of the number of participants in a program offering; rather, it requires that exercise professionals engage in a continual evaluation of the organization's activity and program offerings.

The Marketing Environment

The next appropriate task is to examine the marketing environment of the commercial fitness organization. The literature suggests that since the rate of change in the environment usually outstrips the rate of change within the organization, the organization is constantly left in a maladapted state. The implication is that the organization must either continually adapt to the changing environment or be overwhelmed by it. A passive organization can face severe conflicts and difficulties; an adaptive organization tends to survive and enjoy a degree of modest prosperity; a creative department most often flourishes and in some instances contributes to the changes occurring in its external environment.

What is meant by the term marketing environment? For a commercial fitness organization, the marketing environment is the totality of forces and entities that surround and potentially affect the marketing of the activity and program offerings. The four layers of the marketing environment for a commercial fitness organization are illustrated in Figure 80.2.

The variety of situational factors attendant to each circumstance makes an inclusive discussion of each potential element in the environment impossible. What is necessary, however, is that exercise professionals attempt to conceptualize what factors constitute the organizational

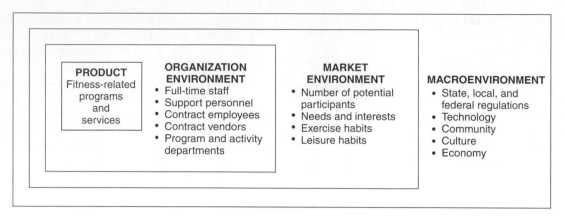

Figure 80.2. The four layers of the marketing environment for a commercial fitness organization.

environment. As the environment changes, the organization must adapt or respond to these changes creatively. Too often, organizations are excessively rigid in actions and approaches to selling products. As the environment changes, more suitable administrative means must be considered and implemented if appropriate.

It is important that exercise professionals view change in a positive light. Change should not be perceived as a threat. Rather (as the literature suggests), change should be regarded as a veiled opportunity, rather than a veiled threat. In that regard, such opportunities should be considered as marketing opportunities. To deal effectively with such possibilities requires an administrative effort at what is collectively referred to as opportunity analysis. To accomplish this objective, the exercise professional should develop procedures for identifying, appraising, and responding to these opportunities. This task is facilitated greatly when an organization has a clear sense of its goals, resources, and capabilities.

The Commercial Market

The term market has various meanings and uses. To a stockbroker, the market is the place where stocks are traded. To a produce merchant, the market is a location in a city where produce is received and sold. To a market theorist, the market is all individuals and organizations who are actual or potential customers for a product or service. It is in the last sense that this section examines the dimensions of a fitness market. A fitness market consists of all members of the community (and in some cases, adjacent communities) who are actual or potential participants in the activity and program offerings of the organization.

Although markets for fitness organizations frequently exhibit vast differences from one geographical location to another, some commercial elements that are common to all markets can be examined to determine how to approach specific markets effectively. The literature suggests that the major elements of a market can be categorized

into mnemonics: the four O's (marketing objects, objectives, organizations, and operations). The four O's answer these questions:

1. What does the market buy?
2. Why does it buy?
3. Who buys?
4. How does the market buy?

In turn, the four O's are interrelated with another set of mnemonics: the four P's of the marketing mix (price, product, promotion, place). The marketing mix consists of the major market decision variables.

Figure 80.3 illustrates the relationship between the four O's and the four P's in the setting for a commercial fitness organization. Collectively, these elements provide an organization with the framework for accomplishing specific marketing objectives. In this regard, exercise professionals face at least two main tasks within the commercial fitness market. First, the target markets must be selected, a task that requires the ability to measure opportunities and assess responsibilities in different segments (the four O's). Second, the appropriate market mix (the four P's) must be selected, a task that entails the ability to assess the requirements of various market segments.

ORGANIZING FOR MARKETING

The previous two sections of this chapter identified and defined several of the parameters of marketing management and examined some dimensions of market opportunities. Having discussed the need and potential benefits of marketing input in the organization, this section addresses how a commercial fitness organization can provide for such input.

Not all fitness-related organizations have the resources to employ a staff member assigned full-time to monitor marketing input. On the other hand, some arrangement should be made to ensure that the structure of an organization does not inhibit (as opposed to actively facilitate) the influence of sound marketing principles. A host of factors can affect organizational structure to ensure that marketing efforts are successful. They include the following:

- Company objectives
- Management philosophy
- Management view of marketing
- Utility of marketing tools
- Products, services, and programs offered by the organization
- The unique character of the competition

Within commercial fitness organizations, at least three arrangements that can provide marketing input seem

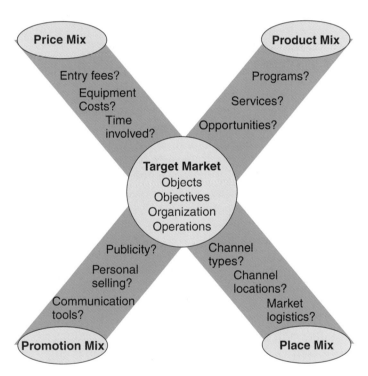

Figure 80.3. The four O's and the four P's in a commercial fitness organization.

plausible. Each of these three marketing arrangements (by program offering, by target market, and by function) can achieve certain advantages for an organization while exposing it to a few disadvantages.

In program offering, a staff member assigned to a specific area of activities or programming (e.g., aerobics, spinning, weight training) is held responsible for marketing strategy within that bailiwick. Interactivity or inter-program marketing strategy is coordinated by the managing director, by staff meetings, by departmental policies, or by some other method of direct communication.

When marketing input is solicited on the basis of target markets, organization staff who are most familiar with a particular target market are usually assigned this responsibility. A staff member with experience working with the elderly, for example, would help analyze the older adult market; a certified athletic trainer, the rehab market, and so on.

The final arrangement, for organizing marketing input by function, is to assign someone on a full- or part-time basis to coordinate marketing efforts for all activity and program offerings. This could be a staff member with a business orientation or experience or someone specifically trained or educated in marketing principles.

Regardless of who is assigned the responsibility for marketing within an organization, the arrangement must include a system or procedure for the orderly collection and use of marketing information. Figure 80.4 presents an overview of the primary elements of a marketing information system constructed within the setting for a commercial fitness organization. On the basis of information obtained, professionals can develop plans and programs that are consistent with organizational goals.

TARGETING A PARTICULAR MARKET

Of all the marketing tasks that a commercial fitness organization must undertake, perhaps none is more important than delineating appropriate target markets. Obviously, if an organization is unable to reach its market, its ability to operate effectively and profitably is severely hindered. Target markets are broadly defined as segments of

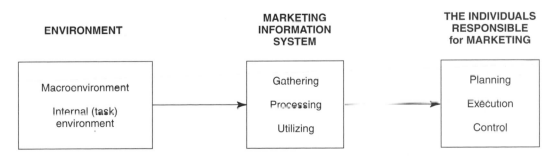

Figure 80.4. Components of a marketing information system.

the market with people having the necessary purchasing power and the general willingness to buy specific products and services.

Taking steps to ensure that a business operates in an environment where enough customers are willing and able to pay for products and services is the essence of the consumer-oriented philosophy known as the marketing concept. This philosophy focuses efforts on determining the needs and wants of target markets and satisfying customers in those markets while meeting its profit goals.

The implications of the marketing concept to fitness professionals are both simple and profound. All successful marketing efforts reach out to satisfy the needs and wants of customers, whether purposefully or blindly. Consequently, such efforts should initially attempt to convert interest to an intent to purchase a particular item (e.g., a service or a product) and then to an actual sale. In other words, all marketing efforts should be geared to produce satisfied customers at a profit for the organization. Before exercise professionals can make this goal a reality by selecting and developing a strategy to satisfy a particular target market, appropriate target markets must be identified and segmented.

Identifying General Markets

People are the key element in market identification. Exercise professionals must remember that potential customers include individuals, groups, and organizations. Collectively, everyone is a potential customer in two broad types of markets, commonly referred to as the **consumer market** and the **industrial market**. Fitness professionals need to keep in mind that products and services may be perceived quite differently within each broad market.

The consumer market is composed of individuals who buy products and services for personal use and satisfaction. For most fitness and health clubs, this broad market constitutes the vast majority of both membership and income. The consumer market is complex, with so many characteristics and influences (e.g., age, occupation, income level, lifestyle, attitude, educational background, and social group) that most successful marketing efforts only attempt to reach and focus on parts. The industrial market, on the other hand, is made up of businesses and organizations that may only require specific products and services to satisfy a particular need or objective. For the fitness and health club, the industrial market may be an important (yet relatively untapped) market. Lowering health and medical costs, serving as a recruiting tool, and offering employees specific benefits are among the reasons most commonly advanced for business involvement in commercial fitness programs.

Segmenting Markets

Market segmentation is the process of dividing the total market into smaller homogeneous buyer groups, including customers with similar characteristics. In recent years, segmenting the market into target markets has emerged as the dominant feature of marketing, because organizational resources can be more efficiently channeled to meet expectations and needs of a specific group. Each targeted segment consists of individuals who share more similar behaviors, lifestyles, and goals than the overall market. For example, the older adult population is usually more concerned with the benefits of regular exercise relating to the maintenance of an independent lifestyle than younger individuals.

To a fitness professional interested and involved in marketing, the question is not whether to segment the market, but to what degree it should be segmented. The literature suggests four questions than can be used to select target market segments:

- Is the segment measurable?
- Is it large enough?
- Is it reachable?
- Is it responsive?

Each potential target market can be rated on the basis of these criteria (Fig. 80.5) The most desirable segments are those with a positive answer to all four questions.

Some factors for segmentation are easily identified and measured; some are not. Age, gender, income level, educational background, and occupation are examples of relatively easy-to-measure parameters. Lifestyles, attitudes, and self-concepts, on the other hand, are difficult to quantify.

A target segment must have a sufficient number of potential customers to permit a profitable sales volume. Competition and market share must also be considered. For example, someone interested in opening and operating a commercial fitness establishment takes into account

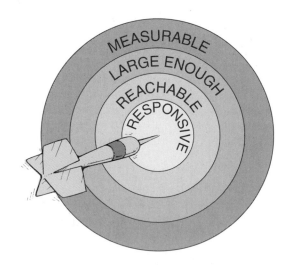

Figure 80.5. Four criteria for a targetable market.

size of the market and growth potential before deciding to build a fitness club in a community that already has several similar facilities. The key factor is the number of customers an organization can attract to its product and services. All identifiable target segments can be reached. Exercise professionals must be able to answer two basic questions in this regard, however:

1. What is the best method for communication with a specific target segment?
2. How much will it cost?

In the final analysis, the ultimate decision involves the key criterion: profitability.

Are the people in this target segment willing to buy the products and services? Is it feasible to develop a marketable product or service and a strategy for selling these products and services that will give an organization a perceived advantage over other organizations with similar products and services? The challenge is to identify consumer needs and wants and then to provide it at a price they are willing to pay. Marketing studies document the fact that people are responsive when needs and wants are satisfied. For example, some individuals question the wide popularity of independent stair climbing machines. Several of the reasons advanced, including safety, convenience, enjoyment, and variety illustrate the concept of consumer responsiveness in action.

Even with satisfactory answers to questions imposed by the four criteria for market segmentation, the process of identifying appropriate market segments can be a challenging task. At best, markets are complicated, constantly changing entities. To be successful, exercise professionals need to employ the best methods available to identify and define markets. The relatively popular methods of trial and error, intuition, and copying the techniques and focuses of other individuals are often ineffective. Although no single method has been found to work in all situations, the literature suggests at least four effective approaches to market segmentation:

- Demographic
- Geographic
- Psychographic
- Behavioral

Demographic Segmentation

When the market is divided demographically, target groups are identified by variables such as age, gender, income, occupation, education, and household. Such variables are relatively accessible and easy to quantify. Demographic variables are often used to shape the size and features of a market segment even when nondemographic factors, such as lifestyle, are also used. In fact, demographic variables often need support from other factors to identify an appropriate segment. For example, a physi-

cally active group of individuals with a high degree of disposable income may constitute an excellent target market.

Geographic Segmentation

Where consumers live and work strongly affects needs, wants, and behavioral patterns. Subdivision, urban living, commuting distance, county, state, and related variables become the basis for geographic segmentation. If convenience is an important factor in deciding where and when someone exercises, the location of the fitness center relative to the workplace and the residence becomes a marketing consideration. By the same token, if a fitness center is in a geographic region where either snow or sunshine is present for most of the year, the organization should (and probably will) gear some products and services to the climate.

Psychographic Segmentation

Psychographic variables include such factors as lifestyle, personality, attitudes, self-concept, and other psychological influences on consumer behavior. Although such variables are fairly difficult to obtain and measure, psychographic information is critical to understanding consumer interests, traits they possess that influence behavior, and how they see themselves.

Behavioral Segmentation

In this approach, consumers are grouped behaviorally according to response to specific features of products and services and to benefits they may desire from those products and services. In the fitness and health club arena, several examples illustrate behavioral segmentation, including the 30-minute workout, the $99 yearly membership, and exercise programs focused on losing weight.

Identifying Target Markets

Marketing strategies aimed at everyone and all groups in a total market seldom succeed. Results-oriented marketers understand the importance of knowing the characteristics of potential markets. Concurrently, they can successfully implement techniques to identify important target segments within the total market and design a specific marketing mix to appeal to each target segment. The fundamental benefit to the fitness and health club is more aggregate sales and profits from satisfying selected segments than from unfocused attempts on the total market.

PLANNING A SUCCESSFUL MARKETING PROGRAM

Proper planning and preparation must occur before exercise professionals can act purposefully and effectively to achieve organizational goals. Planning is deciding in the present what to do in the future. It involves both determining a desired future and taking the necessary steps to bring it about. Collectively, it is a process whereby the decision makers of an organization reconcile resources with goals and opportunities. All organizations carry out some planning. The preparation of an annual budget, for example, is planning.

Commercial fitness organizations vary considerably in how extensively, thoroughly, and formally they plan marketing. It is indisputable, however, that proper planning for a marketing program can yield positive results. Though planning can be overdone, excessive efforts are usually not a problem in a commercial fitness organization. Rather, the main issue is the development of appropriate planning procedures and systems to enhance organizationwide participation and to find the competence to carry out these procedures.

If proper procedures are identified and implemented, several distinct benefits from such planning accrue:

- Systematic, before-the-fact thinking by management
- Better coordination of organizational efforts
- Development of performance standards for control
- Sharpen guiding objectives and policies
- Better preparation for sudden and unexpected situations
- A more vivid sense of interacting responsibilities in staff members who participate in planning

The "Truths" of Human Behavior

A successful marketing plan focuses on several fundamental truths concerning business behavior, including the following:

- Most purchase decisions are made unconsciously. Individuals do not react as quickly to promotional efforts as an organization might prefer. Even when individuals finally act, the reason may be unknown.
- Marketing efforts can be almost twice as effective if they are directed at both right-brained and left-brained individuals. Marketing efforts that do not take into account brain orientation of the audience are irresponsible, outdated, wasteful, and ill-advised. About 45% of people are right-brained (influenced by emotional, aesthetic appeals). A comparable number are left-brained individuals, who respond to logical, sequential reasoning. The remainder (10%) are balanced brained.
- Documented data on individual attitudes and values can provide substantial assistance to marketing efforts. Fitness organizations should address marketing efforts to the value structure of the customer base. Health–fitness organizations must recognize that these values may change periodically.
- Sales can be influenced by two bonds—the human bond and business bond. Both positive relationships and basic business considerations affect sales. If all other factors are equal, people prefer to do business with someone with whom they have a human bond, rather than with someone with whom they do not. A human bond involves any act on the part of the organization that reinforces a caring attitude about the consumer and meets individual specific needs.

- One of the most basic human needs is identity. An organization should recognize that each of its customers is a unique person with special qualities and avoid treating individuals as prospects. Potential clients are more than simply members of a particular demographic group: they are people.
- People have a basic need to belong. Steps should be undertaken to intensify that feeling for members of a health–fitness club (e.g., frequent mailings, personal service, first name greetings).
- Customers buy more than merely an organizational product or service. The organization is selling the total of the organization and its employees. In addition to a specific product, the decision to purchase is often influenced by other factors, including reputation, service policies, status of the offerings, personalities and appearance of employees, and the physical facility.
- People tend to remember the most fascinating element of a marketing effort, not necessarily the product or service being marketed. The organization needs a "share of mind" before it can earn a "share of market." To interest prospective customers, relate offerings directly to them so that the product or service is the most interesting part of the message.

The "Truths" of Marketing

Understanding the disparity between a marketing myth and reality may mean the difference between success and failure in efforts to be competitive. As a result, managers whose goal is to devise and implement a marketing plan designed to transform prospects into customers must be acutely aware of the "truths" of marketing. Exercise professionals should consider that the ever-changing body of knowledge relating to marketing often transforms the marketing reality of today into the marketing myth of tomorrow. Knowing which is myth and which is reality can provide the basis for a successful marketing effort. Accordingly, one of the critical steps for developing insight into an effective approach to marketing involves examining common marketing myths. Some of those are discussed next.

1. *Myth:* Advertisements, brochures, and other printed materials should have a lot of white space.
   Reality: Printed materials should attract attention with substance rather than emptiness. Open space may have aesthetic appeal, but there are more intelligent ways of using marketing space aesthetically than leaving it blank.
2. *Myth:* Customers won't read long copy.
   Reality: People will read whatever interests them. The more it interests them, the more they want. The

last thing an organization wants to deny a reader is sufficient information about products and services.

3. *Myth:* Radio and television time is costly.
   Reality: Advertising time on radio and TV does not have to be costly. In some markets, for example, the cost of such advertising is less than $5 per minute.

4. *Myth:* Sell the sizzle, not the steak.
   Reality: The easiest approach for selling a product (or a service) is to offer it as a solution to a problem. As a result, an organization should focus first on the customer and identify the problem, then sell the solution, not the sizzle.

5. *Myth:* Great marketing should work instantly.
   Reality: Price-sensitive sales may generate instant sales, but successful marketing is geared to a longer-term perspective. Great marketing focuses on creating demand (desire) in the minds of qualified prospects for an offering, not on instant profits.

6. *Myth:* Marketing should entertain and amuse.
   Reality: Marketing efforts should be designed to sell a product. Show business, not marketing, should entertain and amuse.

7. *Myth:* Marketing should be changed periodically to keep it fresh and new.
   Reality: The longer great marketing promotes a product or service, the better it will be. ("You're in good hands with Allstate.")

8. *Myth:* Marketing is successful if it is memorable.
   Reality: The memorability of a marketing effort has nothing to do with the results. Marketing is successful if it facilitates the exchange process with the customer at a profit.

9. *Myth:* Stories of a public relations nature have a short life span.
   Reality: A good public relations story has a short life span only if an organization lets it die. A favorable story about a business has extended marketing value.

10. *Myth:* Bad publicity is better than no publicity.
    Reality: No publicity is a lot healthier for an organization than bad publicity. Bad publicity is bad for business no manner what the circumstance.

11. *Myth:* Word-of-mouth marketing is all a successful business needs.
    Reality: Even if an organization offers so much quality and service that word-of-mouth marketing is a potent source of promotion, it should not be solely relied upon.

12. *Myth:* The main objective of marketing is to generate maximum sales volume.
    Reality: The fundamental underlying purpose of marketing is to generate maximum profits, not maximum sales.

13. *Myth:* Quality is the primary factor that influences sales.
    Reality: Unfortunately, quality alone does not en-

tirely influence sales. Sales are also a byproduct of how well an organization treats the customer.

14. *Myth:* A sale of some kind is a critical element of marketing.
    Reality: Reduced-price sales reduce profit margins, often undermine organizational credibility, and blunt motivation for developing creative marketing ideas.

15. *Myth:* Once a business has a strong customer base, it can cease marketing.
    Reality: While an organization may either reduce marketing thrust somewhat or rechannel marketing focus once it develops a substantial customer base, marketing is an ongoing process that must be an integral part of a business plan during the lifetime of an organization.

16. *Myth:* Effective marketing often requires more than an organization can afford.
    Reality: An organization can market relatively well within any size budget. Effective marketing can be tailored to the financial reality of any budget.

17. *Myth:* An organization's marketing efforts should use as many forms of media as possible.
    Reality: If an organization cannot employ a medium properly, it should not use it. An organization should remember not to spread its message, or its resources, too thinly.

18. *Myth:* The repetition of a marketing message is boring to customers.
    Reality: Repetition implants the benefits of a particular product or service in the unconscious minds of prospective customers. Repetition also reaffirms those messages in the conscious minds of prospective customers.

19. *Myth:* Marketing is too complex to be controlled.
    Reality: Effective marketing is not too complicated to be properly managed. Effective marketing is a relatively straightforward task that enables an organization to channel time, effort, and imagination to take full advantage of opportunities in the marketplace.

20. *Myth:* All that really matters in marketing is selling the product or service and earning an honest profit.
    Reality: Marketing is an ongoing process that should be designed to educate, inform, enlighten, and influence human behavior. Good taste and sensitivity to the customer also count.

► SUMMARY

Some individuals perceive marketing as simply persuading people to do what they were already inclined to do. Conceptually, this definition may make sense to some; however, in operation it fails to address the complexity of the exchange process. In the current marketplace, if an organization does not know who, what, and where the prospective customers are or if it fails to implement a co-ordinated strategy to pursue customers as individuals, it will lose valuable ground to competitors who do.

Adhering to sound marketing practices can help ensure that organizational actions are appropriate to the competitive environment. By enabling an organization to effectively reach out to customers, sound marketing practices allow it to serve members better and to operate at an acceptable level of profitability. What better goal could an organization hope to achieve?

Suggested Reading

Beresford L et. al. Marketing 101: Experts share their newest—and hottest—marketing tips. Entrepreneur 24(5):104, 1996.

Clancy KJ. Marketing Myths That Are Killing Business: The Cure for Death Wish Marketing. New York: McGraw-Hill, 1994.

Edwards P, Edwards S, Douglas LC. Getting Business to Come to You: Everything You Need to Know to Do Your Own Advertising, Public Relations, Direct Mail, and Sales Promotion, and Attract All the Business You Can Handle. New York: Putnam, 1991.

Furlong CB. Marketing for Keeps: Building Your Business by Retaining Your Customers. New York: Wiley, 1993.

Gale BT. Managing Customer Value: Creating Quality and Service That Customers Can See. New York: Maxwell MacMillan, 1994.

Gerson RF. The Fitness Director's Guide to Marketing Strategies and Tactics. Canton, OH: Professional Reports, 1992.

Gumpert DE. How to Really Create a Successful Marketing Plan. Boston: Inc. Publishing, 1994.

Hamper RJ. Strategic Market Planning. Lincolnwood: NTC Business Books, 1990.

Horowitz S. Marketing Without Megabucks: How to Sell Anything on a Shoestring. New York: Simon & Schuster, 1993.

Kotler P, Armstrong. G. Principles of Marketing. 5th ed. Englewood Cliffs, NJ: Prentice-Hall, 1991.

Levinson JC. Guerilla Marketing Attack. Boston: Houghton Mifflin, 1989.

Levinson JC. Lethal Weapons. Entrepreneur 24(6):97, 1996.

Levinson JC, True lies: Clearing up the misconceptions about marketing. Entrepreneur 24(8):82, 1996.

Mullich J. Vertical segmentation gets more emphasis: Survey reveals companies target an average of 20.4 niches. Advertising Age 67(24):S10, 1996.

Peterson JA, Peterson SL. Target marketing. Fitness Manag A3:32, 1991.

Pinson L. Target Marketing: Researching, Reaching, and Retaining Your Target Market. Chicago: Upstart, 1996.

Pride WM, Ferrell OC. Marketing: Concepts and Strategies. 7th ed. Boston: Houghton Mifflin, 1991.

Ries A. The 22 Immutable Laws of Marketing: Violate Them at Your Own Risk. New York: Harper Business, 1993.

Sattler TP, Doniek CA. How to promote your facility through advertising. Fitness Manag H1:43, 1994.

Treacy M, Wiersema F. The Discipline of Market Leaders. Reading, PA: Addison-Wesley, 1995.

Tripps DG, Peterson JA, Bryant CX. Breakthrough strategy for successful marketing. Fitness Manag A4:24, 1992.

Wehling B. The future of marketing: What every marketer should know about being online. Vital Speeches 62(6):170, 1996.

Zaiss CD, Thomas G. Sales Effectiveness Training: The Breakthrough Method to Become Partners with Your Customers. New York: Dutton, 1993.

Ziglar Z. Zig Ziglar's Secrets of Closing the Sale. New York: Berkley Books, 1985.

COMPENDIUM OF PHYSICAL ACTIVITIES: CLASSIFICATION OF ENERGY COSTS OF HUMAN PHYSICAL ACTIVITIES

Barbare E. Ainsworth, William L. Haskell, Arther S. Leon, David R. Jacobs, Jr., Henry J. Montoye, James F. Sallis, and Ralph S. Paffenbarger, Jr.

Division of Epidemiology, School of Public Health (B.E.A., D.R.J., A.S.L.) and Division of Kinesiology.
School of Kinesiology and Leisure Sciences (B.E.A., A.S.L.), University of Minnesota, Minneapolis, MN 55455; Stanford Center for Research in Disease Prevention.
Stanford, CA 94305 (W.L.H); Biodynamics Laboratory, Department of Physical Education.
University of Wisconsin-Madison, Madison WI 53706 (H.J.M.); Child and Family Development Health Studies, Department of Pediatrics.
University of California-San Diego, La Jolla, CA 92093 (J.F.S.); and School of Medicine, Stanford University, Stanford, CA 94305 (R.S.P.)

ABSTRACT

Ainsworth BE, Haskell WL, Leon AS, et al. Compendium of Physical Activities: classification energy costs of human physical activities. Med Sci Sports Exerc 1993;1:71–80.

A coding scheme is presented for classifying physical activity by rate of energy expenditure (i.e., by intensity). Energy cost was established by a review of published and unpublished data. This coding scheme employs five digits that classify activity by purpose (i.e., sports, occupation, self-care), the specific type of activity, and its intensity as the ratio of work metabolic rate to resting metabolic rate (METs). Energy expenditure in kilocalories or kilocalories per kilogram body weight can be estimated for all activities, specific activities, or activity types. General use of this coding system would enhance the comparability of results across studies using self reports of physical activity.

EXERCISE, EXERTION, PHYSICAL ACTIVITY

The proliferation of self-report measures of physical activity reflects growing interest in the study of physical activity and its relation to various health outcomes. A common problem faced by researchers is the coding of physical activities by type and intensity. Each researcher has devised a coding system to fit his or her purposes. While there are similarities across published systems, there are also differences that limit the comparability of results across studies and add confusion to the field. The availability of a comprehensive list of physical activities coded with a standardized system that is flexible enough to meet multiple needs of physical activity researchers would facilitate research in this area.

This Compendium of Physical Activities has been developed to facilitate the coding of physical activities and to promote comparability of coding across studies. The Compendium is designed to be useful for investigators who collect data on physical activity by diary, recall, or direct observation methods. The physical activity data may be used to describe activity patterns of populations, to study determinants of physical activity, or to investigate the relations between physical activity, health, and disease. Because each activity can be coded by function, specific type, and intensity, the same compendium can be used for many different purposes and in both clinical and epidemiologic studies.

The intensity or energy cost values were derived from the best available published and unpublished data. Most sources have been used extensively by investigators in the past, but this Compendium has integrated these sources and offers a single coding system that can serve as a common source for subsequent research.

CODING SCHEME

This activity classification system was a product of a multicenter Request For Applications from the Epidemiology section of the National Heart, Lung, and Blood Institute (NHLBI) for the purpose of validating physical activity measurement techniques. It provides a comprehensive system for

(text continued on page 682)

Appendix A.1 **Compendium of Physical Activities**

ACTIVITY CODING	METs USED	MAJOR HEADING	SPECIFIC ACTIVITY
01009	8.5	Bicycling	Bicycling, BMX or mountain
01010	4.0	Bicycling	Bicycling, < 10 mph, general, leisure, to work or for pleasure (T115)
01020	6.0	Bicycling	Bicycling, 10–11.9 mph, leisure, slow, light effort
01030	8.0	Bicycling	Bicycling, 12–13.9 mph, leisure, moderate effort
01040	10.0	Bicycling	Bicycling, 14–15.9 mph, racing or leisure, fast, vigorous effort
01050	12.0	Bicycling	Bicycling, 15–19 mph, racing/not drafting or >19 mph drafting, very fast, racing general
01060	16.0	Bicycling	Bicycling, > 20 mph, racing, not drafting
01070	5.0	Bicycling	Unicycling
02010	5.0	Conditioning exercise	Bicycling, stationary, general
02011	3.0	Conditioning exercise	Bicycling, stationary, 50 W, very light effort
02012	5.5	Conditioning exercise	Bicycling, stationary, 100 W, light effort
02013	7.0	Conditioning exercise	Bicycling, stationary, 150 W, moderate effort
02014	10.5	Conditioning exercise	Bicycling, stationary, 200 W, vigorous effort
02015	12.5	Conditioning exercise	Bicycling, stationary, 250 W, very vigorous effort
02020	8.0	Conditioning exercise	Calisthenics (e.g., pushups, pullups, situps), heavy, vigorous effort
02030	4.5	Conditioning exercise	Calisthenics, home exercise, light or moderate effort, general (T 150) (example: back exercises), going up & down from floor
02040	8.0	Conditioning exercise	Circuit training, general
02050	6.0	Conditioning exercise	Weight lifting (free weight, nautilus or Universal-type), power lifting or body building, vigorous effort (T 210)
02060	5.5	Conditioning exercise	Health club exercise, general (T 160)
02065	6.0	Conditioning exercise	Stair-treadmill ergometer, general
02070	9.5	Conditioning exercise	Rowing, stationary ergometer, general
02071	3.5	Conditioning exercise	Rowing, stationary, 50 W, light effort
02072	7.0	Conditioning exercise	Rowing, stationary, 100 W, moderate effort
02073	8.5	Conditioning exercise	Rowing, stationary, 150 W, vigorous effort
02074	12.0	Conditioning exercise	Rowing, stationary, 200 W, very vigorous effort
02080	9.5	Conditioning exercise	Ski machine, general
02090	6.0	Conditioning exercise	Slimnastics
02100	4.0	Conditioning exercise	Stretching, hatha yoga
02110	6.0	Conditioning exercise	Teaching aerobic exercise class
02120	4.0	Conditioning exercise	Water aerobics, water calisthenics
02130	3.0	Conditioning exercise	Weight lifting (free, nautilus or universal type), light or moderate effort, light workout, general
02135	1.0	Conditioning exercise	Whirlpool, sitting
03010	6.0	Dancing	Aerobic, ballet or modern, twist
03015	6.0	Dancing	Aerobic, general
03020	5.0	Dancing	Aerobic, low impact
03021	7.0	Dancing	Aerobic, high impact
03025	4.5	Dancing	General
03030	5.5	Dancing	Ballroom, fast (disco, folk, square) (T 125)
03040	3.0	Dancing	Ballroom, slow (e.g., waltz, foxtrot, slow dancing)
04001	4.0	Fishing and hunting	Fishing, general
04010	4.0	Fishing and hunting	Digging worms, with shovel
04020	5.0	Fishing and hunting	Fishing from river bank and walking
04030	2.5	Fishing and hunting	Fishing from boat, sitting
04040	3.5	Fishing and hunting	Fishing from river bank, standing (T 660)
04050	6.0	Fishing and hunting	Fishing in stream, in waders (T 670)
04060	2.0	Fishing and hunting	Fishing, ice, sitting
04070	2.5	Fishing and hunting	Hunting, bow and arrow or crossbow
04080	6.0	Fishing and hunting	Hunting, deer, elk, large game (T 710)
04090	2.5	Fishing and hunting	Hunting, duck, wading
04100	5.0	Fishing and hunting	Hunting, general
04110	6.0	Fishing and hunting	Hunting, pleasants or grouse (T 680)
04120	5.0	Fishing and hunting	Hunting, rabbit, squirrel, prairie chick, raccoon, small game (T 690)
04130	2.5	Fishing and hunting	Pistol shooting or trap shooting, standing
05010	2.5	Home activities	Carpet sweeping, sweeping floors
05020	4.5	Home activities	Cleaning, heavy or major (e.g., wash car, wash windows, mop, clean garage), vigorous effort
05030	3.5	Home activities	Cleaning, house or cabin, general

Appendix A.1 *(continued)*

Activity Coding	METs Used	Major Heading	Specific Activity
05040	2.5	Home activities	Cleaning, light (dusting, straightening up, vacuuming, changing linen, carrying out trash), moderate effort
05041	2.3	Home activities	Wash dishes-standing or in general (not broken into stand/walk components)
	2.3	Home activities	Wash dishes: cleaning dishes from table-walking
05050	2.5	Home activities	Cooking or food preparation-standing or sitting or in general (not broken into stand/walk components)
05051	2.5	Home activities	Serving food, setting table-implied walking or standing
05052	2.5	Home activities	Cooking or food preparation-walking
05055	2.5	Home activities	Putting away groceries (e.g., carrying groceries, shopping without a grocery cart)
05056	8.0	Home activities	Carrying groceries upstairs
05060	3.5	Home activities	Food shopping, with grocery cart
05065	2.0	Home activities	Standing-shopping (non-grocery shopping)
05066	2.3	Home activities	Walking-shopping (non-grocery shopping)
05070	2.3	Home activities	Ironing
05080	1.5	Home activities	Sitting, knitting, sewing, light wrapping (presents)
05090	2.0	Home activities	Implied standing-laundry, fold or hang clothes, put clothes in washer or dryer, packing suitcase
05095	2.3	Home activities	Implied walking-putting away clothes, gathering clothes to pack, putting away laundry
05100	2.0	Home activities	Making bed
05110	5.0	Home activities	Maple syruping/sugar bushing (including carrying buckets, carrying wood)
05120	6.0	Home activities	Moving furniture, household
05130	5.5	Home activities	Scrubbing floors, on hands and knees
05140	4.0	Home activities	Sweeping garage, sidewalk or outside of house
05145	7.0	Home activities	Moving household items, carrying boxes
05146	3.5	Home activities	Standing-packing/unpacking boxes, occasional lifting of household items light-moderate effort
05147	3.0	Home activities	Implied walking-putting away household items-moderate effort
05150	9.0	Home activities	Move household items upstairs, carrying boxes or furniture
05160	2.5	Home activities	Standing-light (pump gas, change light bulb, etc.)
05165	3.0	Home activities	Walking-light, noncleaning (ready to leave, shut/lock doors, close windows, etc.)
05170	2.5	Home activities	Sitting-playing with children-light
05171	2.8	Home activities	Standing-playing with children-light
05175	4.0	Home activities	Walk/run-playing with children-moderate
05180	5.0	Home activities	Walk/run-playing with children-vigorous
05185	3.0	Home activities	Child care: sitting/kneeling-dressing, bathing, grooming, feeding, occasional lifting of child-light effort
05186	3.5	Home activities	Child care: standing-dressing, bathing, grooming, feeding, occasional lifting of child-light effort
06010	3.0	Home repair	Airplane repair
06020	4.5	Home repair	Automobile body work
06030	3.0	Home repair	Automobile repair
06040	3.0	Home repair	Carpentry, general, workshop (T 620)
06050	6.0	Home repair	Carpentry, outside house (T 640), installing rain gutters
06060	4.5	Home repair	Carpentry, finishing or refinishing cabinets or furniture
06070	7.5	Home repair	Carpentry, sawing hardwood
06080	5.0	Home repair	Caulking, chinking log cabin
06090	4.5	Home repair	Caulking, except log cabin
06100	5.0	Home repair	Cleaning gutters
06110	5.0	Home repair	Excavating garage
06120	5.0	Home repair	Hanging storm windows
06130	4.5	Home repair	Laying or removing carpet
06140	4.5	Home repair	Laying tile or linoleum
06150	5.0	Home repair	Painting, outside house (T 650)
06160	4.5	Home repair	Painting, papering, plastering, scraping, inside house, hanging sheet rock, remodeling (T 630)
06170	3.0	Home repair	Put on and removal of tarp-sailboat
06180	6.0	Home repair	Roofing
06190	4.5	Home repair	Sanding floors with a power sander
06200	4.5	Home repair	Scrape and paint sailboat or powerboat
06210	5.0	Home repair	Spreading dirt with a shovel
06220	4.5	Home repair	Wash and wax hull of sailboat, car, powerboat, airplane

(continued)

Appendix A.1 *(continued)*

Activity Coding	METs Used	Major Heading	Specific Activity
06230	4.5	Home repair	Washing fence
06240	3.0	Home repair	Wiring, plumbing
07010	0.9	Inactivity, quiet	Lying quietly, reclining (watch television), lying quietly in bed-awake
07020	1.0	Inactivity, quiet	Sitting quietly (riding in a car, listening to a lecture or music, watch television or a movie)
07030	0.9	Inactivity, quiet	Sleeping
07040	1.2	Inactivity, quiet	Standing quietly (standing in a line)
07050	1.0	Inactivity, light	Recline-writing
07060	1.0	Inactivity, light	Recline-talking or talking on phone
07070	1.0	Inactivity, light	Recline-reading
08010	5.0	Lawn and garden	Carrying, loading or stacking wood, loading/unloading or carrying lumber
08020	6.0	Lawn and garden	Chopping wood, splitting logs
08030	5.0	Lawn and garden	Clearing land, hauling branches
08040	5.0	Lawn and garden	Digging sandbox
08050	5.0	Lawn and garden	Digging, spading, filling garden (T 590)
08060	6.0	Lawn and garden	Gardening with heavy power tools, tilling a garden (see occupation, shoveling)
08080	5.0	Lawn and garden	Laying crushed rock
08090	5.0	Lawn and garden	Laying sod
08095	5.5	Lawn and garden	Mowing lawn, general
08100	2.5	Lawn and garden	Mowing lawn, riding mower (T 550)
08110	6.0	Lawn and garden	Mowing lawn, walk, hand mower (T 570)
08120	4.5	Lawn and garden	Mowing lawn, walk, power mower (T 590)
08130	4.5	Lawn and garden	Operating snow blower, walking
08140	4.0	Lawn and garden	Planting seedlings, shrubs
08150	4.5	Lawn and garden	Planting trees
08160	4.0	Lawn and garden	Raking lawn (T 600)
08170	4.0	Lawn and garden	Raking roof with snow rake
08180	3.0	Lawn and garden	Riding snow blower
08190	4.0	Lawn and garden	Sacking grass, leaves
08200	6.0	Lawn and garden	Shoveling, snow, by hand (T 610)
08210	4.5	Lawn and garden	Trimming shrubs or trees, manual cutter
08215	3.5	Lawn and garden	Trimming shrubs or trees, power cutter
08220	2.5	Lawn and garden	Walking, applying fertilizer or seeding a lawn
08230	1.5	Lawn and garden	Watering lawn or garden, standing or walking
08240	4.5	Lawn and garden	Weeding, cultivating garden (T 580)
08245	5.0	Lawn and garden	Gardening, general
08250	3.0	Lawn and garden	Implied walking/standing-picking up yard, light
09010	1.5	Miscellaneous	Sitting, card playing, playing board games
09020	2.0	Miscellaneous	Standing-drawing (writing), casino gambling
09030	1.3	Miscellaneous	Sitting-reading, book, newspaper, etc.
09040	1.8	Miscellaneous	Sitting-writing, desk work
09050	1.8	Miscellaneous	Standing-talking or talking on the phone
09055	1.5	Miscellaneous	Sitting-talking or talking on the phone
09060	1.8	Miscellaneous	Sitting-studying, general, including reading and/or writing
09065	1.8	Miscellaneous	Sitting-in class, general, including note-taking or class discussion
09070	1.8	Miscellaneous	Standing-reading
10010	1.8	Music playing	Accordion
10020	2.0	Music playing	Cello
10030	2.5	Music playing	Conducting
10040	4.0	Music playing	Drums
10050	2.0	Music playing	Flute (sitting)
10060	2.0	Music playing	Horn
10070	2.5	Music playing	Piano or organ
10080	3.5	Music playing	Trombone
10090	2.5	Music playing	Trumpet
10100	2.5	Music playing	Violin
10110	2.0	Music playing	Woodwind
10120	2.0	Music playing	Guitar, classical, folk (sitting)
10125	3.0	Music playing	Guitar, rock and roll band (standing)
10130	4.0	Music playing	Marching band, playing an instrument, baton twirling (walking)
10135	3.5	Music playing	Marching band, drum major (walking)

Appendix A.1 *(continued)*

Activity Coding	METs Used	Major Heading	Specific Activity
11010	4.0	Occupation	Bakery, general
11020	2.3	Occupation	Bookbinding
11030	6.0	Occupation	Building road (including hauling debris, driving heavy machinery)
11035	2.0	Occupation	Building road, directing traffic (standing)
11040	3.5	Occupation	Carpentry, general
11050	8.0	Occupation	Carrying heavy loads, such as bricks
11060	8.0	Occupation	Carrying moderate loads up stairs, moving boxes (16–40 pounds)
11070	2.5	Occupation	Chambermaid
11080	6.5	Occupation	Coal mining, drilling coal, rock
11090	6.5	Occupation	Coal mining, erecting supports
11100	6.0	Occupation	Coal mining, general
11110	7.0	Occupation	Coal mining, shoveling coal
11120	5.5	Occupation	Construction, outside remodeling
11130	3.5	Occupation	Electrical work, plumbing
11140	8.0	Occupation	Farming, bailing hay, cleaning barn, poultry work
11150	3.5	Occupation	Farming, chasing cattle, nonstrenuous
11160	2.5	Occupation	Farming, driving harvester
11170	2.5	Occupation	Farming, driving tractor
11180	4.0	Occupation	Farming, feeding small animals
11190	4.5	Occupation	Farming, feeding cattle
11200	8.0	Occupation	Farming, forking straw bales
11210	3.0	Occupation	Farming, milking by hand
11220	1.5	Occupation	Farming, milking by machine
11230	5.5	Occupation	Farming, shoveling grain
11240	12.0	Occupation	Fire fighter, general
11245	11.0	Occupation	Fire fighter, climbing ladder with full gear
11246	8.0	Occupation	Fire fighter, hauling hoses on ground
11250	17.0	Occupation	Forestry, ax chopping, fast
11260	5.0	Occupation	Forestry, ax chopping, slow
11270	7.0	Occupation	Forestry, barking trees
11280	11.0	Occupation	Forestry, carrying logs
11290	8.0	Occupation	Forestry, felling trees
11300	8.0	Occupation	Forestry, general
11310	5.0	Occupation	Forestry, hoeing
11320	6.0	Occupation	Forestry, planting by hand
11330	7.0	Occupation	Forestry, sawing by hand
11340	4.5	Occupation	Forestry, sawing, power
11350	9.0	Occupation	Forestry, trimming trees
11360	4.0	Occupation	Forestry, weeding
11370	4.5	Occupation	Furriery
11380	6.0	Occupation	Horse grooming
11390	8.0	Occupation	Horse racing, galloping
11400	6.5	Occupation	Horse racing, trotting
11410	2.6	Occupation	Horse racing, walking
11420	3.5	Occupation	Locksmith
11430	2.5	Occupation	Machine tooling, machining, working sheet metal
11440	3.0	Occupation	Machine tooling, operating lathe
11450	5.0	Occupation	Machine tooling, operating punch press
11460	4.0	Occupation	Machine tooling, tapping and drilling
11470	3.0	Occupation	Machine tooling, welding
11480	7.0	Occupation	Masonry, concrete
11485	4.0	Occupation	Masseur, masseuse (standing)
11490	7.0	Occupation	Moving, pushing heavy objects, 75 lbs or more (desks, moving van work)
11500	2.5	Occupation	Operating heavy duty equipment/automated, not driving
11510	4.5	Occupation	Orange grove work
11520	2.3	Occupation	Printing (standing)
11525	2.5	Occupation	Police, directing traffic (standing)
11526	2.0	Occupation	Police, driving a squad car (sitting)
11527	1.3	Occupation	Police, riding in a squad car (sitting)
11528	8.0	Occupation	Police, making an arrest (standing)
11530	2.5	Occupation	Shoe repair, general

(continued)

Appendix A.1 *(continued)*

ACTIVITY CODING	METs USED	MAJOR HEADING	SPECIFIC ACTIVITY
11540	8.5	Occupation	Shoveling, digging ditches
11550	9.0	Occupation	Shoveling, heavy (more than 16 lbs. min⁻¹)
11560	6.0	Occupation	Shoveling, light (less than 10 lbs. min⁻¹)
11570	7.0	Occupation	Shoveling, moderate (10–15 lbs. min⁻¹)
11580	1.5	Occupation	Sitting-light office work, in general (chemistry lab work, light use of handtools, watch repair or micro-assembly, light assembly/repair)
11585	1.5	Occupation	Sitting-meetings, general, and/or with talking involved
11590	2.5	Occupation	Sitting; moderate (heavy levers, riding mower/forklift, crane operation)
11600	2.5	Occupation	Standing; light (bartending, store clerk, assembling, filing, xeroxing, put up Christmas tree)
11610	3.0	Occupation	Standing; light/moderate (assemble/repair heavy parts, welding, stocking, auto repair, pack boxes for moving, etc.), patient care (as in nursing)
11620	3.5	Occupation	Standing; moderate (assembling at fast rate, lifting 50 lbs, hitch/twisting ropes)
11630	4.0	Occupation	Standing; moderate/heavy (lifting more than 50 lb, masonry, painting, paper hanging)
11640	5.0	Occupation	Steel mill, fettling
11650	5.5	Occupation	Steel mill, forging
11660	8.0	Occupation	Steel mill, hand rolling
11670	8.0	Occupation	Steel mill, merchant mill rolling
11680	11.0	Occupation	Steel mill, removing slag
11690	7.5	Occupation	Steel mill, tending furnace
11700	5.5	Occupation	Steel mill, tipping molds
11710	8.0	Occupation	Steel mill, working in general
11720	2.5	Occupation	Tailoring, cutting
11730	2.5	Occupation	Tailoring, general
11740	2.0	Occupation	Tailoring, hand sewing
11750	2.5	Occupation	Tailoring, machine sewing
11760	4.0	Occupation	Tailoring, pressing
11766	6.5	Occupation	Truck driving, loading and unloading truck (standing)
11770	1.5	Occupation	Typing, electric, manual or computer
11780	6.0	Occupation	Using heavy power tools such as pneumatic tools (jackhammers, drills, etc.)
11790	8.0	Occupation	Using heavy tools (not power) such as shovel, pick, tunnel bar, spade
11791	2.0	Occupation	Walking on job, less than 2.0 mph (in office or lab area), very slow
11792	3.5	Occupation	Walking on job, 3.0 mph, in office, moderate speed, not carrying anything
11793	4.0	Occupation	Walking on job, 3.5 mph, in office, brisk speed, not carrying anything
11795	3.0	Occupation	Walking, 2.5 mph, slowly and carrying light objects less than 25 lbs
11800	4.0	Occupation	Walking, 3.0 mph, moderately and carrying light objects less than 25 lbs
11810	4.5	Occupation	Walking, 3.5 mph, briskly and carrying objects less than 25 lbs
11820	5.0	Occupation	Walking or walk downstairs or standing, carrying objects about 25–49 lbs
11830	6.5	Occupation	Walking or walk downstairs or standing, carrying objects about 50–74 lbs
11840	7.5	Occupation	Walking or walk downstairs or standing, carrying objects about 75–99 lbs
11850	8.5	Occupation	Walking or walk downstairs or standing, carrying objects about 100 lbs and over
11870	3.0	Occupation	Working in scene shop, theater actor, backstage, employee
12010	6.0	Running	Job/walk combination (jobbing component of less than 10 min) (T 180)
12020	7.0	Running	Jogging, general
12030	8.0	Running	Running 5 mph (12 min·mile⁻¹)
12040	9.0	Running	Running 5.2 mph (11.5 min·mile⁻¹)
12050	10.0	Running	Running 6 mph (10 min·mile⁻¹)
12060	11.0	Running	Running, 6.7 mph (9 min·mile⁻¹)
12070	11.5	Running	Running, 7 mph (8.5 min·mile⁻¹)
12080	12.5	Running	Running, 7.5 mph (8 min·mile⁻¹)
12090	13.5	Running	Running, 8 mph (7.5 min·mile⁻¹)
12100	14.0	Running	Running, 8.6 mph (7 min·mile⁻¹)
12110	15.0	Running	Running, 9 mph (6.5 min·mile⁻¹)
12120	16.0	Running	Running, 10 mph (6 min·mile⁻¹)
12130	18.0	Running	Running, 10.9 mph (5.5 min·mile⁻¹)
12140	9.0	Running	Running, cross-country
12150	8.0	Running	Running, general (T 200)
12160	8.0	Running	Running, in place
12170	15.0	Running	Running, stairs, up
12180	10.0	Running	Running, on a track, team practice

Appendix A.1 *(continued)*

ACTIVITY CODING	METs USED	MAJOR HEADING	SPECIFIC ACTIVITY
12190	8.0	Running	Running, training, pushing wheelchair, marathon wheeling
12195	3.0	Running	Running, wheeling, general
13000	2.5	Self-care	Standing-getting ready for bed, in general
13009	1.0	Self-care	Sitting on toilet
13010	2.0	Self-care	Bathing (sitting)
13020	2.5	Self-care	Dressing, undressing (standing or sitting)
13030	1.5	Self-care	Eating (sitting)
13035	2.0	Self-care	Talking and eating or eating only (standing)
13040	2.5	Self-care	Sitting or standing-grooming (washing, shaving, brushing teeth, urinating, washing hands, put on make-up)
13050	4.0	Self-care	Showering, toweling off (standing)
14010	1.5	Sexual activity	Active, vigorous effort
14020	1.3	Sexual activity	General, moderate effort
14030	1.0	Sexual activity	Passive, light effort, kissing, hugging
15010	3.5	Sports	Archery (nonhunting)
15020	7.0	Sports	Badminton, competitive (T 450)
15030	4.5	Sports	Badminton, social singles and doubles, general
15040	8.0	Sports	Basketball, game (T 490)
15050	6.0	Sports	Basketball, nongame, general (T 480)
15060	7.0	Sports	Basketball, officiating (T 500)
15070	4.5	Sports	Basketball, shooting baskets
15075	6.5	Sports	Basketball, wheelchair
15080	2.5	Sports	Billiards
15090	3.0	Sports	Bowling (T 390)
15100	12.0	Sports	Boxing, in ring, general
15110	6.0	Sports	Boxing, punching bag
15120	9.0	Sports	Boxing, sparring
15130	7.0	Sports	Broomball
15135	5.0	Sports	Children's games (hopscotch 4-square, dodgeball, playground apparatus, t-ball, tetherball, marbles, jacks, arcade games)
15140	4.0	Sports	Coaching: football, soccer, basketball, baseball, swimming, etc.
15150	5.0	Sports	Cricket (batting, bowling)
15160	2.5	Sports	Croquet
15170	4.0	Sports	Curling
15180	2.5	Sports	Darts, wall or lawn
15190	6.0	Sports	Drag racing, pushing or driving a car
15200	6.0	Sports	Fencing
15210	9.0	Sports	Football, competitive
15230	8.0	Sports	Football, touch, flag, general (T 510)
15235	2.5	Sports	Football or baseball, playing catch
15240	3.0	Sports	Frisbee playing, general
15250	3.5	Sports	Frisbee, ultimate
15255	4.5	Sports	Golf, general
15260	5.5	Sports	Golf, carrying clubs (T 090)
15270	3.0	Sports	Golf, miniature, driving range
15280	5.0	Sports	Golf, pulling clubs (T 080)
15290	3.5	Sports	Golf, using power cart (T 070)
15300	4.0	Sports	Gymnastics, general
15310	4.0	Sports	Hacky sack
15320	12.0	Sports	Handball, general (T 520)
15330	8.0	Sports	Handball, team
15340	3.5	Sports	Hang gliding
15350	8.0	Sports	Hockey, field
15360	8.0	Sports	Hockey, ice
15370	4.0	Sports	Horseback riding, general
15380	3.5	Sports	Horseback riding, saddling horse
15390	6.5	Sports	Horseback riding, trotting
15400	2.5	Sports	Horseback riding, walking
15410	3.0	Sports	Horseshoe pitching, quoits
15420	12.0	Sports	Jai alai
15430	10.0	Sports	Judo, jujitsu, karate, kick boxing, tae kwon do

(continued)

Appendix A.1 *(continued)*

Activity Coding	METs Used	Major Heading	Specific Activity
15440	4.0	Sports	Juggling
15450	7.0	Sports	Kickball
15460	8.0	Sports	Lacrosse
15470	4.0	Sports	Moto-cross
15480	9.0	Sports	Orienteering
15490	10.0	Sports	Paddleball, competitive
15500	6.0	Sports	Paddleball, casual, general (T 460)
15510	8.0	Sports	Polo
15520	10.0	Sports	Racquetball, competitive
15530	7.0	Sports	Racketball, casual, general (T 470)
15535	11.0	Sports	Rock climbing, ascending rock
15540	8.0	Sports	Rock climbing, rapelling
15550	12.0	Sports	Rope jumping, fast
15551	10.0	Sports	Rope jumping, moderate, general
15552	8.0	Sports	Rope jumping, slow
15560	10.0	Sports	Rugby
15570	3.0	Sports	Shuffleboard, lawn bowling
15580	5.0	Sports	Skateboarding
15590	7.0	Sports	Skating, roller (T 360)
15600	3.5	Sports	Sky diving
15605	10.0	Sports	Soccer, competitive
15610	7.0	Sports	Soccer, casual, general (T 540)
15620	5.0	Sports	Softball or baseball, fast or slow pitch, general (T 440)
15630	4.0	Sports	Softball, officiating
15640	6.0	Sports	Softball, pitching
15650	12.0	Sports	Squash (T 530)
15660	4.0	Sports	Table tennis, ping pong (T 410)
15670	4.0	Sports	Tai chi
15675	7.0	Sports	Tennis, general
15680	6.0	Sports	Tennis, doubles (T 430)
15690	8.0	Sports	Tennis, singles (T 420)
15700	3.5	Sports	Trampoline
15710	4.0	Sports	Volleyball, competitive, in gymnasium (T 400)
15720	3.0	Sports	Volleyball, noncompetitive; 6–9 member team, general
15725	8.0	Sports	Volleyball, beach
15730	6.0	Sports	Wrestling (one match = 5 min)
15731	7.0	Sports	Wallyball, general
16010	2.0	Transportation	Automobile or light truck (not a semi) driving
16020	2.0	Transportation	Flying airplane
16030	2.5	Transportation	Motor scooter, motor cycle
16040	6.0	Transportation	Pushing plane in and out of hangar
16050	3.0	Transportation	Driving heavy truck, tractor, bus
17010	7.0	Walking	Backpacking, general (T 050)
17020	3.5	Walking	Carrying infant or 15-lb load (e.g., suitcase), level ground or downstairs
17025	9.0	Walking	Carrying load upstairs, general
17026	5.0	Walking	Carrying 1- to 15-lb load, upstairs
17027	6.0	Walking	Carrying 16- to 24-lb load, upstairs
17028	8.0	Walking	Carrying 25- to 49-lb load, upstairs
17029	10.0	Walking	Carrying 50- to 74-lb load, upstairs
17030	12.0	Walking	Carrying 74+ lb load, upstairs
17035	7.0	Walking	Climbing hills with 0- to 9-lb load
17040	7.5	Walking	Climbing hills with 10- to 20-lb load
17050	8.0	Walking	Climbing hills with 21- to 42-lb load
17060	9.0	Walking	Climbing hills with 42+ lb load
17070	3.0	Walking	Downstairs
17080	6.0	Walking	Hiking, cross country (T 040)
17090	6.5	Walking	Marching, rapidly, military
17100	2.5	Walking	Pushing or pulling stroller with child
17110	6.5	Walking	Race walking
17120	8.0	Walking	Rock or mountain climbing (T 060)
17130	8.0	Walking	Up stairs, using or climbing up ladder (T 030)

Appendix A.1 *(continued)*

Activity Coding	METs Used	Major Heading	Specific Activity
17140	4.0	Walking	Using crutches
17150	2.0	Walking	Walking, less than 2.0 mph, level ground, strolling, household walking, very slow
17160	2.5	Walking	Walking, 2.0 mph, level, slow pace, firm surface
17170	3.0	Walking	Walking, 2.5 mph, firm surface
17180	3.0	Walking	Walking, 2.5 mph, downhill
17190	3.5	Walking	Walking, 3.0 mph, level, moderate pace, firm surface
17200	4.0	Walking	Walking, 3.5 mph, level, very brisk, firm surface
17210	6.0	Walking	Walking, 3.5 mph, uphill
17220	4.0	Walking	Walking, 4.0 mph, level, firm surface, very brisk pace
17230	4.5	Walking	Walking, 4.5 mph, level, firm surface, very, very brisk
17250	3.5	Walking	Walking, for pleasure, work break, walking the dog
17260	5.0	Walking	Walking, grass track
17270	4.0	Walking	Walking, to work or class (T 015)
18010	2.5	Water activities	Boating, power
18020	4.0	Water activities	Canoeing, on camping trip (T 270)
18030	7.0	Water activities	Canoeing, portaging
18040	3.0	Water activities	Canoeing, rowing, 2.0–3.9 mph, light effort
18050	7.0	Water activities	Canoeing, rowing, 4.0–5.9 mph, moderate effort
18060	12.0	Water activities	Canoeing, rowing, > 6 mph, vigorous effort
18070	3.5	Water activities	Canoeing, rowing, for pleasure, general (T 250)
18080	12.0	Water activities	Canoeing, rowing, in competition, or crew or sculling (T 260)
18090	3.0	Water activities	Diving, springboard or platform
18100	5.0	Water activities	Kayaking
18110	4.0	Water activities	Paddleboat
18120	3.0	Water activities	Sailing, boat and board sailing, windsurfing, ice sailing, general (T 235)
18130	5.0	Water activities	Sailing, in competition
18140	3.0	Water activities	Sailing, Sunfish/Laser/Hobby Cat, keel boats, ocean sailing, yachting
18150	6.0	Water activities	Skiing, water (I 220)
18160	7.0	Water activities	Skimobiling
18170	12.0	Water activities	Skindiving or scuba diving as frogman
18180	16.0	Water activities	Skindiving, fast
18190	12.5	Water activities	Skindiving, moderate
18200	7.0	Water activities	Skindiving, scuba diving, general (T 310)
18210	5.0	Water activities	Snorkeling (T 320)
18220	3.0	Water activities	Surfing, body or board
18230	10.0	Water activities	Swimming laps, freestyle, fast, vigorous effort
18240	8.0	Water activities	Swimming laps, freestyle, slow, moderate or light effort
18250	8.0	Water activities	Swimming, backstroke, general
18260	10.0	Water activities	Swimming, breaststroke, general
18270	11.0	Water activities	Swimming, butterfly, general
18280	11.0	Water activities	Swimming, crawl, fast (75 yards·min^{-1}) vigorous effort
18290	8.0	Water activities	Swimming, crawl, slow (50 yards·min^{-1}), moderate or light effort
18300	6.0	Water activities	Swimming, lake, ocean, river (T 280, T 295)
18310	6.0	Water activities	Swimming, leisurely, not lap swimming, general
18320	8.0	Water activities	Swimming, sidestroke, general
18330	8.0	Water activities	Swimming, synchronized
18340	10.0	Water activities	Swimming, treading water, fast vigorous effort
18350	4.0	Water activities	Swimming, treading water, moderate effort, general
18360	10.0	Water activities	Water polo
18365	3.0	Water activities	Water volleyball
18370	5.0	Water activities	Whitewater rafting, kayaking, or canoeing
19010	6.0	Winter activities	Moving ice house (set up/drill holes, etc.)
19020	5.5	Winter activities	Skating, ice, 9 mph or less
19030	7.0	Winter activities	Skating, ice, general (T 360)
19040	9.0	Winter activities	Skating, ice, rapidly, more than 9 mph
19050	15.0	Winter activities	Skating, speed, competitive
19060	7.0	Winter activities	Ski jumping (climb up carrying skis)
19075	7.0	Winter activities	Skiing, general
19080	7.0	Winter activities	Skiing, cross-country, 2.5 mph, slow or light effort, ski walking
19090	8.0	Winter activities	Skiing, cross-country, 4.0–4.9 mph, moderate speed and effort, general
19100	9.0	Winter activities	Skiing, cross-country, 5.0–7.9 mph, brisk speed, vigorous effort

(continued)

Appendix A.1 *(continued)*

ACTIVITY CODING	METs USED	MAJOR HEADING	SPECIFIC ACTIVITY
19110	14.0	Winter activities	Skiing, cross-country, > 8.0 mph, racing
19130	16.5	Winter activities	Skiing, cross-country, hard snow, uphill, maximum
19150	5.0	Winter activities	Skiing, downhill, light effort
19160	6.0	Winter activities	Skiing, downhill, moderate effort, general
19170	8.0	Winter activities	Skiing, downhill, vigorous effort, racing
19180	7.0	Winter activities	Sledding, tobogganing, bobsledding, luge (T 370)
19190	8.0	Winter activities	Snow shoeing
19200	3.5	Winter activities	Snowmobiling

coding physical data on physical activity by purpose and energy cost. The energy cost of specific activities listed in this Compendium were obtained primarily from the following previously published physical activity energy expenditure lists: Tecumseh Occupational Questionnaire (13, 14), Minnesota Leisure Time Physical Activity Questionnaire (LTPA) (5, 10), McArdle, Katch, and Katch's physical activity lists (7, 9), the 7-Day Recall Physical Activity Questionnaire (2), and the American Health Foundation's physical activity list (8). Activities from the LTPA were identified by a T followed by a number (e.g., T115). By retaining the LTPA designator codes, the new list may be used to score the LTPA with its original physical activity intensity codes.

As would be expected, there was considerable overlap in energy expenditure values among the supplied lists. For example, the Minnesota LTPA, which was developed from the Tecumseh Leisure Time Questionnaire, identifies similar activities; while the list of activities from the 7-Day Physical Activity Recall questionnaire is nearly identical to that of McArdle, Katch, and Katch (9). In general, the majority of the energy expenditure lists were generated from Passmore and Dumin (11), while McArdle, Katch, and Katch (9) also used data derived from Bannister and Brown (1) and Howley and Glover (6). The intensity assigned to activities in this publication were determined by selecting a mean energy expenditure value from the eight sources mentioned previously. The representative intensity levels were determined by consensus of the authors.

Organization

The Compendium of Physical Activities is organized to maximize flexibility in coding, data entry, and interpretation of energy cost for each class and type of activity.

The coding scheme for the Compendium of Activities employs a five-digit code in order to categorize activities by their major heading (first two digits on the left), specific activity (last three digits on the right), and intensity (3-digit column). The coding scheme is organized in the following way:

00 major headings	000 specific activity	0.0 intensity

For example:

01 bicycling	009 bmx	08.5 METs

The Compendium is organized by activity types or purpose and includes activities of daily living or self care, leisure and recreation, occupation, and rest (Table A.1). The major headings explain the reason a person is engaging in a specific activity and is useful in categorizing activity types.

Identification of the proper major heading is the initial step in classifying an activity. However, it is possible that there may be more than one reason for performing an activity; thus, a specific activity may be listed under more than one major heading. For example, an individual may sit and read a book for pleasure in one situation and at another time read a document as a job requirement. These may be classified under the major headings of rest or inactivity and occupation depending on their purpose. Assumptions made for the placement of activities into major headings are listed in Appendix A.2.

The specific activity descriptions range from a general classification of an activity (e.g., tennis, general) to a detailed description that includes the form and intensity of the activity (e.g., tennis, singles, vigorous effort) depending on

Table A.1. Major Types of Activities

Bicycling	Lawn and garden	Sexual activity
Conditioning exercises	Miscellaneous	Sports
Dancing	Music playing	Transportation
Fishing and hunting	Occupation	Walking
Home activities	Running	Water activities
Home repair	Self-Care	Winter activities
Inactivity		

Appendix A.2. Guidelines for Assigning Activities by Major Purpose or Intent

1. Conditioning exercises include activities with the intent of improving physical condition. This includes stationary ergometers (bicycling, rowing machines, treadmills, etc) health club exercise, calisthenics, and aerobics.
2. Home repair includes all activity associated with the repair of a house and does not include housework. This is not an occupational task.
3. Sleeping, lying, sitting, and standing are classified as inactivity.
4. Home activities include all activities associated with maintaining the inside of a house and includes house cleaning, laundry, grocery shopping, and cooking.
5. Lawn and garden includes all activity associated with maintaining the yard and includes yard work, gardening, and snow removal.
6. Occupation includes all job-related physical activity where one is paid (gainful employment). Specific activities may be cross-referenced in other categories (such as reading, writing, driving a car, walking) and should be coded in this major heading if related to employment. Housework is occupational only if the person is earning money for the task.
7. Self-care includes all activity related to grooming, eating, bathing, etc.
8. Transportation includes energy expended for the primary purpose of going somewhere in a motorized vehicle.

the information gathered by the survey method. Activities without a specified intensity are classified as "general". More detailed descriptions of activities are preferred since an appropriate intensity can be assigned. Guidelines for coding specific activities within major headings are listed in Appendix A.3.

All activities are assigned an intensity unit based on their rate of energy expenditure expressed as METs. The intensity of activities in the Compendium are classified as multiples of one MET or the ratio of the associated metabolic rate for the specific activity divided by the resting metabolic rate (RMR). For example, a 2-MET activity requires two times the metabolic energy expenditure of sitting quietly. One MET is also defined as the energy expenditure for sitting quietly, which for the average adult is approximately 3.5 ml of oxygen·kg body wt^{-1}·min^{-1} or 1 kcal·kg^{-1} body wt·h^{-1}.

A MET value was assigned to each activity in the Compendium and was based on the "best representation" from published lists and selected unpublished data as was previously mentioned. For activities not in the original lists, intensity was obtained from published literature, if possible, and assigned a MET value or estimated from similar known activities (3, 4, 11, 16).

Only data for adults were included in this Compendium. When children's games are listed in the Compendium, the intensity level is for adults participating in children's activities. Further, the Compendium is not intended to be used for adults with major neuromuscular handicaps or other conditions that would significantly alter their mechanical or metabolic efficiency.

Calculation of Energy Cost

Energy expenditure values can be expressed in kcal·kg^{-1} body wt·h^{-1}, kcal·min^{-1}, kcal·h^{-1} or kcal·24^{-1}. The most accurate way to determine the kilocalorie energy cost of an activity is to measure the kcal expended during rest (i.e., the RMR) and multiply that value by the MET values listed in the Compendium. Because RMR is fairly close to 1 kcal·kg body wt^{-1}·h^{-1}, the energy cost of activities may be expressed as multiples of the RMR (15). By multiplying the body weight in kg by the MET value and duration of activity, it is possible to estimate a kcal energy expenditure that is specific to a person's body weight. For example, bicycling at a 4 MET value expends 4 kcal·kg^{-1} body wt·h^{-1}. A 60 kg individual bicycling for 40 min expends the following: (4 METs × 60 kg body wt) × (40 min/60 min) = 160 kcal. Dividing 160 kcal by 40 min equals 4 kcal·min^{-1}. Using the same formula for an 80 kg person would yield an energy expenditure of 213 kcal or 5.3 kcal·min^{-1}. However, it is important to note that to the extent the RMR is not equal to 1 kcal·kg body wt^{-1}·h^{-1} for individuals, then estimates of energy expenditure that include weight will more closely reflect body weight than the metabolic rate (2).

Use of the Compendium for PA Records or Diaries

For records or diaries the data collection forms should be organized in a way to identify each activity's major heading, classify the intensity level, and record the duration to ensure accurate data entry.

It is important the participant complete all questions except the space labeled "for clinic use only." The clinic staff will use this space to record the activity code or MET value for data analysis. The space labeled "reason for activity" is to help the coder decide under which major heading to place the activity. The intensity rating is designed to help the coder in assigning the appropriate MET value. Intensity terms of light, moderate, heavy or vigorous, and very heavy or very vigorous should be used in classifying intensity. In the case of walking, the corresponding intensity terms are very slow, slow, moderate, brisk, and very brisk. If a coder does not plan to use the five digit code for data analysis, a space can be provided on the questionnaire to record the MET values to calculate kcal scores.

Discussion and Limitations

The Compendium of Activities is a classification system that groups physical activities by purpose and provides flexibility in determining energy cost. However, there are several factors that may limit the use of the Compendium for determining the precise energy cost of PA. The activity classification system was primarily based on previously published data and as such may not reflect the exact energy cost of all physical activities. Since often the values are merely averages, they do not take into account that some people perform activities more vigorously than others. In addition, the MET values of some activities were not derived from actual mea-

Appendix A.3. Guidelines for Coding Specific Activities

A. General guidelines: All activities should be coded as "general" if no other information about the activity is given. This applies primarily to intensity ratings. If any additional information is given, activities should be coded accordingly.

B. Specific guidelines

1. Bicycling
   a. Stationary cycling using cycle ergometers (all types), wind trainers, or other conditioning devices should be classified under the major heading of Conditioning Exercise, stationary cycling specific activities (codes 02010 to 02015).
   b. The list does not account for differences in wind conditions.
   c. If bicycling is performed in a race, classify it as general racing if no descriptions are given about drafting (code 01050). If information is given about the speed or drafting code as 01050 (bicycling, 16–19 mph, racing/not drafting or > 19 mph drafting, very fast) or 01060 (bicycling, ≤ 20 mph, racing, not drafting).
   d. Using a mountain bike in the city should be classified as bicycling, general (code 01010). Cycling on mountain trails or on a BMX course is coded 01009.

2. Conditioning Exercises
   a. If a calisthenics program is described as a light or moderate type of activity (e.g., performing back exercises) but indicates a vigorous effort on the part of the participant, code the activity as calisthenics, general (code 02030).
   b. Exercise performed at a health club that is not described should be classified as health club, general (code 02060). Other activities performed at a health club (e.g., weight lifting, aerobic dance, circuit training, treadmill running, etc. at a health club) should be classified under separate major headings.
   c. Regardless of whether aerobic dance, conditioning, circuit training, or water calisthenics programs are described by their component parts (i.e., 10 min jogging in place, 10 min sit-ups, 10 min stretching, etc.), code the activity as one activity (e.g., water aerobics, code 02120).
   d. Effort, speed, or intensity breakdowns for the specific activities of stair-treadmill ergometer (code 02065), ski machine (code 02080), water aerobics or water calisthenics (code 02120), circuit training (code 02040), and slimnastics (code 02090) are not given. Code these as general, even though effort or intensities may vary in the descriptions of the activity.

3. Dancing
   a. If the type of dancing performed is not described, code it as dancing, general (code 03025).

4. Home Activities
   a. House cleaning should be coded as light (code 05040) or heavy (code 05020). Examples for each are given in the description of the specific activities.
   b. Making the bed on a daily basis is coded 05100. Changing the bed sheets is coded as cleaning, light (code 05040).

5. Home Repair
   a. Any painting outside of the house (i.e., fence, the house, barn) is coded, painting, outside house (code 60150).

6. Inactivity
   a. Sitting and reading a book or newspaper is listed under the major heading of Miscellaneous, reading, book, newspaper, etc. (code 09030).
   b. Sitting and writing is listed under the major heading of Miscellaneous, writing (code 09040).

7. Lawn and Garden
   a. Working in the garden with a specific type of tool (e.g., hoe, spade) is coded as digging, spading, filling garden (code 08050).
   b. Removing snow may be done by one of three methods: shoveling snow by hand (code 08200), walking and operating a snow blower (code 08130), or riding a snow blower (code 08180).

8. Music Playing
   a. Most variation in music playing will be according to the setting (i.e., rock and roll band, orchestra, marching band, concert band, standing on the stage, performance, practice, in a church etc.). The compendium does not consider differences in the setting (except for marching band and guitar playing).

9. Occupation
   a. Types of occupational activities not listed separately under specific activities (e.g., chemistry laboratory experiments), should be placed into the types of energy expenditure classifications best describing the activity. See sitting: light (code 11580), sitting: moderate (code 11590), standing; light (code 11600), standing: light to moderate (code 11610), standing; moderate (code 11620), standing: moderate to heavy code 11630).
   b. Driving an automobile or a light truck for employment (taxi cab, salesman, contractor, ambulance driver, bus driver), should be listed under the major heading of Transportation, automobile or light truck (not a semi) driving (code 06010).
   c. Performing skin or SCUBA diving as an occupation is listed under the major heading of Water Activities, and the specific activity of skindiving or SCUBA diving as a frogman (code 18170).

10. Running
    a. Running is not classified as treadmill or outdoor running. Running on a treadmill or outdoors should be coded by the speed of the run (codes 12030 to 12130). If speed is not given, code it as running, general (code 12150).

11. Self-care
    a. The compendium does not account for effort ratings. All items are considered to be general.

12. Transportation.
    a. Being a passenger in an automobile is coded under the major heading of inactivity, sitting quietly (code 07020).

Appendix A.3. *(continued)*

13. Walking
    a. Household walking is coded 17150, regardless if the subject identified a walking speed.
    b. If the walking speed is unidentified, use 3.0 mph, level, moderate, firm surface as the standard speed (code 17190). This should not be used for household walking.
    c. Walking during a household move, shopping, or for household work is coded under the major heading of Home Activities. Walking for job-related activities is coded under Occupational Activities.
    d. If a subject is backpacking, regardless of descriptors attached, the code is backpacking, general (code 17010).
    e. The compendium does not account for variations in speed or effort while carrying luggage or a child.
    f. Mountain climbing should be classified as general (rock or mountain climbing, code 17120) if no descriptors are given. If the weight of the load is described, code the activity as climbing hills with the appropriate load (codes 17030 to 17060)
    g. Walking on a grassy area (golf course, in a park, etc.) should be coded as walking, grass track (code 17260). The compendium does not account for variations in walking speed on a grassy area, so ignore recording walking speed or effort. It the walking is not on a grassy area, code activity according to the walking speed (codes 17150 to 17230).
    h. Walking to work or to class should be coded as 17270. The compendium does not account for walking speed or effort in this activity.
    i. Hiking and cross-country walking (code 17080) should be used when the walking activity lasted 3 h or more. Do not use this category for backpacking, but for day hikes.

14. Water Activities
    a. Swimming should be coded as leisurely, not lap swimming, general (code 18130) if descriptors about stroke, speed, or swimming location are not given.
    b. Lap swimming should be coded as swimming laps, freestyle, slow (code 18240) if the activity is described as lap swimming, light or moderate effort, but stroke or speed are not indicated. Swimming laps should be coded as swimming, laps, freestyle, fast (code 18230) if the activity is described as lap swimming, vigorous effort, but stroke or speed are not given.
    c. Swimming crawl should be coded as swimming, crawl, slow (50 yards/min^{-1}) if speed is not given and the effort is rated light or moderate (code 18290). Swimming crawl should be coded as swimming, crawl, fast (yards/min^{-1}) if speed is not given, but the effort is rated as vigorous (code 18280).
    d. The swimming strokes of backstroke (code 18250), breaststroke (code 18260), butterfly (code 18270), and sidestroke (code 18230) are coded as general for speed and intensity.
    e. If a swimming activity is not identified as lake, ocean, or river swimming (code 18300), assume that the swimming was performed in a swimming pool.
    f. If canoeing is related to a canoe trip, code as canoeing, on a camping trip (code 18020). Otherwise, code it according to the speed and effort listed.

surements of oxygen consumption; instead they were estimated from the energy cost of activities having similar movement patterns. Therefore, the estimates may have ill-defined confidence limits around the mean MET values. For activities in which the parameters are undefined, individual differences in energy expenditure can be large and the true energy cost for a person may or may not be close to the stated mean. This does not reduce the value of the standard intensity codes, but it is an important perspective from which to view the Compendium. Calculation of kcal energy expenditure from body weight and MET values may also affect the energy cost of activities. Therefore, the kcal scores should be used with caution in correlation analyses since coefficients may reflect body weight rather than the actual energy cost of activities. Expression of energy expenditure scores as kcal·k^{-1} body weight·h^{-1} or kcal·kg^{-1} body weight·day^{-1} will eliminate this effect. Individual variation in movement patterns and differences in the way activity is reported (i.e., effort, pace, age, and gender differences) may influence the energy cost of activities also. For example, one person may rate his or her walking pace as "brisk" while another classifies the same pace as "slow". The Compendium cannot account for individual differences in movement efficiency; however, variation in how physical activities are recorded can be reduced by providing instruction to partici-

pants on how to classify energy expenditure (i.e., 3 mph is moderate walking), standardizing data recording techniques, and having trained interviewers review the data with participants for clarity before energy costs are calculated.

► SUMMARY

The Compendium of Physical Activities is a unique coding system that classifies the energy cost of physical activities. Based on previously published data, it groups activities by purpose and intensity expressed as METs. The Compendium is easy to use and provides flexibility in calculating the energy cost of various types of physical activities. Despite its possible limitations, the Compendium of Physical Activities is useful for coding physical activity questionnaires or records used in physical activity research, education, and clinic settings.

We wish to thank M. Carl McNally, Mark Richardson, Terri Hartman, and Yvonne Guptill (University of Minnesota) and Martin Yee (Stanford University) for their contributions in creating and organizing the Compendium of Physical Activities. We offer a special thank you to Carl McNally for writing the SAS data analysis program to score the Compendium of Physical Activities.

This work was supported by grant NHLBI (RFA-86-90-P) to Drs. Leon and Jacobs; NHLBI (5-R01-HL-37561) to Dr. Montoye; NHLBI (HL-362-72) to Dr. Haskell; and NHLBI (RFA-86-HL-9-P) to Dr. Sallis.

Dr. Barbara Ainsworth was a post-doctoral associate in the Division of Epidemiology, School of Public Health, University of Minnesota at the time of this project. Dr. Ainsworth is currently with the Applied Physiology Laboratory, Department of Physical Education, Exercise and Sport Science, University of North Carolina at Chapel Hill.

References

1. Bannister EW, Brown SR. The relative energy requirements of physical activity. In: Falls HB, ed. *Exercise Physiology*. New York: Academic Press, 1968.
2. Blair SN, Haskell WL, Ho P, et al. Assessment of habitual physical activity by a 7-day recall in a community survey and controlled experiment. *Am J Epidemiol* 1985; 122:794–804, 1985.
3. Burke EJ, Auchinachie JA, Hayden R, et al. Energy cost of wheelchair basketball. *Physician Sportsmed*;13:99–105.
4. Fisher SV, Patterson RP. Energy cost of ambulation with crutches. *Arch Phys Med Rehabil* 1981;62:250–256.
5. Folsom AR, Caspersen CJ, Taylor HL, et al. Leisure time physical activity and its relationship to coronary risk factors in a population-based sample: the Minnesota Heart Survey. *Am J Epidemiol* 1985;121:570–579.
6. Howley ET, Glover ME. The caloric costs of running and walking one mile for men and women. *Med Sci Sports Exerc* 1974:6:235.
7. Katch FI, McArdle WD. *Nutrition, Weight Control and Exercise*. 3rd Ed. Philadelphia: Lea & Febiger, 1988.
8. Leon AS. Approximate energy expenditures and fitness values of sports and recreational and household activities. In: Wynder EL, ed. *The Book of Health Physical Fitness*.1981;283–341.
9. McArdle WD, Katch FI, Katch VL. *Exercise physiology: Energy, Nutrition, and Human Performance*, 2nd Ed. Philadelphia: Lea & Febiger, 1988;642–649.
10. Minnesota Leisure Time Physical Activity Questionnaire Manual. Division of Epidemiology. School of Public Health. University of Minnesota, Minneapolis, MN 55455.
11. O'Connell ER, Thomas PC, Cady LD, et al. Energy costs of simulated stair climbing as a job-related task in fire fighting. *J Occup Med* 1986;28:282–284.
12. Passmore R, Durnin JVGA. Human energy expenditure. *Physiol Rev* 1955;35:805–840.
13. Reiff GG, Montoye HJ, Remington RD, et al. Assessment of physical activity by questionnaire and interview. In: Karvonen MJ, Barry AJ, eds. *Physical Activity and the Heart*. Springfield, IL: Charles C Thomas, 1967;336–371.
14. Reiff GG, Montoye HJ, Remington RD, et al. Assessment of physical activity by questionnaire and interview. *J Sports Med Phys Fitness* 1967;7:1–32.
15. Taylor H, Jacobins DR Jr., Schucker B, et al. A questionnaire for the assessment of leisure time physical activities. *J Chronic Dis* 1978;31:741–755.
16. Town GP, Sol N, Sinning WE. The effect of rope skipping rate on energy expenditure of males and females. *Med Sci Sport Exerc* 1980;12:295–298.

COMMON MEDICATONS

Table B.1. Generic and Brand Names of Common Drugs by Class

GENERIC NAME	BRAND NAME	GENERIC NAME	BRAND NAME
Beta Blockers		Verapamil	Calan, Isoptin
Acebutolol	Sectral	Nicardipine	Cardene
Atenolol	Tenormin	Amlodipine	Norvasc
Bisopropolol	Zebeta	Felodipine	Plendil
Esmolol	Brevibloc (IV)	Isradipine	DynaCirc
Metoprolol	Lopressor, Toprol	Nimodipine	Nimotop
Nadolol	Corgard	Bepridil	Vascor
Pindolol	Visken	**Cardiac Glycosides**	
Propranolol	Inderal	Digitalis	Digoxin, Lanoxin
Sotalol	Betapace	**Diuretics**	
Timolol	Blocadren	Thiazides	
Carteolol	Cartrol	Chlorthiazide	Diuril
Betaxolal	Kerlone	Hydrochlorothiazide (HCTZ)	Esidrix, Hydrodiuril
Bisoprolol	Zebeta	Indapamide	Lozol
Penbutolol	Levatol	"Loops"	
Alpha₁ Blockers		Furosemide	Lasix
Prazosin	Minipress	Bumetanidine	Bumex
Terazosin	Hytrin	Ethacrynic acid	Edecrin
Doxazosin	Cardura	Torsemide	Demadex
Alpha and Beta Blockers		Potassium-Sparing	
Carvedilol	Coreg	Spironolactone	Aldactone
Labetalol	Trandate, Normodyne	Triamterene	Dyrenium
Antiadrenergic Agents Without		Amiloride	Midamor
Selective Receptor Blockade		Combinations	
Clonidine	Catapres	Triamterine and	
Guanabenz	Wyntensin	hydrochlorothiazide	Dyazide, Maxzide
Guanethidine	Ismelin	Amiloride and	
Guanfacine	Tenex	hydrochlorothiazide	Moduretic
Methyldopa	Aldomet	Others	
Reserpine	Serapasil	Metolazone	Zaroxolyn
Guanadrel	Hylorel	**Peripheral Vasodilators**	
Nitrates and Nitoglycerin		**(Nonadrenergic)**	
Isosorbide dinitrate	Isordil, Diltrate	Hydralazine	Apresoline
Nitroglycerin	Nitrostat, Nitrolingual spray	Minoxidil	Loniten
Nitroglycerin ointment	Nitrol ointment	**Angiotensin-Converting Enzyme**	
Nitroglycerin patches	Transderm Nitro, Nitro-Dur II, Nitrodisc	**(ACE) Inhibitors**	
Isosorbide mononitrate	Ismo, Monoket, Imdur	Captopril	Capoten
Calcium Channel Blockers		Enalapril	Vasotec
Diltiazem	Cardizem, Dilacor, Tiazac	Lisinopril	Prinivil, Zestril, Prinzide
Meberfradil	Posicard	Moexipril	Univasc
Nifedipine	Procardia, Adalat	Ramipril	Altace
Nisoldipine	Sular	Benazepril	Lotensin

(continued)

Table B.1. *(continued)*

GENERIC NAME	BRAND NAME	GENERIC NAME	BRAND NAME
Fosinopril	Monopril	Class IV	
Quinapril	Accupril	Calcium channel blockers	
Trandolapril	Mavik	Verapamil	Procardia
		Diltiazem	Cardizem
Angiotensin II Receptor Antagonist		Other	
Losartan	Cozaar	Digoxin	Digitalis
Valsartan	Diovan	Adenosine	Adenocard (IV), Adenoscan (IV)
		Sympathomimetic Agents	
Antiarrhythmic Agents		Ephedrine	Adrenalin
Class I		Epinephrine	Alupent
IA		Metaproterenol	Proventil, Ventolin
Quinidine	Quinidex, Quinaglute	Albuterol	Bronkosol
Procainamide	Pronestyl, Procan SR	Isoetharine	Brethine
Disopyramide	Norpace	Cromolyn sodium	Intal
IB		**Antihyperlipidemic Agents**	
Tocainide*	Tonocard*	Atorvastatin	Lipitor
Mexiletine	Mexitil	Cerivastatin	Baycol
Phenytoin	Dilantin	Cholestyramine	Questran
Lidocaine	Xylocaine, Xylocard	Clofibrate	Atromid-S
IC		Colestipol	Colestid
Flecainide	Tambocor	Gemfibrozil	Lopid
Propafenone	Rythmol	Lovastatin	Mevacor
Multiclass		Nicotinic acid (niacin)	Nicobid, Nicolar, Slo-Niacin
Moricizine	Ethmozine	Pravastatin	Pravachol
Class II		Simvastatin	Zocor
β-Blockers		Fluvastatin	Lescol
Propranolol	Inderal	**Anticoagulants**	
Acebutolol	Sectral	Ticlopidine Hydrochloride	Ticlid
Esmolol	Brevibloc	Warfarin	Coumadin
Class III		Pentoxifylline	Trental
Amiodarone	Cordarone	Dypridamole	Persantine
Bretylium	Bretylol	Abcixamab	Reo-pro
Ibutilide	Corvet	**Oral-antihyperglycemics**	
Sotalol	Betapace	Glyburide	DiaBeta, Glynase, Micronase
		Metformin hydrochloride	Glucophage
		Troglitazone	Rezulin

*limited clinical use

INDEX

Page numbers in *italics* denote figures; those followed by t denote tables.

Inflammatory phase of healing, 497, 498
Information management, 651
Information resources
on anatomy, 91, 91t
on body composition, 399
effectiveness of, 557
on exercise for older adults, 529, 530t, 531, 532
Informed consent, 627, 628–629
for exercise testing, 367, 627
of children, 526
Initial claudication distance (ICD), 293, 294
Initiation stage, of training, 455
Injuries, 492–499, 501, 502t, 654–658. *See also* Emergencies;
Safety
healing, 497–498
incidence, 492
legal considerations, 626, 628, 629, 630, 631
low back, 121–124, *122–123. See also* Low back pain
abdominal belts and, 127–128
flexibility training for, 120, 125
management, 496, 497t, 498–499, 655, 656t, 657t,
657–658
to older adults, 207
prevention, 494t, 494–495, 658, *659,* 660–661, 661t
flexibility and, 384, 388, 495
resistance training for, 377
recognition, 495, 495t, 496t
risk factors, 492–494, 493t, 655
secondary hypoxic injury, 497, 498
stabilization of, 497, 498
Injury current, 422
Inotropic effect, 69
Inspiration, 74, 77–78, 78
pleural space and, 79, *79*
Insulin. *See also* Diabetes mellitus
arterial receptors for, 228
blood glucose and, 277–278, *278*
medications and, 280, 280t
exercise and, 278–279, 279t
resistance training, 376
fat metabolism and, 135
hypertension and, 285
preparations of, 279t
Insulin resistance, 8, 10, 36, 277. *See also* Hyperinsulinemia
coronary artery disease and, 233
hypertension and, 287, 289
physical activity and, 11
tissue plasminogen activator and, 9
treatment, 287
Insulinlike growth factor I (IGF-I), 181
Insurance, liability, 629
Integrilin, 257
Intensity. *See* Exercise intensity
Interatrial septum, 66
Intercostal muscles, 77, 78, *78*
Interferon-gamma, in atherogenesis, 241
Intermediate-density lipoprotein (IDL), 231
Intermittent claudication. *See* Claudication
Internal oblique muscle, expiration and, 78, *78*
Internal respiration, defined, 319
Internal thoracic artery conduit, 234

Internet sites
on anatomy, 91, 91t
on benefits of exercise, 530t
Interpersonal skill training, 564
Interspinous ligament
forces generated by, 124
injury to, 122–123, *123*
Interstitial lung disease, 332, 343
Interval training, 457, 485
metabolic responses, 488–489, *489*
Interventricular artery, 67, 69
Interventricular septum, 66, 67, *68*
Interventricular sulcus, 65, *66, 69*
Intima, 228, *228*
Intra-aortic balloon pump, 243
Intramyocardial arteries, 238, *239*
Intraventricular conduction delay, nonspecific, 436
Intrinsicoid deflection, 439, 440t
Inversion, 87t, 90t
range of motion, 382, 382t
Iron supplementation, at altitude, 219
Ischemic cascade, 240
Isocitrate dehydrogenase, 135
Isodynamic exercise, cardiovascular response to, 150,
154–155, *155*
Isoelectric lead, 419
Isokinetic dynamometers, 378–379
Isokinetic machines, 643
Isokinetic muscular endurance, 380
Isokinetic training, 169, 170, 174, 376, 462
body composition and, 182
in children, 525
defined, 377
enzymatic adaptations, 178
Isolation exercises, 171
Isometric contraction, 109, 110
neural inhibition of, 206
Isometric (static) exercise
cardiovascular response to, 147, 147t, 148, 150, 154–155,
155
in hypertensive patient, 156, *157*
Isometric side bridge, 126t, 126–127, *127*
Isometric (static) training, 174, 376, 377, 461–462
enzymatic adaptations, 178
specificity of, 174, 488
Isotonic exercise. *See* Dynamic (isotonic) exercise

J
J point, 415, *417*
Job stress, 48
Jogging
deaths, 501
injuries, 492
Joint angle specificity, 174, 377, 378, 488
Joint reaction force, 108, 112
Joints. *See also* Flexibility; Range of motion (ROM)
aging and, 516
blood supply, 87
classification, 82, 89t
impact loading and, 110
injuries, 495t, 498, 655, 656t

Quality control, facility, 633, *635–637*, 638
Quantitative ultrasound (QUS), of bone density, 301
Quetelet equation, 404
Quinidine, ECG changes caused by, 440
Quinine, glucose-altering effects, 280t

R
R wave, 415, 418, 419, 420
  absent
    in CAD, 247
    myocardial infarction and, 422
RA (right atrium), 65, *66*, 66–67, *68–71*
Rabbit ears, on ECG, 436
Racquet sports, warm-up for, 457
Radial pulse, 97–98, *98*
Radiative heat transfer, 210, 211, 213, 214
  aging and, 516
Radionuclide imaging
  in CAD diagnosis, 248, 249–250, 373
  in myocardial infarction, 243
  after risk factor modification, 264–265
  after treadmill vs. cycle, 369
Raloxifene, for osteoporosis, 300
Ramipril, 256
Ramp treadmill protocols, 370
  aerobic capacity measured with, 145
Range of motion (ROM), 87, 381–389. *See also* Joint angle
    specificity; Movement(s)
  active vs. passive, 87, 383
  activity limitations associated with, 388–389
  aging and, 381, *382*, 516
  asymmetry in individual, 381–382, *383*
  evaluation of, 383–384, *385–389*
  factors affecting, 381
  fitness and, 384, 388
  of hypermobile individuals, 468
  muscle force and, 379
  normal values, 381–382, 382t
  resistance training and, 377, 463, 464, 465
  strength testing and, 378, 379
Rapid smoking method, 595
Rate of perceived exertion (RPE), 364, 364t, 372
  in cardiac patients, 369
    during resistance training, 466
  in children, 522t
  in diabetics, 281–282
  in older adults, 531
  in sedentary participants, 579
  training intensity and, 453, 454, 455
Rate-pressure product, 147, 148–149, 154, *155*
  limb-specific aerobic conditioning and, 163
  resistance training and, 181, 289
RCA (right coronary artery), 67, *68–70*
Record keeping
  in exercise program, 451
  in exercise testing, 630
Recovery from exercise, 138
  in resistance training, 463
Recreation centers, 601–602
Recruitment threshold. *See* Motor unit recruitment

Rectal cancer
  alcohol and, 35
  diet and, 34
  physical activity/fitness and, 20, 23, 24t
Rectus abdominis muscle
  exercises for, 126t, 126–127
  expiration and, 78, *78*
Rectus femoris length, *387*
Recumbent bikes, 642
Red blood cells, altitude and, 217, 218
Re-entrant arrhythmias, 427, *428*
  AV nodal re-entrant tachycardia, 430–431, *431*, 505
  AV re-entrant tachycardia, 431, *431*, 441–442, *443*
  ventricular tachycardia as, 433
Refractory period, of cardiac myocyte, 411, 415
Regression, 449. *See also* Detraining
Regression analysis, of body composition, 392
Rehabilitation. *See also* Cardiac rehabilitation; Pulmonary
    rehabilitation
  of bed-rested individuals, 201, 201t
  proprioceptive exercises in, 655
  after reduced muscular activity, 206–207
  resistance training in, 376, 462
  of SCI patients, 207
  after surgery, 529
Reinforcement, 559
Relapse prevention, 559, 575
  in smoking cessation, 595
  in weight management, 589
Relative risk, 42, 247
Relaxation techniques, 562, 564
  in asthma management, 50
  outcomes, 565
Releases, 628
Remodeling phase of healing, 497–498
Renal function, aging and, 516
Renal insufficiency, homocysteine and, 9
Renin-angiotensin system, CAD and, 234
Reperfusion therapy. *See* Angioplasty; Thrombolytic therapy
Repetition maximum (RM), 173, *173*
  one-RM test, 378, 490
  training intensity and, 461
Repetitions, 170, 172, 461, 463
  for cardiac patients, 465
  for elderly, 464
  specificity of training and, 488–489, *489*
Repolarization, cardiac, 411, *412*, 415, 417t, 418
Repolarization variant, benign, 422, *425*
RER (respiratory exchange ratio), 319, *320, 321*
  in children, 527
  endurance training and, 187
Residual volume (RV), 339
  aging and, 514
  in obstructive airway diseases, 328, 329
Resistance training. *See also* Isokinetic training; Isometric
    (static) training; Weight training
  for bedridden patient, 207
  benefits, 376–377, 460
  caloric cost, 175
  in cardiovascular disease, 463, 465–466
  for children, 463–464, 464t, 525